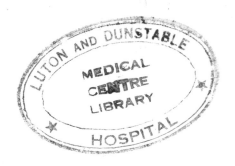

Ophthalmic Surgery

Ophthalmic Surgery
Principles and Techniques

Editor-in-Chief

Daniel M. Albert, MD

Frederick Allison Davis Professor and Chair
Department of Ophthalmology and Visual Sciences
Affiliate Professor
Department of the History of Medicine
University of Wisconsin Medical School
Madison, Wisconsin

Managing Editor

Nancy L. Robinson

Section Editors

Neal P. Barney
Frederick S. Brightbill
Suresh R. Chandra
Henry M. Clayman
Richard K. Dortzbach
Roberta E. Gausas
Paul L. Kaufman
Burton J. Kushner
Bradley N. Lemke
William F. Mieler
Monte D. Mills
Frank L. Myers
T. Michael Nork
Todd W. Perkins
Bryan S. Sires
Thomas S. Stevens

Blackwell
Science

Editorial Offices:

Commerce Place, 350 Main Street, Malden, Massachusetts 02148, USA
Osney Mead, Oxford OX2 0EL, England
25 John Street, London WC1N 2BL, England
23 Ainslie Place, Edinburgh EH3 6AJ, Scotland
54 University Street, Carlton, Victoria 3053, Australia

Other Editorial Offices:

Blackwell Wissenschafts-Verlag GmbH, Kurfürstendamm 57, 10707 Berlin, Germany
Blackwell Science KK, MG Kodenmacho Building, 7-10 Kodenmacho Nihombashi, Chuo-ku, Tokyo 104, Japan

Distributors:
USA
  Blackwell Science, Inc.
  Commerce Place
  350 Main Street
  Malden, Massachusetts 02148
  (Telephone orders: 800-215-1000 or 781-388-8250; fax orders: 781-388-8270)

Canada
  Login Brothers Book Company
  324 Saulteaux Crescent
  Winnipeg, Manitoba, R3J 3T2
  (Telephone orders: 204-224-4068)

Australia
  Blackwell Science Pty, Ltd.
  54 University Street
  Carlton, Victoria 3053
  (Telephone orders: 03-9347-0300; fax orders: 03-9349-3016)

Outside North America and Australia
  Blackwell Science, Ltd.
  c/o Marston Book Services, Ltd.
  P.O. Box 269
  Abingdon
  Oxon OX14 4YN
  England
  (Telephone orders: 44-01235-465500; fax orders: 44-01235-465555)

Acquisitions: James Krosschell
Development: Mike Snider
Production: Karen Feeney
Manufacturing: Lisa Flanagan
Original illustrations: Oxford Illustrators
Cover design: Meral Dabcovich, Visual Perspectives

Typeset by Best-set Typesetter Ltd., Hong Kong
Printed and bound by Walsworth Publishing Company

Library of Congress Cataloging-in-Publication Data

Ophthalmic surgery: principles and techniques / editor-in-chief, Daniel M. Albert; section editors, Frederick S. Brightbill . . . [et al.].
  p.   cm.
  ISBN 0-632-04337-7
  1. Eye—Surgery.   I. Albert, Daniel M.   II. Brightbill, Frederick S.
  [DNLM: 1. Eye Diseases—surgery.   2. Ophthalmologic Surgical Procedures—methods.   WW   16806152   1999]
RE80.064   1999
617.7′1—dc21
DNLM/DLC
for Library of Congress   98-34615
                                                  CIP

This book is dedicated to Matthew D. Davis, MD,
whose contributions as an ophthalmologist are exceeded
only by his contributions as a human being

Contents

Contributing Authors

Stanle
Chairr
Depar
Colun
New Y

Georg
Depar
Unive
Jules
Los A

Henr
Sectio
Volur
Bascc
Univ
Mian

Glen
Assis
Depa
Unif
Silve

Tho
The
Mec
Milv

Joh
Prot
Dep
Uni
Col

Th
Co
Eve
Cli
Un
Pit

Ch
De
Ui
M

Pa
A
D
C
C

R
S
L
N
N

Gary W. Abrams, MD
Professor and Chairman
Department of Ophthalmology
Wayne State University;
Director, Kresge Eye Institute
Detroit, Michigan

Richard M. Ahuja, MD
Fellow
Moorsfield Eye Hospital
London, England

Daniel M. Albert, MD
Editor-in-Chief
Professor and Chair
Department of Ophthalmology and Visual Sciences
University of Wisconsin Medical School
Madison, Wisconsin

Eduardo C. Alfonso, MD
Associate Professor
Bascom Palmer Eye Institute
Department of Ophthalmology
University of Miami School of Medicine
Miami, Florida

Claron D. Alldredge, MD
Department of Ophthalmology and Visual Sciences
University of Wisconsin Medical School
Madison, Wisconsin

O. Claron Alldredge, Jr., MD
Professor of Ophthalmology
University of Utah
Salt Lake City, Utah

C. J. Anderson, MD
Associate Clinical Professor
Department of Ophthalmology and Visual Sciences
University of Wisconsin Medical School
Madison, Wisconsin

Richard M. Auchter, MD
Clinical Assistant Professor
University of Wisconsin–Madison Medicine Center
Holy Family Medical Center
Manitowoc, Wisconsin

Andrew A. Aziz, MD
Corneal and Refractive Surgery Fellow
Hunkeler Eye Centers
Kansas City, Missouri

Neal P. Barney, MD
Section Editor
Associate Professor
Department of Ophthalmology and Visual Sciences
University of Wisconsin Medical School
Madison, Wisconsin

Henry I. Baylis, MD
Director, Oculoplastic Fellowship Program
Department of Ophthalmology
University of California, Los Angeles
Jules Stein Eye Institute
Los Angeles, California

Kevin A. Beadles, MD
Assistant Clinical Professor of Ophthalmology
California Pacific Medical Center;
Clinical Instructor in Ophthalmology
University of California, Davis
Davis, California

Jeremy E. Levenson, MD
Clinical Professor
Department of Ophthalmology
University of California, Los Angeles
Jules Stein Eye Institute
Los Angeles, California

Leonard A. Levin, MD, PhD
Assistant Professor of Ophthalmology and Visual Sciences
Neurology and Neurological Surgery
Neuro-ophthalmologist
Department of Ophthalmology and Visual Sciences
University of Wisconsin Medical School
Madison, Wisconsin

Hilel Lewis, MD
Professor and Chairman
Department of Ophthalmology
Cleveland Clinic Eye Institute
Cleveland, Ohio

John M. Lewis, MD
Clinical Faculty
Department of Ophthalmology
Stanford University School of Medicine
Stanford, California

Jeffrey M. Liebmann, MD
Clinical Associate Professor
Department of Ophthalmology
New York Medical College
New York, New York

Don Liu, MD
Clinical Professor
University of Southern California School of Medicine
Doheny Eye Institute
Los Angeles, California

Mark J. Lucarelli, MD
Instructor
Department of Ophthalmology and Visual Sciences
University of Wisconsin Medical School
Madison, Wisconsin

David B. Lyon, MD
Assistant Clinical Professor
Eye Foundation of Kansas City
Department of Ophthalmology
University of Missouri–Kansas City School of Medicine
Kansas City, Missouri

Elizabeth A. Maher, MD
Assistant Clinical Professor
Department of Ophthalmology
New York Medical College
New York, New York

Curtis E. Margo, MD
Professor of Ophthalmology and Pathology
Department of Ophthalmology
University of South Florida
Tampa, Florida

Craig A. McKeown, MD
Assistant Professor
Department of Ophthalmology
Tufts University
The New England Medical Center
Boston, Massachusetts

William F. Mieler, MD
Section Editor
Professor
The Eye Institute
Medical College of Wisconsin
Milwaukee, Wisconsin

David M. Meisler, MD
Division of Ophthalmology
Cleveland Clinic Foundation
Cleveland, Ohio

Monte D. Mills, MD
Section Editor
Assistant Professor
Department of Ophthalmology and Visual Sciences
University of Wisconsin Medical School
Madison, Wisconsin

Roger C. Mixter, MD
Voluntary Faculty
Department of Ophthalmology and Visual Sciences
University of Wisconsin Medical School
Madison, Wisconsin
Mercy Hospital
Janesville, Wisconsin

Frederic E. Mohs, MD
Mohs Surgery Clinic
Madison, Wisconsin

Michelle Muñoz, MD
Bascom Palmer Eye Institute
Miami, Florida

Michael L. Murphy, MD
Associate Clinical Professor
The Eye Institute
Medical College of Wisconsin
Milwaukee, Wisconsin

Timothy G. Murray, MD
Assistant Professor of Ophthalmology
Department of Ophthalmology
University of Miami School of Medicine
Bascom Palmer Eye Institute
Miami, Florida

Frank L. Myers, MD
Section Editor
Professor
Department of Ophthalmology and Visual Sciences
University of Wisconsin Medical School
Madison, Wisconsin

Jeffrey A. Nerad, MD
Professor
Department of Ophthalmology
University of Iowa Hospitals and Clinics
Iowa City, Iowa

Quan Dong Nguyen, MD
Department of Ophthalmology
Massachusetts Eye and Ear Infirmary
Boston, Massachusetts

T. Michael Nork, MD
Section Editor
Associate Professor
Department of Ophthalmology and Visual Sciences
University of Wisconsin Medical School
Madison, Wisconsin

Stephen G. Nychay, MD
Mohs Surgery Clinic
Madison, Wisconsin

Timothy W. Olsen, MD
Assistant Professor
Department of Ophthalmology and Visual Sciences
University of Wisconsin Medical School
Madison, Wisconsin

Paul Palmberg, MD, PhD
Professor
Bascom Palmer Eye Institute
Miami, Florida

James R. Patrinely
Associate Professor
Department of Ophthalmology
Baylor College of Medicine
Cullen Eye Institute
Houston, Texas

Todd W. Perkins, MD
Section Editor
Associate Professor
Department of Ophthalmology and Visual Sciences
University of Wisconsin Medical School
Madison, Wisconsin

Eric A. Postel, MD
The Eye Institute
Medical College of Wisconsin
Milwaukee, Wisconsin

David V. Pratt, MD
Department of Ophthalmology and
    Department of Plastic Surgery
Baylor College of Medicine
Houston, Texas

Jose S. Pulido, MD
Associate Professor
The Eye Institute
Medical College of Wisconsin
Milwaukee, Wisconsin

Peter A. Rapoza, MD
Assistant Clinical Professor
Harvard Medical School
Cornea Consultants
Boston, Massachusetts

Michael X. Repka, MD
Associate Professor
Department of Ophthalmology
Johns Hopkins University Medical Center
Wilmer Ophthalmological Institute
Baltimore, Maryland

Robert Ritch, MD
Clinical Professor
New York Medical College
New York Eye and Ear Infirmary
New York, New York

Richard M. Robb, MD
Associate Professor
Department of Ophthalmology
Harvard Medical School
Children's Hospital/Ophthalmology
Boston, Massachusetts

Patricia C. Sabb, MD
Department of Ophthalmology and Visual Sciences
University of Wisconsin Medical School
Madison, Wisconsin

Jose A. Sahel, MD
Professor
Faculté de Médicine
Université Louis Pasteur Hôpitaux
Universitaires de Strasbourg
Clinique Ophthalmologique
Hôpital Civil
Strasbourg, France

M. A. Saornil, MD
Associate Professor of Ophthalmology
Ocular Pathology and Oncology Unit
Instituto de Oftalmobiologia Aplicada
Universidad de Valladolid
Valladolid, Spain

Sandeep Saxena, MD
Barnes Retina Eye Institute
St. Louis, Missouri

Robert M. Schertzer, MD
Clinical Assistant Professor
Department of Ophthalmology
University of Michigan School of Medicine
Ann Arbor, Michigan

Joel S. Schuman, MD
Associate Professor
Department of Ophthalmology
Tufts University
The New England Eye Center
Boston, Massachusetts

Stuart R. Seiff, MD
Associate Professor
Department of Ophthalmology
University of California, San Francisco
San Francisco, California

Deborah D. Sherman, MD
Clinical Instructor
Department of Ophthalmology
Vanderbilt University School of Medicine
Nashville, Tennessee

M. Bruce Shields, MD
Professor and Chairman
Department of Ophthalmology
Yale University School of Medicine
New Haven, Connecticut

Jack Kane Shorr, MD
Foundation for Aesthetic Construction and
    Education (FACE)
Beverly Hills, California

Norman Shorr, MD
Clinical Professor of Ophthalmology
Director, Aesthetic Reconstructive Surgery Service
Director, Fellowship in Orbital and Ophthalmic
    Plastic and Reconstructive Surgery
Jules Stein Eye Institute
Los Angeles, California

Joseph P. Shovlin, MD
Associate in Ophthalmology
Geisinger Medical Center
Danville, Pennsylvania

Paul A. Sidoti, MD
Assistant Professor
Department of Ophthalmology
New York Medical College
New York, New York

Bryan S. Sires, MD, PhD
Section Editor
Acting Assistant Professor
Department of Ophthalmology
University of Washington Medical School
Seattle, Washington

Stephen N. Snow, MD
Professor of Surgery
Mohs Surgery Clinic
University of Wisconsin Hospital and Clinics
Madison, Wisconsin

Janet R. Sparrow, PhD
Department of Ophthalmology
Columbia University College of Physicians and Surgeons
New York, New York

David R. Stager, MD
Clinical Professor
Department of Ophthalmology
University of Texas Southwestern Medical Center
Dallas, Texas

George O. Stasior, MD
Clinical Assistant Professor
Albany Medical College
Albany, New York

Orkan George Stasior, MD
Clinical Professor
Albany Medical College
Albany, New York

Roger F. Steinert, MD
Assistant Clinical Professor
Department of Ophthalmology
Harvard Medical School
Boston, Massachusetts

Thomas S. Stevens, MD
Section Editor
Department of Ophthalmology and Visual Sciences
University of Wisconsin Medical School
Madison, Wisconsin

John E. Sutphin, MD
Professor of Clinical Ophthalmology
Department of Ophthalmology
University of Iowa Hospitals and Clinics
Iowa City, Iowa

Francis C. Sutula, MD
Instructor
Harvard Medical School
Boston, Massachusetts

C. A. Swinger, MD
Assistant Professor
Department of Ophthalmology
Mt. Sinai Medical Center
New York, New York

Nasreen A. Syed, MD
Assistant Professor
Department of Ophthalmology
University of Pennsylvania School of Medicine
Philadelphia, Pennsylvania

William M. Tang, MD
The Eye Institute
Medical College of Wisconsin
Milwaukee, Wisconsin

Matthew A. Thomas, MD
Assistant Clinical Professor
Washington University School of Medicine
St. Louis, Missouri

Michael T. Trese, MD
Associated Retinal Consultants, P.C.
Associate Clinical Professor, Krege Eye Institute
Wayne State University
Detroit, Michigan;
Clinical Professor of Biomedical Sciences
Eye Research Institute
Oakland University
Rochester, Michigan

Gregory J. Vaughn, MD
Voluntary Faculty
Emory University School of Medicine
Atlanta, Georgia

Michael P. Vrabec, MD
Assistant Clinical Professor
Department of Ophthalmology and Visual Sciences
University of Wisconsin Medical School
Madison, Wisconsin

David S. Walton, MD
Associate Professor
Department of Ophthalmology
Harvard Medical School
Boston, Massachusetts

David R. Weakley, Jr., MD
Associate Professor
Department of Ophthalmology
University of Texas–Southwestern
Dallas, Texas

Jayne S. Weiss, MD
Associate Professor
Wayne State University School of Medicine
Kresge Eye Institute
Detroit, Michigan

Jane C. Werner, MD
Associate Clinical Professor of Ophthalmology
Oakland University
Rochester, Michigan

Jacob T. Wilensky, MD
Professor
University of Illinois–Chicago
Illinois Eye and Ear Infirmary
Chicago, Illinois

John J. Woog, MD
Associate Clinical Professor
Tufts University School of Medicine;
Ophthalmic Consultants of Boston
Boston, Massachusetts

Preface

The earliest attempts to record and describe techniques of eye surgery date back centuries before Hippocrates. They include the Egyptian papyri on epilation (from 3500 years ago), the Sanskrit texts of Susruta and Vaghbata on cataract, and the tablets describing priestly attempts at ocular surgery in Sumeria, Babylonia, and Assyria. Among the earliest medical books to follow the introduction of the Gutenberg press in 1448 was *Practica oculorum* by Benevenutus Grassus in 1474. This work contained a précis of Greco-Roman and Arabian ophthalmic knowledge.

In 1588, the itinerant barber-surgeon and oculist Georg Bartisch published the first "modern" work on ophthalmology with instructions on how to remove an eye and how to treat cataracts. The work also described numerous ingenious ophthalmologic instruments and devices. A posthumous second edition was published in 1687. In 1790, Guillaume de Quengsy wrote a two-volume textbook, the first devoted exclusively to ophthalmic surgery. The first volume dealt with the author's cataract operations and those of many of his contemporaries. The second discussed diseases of the lid and lacrimal sac, diseases of the vitreous, and removal of the eye.

During the 19th century, ophthalmologists on the European continent increasingly produced surgical texts and treatises distinct from those dealing with medical considerations of the eye. In Great Britain, where ophthalmology was more gradually accepted as a surgical specialty, the medical and surgical treatments of the eye were usually considered jointly for most of the century. In the United States, eye surgery was described in texts of general surgery. Samuel Gross's *A System of Surgery*, first published in 1859, and D. Hayes Agnew's *The Principles and Practice of Surgery* (1878) served as major authoritative texts until nearly the end of the century. The 20th century, particularly the latter half, has seen a predominance of specialized texts dealing in ophthalmic surgical detail, with the individual facets of ocular surgery collaboratively written by experts in the field.

The purpose of *Ophthalmic Surgery: Principles and Techniques* is to provide practicing ophthalmologists with a single set of volumes that cover in a lucid, authoritative, and well-illustrated manner the major ophthalmic operations performed today. The time has long passed when a single gifted ophthalmologist could speak knowledgeably on each type of eye operation. We are grateful to have been able to attract a dedicated group of outstanding section editors, each a leader in his or her field, who in turn put together teams of recognized authorities to write the individual chapters in each section. We have striven to achieve a clear and relatively uniform style and a degree of detail that is appropriate for the needs of the specialist.

In addition to the section editors and the authors, this book could not have been published without the efforts of a gifted group of individuals: Nancy Robinson, Managing Editor for the book; Jim Krosschell, Senior Vice President of Blackwell Science; Mike Snider, Book Development Editor and now head of Snider Publishing Services; Karen Feeney, Book Production Manager; Lisa Flanagan, Manufacturing Coordinator; Irene Herlihy, Production Editor; and Oxford Illustrators. It is the hope of all who participated in the writing and production of this work that it will provide important information to ophthalmic surgeons and aid them in the treatment of their patients.

Daniel M. Albert, MD, MS
Madison, Wisconsin
May 5, 1998

Part

I

Cornea and Anterior Segment Surgery

FREDERICK S. BRIGHTBILL, NEAL P. BARNEY, AND HENRY M. CLAYMAN
Section Editors

Indications and Contraindications for Penetrating Keratoplasty

John E. Sutphin

Penetrating keratoplasty (PKP) is the most frequently performed and most successful organ or tissue transplantation, with the exception of blood transfusions, in the United States. Table 1-1 shows the number of transplantations performed in 1995. These statistics pertain to allografts or homografts, which are transplanted tissues or organs from one member of a species to another member of the same species. PKP may also involve isografts, using tissue from the contralateral eye (autograft) or rotating the transplant within the same eye (rotating autograft), or less frequently, using tissue from a genetically identical twin. Xenografts are tissues transplanted between species and have not been used since the advent of transplantation in the nineteenth century.

The exponential growth in the frequency of PKP is due to two principal developments. Prior to the mid 1930s, corneal transplantation was reported infrequently and occurred in small numbers because the requirement for diseased eyes with clear corneas as sources of tissue limited the availability of the operation. During the 1930s, Filatov in Odessa, Russia, popularized the use of cadaveric donors. The use of refrigerated donor eyes was expanded by the organization of eye banks, with the first American bank, the Eye Bank for Sight, established by R. Townley Paton in 1944 in New York City. The Eye Bank Association of America (EBAA) was organized in 1961 and reported 2000 transplantations that year. In 1995, the EBAA reported 44,169 corneal transplantations (1). The second major contribution to this rapid growth has been the availability of preservation media, allowing for the maintenance of the donor cornea for periods up to 1 week with satisfactory clinical results. The first description of preservation was by Magitot in 1912 (2). But the modern era began with the use of McCarey-Kaufman media, described in 1974 (3). There have been numerous improvements in the technology and technique of PKP since Zirm first performed the procedure in a

patient in 1905, but there have been no major changes in the underlying principles (4).

INDICATIONS

The indications for a procedure are the reasons why that surgery is particularly desirable for the condition to be treated. The decision to perform the surgery balances the benefits and the risks in the specific patient. This section covers the general benefits of corneal transplantation, including the common diagnoses for which it is performed.

The indications for keratoplasty fall into four broad categories (5,6):

1. Optical: The prime purpose is to improve visual acuity.
2. Tectonic: The prime purpose is to restore altered corneal structure including extreme thinning, perforation, and traumatic loss of tissue.
3. Therapeutic: The prime purpose is to relieve pain, to remove tissue for progressive keratitis after failure of specific antimicrobial or anti-inflammatory therapy, or to be an adjunct to other surgery such as temporary keratoprosthesis and pars plana vitrectomy for ocular trauma.
4. Cosmetic: The prime purpose is to restore a normal appearance to an eye with limited vision potential.

Optical or visual indications have become the principal reasons for transplantation, accounting for over 90% of 3089 transplantations recorded in the Australian Corneal Graft Register (7). Therapeutic indications, primarily pain relief, were one of the immediate reasons for grafting in 17%, tectonic indications were listed in 3.5%, and cosmesis was included as an indication in 1.5%. Figures 1-1 to 1-4 show examples of the general indications. In the first series of

Table 1-1.   U.S. Transplantation Statistics

Tissue/Organ	Initial Year	No. in 1995
Cornea	1905	44,169
Kidney	1954	11,807
Heart	1967	2361
Liver	1967	3923
Pancreas	1969	1024
Lung	1981	871
Heart/lung	1981	67

Source: United Network for Organ Sharing Facts and Statistics compiled for the National Organ Procurement and Transplantation Network under contract with the U.S. Department of Health and Human Services.

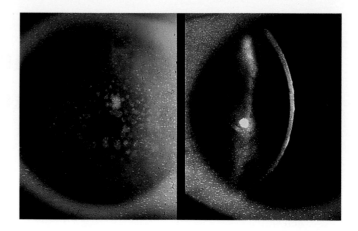

FIGURE 1-1.   *Optical indication for penetrating keratoplasty (PKP). This montage shows two views of an eye of a patient with macular corneal dystrophy and decreased vision from opacity and irregular astigmatism.*

transplantations reported by Elschnig and Vorisek (8), 35 (20%) of 174 of the procedures were for staphylomas or frank corneal perforations (tectonic). With the advent of more specific diagnoses as indications, the general indications are not always reported in large series (9–12). Typically, a transplantation done for visual reasons will have salutary effects to restore the appearance of the eye or to reduce comorbidity such as pain. But more importantly, transplantation done to preserve the globe both tectonically and therapeutically will often have the benefits of improved clarity and subsequently improved visual acuity. Eighty percent of all transplantations resulted in improvement of at least one Snellen level (7). Therapeutic keratoplasties will often have the secondary effect of restoring a more normal appearance.

Optical indications for PKP (see Fig. 1-1) generally follow the same guidelines as those for cataract surgery. There is no absolute level of vision below which a patient requires cataract surgery. The indication for surgery is based on the patient's visual function and visual needs, a finding of intrinsic disease of the lens, or a need for visualizing the fundus. Recently, several national organizations clarified the indications for cataract surgery (13). If both eyes are impaired by the underlying disease and the recipient is an acceptable candidate, then the indication for surgery is usually unequivocal. However, with the advent of managed care and the economic considerations of third parties, all indications for surgery have come under increasing scrutiny. Javitt et al (14,15) showed a correlation between improved quality of life and improved visual function in a prospective, nationwide trial of 1021 patients with cataracts and other degenerative eye diseases, by measuring visual, social, and psychological end points. Others also showed unequivocally the benefit of improved visual function in improving the overall health of the elderly (16–20).

Although PKP shares visual indications with cataract surgery, the prognosis for corrected visual acuity is poorer. Based on series of 4499 records, the Australian graft registry reported an overall 1-year survival rate of 91% and a 5-year survival rate of 72%, with the best vision being 20/40 on

the Snellen chart in 43% of the recipients (7). Fifty-two percent had acuities of 20/60 or better and 20% had acuities worse than 20/200. Better visual outcomes occurred when the indications were limited to dystrophies [20/40 in 64% of patients with Fuchs' dystrophy (21) and 20/40 in 79% of those with keratoconus (7)].

Patients' perception of the value of PKP to themselves was rated in a smaller series; 75% of patients reported overall satisfaction with the operation and results. Satisfaction was associated with better vision in the grafted eye versus the other eye, clarity of the graft, and improvement in lifestyle. Dissatisfaction was primarily related to graft failure or problems with contact lens wear (22).

But in unilateral transplantation or that in the second eye after successful first eye transplantation, there is more controversy. Javitt et al (14) confirmed the value of second eye surgery for cataract in a preliminary study but that study did not look at individual patient outcomes. In a subsequent study, the value of second eye surgery for cataract was confirmed by a 61% increase in VF-14 results (a validated measure of visual function), a 27% decline in trouble with vision, and a 24% improvement in satisfaction with vision (23). These findings are generalizable to the situation involving corneal transplantation, although there is a longer rehabilitation involved with corneal transplants.

The indication for the second eye to receive a transplant involves assessing the specific risk of implanting a second graft. Early work indicated a possible trend toward more rejections in keratoconus patients who underwent surgery in the second eye (24–32). Others found no change in risk to either eye (33–37). Two large graft registries, using multivariate analysis, recently reported an increased survival rate for the second eye graft (38,39). One center did report an increased risk for rejection and failure in the first eye (39), but the risk to both eyes decreased as the interval between surgeries increased, with best survival occurring when there was no rejection for 3 years in the first eye prior to surgery on the second. The reason for the increased survival in the second eye is unclear but there are several possibilities: patient selection bias and an underlying good prognosis for many bilateral conditions (corneal dystrophies); negative bias in avoiding second eye surgery after a poor outcome in the first eye; patient education and experience with medications; use of steroid in the second eye and not the first eye at time of second surgery; immune modulation following first eye surgery; or relative anergy in patients who accept one graft without rejection (39). At this time, second eye surgery that is indicated by the patient's visual requirements is not contraindicated by the risk of rejection if the patient receives proper education and management, including the use of topical steroids in both eyes perioperatively.

Therapeutic and tectonic reasons (see Figs. 1-2 and 1-3) for doing surgery are almost always imperative and are not subject to the same controversy. Therapeutic indications may be involved in the rare circumstance where visualization of the posterior segment is required, for example, following placement of a temporary keratoprosthesis for complicated retinal detachment repair including pars plana vitrectomy, or to allow for photocoagulation of diabetic retinopathy. Alternatives to corneal transplantation should be sought where applicable. Hard or soft contact lenses may be used in patients with irregular astigmatism or for thin scars subject to glare and photophobia. Lamellar keratoplasty or use of tissue glues may be appropriate in the management for tectonic indications. Limbal autografting or allografting may be appropriate for primary restoration of the ocular surface or as preparation for subsequent PKP (40). Optical

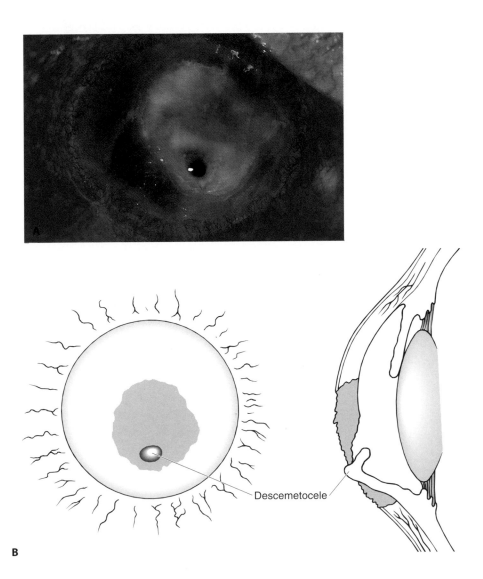

FIGURE 1-2.   A. *Tectonic indication for PKP. This patient has chronic herpes simples keratitis with an area of thinning and descemetocele formation with iris lining the descemetocele. Transplantation is needed to restore ocular integrity.* B. *Diagram showing same patient, with a central and side view to illustrate the zone of thinning and anterior synechiae to the descemetocele.*

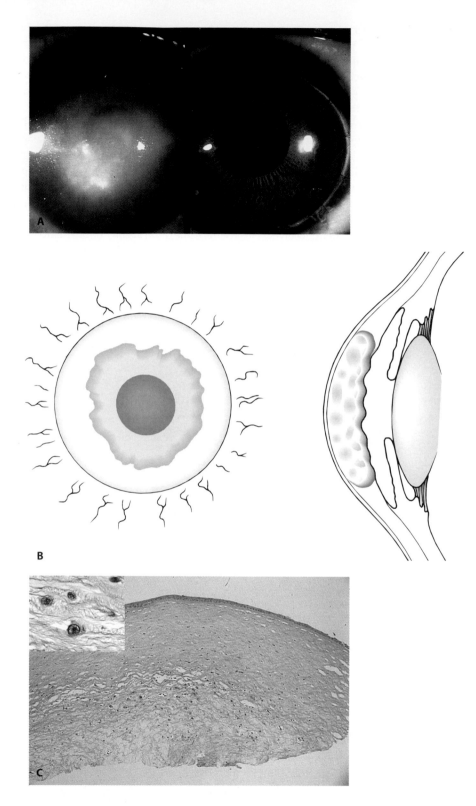

FIGURE 1-3.   A. *Therapeutic indication for PKP. This montage shows a preoperative image of a patient with persisting inflammation despite 6 months of treatment for acanthamoeba keratitis. The image on the right shows the clear corneal transplant. B. Same cornea. The ongoing inflammatory nature of the infection required therapeutic transplantation to reduce the load of organisms and allow the immune system to contain any residual infection from the amoeba. C. Corneal button from A. The relative absence of acanthamoeba in the anterior stroma with an intact epithelium and a concentration of trophozoites and cysts in the deep stroma suggest poor drug penetration. There is artifactual loss of Descemet's membrane. The inset shows acanthamoeba cysts and macrophages.*

iridectomy for Peters' anomaly or other central scarring may provide better long-term visual results than can PKP, which is associated with a poor prognosis (41). Corneal tattooing has been used to improve cosmesis as well as to reduce the glare and photophobia from corneal scarring. Tarsorrhaphy and conjunctival flaps can be successful in treating persistent corneal ulceration. Pharmacologic means including metalloproteinase inhibitors, growth factors, antiviral agents, and oral antibiotics such as tetracycline have also been used with varying degrees of success.

Transplantation done for cosmetic reasons (see Fig. 1-4) is very rare with the advent of the Narcissus Foundation Program, which provides painted soft contact lenses, and of other producers of tinted contact lenses or painted cosmetic shells. Although rare, cosmesis may still be justifiable in circumstances where the cornea is white from a long-standing injury and vision potential is limited by amblyopia.

Recipient Diagnosis

In 1994, the EBAA introduced a grouping of recipient diagnoses in order to improve the tracking of the indications of keratoplasty (12). The intent was to identify trends early to allow for planning at the level of the EBAA and to direct research to appropriate areas. Table 1-2 lists the diagnoses as updated by Lindquist at the annual meeting of the EBAA in Santa Barbara, California (personal communication, 1996). Many patients fall into more than one category and it is difficult for surgeons to know precisely which is the principal indication. A prime example is pseudophakic bullous keratopathy in the presence of Fuchs' corneal dystrophy. The EBAA indicates that in this case Fuchs' dystrophy should be the principal indication.

The aging of the population and the advent of intraocular lenses have led to a rapid rise in the performance

of cataract surgery and also to changes in the indications for transplantation. In the 1950s the more common indications for grafting were the need for regrafting, herpetic scarring, and keratoconus (9,10). Indeed, until Max Fine reported success in 49 eyes at the Cornea World Congress in 1964, PKP was infrequently performed for aphakic bullous keratopathy of Fuchs' corneal dystrophy (42).

In the 1980s pseudophakic bullous keratopathy became the leading indication for corneal transplantation in the United States, peaking at approximately 29% in 1988 (43,44). In the 1990s, excluding nonspecified causes, pseudophakic corneal edema remained the number one cause but was decreasing in frequency (Table 1-3). There was an increase in the number of regraft procedures, both those related to rejection and those not. The rise in regrafting may reflect the larger pool of completed grafts as the total number of transplantations and the longevity of the population have increased. The decline in pseudophakic corneal edema is probably related to improvements in technique of lens extraction and in the design of intraocular lenses.

Although groupings of indications are not precise from study to study, European authors reported increases in grafting for pseudophakic bullous keratopathy from the 1970s to the 1990s (45–47). United Kingdom registries indicated, however, that keratoconus remained the number two reason for transplantation at one center, second to regrafting (46). In a similarly sized series involving more than tertiary-care hospitals, keratoconus was the number one reason for grafting (20%), followed by regrafts (16%) and pseudophakic bullous keratopathy (15%) (45). In Denmark, pseudophakic bullous keratopathy was the most frequent indication (at 28%), followed by keratitis and endothelial dystrophy at 14% each and regrafting at 11%. As in the United States, keratoconus was an infrequent indication for transplantation, perhaps reflecting the underlying population. The Australian graft registry found that keratoconus was the most common indication, at 31%, followed by bullous keratopathy at 25% and regrafting at 14% (22). These indications affirm the similar genetic makeup of Australia and the United Kingdom. Despite improvements in the diagnosis and therapy of viral and other microbial keratitis, there has not been a substantial decline in the relative percentage of corneal transplantations done for these indications.

CONTRAINDICATIONS

Absolute Contraindications

Absolute contraindication refers to the absence of any indication to do the procedure. The operation should not be done in a patient with a high probability of not surviving the procedure. The patient's or their legal surrogate's decision not to have surgery should be respected. The procedure should not be attempted in patients with no light perception vision for whom there is no hope for return of vision unless there

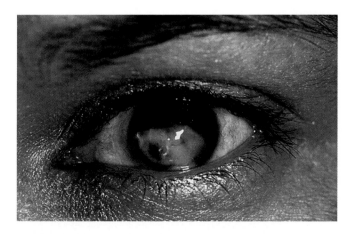

FIGURE 1-4. *Optical indication for PKP. This young Asian female with a history of a fork injury to the left eye at the age of 2, for which she received minimal medical intervention, desires improvement in her appearance. Improvement in vision from corneal transplantation is unlikely due to amblyopia.*

Table 1-2. Clinical Indications for Penetrating Keratoplasty, 1996

1. *Pseudophakic corneal edema*
   Pseudophakic bullous keratopathy
     Anterior-chamber lens implant
     Iris-fixated lens implant
     Posterior-chamber lens implant
2. *Aphakic corneal edema*
   Aphakic bullous keratopathy
   Vitreoendothelial touch syndrome
3. *Stromal corneal dystrophies*
   Granular and Avellino dystrophies
   Lattice dystrophy
   Macular dystrophy
   Central crystalline dystrophy of Schnyder
   Central cloudy dystrophy of François
   Recurrent stromal dystrophy
4. *Primary corneal endotheliopathies*
   Fuchs' endothelial dystrophy
   Congenital hereditary endothelial dystrophy
   Posterior polymorphous dystrophy
   Iridocorneal endothelial syndrome
     Chandler syndrome
5. *Ectasias/thinnings*
   Anterior keratoconus
   Pellucid marginal degeneration
   Keratoglobus
   Posterior keratoconus
6. *Congenital opacities*
   Peters' anomaly
   Glaucoma/buphthalmos
   Aniridia
   Sclerocornea
7. *Viral/postviral keratitis*
   Herpes simplex virus
   Varicella zoster virus
   Epstein-Barr virus
   Adenovirus
     Epidemic keratoconjunctivitis
8. *Microbial/postmicrobial keratitis*
   Bacterial
     Infectious crystalline keratopathy
   Spirochete
     Luetic (syphilitic) interstitial keratitis
   Chlamydial
     Trachoma
   Fungal
   Parasitic
     Acanthamoeba
9. *Optical/refractive*
   Ammetropias
     High and/or irregular astigmatism
     Myopia
     Hyperopia
     Previous refractive surgery
     Epikeratophakia, radial keratotomy, astigmatic keratotomy, automated lamellar keratoplasty, photoreactive keratoplasty, laser-assisted in situ keratomileusis, etc.
10. *Noninfectious ulcerative keratitis or perforation*
    Keratoconjunctivitis sicca
      Sjögren syndrome
    Neuroparalytic/neurotrophic keratopathy
    Exposure keratopathy
    Systemic vasculitides
    Bullous oculocutaneous diseases
    Mooren's ulcer
    Thyroid eye disease
    Rheumatoid disease
      Rheumatoid arthritis
    Cocaine-induced keratopathy
11. *Corneal degenerations*
    Terrien's marginal degeneration
    Calcific band keratopathy
    Polymorphic amyloid degeneration
12. *Chemical injuries*
    Alkaline
    Acid
    Petroleum
    Tear gas
13. *Mechanical trauma, nonsurgical*
    Traumatic opacity
    Traumatic corneal edema
14. *Regraft related to allograft rejection*
    (Include triggers as secondary indication)
15. *Regraft unrelated to allograft rejection*
    Primary tissue failure
    Vitreoendothelial touch
    Glaucoma
    (Include indications listed elsewhere)
16. *Other causes of corneal opacification/distortion*
    Uveitis
    Glaucoma
    Detached Descemet's membrane
    Thermal injury
    Fundus laser keratopathy
    Intraocular silicone keratopathy
    Epithelial downgrowth

Source: Eye Bank Association of America, annual meeting, Santa Barbara, California, June 1996.

Table 1-3.   Corneal Transplant Recipient Diagnoses

Recipient Diagnosis	1991 %	1991 Relative Rank	1995 %	1995 Relative Rank
Nonspecified	18.9	2	21.5	1
Pseudophakic corneal edema	25.1	1	20.5	2
Ectasias/thinnings	11.4	3	12.3	3
Endothelial corneal dystrophies	11.1	4	11.9	4
Regraft unrelated to allograft rejection	2.41	11	5.6	5
Aphakic corneal edema	8.5	5	5.6	6
Regraft related to allograft rejection	4.7	6	4.8	7
Stromal corneal dystrophies	4.1	8	4.1	8
Noninfectious ulcerative keratitis	3.1	9	3.8	9
Corneal degenerations	4.2	7	3.4	10
Congenital opacities	0.6	14	1.5	11
Mechanical trauma	2.6	10	1.5	12
Viral/postviral keratitis	1.5	12	1.4	13
Syphilitic/postsyphilitic keratitis	0.4	16	1.0	14
Microbial/postmicrobial keratitis	0.9	13	0.6	15
Chemical injuries	0.5	15	0.4	16

Source: Eye Banking Statistics for 1991 and 1995, Eye Bank Association of America.

is a psychological contraindication to either enucleation or evisceration and there are no other suitable alternatives. Patients who are satisfied with their current vision with their usual type of correction (glasses or contact lenses) or whose lifestyles are not compromised should not have surgery.

Relative Contraindications

Relative contraindications include the risk factors for failure of the transplant to remain clear or for the patient to obtain significant improvement in vision. Many of these risk factors have been based on clinical experience (43,48). Several large, single-center and multicenter trials applied univariate and multivariate analyses to the more commonly considered causes of graft failure (38,45,49–54). Not every study assessed the same risk factors and not all potential risk factors were studied rigorously. Most studies found that when the data were adjusted for various factors, many of the commonly accepted risk factors were not significant. Table 1-4 outlines many of the risk factors found to be significant by authors of large series (43,45–47,50).

In the largest study from Australia, the factors that influenced survival in a univariate analysis were the transplant center (centers performing more than 20 grafts per year showed increased survival rates), indication for the graft (keratoconus was associated with the best survival), graft number in the ipsilateral eye, history of pregnancy or blood transfusion, inflammation before or at the time of grafting, corneal vascularization at the time of grafting, history of raised intraocular pressure, the source of the donor cornea

(eye bank eyes showed a poorer survival than those obtained by individual surgeons), the time from death to donor enucleation (cutoff at 6 hours), graft smaller than 7 mm or larger than 8.5 mm in diameter or with more than 0.5-mm difference between host and recipient, and lens status (aphakic grafts have the shortest survival time followed by pseudophakic then phakic grafts; and posterior-chamber intraocular lenses had the best survival followed by anterior-chamber intraocular lenses, iris clip, or other style) (38). Evaluation of risk factors for failure in the postoperative period disclosed that the risk of failure increased with early removal of the graft sutures, neovascularization of the graft, herpetic recurrence in the graft, and a rejection episode. Following adjustment for the various factors using Cox proportional hazards regression analysis, the Australian graft registry found the significant factors to be aphakia or the presence of an anterior-chamber or iris-clip lens, very small or very large grafts, prior history of transplantation on the ipsilateral side, an indication for transplantation other than keratoconus or corneal dystrophy, active inflammation at the time of the transplantation, and a postoperative rise in intraocular pressure. The registry found specifically that there was no effect on outcome of donor age, donor cornea storage medium, or whether the transplantation was performed simultaneously with cataract surgery or in a staged manner.

Yamagami et al (53) found six preoperative risk factors that were associated with poor outcome, using Cox multiple regression analysis: corneal endothelial damage, the presence of anterior synechiae, glaucoma, older donor, area of vascularization, and aphakia or pseudophakia.

Table 1-4.   Risk Factors for Graft Failure*

Risk Factor	Australian Corneal Graft Registry (50)	Collaborative Corneal Transplant Study (43)	United Kingdom Transplant Study (46)	Indiana Study (45)	Japanese Study (47)
No. of transplants in study	3608	457	2242	1819	698
No. (%) failure/time of follow-up	28%/5 yr	32%/3 yr	9%/3–12 mo	9%/5 yr	—
Characteristics of the host cornea					
Not keratoconus or other central corneal disease	Yes	Yes	Yes	Yes	Yes
Previous ipsilateral graft	Yes	Yes	—	Yes	—
Vascularization before PKP	Yes	Yes	—	Yes	Yes
Anterior synechiae	—	Yes	No	—	Yes
Previous increase in IOP	Yes	Yes	No	—	Yes
Not phakic	—	Yes	—	—	Yes
Aphakic	Yes	—	—	Yes	—
Pseudophakic	Yes	—	—	Yes	—
Previous surgery, not PKP	—	Yes	—	—	—
Inflammation at time of PKP	Yes	—	No	—	—
Characteristics of the recipient					
Previous blood transfusion	Yes	No	—	—	—
Previous pregnancy	Yes	No	—	—	—
Smoker	—	Yes	—	—	—
Younger than 40 yr	Yes	Yes	—	—	—
Characteristics of the donor or surgery					
Older donor age	No	No	—	—	Yes
Graft size	Yes (<7.0 or ≥8.5 mm)	Yes (<8.0 mm)	Yes (trephine sum ≤14.5 mm)	—	—
Time to preservation					
≤6.0 hr	No	No	—	—	—
>6.0 hr	Yes	Yes	—	—	—
Method of donor storage	No	—	—	—	—
Time to surgery (up to 96 hr)	No	No	—	—	—
Suture technique					
Interrupted	—	Yes	No	—	—
Running	—	No	No	—	—
Both	—	No	Yes	—	—
Viscoelastic substance					
Not used	—	Yes	—	—	—
Blood group ABO incompatibility	—	Yes	—	—	—

PKP = penetrating keratoplasty; IOP = intraocular pressure.
* Risk factors assessed by univariate analysis. Yes = statistically significant risk factor in the reference; No = tested risk factor that is not statistically significant in that study; — = risk factor not reported.

Price et al (51,54), in a consecutive series of transplantations from a single practice, found immunologic allograft reaction as the most common cause of failure, followed by problems with the external surface of the transplant. They indicated that the risk of failure decreased with increasing postoperative time. The significant risk factors for secondary failure included a previous failed graft, race, age, iris color, use of preoperative glaucoma medicines, deep stromal vascularization, and horizontal diameter of the host cornea (54). Price et al further indicated that the risk factors for immunologic allograft rejection included the patient's horizontal corneal diameter, donor size, the difference between the host cornea and the donor diameters, and the difference between the host diameter and the recipient trephine size.

In a study of high-risk transplant patients, Maguire et al (49), using multivariate survival analysis, found that many risk factors did not show a significant association in the very-high-risk recipient. They found the strongest risk factors identified with graft failure to be a young recipient, number of prior transplantations, history of prior anterior-segment surgery, preoperative glaucoma, number of anterior synechiae, amount of stromal vascularization, diagnosis of chemical burn, and blood group ABO incompatibility. They found no association between donor and corneal preservation characteristics with outcome. After multifactorial analysis Vail et al (52) found the following risk factors to be significant: surgeons who performed fewer than 50 transplantations during the study period (1986–1992), recipients under 10 years old, prior failed transplant, grafting for nonvisual indications, vascularization of the corneal bed, eccentric edema of the cornea as opposed to central edema, smaller trephine diameter, and differences between the donor and recipient diameters of more than 0.25 mm.

HLA matching is discussed in another section of the book (graft rejection). Other factors considered to be detrimental to a good prognosis but not specifically assessed in these various analyses are corneal anesthesia, exposure keratitis, severe dry eye, systemic conditions of the patient, and patient compliance. Many of these conditions would fall under the sobriquet of inflammation at the time of transplantation and are associated with a poor outcome. The mechanism by which many of the ocular surface conditions have interfered with the long-term success of transplantation has been clarified with better understanding of the limbal stem cell (40,55–58). Stem cells are lost as a result of

alkaline and severe acid injuries, following Stevens-Johnson syndrome or other severe conjunctivitides, and in specific ocular conditions such as aniridia and ectodermal dysplastic syndromes. To date no study has examined the absence of limbal stem cells as a separate risk factor for PKP failure, in part owing to the lack of a good clinical marker. Absence of the palisades of Vogt, superficial conjunctival vessels crossing the limbus, and presence of goblet cells on the corneal surface are nonspecific markers for loss of stem cells and conjunctivalization of corneal epithelium. Holland et al (40) suggested an improved outcome when the stem cells are replaced before PKP is performed.

Table 1-4 shows the statistically significant risk factors for the long-term success of transplantation as determined in five large studies using univariate analysis (43,45–47,50). Not all potential risk factors have been studied and these reports vary widely in terms of definitions, length of follow-up, baseline characteristics, number of surgeons, and number of factors assessed. These risk characteristics are based on a much larger experience than that of the early pioneers who

Table 1-5.   Relative Risk of Graft Failure by Specific Factors*

	Value	Australian Corneal Graft Register (50) (n = 936 transplants) Relative Risk (Confidence Interval)	Clear at 1 yr/3 yr	Collaborative Corneal Transplant Study (49) (n = 457 transplants) Relative Risk (Confidence Interval)	Clear at 1 yr/3 yr	Anatomic Basis for Risk [Paton (48) and Buxton (43)] Group	Clear at 1 yr
Percent of total	—	—	91%/79%	—	89%/68%	—	—
Risk factor							
Indication	Keratoconus/ corneal dystrophy	1.00	98%/81%	—	—	I	90%
	Other condition	4.38 (2.04, 7.18)	83%/68%	—	—	II, III, IV	0%–85%
Recipient age	≥40 yr	—	—	1.00	95%/77%	—	—
	<40 yr	—	—	2.50 (1.75, 3.58)	81%/47%	—	—
Previous failed PK	None	1.00	92%/83%	1.00	93%/77%	—	—
	≥1	1.43 (1.07, 1.91)	77%/50%	1.20 (1.09, 1.32)	88%/64%	II, III	75%–85%
Lens status	Not aphakic	1.00	93%/83%	—	—	—	—
	Aphakic	1.98 (1.24, 3.18)	82%/65%	—	—	II	85%
Inflammation	None at graft	1.00	97%/94%	—	—	—	—
	Present at graft	2.05 (1.38, 3.03)	80%/46%	—	—	—	—
Vascularization	None	1.00	95%/85%	1.00	93%/77%	—	—
	After grafting	5.03 (3.33, 7.56)	83%/70%	1.14 (1.01, 1.28)	90%/67%	II, III	75%–85%
Anterior synechia	None	—	—	1.00	Not available	—	—
	Present	—	—	1.19 (1.07, 1.32)	Not available	IV	0%–50%
Glaucoma	None	—	—	1.00	92%/77%	—	—
	Preoperative	—	—	1.58 (1.14, 2.21)	85%/64%	I–IV	Reduce by 10%–50%
Graft size	7.0–7.9 mm	1.00	95%/85%	—	—	—	—
	Other	1.89 (1.28, 2.80)	86%/65%	—	—	II, IV	50%–75%
Intraocular lens (IOL)	No anterior-chamber or iris-clip IOL	1.00	93%/86%	—	—	—	—
	Anterior-chamber IOL	1.74 (1.03, 2.94)	89%/57%	—	—	—	—
	Iris-clip IOL	3.59 (1.90, 6.79)	74%/30%	—	—	—	—

* Percentages estimated from published graphs.

Table 1-6.   Prognosis for Graft Clarity at 1 Year

Group	Diagnosis	Morphology	Prognosis*
Group I	Keratoconus Early Fuchs' dystrophy Stromal dystrophy Other central opacity	Central corneal disease with normal peripheral architecture, limbal anatomy, and sensation, and healthy microenvironment of eyelids and tear film	92%–98%
Group II	Pseudophakic bullous keratopathy Aphakic bullous keratopathy Diffuse Fuchs' dystrophy Inactive peripheral scarring	Disease that crosses the graft-host junction with an intact surface, and minimal vascularization	85%–90%
Group III	Keratoglobus Pellucid degeneration Corneal perforation Pseudophakic bullous keratopathy with an iris-clip intraocular lens	Extremes of peripheral corneal contour or thickness involving a large part of the recipient zone adjacent to limbus and Langerhans' cells	70%–85%
Group IV	Ocular pemphigoid Aniridia Stevens-Johnson syndrome Anterior-chamber cleavage syndrome Neuroparalytic or neurotrophic disease	Absence of normal limbal stem cells and normal maturation of corneal epithelium, loss of corneal sensation, loss of anterior chamber	40%–70%

* Prognoses are estimates only and must be modified by any significant cofactors such as the ones included in Table 1.7.

Sources: Buxton JN, Buxton DF, Westphalen JA. Indications and contraindications. In: Brightbill FS, ed. *Corneal surgery: theory, technique and tissue.* 2nd ed. St. Louis: Mosby, 1993:77–104; and Paton D, Jones DB. *Penetrating keratoplasty.* Outcome monographs. Alcon monograph series 1(1). Fort Worth, TX: Alcon Laboratories, 1976.

Table 1-7.   Ancillary Factors Modifying Prognosis of 1-Year Graft Survival*

Factor	Reduction in Prognosis
Vascularization	7% for each quadrant of vessels
Prior pregnancy or blood transfusion	2%–5%
Active inflammation in past	10%
Active inflammation at time of transplantation	20%
Donor size <7.0 mm	25%
Donor size >8.5 mm	20%
Difference between donor and host trephines >0.5 mm	35%
Increased intraocular pressure	10%–25%
Poor patient compliance	5%–20%

* Prognosis reduction is estimate only. Factors are not intended to be algebraically additive.

Source: Modified from Paton D, Jones DB. *Penetrating keratoplasty.* Outcome monographs. Alcon monograph series 1(1). Fort Worth, TX: Alcon Laboratories, 1976.

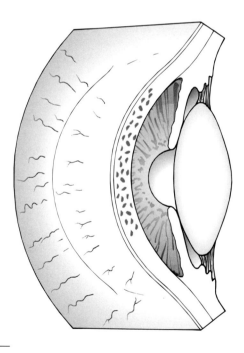

FIGURE 1-5.   *Prognostic group I. Normal peripheral architecture with central corneal disease carries a 92% to 98% 1-year graft survival rate.*

grouped corneal prognosis primarily by anatomic factors. However, there is much in common between Paton's (48) and Buxton's (43) groupings and these later studies. Some authors reduced the confounding variables and biases of these uncontrolled studies using stepwise, multivariate analysis. Table 1-5 (43,48–50) shows the relative risks, confidence intervals, and percentage of failed grafts as determined in two studies related to the accepted prognostic groupings of Paton and Buxton.

Table 1-6 outlines a modified prognostic chart generated from these large registries (5,59). Figures 1-5 to 1-8 show the morphologies and corresponding prognoses for 1-year survival of corneal transplants. The prognosis can be reduced further by the presence of the cofactors listed in Table 1-7.

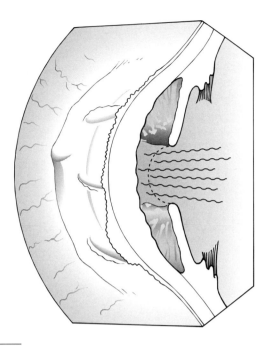

FIGURE 1-6. *Prognostic group II. Corneal edema that extends to the periphery, other lesion that involves the peripheral cornea, aphakia, and corneal neovascularization carry an 85% to 90% 1-year graft survival rate.*

Combining these estimates can provide a useful estimate of the initial success for a clear transplant to a patient considering transplantation.

CONSENT

When explaining the risks and benefits of PKP to the patient and assessing the risk factors for determining the best operation, the surgeon must keep in mind that risk is not the same as risk factors. The risks of corneal transplant surgery include nonimmunologic allograft failure, allograft rejection, expulsive choroidal hemorrhage, infection (both keratitis and endophthalmitis), loss of the eye, donor-to-host transmission of disease, glaucoma, retinal detachment and retinal cystoid macular edema, repeat transplantation, fixed pupil, and astigmatism. In addition, the major risks of anesthesia including stroke, myocardial infarction, and death have to be considered but rarely play a role in the patient's decision for surgery. The benefits represent the positive outcome and risk represents the negative outcome of transplantation or, alternatively, the consequences of not performing the transplantation. In balancing these opposing forces, the surgeon makes a recommendation to the patient and when both are in agreement to proceed, a long-term relationship of careful attention and nurturing ensues.

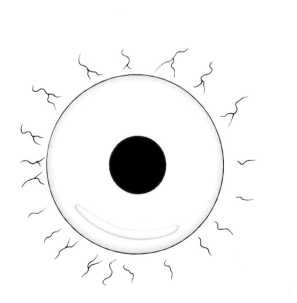

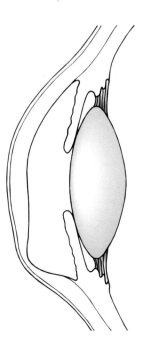

FIGURE 1-7. *Prognostic group III. Abnormal peripheral cornea with extreme thinning or variations in peripheral thickness carries a prognosis of a 70% to 85% 1-year survival rate.*

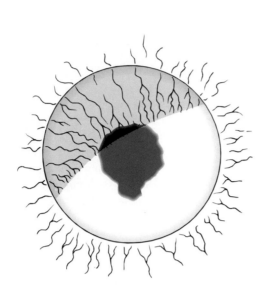 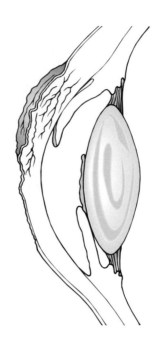

FIGURE 1-8. *Prognostic group IV. Ocular surface disease with diffuse loss of limbal stem cells, extensive peripheral anterior synechiae, or neurotrophic keratitis carries a prognosis of 40% to 70% 1-year survival rate.*

REFERENCES

1. Eye Bank Association of America. *Eyebanking statistical report.* Washington, DC: Eye Bank Association of America, 1995.
2. Magitot A. Transplantation of the human cornea previously preserved in an antiseptic fluid. *JAMA* 1912;59:18–21.
3. McCarey BE, Kaufman HE. Improved corneal storage. *Invest Ophthalmol* 1974;13:165–173.
4. Laibson PR, Rapuano CJ. 100-Year review of cornea. *Ophthalmology* 1996;103:S17–S28.
5. Paton D, Jones DB. *Penetrating keratoplasty.* Outcome monographs. Alcon monograph series 1(1). Fort Worth, TX: Alcon Laboratories, 1976.
6. Buxton JN. Corneal surgery. In: Collins JF, ed. *Handbook of clinical ophthalmology.* New York: Masson, 1982:356–363.
7. Williams KA, Muehlberg SM, Lewis RF, Coster DJ. How successful is corneal transplantation? A report from the Australian Corneal Graft Register. *Eye* 1995;9(Pt2):219–227.
8. Elschnig A, Vorisek EA. Keratoplasty. *Arch Ophthalmol* 1930;4:165–173.
9. Arentsen JJ, Morgan B, Green WR. Changing indications for keratoplasty. *Am J Ophthalmol* 1976;81:313–318.
10. Smith RE, McDonald HR, Nesburn AB, Minckler DS. Penetrating keratoplasty: changing indications, 1947 to 1978. *Arch Ophthalmol* 1980;98:1226–1229.
11. Mamalis N, Craig MT, Coulter VL, et al. Penetrating keratoplasty 1981–1988: clinical indications and pathologic findings. *J Cataract Refract Surg* 1991;17:163–167.
12. Lindquist TD, McNeill JI, Wilhelmus KR. Indications for keratoplasty. *Cornea* 1994;13:105–107.
13. American Academy of Ophthalmology and American Society of Cataract and Refractive Surgery. White paper on cataract surgery. *Ophthalmology* 1996;103:1152–1156.
14. Javitt JC, Brenner MH, Curbow B, et al. Outcomes of cataract surgery. Improvement in visual acuity and subjective visual function after surgery in the first, second, and both eyes. *Arch Ophthalmol* 1993;111:686–691.
15. Brenner MH, Curbow B, Javitt JC, et al. Vision change and quality of life in the elderly. Response to cataract surgery and treatment of other chronic ocular conditions. *Arch Ophthalmol* 1993;111:680–685.
16. Applegate WB, Miller ST, Elam JT, et al. Impact of cataract surgery with lens implantation on vision and physical function in elderly patients. *JAMA* 1987;257:1064–1066.
17. Mangione CM, Phillips RS, Lawrence MG, et al. Improved visual function and attenuation of declines in health-related quality of life after cataract extraction. *Arch Ophthalmol* 1994;112:1419–1425.
18. Lundstrom M, Fregell G, Sjoblom A. Vision related daily life problems in patients waiting for a cataract extraction. *Br J Ophthalmol* 1994;78:608–611.
19. Steinberg EP, Tielsch JM, Schein OD, et al. National study of cataract surgery outcomes. Variation in 4-month postoperative outcomes as reflected in multiple outcome measures. *Ophthalmology* 1994;101:1131–1140; discussion, 1140–1141.
20. Legro MW. Quality of life and cataracts: a review of patient-centered studies of cataract surgery outcomes. *Ophthalmic Surg* 1991;22:431–443.
21. Pineros O, Cohen EJ, Rapuano CJ, Laibson PR. Long-term results after penetrating keratoplasty for Fuchs' endothelial dystrophy. *Arch Ophthalmol* 1996;114:15–18.
22. Williams KA, Ash JK, Pararajasegaram P, et al. Long-term outcome after corneal transplantation. Visual result and patient perception of success. *Ophthalmology* 1991;98:651–657.
23. Javitt JC, Steinberg EP, Sharkey P, et al. Cataract surgery in one eye or both. A billion dollar per year issue. *Ophthalmology* 1995;102:1583–1593.
24. Buxton JN, Schuman M, Pecego J. Graft reactions after unilateral and bilateral keratoplasty for keratoconus. *Ophthalmology* 1981;88:771–773.
25. Young SR, Olson RJ. Results of a double running suture in penetrating keratoplasty performed on keratoconus patients. *Ophthalmic Surg* 1985;16:779–786.
26. Meyer RF. Corneal allograft rejection in bilateral penetrating keratoplasty: clinical and laboratory studies. *Trans Am Ophthalmol Soc* 1986;84:664–742.
27. Ruedemann AD Jr. Clinical course of keratoconus. *Trans Am Acad Ophthalmol Otolaryngol* 1970;74:384–398.
28. Pouliquen Y, Rocher C. Keratoplasties successives et maladie du greffon. *Arch Ophthalmol Rev Gen Ophtalmol* 1975;35:847–864.
29. Donshik PC, Cavanagh HD, Boruchoff SA, Dohlman CH. Effect of bilateral and unilateral grafts on the incidence of rejections in keratoconus. *Am J Ophthalmol* 1979;87:823–826.
30. Khodadoust AA, Karnema Y. Corneal grafts in the second eye. *Cornea* 1984;3:17–20.
31. Kirkness CM, Ficker LA, Steele ADM, Rice NSC. The success of penetrating keratoplasty for keratoconus. *Eye* 1990;4:673–688.
32. Vail A, Gore SM, Bradley BA, et al. Corneal graft survival and visual outcome. A multicenter study. *Ophthalmology* 1994;101:120–127.

33. Musch DC, Meyer RF. Risk of endothelial rejection after bilateral penetrating keratoplasty. *Ophthalmology* 1989;96:1139–1143.

34. Payne JW. Primary penetrating keratoplasty for keratoconus: a long term followup. *Cornea* 1982;1:21–27.

35. Malbran ES, Fernandez-Meijide RE. Bilateral versus unilateral penetrating graft in keratoconus. *Ophthalmology* 1982;89:38–40.

36. Chandler JW, Kaufman HE. Graft reactions after keratoplasty for keratoconus. *Am J Ophthalmol* 1974;77:543–547.

37. Arentsen JJ. Corneal transplant allograft reaction: possible predisposing factors. *Trans Am Ophthalmol Soc* 1983;81:361–402.

38. Williams KA, Muehlberg SM, Wing SJ, Coster DJ, eds. The Australian corneal graft registry: 1990 to 1992 report. *Aust N Z J Ophthalmol* 1993;21(2 suppl):1–48.

39. Tuft SJ, Gregory WM, Davison CR. Bilateral penetrating keratoplasty for keratoconus. *Ophthalmology* 1995;102:462–468.

40. Holland EJ, Schwartz GS. The evolution of epithelial transplantation for severe ocular surface disease and a proposed classification system. *Cornea* 1996;15:549–556.

41. Junemann A, Gusek GC, Naumann GOH. Optical sector iridectomy: an alternative approach to penetrating keratoplasty in Peters anomaly. *Klin Monatsbl Augenheilkd* 1996;209:117–124.

42. Fine M. Keratoplasty in aphakia. In: King JG Jr, McTigue JW, eds. *The Cornea World Congress*. Washington, DC: Butterworths, 1964:538–552.

43. Buxton JN, Buxton DF, Westphalen JA. Indications and contraindications. Part II, Section One: preoperative considerations. In: Brightbill FS, ed. *Cornea surgery: theory, technique, and tissue*. 2nd ed. St. Louis: Mosby, 1993:77–104.

44. Hyman L, Wittpenn J, Yang C. Indications and techniques of penetrating keratoplasties, 1985–1988. *Cornea* 1992;11:573–576.

45. Bradley BA, Vail A, Gore SM, et al. Penetrating keratoplasty in the United Kingdom: an interim analysis of the corneal transplant follow-up study. In: Terasaki PI, Cecka JM, eds. *Clinical transplants*. Los Angeles: UCLA Tissue Typing Laboratory, 1993:293–315.

46. Sharif KW, Casey TA. Changing indications for penetrating keratoplasty, 1971–1990. *Eye* 1993;7:485–488.

47. Haamann P, Jensen OM, Schmidt P. Changing indications for penetrating keratoplasty. *Acta Ophthalmol Scand* 1994;72:443–446.

48. Paton D. The prognosis of penetrating keratoplasty: based upon corneal morphology. *Ophthalmic Surg* 1976;7(3):36–45.

49. Maguire MG, Stark WJ, Gottsch JD, et al. Risk factors for corneal graft failure and rejection in the collaborative corneal transplantation studies. *Ophthalmology* 1994;101:1536–1547.

50. Williams KA, Roder D, Esterman A, et al. Factors predictive of corneal graft survival: report from the Australian corneal graft registry. *Ophthalmology* 1992;99:403–414.

51. Price FW, Whitson WE, Collins KS, Marks RG. Five-year corneal graft survival: a large, single-center patient cohort. *Arch Ophthalmol* 1993;111:799–805.

52. Vail A, Gore SM, Bradley BA, et al. Clinical and surgical factors influencing corneal graft survival, visual acuity, and astigmatism. *Ophthalmology* 1996;103:41–49.

53. Yamagami S, Suzuki Y, Ohya T, et al. Statistic evaluation of prognostic risk factors in penetrating keratoplasty using Cox multiple regression model. *Nippon Ganka Gakkai Zasshi* 1994;98:777–781.

54. Price FW. Risk factors for corneal graft failure. In: *World Congress on the Cornea IV*. Orlando, FL: Castroviejo Society, 1996. Abstract.

55. Davanger M, Evensen A. Role of the pericorneal papillary structure in renewal of corneal epithelium. *Nature* 1971;229:560–561.

56. Kinoshita S, Kiorpes TC, Friend J, Thoft RA. Limbal epithelium in ocular surface wound healing. *Invest Ophthalmol Vis Sci* 1982;23:73–80.

57. Thoft RA. Keratoepithelioplasty. *Am J Ophthalmol* 1984;97:1–6.

58. Pfister RR. Corneal stem cell disease: concepts, categorization, and treatment by auto- and homotransplantation of limbal stem cells. *CLAO J* 1994;20:64–72.

Preoperative Tests and Evaluations

ROBERT E. BRASS   FREDERICK S. BRIGHTBILL

IMPORTANCE OF THE PREOPERATIVE EVALUATION

A thorough preoperative evaluation should take into account the factors making each case unique. Each underlying indication for keratoplasty has distinctive features that the surgeon must identify prior to keratoplasty, to avoid problems during the procedure and to decrease the incidence and severity of problems postoperatively. A thorough ocular history will often provide an indication as to what level of visual acuity will be feasible after the procedure. A patient with a failed graft secondary to uncontrolled glaucoma has a different prognosis than a patient undergoing keratoplasty for Fuchs' endothelial dystrophy. Systemic history is also important, as it can indicate the type of anesthesia to use as well as the feasibility of performing the proposed procedure. Finally, the slit-lamp examination combined with other forms of ocular assessment provides the cornerstone of diagnosis and management. Proper patient selection, preparation, and evaluation maximize the potential for a favorable outcome.

MEDICAL HISTORY

When one is obtaining the patient's history and review of the systems, the main questions to be answered ultimately relate to the ability of the patient to undergo the proposed operative procedure. Regarding local anesthesia, for example, the ability of the patient to lie flat for the duration of the procedure could be compromised by pulmonary or cardiac abnormalities. Severe arthritis may make it impossible for the patient to comfortably remain in any one position for an extended period of time and may warrant general anesthesia. Through consultation with the patient's primary-care physician, preexisting medical problems such as hypertension and diabetes should be stabilized prior to the keratoplasty. Because preoperative anxiety is common, patients should be advised to take their normal dose of antihypertensive medication on the morning of surgery. Insulin-dependent diabetics should undergo surgery early in the day if possible, and use one-half their normal dose prior to surgery, with the other one-half given postoperatively along with breakfast. Allergies to such medications as antibiotics, systemic agents, and anesthetics should be directly questioned, noted in the chart, and reviewed to avoid subsequent complications. With regard to topical agents, patients may be allergic to the preservative in the medication rather than the drug itself. If this is suspected, one can perform skin testing to identify such allergies before deciding to exclude use of an entire class of medications. The presence of cardiopulmonary disease should be noted, as it may limit the use of β-blockers postoperatively.

Patients taking aspirin, nonsteroidal anti-inflammatory drugs, and other medications interfering with blood coagulability deserve special preoperative consideration. It has been traditional practice to discontinue anticoagulants 10 to 14 days prior to surgery in consultation with the prescribing physician, with or without heparinization perioperatively. Relative safety has been demonstrated in patients undergoing intraocular procedures who have remained on medications that affect their coagulation. McCormack et al (1) demonstrated that procedures such as extracapsular cataract extraction with intraocular lens implantation, vitreoretinal surgery, and trabeculectomy can be performed safely without changing the anticoagulation status of the patient. Gainey et al (2) concluded that "if anticoagulants are necessary for a patient's well being, they should not be discontinued for cataract surgery." For patients with prothrombin times in a reasonably good range, we have had good success with simply discontinuing anticoagulation 48 hours prior to keratoplasty and resuming treatment the first postoperative day. If temporary cessation of anticoagulation is deemed inadvisable, patients taking warfarin (Coumadin) may require heparinization 24 to 48 hours preoperatively.

The patient's social and family support systems also need to be reviewed. As there will be a need for consistent use of postoperative medications and follow-up, the patient's compliance and reliability are important to the ultimate success of the graft. The patient's compliance with appointments and preoperative testing will have a direct bearing on postoperative compliance. However, even a compliant patient may not be physically able to self-administer topical eye medications. Family and local medical support, such as a visiting nurse, should be arranged prior to performing surgery. A history of substance abuse, or abrupt changes in family conditions that may interfere with patient follow-up may be a relative contraindication to surgery until the conditions stabilize.

OCULAR HISTORY

When contemplating keratoplasty, the ophthalmologist needs to have a complete understanding of the events that led to the patient's current status. The nature of the patient's ocular complaints helps guide the physician during the ocular examination and often leads to the diagnosis. As confirmed by a careful history, the presence of good visual acuity in the affected eye at some time prior to the current condition is associated with a better prognosis (e.g., good acuity after cataract surgery in eyes later developing pseudophakic bullous keratopathy). The presence of a corneal scar since childhood may have resulted in amblyopia, limiting potential visual acuity in the affected eye. A patient with a failed corneal graft secondary to uncontrolled glaucoma may have a poorer prognosis, even though good visual acuity was once present. Information should be obtained pertaining to the onset of the visual disturbance and to whether it was preceded by a prior intraocular procedure or infection or whether it simply deteriorated over time. The presence of pain should be determined, and if present, quantified as to occurrence and severity. Changes in quality of vision as the day progresses should also be ascertained; for example, in Fuchs' dystrophy, vision is often worse immediately upon awakening, with gradual improvement as the day progresses.

EVALUATION FOR KERATOPLASTY

The factors that affect the timing of keratoplasty are myriad. The patient's subjective complaints are very important during an evaluation for surgery. An active 55-year-old woman with painful bullae and decreased vision secondary to Fuchs' endothelial dystrophy or a 24-year-old keratoconus patient with an enlarging cone, diplopia, contact lens intolerance, and difficulty with night vision may be in greater need of intervention than an 80-year-old patient with pseudophakic bullous keratopathy who has 20/100 visual acuity, has no

pain, and is functioning well in the home environment. The rheumatoid patient with acute corneal melting and impending perforation may require emergency patch grafting. At times the status of the other eye must be considered. For example, a patient with pseudophakic bullous keratopathy in one eye, poor visual acuity, and the same closed-loop anterior chamber lens in the other eye is in a greater need of a keratoplasty than the keratoconus patient with asymmetric involvement and good contact lens tolerance.

Old medical records are invaluable and can alert the physician to potential operative problems and confirm important information such as prior best-corrected visual acuity, past intraocular pressure control, and previous intraocular lens powers. Patients often carry intraocular lens identification cards containing the desired information, which we find useful in computing the replacement intraocular lens power. A history should be ascertained of prior ophthalmic surgical procedures such as cataract extraction, filtering procedures, or use of the neodymium:yttrium-aluminum-garnet (Nd:YAG) laser for posterior capsular opacification. Knowledge of complications during the previous procedures will help to prevent potential surprises during keratoplasty.

Glaucoma and its control must be carefully evaluated before keratoplasty. Elevated pressure postoperatively can have deleterious effects on graft survival (3), and will ultimately lead to graft failure. Investigators demonstrated that elevated intraocular pressure leads to thinning of the corneal endothelium, morphologic signs of damage, and decreased endothelial cell count (4,5).

The prognosis for a successful outcome is ultimately linked to a knowledge of the patient's preoperative history. A corneal leukoma in the visual axis has important implications worthy of consideration: Was it the result of bacterial keratitis in a soft contact lens wearer, or was it of viral origin (i.e., herpes simplex), with the potential for graft rejection, perhaps requiring administration of a topical antiviral drug or oral acyclovir (6) after keratoplasty?

PREOPERATIVE EXAMINATION

Visual Acuity

Good history taking should confirm when in the past, visual acuity was better. One should rule out any amblyopia secondary to anisometropia, strabismus, or corneal scarring during childhood. The patient's best-corrected visual acuity should be determined initially. Standard Snellen testing is the normal mode of assessing visual acuity. If the patient cannot read the chart at 20 feet, poorer acuity such as the ability to only see and count fingers, to see hand motions, and to perceive light or no light needs to be documented. One of the most important acuity factors involves the careful testing of an eye for light projection. For eyes with corneal opacity and light-perception vision, the ability of the patient to discern the direction from which a light is projected is an important indicator of retinal and optic nerve function. A patient with good retinal function should be able to appreciate the light emitted from a standard muscle lamp in all quadrants (Fig. 2-1). In some patients with severe central visual loss, the light emitted from the indirect ophthalmoscope may be required. Testing visual acuity in a darkened room to compensate for light scattering and glare may also be beneficial.

The importance of good refraction cannot be overemphasized. In patients with keratoconus, for example, in whom retinoscopy is impossible due to scissoring light reflexes, one should consider checking keratometry values and performing a manifest refraction by dialing in the high astigmatic components (e.g., +3.00 first at 90 degrees, then 180 degrees and refining) and then progressively changing the sphere. It is also helpful to test for visual acuity with a rigid gas-permeable lens on the eye after a topical anesthetic is instilled. Even if not practical for long-term management, a contact lens can often eliminate irregular corneal astigmatism and provide an indication of better-corrected visual acuity and visual potential. In our experience, pinhole visual acuity, potential-acuity-meter, and glare tests have limited value in predicting best visual acuity, probably because of severe light scattering from the corneal pathology. One study (7) suggested that the placement of a hard contact lens over the cornea prior to performing potential-acuity-meter tests may be of benefit.

When there is a question as to whether there will be improvement in visual acuity after keratoplasty in eyes with corneal edema, one can instill topical glycerin after topical anesthesia and wait 20 to 30 minutes for corneal clearing; this may improve the patient's acuity and facilitate retinal viewing. Epithelial debridement with intravenous fluorescein injection may also be utilized preoperatively for evaluating preexisting cystoid macular edema (8) (Fig. 2-2).

External Examination

A preoperative evaluation of the bony structures of the orbit and prominence of the brow should be undertaken. For the patient with deep-set eyes or abnormally thin palpebral fissures, the proper position of the patient's head and the appropriate lid speculum to use during surgery should be determined in advance. If the patient has active acne rosacea with staphylococcal blepharitis, appropriate treatment should be instituted prior to the procedure. Herpes zoster, trauma, and radiation may account for lid scarring or neurotrophic keratitis and ultimate graft failure.

Slit-Lamp Examination

Lids, Lashes, and Lacrimal Gland

Lid disease such as blepharitis or meibomitis should be identified and controlled prior to keratoplasty. If the patient has an ectropion, entropion, or trichiasis, all of which can lead to epithelial scarring, permanent correction, usually surgical, prior to the keratoplasty is advised. Mild spastic entropion is frequently subclinical until surgery and should be treated rapidly when noted postoperatively.

Because normal tear production is crucial to graft re-epithelialization, the examiner must note tear-film abnormalities and dryness during the preoperative examination. The fluorescein or rose bengal test and Schirmer's test will give the ophthalmologist an indication as to the extent of dryness and epitheliopathy. When there is significant evidence of dryness, consideration should be given to partial or complete punctal occlusion preoperatively or at keratoplasty, sometimes in combination with partial medial or lateral tarsorrhaphy, particularly when lagophthalmos or exposure keratitis is suspected.

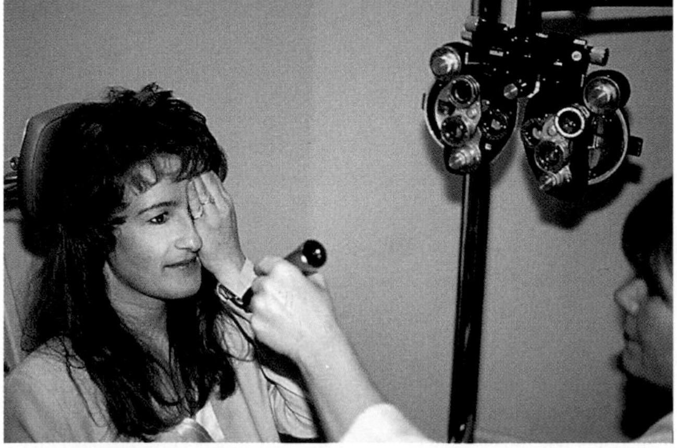

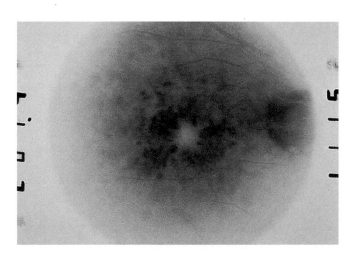

FIGURE 2-1.   *Evaluation of light projection. Note the patient is looking straight ahead, with the other eye completely covered.*

FIGURE 2-2.   *Cystoid macular edema viewed through a cornea with Fuchs' endothelial dystrophy 20 minutes after topical glycerin was applied.*

Conjunctiva and Limbus

A history of Stevens-Johnson syndrome, ocular cicatricial pemphigoid, or chemical burn should alert the ophthalmologist to look for scarring and symblepharon. These patients are at significant risk for dry eyes, nonhealing epithelial defects (Fig. 2-3), and infections postoperatively, as the normal external immune defense mechanisms of IgA and lysozyme are compromised. Procedures such as punctal occlusion, conjunctival transplantation, and limbal stem-cell transplantation (9,10) done prior to keratoplasty may improve the prognosis for graft survival in these high-risk patients (Fig. 2-4). On the day of surgery, the patient should be evaluated for blepharitis and conjunctivitis. If either is present, the surgery should be canceled and undertaken only after treatment and complete resolution.

Cornea

The underlying corneal problem necessitating transplantation is of obvious importance to planning for keratoplasty. The causes of corneal opacification requiring transplantation can be divided broadly into ectatic and stromal dystrophies, such as keratoconus, lattice, granular, and macular dystrophy; postinfectious corneal scarring with or without corneal vascularization, such as bacterial or viral ulcers; endothelial dysfunction with secondary stromal or epithelial edema, or both, such as Fuchs' dystrophy; and endothelial degeneration such as pseudophakic bullous keratopathy. These causes are associated with the prognosis for graft success (Table 2-1).

The diameter of the graft will be determined in part by the diameter of the corneal irregularity and its proximity to the central visual axis. For example, if possible, the diameter of the cone in keratoconus should be completely surrounded by the trephine so as to avoid suturing a thick edge to a thin edge and progressive thinning of the recipient bed postoperatively. Cone diameter is best determined by direct ophthalmoscopic viewing at +6.00 diopter (D) following

maximum mydriasis or by viewing the Fleischer ring intraoperatively. The Fleischer ring can be seen well at the slit lamp using the cobalt blue light. Preoperative sketching is also of value. Leukoma need not necessarily be totally surrounded by the trephine except when there are scars caused by herpes simplex virus, in which case removal of latent virus is desirable.

Consideration must also be given to the condition of the host graft bed, its corneal thickness or peripheral thinning. Ultrasonic pachymetry should be performed to quantify thinning or thickening. The presence of corneal vascularity will dictate the graft sizing and suturing technique to best minimize the propensity toward vascularization of the graft and possible rejection. In eyes with a postinfectious leukoma without vascularization, or with corneal edema secondary to Fuchs' dystrophy or bullous keratopathy, the central visual axis should be the center of the donor button with an average diameter ranging from 7.5 to 8.5 mm. A diameter

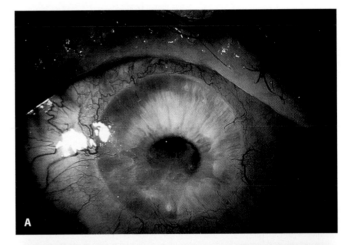

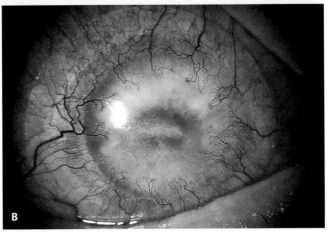

FIGURE 2-4. A. Corneal graft in a patient with severely dry eyes secondary to sulfuric acid burns. Early vascularization and clouding are seen 15 months after corneal transplantation. B. Same eye 2½ years later. The patient had numerous bouts with persistent epithelial defects. This patient may have benefited from limbal transplantation prior to penetrating keratoplasty.

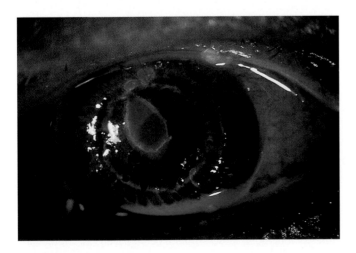

FIGURE 2-3. Nonhealing epithelial defect in the corneal graft of a patient with dry eye.

Table 2-1.   Prognosis for Graft Success*

Prognosis	Diagnosis
Excellent, 90% or more	1. Keratoconus
	2. Central Fuchs' dystrophy (early)
	3. Granular dystrophy
	4. Central or paracentral inactive scars
	5. Rotating grafts or autografts
Very good, 80%–90%	1. Advanced Fuchs' dystrophy
	2. Pseudophakic bullous keratopathy
	3. Aphakic bullous keratopathy
	4. Inactive herpes simplex keratitis
	5. Macular dystrophy
	6. Interstitial keratitis
	7. Iridocorneal endothelial syndromes
Fair, 50%–80%	1. Active bacterial keratitis
	2. Active herpes simplex keratitis
	3. Congenital hereditary endothelial dystrophy and breaks in Descemet's membrane associated with birth trauma
	4. Active fungal keratitis
	5. Mild chemical burns
	6. Moderate keratitis sicca
	7. Lattice dystrophy
	8. Congenital glaucoma
Poor, 0%–50%	1. Severe chemical burns
	2. Radiation burns
	3. Ocular pemphigoid
	4. Stevens–Johnson syndrome
	5. Neuroparalytic disease
	6. Epithelial downgrowth
	7. Anterior-chamber cleavage syndromes
	8. Multiple graft failures

* This table is meant as a guideline and is certainly not absolute. The prognosis for each group is worsened by the presence of elevated intraocular pressure, intraocular inflammation, lid or conjunctival defects, or other ocular surface disorders. Failed grafts are generally considered to possess the prognosis for the group of their primary diagnosis, or slightly less.

Source: Buxton JN, Buxton DF, Westphalen JA. In: Brightbill FS, ed. *Corneal surgery, theory, technique, and tissue.* 2nd ed. St. Louis: Mosby, 1993:81.

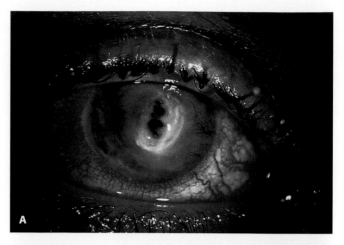

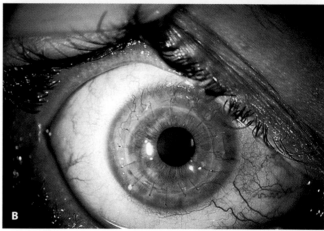

FIGURE 2-5.   A. *Stromal necrotizing keratitis secondary to herpes simplex infection with descemetocele and deep vascularization. B. Same eye 6 months after penetrating keratoplasty, demonstrating crystal clear graft with interrupted-suture placement. Note the absence of vessels in the donor tissue.*

of 8 mm is usually a good average size for trephination, but the total corneal diameter must be considered and when the overall corneal diameter is large, the surgeon should consider larger grafts. In most of our patients, the donor cornea is oversized by 0.25 mm. In the keratoconus patient, some surgeons will not use an oversized donor button in order to avoid inducing more myopia and may even use a smaller donor cornea (11,12). In patients with postinfectious scarring with thinning and vascularization, or displaced corneal ectasias as in pellucid marginal degeneration, sizing and placement of the graft may be less straightforward and some decentering may be required. The surgeon will need to decide the optimal size of the graft to avoid areas of vascularization and peripheral thinning. Interrupted sutures may be indicated to allow for selected removal of sutures from areas of vascularization aggravated by the sutures (Fig. 2-5).

In patients with corneal edema, an increased depth of trephination and deep suturing into the host bed to allow graft-host approximation of Descemet's membrane is important.

Anterior Segment and Iris

Perhaps most important in this part of the ocular examination is to rule out active inflammation. In patients undergoing elective transplantation, the chance for the best outcome is in a quiet, noninflamed eye. A ciliary flush, keratitic or intraocular lens precipitates, anterior synechiae, and iridocorneal adhesions are all signs of past or present inflammation and should be noted. The presence of an anterior-chamber lens necessitates identification as to whether it is an open- or closed-loop lens. Iris-supported and closed-loop anterior-chamber lenses should be replaced, as should any open-looped anterior-chamber lens when movement is suspected (13,14) (Fig. 2-6). Gonioscopy should be considered to examine iridocorneal adhesions and peripheral iridec-

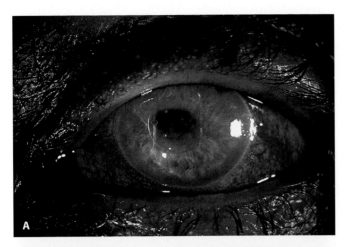

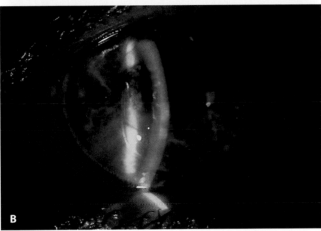

FIGURE 2-6.   A. *Patient with an iris-supported lens and pseudophakic bullous keratopathy.* B. *Magnified slit-beam view of the same eye, demonstrating stromal edema.*

tomies, as well as to locate the position of lens haptics if an anterior-chamber lens is present. In a cornea with dense corneal scarring precluding direct visualization, ultrasound biomicroscopy can aid in the evaluation of the iris, lens, iridocorneal adhesions, and peripheral anterior synechiae (15). If the anterior-chamber lens needs to be replaced, consideration of the patient's anterior-chamber anatomy (e.g., location of posterior and anterior synechiae and residual lens capsule) will play a role in deciding the appropriate type of lens to use. A thorough evaluation of the iris is important. The presence of rubeosis and fibrovascular membranes obscuring the pupil, and the location of peripheral iridectomies need to be noted.

If the pupil can be well visualized, the presence or absence of a relative afferent pupillary defect should be documented. Presence of color visual perception will also help to rule out optic nerve damage.

Lens

Prior to keratoplasty, the patient's lens should be examined with the slit-lamp microscope. The lens may have weakened

zonules and exhibit phakodinesis. In many elderly patients, especially eyes with Fuchs' dystrophy, the lens may exhibit early cataractous changes, which may signal the need for a combined keratoplasty and cataract extraction. It is our belief that keratoplasty, perhaps aided by high-dose postoperative corticosteroids, is frequently a cataractogenic procedure. Triple procedures should be performed when even minimal lens opacities are present, to avoid the need for future cataract extraction, which can damage the endothelium and threaten the integrity of the graft. Patients with chronic, luetic, inactive interstitial keratitis and scarring frequently do not present to the corneal surgeon until progressive cataract occurs. When combined with the leukoma this produces a significant inability to function, necessitating a combined procedure.

In eyes that have had prior cataract extraction, knowledge of the intraocular lens design (anterior chamber, iris supported, or posterior chamber) or of aphakia is critical to operative planning. The type of lens implanted will dictate whether it should be replaced.

Intraocular Pressure

The presence of borderline controlled or uncontrolled glaucoma is a contraindication to keratoplasty. Accurate applanation pressures in corneas with epithelial edema are difficult to obtain and falsely low readings may be generated. A Tonopen, pneumotonometer, and MacKay-Marg tonometer are considered to provide more accurate values (16,17). We believe that the intraocular pressure should be no higher than the low 20s when no more than two topical medications are used. If not, primary filtering, combined filtering and penetrating keratoplasty or seton surgery should be considered. Because all keratoplasty patients receive intraoperative viscoelastic agents to coat the donor endothelium, to aid in the control of bleeding, and to help prevent synechiae (18), eyes with preexistent glaucoma will usually require immediate postoperative oral ocular hypotensives and topical aqueous inhibitors to control intraocular pressure. The use of a lower-viscosity viscoelastic agent such as Healon and its removal or dilution with balanced salt solution in the anterior chamber prior to button placement and suturing are recommended. The long-term use of a topical steroid to prevent rejection may lead to steroid-induced glaucoma and requires careful monitoring of intraocular pressure for the entire postoperative period. In our experience, long-standing chronic glaucoma with intraocular pressures in the low to mid 20s is a common cause of slow graft failure.

Retina and Vitreous

An evaluation of retinal function and the vitreous is required to ensure that decreased vision is secondary to problems with the cornea alone. Macular degeneration, cystoid macular edema, macular holes, and an opaque or hazy vitreous among other maladies will not improve after keratoplasty. Knowledge of such conditions prior to keratoplasty will help in the prognostication, and can often be obtained during examination of old records and discussions with the referring ophthalmologist. When there is a question regarding the presence of these conditions, potential-acuity-meter testing, or electrophysiological testing can be tried but have limited sensitivity. If the retina and vitreous cannot be visualized by direct or indirect ophthalmoscopy, ultrasonography should be undertaken to rule out a retinal detachment, retinal mass, or vitreous hemorrhage.

COMMUNICATION WITH PATIENT

Once the evaluation has been completed, the diagnosis and plans for keratoplasty should be discussed with the patient. The procedure should be clearly explained using handouts, models, or videotapes as indicated. Our videotape, "Patient Eye View," is available through the Eye Bank Association of America and offers prior recipients' evaluations of their surgery, preoperative and postoperative instructions, and education on drop instillation, eye care, and signs of rejection. The risks of the procedure specifically regarding the long healing time, need for antiglaucoma treatment, and rejection rates should be addressed. The patient should be given realistic expectations for potential visual acuity and the time it may take to reach that acuity. The possible use of a contact lens, relaxing incisions, or wedge resection to reach best visual acuity should be understood by the patient prior to the procedure, to ensure patient satisfaction in the postoperative period. The keratoplasty patient is entering into a lifelong physician-patient relationship. Sound preoperative planning and explanation between the surgeon and the patient will help to make this relationship a fruitful one.

REFERENCES

1. McCormack P, Simcock PR, Tullo AB. Management of the anticoagulated patient for ophthalmic surgery. *Eye* 1993;7:749–750.
2. Gainey S, et al. Ocular surgery on patients receiving long term warfarin therapy. *Am J Ophthalmol* 1989;108:142–146.
3. Maguire MG, et al. Risk factors for corneal graft failure and rejection in the Collaborative Corneal Transplant Studies. Collaborative Corneal Transplantation Studies Research Group. *Ophthalmology* 1994;101:1536–1547.
4. Svedbergh B. Effects of artificial intraocular pressure elevation on corneal endothelium in the vervet monkey. *Acta Ophthalmol* 1975;53:839.
5. Vannag A, Setala K, Ruusuvaana P. Endothelial cells in capsular glaucoma. *Acta Ophthalmol* 1977;55:951.
6. Barney NP, Foster CS. A prospective randomized trial of oral acyclovir after penetrating keratoplasty for herpes simplex keratitis. *Cornea* 1994;13:231–236.
7. Smiddy WE, et al. Potential acuity meter for predicting postoperative visual acuity in penetrating keratoplasty. A new method using a hard contact lens. *Ophthalmology* 1987;94:12–16.
8. Brightbill FS, Dudley SS. Aphakic bullous keratopathy: preoperative fluorescein angiographic screening for macular edema. *Contact Intraocular Lens Med J* 1981;7:144–149.
9. Tan DT, Ficker LA, Buckley RJ. Limbal transplantation. *Ophthalmology* 1996;103:29–36.
10. Kenyon KR, Tseng SC. Limbal autograft transplantation for ocular surface disorders. *Ophthalmology* 1996;96:709–722 (discussion, 722–723).
11. Lanier JD, Bullington RH Jr, Prager TC. Axial length in keratoconus. *Cornea* 1996;11:250–254.
12. Girard LJ, et al. Use of grafts smaller than the opening for keratoconic myopia and astigmatism. A prospective study. *J Cataract Refract Surg* 1992;18:380–384.
13. Doren GS, Stern GA, Driebe WT. Indications for and results of intraocular lens explantation. *J Cataract Refract Surg* 1992;18:79–85.
14. Kornmehl EW, et al. Penetrating keratoplasty for pseudophakic bullous keratopathy associated with closed-loop anterior chamber lenses. *Ophthalmology* 1990;97:407–412.
15. Milner MS, et al. High-resolution ultrasound biomicroscopy of the anterior segment in patients with dense corneal scars. *Ophthalmic Surg* 1994;25:284–287.
16. Rootman DS, et al. Accuracy and precision of the Tono-Pen in measuring intraocular pressure after keratoplasty and epikeratophakia and in scarred cornea. *Acta Ophthalmol* 1988;106:1600–1700.
17. Wind CA, Irvine AR. Electronic applanation tonometry in corneal edema and keratoplasty. *Invest Ophthalmol* 1969;8:620–624.
18. Liesegang TJ. Viscoelastics. *Int Ophthalmol Clin* 1969;33:127–147.

Phakic Corneal Transplantation

Michael P. Vrabec

Corneal transplantation represents one of the most successful and most commonly performed operations in all of medicine. The Eye Bank Association of America (EBAA) estimates that over 40,000 transplant procedures were performed in 1994 (1). There are multiple factors in the overall success rate of the restoration of vision after corneal transplantation. This chapter covers the surgical technique of phakic corneal transplantation. Just as a pilot would not enter the cockpit of a plane without a specific flight plan, the surgeon must have a plan prior to entering the operating room. Hence, a section on preoperative considerations is included.

PREOPERATIVE CONSIDERATIONS

The Eye Examination

The surgeon needs to begin the surgical plan while the patient is being examined in the office. A complete ophthalmologic examination is required, with special attention to eyelid anatomy, function, and disease. For example, an incomplete blink due to a prior Bell's palsy may result in delayed epithelial healing after transplantation. This could ultimately affect the clarity of the graft. In this situation a temporary tarsorrhaphy should be performed at the completion of the operation to encourage healing. This should be discussed prior to surgery and included in the operative consent. Blepharitis must be managed and controlled prior to surgery, to prevent secondary ulceration of the cornea. The presence of keratitis sicca and its severity should also be determined. In patients with significantly dry eyes, either temporary or permanent punctal occlusion with plugs or cautery should be achieved at the conclusion of the procedure. Multiple techniques for achievement of punctal occlusion have been described (2,3). Any active keratitis should

be controlled prior to surgery, unless there is an associated perforation of the cornea. If the cornea is anesthetic, the likelihood of the graft remaining clear in the long term is significantly reduced and the patient should be informed of this possibility. There should not be any active uveitis at the time of surgery. This chapter assumes that the patient's lens is clear and will not be removed at the time of surgery. If there is associated glaucoma, it should be under control prior to surgery. The factors important in the preoperative evaluation are as follows:

Lid function (lagophthalmos, ectropion, entropion)
Lid disease (blepharitis)
Tear quality and quantity (keratitis sicca, vitamin A deficiency)
Keratitis
Corneal sensation
Uveitis/iritis
Lens status
Glaucoma

Careful examination of the recipient's cornea cannot be overemphasized. The location and depth of the disease process can be better determined prior to the operation with a slit lamp than under the operating microscope. It is important to include as much of the pathology as possible when choosing the size of the recipient bed, but as important, the surgeon should always attempt to sew the donor button into a recipient bed of the same thickness. Improper apposition between the host and donor can lead to wound displacement with resultant wound-healing problems as well as astigmatism (Fig. 3-1).

In general, the larger the recipient bed, the better the optical results of a penetrating keratoplasty. However, the risk of transplant rejection also increases, owing to the closer approximation of the donor tissue to the vascularized

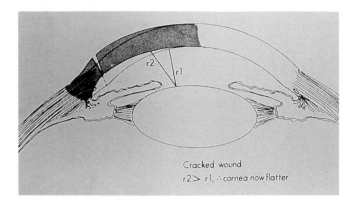

Cracked wound
r2> r1, ∴ cornea now flatter

FIGURE 3-1.   *Wound gape between the donor cornea and host site results in flattening of the donor cornea in this meridian and induced astigmatism.*

limbus. A larger graft may be associated with a higher risk of postoperative glaucoma because of compression of the anterior-chamber angle. The final size of the host bed is determined at surgery, but again the surgeon should have a clear idea of the necessary size of the transplant prior to entering the operating room.

Informed Consent

In this increasingly litiginous atmosphere, it behooves the surgeon to document that the patient has been fully informed of the potential risks, benefits, and alternatives to surgery. I have found the form in Figure 3-2 to be of help in documenting that the patient has indeed been through the informed consent process, as the general informed consents used by hospitals do not document a thorough discussion with the patient. Our clinic also uses a videotape as part of this process.

Preoperative Antibiotics

Most corneal surgeons will use topical antibiotics preoperatively to reduce the risk of postoperative infection. I typically start ofloxacin 2 hours prior to surgery, giving one drop every 30 minutes for a total of four doses. This medication could be given the night before, but then the surgeon must count on the patient remembering to take the medication. The patient continues to take this medication postoperatively as well. I tend to avoid ciprofloxacin because of the risk of plaque formation in patients in whom the graft epithelializes slowly.

Pupil Considerations

For patients who are phakic and are to remain phakic, pilocarpine is critical to protect the lens during the procedure. Additional benefits include help in determining the patient's visual axis, and keeping the lens back in the setting of posterior vitreous pressure. One drop of a 2% concentration of

Patient Name _____

This patient was informed of potential risks, complications, benefits, and alternatives to treatment of the recommended surgery. These include infection, lid droop (ptosis) bleeding, swelling of the cornea (resulting in the need for a corneal transplant), glaucoma, retinal swelling, retinal detachment, loss of best corrected vision, and loss of the eye. These complications can occur immediately, days, weeks, months

or years after surgery. In addition, the procedure of _____

_____

may also result in the following complications: _____

_____

of which the patient was informed.

The patient had the opportunity to have all of their questions answered and understands no guarantee has been made regarding the outcome of the operation.

The patient was also informed that the doctor can not possibly predict and discuss every possible complication that might occur with the planned operation.

_____   _____

DATE   DOCTOR

FIGURE 3-2.   *Informed consent document that becomes part of the patient's chart.*

pilocarpine given three times an hour before surgery will suffice in maintaining a small pupil during surgery. The same arguments can be used in the pseudophakic patient with a posterior-chamber lens and an intact posterior capsule in whom only a corneal transplantation will be performed.

Tissue Concerns

It is beyond the scope of this chapter to discuss in detail factors to consider in tissue selection for a particular patient. However, the surgeon must bear in mind that he or she carries the ultimate responsibility for the tissue being used. The eye bank makes it clear in the tissue information forms that come with the cornea that no guarantee or warrantee is made regarding the quality of tissue. Surgeons who work with EBAA-certified eye banks will not be offered tissue that does not meet certain standards; nonetheless the surgeon should consider the following factors when accepting tissue.

Donor Age

There is no upper limit in terms of donor age and acceptability of the cornea for transplantation. For tissue over the age of 65, specular microscopy should be done. The absolute cell count and the degree of polymorphism and polymegathism are important. A cell count of more than 2000 cells/mm^2 is acceptable. Although most surgeons would prefer that the donor age be similar to the recipient age, there are no studies to indicate that this is necessary. Tissue life will also be lengthened when the interval from death to preservation is as short as possible and the body is refrigerated with ice placed over the eyes, prior to in situ removal or enucleation. Infant corneas should be used with caution as reports of large myopic shifts in recipients of such corneas have been reported (5).

Cause of Death

Again, the EBAA medical standards are clear in terms of acceptable causes of death. Of note, if there is an unclear cause of death, or if the donor exhibited high-risk behavior for the presence of diseases such as human immunodeficiency virus (HIV) infection or hepatitis, the surgeon should take this into consideration and possibly decline the tissue being offered. It is rare that such tissue would be offered to the surgeon, but it has occurred.

Serology

Current (1996) EBAA standards require the testing of every donor for HIV, hepatitis B, and hepatitis C. Syphilis testing is no longer required. The surgeon should carefully review the paperwork that accompanies each cornea to make sure the results of all serology tests are in fact negative.

Tissue Quality

If a surgeon anticipates potential epithelial healing problems during the postoperative period, donor tissue with minimal changes due to exposure of the epithelial surface and without actual defects should be requested. This is an important consideration as the eye bank will have very limited information on the recipient. If the tissue being offered has a broad band of arcus and the surgeon anticipates the need for a large graft in a young recipient (i.e., keratoconus), he or she may elect not to accept the particular tissue because of the potentially unacceptable cosmetic result.

The surgeon should inspect the tissue in the operating room prior to the operation. If this is done prior to the day of surgery and there are problems with the tissue, another donor might be obtained without the need to postpone the surgery. Slit-lamp examination of the tissue is preferred but may not be possible. The color and clarity of the storage media should be evaluated; any change of color from the typical orange-pink hue (assuming Optisol GS is the storage media) indicates a change in the pH of the solution. This signals a potential for contamination, and the tissue should be returned to the eye bank. A careful review of the paperwork is recommended to make sure the I.D. number on the tissue label matches that on the recipient form.

Anesthesia

The decision on the type of anesthesia to be employed during the operation should be discussed in advance with the patient. For most adult patients, a local anesthetic with intravenous conscious sedation and supplemental oxygen will suffice. This represents a safer alternative and a faster recovery time than a general anesthetic allows. Because the globe will be soft and the risk for extrusion of intraocular contents is high, the block must be solid and should be checked by the surgeon. For this reason, a retrobulbar anesthetic including a long-acting agent [i.e., 2% lidocaine with 0.75% bupivacaine (Marcaine)] is preferable over a peribulbar anesthetic. The other advantage of a retrobulbar block over a peribulbar injection is less risk of chemosis of the bulbar conjunctiva. Chemosis can make placement of a scleral fixation ring much more difficult. A facial nerve block (i.e., van Lint's or O'Brien's) is required for the same reason. Blocking the superior oblique muscle is optional. The eye should also be softened for 10 to 20 minutes with a pressure-reducing device (Honan balloon or SuperPinky) to reduce posterior vitreous pressure. In the era of topical anesthesia for no-stitch cataract surgery, the anterior-segment surgeon performing corneal transplantation must not be lulled into accepting an incomplete block for corneal transplantation.

General anesthetic should be reserved for children, patients with severe anxiety, and those who are unable to lay still during the operation.

THE PROCEDURE

Patient Positioning

Before the patient is draped, the position of the patient's head should be adjusted in such a manner that the corneal plane is parallel to the floor. If the cornea is not in this position (i.e., straight up), there is a greater chance of inducing postoperative astigmatism, due to either uneven trephination or distortion of intraoperative keratoscopic mires owing to errors of parallax. The best way to see if this is in fact the case is to view the patient from the side at an eye-to-eye level. The effectiveness of the local anesthetic should be verified one more time in terms of both anesthesia and akinesia prior to the preparation and draping of the patient.

Draping

I have found that trimming the lashes prior to surgery is unnecessary for corneal transplantation. In fact, it may prove more difficult to completely cover the ends of trimmed eyelashes with a drape than it would otherwise be to cover long lashes. However it is achieved, the lashes must be carefully covered to avoid contamination of suture as it is being placed in the cornea. Even with careful cleansing of the lashes preoperatively, they can be the source of serious postoperative ocular infections.

Lid Support

Lid support must be consistent throughout the procedure with as little disruption to the globe as possible. Poor lid support may lead to increased intraocular pressure and distortion of the globe, leading to postoperative astigmatism. This generally results from the host wound becoming oval in shape from the additional pressure. Several choices are available. I prefer the Barraquer wire speculum because of its small size. The McNeill-Goldman ring combines the blepharostat with the scleral support ring and is less likely to distort the eye during surgery.

Scleral Support

There are multiple ways to ensure adequate support of the sclera during corneal transplantation. For the phakic patient who is to remain phakic, two 4-0 silk sutures placed through the rectus superior and inferior tendons will provide adequate support of the globe during the operation. The needle should be tapered to lessen the risk of inadvertent perforation of the sclera. When compared to metal rings (i.e., Flieringa ring) fixated to the episclera, rectus traction sutures can be placed in less time and cause less corneal distortion. However, in patients who are pseudophakic and are going to keep their intraocular lens implant, patients who are highly myopic with extremely flaccid sclera, obese patients with a short neck in whom the surgeon may anticipate problems with excessive posterior vitreous pressure, or if an unusually large graft is contemplated, a metal ring should be used. The ring is typically anchored by four interrupted 5-0 Mersilene or Vicryl sutures on a spatulated needle. The sutures should be placed 3.5 to 4.0 mm posterior to the limbus so if inadvertent perforation of the sclera occurs, the retina will not be damaged (Fig. 3-3). With the ring resting at this distance, it is possible to gain rapid access to the vitreous cavity. When I anticipate excessive posterior pressure, I perform a small conjunctiva resection followed by a partial-thickness cutdown through the sclera 3.5 mm posterior to the limbus. This can provide rapid access to aspirate a pocket of liquid vitreous if other maneuvers to relieve posterior pressure have failed and the patient is in jeopardy

of losing the lens. It is important to place all four sutures at the same depth, tension, and distance from the limbus to minimize distortion that could lead to postoperative astigmatism (6).

Host/Donor Trephination and Host Centration

In a previous section, I discussed factors to consider when determining the size of the host bed. I begin by using calipers to measure the cornea in at least two directions (Fig. 3-4). Many times, the desired wound may be good in one meridian, but too close to the limbus in another, so that a compromise is necessary. A sterile marking pen or sponge saturated with gentian violet can be used to mark the trephine. If the trephine is then gently placed on the cornea (Fig. 3-5A), a mark is left behind to allow the surgeon to see where the wound will lie in relation to the limbus (Fig. 3-5B). This allows for recentration of the trephine or exchanging the size of the trephine based on the mark.

I generally place the host mark to cover the visual axis (center of the constricted pupil) evenly. However, it is

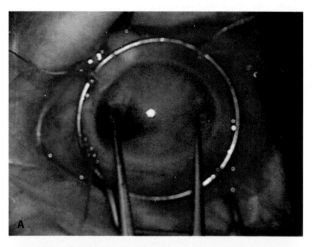

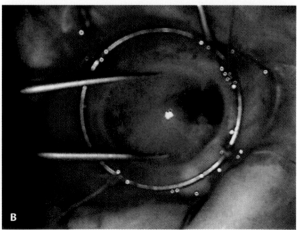

FIGURE 3-4.   A. *Horizontal measurement of the host cornea to determine trephination size.* B. *Vertical measurement of the host cornea to determine trephination size.*

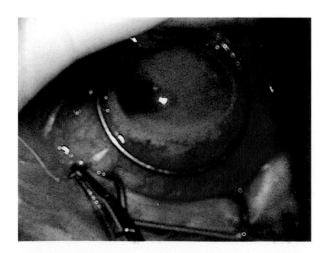

FIGURE 3-3.   *Placement of 5-0 Mersilene suture to fixate the scleral support ring. The suture is 3 to 4 mm posterior to the limbus.*

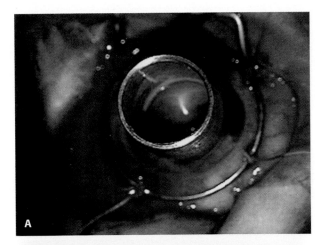

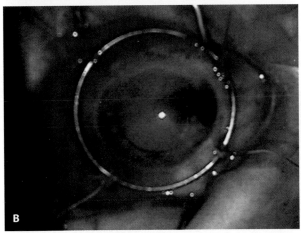

FIGURE 3-5. A. *Trephine gently resting on the cornea to mark the site of trephination.* B. *Gentian violet mark left behind from the trephine.*

important to try to leave 1 to 2 mm of peripheral cornea for 360 degrees. Many times this means the final location of the wound will be slightly nasal and inferior in terms of the geometric center of the host cornea.

When the surgeon is satisfied that the position of the wound will be acceptable, a choice for the size of the donor button must be made. *The donor button should always be punched and placed aside prior to any trephination of the host cornea.* If the button is not successfully punched, the procedure can be aborted with no harm to the host cornea.

The corresponding size of the donor button depends on several factors. The size of the recipient bed itself must be considered. In small recipient beds (i.e., 6.0–6.5 mm), the donor button should be 0.5 mm larger to ensure adequate tissue distribution over the host surface area. In the mid-range recipient beds (i.e., 7.0–8.0 mm), the donor button is usually oversized 0.2 mm. In large recipient beds (i.e., 9.0 mm or more), the donor button should be the same size as the recipient site. These guidelines are appropriate when the surgeon plans to bevel the recipient wound, leaving a

small posterior shelf of tissue to support the donor button. This technique allows the surgeon to use minimum tension to create a watertight closure. If a surgeon chooses not to bevel the wound, the sutures may need to be tighter and the donor tissue may need to be oversized for a larger recipient bed.

Special circumstances may alter the general guidelines listed here. For example, in a patient with keratoconus who is also highly myopic, the surgeon may use donor tissue that is the same size as the host bed. This would stretch the tissue and tend to induce flattening of the cornea, thereby reducing the amount of myopia.

Other factors determining the size of the recipient bed have been discussed (see Preoperative Considerations, The Eye Examination).

Most surgeons will cut the donor tissue from the endothelial surface. Care must be taken not to touch the endothelium during this process. Several different systems are available to the surgeon. Three commonly used punches include the Iowa PK Press (7), the Lieberman punch, and the Hanna trephine (8). Few surgeons perform the trephination freehand with the tissue placed in a concave Teflon well. Care must be taken to dry the tissue prior to placing it in the well, to avoid the accumulation of fluid under the cornea and inducing an irregular cut.

The Iowa PK Press uses disposable Weck trephines. The Teflon disk has a red center of 8.0 mm to help center the donor button. The disk automatically centers in a circular depression in the base of the trephine. The properly sized trephine is fixated to the end of the trephine and the piston driven completely through the donor tissue. The piston is then lifted, making sure the button has been successfully cut. If the cut is incomplete, it can be completed with corneal scissors. Care must be taken not to damage the corneal endothelium. If the tissue remains in the barrel of the trephine, the trephine should be removed from the barrel of the punch. Saline solution is then gently placed inside the trephine to dislodge the tissue. The Hanna system employs an artificial chamber to allow trephination from the epithelial side.

When it is determined that the button has been successfully created, it can be left in the Teflon cutting disk immersed in preservation media and covered with a medicine glass until needed.

Attention can now be given to cutting the recipient cornea. Several techniques are possible, the simplest being that of holding a disposable trephine by hand. The trephine is placed over the host cornea, guided by the previously placed gentian violet mark. Placing one or two drops of saline solution on the cornea prior to trephination will allow the cutting to proceed more smoothly. If trephination is to be performed by hand, large rotations of the trephine (of at least 180 degrees) will allow for more even wound edges (Fig. 3-6). This technique allows for the best visualization of the exact location of the incision, but may also result in uneven wound edges or unequal depth of

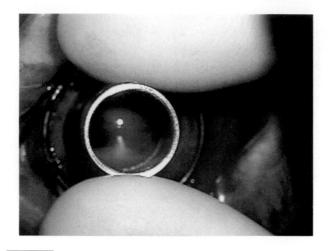

FIGURE 3-6.   *Cutting of the host cornea by hand with a disposable trephine.*

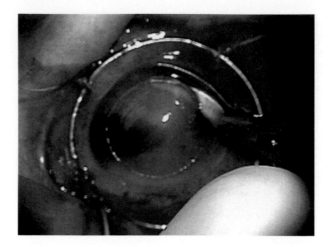

FIGURE 3-8.   *Cutting the host tissue with corneal scissors. Upward force is applied to the scissors so as not to damage the iris or induce a cataract.*

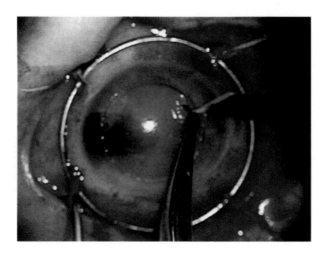

FIGURE 3-7.   *Entry into the anterior chamber with a super-sharp blade at the 9-o'clock position.*

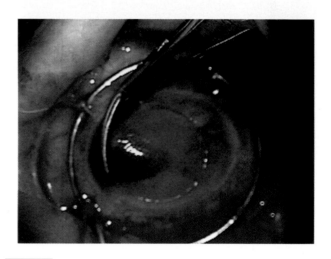

FIGURE 3-9.   *Cutting host tissue past the 3-o'clock meridian with corneal scissors.*

penetration into the stroma. Alternatively, the trephine can be placed on a handle with an internal obturator to prevent complete penetration of the cornea.

The Barron-Hessburg vacuum trephine is another popular tool used to cut the host cornea (9). This fixates the cornea with suction during trephination. There is a spring-loaded syringe connected by a plastic tube to a vacuum chamber. The blade is next to the inner wall of the chamber. It may be particularly well suited for perforated corneas, as it may avoid any undue pressure on the eye.

Some surgeons prefer to trephine a partial thickness (perhaps 85%–90% of the stroma) of the cornea, which will allow for the creation of a small posterior ledge of tissue. This can provide support for the donor button in addition to the suture, allowing for less tension on the suture. Tight sutures can result in irregular astigmatism. With a partial-depth cut, entry into the anterior chamber is achieved with a sharp-point blade, typically at the 9-o'clock position (Fig.

3-7). Other surgeons prefer to cut completely through the cornea. It is their contention that the additional tissue in the posterior aspect of the wound makes it more difficult to distribute donor tissue equally, resulting in postoperative astigmatism.

Cautery may be applied to the apex of a cone prior to trephination in severe keratoconus, to shrink the tissue in an attempt to create a more normal contour.

The host cornea can now be removed with corneal scissors. Care must be taken to ensure that the scissors have been completely inserted into the anterior chamber so as to not leave Descemet's membrane behind. Slight upward traction and cutting near the heal of the scissors will allow for the smoothest possible cut (Fig. 3-8). For righthanded surgeons, scissors to the left are initially used, and continued to the 2-o'clock meridian (Fig. 3-9). By carrying the incision beyond the 3-o'clock meridian, it is much easier to complete the incision with left-cutting scissors (Fig. 3-10). With forceps, tension should be maintained at 90 degrees from the scissors, to allow for a smooth cut. A cellulose sponge is often useful in drying the wound just before the scissors are used, to allow for better visualization (Fig. 3-11).

The surgeon must keep a careful eye on the intraocular contents during the incision. Obviously, care must be taken not to damage the iris with scissors. For the novice surgeon, a viscoelastic agent can be injected into the anterior segment after initial entry with the super-sharp blade (Fig. 3-12). This will keep intraocular contents back and allow for easier cutting.

Excessive vitreous pressure can result in endothelial cell damage (10). Certain patients (obese patients, short-necked patients, and those with emphysema) may be expected to present with this problem. A series of steps should be taken to control excessive vitreous pressure:

Check the speculum for proper positioning.
Consider hyperventilation to relieve the pressure (if patient is under a general anesthetic).
Control blood pressure if elevated.
Consider intravenous administration of mannitol.
Consider aspiration of liquid vitreous through the pars plana.

If the vitreous pressure remains elevated, the surgeon may wish to abandon the procedure and resuture the patient's own cornea. Another technique that has been described involves fixating the donor cornea onto the host before the host tissue has been completely removed. Initially, a small amount of viscoelastic substance is placed on the host epithelium to protect the donor endothelium. The donor button is then placed on top of the host and sutured in as the underlying host cornea is cut and removed. After the first three cardinal sutures are in place, the host cornea is completely excised and slid out from under the donor.

After removal of the host cornea, the wound should be inspected. Any excessive tissue can be carefully excised with corneal or Vannas scissors; however, in general it is best to err on the side of leaving extra tissue to avoid any potential for a wound leak or tissue distortion due to a lack of tissue (Fig. 3-13).

Transfer of the Donor Button to the Recipient

The transfer of the donor button to the host bed should be done as quickly but carefully as possible. Cellulose sponges can be used to remove the storage media and gently push the button to the edge of the Teflon disk where it can be grasped with toothed forceps (Fig. 3-14). The forceps should grasp nearly the entire thickness of the cornea. Alternatively, a Paton spatula can be used to transfer the button. As it is placed in the host, it should be rotated in such a way as to equally distribute tissue in all four quadrants (Fig. 3-15). If

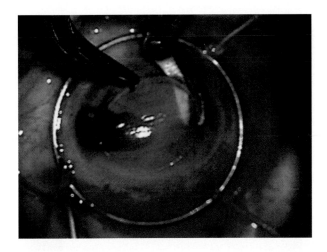

FIGURE 3-10. *Cutting the host tissue in the opposite direction. Traction is applied 90 degrees from the scissors to avoid uneven cutting of the tissue.*

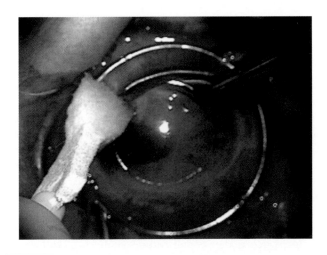

FIGURE 3-11. *Use of a cellulose sponge to dry the wound before employing the scissors improves visualization.*

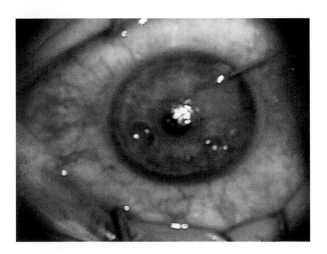

FIGURE 3-12. *Viscoelastic substance being placed in the anterior chamber to protect the intraocular contents while scissors are used to cut the cornea.*

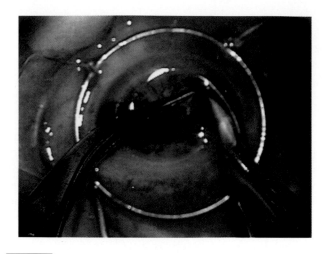

FIGURE 3-13.   *Trimming excessive posterior tissue with corneal scissors.*

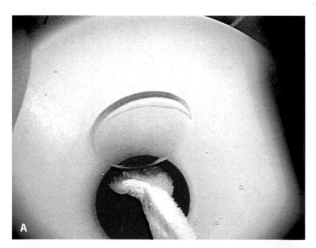

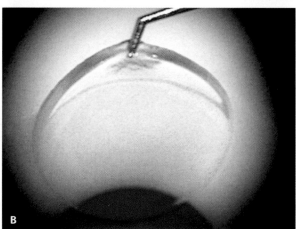

FIGURE 3-14.   A. *Donor button on the edge of the Teflon disk.* B. *Holding the button with 0.12 forceps prior to transfer.*

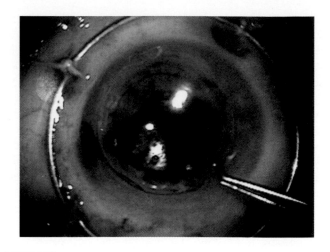

FIGURE 3-15.   *Rotating the donor button to equally distribute the tissue.*

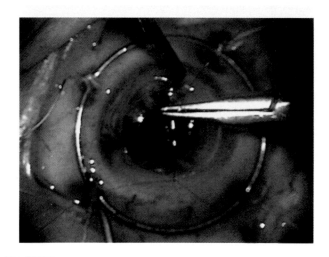

FIGURE 3-16.   *Placement of the second cardinal suture.*

there happens to be part of an arcus on the donor button, it can be hidden under the upper lid.

Suturing the Donor

The next step in a phakic penetrating keratoplasty is to place the donor tissue into the host bed and fixate the tissue with suture. Multiple types of sutures have been used, but the most common is 10-0 nylon. Nylon has the advantage of elasticity and as such is easier to handle when compared to Mersilene, but nylon may dissolve unpredictably, resulting in induced astigmatism. The 11-0 suture is popular with some surgeons, but may be difficult to handle as well.

Common to all suturing techniques is placement of the first four cardinal sutures. The placement of these sutures, and in particular the second suture (at the 6-o'clock position), is critical in minimizing postoperative astigmatism (Fig. 3-16). Care should be taken to ensure adequate and equal distribution of tissue in each of the four quadrants. Usually at this time, a ring light or intraoperative keratometer can be used to detect astigmatism, which should be corrected by suture replacement and tissue readjustment. It is nearly impossible to correct astigmatism detected at this point with additional "compensatory" sutures. Rather, the four sutures should be replaced as necessary until the astigmatism appears minimal. The scleral ring can be removed at this time if there is concern that it might be inducing corneal distortion leading to astigmatism.

Multiple suturing techniques have been described. These include a single running suture, a double running suture, a combination of interrupted and running sutures, and all interrupted sutures. There are advantages and disadvantages to all techniques. A running suture tends to be faster to place, hence shortening the operating room time. It tends to allow for faster recovery of vision when compared to all interrupted sutures. However, there is less ability to manipulate sutures in the early postoperative period to decrease astigmatism. Many surgeons use a combination of interrupted and a single running suture, typically a 12 interrupted suture with a 12-bite running suture pattern (Fig. 3-17). Alternatively, an 8-bite interrupted–8-bite running technique can be employed. However, in special circumstances, the surgeon may prefer to use all interrupted sutures. These circumstances include a vascularized peripheral host, pediatric recipients, and large (>10 mm) donor buttons. In these situations sutures have a high likelihood of eroding at an unpredictable rate, and using just a running suture technique could result in segments of the suture eroding prior to wound stabilization, risking wound dehiscence.

Whatever pattern is employed, there are several principles that should be followed with each suture bite. Sutures should be passed under the fixation forceps with minimal torque on the tissue. Suture length should be minimized to 1 mm or less on each side of the wound to prevent irregular astigmatism. They should be at least three-fourths the depth of the cornea to allow for secure fixation. The depth of the suture should be equal on the host and recipient side to prevent tissue disparity, wound override, and secondary astigmatism (Fig. 3-18). Suture tension should be minimized to prevent astigmatism but still maintain a watertight closure.

Tieing of the suture knots can be achieved in one of several fashions. Using a one throw–one throw–one throw slip knot allows the surgeon excellent control of the tension of the knot. The second throw creates a "granny" knot, which can be adjusted to the desired tension. The third throw squares the second so that the knot will not slip. It is important to orient the suture ends correctly to avoid the knot becoming overly tight when the last throw is placed.

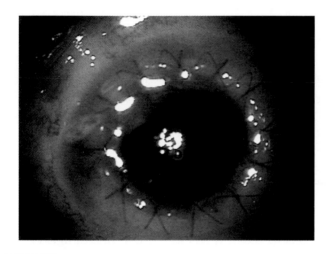

FIGURE 3-17. *A 12 interrupted and 12-bite running suture pattern.*

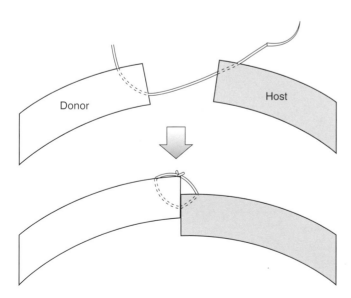

FIGURE 3-18. *Wound displacement resulting from an unequal depth of suture bites in the host and donor.*

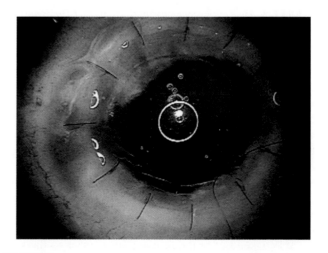

FIGURE 3-19. *Minimal astigmatism detected with a ring light during suturing.*

GUIDELINES FOR HOME CARE FOLLOWING CORNEAL TRANSPLANT SURGERY

1. YOU SHOULD HAVE SPECTACLES OR A SHIELD OVER THE OPERATED EYE AT ALL TIMES. GLASSES ARE SUFFICIENT DURING THE DAY, BUT YOU SHOULD USE A SHIELD AT NIGHT. AN EYE PATCH IS/IS NOT NECESSARY UNDER THE SHIELD. YOU WILL NEED TO WEAR EITHER GLASSES OR A SHIELD TO PROTECT THE EYE FOR THREE MONTHS. CLEAN GAUZE MOISTENED WITH EYE WASH (WHICH CAN BE OBTAINED AT YOUR PHARMACY) IS THE BEST WAY TO REMOVE MUCUS FROM THE EYELIDS. CLEAN GENTLY AROUND THE EYE, NEVER TOUCH THE EYE DIRECTLY. DO NOT USE ANYTHING BUT CLEAN GAUZE TO WIPE THE EYE.

2. PLEASE DO NOT BEND OVER SO THAT YOUR HEAD IS BELOW THE LEVEL OF YOUR HEART. IF YOU NEED TO PICK SOMETHING UP OFF THE FLOOR, PLEASE SIT DOWN AND BEND FROM THE WAIST. THIS RESTRICTION IS FOR THE FIRST MONTH FOLLOWING SURGERY.

3. PLEASE DO NOT WASH YOUR OWN HAIR FOR TWO WEEKS. IF YOU WANT YOUR HAIR WASHED, PLEASE HAVE SOMEONE ELSE DO IT WITH YOUR HEAD TIPPED BACK OVER A SINK, SO THAT ALL WATER, SOAP, ETC. WILL DRAIN BACKWARDS AND NOT INTO THE OPERATED EYE.

4. PLEASE TAKE THE FOLLOWING MEDICATIONS IN THE OPERATED EYE:

_____ TIMES A DAY

_____ TIMES A DAY

_____ TIMES A DAY

_____ TIMES A DAY

WAIT FIVE MINUTES BETWEEN EACH DROP SO THAT THE DROPS WILL NOT WASH EACH OTHER OUT.

5. PLEASE TAKE ALL MEDICATIONS THAT YOU WERE TAKING BY MOUTH BEFORE SURGERY AND ALSO ANY EYE DROPS TAKEN IN THE UNOPERATED EYE.

6. LIGHT READING IS PERMITTED THE FIRST WEEK FOLLOWING SURGERY; HOWEVER, PLEASE DO NOT SIT DOWN TO READ FOR A LONG PERIOD OF TIME. IT IS OKAY TO WATCH TELEVISION.

7. PLEASE DO NOT DO ANY HEAVY LIFTING FOR THE FIRST THREE MONTHS. YOU SHOULD ALSO NOT DO ANY ACTIVITIES WHERE YOU EXERT YOURSELF TO THE POINT WHERE YOU GET "RED IN THE FACE" OR ARE BREATHING HEAVILY. A SCRATCHY SENSATION LIKE "SOMETHING IN YOUR EYE" IS EXPECTED DUE TO THE RUBBING OF STITCHES. STEADY ACHING, INCREASING REDNESS, OR DECREASING VISION IS ABNORMAL AT ANYTIME AND A REASON FOR YOU TO CALL THE OFFICE FOR ADVICE.

8. PLEASE SLEEP ON YOUR UNOPERATED SIDE. DO NOT SLEEP ON THE SIDE ON WHICH THE EYE WAS OPERATED. THIS HOLDS TRUE FOR THE FIRST THREE MONTHS.

9. PLEASE DO NOT HESITATE TO CALL ME SHOULD YOU HAVE ANY QUESTIONS.

MICHAEL P VRABEC, M.D., F.A.C.S.

DOC #2/PKSXGUI-JW   REV 10–94

FIGURE 3-20.   *Postoperative instruction sheet. Drops are color coded.*

The ends of the suture knots should be left slightly long, to avoid having the knot come undone when it is buried. This type of knot tends to bury much more easily than does a larger knot and will also come out of the wound postoperatively more easily without breakage. This knot will not work when there is excessive positive vitreous pressure. In such cases two or three throws for the first knot component are necessary. If a running suture is employed, the knot can be started in the wound, or it can be tied close to the end of the wound where it will be buried. All slack should be taken out of the running suture prior to the knot being tied. A viscoelastic substance can be placed on the epithelium for protection during placement of the running suture.

During placement of sutures, the reflex of a surgical keratometer should be observed and sutures adjusted to minimize astigmatism (Fig. 3-19). If a keratometer is not available, the reflex of a safety pin can be used. Also, care should be taken that no iris is included in the wound, and if it is, it should be swept out of the wound with a blunt spatula.

At the completion of the procedure, the wound should be carefully checked for any leaks. If found, supplemental sutures are placed to make the wound watertight. The chamber should be deep, and no synechiae should be present.

Additional procedures to enhance the outcome of the graft can be performed at this time. For example, patients with dry eyes can have their puncta either temporarily or permanently occluded. A temporary tarsorrhaphy would be indicated for patients in whom epithelial healing problems (i.e., a patient with herpes simplex with a dysesthetic cornea or a patient who previously had an alkali burn) might be anticipated.

At the conclusion of the procedure, subconjunctival injections of antibiotics (typically cefazolin and gentamicin) and corticosteroids are given. One should always verify that the patient is not allergic to any of these medications prior to injection. In patients with herpes simplex, a subconjunctival corticosteroid injection should be avoided. A topical antibiotic–corticosteroid ointment is put on the eye prior to placement of a patch and shield. For the phakic transplantation patient, cycloplegia is typically not indicated.

The surgeon should make sure all recipient and surgical information is included in the eye bank forms that came with the tissue.

Giving written postoperative instructions to the patient (Fig. 3-20) and having the patient view a videotape will help ensure that graft survival is maximized.

REFERENCES

1. *1995 Eye banking statistical report.* Eye Bank Association of America. 1001 Connecticut Ave., N.W., Suite 601, Washington, D.C. 20036.
2. Vrabec MP, Elsing SH, Aitken PA. A prospective randomized comparison of thermal cautery and argon laser for permanent punctal occlusion. *Am J Ophthalmol* 1993;116:469–471.
3. Freeman JM. The punctum plug. Evaluation of a new treatment for the dry eye. *Trans Am Acad Ophthalmol Otolaryngol* 1975;79:874–879.
4. Wilhelmus KR, Hyndiuk RA, Caldwell DR, et al. 0.3% Ciprofloxacin ophthalmic ointment in the treatment of bacterial keratitis. *Arch Ophthalmol* 1993;111:1210–1218.
5. Koenig S, Graul E, Kaufman HE. Ocular refraction after penetrating keratoplasty with infant donor tissue. *Am J Ophthalmol* 1982;94:534–539.
6. Olson RJ. The effect of scleral fixation ring placement and trephine tilting on keratoplasty wound size and donor shape. *Ophthalmic Surg* 1981;12:23–26.
7. Vrabec MP, Krachmer JH. Florakis GJ. Iowa PK Press for donor corneas—a comparative study of donor corneal shape. *Refract Corneal Surg* 1992;8:475–477.
8. Pouliquen Y, Ganem J, Hanna K, et al. New trephine for keratoplasty (Hanna trephine). *Dev Ophthalmol* 1985;11:99–102.
9. Hessburg P, Barron M. A disposable trephine. *Ophthalmic Surg* 1980;11:730–733.
10. Bourne WM. Reduction of endothelial cell loss during phakic penetrating keratoplasty. *Am J Ophthalmol* 1980;89:787–790.

Aphakic and Pseudophakic Keratoplasty

John Irvine

Aphakic or pseudophakic patients requiring corneal transplantation represent a unique keratoplasty subgroup characterized by 1) their requirement for careful preoperative evaluation and 2) their potential need for extensive or surgically demanding adjunctive procedures.

INDICATIONS

Pseudophakic bullous keratopathy (PBK) is the leading indication for corneal transplantation in the United States (1). Less frequent indications include previously failed transplants, corneal scarring secondary to recurrent herpes simplex, old bacterial keratitis, interstitial keratitis, and ocular-surface disorders.

Preoperative Considerations

Pseudophakic patients with corneal edema may have any style of intraocular lense (IOL) in place: iris fixated, anterior chamber, or posterior chamber. Patients for whom keratoplasty is indicated include those with a posterior-chamber IOL whose cornea is edematous (usually individuals with preexisting Fuchs' dystrophy) and those with a history of corneal infection with subsequent scarring or traumatic lens extraction. As almost all routine cataract surgeries now include placement of a posterior-chamber lens, the presence of PBK in an eye with an anterior-chamber IOL usually indicates that a complication (vitreous loss) occurred and a vitrectomy was performed and an anterior-chamber IOL placed. Some patients still have old-style, closed-loop or iris-clip lenses, which should be removed during keratoplasty. However, if the IOL is a modern, open-loop, "Kelman"-style IOL, and if there is no vitreous present in the anterior chamber, then a penetrating keratoplasty can be performed without removal of the IOL. A vitrectomy,

anterior synechiolysis or pupilloplasty, and anterior-segment reconstruction may be required in conjunction with the keratoplasty in order to improve the surgical outcome.

The style of the replacement IOL depends on the anatomy of the angle, the surgeon's expertise, and the patient's ocular history. A posterior-chamber lens is preferred if there is adequate peripheral capsular support; however, a modern anterior-chamber lens is satisfactory if the posterior capsule is absent. Some surgeons fixate the posterior-chamber lens into the sulcus by transscleral fixation if the posterior capsule is absent and if the anterior-chamber angle is extensively compromised.

Aphakic keratoplasty is performed in patients in whom a cataract extraction was performed without IOL implantation (e.g., in young patients, in patients with uveitis or trauma). Examination will reveal either complete absence of the lens capsule or some residual lens capsule, which may allow easy sulcus placement of a posterior-chamber IOL. If the peripheral capsule is not intact and vitreous is present, placement of a posterior-chamber lens requires vitrectomy and sulcus fixation with either transscleral or iris fixation. However, potential problems exist with both the transscleral and iris fixation techniques: operative time, infection, chronic inflammation, as well as possible subsequent dislocation of the IOL. Anterior-chamber lens placement may require vitrectomy, synechiolysis, or pupiloplasty. Careful placement of haptics is critical to avoid haptic migration through a peripheral iridectomy. A special lens, such as a three-piece, open-loop, anterior-chamber lens, may be required if the iris or angle is compromised in a focal manner (Fig. 4-1).

Aphakic keratoplasty is also performed in patients who have undergone repair of a corneal laceration and lensectomy for a traumatic cataract. Preoperatively, it is important to rule out the traumatic scar as a source of the poor vision.

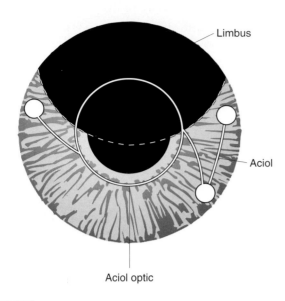

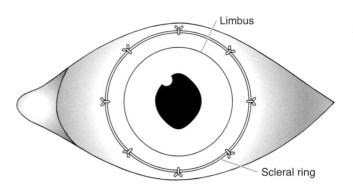

FIGURE 4-2. *Distorted host bed due to tight sutures on the fixation ring at 12- and 6-o'clock positions.*

FIGURE 4-1. *An anterior-chamber intraocular lens with three-point fixation may be used in eyes with partial iris loss and otherwise open angles in the areas of point fixation.*

Use of a preoperative hard contact lens and overrefraction is important in such patients. If the posterior capsule is intact, placement of a posterior-chamber lens is recommended. If not, the surgeon must decide whether to suture the IOL to the sulcus or implant an anterior-chamber lens.

SURGICAL TECHNIQUES

Draping

A key intraoperative consideration in aphakic or pseudophakic keratoplasty is to avoid pressure from the drape on the peripheral part of the operative field. Additionally, it is imperative to ensure that pressure from the surgeon's or assistant's hands does not transfer to the globe, causing the intraocular contents to bulge through the trephine site. Similarly, selection of a speculum that will not rest heavily on the globe is important.

Scleral Support

Because the aphakic or pseudophakic eye is lacking crystalline lens support, and may require vitrectomy and IOL manipulation, it is important to provide scleral support. Various scleral support rings are available. These are usually composed of a single ring although double rings may provide a broader level of scleral support. The selection of these support devices is left to each surgeon's preference, but the principle is to provide support while minimizing distortion of the globe. Such distortion can cause host bed "ovality," a distortion of the host bed due to meridional distortion by the scleral ring (Figs. 4-2 to 4-4). This distortion leads to inaccurate placement of the donor graft in the host bed. It is

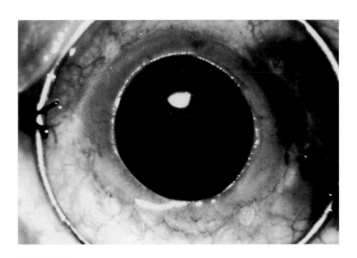

FIGURE 4-3. *Proper tension of the fixation ring sutures helps to make the host bed round making donor placement more accurate.*

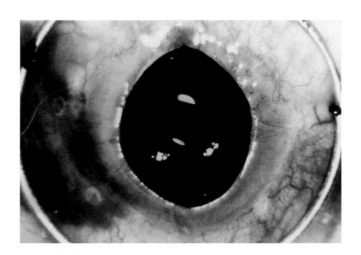

FIGURE 4-4. *The host bed is distorted and oval resulting from relative tightness of several fixation ring sutures.*

important that the ring be the appropriate size for the eye and adnexa and that it be secured to the eye with equal pressure at the points of fixation. This will help not only with accurate placement of the donor button on the eye but also with decreased postoperative astigmatism once the sutures are removed. Sutures (e.g., 4-0 silk) are passed through the episclera in a posterior to anterior direction. Generally, four to eight sutures are placed, but the number of sutures may vary if there are filtration blebs or areas of scleral thinning to be avoided. It is frequently helpful to have traction sutures fixated to the scleral ring. The 12- and 6-o'clock scleral fixation sutures may be placed, tied, and trimmed, leaving one end long to be secured to the drape for traction. Alternatively, if these cardinal sutures are not present owing to unusual placement of the scleral fixation sutures, traction sutures may be fashioned by passing a double loop of suture around the ring without scleral fixation and tying the two ends to the drape for traction (Fig. 4-5A). The needle is passed

around the ring, with the swaged end first to avoid inadvertent perforation (Fig. 4-5B).

Trephination Bed Size

Determination of the corneal trephination size in the host depends on the amount of pathology tissue to be removed as well as whether any adjunct procedures are anticipated. In general, recipient graft sizes from 7.0 to 8.5 mm are utilized in pseudophakic and aphakic keratoplasty, depending on the extent of corneal scarring, irregular thinning, and other factors. For corneal edema alone, recipient sizes from 7 to 8 mm are suggested. These sizes allow enough room for removal, placement, and suturing of IOLs and for other various required intraocular manipulations. The size of the donor graft in an aphakic or pseudophakic individual is usually 0.25 to 0.50 mm larger than the size of the host bed. Should cataract extraction with lens implantation be planned in conjunction with transplantation, such as for Fuchs' dystrophy, the surgeon must select an adequately sized trephine to facilitate the type of IOL anticipated. On the other hand, if a temporary operating keratoprosthesis is to be utilized during a combined procedure with a vitreoretinal surgeon, the usual keratoprosthesis is 7.0 mm in diameter, thus requiring a 6.5-mm host trephination. (Note: Operating keratoprosthesis manufacturers often recommend a donor size 0.75 mm larger than the host bed because of "stretching of the wound" during keratoprosthesis placement.)

Trephination Alignment and Technique

Centering the trephine on the host cornea depends on several factors: the existing pathology to be excised, areas of corneal thinning to be avoided, and pupil position. In an edematous cornea, the center of trephination is usually determined by judging the position of the pupillary aperture as well as the measured center of the cornea. The latter can be determined by measuring the vertical and horizontal diameters of the cornea and then marking the point of the cornea where the "radii" intersect. These radii are usually measured from nasal and inferior limbal margins. This cross-point can then be judged with respect to its position relative to the pupil (Fig. 4-6). This central mark in the cornea can also be used as a target for trephines that utilize cross-hairs for alignment purposes (e.g., the Hessburg vacuum trephine). If a handheld, manual trephine is employed, the blade is lightly applied to mark the cornea to ensure centration and size adequacy.

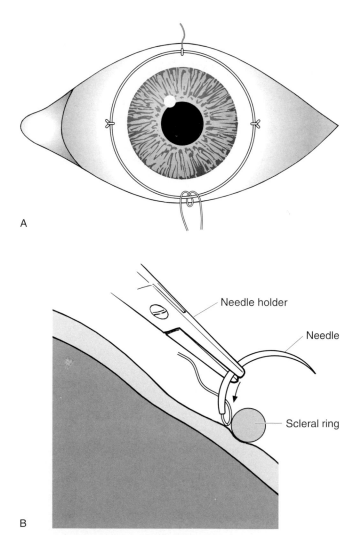

A

B

FIGURE 4-5. A, B. *In eyes with filtration blebs, a traction suture may be looped around the scleral fixation ring, butt end first, without engaging conjunctival or episcleral tissue.*

Cardinal Suture Placement

The cardinal meridians can be marked to guide the accurate placement of the initial four cardinal sutures, thus minimizing astigmatism. An eight-point radial keratotomy (RK) marker can be applied gently on the center of the cornea,

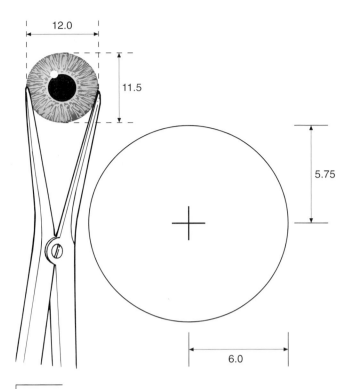

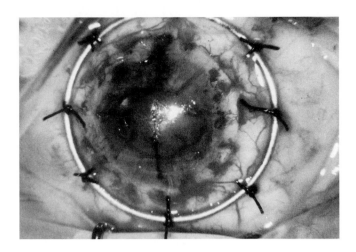

FIGURE 4-8. *Placement of the cardinal sutures is facilitated by the marks from the painted radial keratotomy marker teeth.*

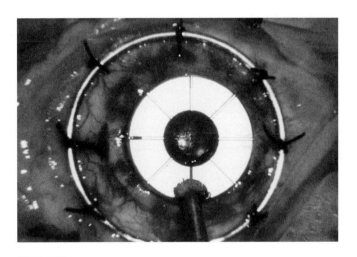

FIGURE 4-6. *The intersection of the horizontal and vertical diameters can be used to center the trephine.*

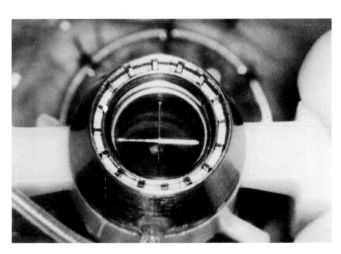

FIGURE 4-9. *The small teeth in the outer barrel of this vacuum trephine ensure the proper alignment of the sutures relative to the trephination.*

FIGURE 4-7. *A radial keratotomy marker is placed on the cornea to indicate the positions of the cardinal sutures.*

leaving radial marks to facilitate cardinal suture placement (Fig. 4-7). The *teeth* can be painted with a marking pen to extend the duration of the visibility of these marks (Fig. 4-8). Limbal cautery can also be used at the various meridians to guide suture placement.

An inherent problem with using an RK marker distinct from the trephine is that the surgeon may not align the trephine exactly as her or she did the RK marker. Thus, the predetermined cardinal suture placement is not as valid if

the trephine is decentered from the center where the RK marker was placed. One solution is the use of vacuum trephines, which have small teeth in the outer barrel that coincide with the placement for sutures and can be painted with a marking pen (Fig. 4-9). Thus, the only centration required is that of the trephine over the predetermined area of trephination. In this fashion, cardinal suture placement is accurately linked to the center of centration and donor placement.

Trephination of the Host Bed

Trephination of the host cornea can be done in several ways, depending on the type of trephine utilized and the goal of surgery. Specifically, the trephination can be partial or full thickness, depending on the surgeon's preference. The very sharp nature of the blades in a nonguarded disposable trephine makes it almost impossible to perform a consistent partial-thickness trephination. Surgeons will generally trephine carefully until they see aqueous on the surface of the eye. It is important that any areas of iris adhesion or pathology be noted during the preoperative assessment, in order to avoid a full-thickness penetration in that location (Fig. 4-10). In those instances, a partial-thickness trephination is preferable, with entrance into the anterior chamber away from the area of iris-corneal touch. After the anterior chamber is entered with a sharp blade, viscoelastic substance

can be introduced to spare areas of iris adhesion by creating planes between the cornea and the iris or IOL material so that no major damage is done (Fig. 4-11).

If a nondisposable or vacuum trephine that allows partial-thickness trephination is used, the goal is to achieve a deep trephination of at least 80% of the corneal bed. The anterior chamber is then entered with a sharp blade, and viscoelastic substance is introduced to keep the lens and iris away from the cornea during further excision of the host cornea. This allows the surgeon to proceed safely in removing the host tissue with scissors without causing damage to the iris. The deep partial-thickness trephination also allows the surgeon to determine what, if any, bevel to create. Curved corneal scissors are useful in removing the cornea; it is desirable to minimize piecemeal removal of tissue, which would leave small jagged edges within the bed. Large, curved corneal scissors allow for smooth host edges. One must also be careful to maintain a consistent cutting angle of the blades as the hands change position during the circumferential placement of the scissors.

A technique has been described as a safety precaution in the event of an expulsive hemorrhage: All but one-half of one clock hour is cut and the host cornea is hinged back onto the bulbar surface (2) (Fig. 4-12). If necessary, one can quickly swing the hinged tissue back into place and secure it with a suture. This technique may be helpful if a temporary operating keratoprosthesis (e.g., Cobo lens) is not available and other open sky intraocular procedures are to be performed.

After the host tissue has been removed and placed to the side, the wound is inspected for uniformity, and excess tissue

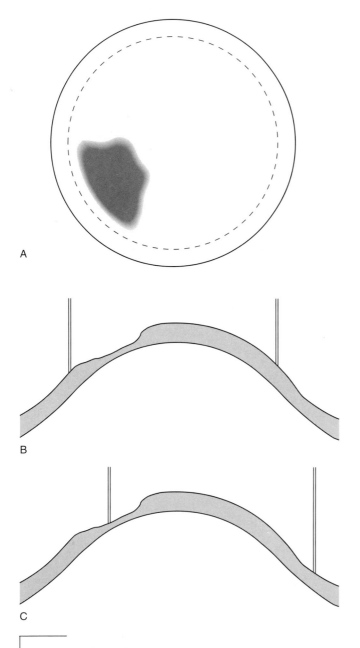

FIGURE 4-10.   *The size and location of the trephination site are selected so as to remove focal pathology and to avoid cutting through areas of corneal thinning, if possible.*

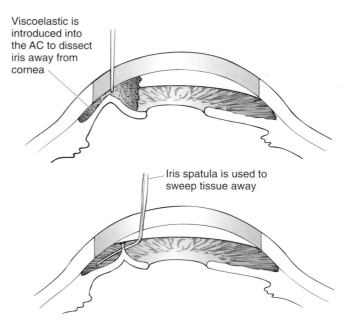

Viscoelastic is introduced into the AC to dissect iris away from cornea

Iris spatula is used to sweep tissue away

FIGURE 4-11.   *A viscoelastic substance is injected into the anterior chamber to dissect the iris away from the cornea. An iris spatula may be used to help sweep tissue away.*

is trimmed with Vannas or other scissors. It is important to avoid distortion of the tissue as well as excessive tissue excision during this process, to lessen the chance of poor wound apposition and wound leak.

If necessary, additional adjunctive procedures are performed at this time. These can include anterior-segment reconstruction (pupiloplasty, pupillary membrane removal, synechiolysis, and repair of iridodialysis), anterior vitrectomy, IOL removal or exchange, and placement of an operating keratoprosthesis to facilitate vitreoretinal surgery.

Donor Placement

Once the host bed is prepared to the surgeon's satisfaction and any adjunct procedures (e.g., cataract extraction, anterior vitrectomy) have been performed, a small amount of viscoelastic material is placed in the angle, on the IOL if one is present, and on the iris surface. The donor button is lifted off the trephine block with a spatula and placed on the host bed. The donor may slide on the host surface, and thus a generous application of the viscoelastic substance on the peripheral ocular surface affords extra protection to the endothelial cells. The lip of the corneal button is then grasped with a fine (0.12) forceps on the epithelium and stromal surfaces, taking care to avoid full-thickness purchase. A 10-0 nylon suture needle is then passed directly beneath this area of fixation, through approximately 80% to 90% of the corneal thickness (Fig. 4-13). The assistant can facilitate the placement of the first sutures in each meridian (12-, 6-, 3-, and 9-o'clock positions) by fixating the tissue on the opposite side to provide countertraction. Approximately

1 mm of tissue purchase is desired on both the donor button and the host cornea. The initial cardinal sutures are tightened to a tension that allows secure apposition of donor to host tissue but not to the point of bunching up the corneal tissue. A faint crease may be present on the cornea between adjacent sutures. Thus, a line extending from each suture will impart a "diamond" pattern between the first four cardinal sutures (Fig. 4-14). Following placement of the four cardinal sutures, the anterior chamber is formed with balanced salt solution and the suture tension is assessed and deemed either to be adequate or to require replacement. The intervening sutures will then be placed to give a similar tension on the corneal surface.

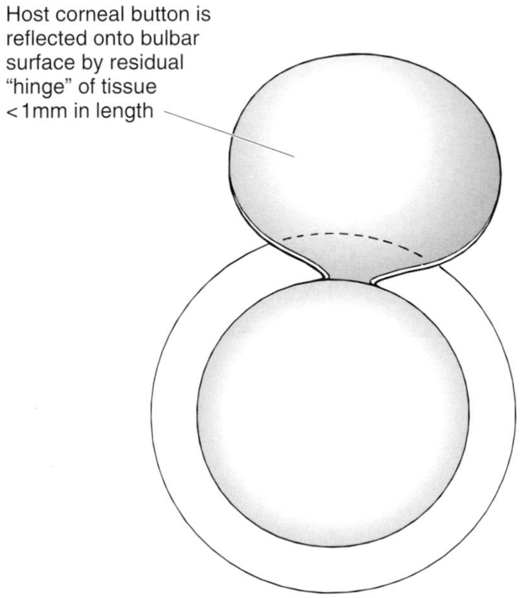

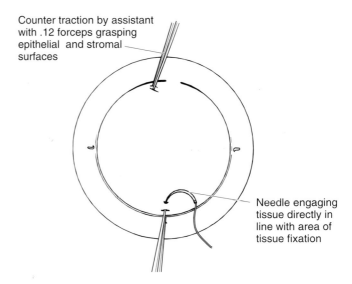

Counter traction by assistant with .12 forceps grasping epithelial and stromal surfaces

Needle engaging tissue directly in line with area of tissue fixation

FIGURE 4-13. *While the surgeon engages the tissue with the needle directly in line with the point of tissue fixation, the assistant facilitates with countertraction using 0.12 forceps to grasp epithelial and stromal surfaces of the button 180 degrees away.*

Host corneal button is reflected onto bulbar surface by residual "hinge" of tissue <1mm in length

FIGURE 4-12. *Host corneal button is reflected back onto the bulbar surface by a "hinge" of residual tissue less than 1 mm long.*

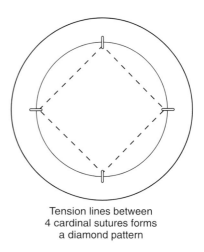

Tension lines between 4 cardinal sutures forms a diamond pattern

FIGURE 4-14. *The tension lines between the anterior insertion of the four cardinal sutures form a diamond pattern.*

At this point, the surgeon is faced with the decision of a final closure technique (i.e., all interrupted sutures, a combination of running and interrupted sutures, or complete running suture closure). The latter requires the placement and subsequent removal of the interrupted sutures after the running suture is secure. The usual number of sutures for an interrupted suture closure is 16, four per quadrant. A combination interrupted and running suture closure can be done in several ways. One method is to use 8 interrupted sutures with a 16-bite running suture, necessitating two passes of the running sutures between each of the 8 interrupted sutures; alternatively, 12-12 and 8-24 patterns are popular and work very well for some surgeons. The choice is determined by the surgeon, based on personal expertise and on the assessment of best postoperative astigmatism results (Fig. 4-15).

The decision of whether or not to use a running suture should be made on the basis of the patient's age and corneal pathology. While a running suture is aesthetically pleasing to view at the slit lamp and may afford postoperative adjustment of suture tension, there are relative contraindications for its use. Specifically, these include pediatric patients whose wounds heal very rapidly, causing the suture to buckle up

through the epithelium faster than in adults (Fig. 4-16). This can lead to persistent irritation, suture abscess, and even graft failure if the child does not communicate well or the family is not educated about the potential problems. Significant stromal neovascularization is also a relative contraindication for a running suture, because the wound will heal more rapidly in vascularized areas than it will in nonvascularized portions. This can lead to loosening of the suture in one quadrant, prompting the physician to remove it completely because once it is cut, the remaining suture loses its tensile strength to support the wound and will quickly become loosened. Removal of the entire running suture may be deleterious because the unvascularized areas of the adult corneal wound may not have healed sufficiently to main-

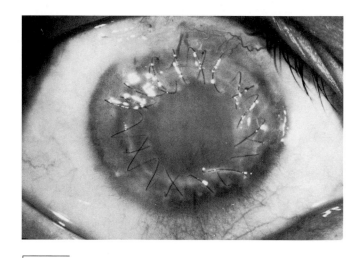

FIGURE 4-16.   *Running suture in a pediatric transplant is diffusely loose and exposed, causing irritation, vascularization, and graft failure.*

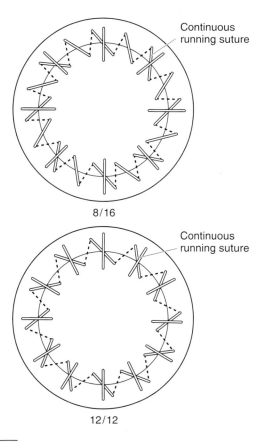

FIGURE 4-15.   *Patterns of combined interrupted and running sutures vary. Two popular patterns are 8 interrupted sutures with a 16-bite running suture or 12 interrupted sutures with a 12-bite running closure.*

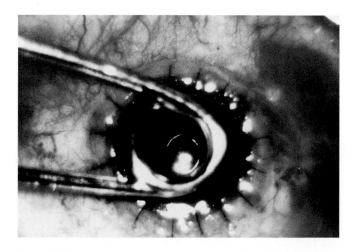

FIGURE 4-17.   *Corneal topography can be estimated by holding the back end of a safety pin over the cornea and viewing the resultant mires.*

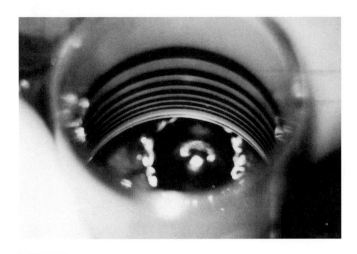

FIGURE 4-18.   *Disposable keratoscope with circles on the cylinder allow light from the operating microscope to be projected as mires onto the fresh cornea surface.*

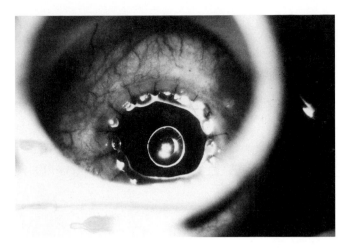

FIGURE 4-19.   *The projected mires of a disposable keratoscope are viewed by focusing down through the cylinder onto the cornea.*

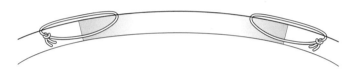

FIGURE 4-20.   *The suture knot is buried on the host side of the wound with the tails pointing centrally toward the graft.*

tain their integrity, thus leading to corneal wound slippage or dehiscence.

Intraoperative Astigmatism Control

Postoperative astigmatism depends on a number of factors, including host astigmatism due to peripheral preoperative scarring, donor astigmatism, variable suture tension, and wound-healing factors. Intraoperative adjustment of suture tension to minimize distortion of the corneal topography at the conclusion of the operation may well mask "non-suture-related factors" that become manifest after suture removal. Any measurement and adjustment of the topography should be made only after the scleral ring has been removed, to avoid any distortion due to the ring sutures. The cornea should be wetted with balanced salt solution and excess fluid removed with a sponge just prior to viewing the mires of the keratoscope, which can be as simple an instrument as a safety pin (Fig. 4-17) or a disposable keratometer (Figs. 4-18 and 4-19). Gross distortions of the circle should be corrected with suture replacement and tension titration. A useful knot to employ in this situation is a slipknot, which

can be adjusted to minimize distortion and then secured with a square knot. The knots should be buried on the host side of the wound with their tails pointing toward the graft-host interface (Fig. 4-20).

Intraoperative Medications

At the conclusion of the operation, antibiotic and steroid medications are usually administered. Subconjunctival injections are frequently used but often cause subconjunctival hemorrhages and may be uncomfortable. Alternatively, combination antibiotic-steroid ointments or collagen shields soaked in the steroid-antibiotic drops are sometimes used. It is wise not to give long-acting depo steroids in case the patient proves to be a steroid responder.

CONCLUSIONS

Aphakic and pseudophakic keratoplasty provides the surgeon with challenges requiring special attention to planning as well as execution. A careful surgical plan minimizes the time the globe is "open" and therefore decreases the risk of disastrous complications in these eyes that have already undergone surgery.

REFERENCES

1. Flowers CW, Chang K, McLeod SD, et al. Changing indications for penetrating keratoplasty, 1989–1993. *Cornea* 1995;14:583–588.
2. Weiss, JS. Hinge keratoplasty. *Ophthalmic Surg Lasers* 1995;27:156–157.

Combined Penetrating Keratoplasty and Cataract Extraction

O. Claron Alldredge Jr.   Claron D. Alldredge

GENERAL CONSIDERATIONS

Whenever penetrating keratoplasty is indicated, the status of the crystalline lens must be assessed, and conversely, whenever cataract extraction is indicated, the status of the cornea must be assessed. Let us first give attention to those patients in whom the cornea is the main cause of decreased visual acuity, a cataract is present, and a penetrating keratoplasty is clearly indicated. The question arises, Should the cataract also be removed? Cataract formation is more common in patients with Fuchs' dystrophy or in patients in whom inflammation or trauma has been a factor. Cataract formation is less common in younger patients needing penetrating keratoplasty, such as for keratoconus. The indication for removal of the cataract along with penetrating keratoplasty is determined by the visual significance of the cataract. This is more difficult to determine than when the cornea is normal, because the evaluation of the cataract is impaired when there is a loss of corneal clarity. Nevertheless, a reasonable estimation of the visual significance of the cataract can usually be obtained before penetrating keratoplasty is performed. A general rule of thumb indicating removal of nuclear sclerotic cataracts is a cataract of more than 2+ (on a scale of 1+ to 4+). A guideline for removal of posterior subcapsular cataracts is a cataract of 1+ or more. However, each case must be individualized according to the visual needs of each patient and the status of the rest of the eye. One must bear in mind that corneal transplantation can hasten the development of cataracts (1,2).

Now, let us consider those situations where cataract extraction is indicated in the presence of corneal pathology, such as guttata or Fuchs' dystrophy. If there is no stromal edema on morning slit-lamp examination or the central corneal pachymetry reading is 0.60 mm or less, cataract surgery alone can usually be performed without corneal decompensation. When cataract surgery is performed in the setting of significant corneal guttata, a viscoelastic substance that gives maximum protection to the endothelium (such as Viscoat) should be used (3,4). When there is frank stromal edema and a corneal thickness of more than 0.60 mm, it is usually best to perform a triple procedure. When corneal scarring is present and cataract extraction is indicated, one must bear in mind that the anterior corneal surface is the largest contributor to the refractive power of the eye. Significant corneal scarring can be present with little effect on the visual acuity (a specific example would be interstitial keratitis). Assessing the smoothness or irregularity of the anterior corneal surface with keratometry or computerized topography and a rigid contact lens plus overcorrection is necessary to diagnose irregular astigmatism.

When both corneal transplantation and cataract surgery are needed to give the best visual acuity, the surgeon may choose between a combined procedure or two separate operations.

The factors suggesting an advantage to a combined procedure are as follows: 1) single surgery, hence, less cost; 2) endothelial preservation of the donor cornea by limiting the intraoperative loss of endothelial cells (5–7); and 3) some evidence that posterior capsular opacification occurs less when a combined procedure is performed than when cataract extraction is performed first (8).

The advantages of doing two separate procedures are that there is a more precise calculation of the intraocular lens (IOL) power and elimination of significant anisometropia. The difficulty of accurately predicting the IOL power in combined procedures stems from the fact that the postoperative keratometry readings can only be estimated. If the decision is made to do the procedures separately, it is recommended that the second procedure be done at least 2 or 3 months after the penetrating keratoplasty, to allow for stabilization of the keratometry readings. This approach makes the assumption that the corneal curvature, specifically the mean keratometry reading, will not change significantly with suture removal. We recommend against a tight suturing technique, which may induce corneal steepening on removal. This is described later in the chapter.

PREOPERATIVE EVALUATION

Prior to performance of a combined procedure, a thorough preoperative work-up must be done and includes a complete eye examination, with special attention given to measurement of the intraocular pressure (IOP), and retinal examination. Poorly controlled IOP can greatly complicate the postoperative course (9,10). This may require the use of antiglaucomatous drops, argon laser trabeculoplasty, or even trabeculectomy. Macular function should also be assessed so that the patient can be counseled as to postoperative visual acuity expectations. A potential-acuity-meter (PAM) reading can often be obtained and be very helpful. When corneal as well as lens opacity is present, a favorable PAM reading is less likely; however, when a favorable reading is obtained, a good visual outcome can be expected. The converse, a poor PAM reading means a poor visual outcome, is not always true. Sometimes therefore, macular function must be assessed more on the basis of the appearance of the macula.

Since most combined procedures are performed in older patients, it is advisable to have the patient's general medical health assessed, and this can be done by an internist or family physician. Special attention should be given to blood pressure as well as any blood abnormalities, as there is some risk for expulsive hemorrhage with "open-sky" combined procedures.

Axial length should be determined and IOL power calculated. Various ways of determining the keratometry readings to use for IOL calculations are employed by different surgeons (11). One technique is to average the keratometry readings for a particular surgeon based on a large series of patients who have undergone penetrating keratoplasty. Some surgeons also tend to modify this depending on the preoperative keratometry readings of the patient's eye or the fellow eye if adequate readings cannot be obtained for the operative eye. Some surgeons believe that if a patient has a relatively steep cornea, the results may be steeper-than-average keratometry readings, or, if the patient has a relatively flat cornea, the keratometry readings may be flatter postoperatively. Other surgeons try to use an average change in keratometry in readings, using the preoperative readings from the operated eye or the fellow eye if accurate keratometry is not possible in the operated eye, and then adding or subtracting the average change in readings determined by averaging the change of keratometry readings in a large series of patients. McCulley (unpublished

data) reported a small series of patients for whom keratometry readings of the donor were determined before the donor cornea was removed. There was a fairly high correlation of keratometry readings in the recipient cornea postoperatively. This merits further study and may be a very helpful tool in selecting the appropriate keratometry readings to use for IOL power calculations in combined procedures.

It is also appropriate to have alternative IOLs. If in-the-bag or ciliary sulcus placement of the IOL is not possible, it is important to determine preoperatively which lens can be sewed into the posterior chamber and which anterior-chamber IOL would be appropriate. However, one should bear in mind that even when the posterior capsule has been torn, it is rare that enough capsular remnants cannot be found to place a lens in the ciliary sulcus (12).

DETERMINE THE APPROPRIATE PROCEDURE

The conventional method of removing the cataract with a combined procedure is to proceed with the corneal transplantation to the point of removing the recipient button. Open-sky extracapsular cataract extraction can then be used to remove the cataract. The IOL can be placed in the capsular bag and the donor corneal button sewed in place.

The other alternative is to do the cataract extraction first using a technique of small-incision phacoemulsification, as one would in a phakic eye, followed by keratoplasty. Some authors believe the procedure of choice to be first cataract extraction by phacoemulsification, followed by penetrating keratoplasty (13,14). The advantage to this method is that the operation is done in a closed system, which makes cataract surgery much safer. With the intercapsular space being maintained during phacoemulsification, the risk of ruptured capsule and posterior vitreous pressure is much less. The procedure is much more controlled in this fashion and the risk of choroidal hemorrhage and other complications is certainly much less (15–19). All corneal surgeons who do cataract extractions along with corneal transplantation can attest to the fact that the most worrisome time during the procedure is the open-sky removal of the cataract and placing the IOL in position, because of the difficulties of vitreous pressure and possible posterior capsular rupture. The procedure becomes much more controlled and less worrisome when the cataract is removed first by phacoemulsification. Of course, this is not always possible because some corneas lack sufficient clarity for visualization of the lens. The microscope can be focused down through the scarred and cloudy cornea, sometimes providing an adequate view for capsulorrhexis. Epithelial removal in edematous eyes may also improve the surgeon's view. However, this technique should not be tried by surgeons inexperienced with phacoemulsification.

REMOVAL OF THE CATARACT BY PHACOEMULSIFICATION

The procedure is usually performed under local anesthesia. It is recommended that a retrobulbar injection of lidocaine hydrochloride be given, with bupivacaine hydrochloride added for longer anesthesia time as well as for some relief of postoperative pain. Some surgeons prefer to use a peribulbar anesthetic (20,21), although the degree of anesthesia is more variable. A block of the seventh nerve is also desirable to suppress orbicularis function during keratoplasty.

A small incision should be made at the superior limbus in the conjunctiva and the conjunctiva reflected slightly back away from the limbus. Episcleral vessels showing any bleeding should be lightly cauterized. It is important not to cauterize too much because the sclera can actually shrink, causing some difficulties with the wound. The incision into the eye should be by a "scleral tunnel" approach. A clear corneal approach would not be appropriate when transplantation is also being performed. With a diamond knife an incision 2 mm posterior to the limbus is made to half thickness of the sclera; the incision should be performed in a "frown" fashion. A lamellar dissection up into the peripheral cornea should then be done. It is important not to go too far into the cornea as this may interfere with the transplant itself. But for the wound to seal properly, the dissection does need to be carried out in the peripheral aspect of the cornea just into the limbal vascular palisades. A stab incision is then performed at the 2-o'clock position right at the limbus to facilitate a second instrument and also to inject fluids. Once the incision has been made from the inner aspect of the wound into the anterior chamber using a 3.0-mm or 3.2-mm keratome, then a viscoelastic substance should be injected into the anterior chamber. A continuous-tear capsulotomy should then be performed. Care must be taken not to allow the capsulotomy to tear out into the periphery. If it does, proceeding with the capsulotomy in the other direction from the starting point or a straight cut with a Vannas scissors to redirect the tear can prevent the capsular tear from extending out to the equator. After the capsulotomy has been made, hydrodissection should be carried out. Phacoemulsification of the nucleus is then accomplished in the usual fashion. A fractionation technique works well: Deep grooves are made into the four quadrants, then each fragment is fractured using the second instrument; the four quarters are then brought into the plane of the anterior capsule and are removed by phacoemulsification. It is particularly helpful, when making the grooves, to use zero-millimeter vacuum with the phacoemulsifier (22). By using a low phacoemulsification power such as 50% or 60% along with zero-millimeter mercury vacuum and an aspiration flow rate of approximately 20 to 25, one can make the grooves with much less risk of posterior capsule rupture. With quadrant removed, high vacuum powers are employed, particularly with the newer machines which have the fluidics that allow the anterior chamber to be properly

maintained. Once the nuclear fragments are removed, irrigation and aspiration of the remaining cortical material are accomplished. At this point, the posterior capsule can be polished with a capsule polisher, which helps to prevent opacification of the posterior capsule. Following this, a single-piece or foldable IOL can then be passed through a 5.5-mm or 3.0-mm incision and placed into the capsular bag.

If the posterior capsule has been ruptured and vitreous loss occurs, the vitreous must be dealt with appropriately (23). A vitrectomy should be performed, and the vitreous must be meticulously cleaned from the iris and anterior chamber. A posterior-chamber IOL can usually be used, but if there is a significant tear in the posterior capsule, the IOL should usually be placed in the sulcus. Once this is done, the pupil should be constricted with acetylcholine chloride (Miochol).

Usually, one interrupted 10-0 Vicryl suture placed in a horizontal mattress fashion is used to close a 3-mm wound or a 10-0 nylon suture placed in mattress or "shoelace" fashion is used to close larger wounds. With the pupil constricted and the IOL in good position, the transplant surgery can then proceed.

REMOVAL OF THE CATARACT USING AN OPEN-SKY APPROACH

If it is determined that phacoemulsification is not advisable or possible, extracapsular cataract extraction should be performed with the corneal transplant procedure. Preoperative softening of the eye using a super-pinky, Honan balloon, or digital massage to minimize posterior pressure is very important. The combined procedure can be made infinitely more difficult when there is significant vitreous pressure. The procedure should be carried out to the point of removing the recipient corneal button. If excessive posterior pressure is encountered at this point, it is best to perform a posterior sclerotomy 4 mm posterior to the limbus, with aspiration of liquid vitreous to allow the iris-lens diaphragm to fall back. If cataract removal is attempted in the setting of significant posterior pressure, posterior capsular rupture with its attendant complications can often result. At this point, one can then proceed with extracapsular cataract extraction.

It is still advantageous to perform a continuous-tear capsulotomy to begin the cataract removal. This is more difficult than it is under a closed system, but with some practice it can be done quite nicely (24,25). A rent should be made in the anterior capsule fairly near the center (Fig. 5-1); then a tear at one edge should be started (Fig. 5-2). With a smooth-tipped instrument or a Utrata forceps, a continuous-tear capsulotomy can be performed. This should be placed or positioned as far out into the periphery as possible, but one must bear in mind that the tendency for a capsule to tear out toward the equator is greater using the open-sky approach. The trick to doing a continuous-tear capsulotomy

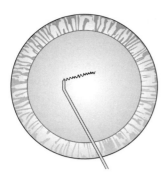

FIGURE 5-1.   *A horizontal rent is made in the capsule with a sharp instrument.*

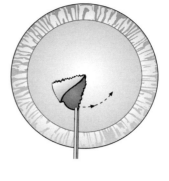

FIGURE 5-3.   *The edge of the tear is grasped with a Utrata forceps. The tear is propagated by folding the torn capsule over the part of the capsule to be torn.*

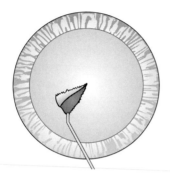

FIGURE 5-2.   *At one edge of the rent, a tear is started by pulling toward the 12-o'clock position.*

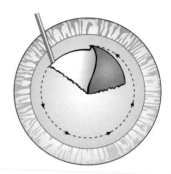

FIGURE 5-4.   *The continuous tear is made by pulling the torn edge around a continuation of the curvilinear line made by the already torn edge of the capsule.*

in an open-sky fashion is to begin the capsular tear and then to fold the flap of the torn capsule over the part of the capsule to be torn next (Fig. 5-3). The tear proceeds along the line made by the torn edge of the capsule (Figs. 5-4 and 5-5). If the capsule begins to tear out toward the periphery, that tear should be stopped and one should start again from the starting point going around the opposite way. The use of a Vannas scissors to start the tear in the other direction can facilitate this. Since it is an open-sky approach, it is possible to perform a circular capsulotomy using only scissors. However, even though this theoretically may appear to be easy, the continuous-tear method is much more reliable. In some cases there is too much posterior pressure, with the nucleus of the lens pushing forward, and no matter what is done, the capsule will tend to tear toward the periphery. If this happens, scissors should be used to complete the capsulotomy with as smooth an edge as possible.

Once a capsulotomy has been performed, the nucleus can simply be expressed. It is often helpful to perform hydrodissection by injecting balanced saline solution just under the anterior capsular edge, and in some cases, the nucleus will almost deliver itself after the hydrodissection has been performed. Sometimes this process will require pressure with one instrument at the limbus and then counterpressure with a second instrument applied 180 degrees from the first about

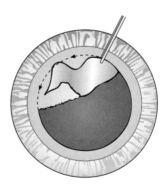

FIGURE 5-5.   *The edge must be regrasped several times a slight distance away from the actual site of tearing.*

4 mm posterior to the limbus. The nucleus can be easily delivered in this fashion. If the nucleus is too large to pass through the capsular opening, one must perform a relaxing incision out toward the periphery of the capsule. If a relaxing incision must be made, it is best to have only one because this facilitates in-the-bag capsular placement.

Following expression of the nucleus, the cortical material can be removed using either the automated irrigation and aspiration machine or a manual aspiration system. With an automated approach, very little or no irrigation can be used and the cortical material can be removed by engaging the anterior aspect of the material and then peeling out the residual cortex. Often it is helpful to place the irrigation and aspiration tip against the posterior cortex and posterior capsule, pushing it slightly away from the anterior cortex, enabling the engagement of the anterior cortex which will then strip out nicely. This can also be done with the manual aspiration approach. However, one must use a tip that has the opening on the side and not on the end. Once all the cortical material has been removed, the posterior capsule should be polished. This can be accomplished nicely using a capsule polisher. An olive-tipped cannula with a sandblasted tip works well, but other capsule polishers or even a moistened Weck sponge can be used.

At this point the capsule should be filled with a viscoelastic substance and then the inferior haptic of the posterior-chamber IOL can be introduced into the capsular space. Care must be taken to make sure that the haptics go into the capsular bag. This can be done by placing the haptic against the posterior capsule centrally and then gently pushing the IOL inferiorly. Once the inferior haptic is in place, the optic of the lens should be introduced through the capsular opening. With a second instrument, pressure can be maintained on the optic of the IOL to prevent it from moving, and the trailing haptic of the IOL can then be grasped with a forceps. With a pronation movement of the wrist, one can introduce the trailing haptic into the capsular bag superiorly. Once the IOL is in the capsular bag, it is worthwhile to "dial" the lens slightly to make sure the lens is securely in the capsular bag. If there have been significant tears in the anterior capsule, or if difficulty is encountered in determining how much of the anterior capsule is present, it is preferable to insert the IOL in the ciliary sulcus. It is much better to have the haptics in the ciliary sulcus than to have one in the bag and one out of the bag. This will often result in decentration of the IOL. In the past, it was thought that a very long IOL was needed for sulcus fixation. However, work done by Holland and Orgul et al showed that the average diameter of the ciliary sulcus is such that a 12.5-mm IOL will center nicely (26). If one decides to put the implant in the ciliary sulcus, a viscoelastic substance should be injected just under the iris. The cannula tip of the viscoelastic can be used to lift up the edge of the iris so the substance can be injected directly under the iris, making sure that the anterior capsule or any remnants from it go back. A similar procedure to placing the haptics as that described for capsular fixation can be used. Once the lens is in good position in either the capsular bag or the ciliary sulcus, acetylcholine chloride should be injected into the anterior chamber to constrict the pupil. Administration of carbachol (Miostat) is also worthwhile to maintain pupillary constriction through the rest of the procedure.

If the posterior capsule tears during any part of the procedure, it must be managed. If the tear is fairly central and is a small one, the tear can be made to be a continuous tear in the same manner as previously described for the anterior capsule. If vitreous is presenting through the tear, a small vitrectomy should be performed. If the tear is larger and extends toward the periphery, it is usually not possible to end up with a circumscribed continuous tear. In this case care must be taken to preserve as much of the posterior capsule as possible. A vitrectomy is almost always required, and an automated vitrectomy will usually preserve more of the capsule. The vitreous must be removed from the anterior chamber and no vitreous strands can be left coming through the capsular tear. Once all the vitreous is removed from the anterior chamber and around the iris and capsular tear, the capsule that remains must be inspected. This can be done by gently retracting the iris. It is rare, in our experience, that there will not be enough capsule to support a posterior-chamber IOL. When a larger posterior capsular tear is present, it is best to place the haptics in the ciliary sulcus in areas where there is more capsular support. A continuous-tear anterior capsulotomy is a great advantage in the setting of posterior-capsule tears, because invariably a posterior-chamber IOL can be placed in the ciliary sulcus. In those instances where most or all of the capsule is lost or where there is little zonular support, a posterior lens can be sewn into the sulcus transsclerally, or can be sewn to the iris, or alternatively, an anterior-chamber IOL can be used.

Once the IOL is in good position and the cataract part of the operation has been completed, corneal transplantation can proceed.

CORNEAL TRANSPLANT PROCEDURE

When corneal transplantation and cataract surgery are indicated, our current preference is to do the corneal transplantation first, wait for 2 or 3 months to allow the keratometry readings to stabilize, and then to remove the cataract by a small-incision phacoemulsification technique. This approach presupposes that the mean keratometry readings will not change significantly after 2 or 3 months. The only way to make that supposition is to use a technique where the keratometry readings actually do not change. To do this, sutures must be adjusted and tied very loosely so as not to bunch up the tissue. To make it possible to close the wound effectively, other alterations in technique are required. When trephination and the excision of the recipient cornea are completed, a posterior shelf must be left, to act as a valve to close the posterior aspect of the wound without putting undo tension on the sutures.

Recipient Wound Construction

After adequate anesthesia is obtained with a retrobulbar injection and adequate akinesia is obtained with a seventh-nerve block, a McNeil-Goldman ring (this ring is a combination of a double Flieringa ring and a blepharostat) is placed in the palpebral fissure. The ring is secured to the globe using a 6-0 or 7-0 silk suture on a spatula needle; four sutures are used, one in each quadrant. Care must be taken to use shallow bites in the episclera and to avoid excessive traction on these sutures, which can distort the globe and give rise to astigmatism. The center of the intended trephination is marked, usually directly over the pupil. (One should remember that the pupil is usually somewhat nasal.) The trephination is carried out to about three-fourths depth in the cornea. A diamond knife is then used to enter the anterior chamber—this incision is made with the diamond blade angled toward the pupil so that a posterior bevel is created. Corneal scissors are then used to complete the removal of the recipient button. Instead of holding the scissor blades vertically, the top blade is angled toward the limbus and the bottom blade is angled toward the pupil. This will result in a posterior shelf being created (Fig. 5-6).

Placement of Donor Button and Suturing

Viscoelastic substance is placed into the anterior chamber. The donor button, which was previously prepared using a trephine that is generally 0.25 mm larger than the recipient button, is then sutured in place. A combined interrupted and running suture technique works well, although any desired suture technique may be used. Twelve interrupted sutures of 10-0 nylon should be placed at about two-thirds depth and above the posterior shelf. Alignment of the anterior surfaces of the donor and recipient cornea should be the goal (remember that the anterior surface of the cornea is by far the most important refractive surface of the eye). When these sutures are tied, the first throw should have three loops and the donor and recipient edges are brought together so that they just touch. Care must be taken not to tie this first throw too tightly. The second throw is then performed with one loop. This second throw results in a slight tightening of the knot. A third throw is then made to lock the knot. The knot should not tighten any more on this third throw. The twelve interrupted knots are then buried in the recipient cornea and the anterior chamber is filled with balanced salt solution. If the suturing has been done properly, the wound will be watertight at this point. A handheld or microscope-mounted keratoscope is utilized at this point to control astigmatism. If some sutures are too tight, they can be stretched or replaced. If some sutures are too loose, they can

be replaced. Once the mires are round, the second set of sutures can be placed.

A twelve-bite running 11-0 nylon suture is used for the second set, with each bite going between the interrupted sutures. These running sutures are placed at half depth. After all these sutures have been placed, the running suture is tightened just enough to produce a secure wound but not tight enough to loosen any of the interrupted sutures. The knot of the running suture is also buried in the cornea. A keratoscope is again utilized to inspect for astigmatism, and if any is found it can be adjusted easily by tightening or loosening sections of the running suture.

A double running suture technique, an all interrupted suture technique, or even a single running suture technique can be used as well. The important goals of this technique are to make a posterior shelf and to not tie the sutures too tightly. Most surgeons tie the sutures tightly in an effort to make the wound watertight, which results in a gutter being formed approximately 1 mm inside the wound. This gutter makes contact lens fitting difficult as long as the sutures are present and can contribute to irregular astigmatism, which makes refraction difficult and delays the possibility of glasses being prescribed.

CONCLUSION

When a triple procedure (penetrating keratoplasty, cataract extraction, and IOL implantation) is performed, consideration may be given to performing the cataract extraction first by small-incision phacoemulsification techniques. This makes the procedure safer with less chance of posterior-capsule rupture. It is very helpful to use a continuous-tear capsulotomy whether the cataract is removed first by phacoemulsification or by the traditional open-sky approach.

When the open-sky cataract extraction method is used, making sure the eye is soft is very important. When there is significant posterior vitreous pressure in spite of preoperative efforts to lower the pressure, a posterior sclerotomy with aspiration of vitreous is a prudent course to follow.

When both corneal transplantation and cataract extraction need to be performed, it may be advisable to perform the transplantation first, followed by cataract surgery a few months later. This allows for more accurate selection of the IOL power and avoids undesirably large amounts of anisometropia.

REFERENCES

1. Martin TP, Reed JW, Legault C, et al. Cataract formation and cataract extraction after penetrating keratoplasty. *Ophthalmology* 1994;101:113–119.
2. de Charnace B, Guidi M, Valiere-Vialeix JP. [Short-, medium- and long-term postoperative complications in 150 patients undergoing penetrating keratoplasty after one year.] *Ophtalmologie* 1989;3:11–12.
3. Craig MT, Olson RJ, Mamalis N. Air bubble endothelial damage during phacoemulsification in human eye bank eyes; the protective effects of Healon and Viscoat. *J Cataract Refract Surg* 1990;16:597–602.

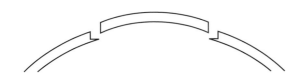

FIGURE 5-6.   *Note the posterior lip on the recipient.*

4. Koch DD, Liu JF, Glasser DB, et al. A comparison of corneal endothelial changes after use of Healon or Viscoat during phacoemulsification. *Am J Ophthalmol* 1993;115:188–201.

5. Bourne WM, Nelson LR, Hodge DO. Continued endothelial cell loss ten years after lens implantation. *Ophthalmology* 1994;101:1014–1022.

6. Zacks CM, Abbott RL, Fine M. Long-term changes in corneal endothelium after keratoplasty. *Cornea* 1990;9:92–97.

7. Binder PS. Intraocular lens implantation after penetrating keratoplasty. *Refract Corneal Surg* 1989;5:224–230.

8. Dangel ME, Kirkham SM, Phipps MJ. Posterior capsule opacification in extra capsular cataract extraction and the triple procedure. *Ophthalmic Surg* 1994;25:82–87.

9. Yamagami S, Suzuki Y, Ohya T, et al. [Statistic evaluation of prognostic risk factors in penetrating keratoplasty using Cox multiple regression model.] *Nippon Ganka Gakkai Zasshi* 1994;98:777–781.

10. The Australian Corneal Graft Registry. 1990 to 1992 report. *Aust N Z J Ophthalmol* 1993;21:1–48.

11. Vajpayee RB, Angra SK, Honavar SG. Combined keratoplasty, cataract extraction, and intraocular lens implantation after corneolenticular laceration in children. *Am J Ophthalmol* 1994;17:507–511.

12. Donnenfeld ED, Ingraham HJ, Perry HD, et al. Soemmering's ring support for posterior chamber intraocular lens implantation during penetrating keratoplasty. Changing trends in bullous keratopathy. *Ophthalmology* 1992;99:1229–1233.

13. Keates RH, Rothchild EJ, Bloom R. Endocapsular triple procedure—a new triple procedure technique. *J Cataract Refract Surg* 1989;15:332–335.

14. Malbran ES, Malbran E, Buonsanti J, Adroque E. Closed-system phacoemulsification and posterior chamber implant combined with penetrating keratoplasty. *Ophthalmic Surg* 1993;24:403–406.

15. Gloor B, Kalman A. [Choroidal effusion and expulsive hemorrhage in penetrating interventions—lessons from 26 patients.] *Klin Monatsbl Augenheilkd* 1993;202:224–237.

16. Aiello LP, Javitt JC, Canner JK. National outcomes of penetrating keratoplasty. Risks of endophthalmitis and retinal detachment. *Arch Ophthalmol* 1993;111:509–513.

17. Egger SF, Huber-Spitzy V, Scholda C, et al. Bacterial contamination during extra capsular cataract extraction. Prospective study on 200 consecutive patients. *Ophthalmologica* 1994;208:767–781.

18. Boke W. [Phacoemulsification. Why?] *Klin Monatsbl Augenheilkd* 1990;197:100–105.

19. Ohrloff C. [Comparison of phacoemulsification and planned extracapsular cataract extraction.] *Klin Monatsbl Augenheilkd* 1993;203:93–98.

20. Loots JH, Venter JA. Posterior peribulbar anaesthesia for intra-ocular surgery. *S Afr Med J* 1988;74:507–509.

21. Davis DB, Mandel MR. Posterior peribulbar anesthesia: an alternative to retrobulbar anesthesia. *J Cataract Refract Surg* 1986;12:182–184.

22. Johnson SH. Split and lift: nuclear quadrant management for phacoemulsification. *J Cataract Refract Surg* 1993;19:420–424.

23. Wang HS. Management of a posterior capsule rupture in planned extra capsular cataract extraction and posterior chamber lens implantation. *J Cataract Refract Surg* 1986;12:73–76.

24. Galand A. [Capsulorrhexis and manual extracapsular extraction.] *Bull Soc Belge Ophtalmol* 1993;247:43–45.

25. Groden LR. Continuous tear capsulotomy and phacoemulsification cataract extraction combined with penetrating keratoplasty. *Refract Corneal Surg* 1990;6:458–459.

26. Orgul SI, Daicker B, Buchi ER. The diameter of the ciliary sulcus; a morphometric study. *Graefes Arch Clin Exp Ophthalmol* 1993;231:487–490.

Chapter

6

Intraocular Lens Management in Penetrating Keratoplasty

DEBORAH S. JACOBS

PRINCIPLES

Intraocular lens (IOL) management in keratoplasty is a complex issue. Successful visual rehabilitation is contingent on many factors. First, there must be anatomic success with a clear graft and optical correction of aphakia. Second, there must be physiologic success with an eye that is free of escalating glaucoma and has no inflammation or cystoid macular edema. Finally, there must be refractive success, with no high or irregular astigmatism in the graft and with a good spherical result from the combined effects of the IOL and the graft. IOL management can have an impact on the anatomic, physiologic, and refractive result, and thus is critical to outcome.

In choosing whether or not to exchange an IOL or to place a secondary IOL in the setting of keratoplasty, one must consider what factors led to corneal decompensation or opacification in the first place, whether there are surgically induced anatomic changes limiting the choice of IOL style and implantation technique, and whether there are coexisting ocular diagnoses. The surgeon must assess the adequacy of the current lens. If IOL exchange is indicated, then the surgeon must decide what sort of lens it should be replaced with and what surgical technique should be used. The age and health of the patient, the patient's ability to cooperate for a longer procedure, and the skill of the surgeon must also be considered.

TECHNIQUES

The Preoperative Evaluation

The preoperative evaluation is critical. In eyes under consideration for keratoplasty, the view of the anterior segment is often limited by corneal edema or opacification. One must attempt to treat or control the reversible factors that can contribute to corneal decompensation or opacification, such as high pressure or acute inflammation, so as to gather as much information preoperatively as possible. Uncontrollable glaucoma or uncontrollable inflammation mandates IOL removal. If underlying inflammatory disease is thought to be contributory, then placement of a secondary IOL may be contraindicated. If the lens style or position is thought to be the likely source of glaucoma or inflammation, then a lens exchange rather than lens removal alone is a reasonable option. For these reasons, an attempt should be made to control inflammation and glaucoma medically preoperatively. The degree of success and the information obtained through an improved view of the anterior segment will guide the surgeon through appropriate management decisions.

The following questions are asked: Is the IOL contributing to inflammation, glaucoma, or corneal decompensation? If an anterior-chamber IOL (ACIOL) is present, is it of a one-piece, open-loop design and is it sized and positioned well? If a posterior-chamber IOL (PCIOL) is present, is it positioned well? The optic edge should not be visible through an undilated pupil. Are there peripheral anterior synechiae (PAS) that will complicate removal of an ACIOL or preclude placement of an ACIOL? Is there vitreous in the anterior chamber? Is the vitreous face intact? Are there large iris defects or PAS that would preclude safe placement of an ACIOL?

Based on the answers to these questions the surgeon should decide if the eye is to be left aphakic, if the current lens is satisfactory, if vitrectomy is necessary, and if IOL exchange is indicated. If secondary lens implantation or lens exchange is planned, the lens style and insertion technique (open-loop ACIOL, iris fixation of PCIOL, or scleral fixation of PCIOL) should be selected. (The current literature on lens style and insertion technique is reviewed later, in

Complications and Outcomes.) These decisions are best made in advance of surgery so that axial length and K values (corneal curvature) may be determined for lens power calculations, so that the vitrectomy machine will be at the ready if needed, so that a plan is made to measure white-to-white (anterior chamber diameter) before entering the eye if an ACIOL is selected, and so that a plan is made for dissection of scleral flaps before entering the eye if scleral fixation of PCIOL under flaps is selected. A decision tree

showing how one might make a plan for IOL management in the setting of keratoplasty is provided in Figure 6-1.

Regarding IOLs, not only are style and insertion technique a consideration, but also IOL power is important. In calculating IOL power, one should use the same formula that one uses for cataract extraction; I use the SRK II formula. IOL A-constant and axial length should be entered into the formula as usual. Mean K can be arbitrarily chosen at 44 if one does not use an oversized graft, or at a slightly

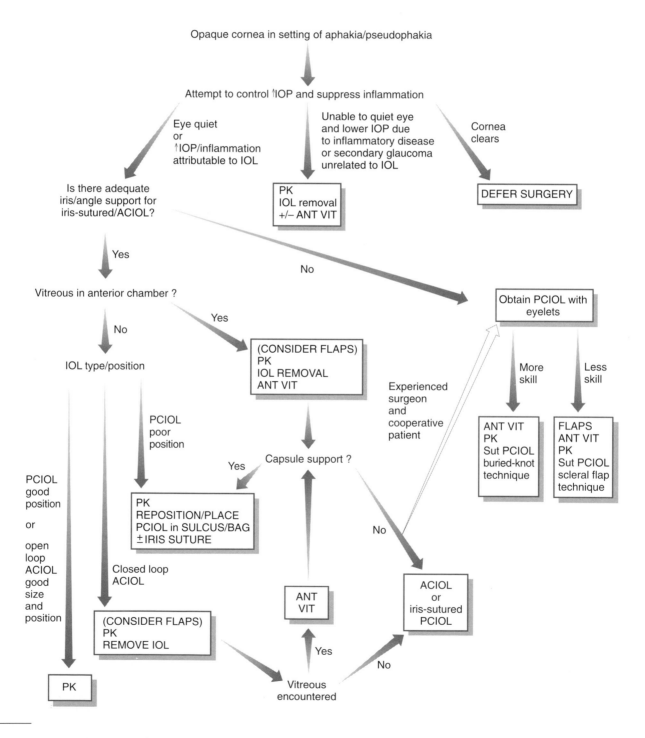

FIGURE 6-1. *Decision tree for intraocular lens management in keratoplasty.*

higher value if one does. Alternatively the surgeon may use the mean K from the eye to be operated on if it is measurable or the mean K from the fellow eye; this latter approach may be preferable if the eye to be operated on is particularly flat or steep. The surgeon should periodically review his or her keratometric and refractive results, in light of the surgical technique used (whether graft is oversized or not, IOL style and placement, and corneal suture technique), and empirically modify the selection of mean K, A-constant, or the final lens power on the basis of refractive outcomes. Mattax and McCulley (1) reported that a single surgeon using a standardized keratoplasty can achieve good results in the triple procedure combining penetrating keratoplasty, cataract extraction, and IOL implantation. Consistent keratoplasty technique should also yield good refractive results in cases of secondary IOL placement or IOL exchange.

The Initial Steps of Keratoplasty

IOL management should not alter the initial steps of keratoplasty, including measurement and marking of the cornea, surgical preparation and drape, trephination, and entrance into the globe. There is less consensus on the use of Flieringa rings than ever before. The traditional approach is that they should be used for all keratoplasty procedures except phakic keratoplasty and certainly in patients in whom vitrectomy is planned, to avoid positive vitreous pressure and to avoid collapse and distortion of the globe, all of which might contribute to postoperative astigmatism. Many surgeons including myself believe that there is no assurance that the ring will accomplish these ends, that application of the ring adds to operative time, and that the ring may distort the globe. With careful attention to alignment of the globe, to the pressure applied by the lid speculum and drape, and to tissue distribution and tension at the time of placement of the four cardinal sutures, the ring may not be necessary.

If the surgeon is fairly certain that vitrectomy will either be needed or not be necessary, then one should instill viscoelastic substance in the anterior chamber at the time the chamber is entered. If the decision for vitrectomy depends on intraoperative findings, then it may be reasonable to maintain the chamber with balanced salt solution so the presence or absence of vitreous can be ascertained more easily without the confounding presence of viscoelastic substance. If the lens is to be left in place, then lack of vitreous, good lens position in the case of a PCIOL, and adequate sizing and placement in the case of ACIOL should be verified.

Assessing the IOL and Angle

In an eye with a PCIOL, the optic edge should not be visible through an undilated pupil and the lens should lie parallel to the iris plane. In an eye with an ACIOL, the pupil margin should not extend beyond the optic edge, the foot-plates should be no more than partially visible, the lens should lie flat and parallel to the iris plane, and there should be no iris touch or incarceration of footplates in iridectomies. The patency of at least one iridectomy should be verified. Some believe that every eye with an ACIOL should have two iridectomies to avoid segmental block; a second iridectomy could be made at this time.

Distortion of the globe suggests a lens that is too large. One should perform the "nudge" test, pushing toward the 6-o'clock from the 12-o'clock position on the optic of the ACIOL to be sure it is not too easily displaced; a lens that is too small may undergo excessive movement and contribute to corneal decompensation on that basis. One should perform the "tap" test, tapping at the limbus 90 degrees away from the axis of the lens; there should be iris movement but no lens movement. Lack of iris movement suggests the lens is too large, putting traction on the iris. Lens movement suggests the lens is sitting on the iris itself, not at the scleral spur, and is too small.

If PAS are present, an attempt should be made to lyse them first with "viscodissection" and then with a cyclodialysis spatula. Significant iris trauma and hemorrhage can lead to inflammation and perhaps progressive PAS formation, so if bleeding is encountered it may be best to avoid further manipulation of preexisting PAS. An attempt should be made to irrigate and then strip clot from the angle. If the lens size and position are deemed adequate, then a small amount of viscoelastic substance should be placed over the center of the optic and the donor cornea placed over the wound and sutured as usual.

IOL Removal

Removal of a failed IOL requires judgment and skill; no universal rules apply in all cases. Most failed IOLs are closed-loop ACIOLs. Some basic guidelines for removal of ACIOLs are to sever vitreous bands as soon as they are detected and to avoid traction on the haptics to the extent that that could cause tearing of the iris root. Haptics can be cut or amputated close to the angle, to facilitate optic and haptic removal. If there is to be much manipulation of haptics in the angle, then viscoelastic substance should be placed in the angle prior to this manipulation so that the endothelium and angle structures are protected. A useful instrument for the cutting or amputation of haptics is the Rapazzo scissors. DeWecker or Wescott scissors may also be used but require more force and are less precise in their cutting action because torque is applied. Vannas scissors are not likely to transmit enough cutting force. Use of tying forceps or serrated tissue forceps for grasping haptics is preferred over use of toothed forceps or jeweler's forceps, both of which are likely to cause the haptic to torque and snap uncontrollably because the area of contact is too limited. Toothed forceps with a tying platform may be useful if the teeth are used clenched to lift upward on the haptic.

In some cases, the lens, regardless of the style, can simply be grasped and lifted out of the sulcus with no surgical maneuvers required. This should be attempted first. If resistance is encountered, if there is iris or scleral movement, or if bleeding occurs, the lens should be released. These latter findings all suggest incarceration of the haptics by PAS. With small lifting and rotating movements, one should determine if one or both haptics are incarcerated. Attention is directed toward the incarcerated haptic(s). It should be cut close to the angle and an attempt made to tunnel the remaining attached and incarcerated piece out of the tunnel. If this is not easily accomplished, then the haptic should be cut on the other side of the tunnel, close to the angle, but leaving a long-enough end to grasp. The optic should be lifted out of the wound and then a final attempt made to remove the encarcerated piece of haptic. If there is significant iris trac-

tion or more than minimal bleeding, then the piece of haptic, which is generally made of polypropylene or polymethylmethacrylate (PMMA), being inert, may be left in place. It is reasonable then to ascertain that the exposed end is not excessively long, ragged, or deflected toward the endothelium or iris, and to trim it, if necessary.

Figure 6-2 portrays many of the ACIOL styles and my preference as to where haptics are best cut and grasped.

The removal of a PCIOL is accomplished by grasping the IOL, typically at the junction of the optic and haptic, lifting, and severing vitreous bands as soon as they are detected. Sometimes a dialing motion can facilitate delivery into the anterior chamber. It may be necessary to use a vitrectomy probe or scissors to lyse capsular adhesions to the optic or haptic if it is thought that these adhesions preclude easy lens removal. If a posterior-chamber lens is problem-

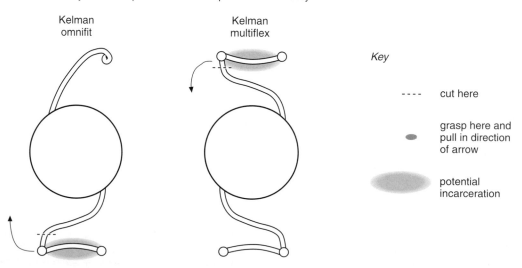

FIGURE 6-2. *Anterior-chamber intraocular lenses.*

atic only in that it is poorly positioned, it may be possible to dial it into place if there is adequate capsule support. If there is not, and if the lens has an eyelet on the haptic or a positioning hole on the optic, it may be possible to reposition it, using a polypropylene suture to secure it to the iris as described in the section on iris-fixation IOL. The surgeon should consider dislocating the optic into the anterior chamber to stabilize it for the passing of the suture and to ascertain that it will remain centered. If vitreous is encountered, it is best to remove the lens entirely, perform vitrectomy, and proceed with one of the techniques for secondary IOL placement as outlined later.

Vitrectomy

Vitrectomy should be performed if vitreous in the anterior chamber is noted preoperatively, or at the time that the corneal button or IOL is removed. Vitrectomy is also necessary in eyes in which scleral fixation of a PCIOL is planned. Automated vitrectomy is generally preferred to manual vitrectomy. Manual vitrectomy is not sufficient if suturing a posterior-chamber lens to the sclera is planned, because there is no way to remove vitreous scaffolding behind the iris by manual vitrectomy. If the eye is to be left aphakic or placement of an ACIOL is planned, then manual vitrectomy may be adequate because the open-sky approach does allow clear visualization and testing of the entire anterior chamber for vitreous.

Manual Vitrectomy

The technique for manual vitrectomy through an open-sky keratoplasty wound is to use a sponge spear to engage vitreous at the pupil plane, to apply a small amount of traction axially, and then to amputate the strand just posterior to the iris plane by holding Wescott scissors with blades parallel to the iris. This maneuver should be repeated several times. Adequate vitrectomy has been performed when the iris plane is somewhat concave and when testing with cellulose sponge reveals that there is no vitreous at the wound, on the iris, at the pupillary plane, or at the plane of any peripheral iridectomies. Acetylcholine (Miochol) or carbachol (Miostat) should be instilled in the chamber after the initial bulk of vitreous is removed.

Automated Vitrectomy

Automated vitrectomy through an open-sky keratoplasty wound can be performed dry, which is my preference, or with irrigation. If irrigation is used, the goal is to minimize turbulence and stirring up of vitreous. For this reason, many choose not to use the coaxial irrigation sleeve that most vitrectomy probes are equipped with, but rather to separate off the irrigation tubing and clamp it shut or remove the sleeve, and allow the irrigation to drip in at 1 to 2 drops per second from a butterfly needle held at the plane of the iris. The bottle should be lowered so that the drip rate simply maintains the volume of the globe, no more. The cutting rate

should be high and the aspiration flow rate and vacuum suction should be low. If placement of an ACIOL is planned, core vitrectomy is adequate. The probe should be placed in the pupil to a few millimeters' depth and vitrectomy performed just until the iris drops back. The probe aperture can be slowly rotated 180 degrees in each direction to ensure that no strands of vitreous remain in the pupillary axis. If the plan is to suture a PCIOL to iris or sclera, then the entire posterior chamber must be cleared of vitreous to avoid encarceration of vitreous along sutures or haptics as sutures are passed and tied. In this instance, the probe must be passed into the pupil as near as parallel to the iris plane as possible and swept slowly through the entire 360 degrees. This maneuver may be difficult to perform dry because of posterior collapse of the iris. The surgeon can just maintain globe volume with the use of iris-plane irrigation. Vitrectomy is complete when the pupillary plane and, in the case of scleral or iris fixation, the posterior chamber are clear of vitreous, and when the iris has fallen back into concave configuration. At that point acetylcholine or carbachol can be instilled in the anterior chamber and with a cellulose sponge, the pupillary plane, iris surface, and iridectomies are checked for the presence of vitreous.

After vitrectomy viscoelastic material should be instilled over the pupil so that it falls into the posterior chamber, keeping the vitreous back. More should probably be used if suturing a lens is planned or if there is significant collapse of the globe; less should be used with substitution of miotic or balanced salt solution, if ACIOL placement is planned, or if there is glaucoma, in which case the use of viscoelastic material that cannot be removed is to be minimized.

Iris Defects

Iris defects should be repaired with the goals of creating a flat, taught, iris diaphragm; of eliminating flaps of iris that could adhere to the wound; and of eliminating exposure of the optic edge through or in front of the pupil. Sector iridectomies should be repaired to form peripheral iridectomies. The goal is a round central pupil of 3 to 5 mm.

Aphakia

If the eye is to be left aphakic, then one might use a graft that is oversized by 0.5 mm to increase the corneal power, resulting in less hyperopia. An infant donor cornea might be obtained. These corneas often steepen, increasing corneal power and yielding a less hyperopic result.

Placement of the IOL

If there is sufficient capsule remaining to support a posterior-chamber lens, either in the bag or in the sulcus, then conventional placement of a PCIOL should be attempted. Viscoelastic material and an iris hook can be used to aid in visualization during assessment of capsular sufficiency and for lens placement. In the absence of sufficient capsular support, three options for lens placement remain.

ACIOL

Only ACIOLs that are one piece, made of PMMA, and with open haptics should be used. The choice between a lens with three or four footplates for three- or four-point fixation can be left to the surgeon's preference. A lens with a diameter at least 1 mm greater than the white-to-white measurement should be selected. The lens should vault anteriorly, which in the case of a three-point IOL means that the open portion of the haptics should face in the clockwise direction. This is opposite of a PCIOL. Back-to-front placement of the ACIOL with the lens vaulting posteriorly has been proposed as a way of preventing PAS and increasing the distance between the endothelium and the IOL, which is thought to reduce the likelihood of damage to the endothelium (2). This approach could be considered in an especially short eye or in an eye with PAS that cannot be lysed. This approach has never been tested in a controlled trial. A small amount of viscoelastic substance can be placed in the angle to reduce the trauma of lens placement. A sheets glide is not necessary in this open-sky situation. Care should be taken to avoid incarceration of haptics in preexisting iridectomies. For ACIOL exchange, the new lens should be placed in the same orientation as the old lens if possible. Proper lens placement should be verified according to the criteria listed in the section, Assessing the IOL and Angle. The presence of at least one patent iridectomy should be verified.

Iris Fixation of PCIOL

A lens style with a positioning hole on or adjacent to the optic should be selected. Vitrectomy is performed as indicated and as described previously. The suture selected should be double-armed 10-0 polypropylene on a curved needle. A taper or vascular needle is sufficient to pass through iris and may minimize trauma to iris vessels. Two double-armed sutures are used. The suture is passed through the positioning holes with the lens on the field and the two needles are passed through the peripheral iris. A single, double, or triple throw can be used to temporarily secure the first knot while the second pair of needles is passed. A single throw and similar tension can be placed on the second knot. The resulting anterior traction on the lens will result in the optic and haptic impinging on the iris, and axial position and plane of fixation can be ascertained. The initial throws can be tightened or loosened as necessary. Each suture is secured with at least three throws and the knot is trimmed short.

Scleral Fixation of PCIOL

There are many techniques used for scleral fixation. There are variations in the technique for avoiding exposed knots, for attaching the suture to the lens, and for passing the needles through the sclera. Knots should not be left exposed

at the surface or covered by conjunctiva alone, so either scleral flaps are carved prior to entering the globe or a technique in which the knot can be buried is selected. Vitrectomy is performed as described already. Regarding attachment of suture to the lens, a double-armed suture can be used with the suture knotted or hitched to the eyelet or haptic or the suture can be passed through the eyelet. A single-armed suture can be used with the suture knotted to the eyelet. Regarding the passage of needles, if both arms are passed through the sclera, the two entrance or exit sites should be at least 1 mm apart. If single-armed fixation is used, the needles can be passed from the inside out or the outside in; for double-armed fixation the sutures must be passed from inside out. Some use a hollow needle, 25-, 26-, or 28-gauge, placed from outside in to guide the passage of the suture needle from inside out. The needle entrance or exit site at the sclera should be 1 mm posterior to the limbus. If single-armed fixation is used, one arm is passed through full thickness and then a second pass is through partial thickness of the sclera and the suture is tied to itself. If double-armed fixation is used, both arms are passed through the sclera and the two ends are used to secure a knot.

I prefer double-armed fixation that accomplishes four-point fixation, reducing the chance of torque on the IOL. I have also observed a tendency for the knot in the single-armed technique to loosen in the process of tying the suture to itself, again resulting in a malpositioned lens. I advocate the use of flaps for the less experienced surgeon, to avoid the need for burying a critical knot. If the surgeon is not comfortable with his or her ability to ensure that an inside-to-out "blind" pass of the needle will end up 1 mm from the limbus under the flap, then a hollow-bore needle passed from outside to in should be used. Thus, the surgeon with less experience in these techniques may find it advisable to use the more conservative approach employing flaps and passing hollow-bore needles, resulting in longer operative time and more potential for complications. The surgeon less experienced in these techniques may simply choose ACIOL or iris fixation unless the angle and iris configuration absolutely preclude that approach.

My preferred technique is as follows: Conjunctival peritomies are made at 1- and 7-o'clock positions. The flaps and sutures are oriented obliquely so as to avoid suturing at the 3- and 9-o'clock positions where the long posterior ciliary nerves and vessels are located. A blade of the sort used to make a trabeculectomy flap is used to make triangular scleral flaps of 50% depth and 1.5 to 2.0 mm long on each side. The 1-o'clock flap is hinged at the limbus. The 7-o'clock flap is hinged on the inferior not the limbal side, to facilitate visualization under the flap from the surgeon's position. Two 10-0 polypropylene sutures double armed with long curved cutting needles are used. The long needle avoids distortion of the globe and thus allows more confident localization of the tip. The cutting design facilitates the passage through the sclera. The sutures are fixated to the haptics using a girth hitch with each half hitch on either side of the eyelet (Fig. 6-3). This accomplishes four-point fixation and does not require the tying of knots. The needles are placed back into the foam or cardboard in which they are packed, to avoid tangles. Both arms of the 7-o'clock suture are passed internally to externally so as to exit 1 mm apart and 1 mm posterior to the limbus under the flap. The needles are cut off and a single triple throw is used to secure the haptic; this throw is left somewhat loose to facilitate positioning the second haptic. The two arms of the 1-o'clock suture are passed inside to out 1 mm apart and 1 mm posterior to the limbus while ensuring that the sutures are 180 degrees from the 7-o'clock suture. A triple throw is made. Prior to tightening up completely on the sutures, the lens is placed over the pupil and the superior haptic tucked under the iris. The tension in the triple throw is adjusted so that the globe is not distorted and so the lens is in the visual axis, in a flat plane just posterior to the iris. If the lens appears torqued or off axis, the cause should be identified and, if necessary, the problem haptic should be loosened and

brought out of the eye, the suture cut, and a new suture passed. Once the lens is positioned well, two additional throws should be placed over the triple throw and the knots trimmed. The flaps should be brought down and covered with the conjunctival flap, to keep them moist until after the cornea is sutured in place. At that time the flaps should be secured with an interrupted 10-0 nylon suture through the apex and the knot buried. The conjunctiva should then be closed with polyglactin (Vicryl) suture. I recommend using different suture material for the lens, scleral flap, and conjunctiva so that in the event of an exposed knot or irritation, the IOL suture is not inadvertently cut.

In the flapless technique, conjunctival peritomies are made and the suture is passed through the eyelet but not knotted or hitched. The needles are passed through the full thickness of the sclera, 1.5 to 2.0 mm apart and 1 mm posterior to the limbus, and the lens is positioned as described previously. The knot is tied using three single throws to minimize the bulk of the knot and the knot is buried using a tying forceps. The conjunctiva is closed with polyglactin suture.

COMPLICATIONS AND OUTCOMES

Management techniques for the specific complications of keratoplasty such as graft failure, endophthalmitis, choroidal hemorrhage, and glaucoma are discussed elsewhere in this volume. It is possible that the rate of certain surgical or postoperative complications in the surgical rehabilitation of aphakic or pseudophakic bullous keratopathy, such as endophthalmitis or glaucoma, may be related to the lens style or implantation technique chosen. Outcome as measured by graft clarity, visual acuity, and incidence of complications may also correlate with lens style or implantation technique.

Here it is appropriate to discuss what is known regarding complications and outcomes as they relate to IOL management. With one exception, all reports on complications or outcome are based on series that are retrospective and in which lens management was not randomized. The validity of the findings from these series may be limited by selection bias as far as which patients were treated and what treatment option was chosen. For example, in several of the retrospective series, eyes with PAS were excluded from receiving an ACIOL; these eyes may be more predisposed to glaucoma and then in a biased way show an association of glaucoma with PCIOL use.

Sugar (3), in a retrospective series published in 1989 of 469 patients in whom he studied outcomes, broke the patients down into seven groups: IOL removed; ACIOL retained; PCIOL retained; iris-supported IOL retained; IOL exchanged for PCIOL; IOL exchanged for one-piece, open-loop ACIOL; and IOL exchanged for closed-loop ACIOL. He found that when the original IOL was retained in the eye for keratoplasty, the failure rate (loss of graft clarity) was significantly lower for PCIOLs (6%–7%) than for anterior-

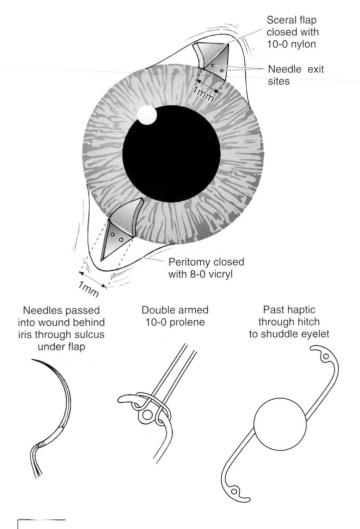

FIGURE 6-3. *Scleral fixation of a posterior-chamber intraocular lens.*

chamber (34%) and iris-supported IOLs (29%). Retained ACIOLs were not broken down by lens type into open- and closed-loop lenses; closed-loop lenses were still in use at the time. The failure rates for exchanged lenses were 8% and 11% for sutured and capsule-supported PCIOLs, respectively, and 24% for closed-loop ACIOLs. Of note, with the one-piece, open-loop ACIOLs the failure rate was lowest, at 5%, although the sample was very small. Endothelial cell loss over the first postoperative year was consistent with the outcome measure of graft clarity in that the lowest cell loss was for retained and exchanged PCIOLs and for one-piece exchanged ACIOLs; again retained ACIOLs were not broken down as to lens type. Visual acuity results were best for eyes with a retained PCIOL and for those eyes that underwent exchange for one-piece, open-loop ACIOLs. Exchange for one-piece ACIOLs or capsule-supported PCIOLs resulted in significantly better visual acuity than did exchange for sutured PCIOLs.

Sugar (3) summarized by stating, "From a visual, functional, graft survival, and endothelial maintenance standpoint, it would be reasonable to recommend that posterior chamber IOLs be retained at PKP [penetrating keratoplasty], that flexible one-piece anterior chamber IOLs be retained if they are stable and well positioned, and that all other IOLs be removed and replaced with posterior chamber lenses, sutured if necessary, or one-piece flexible anterior chamber IOLs at keratoplasty for PBK [pseudophakic bullous keratopathy]." Of note Sugar studied only outcomes and not complications, so nothing can be learned as far as what complications might influence outcome and whether any of these complications are associated with lens style or implantation technique.

Lass et al (4), in a retrospective series of 49 cases reported in 1990, found no advantage of iris-sutured IOL to ACIOL as far as graft clarity, visual outcome, intraocular pressure control, and endothelial survival. Davis et al (5), in a retrospective study of 41 cases reported in 1991 in which keratoplasty, anterior vitrectomy, and placement or exchange of the IOL was performed, found no difference between eyes with an ACIOL, iris-sutured IOL, or sulcus-sutured IOL as far as postoperative acuity, corneal thickness, or intraocular pressure. Of note, 6 of 23 eyes with a sulcus-sutured lens had new-onset secondary glaucoma, which was uncontrollable in 3. No patients had more than 90 degrees of PAS preoperatively. There was a preoperative history of glaucoma in 11 of 41 eyes and postoperative glaucoma in 19 of 41.

Hassan et al (6), in a retrospective series reported in 1991, compared 40 eyes with an exchanged or secondary open-loop ACIOL placed at the time of keratoplasty, with 400 eyes with an iris-sutured lens placed for the same indications. Visual outcomes and complication rates were similar for the two groups. Endothelial attrition at 1 and 2 years was greater for the sutured PCIOLs than for the ACIOLs.

Brunette et al (7), in a retrospective series of 122 cases reported in 1994, found a trend toward better graft survival and acuity in eyes receiving an iris- or scleral-sutured PCIOL compared to an open-loop ACIOL as well as better control of pressure, although the difference in intraocular pressure between the two groups after surgery was not statistically significant. These trends emerged over the second follow-up year, suggesting that any randomized trial may require long follow-up to uncover differences between lens styles and implantation techniques.

Schein et al (8) reported in 1993 the only prospective randomized trial addressing lens style and fixation in keratoplasty, in which 176 consecutive patients underwent surgery for pseudophakic bullous keratopathy. They found a higher complication rate with scleral fixation of a PCIOL than with iris fixation. The complication rate with ACIOL was intermediate and not statistically different from the rate for either of the other two groups. The complications or adverse outcomes that they monitored were escalation of glaucoma therapy, loss of graft clarity, iridocorneal synechiae, inadequate lens centration, and cystoid macular edema. Monitoring extended for 18 months after surgery. These investigators found no difference in the escalation of glaucoma between the three groups, and noted that there was less synechial progression in the ACIOL group. They had no instances of endophthalmitis, thought to be associated with the longer intraoperative times and external fixation techniques used for scleral-sutured lenses. There were three retinal detachments, two in the ACIOL group and one in the scleral-sutured lens group. Lens dislocation requiring repeat surgery occurred once with an ACIOL and three times with a scleral-sutured lens. Outcomes such as endophthalmitis, vitreous hemorrhage, effects on the corneal endothelium, flap necrosis, and suture erosion were not addressed in their trial. The authors (8) concluded that "in those rare instances where iris atrophy, distortion or absence render iris fixation of a PCIOL or flexible ACIOL insertion problematic, scleral fixation of a PCIOL remains a reasonable option."

In an editorial published in 1994, Olson (9) reviewed the arguments for and against ACIOL, iris-sutured PCIOL, and sulcus-sutured PCIOL, in light of the findings of Brunette et al (7) and Schein et al (8). He concluded that more long-term data are needed to determine if early differences detected in these two series are borne out over time and to provide hard evidence against use of the open-loop, one-piece ACIOL. Newer long-term data would also determine whether techniques for scleral fixation have improved the complication rate for that mode of fixation.

CONCLUSIONS

IOL management in keratoplasty is not a simple issue. Eyes with aphakic or pseudophakic bullous keratopathy have already had one complication related to surgery, and may have other associated problems, such as vitreous prolapse, cystoid macular edema, or glaucoma. The preoperative assessment is critical for identifying these anatomic and physiologic problems, so that the surgical plan can be formulated and the appropriate prognosis conveyed to the patient. The flow diagram in Figure 6-1 may serve as a useful guide to IOL management but cannot possibly take into account all the variables in an individual patient. Lens removal presents the potential for unanticipated intraoperative complications and must be approached systematically and cautiously, as described. Finally, the selection of lens type and fixation remains controversial. On the basis of personal experience and the published data reviewed here, I recommend the use of ACIOLs in eyes in which vitrectomy is not planned and where there is adequate iris support. The advantage of this approach is technical simplicity with subsequent reduced operative time and risk of complications. If vitrectomy is planned or iris support is insufficient, then iris or scleral fixation may be considered, with options as far as technique based on the surgeon's skill and experience. Recommendations are likely to change as series with follow-up longer than 1 to 2 years using improved fixation techniques are published. Attention must be paid equally to anatomic, physiologic, and refractive issues in order to achieve successful surgical rehabilitation.

REFERENCES

1. Mattax JB, McCulley JP. The effect of standardized keratoplasty technique on IOL power calculation for the triple procedure. *Acta Ophthalmol* 1989;67:24–29.
2. Sandboe FD, Medin W, Anseth A. Back to front ACIOL implantation combined with penetrating keratoplasty. *Acta Ophthalmol* 1994;72:381–383.
3. Sugar A. An analysis of corneal endothelial and graft survival in pseudophakic bullous keratopathy. *Trans Am Ophthalmol Soc* 1989;87:762–801.
4. Lass JH, DeSantis DM, Reinhart WJ, et al. Clinical and morphometric results of penetrating keratoplasty with one-piece anterior-chamber or suture-fixated posterior-chamber lenses in the absence of lens capsule. *Arch Ophthalmol* 1990;10:1427–1431.
5. Davis RM, Best D, Gilbert GE. Comparison of intraocular lens fixation techniques performed during penetrating keratoplasty. *Am J Ophthalmol* 1991;111:743–749.
6. Hassan TS, Soong HK, Sugar A, Meyer RF. Implantation of Kelman-style open-loop anterior chamber lenses during keratoplasty for aphakic and pseudophakic bullous keratopathy. *Ophthalmology* 1991;98:875–880.
7. Brunette I, Stulting RD, Rinne JR, et al. Penetrating keratoplasty with anterior or posterior chamber intraocular lens implantation. *Arch Ophthalmol* 1994;112:1311–1319.
8. Schein OD, Kenyon KR, Steinert RF, et al. A randomized trial of intraocular lens fixation techniques with penetrating keratoplasty. *Ophthalmology* 1993;100:1437–1443.
9. Olson RJ. Pseudophakic bullous keratopathy and intraocular lens fixation. *Arch Ophthalmol* 1994;112:1289–1290.

Corneal Sutures, Trephines, and Cutting Blocks

CATHERINE H. LEE

The ideal penetrating keratoplasty results in rapid visual recovery and minimal to no residual astigmatism. Unfortunately, the mechanical principles of cutting, removing, and suturing tissue limit the ophthalmologist's ability to achieve this goal. A number of different trephine systems and suture techniques have been utilized in an attempt to achieve the ideal postoperative result. In this chapter, the fundamental principles, optional trephine systems, suture materials, and suture techniques are discussed.

FUNDAMENTAL PRINCIPLES

In penetrating keratoplasty a recipient bed is created by the removal of a cylindrical piece of tissue from a theoretically spherical structure. The surgeon's task is to recreate a spherical structure by replacing the cylindrical piece of tissue. The surgeon is limited by inevitable incongruity, decreased tissue sectility, and the influence of sutures.

Congruity refers to the precision of the trephination. Ideally, a perfectly cylindrical instrument will consistently create a cylindrical tissue of the exact same diameter and profile for each piece of tissue that is cut. Movement of tissue while the recipient bed is being cut, with subsequent distortion; the use of two different cutting instruments to create the recipient bed; and the change in sectility of tissue during the cutting process contribute to a less than perfect trephination.

During trephination, two motions occur. One is a downward pushing or thrusting motion and the other is a rotational, circular motion (Fig. 7-1). The thrusting motion of a trephine serves to deepen the cut (1). When the trephine is initially applied to the surface of the cornea, the tissue resistance to the lateral edge of the trephine is asymmetric and tissue deformation occurs. The rotational motion guides the profile of the cut and creates a shearing force between the

corneal disk within the trephine and the recipient bed (1), which causes tissue to move in front of the blade (Fig. 7-2). Both motions limit the precision of the cut profile. A small cutting error can result in a significant amount of astigmatism (2).

To minimize distortion and improve precision, the downward thrusting motion should be minimized and a rotational motion should be applied at the surface (1,3–5). As the trephine deepens, the lateral resistance of tissue increases and is distributed evenly along the circumference of the blade. Both the rotational and the thrusting motion are used to deepen the cut. The intraocular contents are exposed to the cutting edge of the trephine and are at risk of damage; in most cases, it is difficult to remove an entire corneal button by trephination alone (6) (Fig. 7-3). This necessitates the use of a second instrument to completely remove the tissue.

The trephine is used to create as precise and deep a profile as possible. The second instrument, either a sharp blade or a scissors, can be used to complete the cut. A sharp blade can provide a sharp, precisely cut profile (7). The amount of manipulation from scissors should be minimized (8) because these are crushing instruments (7–9) and poor technique with corneal scissors can produce irregular wound margins (9). The less tissue distortion in front of the scissors, the more precise the cut (6). An optimal profile can be obtained with corneal scissors if the radius of curvature of the blade is the same as the radius of the trephine (1). Corneal scissors can be held vertically and used to achieve a regular curve that conforms to the trephine incision (6). In most cases, however, a ledge of tissue, also known as a posterior lip, is left behind.

Sectility is the ability to cut the tissue. The sectility decreases during the cutting process as the pressure from the tissue against the instrument decreases. With continued rota-

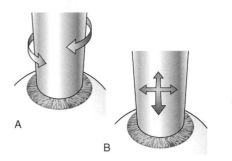

FIGURE 7-1. *Direction of trephine motion. (Reproduced by permission from Penetrating keratoplasty. In: Bruner WE, Stark WJ, Maumenee AE, eds. Manual of corneal surgery. New York: Churchill Livingstone, 1987:21.)*

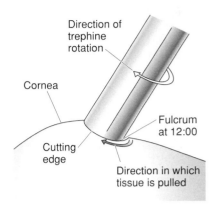

FIGURE 7-2. *Rotation occurs about a fulcrum, and the cornea is compressed ahead of the trephine's cutting edge. (Reproduced by permission from Cohen KL, Holman RE, Tripoli NK, Kupper LL. Effect of trephine tilts on corneal button dimensions. Am J Ophthalmol 1986;101:725.)*

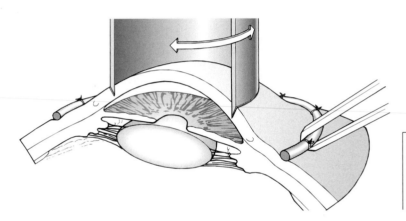

FIGURE 7-3. *The trephine is used to make an incision to approximately 80% depth. (Reproduced by permission from Waltman SR. Penetrating keratoplasty. In: Waltman SR, Keates RH, Hoyt CS, et al, eds. Surgery of the eye. New York: Churchill Livingstone, 1988:202.)*

tional and thrusting motions in less sectile tissue, asymmetric tissue resistance and distortion result, and it becomes more difficult to remove perfectly cylindrical tissue. The precision of the cut is not optimal if the anterior chamber is open. Furthermore, incongruity and change in sectility limit the ability to remove a perfectly cylindrical piece of tissue. Trephines have been developed to provide an even cut (3), minimize the effects of the instrument on incongruity, and minimize the change in sectility.

TREPHINE SYSTEMS

The ideal trephine system allows for accurate and reproducible centration; provides a sharp (10), perpendicular cut (6) with minimal tissue incongruity; allows for visualization of the circumference of the cutting edge, limbal area, and central pupillary zone under the operating microscope; and provides a mechanism for offering stable fixation and for preventing damage to intraocular structures (9–11). Centration is important (6) because eccentric grafts can produce severe astigmatism (12). Uneven, downward pressure and

side-to-side movement can shift the fulcrum during rotation and lead to asymmetric cuts (5) and unpredictable shapes (13). Slight tilting of a manually guided trephine can result in an oval recipient bed, undercutting of the profile, or formation of a posterior lip in the wound (9). A 1-mm cutting error can result in as much as 10 diopters of astigmatism (2,9,14). A manual system using a free hand to manually guide the cut has been used; however the handle often interferes with the surgeon's view during the cutting process (10) (Fig. 7-4). Usually, however, the experienced surgeon can guide a precise cut.

Suction trephine devices, such as the Hessburg-Barron vacuum trephine, decrease the asphericity of the button's epithelial trephine and avoid the unpredictably misshapen wounds produced by handheld trephines (13). These systems provide an outer corneal suction ring for fixation and an inner circular blade. A spring-loaded disposable syringe creates negative pressure to allow for fixation of the trephine system by suction (4,9,15) (Fig. 7-5). These features provide stability, minimize distortion (7), and therefore allow for an exact trephination perpendicular to the limbus, even if the

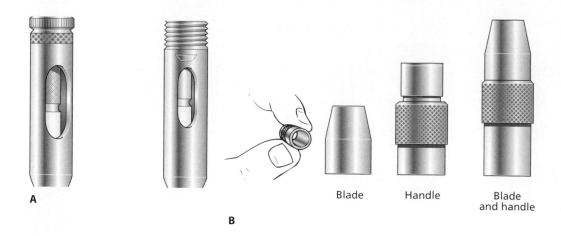

Blade   Handle   Blade
and handle

A

B

FIGURE 7-4. *A. Castrovié jo corneal trephine. Modified trephine also used with the corneal graft punch, shown here with a Weck disposable blade. (Reproduced by permission from Brightbill FS, Pollack FM, Slappey T. A comparison of two methods for cutting donor corneal buttons. Am J Ophthalmol 1973;75:501.) B. A "see-through" handle is available for each size to allow the surgeon to fully visualize the cutting process through the center of the blade and handle. (Reproduced by permission from Katena Products, Inc., 1996 catalog, p. 16.)*

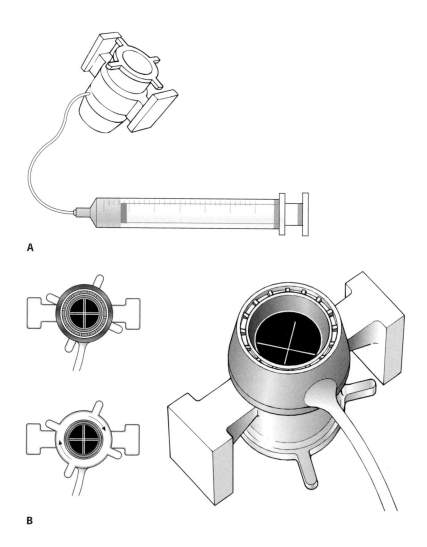

A

B

FIGURE 7-5. *A. Diagram of a Hessburg-Barron vacuum trephine. (Reproduced by permission from Penetrating keratoplasty. In: Bruner WE, Stark WJ, Maumenee AE, eds. Manual of corneal surgery. New York: Churchill Livingstone, 1987:22.) B. Corneal distortion is reduced by this suction chamber device. Extra-fine cross hairs are centered inside the trephine blade for accurate alignment with the visual axis of the recipient. A precisely calibrated rotating mechanism allows the surgeon to advance the blade depth 0.25 mm with each 360-degree rotation for lamellar or penetrating keratoplasty. (Reproduced by permission from Katena Products, Inc., 1996 catalog, p. 17.)*

system is angled or tilted. The suction allows the forces of the trephine to be evenly distributed and as long as suction is maintained, presssure is equally distributed—resulting in a deep, uniform, circular cut (16).

Complete visualization of the trephination can be achieved with a cone-shaped instrument (10,17) that utilizes either a single-point blade or a circular blade. Stabilization of tissue is achieved more readily with a cylindrical trephine than with a small, single-point blade. Lateral tissue resistance to a single-point blade is very low and so the blade can easily deviate from the intended path. Single-point cutting trephines have been developed by Lieberman (2,10,18), Crock (6,10,11), Kadesky (19), and others (9). Although these systems maximize visibility, offer less corneal distortion, and increase the potential for reproducible corneal cutting (9), the Hanna corneal trephine system provides the increased lateral resistance in a conical system by using a circular cutting blade (Fig. 7-6). A limbal suction ring is used to fixate the corneal trephine regardless of eye position. The anterior chamber is protected from inadvertent entry by the ability to preset the depth of trephination. Laser trephination allows for complete corneal visualization, minimal distortion, and improved centration but its use is limited because of the potential for endothelial injury (9).

CUTTING BLOCKS

The tissue that has been removed must be replaced with a corneal button from a human donor cornea. After the tissue is evaluated and approved, it is placed on a cutting block with the epithelial side down at the time of surgery, to minimize both endothelial damage and irregularities in the tissue profile (2,5,7,20–22).

The same mechanical principles of cutting tissue apply to cutting the donor button. In contrast to the need for two instruments in preparation of the recipient bed, a full-thickness cut can be made with a single instrument because there is no danger of damaging intraocular structures. Poor centration can produce incomplete cuts, eccentric cuts, and elliptical configurations (7). Tissue movement can contribute to a less precisely cut profile and lead to astigmatism (23).

Cutting blocks have been designed to improve centration and tissue stability. Manual cutting blocks often have tissue wells of different concavities or of different diameters and radii of curvature designed to match the donor corneal shape to the shape of the cutting block (9). The Brightbill corneal cutting block has three wells of different radii of curvature and diameters to allow for approximation between the donor corneal shape and the cutting block (Fig. 7-7). The central red target is designed to improve centration.

The manual systems, however, occasionally lead to eccentric cuts with elliptical configurations if the tissue slips within the well during cutting (24). Other cutting blocks have a central air-escape hole to stabilize tissue (24). The Tanne cutting block combines a single well with multiple radii of curvature and a central air-escape hole (9). Suction helps hold tissue in place as well as mark the donor epithelium. These systems decrease the movement within the well and therefore, minimize tissue distortion (Figs. 7-8 and 7-9). Marking improves host-donor alignment (24).

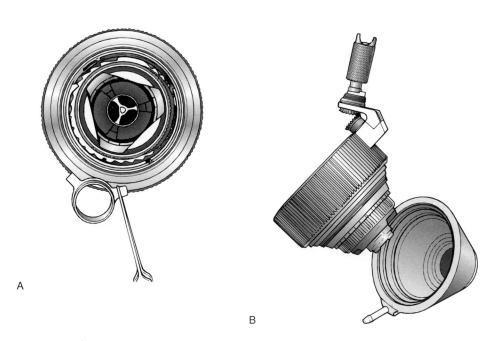

A

B

FIGURE 7-6.   A, B. *The trephine features a 360-degree limbal suction ring that secures the trephine to the eye; support surfaces on both sides of the trephine blade that stabilize the cornea during trephination; a manually operated gear mechanism for smooth, uniform cutting; and a calibration device that governs the blade extension and also allows cutting without descent. The trephine produces a symmetric and nearly vertical incision. (Reproduced by permission from the Moria 1996 catalog, on the Hanna corneal trephine system, France.)*

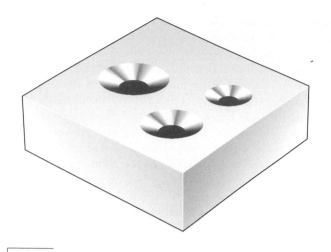

FIGURE 7-7.   *The Brightbill corneal cutting block incorporates three wells of various sizes with red 8-mm centering dots. (Reproduced by permission from Storz Ophthalmics 1996 catalog, p. 259.)*

Piston systems also have been designed to improve the precision of the cut and provide a round button with vertical sides (8,21). Stability is achieved by using a base plate that holds the Teflon cutting block. A hole in the center of the Teflon cutting block allows for drainage of fluid from the donor tissue, which minimizes the amount of tissue movement (2). A piston sleeve is fit over the cutting block and a piston with the appropriately sized blade is guided within the piston sleeve to achieve a more precise vertical cut (2,9). The Iowa P.K. press punch (Fig. 7-10) (10) uses a rack-and-pinion principle to guide a straight downward path, which minimizes the possibility of tilting, turning, or slipping of the trephine (25).

SUTURE MATERIAL

Although the primary cause of astigmatism is related to the profile of the cut tissue and the tissue-healing pattern (2,15,16,26–28), and the actual suture technique does not contribute to post–penetrating keratoplasty (post-PKP) astigmatism (5,26,29–31), the removal of sutures changes the final amount of astigmatism (5,26,32,33). Hence, proper application of the principles of suturing can help reduce post-PKP astigmatism. Use of appropriate suture materials as well as technique is important in ensuring optical control of post-PKP astigmatism (2). The ideal suture material is not biodegradable, is easy to manipulate, has tensile strength that is maintained over time, induces minimal tissue reactivity, and achieves perfect wound apposition (9,34–37). Nonabsorbable sutures, such as nylon, polyester (Mersilene), and polypropylene (Prolene), produce less inflammatory reaction (38) and are less elastic than other suture materials. Suture material with elasticity and biodegradability imposes a torque on the tissue. The elastic properties of nylon require deep and tight placement of sutures to ensure

adequate wound closure and prevent postoperative leaks (39) (Fig. 7-11). This manner of closure, however, distorts the wound and leads to irregular corneal astigmatism and decreased postoperative visual acuity (39).

Nylon monofilament hydrolyzes and loses tensile strength when bathed in tissue fluids (39,40). The 10-0 nylon suture has greater tensile strength than 11-0 nylon (26) and therefore can be tied more tightly and be placed at full-thickness depth. Alternatively, the smaller, 11-0 running suture allows for less wound compression and distortion. Nylon suture has low tissue reactivity and is easy to handle (9). The disadvantage of using nylon is that the wound-healing process is slower because of the low tissue reactivity (41), and thus sutures must be left in the wound for prolonged periods of time to prevent wound dehiscence.

Other suture materials such as polyester (Mersilene) are stronger and less elastic than nylon; control of wound tension is better with polyester than with nylon (9). Although polyester is not biodegradable, it imposes significant tissue reactivity, is difficult to handle, and tends to cheesewire (9,33). Monofilament polypropylene (Prolene) is nonabsorbable, has high tensile strength, and is elastic (9,38). The tissue reactivity as well as the tensile strength of polypropylene is comparable to that of nylon (34,38). Polypropylene maintains its tensile strength for a longer period of time compared to nylon (34,35,38,40), but it is more difficult to handle. The ideal suture material has properties that facilitate suture adjustment, such as elasticity comparable to that of nylon, resistance to biodegradation, and nonreactivity (33,35).

SUTURE TECHNIQUE

Firm, prolonged apposition of graft edges produces a more regular scar and a more stable cornea (29). The function of sutures, to appose the wound edges (6), can be achieved with full-thickness or through-and-through closure of the corneal wound (2). The ideal suturing technique involves apposition of wound edges without any tension. Tissue distortion during suturing can lead to high degrees of astigmatism, and therefore all efforts must be made to minimize the amount of distortion during suturing. Techniques include single continuous, double continuous, simple interrupted, or a combination of interrupted and continuous techniques. The use of interrupted sutures in a circular configuration flattens the donor cornea (26) and allows for localized areas of tension; the tension is confined to the area of the individual loop of thread. Tension can increase incongruity, thereby resulting in suboptimal amounts of post-PKP astigmatism. To minimize the amount of distortion from suture tension, the needle must pass directly under the tissue forceps. Furthermore, the needle must be perpendicular to the tissue when passing through the lamellae and parallel to the tissue when passing across the lamellae. A reverse-cutting spatula-type needle divides the lamellae at whatever level the needle is placed (6,9,22), tends to stay in

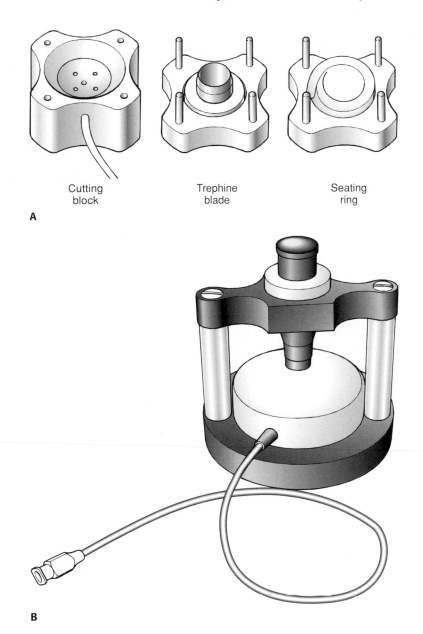

FIGURE 7-8. A. *The base of the Barron vacuum punch features a circular groove for aspirating the epithelial side of the cornea and immobilizing it for cutting the button. The seating ring is used to ensure complete contact between the peripheral part of the cornea and the aspirating groove, for positive vacuum. Immobilizing the donor cornea in this manner allows the surgeon to cut a perfectly round button from the center of the cornea every time. (Reproduced by permission from Katena Products, Inc., 1996 catalog, p. 2.) B. The Rothman-Gilbard corneal punch utilizes a specially designed suction cutting block with eight precisely placed suction holes. These holes are inked, the cornea is placed in the well, suction is applied, and the button is punched. (Reproduced by permission from Storz Ophthalmics 1996 catalog, p. 257.)*

the planned tissue plane, and follows the required curve of the needle. Suture bites of equal depth and equal length will result in optimal tissue apposition, minimal tension, and minimal astigmatism.

An ideal needle should be rigid, long, sharp, and atraumatic (7,24,42) (Fig. 7-12). A sharp needle requires minimal effort to fixate the tissue because it meets little resistance and creates less tissue distortion while it is passed through the stroma.

Continuous suture techniques do not flatten the cornea as much as interrupted sutures do (4), and therefore straighten out the curved incision. The disadvantage of a continuous suture is that suture tension must be evenly distributed around the entire graft to avoid graft displacement (6). A continuous running suture can minimize the amount of residual astigmatism and result in more rapid visual recovery (9,33) when a cylindrical piece of tissue is cut and placed into a cylindrical bed. Continuous sutures will

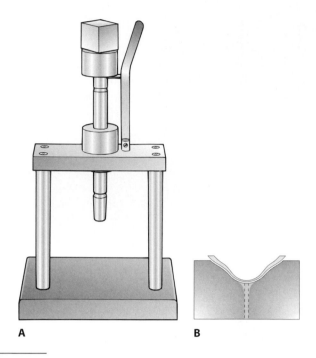

A

B

FIGURE 7-9. A. *The Lieberman gravity action corneal donor button punch is made of solid stainless steel and produces a symmetric, smooth, vertical cut. The punch accepts blade sizes 7.5 to 9.0 mm. The cutting block is made of black nylon and its concavity features multiple radii to most closely approximate the shape of the average of the corneoscleral surface. A black nylon cutting block was chosen for better visualization of the clear cornea. The block is vented to the outside to release air and fluid beneath the donor button. B. Lieberman donor button cutting block features multiple radii to closely approximate the corneoscleral profile. (Reproduced by permission from Katena Products, Inc., 1996 catalog, p. 16.)*

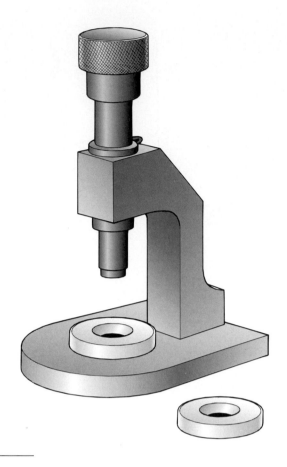

FIGURE 7-10. *The Iowa P.K. press punch was designed for precise punching of the donor corneal button. A unique two-color cutting block aids in centration of the donor tissue. A recessed base ensures that the block is held centrally under the trephine blade. (Reproduced by permission from Storz Ophthalmics 1996 catalog, p. 258.)*

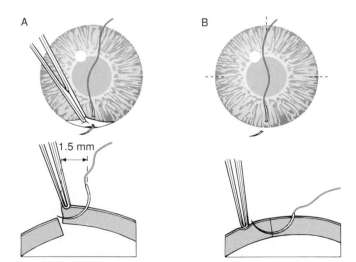

A

B

1.5 mm

FIGURE 7-11. *Deep suture bites allow for appropriate wound apposition. (Reproduced by permission from Penetrating keratoplasty. In: Bruner WE, Stark WJ, Maumenee AE, eds. Manual of corneal surgery. New York: Churchill Livingstone, 1987:24.)*

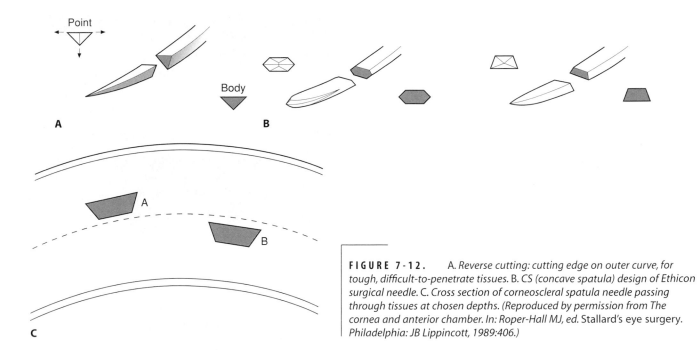

FIGURE 7-12.   A. *Reverse cutting: cutting edge on outer curve, for tough, difficult-to-penetrate tissues.* B. *CS (concave spatula) design of Ethicon surgical needle.* C. *Cross section of corneoscleral spatula needle passing through tissues at chosen depths. (Reproduced by permission from The cornea and anterior chamber. In: Roper-Hall MJ, ed.* Stallard's eye surgery. *Philadelphia: JB Lippincott, 1989:406.)*

deform the surface when stitches are placed at unequal distances from the wound line or at unequal depth. Although continuous, radially placed sutures introduce a rotational torque (9,29,39), one can adjust the suture tension at the slit lamp or under the microscope (6,9). As the suture is tightened, the tension shifts and can be distributed uniformly (32,41). Unfortunately, this technique also flattens the central part of the cornea, resulting in a more drumhead, less spherical configuration. A single, continuous, no-torque technique, in which 8 bites are placed at 45 degrees from the radial plane angled in the direction of suture advancement, compensates for induced torsion (6,9). A double, continuous-torque, antitorque technique, in which 10-0 nylon is placed in a clockwise, continuous radial pattern and a second 10-0 nylon suture is placed counterclockwise to but parallel to the first clockwise suture, allows the tension from the second suture to compensate for the torque and to produce a firmer, more secure closure (9,29,43). A double, continuous, same-direction technique is used with 10-0 nylon placed at Descemet's membrane and 11-0 nylon placed at one-third to one-half the depth. The advantage of this technique is earlier visual rehabilitation (9,27,33,39,43,44). The deep, tight suture allows for appropriate wound apposition, and the looser, smaller suture allows for good visual acuity while preventing wound dehiscence (16,39,42). The interrupted suture combined with a single running suture allows for selective removal of interrupted sutures early in the postoperative period to decrease the postoperative astigmatism. Although both techniques—single, interrupted sutures and continuous running sutures—have advantages, the best visual acuity is not achieved until

all sutures are removed completely; removal of sutures produces unpredictable changes in astigmatism (26,27,33) regardless of which technique is used.

NEWER SYSTEMS

To achieve the original goals—to minimize residual (9) astigmatism and facilitate rapid visual recovery—systems that combine newer trephination and suturing techniques have been designed. Many surgeons use an individual combination of techniques that results in precision, congruity, and adequate sectility with minimal postoperative astigmatism. The laser has been introduced to improve the precision of the cut.

Newer techniques continue to evolve. The Tampa trephine (Fig. 7-13) provides a precision cut in both the recipient bed and the donor. This technique offers a more stable donor-host interface by creating tabs on the donor tissue that are inserted into intrastromal pockets within the host bed (Fig. 7-14). The need for fewer sutures (12 interrupted) and the earlier removal of sutures would allow for rapid visual recovery with minimal astigmatism (45).

Future clinical trials will identify the advantages of the Tampa trephine over standard penetrating keratoplasty. In years to come, application of biologic glues may provide for a sutureless penetrating keratoplasty and eliminate postoperative astigmatism.

The author has no proprietary interest in any of the companies or devices mentioned in this article.

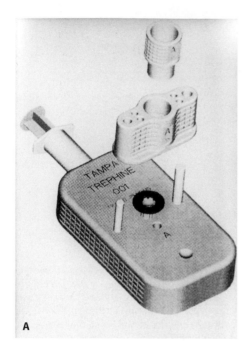

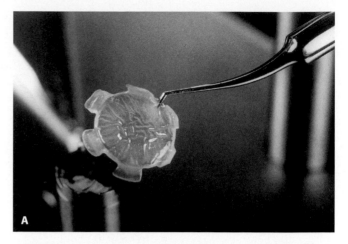

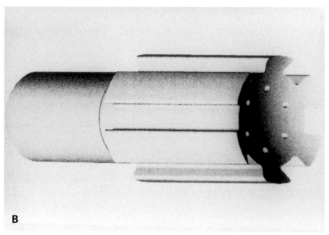

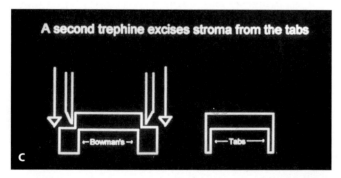

A second trephine excises stroma from the tabs

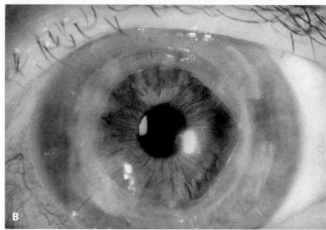

FIGURE 7-14. A. *The final corneal donor is a 7.0-mm button with six tabs. B. The donor-recipient interface after most sutures have been removed. (Courtesy of J. James Rowsey, MD.)*

FIGURE 7-13. A. *Tampa trephine (Martin Marietta Speciality Components, Largo, FL) consists of two metallic bases on which the donor corneoscleral rim is submitted for trephination. B. A six-tab donor punch is initially performed, providing six full-thickness tabs. C. A second trephination shaves excess tab tissue and leaves Bowman's layer and anterior stroma for subsequent imbrication into the recipient bed. (Courtesy of J. James Rowsey, MD.)*

REFERENCES

1. Eisner G. *Eye surgery. An introduction to operative technique.* 2nd ed. Fort Worth, TX: Springer 1990.
2. Troutman RC. Astigmatic considerations in corneal graft. *Ophthalmic Surg* 1979;10:21–26.
3. Arato S. A new electro-motor cornea-trephine for keratoplasty. *Ophthalmologica* 1950;120:38–40.
4. Hessburg PC, Barron M. A disposable corneal trephine. *Ophthalmic Surg* 1980;11:730–733.
5. Perlman EM. An analysis and interpretation of refractive errors after penetrating keratoplasty. *Ophthalmology* 1981;88:39–45.
6. The cornea and anterior chamber. In: Roper-Hall MJ, ed. *Stallard's eye surgery.* Philadelphia: JB Lippincott, 1989:392–423.
7. Instruments in corneal grafting. In: Casey TA, Mayer DJ, eds. *Corneal grafting: principles and practice.* Philadelphia: WB Saunders, 1984:87–96.
8. Waltman SR. Penetrating keratoplasty. In: Waltman SR, Keates RH, Hoyt CS, et al, eds. *Surgery of the eye.* New York: Churchill Livingstone, 1988:193–216, 285–297.
9. Brightbill FS. *Corneal surgery: theory, technique, and tissue.* St. Louis: Mosby, 1993.
10. Smirmaul H, Casey TA. A clear view trephine and lamellar dissector for corneal grafting. *Am J Ophthalmol* 1980;90:92–94.
11. Crock GW, Pericic L, Chapman-Smith JS, et al. A new system of microsurgery for human and experimental corneal grafting. 1. The contact lens corneal cutter stereotaxic eye holder, donor disc chuck and frame. *Br J Ophthalmol* 1978;62:74–80.

12. Van Rij G, Cornell M, Waring GO III, et al. Postoperative astigmatism after central versus eccentric penetrating keratoplasties. *Am J Ophthalmol* 1985;99:317–320.

13. Cohen KL, Holman RE, Tripoli NK, Kupper LL. Effect of trephine tilts on corneal button dimensions. *Am J Ophthalmol* 1986;101:722–725.

14. Olson RJ. Corneal curvature changes associated with penetrating keratoplasty: a mathematical model. *Ophthalmic Surg* 1980;11:838–842.

15. Duffin RM, Olson RJ, Ohrloff C. Analysis of the Hessburg-Barron vacuum trephine. *Ophthalmic Surg* 1984;15:51–54.

16. Insler MS, Cooper HD, Caldwell DR. Final surgical results with a suction trephine. *Ophthalmic Surg* 1987;18:23–27.

17. Drews RC. Corneal trephine. *Trans Am Acad Ophthalmol Otolaryngol* 1974;78:223–224.

18. Lieberman DM. A new corneal trephine. *Am J Ophthalmol* 1976;81:684–685.

19. Kadesky D. An electric automatic trephine. *Am J Ophthalmol* 34:1038.

20. Brightbill FS, Pollack FM, Slappey T. A comparison of two methods for cutting donor corneal buttons. *Am J Ophthalmol* 1973;75:500–506.

21. Michaelson IC. Slope of sides of corneal grafts and recipient beds. *Br J Ophthalmol* 1954;38:19–21.

22. Polack FM, ed. *Corneal transplantation*. New York: Grune & Stratton, 1977.

23. Penetrating keratoplasty. Bruner WE, Stark WJ, Maumenee AE, eds. In: *Manual of corneal surgery*. New York: Churchill Livingstone, 1987:19–28.

24. Gilbard JP, Rothman RC, Kenyon KR. A new donor cornea marker and punch for penetrating keratoplasty. *Ophthalmic Surg* 1987;18:908–911.

25. Bourne WM. A corneal trephine press. *Trans Am Acad Ophthalmol Otolaryngol* 1973;77:479–480.

26. Stainer GA, Perl T, Binder PS. Controlled reduction of postkeratoplasty astigmatism. *Ophthalmology* 1982;89:668–676.

27. Musch DC, Meyer RF, Sugar A. The effect of removing running sutures on astigmatism after penetrating keratoplasty. *Arch Ophthalmol* 1988;106:488–492.

28. Van Rij G, Waring GO III. Suture-induced astigmatism after a circular wound in the rhesus monkey. *Cornea* 1986;5:25–28.

29. Troutman RC, Meltzer M. Astigmatism and myopia in keratoconus. *Trans Am Ophthalmol Soc* 1972;70:265–267.

30. Baum JL. [Comment on: Troutman RC. Astigmatism and myopia in keratoplasty. *S Afr Arch Ophthalmol* 1974;1:29–35.] *Surv Ophthalmol* 1976;20:294.

31. Jensen AD, Maumenee AE. Refractive errors following keratoplasty. *Trans Am Ophthalmol Soc* 1974;72:123–131.

32. Van Meter WS, Gussler JR, Soloman KV, Wook TO. Postkeratoplasty astigmatism control. Single continuous suture adjustment versus selective interrupted suture removal. *Ophthalmology* 1991;98:177–183.

33. Lin DTC, Wilson SE, Reidy JJ, et al. An adjustable single running suture technique to reduce postkeratoplasty astigmatism. *Ophthalmology* 1990;97:934–938.

34. Kelly SE, Ehlers J, Llovera I, Troutman RC. Comparison of tissue reaction to nylon and Prolene sutures in rabbit iris and cornea. *Ophthalmic Surg* 1975;6:105–110.

35. Miller JM. Evaluation of a new surgical suture (Prolene). *Am Surg* 1973;39:31–39.

36. Herrmann JB. Tensile strength and knot security of surgical suture materials. *Am Surg* 1971;37:209–217.

37. Basu PK, Hasany SM. A histochemical study on corneal suture reaction. *Can J Ophthalmol* 1971;6:328–341.

38. Miller JM, Kimmel LE Jr. Clinical evaluation of monofilament polypropylene suture. *Am Surg* 1967;33:666–670.

39. Davison JA, Bourne WM. Results of penetrating keratoplasty using a double running suture technique. *Arch Ophthalmol* 1981;99:1591–1595.

40. Postlethwait RW. Long-term comparative study of nonabsorbable sutures. *Ann Surg* 1970;171:892–898.

41. Boruchoff SA, Jensen AD, Dohlman CH. Comparison of suturing techniques in keratoplasty for keratoconus. *Ann Ophthalmol* 1975;7:433–436.

42. Pollack FM, Sanchez J, Eve FR. 10-0 Microsurgical sutures. 1. Evaluation of various types of needles and sutures for anterior segment surgery. *Can J Ophthalmol* 1974;9:42–47.

43. McNeill JI, Kaufman HE. A double running suture technique for keratoplasty: earlier visual rehabilitation. *Ophthalmic Surg* 1977;8:58–61.

44. Young SR, Olson RJ. Results of a double running suture in penetrating keratoplasty performed on keratoconus patients. *Ophthalmic Surg* 1985;16:779–786.

45. Rowsey JJ, Thoren JCS, Rocha G, Stevens S. Tampa trephine penetrating keratoplasty: preliminary patient insights. Presented at the American Academy of Ophthalmology annual meeting, Atlanta, November 1995.

Corneal Transplantation: Early Postoperative Management

Jeremy E. Levenson

The advent of modern cataract surgery has made most ophthalmic surgeons skilled in the use of the operating microscope, delicate surgical instruments, and fine sutures. As a result, many surgeons feel comfortable with the technical aspects of performing corneal transplantation. However, in contrast to cataract surgery, it is the appropriateness of the care provided in the postoperative period that determines the outcome of corneal transplant surgery (1). Identifying the minor as well as the major complications that can and often do occur in the postoperative period can make the difference between surgical success and failure. This chapter provides an approach to the care of the corneal transplant patient in the early postoperative period, focusing on the identification and treatment of potential complications.

POSTOPERATIVE CARE

There are probably as many postoperative care regimens as there are surgeons performing corneal transplantation. Each surgeon will be influenced by his or her training and experience, the nature of the condition requiring surgery, and even the availability of the patient for follow-up care. Whatever the specific approach taken, the following must be monitored in the early postoperative period:

1. Signs of infection
2. Evidence of a wound leak
3. Thickness of the graft
4. Status of the corneal epithelium
5. Depth of the anterior chamber
6. Intraocular pressure
7. Degree of inflammation
8. Presence of synechiae
9. Pupillary block

Schedule of Examinations

The patient must be examined on the first postoperative day, as this is the appropriate time to discover any major surgical complications. During this examination, the patient should be questioned about the presence and degree of any pain being experienced. The visual acuity should be determined, a careful slit-lamp examination undertaken, the intraocular pressure measured, and if possible, indirect funduscopy performed. Based on the findings at this examination, the frequency of the visits for the next week or two will be decided. Even in an entirely uncomplicated case, the corneal epithelium will probably not be completely healed (2). Because, as discussed in detail later, establishing complete corneal epithelialization is a major step in securing a clear corneal graft, the patient should be seen again in 1 or 2 days, and then followed frequently until this condition has been achieved. Once a stable state has been reached, a reasonable schedule of postoperative visits would include seeing the patient every week or two for the first month and then every 2 to 4 weeks for the next 3 months. By this time, patients can often by visually rehabilitated. It is necessary, however, to be flexible in providing postoperative care because if any problem is discovered, much more frequent, even daily visits, may be needed. Since complications can develop between visits and their early treatment can be critical to a successful surgical result, patients must be instructed to notify their surgeon quickly if they note any change in the status of their operated eye, such as increased pain, redness, or decreased vision.

Patching

The surgical dressing is removed on the first postoperative visit. Many surgeons will then continue full-time patching until the epithelial layer on the corneal transplant has completely healed. For the majority of patients, this will take 1 to 3 days (2). Although there is a trend toward not patching traumatic corneal abrasions and at least one study found that patching does not speed up healing (3), the immediate postoperative transplant is anesthetic, and the protection of mild, but effective, pressure patching may be beneficial. The eye must be protected in the longer term with protective eye wear during the day and a shield at night (4). This regimen should be continued for 2 to 3 months.

Graft Thickness

Most corneal grafts will show a certain amount of edema in the immediate postoperative period. This edema will be manifested by increased corneal thickness with pachymetry readings higher than 0.6 mm (5). The amount of swelling will be affected by the age of the donor, the death to preservation time, the duration of preservation, the type of storage medium, the amount of surgical trauma, the nature of the condition requiring transplantation, the status of the endothelium and epithelium, and the intraocular pressure. The edema is caused by endothelial "pump" dysfunction resulting from a combination of metabolic insult and actual endothelial cell loss. Epithelial edema may not be present because of the absence or thinning of the epithelial layer. Classically, corneal transplants in phakic eyes tend to have more endothelial cell loss than do transplants in aphakic eyes, presumably due to the "washboarding" effect of rubbing the donor button against the lens-iris diaphragm during surgery in the former (5). The use of viscoelastic agents during surgery has removed this difference (6). In the uncomplicated case, a gradual thinning of the graft should be anticipated, with most of the folds in Descemet's membrane gone by 2 to 3 weeks after surgery. Peripheral circumferential folds may persist near the wound margin owing to the compression of tissue by the corneal sutures and possibly the use of an oversized donor graft. These folds will tend to disappear with time or with removal of the corneal sutures. If there is normal endothelium on the patient's own cornea, longer-term thinning of a thicker than normal graft may occur owing to the gradual migration of endothelium from the recipient bed onto the donor graft.

Medications

Routinely, corneal transplant patients will receive a topical steroid and a topical antibiotic eyedrop. On the evening of surgery and the following morning, if a significant amount of viscoelastic agent has been left in the eye or if there is a concern about the possibility of glaucoma, an oral carbonic anhydrase inhibitor can be administered, assuming there are no medical contraindications (7). Starting on the first or second postoperative day a topical steroid such as prednisolone acetate 1% or an equivalent should be prescribed for use four times a day and a topical antibiotic such as tobramycin 0.3% or ciprofloxacin 0.3%, two to four times

a day. Combination steroid-antibiotic drops are popular but have the disadvantage of inflexibility as it is often necessary to use a steroid drop much more frequently than an antibiotic drop. In addition, many of these combination drops include neomycin, which can prove to be especially toxic to the unstable graft epithelium (8). Some surgeons prefer to administer these drugs in ointment form. In the routine, uncomplicated case, the steroid drops can begin to be tapered after the postoperative inflammation is controlled, usually in 3 to 4 weeks. Typically, in phakic grafts, by 2 to 3 months, the steroid drops can be discontinued. For aphakic or pseudophakic eyes, where the complication of cataract formation is not a concern, and the patient is not a steroid responder, many surgeons recommend continuing a drop or two of topical steroid indefinitely in hopes of decreasing the long-term chance of graft rejection (Fig. 8-1). Since not all cases are routine, the use of steroids postoperatively may vary greatly from patient to patient. In addition to the usual steroid side effects of cataract formation and secondary glaucoma, their effect on decreasing wound healing must be kept in mind (9,10). Obtaining a wound of adequate tensile strength, especially in the elderly, is already a concern in corneal transplantation, and the intensive and prolonged use of steroids can only exacerbate this problem. The steroidal effect on depressing local immunity can lead to opportunistic infection with bacteria and fungi, and is a known correlate with the development of crystalline keratopathy (11). Still, until a good prospective study determines the relative value of steroids, low-dose, long-term steroid use in nonphakic patients is probably warranted. The use of topical antibiotics can be discontinued once the epithelial layer has stabilized and completely covers the cornea, typically in 3 to 4 weeks.

Many patients will require frequent use of artificial tears to help stabilize and protect the delicate epithelium on the surface of the graft. If artificial tears are used more than four times a day, nonpreserved tears should be prescribed. If ointments are used, these, too, should be nonpreserved.

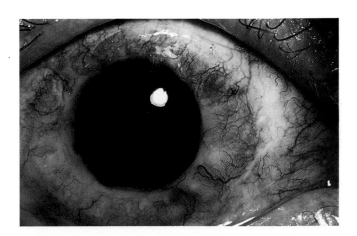

FIGURE 8-1.   *When a graft is placed in a vascularized bed, steroids must be continued indefinitely to prevent rejection.*

A topical cycloplegic is usually not required in routine cases. If it is thought necessary, a short-acting drug such as cyclopentolate hydrochloride 1% (Cyclogyl) or homatropine 5% should be used. Long-acting cycloplegics, such as sco-palamine and atropine, limit the ability to manipulate the pupil pharmacologically, which can be necessary in the post-operative period to break synechiae. In addition, they have been implicated in the development of fixed, dilated pupils postoperatively in eyes that have undergone corneal trans-plantation for keratoconus (12). However, this etiology has been seriously called into question by more recent findings (13), and it seems more likely that the fixed, dilated pupil seen rarely following keratoplasty for keratoconus is due to iris ischemia developing during surgery from posterior pressure.

Although not universally accepted (14), the use of an antiviral agent is recommended for a patient with a history of herpes simplex keratitis (Fig. 8-2). Most surgeons will use a drop of trifluorothymidine four or five times a day while steroids are being applied (15). It must be kept in mind, however, that these agents are metabolic inhibitors and can only be effective if they are continuously present in ade-quate concentration. The studies that have been published concerning the prevention of recurrent herpes infections in patients on topical steroids utilized these agents in full dosage (16). On the other hand, in full dosage these agents can be very toxic to the epithelium (17,18), and since they empirically seem to be effective in lower dosage, this trend will probably continue until findings to the contrary are presented. Once the steroid dosage has been decreased to one drop daily, the antiviral agent can be stopped. To avoid the toxicity of topical antivirals, oral acyclovir can be used, as it is effective prophylaxis against recurrent herpes simplex keratitis in patients receiving topical steroids postoperatively (19). Starting initially with 800 to 1000 mg in divided doses, acyclovir can be gradually tapered over 12 months or more. Presumably, the newer oral antiviral agents famciclovir and valacyclovir are at least as effective.

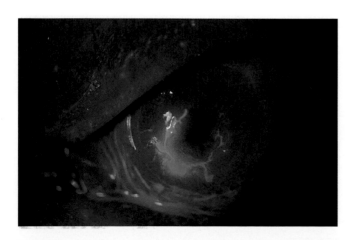

FIGURE 8-2. *Recurrent herpes dendritic keratitis in a graft. The patient was on steroids without antiviral coverage.*

The other class of drugs commonly utilized in the post-operative period are antiglaucomatous agents. These drugs are discussed later.

Instructing patients in the proper technique of eyedrop instillation can help avoid the occasional complication of eye trauma from a medication bottle. This is a particular risk in the elderly who may have unsteady hands.

Activity

Modern corneal transplant techniques, primarily by producing wounds of sufficient integrity, have allowed early ambulation of the patient beginning on the day of surgery. Patients may resume taking care of their personal needs as soon as they have recovered from the effects of anesthesia. They need to be reassured that the sutures holding their wound are sufficiently strong to permit then to return to the activities of normal living. Most wounds can withstand the stress of coughing, sneezing, and usually even vomiting. Activities such as reading or watching television are per-mitted, only limited by the patient's level of comfort. At the same time, patients must be made to understand that the sutures used are finer than human hair and cannot withstand a direct blow to the eye. Many patients, unless the risk of trauma is stressed, do not fully understand this danger. Eye protection should be worn at all times, even when sitting at home. Protective eye wear usually consists of a sturdy pair of glasses during the day and a taped-on shield at night. This practice should be continued for the first 2 to 3 months after surgery. Patients should be instructed to avoid situations where there is a risk of trauma to the eye, such as large crowds, contact or racquet sports, skiing, and so on. Heavy lifting or straining that could lead to increased intraocular pressure through the Valsalva maneu-ver or eyelid squeezing should be avoided for the first 2 to 3 months. Although often not asked, many patients, partic-ularly younger ones, are concerned about when they can return to sexual activity. Usually an explanation about the type of risks to avoid will be sufficient to allow them to proceed safely.

Patients should be made aware of the need to protect their eye from potential sources of infection during the initial weeks following surgery. Wearing an eye patch until the epithelium is healed is part of this protection. Patients can have their hair washed but this should be done with the head back so that the soapy water does not enter the eye. Bathing is permitted, but again dirty water should be kept out of the eye. Care must be taken in getting in and out of the bathtub because of the real danger of slipping. Once the surface of the graft has fully epithelialized, usually by 2 to 3 weeks, these restrictions can be eased. During this same period, patients should be discouraged from working on their hands and knees in a garden and from swimming. If there are any exposed knots in the graft, these restrictions must be extended because these knots can allow infectious agents access to the graft.

The amount of time a patient takes off from work must be tailored to his or her individual situation and will be determined in large part by the individual's type of work and the level of vision in the unoperated eye. In practice, most patients who are not engaged in heavy manual labor or work in a dusty, contaminated environment, and who have adequate vision in their opposite eye, can return to work as soon as their level of comfort permits, usually a week or less. For those who do manual labor, 6 to 8 weeks of leave may be required. For those requiring the vision of the operative eye to be able to work, a number of months may be needed.

Suture Adjustment

In suturing the corneal donor button into the recipient bed, the corneal surgeon has two opposing goals. On the one hand, the surgeon wants the suture tight enough so that there is no wound leak. On the other hand, the suture should be loose enough so that there is minimal distortion, the tension created by the suture being evenly distributed leaving a spherical graft. Occasionally, the proper balance between these two goals is achieved, allowing early visual rehabilitation of the patient. Often, however, rehabilitation awaits wound healing and suture removal. Suturing techniques utilizing either a single running 10-0 nylon suture with 20 to 24 bites or a combination of 12 to 16 interrupted 10-0 nylon sutures with a running 10-0 or 11-0 suture have been devised. The adjustment of these sutures is performed early in the postoperative course to reduce graft astigmatism.

Adjustment of the running 10-0 nylon suture is begun as soon as there is adequate healing of the epithelial surface to allow reliable manifest refraction, keratometry, or a computer-assisted corneal topography study (20). Practically speaking, even with a drop of artificial tears to temporarily improve the optical quality of the graft surface, adjustment usually cannot begin before 2 to 4 weeks postoperatively. The steeper and flatter meridians of the graft are determined as accurately as possible. Topical anesthesia is applied and the patient placed in a comfortable position at the slit lamp. Placing a small wire speculum may be helpful for some patients, whereas others may be able to cooperate more fully without a speculum in place. A sterile, fine, smooth-edged tying forceps is used to tighten the suture in the flattest meridian by carefully pulling in a radial fashion on the surface loop. The slack in the suture is then passed, loop by loop, to the steepest meridian, relieving some of the tension in this area. The maneuver is then repeated going in the opposite direction from the flattest to the steepest meridian. Further adjustment is obtained by repeating this procedure on the opposite side of the graft. A measurement of the corneal graft topography is again taken, utilizing a drop of sterile artificial tears, and the procedure repeated until a near spherical pattern is obtained or until the surface is too distorted to permit a meaningful measurement. This procedure

is more effective, if, prior to the adjustment, the tying forceps is used to break the epithelial and anterior stromal adhesions throughout the circumference of the graft wound. The obvious risk of this procedure is the inadvertent breaking of the suture. This risk can be minimized by having the patient well anesthetized, well positioned at the slit lamp, and properly informed as to what to expect with the procedure. Traction on the suture should only be in the direction of the suture using a fine-quality forceps best dedicated to this purpose. A jeweler's forceps, which is adequate for removing interrupted sutures, is too sharp edged to be used safely. Following the adjustment, topical antibiotic drops are applied and the patient then continues his or her regular regimen of antibiotics and steroids. The patient is seen again in 2 to 4 weeks and the degree of corneal astigmatism determined. The procedure can be repeated if the astigmatism is thought to be excessive, usually 3 diopters (D) or more.

Where a combination suturing technique has been utilized, the first interrupted 10-0 nylon sutures can be removed starting 2 to 3 months postoperatively. Once the steep meridian has been determined, the interrupted suture closest to this axis is identified. This identification can be helped by computer-assisted corneal topography. The patient is placed at the slit lamp as noted previously and the appropriate suture is cut with a sterile blade such as a No. 11 Bard Parker or the side of a No. 25 needle. The end of the suture on the side of the wound where the knot is buried is teased out, and the suture grasped with forceps and removed. Although not usually a problem in the first few months after surgery, healing may make it difficult to remove the suture because the knot acts like a barb. Making the initial cut in the elbow of the suture on the side opposite the knot will allow the deep end to retract into the corneal stroma. Then, if the suture is not easily removed, it can be cut flush to the surface on the opposite side under slight tension, which will allow this end of the buried segment of suture to retract into the stroma as well. The epithelium will then heal over the surface and the buried segment can remain safely in the cornea until it eventually reabsorbs years later. The suture should never be pulled in the opposite direction because the knot would be pulled across the wound, very likely causing disruption. Antibiotic drops are applied and the patient is seen again in 3 to 4 weeks. The procedure can be repeated until the desired result is obtained, that is, a cornea with less than 2 to 3 D of astigmatism, or until there are no additional appropriate sutures to remove.

COMPLICATIONS IN THE EARLY POSTOPERATIVE PERIOD

Complications in the period following corneal transplantation can vary from the minor to the true ophthalmic disaster resulting in the loss of the eye. What is certain for all the potential complications is that the best chance for a successful outcome occurs with early intervention. It is for this reason that close and meticulous follow-up of the corneal transplant patient is essential. Recognition and treatment of the following complications, not necessarily in the order of frequency or potential severity, are discussed in this section:

1. Endophthalmitis and infectious keratitis
2. Wound leak
3. Epithelial defects
4. Filamentary keratitis
5. Synechial formation
6. Hyphema
7. Excessive iritis
8. Pupillary block
9. Glaucoma
10. Vascularization
11. Retained Descemet's membrane
12. Primary graft failure

Endophthalmitis and Infectious Keratitis

The risk of infection is inherent in the nature of corneal transplant surgery. Certain risk factors can, however, significantly increase the possibility of postoperative infection (Table 8-1).

Endophthalmitis can occur both immediately after and late in the course following corneal transplantation. The incidence, which has been reported to be between 0.1% (21) and 2% (22), is low and seems to be about the same as that for cataract surgery (23). This is surprising since between 12.4% (21) and 100% (24) of cultures taken from donor eyes prior to processing are positive for contamination. A wide variety of gram-positive bacteria as well as gram-negative bacteria and fungi have been isolated from patients with postkeratoplasty endophthalmitis.

The presentation of endophthalmitis following corneal transplantation is similar to that occurring after cataract surgery. Patients may present with intense pain, a swollen lid, marked conjunctival hyperemia, and hypopyon with even more corneal edema and clouding than typically found in the cataract surgery patient (23). At other times, endophthalmitis can present more insidiously (22). There may be little pain. The vision may be poorer than expected and the vitreous progressively more cloudy with loss of the red reflex, as much of the inflammation is masked by the intensive steroid use. Since vision is often poor in the initial postoperative period, and graft edema may limit intraocular visualization, the diagnosis of endophthalmitis can be difficult to make and, therefore, is more delayed in the corneal transplant patient. It, therefore, behooves the surgeon to keep in mind the possibility of infection when the postoperative course is not as expected. B-Scan ultrasonography is useful in demonstrating the presence of vitreous vials when visibility is poor.

Table 8-1. Risk Factors for Postoperative Infection

Preoperative conditions
  Keratitis sicca
  Blepharitis
  Acne rosacea
  Cicatricial conjunctival disease (ocular pemphigoid, alkali burns, Stevens-Johnson syndrome)
  Trichiasis
  Trachoma
  Graft failure
  Previous herpetic keratitis
  Ocular adnexa and lid abnormalities
  Preexisting corneal or external infection
  Systemic diseases (atopic disease, systemic immunosuppression, diabetes, rheumatoid disease)
Intraoperative factors
  Contaminated instruments or solutions
  Contaminated donor tissue or storage media
  Extensive tissue manipulation
  Aphakia
Postoperative factors
  Epithelial defects or severe punctate keratopathy
  Exposed or loose sutures
  Soft contact lens use
  Wound dehiscence
  Corticosteroid use

Although no series in corneal transplantation has been reported to date, the laboratory diagnosis and treatment of endophthalmitis should probably follow the recommendations of the Endophthalmitis Vitrectomy Study Group (25): early vitreous aspiration followed by intravitreal antibiotics and possibly vitrectomy in nonresponding patients. Since the donor graft can be a potential source of infection (26), all donor cornea-scleral rims should be cultured at the time of surgery. Information obtained from these cultures may provide a head start in choosing appropriate therapy should an infection develop postoperatively. Unfortunately, the prognosis for endophthalmitis following corneal transplantation has been very poor despite treatment (22). Whether the outcome will improve following the newer guidelines for therapy remains to be seen.

Given the high incidence of positive cultures from donor rims and the low incidence of actual postoperative infection, the surgeon not infrequently faces the situation a day or two postoperatively of being informed that the rim culture is growing a contaminant (most often *Staphylococcus epidermidis*, but occasionally even a fungus). Having already seen the patient and feeling that the postoperative course is uncomplicated, the surgeon is unsure how to proceed. Since most positive rim cultures do not translate into active infection (23), in most cases, nothing more than continued observation is required, perhaps increasing the frequency of visits for the next week or two.

Infectious keratitis can develop after corneal transplantation, with an incidence between 1.8% (27) and 4.9% (28) in the United States. With this significant rate of infection in mind, all preoperative conditions that can lead to corneal infections, such as lid abnormalities (blepharitis, trichiasis, lagophthalmos, entropion or ectropion), lacrimal system infection, or dry eye problems, should be treated and corrected to the greatest extent possible. Unfortunately, a number of the conditions that have associated corneal problems requiring transplantation, such as keratoconus in atopia or corneal scarring in various conjunctival cicatricial diseases, cannot be cured and must be dealt with postoperatively. Anticipating the problems these conditions may present postoperatively allows precautionary measures to be taken. Closing off the lacrimal puncta permanently with cautery or reversibly with punctal plugs before or at the time of surgery is an example of this approach. Similarly, performing a lateral or even a medial and lateral intermarginal tarsorrhaphy in a patient with rheumatoid disease can help prevent postoperative problems with melting and infection.

Postoperative factors that can predispose the corneal transplant to infection include the presence of corneal sutures, epithelial defects, and punctate erosions; the use of a bandage contact lens; and the general depression in the local immune state from the use of steroids and occasionally other immunosuppressive drugs. Corneal sutures should always be considered potential "time bombs." Whenever a suture is not completely covered with epithelium, the exposed knot or suture loop causes a break in the normal barrier function of the corneal surface, allowing access of infectious organisms to the corneal stroma (29). At the time of surgery, all exposed knots should be buried and care taken that all suture material is flush to the surface to allow rapid epithelialization. When knots must be left exposed, the patient should be left on prophylactic antibiotic coverage until wound healing permits suture removal. All loosened or broken sutures should be removed as soon as they are found, as they are no longer affording any strength to the wound, but rather collect mucus, allow bacteria to adhere, and offer a pathway for infection (30). Any foreign material, such as a lint fiber, should be carefully removed at the slit lamp. Following removal, coverage with a topical antibiotic such as tobramycin 0.3% or ciprofloxacin 0.3% every 2 hours for the next 2 to 3 days is indicated.

Epithelial defects and erosions are a frequent precursor of corneal infection (Fig. 8-3). Their specific management is discussed later. To the extent that they may be the result of topical prophylactic antibiotics, epithelial-friendly agents should be used, avoiding drugs that contain neomycin. Although occasionally helpful in allowing healing of the corneal surface, the routine use of extended-wear soft contact lens is not recommended because of their known propensity to cause corneal infections. When their use is believed to be necessary, these patients should be kept on

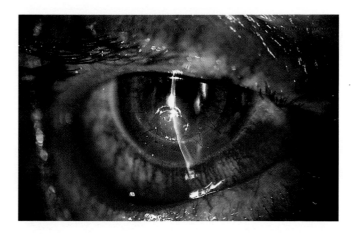

FIGURE 8-3. *Corneal epithelial defect that has become infected.*

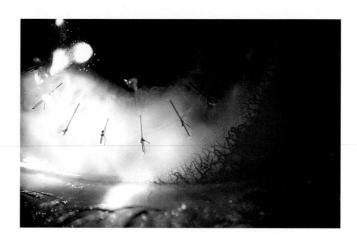

FIGURE 8-4. *Fungal keratitis developing in the wound margin, with a mass of hyphae extending into the anterior chamber.*

topical prophylactic antibiotics. They should be made aware of the potential risks of this treatment modality so that they can report the earliest signs of a problem. Because of their immunosuppressive side effect, steroids should be used in the least amount required for the shortest period of time necessary to achieve the desired result. Since all the risk factors for infection cannot be eliminated, every patient must be made aware of the need to report any change in status, such as a new foreign body sensation, increasing redness, and a white spot on the cornea, keeping in mind that the usual symptoms of infection, including pain and photophobia, may be masked by the use of steroids.

The majority of the agents causing postkeratoplasty infectious keratitis are gram-positive bacteria, but the full spectrum of agents associated with corneal ulceration has been described (28,31,32) (Table 8-2) (Fig. 8-4). The approach to therapy should follow generally accepted practice, including the standard culturing and scrapping of

Table 8-2.   Organisms Isolated from Postkeratoplasty Ulcers

Gram positive
   Coagulase-negative staphylococci
   Staphylococcus aureus
   Streptococcus pneumoniae
   β-Hemolytic streptococci
   α-Hemolytic streptococci
   Corynebacterium diphtheriae
Gram negative
   Pseudomonas aeruginosa
   Serratia marcescens
   Klebsiella species
   Proteus mirabilis
   Hemophilus species
   Moraxella species
   Escherichia coli
   Bacillus species
Fungi
   Candida species
   Other fungi

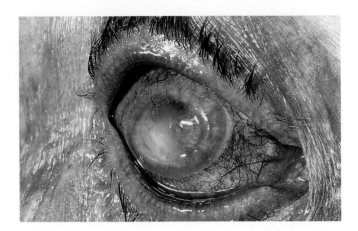

FIGURE 8-5.   *Neglected corneal ulcer that has led to perforation. Note the relatively mild inflammatory reaction due to use of topical steroids.*

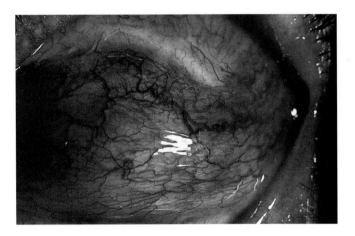

FIGURE 8-6.   *Conjunctival flap pulled to save an eye with an ulcer on an alkali-burned cornea.*

material from the ulcer bed (remembering to send any removed suture material for culture) and the use of intensive, broad-spectrum, topical antibiotics (33). The decision on whether or not to hospitalize a patient depends on the extent of the infection, the status of the patient's other eye, and the patient's ability to comply with the treatment schedule. The prognosis for corneal graft infections that have progressed beyond a localized stitch abscess is very guarded (28,34). Scarring or the associated irregular astigmatism, even when the scarring is not directly in the visual axis, can have a profound deleterious effect on the final vision. Corneal perforation, wound dehiscence, and endophthalmitis occur more frequently than what is usually seen with corneal infections in otherwise normal corneas (31) (Fig. 8-5). Regrafting, on either an emergent or an elective basis, is a common outcome (35). The decision regarding the continued use of topical steroids presents the surgeon with a difficult choice. On the one hand, steroids may be necessary to prevent graft rejection and preserve graft clarity, or, at least, to prevent or limit vascularization of the graft bed, allowing a better prognosis for a regraft. On the other hand, infection can develop in many of these patients because they are immunosuppressed by the steroids. Most treating physicians in this situation take the middle road of decreasing the steroid dosage, but not stopping it, at least initially. If steroids are stopped, an initial, and at times marked, worsening of the inflammation is to be expected; this change does not necessarily indicate a worsening of the infection. Whatever approach to steroid use is selected, it must be kept in mind that the ultimate goal has to be to save the eye in this potentially disastrous situation (Fig. 8-6).

Other white lesions that are not infectious in origin can develop in the graft postoperatively. The most common are the myriad of tiny, discrete white dots that frequently appear in the epithelium in the furrow at the base of the ridge created by the corneal sutures (Fig. 8-7). These dots are composed of degenerating epithelial cells (36). They appear several weeks after surgery and usually persist until the sutures are removed or until the cornea assumes a more normal contour. The dots do not take up fluorescein and the patients are asymptomatic. Their importance lies only in recognizing their benign nature.

Of greater significance are the white to gray-white infiltrates that occasionally appear along the corneal sutures early in the postoperative course. They seem to be an immune response to the suture material or to a substance on its surface. Unlike the usual isolated stitch abscess, these infiltrates are minute foci of white blood cells located along many or all of the suture loops. Affected eyes tend to be moderately inflamed. The epithelium, unlike the situation found with a stitch abscess, is usually intact over the sutures.

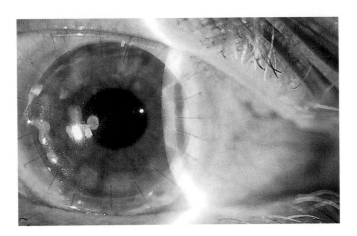

FIGURE 8-7. *Minute white dots, sometimes referred to as Kaye dots, frequently develop in the epithelium in the base of the furrow near the wound margin. They are best seen here in the slit beam light.*

Treatment consists of increasing the steroid dosage to a drop every hour or two until the inflammatory response is brought under control, followed by a slow taper.

Wound Leak and Suture Problems

Wound leaks and suture problems are uncommon with modern suturing techniques but often are related when they do occur. A patient presenting with a broken running 10-0 nylon suture in the immediate postoperative period before there is significant wound healing will need to have the suture repaired. This should be completed quickly, even if there is no leak, because of the great risk of further unraveling of the suture with loss of the anterior chamber or the development of graft override. The repair should be done under the microscope in a sterile setting because of the danger of infection. With a cooperative patient the repair can be made using topical anesthesia, with mild sedation as needed. Subconjunctival injection, sub-Tenon's injection, or even general anesthesia may be required for certain patients. Retrobulbar or peribulbar injections should be avoided because of the risk of a retrobulbar hemorrhage in an open eye. A new segment of 10-0 nylon suture must be added, making several bites across the wound. It is then tied to both ends of the broken suture, which have been withdrawn a loop or two on either side to provide enough suture for tying. This maneuver is made easier if the new suture is passed for several bites before the original suture is disturbed, to lessen the chance of anterior-chamber loss, if it is still formed. Prior to tying the final knot, tension on the sutures is adjusted appropriately. An attempt can be made to bury the knots. An alternative is to tie the suture in the wound, but in this case it will never be possible to remove all the suture material because the knot becomes trapped in the wound scar. A broken running suture occurring a few months after surgery, as from mild trauma, does not neces-

sarily need to be repaired. If it shows signs of loosening, the suture can be protected from the movement of the eyelids by a bandage soft contact lens. A broken interrupted suture can usually be removed without replacement unless there is evidence of wound gape.

A wound leak may be found on the first or second postoperative visit even with an intact suture or sutures, particularly when an attempt has been made to avoid an excessively tight suture. Checking for wound leaks is an important part of the postoperative examination and is done by placing a concentrated drop of fluorescein over the graft wound. A positive result on Seidel's test occurs when a rivulet of fluorescing yellow-green dye is seen emanating from the wound under cobalt blue light. This leak may be either from the wound itself or along a suture track. If the anterior chamber is of normal or near-normal depth, the patient can be treated with mild-pressure patching or a bandage soft contact lens for a few days. Many small leaks, particularly those around sutures, will spontaneously close as the epithelial plug grows into the wound. If there is a running suture in place, a persistent leak can often be managed with a suture adjustment, as described already, tightening the suture in the area of the leak and distributing the released suture tension evenly about the wound. Occasionally, if the entire running suture seems too loose, the suture can be saved by tightening the suture all around, leaving one large loop of excess suture material. This loop is then attached to the peripheral cornea near the limbus with a single suture of 10-0 nylon whose knot is buried. A mattress suture of 10-0 nylon can be placed as a compression suture about a leaking suture track but should rarely be necessary. A leaking interrupted suture track can be cured by removing the suture and replacing it if needed. Interrupted sutures can always be added to close the graft wound if all else fails. These can be placed under sterile conditions, taking great care that the side of the needle does not cut a running suture, if present.

If the anterior chamber is very shallow, the wound leak should be repaired without waiting more than a day or two, depending on the level of inflammation, because of the risk to the angle of permanent synechial formation. A totally flat chamber requires an immediate wound repair because of the additional risk to the graft endothelium.

Epithelial Defects

Obtaining an intact, stable epithelial surface covering the fresh transplant is the first step in obtaining a successful outcome of surgery. Unfortunately a number of factors operate to interfere with this goal. First, the donor cornea may have had epithelial sloughing during the period of time from death to preservation, particularly if the eyes were not taped shut and cooled with eye bags while waiting for the corneas to be harvested. Second, depending on the storage media and the length of storage time, epithelial viability can be compromised (37). Third, intraoperative trauma, either mechanical or through drying under the bright microscope light, can lead to further loss. For these and other reasons, the majority of patients will not have an intact epithelial layer when seen at the first postoperative visit (38). The new transplant has several factors interfering with rapid healing. First, the center of the graft tends to be flat and is surrounded by a ridge of tissue created by the sutures used to make a watertight closure. This ridge can interfere with the normal lid function of spreading the tear film across the corneal surface. In the extreme case, where the sutures have been drawn excessively tight, a dellen can form in front of this ridge. Second, the new transplant is devoid of all innervation, creating in essence a neurotrophic state that interferes with epithelial healing (39). Third, the transplant is assaulted with a variety of eyedrops which, either of themselves or through their preservatives, can be damaging to the epithelium and retard healing (40) (Fig. 8-8). Fortunately, despite these obstacles, most transplants will epithelialize in a timely fashion.

A delayed or incomplete epithelialization of the corneal transplant can lead to potentially disastrous results (Fig. 8-9). After about a week, there can be damage to Bowman's membrane, which, even if epithelialization occurs later, may leave the transplant with superficial haze and scarring. With a further delay, melting of the stroma begins, leaving the graft with a depressed scar that is even more optically disturbing. If the problem is still not corrected, continued melting will lead to perforation, necessitating additional surgery. In addition, as noted already, epithelial defects are often the precursor of infection. Active and aggressive treatment of all epithelial defects, whether present initially or developing during the postoperative period, is mandatory.

Prevention of epithelial problems begins in the preoperative period. Lid problems, such as entropion, ectropion, trichiasis, lagophthalmos, and blepharitis, should be corrected. If tear production is deficient, punctal occlusion should be considered. Certain conditions, such as ocular pemphigoid, Stevens-Johnson syndrome, and alkali, acid, and other chemical burns, are notorious for their association with postoperative epithelial problems. Unless such steps as limbal stem cell transplantation can be undertaken (41), the prognosis for these conditions is very guarded. Intraoperatively, the epithelium should be left on the transplant, even though there are conflicting findings at to whether its removal lessens the long-term risk of graft rejection (42,43). During surgery, the epithelium should be protected from drying with a blob of viscoelastic substance (44). When epithelial problems are anticipated, as in dry-eye patients or patients with rheumatoid disease, punctal occlusion or a tarsorrhaphy can be done at the conclusion of the operation.

Postoperatively, treatment of epithelial defects can be approached in a stepwise fashion. Initially mild-pressure patching can be tried, even though one study found that small defects healed as fast without patching (3). Care must be taken to ensure that the lids do not open under the patch, and this may be helped by directly taping the lids together before the patch is applied. The patch may be left in place for 24 to 48 hours without being disturbed, if active infection is not a concern. Sutures with exposed ends should be removed or the exposed suture material amputated (45). Aberrant lashes or lint trapped under a suture should be removed. Topical lubrication with frequently administered (every 30–60 minutes) nonpreserved artificial tears or nonpreserved bland ophthalmic ointment can be used. If not already performed, in the dry-eye patient, punctal occlusion either permanently with cautery or reversibly with punctal plugs should be tried (Fig. 8-10).

Since topical medications can contribute to poor epithelial healing, a re-evaluation of all eyedrops the patient is receiving is in order. Any medication containing neomycin should be switched to a less epithelial-toxic antibiotic such as tobramycin 0.3% (46) [remember that longer-term use of

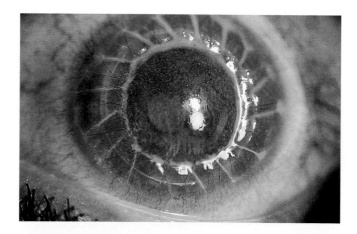

FIGURE 8-8.   Heavy punctate fluorescein staining on a graft due to medication-induced epithelial desiccation. When more severe, this staining pattern has been referred to as hurricane keratitis, owing to its spiral appearance.

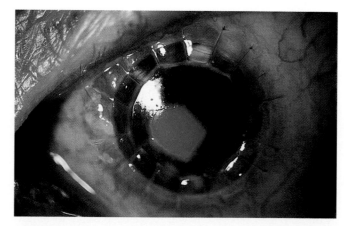

FIGURE 8-9.   An epithelial defect requires prompt treatment to prevent secondary complications.

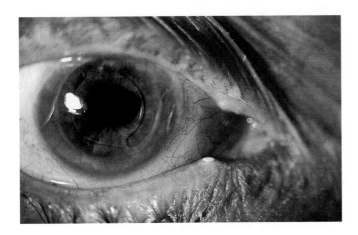

FIGURE 8-10.   *Punctal plug placed to help protect the graft epithelium in a dry-eye patient.*

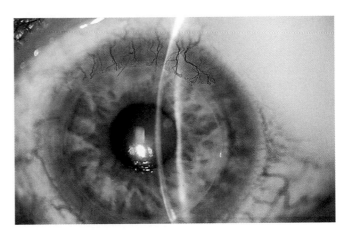

FIGURE 8-11.   *Superficial vascularization of the cornea following placement of a bandage soft contact lens for chronic filamentary keratitis.*

ciprofloxacin can cause white deposits in chronic epithelial defects (47)]. The need and the frequency of dosage of topical antiviral agents should be considered carefully. Topical antiglaucomatous medications, in part due to their preservatives, can be toxic (48), and, if possible, switching to a nonpreserved agent (unit dose timolol) or using an oral antiglaucomatous agent should be tried. Topical steroids can retard epithelial healing and their dose should be kept to the minimum. In short, one should use the least number of drugs possible, in the least dosage.

If epithelial healing has not taken place after conservative management for several days, a more aggressive approach must be adopted. A bandage soft contact lens can be placed over the graft (49). The lens will protect the epithelium from the constant trauma of the eyelids and is particularly helpful where tarsal scarring is present. Low-power (0.5 diopter), disposable, extended-wear soft lenses are readily available and inexpensive. Inserting a very thin soft lens can present a problem in many patients because their eye is tender and their eyelids swollen. Obtaining a proper fit can also be difficult because these corneas do not have a normal curvature, often being flat centrally. A tight-fitting lens will interfere with tear exchange and reduce the amount of oxygen available to the epithelium. A flat-fitting lens will move excessively, causing further epithelial damage. Frequently the lens will rub on the ridge of tissue around the margins of the corneal incision, inducing new defects to appear here. At times it will be necessary to fit a large flat lens in order to obtain centration. In placing a contact lens on the cornea, however, it must be kept in mind that there is a very significant risk of inducing an infection. In addition to the usual factors causing corneal ulceration with extended-wear soft contact lens, there is the increased risk of an already present epithelial defect and the immunosuppression induced by topical steroids (50). These patients should be treated with a topical antibiotic such as ofloxacin 0.3% every 3 to 4 hours and followed carefully. Once the

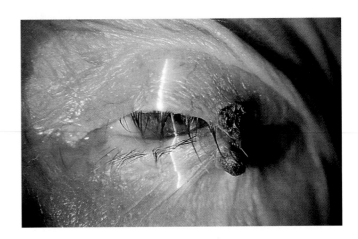

FIGURE 8-12.   *This lateral tarsorrhaphy was extended further medially because of continuing epithelial breakdown.*

defect has healed, an attempt should be made to remove the lens as long-term use of soft lenses in corneal transplant patients has been associated with a high rate of infection as well as corneal vascularization (51) (Fig. 8-11).

In patients whose epithelium cannot be healed with a contact lens or in whom the condition leading to the epithelial problem is ongoing and cannot be corrected, a tarsorrhaphy should be performed. This can be done with a simple frost suture or by forming a temporary adhesion between the eyelashes of the upper and lower lids using cyanoacrylate glue (52), but more likely a permanent lateral tarsorrhaphy will be needed (Fig. 8-12). For patients who have already had a lateral tarsorrhaphy, a medial intermarginal tarsorrhaphy can be added.

Once corneal melting has begun, the optical outcome for the transplant is compromised. At this point, if the condition of the donor tissue itself is believed to have contributed to the epithelial problem, or if any contributing factors can be corrected, consideration should be given to replacing the graft. If it is thought that a further corneal transplant would arrive at the same fate, a conjunctival flap can be pulled in order to save the eye from corneal perforation.

The possibility that a late-appearing or nonresponding epithelial defect actually represents a herpes simplex infection must be kept in mind. These ulcers tend to occur near the wound margin, often do not look like a typical dendrite, and may even occur in a patient without a known previous history of herpetic disease (53) (Fig. 8-13). When herpes infection is suspected, viral cultures and immunofluorescent staining for herpes are indicated. If herpes simplex virus is found, appropriate antiviral treatment can be started.

Filamentary Keratitis

Filamentary keratitis has occurred in at least 25% of postkeratoplasty patients (54). This finding is not surprising since many of the conditions in which filaments occur (inflammation, increased mucus production, anesthetic cornea, patching) are present in the postkeratoplasty eye. Filaments consist of strings of mucus with a few epithelial cells attached to receptor sites on the epithelial surface. They occur most frequently near the wound margin and may come and go over many months.

Patients experiencing filament formation may present with symptoms of irritation and foreign body sensation, particularly if the filaments occur near the edge of the graft. Their eye tends to be slightly injected. The filaments stain poorly with fluorescein and brightly with rose bengal.

Treatment of filamentary keratitis proceeds in a stepwise fashion. For mild symptoms the use of hypotonic artificial tears may give temporary relief. If artificial tears are used frequently, nonpreserved tears are indicated. For more pronounced symptoms, the filaments can be removed under the slit lamp using topical anesthesia and fine jeweler's forceps.

Care should be taken not to pull off surface epithelium with the filament. For recurrent problems, acetylcysteine diluted to a 10% solution in artificial tears can be tried as a mucolytic agent. If all else fails, a bandage soft contact lens can be applied, keeping in mind all the potential risks associated with this treatment modality. Fortunately, the frequency of filament formation decreases after suture removal.

Anterior Synechiae

The significance of anterior synechiae depends on the location, extent, and time frame of their appearance. Anterior synechiae may develop to the peripheral cornea or to the corneal wound itself, or extend from one to the other. The greatest problem with synechial formation occurs when one is operating on inflamed eyes with excessive fibrin in the anterior chamber. Synechiae to the wound found on the first postoperative visit probably were left in place at the time of surgery. It is much easier to deal with this problem on the operating table when the wound can be approached directly and any synechiae pushed back with a viscoelastic agent on a fine cannula. Anterior synechiae may form later as the result of a wound leak with a flat chamber or a persistent shallow chamber, or from trauma with partial or complete iris prolapse. The approach to treatment depends on the location and extent of the adhesions.

Limited synechiae extending directly to the graft wound, especially when the chamber angle is spared, will have only a limited effect on graft survival, though on occasion they can be a source of vascularization and graft rejection (55,56) (Fig. 8-14). It may be possible to free these adhesions pharmacologically, especially if there is no significant tissue incarceration. On the third or fourth postoperative day, when the fibrin begins to break down, the pupil should be aggressively dilated with a series of 3 drops of cyclopentolate hydrochloride 1% alternating every 5 minutes with 3 drops

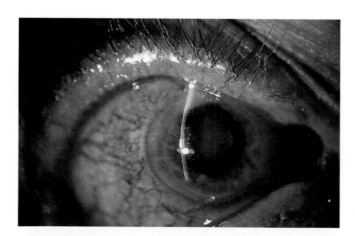

FIGURE 8-13.   *This late-appearing, irregularly shaped epithelial defect on this otherwise clear graft was positive for herpes simplex virus on culture.*

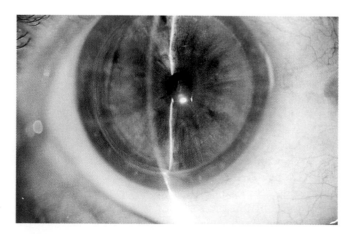

FIGURE 8-14.   *Limited anterior synechia to the graft wound that has been present for years without adversely affecting graft survival.*

of phenylephrine hydrochloride 2.5%, and, if this is not effective, constricted with pilocarpine. Long-acting cycloplegics, such as atropine and scopolamine, should not be used postoperatively in order to preserve this pupillary capacity. If unsuccessful and the intraocular pressure remains under control, these synechiae probably are best left alone. When surgery is believed to be indicated, use of a viscoelastic agent to assist in sweeping iris adhesions from the back of the cornea will help to prevent irreversible damage to the graft endothelium (57).

More extensive anterior synechiae, with broad contact between the iris and the back of the cornea threatening the filtration angle, usually develop in eyes that have been operated on in the inflamed state. Although the potential to develop severe glaucoma in these eyes is very real, surgical intervention is fraught with danger, particularly of bleeding, and usually makes the situation worse by increasing the inflammation. The use of intensive topical steroids (prednisolone 1% hourly) and occasionally systemic steroids for a few days may control the inflammation and allow the iris to drop back. At this point pharmacologic manipulation of the pupil may be helpful.

Iris prolapse usually occurs from trauma and should be repaired immediately under sterile conditions with microscopic control (Fig. 8-15). Depending on the extent of wound disruption, topical or general anesthesia can be used. If the iris tissue prolapse is limited in both extent and duration, and if the tissue appears viable, it can be reposited directly. Exposed, nonviable iris tissue should be excised before repositing the portion of iris incarcerated in the wound. The wound will usually require repair with additional interrupted sutures until a watertight closure is obtained. These wounds should be considered potentially contaminated and appropriate antibiotic coverage administered.

Anterior synechiae can, on occasion, cause a progressive zippering of the chamber angle (Fig. 8-16). This situation most commonly develops in patients who have active inflammation at the time of keratoplasty, particularly if there are preexisting adhesions. These adhesions may have been lysed at surgery, so that the chamber initially seems of good depth. Then several weeks into the postoperative period, broad peripheral anterior synechiae begin to appear. At first, these are localized, but gradually and relentlessly the synechiae progress. Over a period of weeks the angle becomes "zippered" up. Occasionally, the process will stop at a large peripheral iridectomy, which has caused some surgeons to recommend doing an iridectomy in advance of the zippering process in hopes of halting it. Frequently, however, the process will "jump" across the iridectomy site until all or nearly all the angle is closed. As might be expected, there is a gradual elevation of the intraocular pressure until a secondary glaucoma develops, which is very difficult to control medically. At times an anterior-chamber lens will hold the angle open, at least grossly, in the region of the footplates, so that the associated glaucoma may not be quite as difficult to control. There is no proven way to abort this process once it begins other than to attempt to suppress the associated inflammation (58). Surgical intervention is fraught with potential complications. Possible ways to control the glaucoma in these patients are discussed separately.

Hyphema

Blood in the anterior chamber postoperatively is unusual. Even with very vascularized corneas, the vessels are tamponaded by the pressure created by the corneal sutures. When a hyphema does occur, it is usually due to bleeding from the angle occurring when an anterior-chamber lens foot process is being removed, from a vascularized synechiae that is lysed during anterior-chamber reconstruction, or from generalized oozing from the surface of a highly inflamed iris. Usually, these bleeding points can be managed

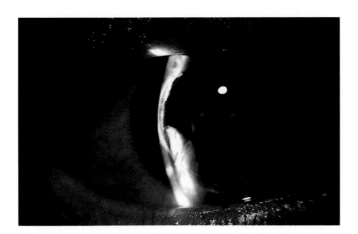

FIGURE 8-15.   *Iris incarceration (without prolapse) and loss of the anterior chamber from trauma in a patient with Down syndrome. It was elected not to repair the wound as the chamber re-formed spontaneously. The graft remained clear for years.*

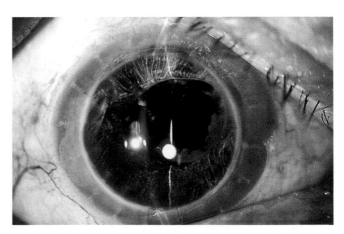

FIGURE 8-16.   *Total angle closure from progressive anterior synechial formation developed in this patient with marked postoperative inflammation. The graft remained clear and the intraocular pressure was controlled with medication.*

at the time of surgery using a viscoelastic agent to tam-panade them or a fine retinal cautery needle for direct cautery (59). Alternatively, the use of thrombin 1:100 or epinephrine 1:1000 may be helpful. A small hyphema post-operatively can be ignored and will spontaneously absorb in a few days if there is no further bleeding. A large hyphema that is causing uncontrollable glaucoma will require sur-gical evacuation. If the bleeding source is thought to be contained, consideration can be given to an open-sky evacuation with replacement of the graft. In most cases, where there is doubt, removal of the blood through small limbal incisions is indicated, leaving replacement of a potentially failed graft to some future intervention.

Excessive Iritis

All corneal transplant patients will show some degree of anterior-chamber reaction immediately following surgery, its extent dependent on such things as the degree of iris manipulation performed and the condition of the eye before surgery. Excessive inflammation including fibrin clot forma-tion and even a hypopyon in the anterior chamber may be encountered postoperatively. Clinical judgment must be exercised in deciding whether this is a sterile inflammatory reaction or whether an infection must be actively ruled out. The presence of excessive white blood cells in contact with the new endothelium can be damaging to the graft as evidenced by the stromal edema and thickening these grafts demonstrate (60). If infection is believed to be unlikely, intensive steroid therapy is warranted. Prednisolone acetate 1% can be administered as often as one drop every hour. A short course of systemic steroids may be needed. The risks of steroids in this intensive dosage, including delayed epithelialization, interference with the development of normal wound tensile strength, and the compromise of local immunity, must be weighed in the decision. Any cornea, but particularly the cornea of an elderly patient that has received an intensive course of topical steroids in the early postoperative period may never achieve normal wound strength and the corneal sutures should be left in place for a longer period of time than usual. A cyclople-gic agent should be given to help prevent the formation of posterior synechiae and pupillary block. Short-acting agents are probably best, as they allow some pupillary movement.

If the fibrin clot does not respond to intensive steroid therapy, and there is a risk of pupillary block from a secluded or occluded pupil as well as damage to the graft endothe-lium, the use of tissue plasminogen activator (TPA) can be considered. A 25-μg dose of TPA given intracamerally has been described (61). This drug will cause complete resolu-tion of the fibrin clot over several hours and appears to be nontoxic to the endothelium (62). This drug can also result in intraocular bleeding, and therefore, its use in any patient who has had intraoperative hemorrhage should be very guarded. Even though discounted initially, the possibility of

infection must be considered in any eye that does not respond to treatment.

Pupillary Block

With the development of pupillary block, aqueous is obstructed in its movement from the posterior to the ante-rior chamber, the anterior chamber shallows as the iris bulges anteriorly, and the angle is thus obstructed, causing an elevation of the intraocular pressure. The incidence of pupillary block must be very low following surgery using modern corneal transplantation techniques. Air, which can be trapped behind the pupil at the time of surgery, has largely been replaced as a tissue separator by various vis-coelastic agents (44). Vitreous, which can adhere to and block the pupil, is either removed by an adequate anterior vitrectomy or held back by an intact posterior capsule or posterior-chamber intraocular lens. Pupillary block can arise when an eye is left aphakic or a secondary anterior-chamber or sewn-in posterior-chamber lens is used. If no iridectomy has been done, or more likely has been blocked with peripheral vitreous, pupillary block may ensue. In a phakic eye, marked inflammation can occlude the pupil with pos-terior synechiae. The elevated intraocular pressure usually will differentiate a shallow chamber due to pupillary block from a shallow chamber secondary to a wound leak. Vigor-ous dilation of the pupil with several drops of cyclopen-tolate hydrochloride 1% alternating with phenylephrine hydrochloride 2.5% will often relieve the situation. When dilation is ineffectual or the block recurs, a peripheral iri-dectomy is indicated. This can usually be done with a laser, but where the peripheral iris cannot be approached through the cornea, perhaps due to a lack of clarity, a surgical iri-dectomy is warranted. This condition should be aggressively treated to avoid the formation of permanent peripheral anterior synechiae.

Glaucoma

Glaucoma following corneal transplantation can be difficult to diagnose and treat. It develops in approximately one-third of patients (63), being unusual in the setting of uncompli-cated phakic grafts and quite common in the presence of pseudophakic or aphakic grafts (64), especially when there are associated anterior-segment abnormalities. A variety of conditions can lead to postkeratoplasty pressure elevation. The most frequent association with postkeratoplasty glau-coma, however, is the presence of preexisting glaucoma (64). Since the inability to successfully control intraocular pres-sure after surgery is frequently associated with graft failure (65), preoperative pressure control is mandatory. Diagnosing glaucoma preoperatively can be difficult because of the problem of accurately measuring intraocular pressure in the presence of a scarred, irregular, or edematous cornea. Corneal opacification can also interfere with visualization of the chamber angle and optic nerve as well as obtaining an accurate visual field. Patients whose pressures are controlled, but only by maximally tolerated medication, should be considered for possible glaucoma surgery prior to keratoplasty, as pressure control will most likely be lost after corneal transplantation. Combining glaucoma surgery and keratoplasty has been reported (66,67). This approach is risky because if the glaucoma procedure fails, the surgeon must deal with the difficult problem of uncontrolled intraocular pressure in a patient with a fresh graft.

Measuring intraocular pressure postoperatively presents a technical problem. The limited corneal area with a smooth surface contour in the immediate postkeratoplasty period limits the ability to utilize applanation tonometry. Makay Marg electronic tonometry (68), pneumatic tonometry (69), and the newer Tono-Pen (70) give more accurate measurements under these circumstances, but even measurements with these instruments can, on occasion, be misleading. At times the surgeon must rely on tactile tensions as the best estimate of intraocular pressure available. These measurements, though not accurate, can allow the determination as to whether the pressure is very low, about normal, or significantly elevated, which is sufficient for management in the immediate postoperative period. Even before the pressure is measured, examination of the eye will give other indications that the pressure is significantly elevated. A very thin and clear corneal transplant on the first postoperative day should raise the possibility of elevated intraocular pressure (71). The high pressure compresses the stroma, but because there is no epithelium or only a thin layer of epithelium, the epithelial barrier is not functioning, and therefore, epithelial edema is not seen. The presence of synechiae or the presence of blood or fibrin or both in the anterior chamber should increase the suspicion of pressure problems. The knowledge of preoperative risk factors or intraoperative problems will allow the anticipation of postoperative glaucoma.

A number of agents are now available for the treatment of postkeratoplasty glaucoma, some so new that their specific use in this situation has not been reported. The approach to glaucoma treatment following keratoplasty is the same as that following other operative procedures, basically using the least amount of medication needed and, when possible, correcting any underlying cause.

On the first postoperative day, it is not unusual to find a significant elevation in intraocular pressure. In fact, pressure elevation may occur within the first 3 hours after keratoplasty (72). Initial treatment utilizes an oral carbonic anhydrase inhibitor, such as acetazolamide 250mg four times a day, supplemented by a topical agent such as timolol 0.5%, apraclonidine 0.5%, or both (73). Latanoprost may prove helpful in some patients (74). The aggressive management of any associated pupillary block, synechiae, or excessive inflammation has already been discussed. Elevated intraocular pressure from the presence of a retained viscoelastic agent will usually clear spontaneously in 24 to 48 hours (6). In the rare instance where the pressure is so high that acute damage to the optic nerve is feared, a hyperosmotic agent can be given orally for a day or two, understanding the difficulty many patients have with these agents. Such an approach can only be considered a temporizing measure until more definitive therapy is instituted.

On a more chronic basis, if elevated intraocular pressure persists, it may be possible to switch patients to dorzolamide hydrochloride 2%, a topical carbonic anhydrase inhibitor. A miotic, such as pilocarpine or carbachol, though initially contraindicated because of their effect on the blood-aqueous barrier, can be added once the postoperative inflammation is brought under control. Topical epinephrine and dipivefrin will only have a limited use because of their known propensity to cause macular edema in the aphakic or pseudophakic patient. As pointed out previously, these agents and their preservatives may adversely affect the status of the corneal epithelium on the surface of the new graft, and this consideration must be taken into account in treating glaucoma.

The possibility that the use of a topical steroid is playing either a primary or a contributing role in the development of a patient's pressure elevation should be considered, particularly when this elevation develops a week or two after the steroids are started. In addition to keeping the use of steroids to the minimal dosage necessary, switching the patient to a steroid with less propensity to pressure elevation, such as fluorometholone or rimexolone 1% (75), is warranted.

In a number of these patients the glaucoma will prove refractory to medical therapy, especially if it is secondary to severe damage to their angle structures. The presence of a corneal transplant makes surgical intervention more risky because of the possibility of causing graft failure. The simplest and safest surgical approach is argon laser trabeculoplasty (76). Most patients will not prove suitable for this procedure either because they are aphakic or pseudophakic, or because visualization of their angle is poor or much of their angle is closed. For the same reasons, a classic trabeculectomy has a low success rate (77). Adding an antimetabolite, such as mitomycin or 5-fluorouracil (5FU), may increase the risk of graft failure (78). In the recent past, for most of these eyes, the best option available was a cyclodestructive procedure. Originally cyclocryotherapy was the procedure of choice for intractable glaucoma (79) and still has a place in the therapeutic armamentarium when access to other treatment modalities is unavailable (58). Significant complications including iritis, hemorrhage, macular edema, graft failure, decreased vision, and especially late-term phthisis bulbi are associated with this treatment (80,81) (Fig. 8-17). For this reason a graded approach to treatment is indicated. Initially 180 degrees of the ciliary body is treated using three applications in each quadrant for 60 seconds at 60 to 80°C. Depending on the response achieved, additional treatment applications can be added, one or two at a time, in the previously untreated quadrants of the globe. It should be kept in mind that the difference in aqueous

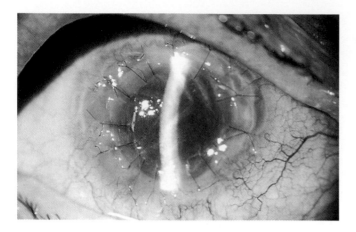

FIGURE 8-17.   *Graft failure following cyclocryotherapy.*

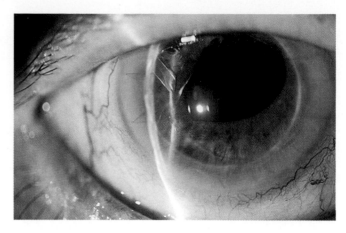

FIGURE 8-18.   *Note that the tube from this valve is positioned well away from the back of the graft.*

production between a high pressure and phthisis is very little in these eyes with minimal outflow. Where available, transscleral neodymium:yttrium-aluminum-garnet (Nd: YAG) laser photocoagulation, either contact (82) or non-contact (83), has supplanted cryotherapy as a means of destroying the ciliary processes and decreasing aqueous production because the associated complication rate appears to be less. A graded approach should be used, keeping in mind that the rate of graft failure appears to go up with multiple treatment sessions. Whether other laser glaucoma procedures, such as transpupil (84) or endoscopic (85) argon laser cyclophotocoagulation, will have a place in the treatment of postkeratoplasty glaucoma remains to be seen.

Currently, the most promising approach to the treatment of refractory postkeratoplasty glaucoma is the placement of a valve, such as the Ahmed (86), Baerveldt (87), or Molteno valve (88). When successful, they appear to give the best chance for long-term pressure control with little or no medication. The surgical approach is essentially the same as in the nontransplant patient. The drainage tube can be placed in the anterior chamber, or where none is present, in the posterior chamber after an adequate vitrectomy. With anterior-chamber placement, particular care must be given to the length, position, and angle of the tube in order to avoid touching the back of the graft (Fig. 8-18). The fact that there is still a significant incidence of graft failure and hypotony postoperatively only underscores the difficulty of treating glaucoma in the postkeratoplasty patient (89).

Vascularization

Vascularization of the graft bed greatly influences the incidence of graft rejection (55), and therefore must be avoided where possible or at least limited. The most important sources of blood vessels extending up to and into a corneal transplant are as follows:

1. Preexisting corneal vascularization
2. Loose sutures and exposed corneal knots

3. Corneal ulcers
4. Bandage soft contact lenses, especially when used on an extended-wear basis

Unfortunately, there is usually no way to remove preexisting vessels from the corneal bed. Rarely a single feeder vessel, if it originates from the surface of the sclera, can be cauterized outside the limbus or is amenable to laser photocoagulation. A fibrovascular pannus can be stripped off the cornea at the time of surgery. Often removal of the diseased recipient button will remove the impetus to vascular ingrowth, and the active vessels present preoperatively will regress after surgery.

Treatment of corneal vascularization involves the suppression of vessel growth by the appropriate use of topical steroids (90), removing loose sutures and exposed knots as discussed already, aggressively treating corneal infections, and limiting the use of bandage lenses to the minimal time necessary to achieve their treatment objective. Timing of suture removal plays a large role in preventing the complications of corneal vascularization. If the donor graft is healthy, preexisting vessels, or vessels approaching the host-graft junction, will tend to grow along the junction and not enter the graft. Once this has happened, the wound in this area has usually healed sufficiently to allow suture removal. If interrupted sutures have been used, the suture at this location should be removed. The flexibility of interrupted sutures in this situation is an indication for their use where preexisting corneal vessels are present. If a running suture has been used, management is more difficult. If the rest of the wound has not sufficiently healed, suture removal can lead to wound dehiscence. The options then are to increase the dose of topical steroids, keeping in mind that this will slow healing in the rest of the wound, or to remove a section of the running suture. Once a section has been removed, the running suture will tend to keep loosening, a loop at a time, due to the action of the eyelids. If this happens, the suture can be stabilized by the placement of a bandage soft contact lens, but the presence of the latter may cause further progression of the vascularization. Superficial vessels crossing the graft-host junction do not indicate wound healing, but fortunately do not carry an increased risk of rejection. On occasion, however, superficial vessels, on reaching the junction, can dip down entering the stroma of the graft and, thereby, pose a risk of rejection.

Retained Descemet's Membrane

Finding a wavy, diaphanous membrane in the anterior chamber creating a false chamber behind a graft on the first postoperative visit indicates that Descemet's membrane has been left behind at the time the recipient button was removed (Fig. 8-19). Retention of Descemet's membrane occurs most commonly in an edematous cornea where, following partial trephination, an opening is made into the anterior chamber and curved corneal scissors are introduced. By accident, the lower blade is not placed into the anterior chamber, but rather anterior to Descemet's membrane, which is only loosely adherent to the corneal stroma. Upon completion of the excision of the recipient button, the button is lifted from the eye, leaving the central portion of Descemet's membrane behind. Because of the opening made with the initial incision, Descemet's membrane then settles down over the iris where it is remarkably difficult to see. For this reason, care should be taken at the time of all graftings, but particularly those done on edematous corneas, to make sure that Descemet's membrane has not been left behind, even if this means gently grasping the surface of the iris with fine forceps.

A retained Descemet's membrane will eventually lead to loss of graft clarity by clouding or by coming into contact with the graft endothelium. Several approaches to dealing with this problem are available. If the membrane has been mostly cut free at the time of surgery leaving only a small

area of connection, its excision can be completed under a viscoelastic agent either through a limbal excision or through the corneal wound. A technique using the Nd: YAG laser to make a central opening in the membrane has been described (91). The long-term outcome of this procedure has not been reported. Perhaps the best long-term solution to this problem is to repeat the keratoplasty, allowing complete and accurate removal of the retained portion of Descemet's membrane.

Primary Graft Failure

Primary graft failure refers to the situation where the donor cornea is thick and edematous from the first postoperative day and never clears (92,93). Technically the term *primary* would imply that the transplanted tissue itself was not healthy. This occurrence should be very rare if the tissue is harvested and utilized under the protocol established by the Eye Bank Association of America. Usually, graft failure in this circumstance is secondary to intraoperative problems. Primary graft failure is best handled by graft replacement with a new donor prior to wound healing (94). In this circumstance, the sutures can be cut and the failed graft removed without the need for trephining. However, haste in making this decision is not warranted, as almost all grafts can be easily removed up to a month or later following surgery. Especially in the elderly, where wound healing may be delayed for many months, graft removal can be carried out with minimal dissection. Because some graft will clear rapidly in the first few weeks, a period of observation is indicated. Most grafts will show some thinning, but if the clearing is not progressive after the first 2 or 3 weeks, timing of the repeat grafting will be dictated by the status of the eye. If the postoperative course is otherwise uncomplicated, regrafting can be undertaken at this point. If the case is complicated by marked inflammation, or if the intraocular pressure is out of control, these problems should be brought under control prior to repeating surgery in order to provide the best chance of success.

CONCLUSION

The road to successful corneal transplantation begins at surgery but only ends with appropriate postoperative management. Though postoperative complications are potentially numerous and at times serious, vigorous follow-up care and aggressive treatment will allow most patients to achieve a successful surgical result.

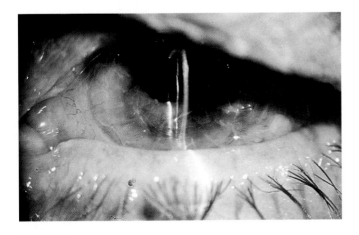

FIGURE 8-19. *Retained Descemet's membrane presenting as a thin, clear, wavy membrane separated by a false anterior chamber from a clear corneal transplant.*

REFERENCES

1. Vail A, Gore SM, Bradley BA, et al. Corneal Graft Survival and Visual Outcome: a multicenter study. *Ophthalmology* 1994;101:120–127.
2. Meyer RF, Robb KC. Corneal epithelium in penetrating keratoplasty. *Am J Ophthalmol* 1980;90:142–147.
3. Sugar A, Meyer RF, Bahn CF. A randomized trial of pressure patching for epithelial defects after keratoplasty. *Am J Ophthalmol* 1983;95:637–640.

4. Raber IM, Arentsen JJ, Laibson PR. Traumatic dehiscence after penetrating keratoplasty. *Arch Ophthalmol* 1981;98:1407–1409.

5. Bourne WM, O'Fallon WM. Endothelial cell loss during penetrating keratoplasty. *Am J Ophthalmol* 1978;85:760–766.

6. Alpar J. The use of Healon in corneal transplant surgery with and without intraocular lenses. *Ophthalmic Surg* 1984;15:757–760.

7. Shrader CE, Thomas JV, Simmons RJ. Relationship of patient age and tolerance to carbonic anhydrase inhibitors. *Am J Ophthalmol* 1983;96:730–733.

8. Lass JH, Mack RJ, Imperia PS, et al. An in vitro analysis of aminoglycoside corneal epithelial toxicity. *Curr Eye Res* 1989;8:299–304.

9. Aquavella JV, Gasset AR, Dohlman CH. Corticosteroids in corneal wound healing. *Am J Ophthalmol* 1964;58:621–626.

10. McDonald TO, Borgman AR, Roberts MD, et al. Corneal wound healing. I. Inhibition of stromal healing by three dexamethasone derivatives. *Invest Ophthalmol Vis Sci* 1970;9:703–709.

11. Stern GA. Infectious crystalline keratopathy. *Int Ophthalmol Clin* 1993;33:1–7.

12. Urrets-Zavalia A. Fixed dilated pupils, iris atrophy and secondary glaucoma. A distinct clinical entity following keratoplasty in keratoconus. *Am J Ophthalmol* 1963;56:257–265.

13. Geyer O, Rothkoff L, Lazar M. Atropine in keratoplasty for keratoconus. *Cornea* 1991;10:372–373.

14. Cobo LM, Coster DJ, Rice MSC, et al. Prognosis and management of corneal transplantation for herpes keratitis. *Arch Ophthalmol* 1980;98:1755–1759.

15. Pavan-Langston D. Viral keratitis and conjunctivitis: herpetic infections. In: Smolin G, Thoft R, eds. *Cornea*. 3rd ed. Boston: Little, Brown, 1993:193–199.

16. Peterson A, Jones BR. The management of ocular herpes. *Trans Ophthalmol Soc UK* 1967;87:59–84.

17. Foster CS, Pavan-Langston D. Corneal wound healing and antiviral medication. *Arch Ophthalmol* 1977;95:2062–2067.

18. Lass JH, Langston RHS, Foster CS, Pavan-Langston D. Antiviral medications and corneal wound healing. *Antiviral Res* 1984;4:143–157.

19. Barney NP, Foster CS. A prospective randomized trial of oral acyclovir after penetrating keratoplasty for herpes simplex keratitis. *Cornea* 1994;13:232–236.

20. Van Meter WS, Gussler JR, Soloman KD, Wood TO. Post keratoplasty astigmatism control. Single continuous suture adjustment versus selective interrupted suture removal. *Ophthalmology* 1991;98:177–183.

21. Pardos GJ, Gallagher MA. Microbial contamination of donor eyes. *Arch Ophthalmol* 1982;100:1611–1613.

22. Guss RB, Koenig S, De La Pena W, et al. Endophthalmitis after penetrating keratoplasty. *Am J Ophthalmol* 1983;95:651–658.

23. Leveille AS, McMullan FD, Cavanagh HD. Endophthalmitis following penetrating keratoplasty. *Ophthalmology* 1983;90:38–39.

24. Polack FM, Locatcher-Khorazo D, Gutierrez E. Bacteriologic study of "donor" eyes. *Arch Ophthalmol* 1967;78:219–225.

25. Endophthalmitis Vitrectomy Study Group. Results of the Endophthalmitis Vitrectomy Study: a randomized trial of immediate vitrectomy and of intravenous antibiotics for the treatment of postoperative bacterial endophthalmitis. *Arch Ophthalmol* 1995;113:1479–1496.

26. Matoba A, Moore M, Merten J, McCulley JP. Donor to host transmission of streptococcal infection by corneas stored in McCarey-Kaufman medium. *Cornea* 1984;3:105–108.

27. Lamensdorf M, Wilson LA, Waring GO, Cavanagh D. Microbial keratitis after penetrating keratoplasty. *Ophthalmology* 1982;89(suppl):124.

28. Tuberville AW, Wood TO. Corneal ulcers in corneal transplants. *Curr Eye Res* 1981;1:479–485.

29. Narankari VS, Karesh JW, Richards RD. Complications of exposed monofilament sutures. *Am J Ophthalmol* 1983;95:515–519.

30. Dana MR, Goren MB, Gomes JA, et al. Suture erosion after penetrating keratoplasty. *Cornea* 1995;14:243–248.

31. Fong LP, Ormerod LD, Kenyon KR, Forster CS. Microbial keratitis complicating penetrating keratoplasty. *Ophthalmology* 1988;95:1269–1275.

32. Al-Hazzaa SAF, Tabbara KF. Bacterial keratitis after penetrating keratoplasty. *Ophthalmology* 1988;95:1504–1508.

33. Abbot RL, Kremer PA, Abrams MA. Bacterial corneal ulcers. In: Tasman W, Jaeger EA, eds. *Duane's clinical ophthalmology*. Philadelphia: Lippincott-Raven, 1995:1–36.

34. Driebe WT, Stern GA. Microbial keratitis following corneal transplantation. *Cornea* 1983;2:41–45.

35. Harris DJ, Stulting RD, Waring GO, Wilson LA. Late bacterial and fungal keratitis after corneal transplantation. *Ophthalmology* 1988;95:1450–1457.

36. Kaye DB. Epithelial response in penetrating keratoplasty. *Am J Ophthalmol* 1980;89:381–387.

37. Kim T, Palay DA, Lynn M. Donor factors associated with epithelial defects after penetrating keratoplasty. *Cornea* 1996;15:451–456.

38. Nelson JD. Epithelial problems. In: Brightbill FS, ed. *Corneal surgery. Theory, technique, and tissue.* 2nd ed. St. Louis: Mosby, 1993:236.

39. Beuerman R, Schimmelpfennig B. Sensory deprivation of the rabbit cornea affects epithelial properties. *Exp Neurol* 1980;69:196–201.

40. Mackman GS, Polack FM, Sydrys L. Hurricane keratitis in penetrating keratoplasty. *Cornea* 1983;2:31–34.

41. Tan DHT, Ficker LA, Buckley RJ. Limbal transplantation. *Ophthalmology* 1996;103:29–36.

42. Stulting RD, Waring GO, Bridges WZ, Cavanagh HD. Effect of donor epithelium on corneal transplant survival. *Ophthalmology* 1988;95:803–812.

43. Tuberville AW, Foster CS, Wood TO. The effect of donor cornea epithelium removal on the incidence of allograft rejection reactions. *Ophthalmology* 1983;90:1351–1356.

44. Levenson JE, Imperia PS. Viscoelastic materials. In: Brightbill FS, ed. *Corneal surgery. Theory, technique, and tissue.* 2nd ed. St. Louis: Mosby, 1993:218–219.

45. Shahinian L, Brown SI. Postoperative complications with protruding monofilament nylon sutures. *Am J Ophthalmol* 1977;83:546–548.

46. Nelson JD, Silverman V, Lima PH, Beckman G. Corneal epithelial wound healing: a tissue culture assay on the effect of antibiotics. *Curr Eye Res* 1990;9:277–285.

47. Kanellopoulos AJ, Miller F, Wittpenn JR. Deposition of topical ciprofloxacin to prevent re-epithelialization of a corneal defect. *Am J Ophthalmol* 1994;117:258–259.

48. Nork TM, Holly FJ, Hayes I, et al. Timolol inhibits corneal wound healing in rabbits and monkeys. *Arch Ophthalmol* 1984;102:1224–1228.

49. Aquavella JV, Shaw EL. Hydrophilic bandages in penetrating keratoplasty. *Ann Ophthalmol* 1976;8:1207–1219.

50. Smith SG, Lindstrom RL, Nelson JD, et al. Corneal ulcer-infiltrate associated with soft contact lens use following penetrating keratoplasty. *Cornea* 1984;3:131–134.

51. Purcell JJ. Extended-wear contact lenses after corneal transplants. *Am J Ophthalmol* 1981;91:119.

52. Donnenfeld ED, Perry HD, Nelson DB. Cyanoacrylate temporary tarsorrhaphy in the management of corneal epithelial defects. *Ophthalmic Surg* 1991;22:591–593.

53. Mannus MJ, Plotnik RD, Schwab IR, Newton RD. Herpes simplex dendritic keratitis after keratoplasty. *Am J Ophthalmol* 1991;111:480–484.

54. Rotkis WM, Chandler JW, Forstat SC. Filamentary keratitis following penetrating keratoplasty. *Ophthalmology* 1982;89:946–949.

55. Arentsen JJ. Corneal transplant allograft reaction: possible predisposing factors. *Trans Am Ophthalmol Soc* 1983;81:361–402.

56. Smolin G, Biswell R. Corneal graft rejection associated with anterior iris adhesion. *Ann Ophthalmol* 1978;10:1603–1604.

57. Campbell DG, Vela A. Modern goniosynechiolysis for the treatment of synechial angle-closure glaucoma. *Ophthalmology* 1984;91:1052–1060.

58. Foulks GN. Glaucoma associated with penetrating keratoplasty. *Ophthalmology* 1987;94:871–874.

59. Parker A, Folk J, Weingeist T, Goldsmith J. Procoagulant effects of intraocular sodium hyaluronate. *Am J Ophthalmol* 1985;100:479–480.

60. O'Brien WJ, Guy J, Taylor JL. Pathogenesis of corneal oedema associated with herpetic disease. *Br J Ophthalmol* 1990;74:723–730.

61. Snyder RW, Sherman MD, Allinson RW. Intracameral tissue plasminogen activator for treatment of excessive fibrin response after penetrating keratoplasty. *Am J Ophthalmol* 1990;109:483–484.

62. McDermott ML, Edelhauser HF, Hyndiuck RA, Koenig SB. Tissue plasminogen activator and the corneal endothelium. *Am J Ophthalmol* 1989;108:91–92.

63. Simmons RB, Stern RA, Teekhasaenee C, Kenyon KR. Elevated intraocular pressure following penetrating keratoplasty. *Trans Am Ophthalmol Soc* 1989;87:79–93.

64. Karesh JW, Nirankari VS. Factors associated with glaucoma after penetrating keratoplasty. *Am J Ophthalmol* 1983;96:160–164.

65. Charlin R, Polack FM. The effect of elevated intraocular pressure on the endothelium of corneal grafts. *Cornea* 1982;1:241–249.

66. Insler MS, Cooper HD, Kastl PR, Caldwell DR. Penetrating keratoplasty with trabeculectomy. *Am J Ophthalmol* 1985;100:593–595.

67. Kirkness CM, Steele AD, Ficker LA, Rice NS. Coexistent corneal disease and glaucoma managed by either drainage surgery and subsequent keratoplasty or combined drainage surgery and penetrating keratoplasty. *Br J Ophthalmol* 1992;76:146–152.

68. Wind CA, Irvine AR. Electronic applanation tonometry in corneal edema and keratoplasty. *Invest Ophthalmol* 1969;8:620–624.

69. West CE, Capella JA, Kaufman HE. Measurement of intraocular pressure with a pneumatic applanation tonometer. *Am J Ophthalmol* 74;1972:505–509.

70. Rootman DS, Insler MS, Thompson HW, et al. Accuracy and precision of the Tono-Pen® in measuring intraocular pressure after keratoplasty and epikeratophakia and on scarred corneas. *Arch Ophthalmol* 1988;106:1697–1700.

71. Klyce SD, Beverman RW. Structure and function of the cornea. In: Kaufman HE, et al, eds. *The cornea.* New York: Churchill Livingstone, 1988:42.

72. Chien AM. Glaucoma in the immediate post-operative period after penetrating keratoplasty. *Am J Ophthalmol* 1993;115:711–714.

73. Stewart WC, Ritch R, Shin DH, et al. The efficacy of apraclonidine as an adjunct to timolol therapy. *Arch Ophthalmol* 1995;113:287–292.

74. Camras CB, for the United States Latanoprost Study Group. Comparison of latanoprost and timolol in patients with ocular hypertension and glaucoma: a six month, masked multicenter trial in the United States. *Ophthalmology* 1996;103:138–147.

75. Leibowitz HM, Bartlett JD, Rich R, et al. Intraocular pressure-raising potential of 1.0% rimexolone in patients responding to corticosteroids. *Arch Ophthalmol* 1996;114:933–937.

76. Van Meter WS, Allen RC, Waring GO III, Stulting RD. Laser trabeculoplasty for glaucoma in aphakic and pseudophakic eyes after keratoplasty. *Arch Ophthalmol* 1985;106:185–188.

77. Gilvarry AME, Kirkness CM, Steele AD, et al. Management of post-keratoplasty glaucoma by trabeculectomy. *Eye* 1989;3:713–718.

78. Knapp A, Heuer DK, Stern GA, Driebe WT. Serious corneal complications of glaucoma filtering surgery with postoperative 5-fluorouracil. *Am J Ophthalmol* 1987;103:183–187.

79. West CE, Wood TO, Kaufman HE. Cyclocryotherapy for glaucoma pre- or postkeratoplasty. *Am J Ophthalmol* 1973;76:485–489.

80. Caprioli J, Straing S, Spaeth GL, Poryzees EH. Cyclocryotherapy in the treatment of advanced glaucoma. *Ophthalmology* 1985;92:947–954.

81. Caprioli J, Sears M. Regulation of intraocular pressure during cyclocryotherapy for advanced glaucoma. *Am J Ophthalmol* 1986;101:542–545.

82. Schuman JS, Puliafito CA, Allingham RR, et al. Contact transscleral continuous wave neodymium : YAG laser cyclophotocoagulation. *Ophthalmology* 1990;97:571–580.

83. Cohen EJ, Schwartz LW, Luskind RD, et al. Neodymium : YAG laser transscleral cyclophotocoagulation for glaucoma after penetrating keratoplasty. *Ophthalmol Surg* 1989;20:713–716.

84. Lee PF. Argon laser photocoagulation of the ciliary processes in cases of aphakic glaucoma. *Arch Ophthalmol* 1979;97:2135–2138.

85. Patel AC, Thompson JT, Michels RG, Quigley HA. Endophotocoagulation of the ciliary body for refractory glaucoma in aphakes. *Ophthalmology* 1985;92(suppl 2):65.

86. Coleman AL, Hill R, Wilson MR, et al. Initial clinical experience with the Ahmed glaucoma valve implant. *Am J Ophthalmol* 1995;120:23–31.

87. Hodkin MJ, Goldblatt WS, Burgoyne CF, et al. Early clinical experience with the Baerveldt implant in complicated glaucomas. *Am J Ophthalmol* 1995;120:32–40.

88. Beebe WE, Starita RJ, Fellman RL, et al. The use of Molteno implant and anterior tube shunt to encircling band (ACTSEB) for the treatment of glaucoma in keratoplasty patients. *Ophthalmology* 1990;97:1414–1422.

89. McDonnell PJ, Robin JB, Schanzlin DJ, et al. Molteno implant for control of glaucoma in eyes after penetrating keratoplasty. *Ophthalmology* 1988;95:364–369.

90. Phillips K, Arffa R, Cintron C, et al. Effect of prednisolone and medroxyprogesterone on corneal wound healing, ulceration, and neovascularization. *Arch Ophthalmol* 1983;101:640–643.

91. Steinemann TS, Henry K, Brown MF. Nd : Yag laser treatment of retained Descemet's membrane after penetrating keratoplasty. *Ophthalmic Surg* 1995;26:80–81.

92. Chipman ML, Slomovic AS, Rootman D, Dixon WS. Changing risk for early transplant failure: data from the Ontario Corneal Recipient Registry. *Can J Ophthalmol* 1993;28:254–258.

93. Wilhelmus KR, Stulting RD, Sugar J, Khan MM. Primary corneal graft failure. A national reporting system. *Arch Ophthalmol* 1995;113:1447–1502.

94. Mondino BJ, Brown SI. Early repeated corneal grafts. *Arch Ophthalmol* 1976;94:1720–1722.

Conjunctival Surgery

Christopher R. Croasdale Neal P. Barney

The main goal of this chapter is to discuss the surgical management of pterygia and conjunctival intraepithelial neoplasia (CIN), including indications for excision, past and current techniques, and possible complications. A secondary goal is to convey the lack of an accepted consensus regarding the best approach for excising pterygia.

PTERYGIA

Patients seldom remember the Greek-based word *pterygium* for the diagnosis of the fleshy growth on their eye. The name comes from *pterygion*, meaning "anything like a wing," (1) and describes the triangular shape of this conjunctival overgrowth as it extends from either the nasal or temporal interpalpebral bulbar conjunctiva onto the cornea (Fig. 9-1). Complaints and problems caused by these lesions range from ocular surface irritation to cosmetic concerns, to decreased vision due to induced astigmatism, or rarely, involvement of the visual axis. Often considered by ophthalmologists to be a low-complexity condition easily remedied by a "simple" operation, pterygia have an annoying tendency to recur, and frequently with greater severity than the primary growth, leaving the patient more symptomatic than when attention was first sought. In addition, a number of sight-threatening complications have resulted from some of the various techniques of pterygia excision. Thus, for the patient's sake, a cavalier attitude toward removing a pterygium is inappropriate.

Review of the literature reveals that many techniques have been developed and employed over the years. Evaluating published results on the efficacy of different techniques can be confusing for various reasons. Use of nomenclature is sometimes inconsistent; for example, some authors defined a bare sclera technique as being an excision with no suturing (2,3), whereas others partially closed the conjunctiva with sutures (4–6). Such modification, depending on the extent of closure, may actually be more accurately described as a type of primary closure or sliding conjunctival autograft. This distinction is important when making comparisons of outcome because the various techniques may actually produce quite different results. Other studies presented impressive results for a specific technique, but lacked a control group to add an extra measure of validity now desired in today's medical scientific community (7–9). In other cases, different authors reported significantly different recurrence rates for the same technique (2,7,9,10). Explanations for such variable results for a single technique likely involve a number of factors, of which the following are a partial list: unstated variations in surgical technique between surgeons; the proportion of primary versus recurrent pterygia included in a series; differences in postoperative medication regimes; the age, race, and location of the population studied; length of follow-up; and differences in the definition of a recurrence (9).

In the sections on pterygia we emphasize some of the above-mentioned limitations when appropriate. Obviously any discussion such as this is likely to include the authors' own biases on the subject and ours is no different; our hope is that we have included sufficient citations to allow the reader to further investigate the subject and draw his or her own conclusions as to the most safe, appropriate, and effective manner in which to treat pterygia.

PATHOGENESIS AND EPIDEMIOLOGY OF PTERYGIA

Probably the two most important factors among those who develop pterygia are geographic location of residence and amount of exposure to environmental risk factors, such as wind, dust, and sunlight. Both of these factors directly influ-

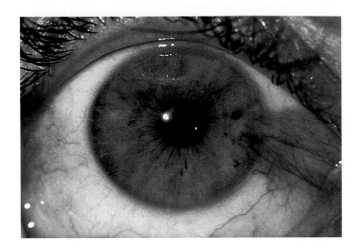

FIGURE 9-1. *Pterygium. Note the broad vascular raised fleshy extension onto the cornea.*

ence the strongest causally related factor, exposure to the ultraviolet (UV) component of sunlight (11,12). Persons from sunnier regions of the world, be it the humid tropics of the Caribbean or the desert regions of the Middle East or Central Australia, have a higher incidence of developing pterygia than do people from less sunny climes. In the same fashion, persons in any climate who spend a significant portion of their time out-of-doors for either work or recreation, such as farmers and fishermen, develop more pterygia than do their indoor counterparts (13).

The age at which a person may first develop a pterygium ranges from teenage years onward, with the prevalence increasing with age. Although difficult to prove, hereditary influences have been considered (14). We found the following excerpt from Duke-Elder's *Diseases of the Outer Eye* (15) to be interesting: "Heredity has an undoubted influence in the occurrence of pterygia although its influence is not crucial. The inheritance is dominant with a low penetrance, but it would appear that it is not the actual lesion which is transmitted but rather the tendency of the eye to react in this way to environmental stimuli." Several studies of families are referenced, but the numbers involved are few. It is an interesting explanation for why only some persons in the same environment develop pterygia. To fully substantiate this theory one must separate the influences of environment from the influences of genetic inheritance. This requires having a control group within a single family whereby some members either live in a substantially different climate than the rest of the family, or are exposed to different environmental risk factors, and for a sufficient length of time. Occasionally such situations occur due to circumstances, but the likelihood of finding a sufficient number of cases to achieve statistical significance makes the feasibility of such a study highly improbable.

Also along the lines of genetic influences, differences in prevalence rates have been reported between different racial

groups in the same geographic locations (16–18). Whether this reflects a true genetic difference in the tendency of different ethnic groups to develop pterygia in response to their environment, or just differences in exposure rates to environmental risk factors between individuals of different races in the same population is not clear.

A final puzzler regarding pathogenesis is the often marked asymmetry of involvement of a patient's eyes. For instance, it is unclear why most pterygia occur on the nasal bulbar surface of the eye as opposed to the temporal surface, or why one eye of a patient will be affected and not the other, when both eyes are presumably exposed equally to the same environmental risk factors. The first issue might be explained on the basis of the anatomy of the eyelid and lashes, with the temporal interpalpebral bulbar surface receiving less exposure to sunlight and irritants than the nasal surface (11,19). The second point remains more enigmatic, though perhaps it is partially answered by another question. Why does anyone develop a unilateral lesion, such as carcinoma of the breast, or eyelid? Although both hereditary predisposition and environmental exposures are factors, random chance still remains as a possible explanation.

HISTOPATHOLOGY OF PTERYGIA

Histopathologically these fibrovascular connective tissue overgrowths contain areas of elastotic degeneration of collagen within the substantia propria of the conjunctiva (*elastotic degeneration*, or *pseudoelastosis*, refers to tissue that stains with elastin but is not degraded by elastase). The overlying epithelium shows various dysplastic features including hyperkeratosis, acanthosis, and dyskeratosis (20), changes that are consistent with the effects of sun-induced UV light damage (12).

Cameron (20) believed that the degenerative changes within the conjunctival portion of a pterygium receive too much emphasis, and proposed that the essential pathology is the invasion by subconjunctival fibroblasts into the cornea, altering or destroying Bowman's layer and variable amounts of the superficial corneal stroma. He contended that degenerative or inflammatory theories of etiology do not explain the often rapid recurrence of a pterygium within months of excision, whereas a fibroblastic cell invasion of the cornea could explain the accelerated reinvasion.

MEDICAL MANAGEMENT OF PTERYGIA

Patients who present to ophthalmologists with pterygia usually do so for one or several reasons: They want to clarify what the growth is and how much concern to have (i.e., "Doctor, is it cancer?"); they are bothered by the cosmetic appearance; or they are experiencing discomfort and irritation. Complaints of affected vision are less common as a presenting symptom in most countries where access to eye-care providers is readily available; when vision is affected it is more often due to induced astigmatism or tear film instability as opposed to actual involvement of the visual axis. For reasons that are unclear, even in less developed regions of the world where access to medical care may be difficult, it is still uncommon to see pterygia that have grown into the visual axis (11). Patients who have had prior surgical excisions with recurrence may experience more severe manifestations of the above. A minority of patients may develop limitation of extraocular movements and diplopia due to mechanical restriction of (usually) the medial rectus muscle from scarring and fibrosis after prior surgery (7).

Medical management for the complaints of surface discomfort and redness ranges from use of artificial tear lubricants and vasoconstrictors to intermittent courses of topical steroids. Minimizing or eliminating the irritating environmental factors that stimulate continued growth and inflammation is also important. Patients should be educated as to the benefit of eye wear with approved UV filters. An appropriate combination of protective glasses, topical lubricants, and medications, if indicated, can improve the patient's comfort while simultaneously reducing the amount of exposure to further harmful environmental risk factors. The few patients who have symptomatic diplopia secondary to recurrence of a pterygium will require a careful re-excision, probably best combined with a free conjunctival autograft (7).

INDICATIONS FOR SURGERY FOR PTERYGIA

There is no standardized scheme for determining when a pterygium is of sufficient size to warrant surgery. Since the growth rate of a pterygium is variable and unpredictable, and the frequency of cases that actually involve the visual axes is low, observation with use of medical treatment as needed is warranted for patients in whom discomfort is controllable, cosmesis is acceptable, visual acuity is not impaired, and there is a safe margin of several millimeters before the visual axis will be affected. Recommending an initial period of observation with or without use of topical agents for a new patient serves several purposes. It develops the relationship between the patient and the ophthalmologist; it allows the physician to gain a better sense of how much the patient is bothered by the pterygium as well as the degree of motivation he or she has to comply with treatment and follow-up. Perhaps most importantly, trial of a medical regimen may provide sufficient relief to allow for delaying surgery or avoiding it altogether.

When discomfort, cosmetic concerns, vision impairment, or a combination thereof reaches significant proportion (a qualitative judgment), the ophthalmologist and patient will discuss surgery. Although the ophthalmologist may consider surgical excision a relatively simple and minor procedure, it can be complicated by recurrence of the lesion, with rates ranging from as low as a few percent to as high as 90%, depending on both the surgeon and the technique used (2,3,7,9,10). This underscores the need for appropriate patient selection regarding timing of surgery, and well-informed consent.

SURGICAL TECHNIQUES FOR EXCISING PTERYGIA

General Aspects

Infections rarely occur after pterygium excisions, so use of preoperative topical antibiotics is not routinely indicated. General surgical antiseptic preparation techniques of cleaning the periocular skin and lashes, and perhaps placing a drop of 5% povidone-iodine solution into the conjunctival cul-de-sac are sufficient. A rigid lid speculum is used to provide maximal exposure of the eye.

Choices for anesthesia vary according to technique and surgeon preference. In many patients the procedure can be done with a combination of topical and subconjunctival anesthesia. A common regimen is administration of several drops of topical anesthetic prior to subconjunctival injection of lidocaine 1% or 2%, with or without epinephrine 1:100,000 to 1:200,000. If one is planning to place a free conjunctival autograft, then avoiding epinephrine may theoretically pose less risk toward inducing ischemia in the graft, though we are not aware of any reports of this being a problem. The subconjunctival injection is performed by placing a small-gauge needle (e.g., 25 gauge, or smaller) tangential to the globe and inserting it under the body of the pterygium so that the injection balloons the pterygium away from the sclera. This facilitates establishment of a dissection plane. The extent of the pterygium to be resected should be marked prior to the subconjunctival injection with either a surgical marking pen or light cautery, to avoid later confusion due to loss of landmarks.

If a free conjunctival autograft technique is employed, or under any circumstances where a longer, more difficult operation is anticipated, then use of a peribulbar or retrobulbar block, with or without a lid block, may provide the best exposure and patient comfort. Without akinesia, one relies on patient cooperation to assist in maintaining the globe in the desired position. In some patients with multiple recurrent pterygia requiring major lid and fornix reconstruction, surgery is best performed with the patient under general anesthesia (21).

We prefer the higher magnification of most operating microscopes as opposed to the lower magnification of surgical loupes. Higher magnification aids both in dissecting the head of the pterygium from the cornea with the least stromal damage and in obtaining conjunctival grafts that are thin and free of underlying Tenon's tissue. Surgical loupes are a viable alternative in situations where an operating microscope is not available.

Opinions differ regarding whether to begin excising a pterygium at the corneal head (apex) or the conjunctival body. We have no strong preference. When one begins with the corneal head, the tissue is grasped with a toothed forceps while a rounded scarifier blade (e.g., Beaver 64) is used to carefully undermine the pterygium with as little damage as possible to Bowman's layer or the underlying corneal stroma. Keeping the cornea dry with a cellulose sponge helps minimize various light reflections that can interfere with visualization and cause an unduly deep incision. Use of sufficient tension when grasping and elevating the pterygia is worth emphasizing; some pterygia can literally be avulsed or peeled from the underlying stroma, resulting in a relatively smooth surface, with minimal use of a sharp instrument.

Alternatively, the conjunctival body of the pterygium can be grasped and elevated to allow an incision to be started at either the upper or the lower edge. Blunt dissection to tunnel underneath the body is performed with Wescott scissors through conjunctiva and Tenon's capsule and down to bare sclera, with care to avoid damaging the insertion of the rectus muscle. The pterygium can be excised close to the insertion of the muscle and reflected forward. As opposed to the above-mentioned approach of removing the apex first, a dissection plane is begun at the limbus, allowing the head to be removed from a peripheral to central direction, using a scarifier blade. Beginning at the limbus after the body is already dissected may offer an advantage in that it may be easier to establish and preserve a superficial plane of cleavage between the lesion and the subjacent corneal stroma (9).

One consideration as to which approach may be preferred is the likelihood for bleeding and interference with visualization. Grasping a fleshy, vascular pterygium with toothed forceps can cause an annoying amount of bleeding. If done as few times as possible, with minimal manipulation, a relatively bloodless dissection from the corneal side can be accomplished. This additionally may relieve tension on the body for a more accurate assessment as to the amount of tissue to be removed from the bulbar surface. If dissection from the cornea cannot be done easily, removing the body first allows for hemostasis to be achieved by use of cautery, which should stop blood flow into any corneal bleeder vessels. Use of cautery is kept to a minimum to avoid excessive scar formation and scleral shrinkage.

Once complete removal of the bulk of the pterygium has been accomplished, any remaining abnormal tissue on the cornea can be gently scraped or polished away with either a scarifier blade or a diamond-encrusted dental burr. However, one should not be overly aggressive in trying to create a smooth corneal surface; the cornea's own healing mechanisms have an amazing ability to resurface and smooth over areas of irregularity. Excessive corneal polishing or scraping risks inducing fibrosis, scar formation, and irregular astigmatism.

The limbus and sclera should also be cleaned of residual Tenon's capsule and subconjunctival tissue. It is reasonable to postulate that pterygium recurrences arise from abnormal subconjunctival tissue inadvertently left behind after excision. Some authors (22) advocated a thorough removal of subconjunctival fibrous tissue for an area larger than the pterygium body itself, even extending to the superior and inferior fornices and caruncle (for nasal pterygia).

Surgical Excision Without Adjunctive Therapy

This section includes pterygium excision with bare sclera, primary conjunctival closure, pterygium transplantation, and placement of free and sliding conjunctival autografts. Some of these techniques have been in use for over 100 years (15), and many of the pioneering techniques with their original eponyms are illustrated nicely in *An Atlas of Ophthalmic Surgery* (23).

Bare Sclera and Primary Conjunctival Closure

A bare sclera technique, in a literal sense, involves leaving the area of denuded sclera uncovered after excision of the pterygium (2,3,10). If the excised pterygium and subconjunctival tissue extend as far back as the insertion of the rectus muscle, then some surgeons will undermine the surrounding conjunctiva and approximate the edges over the exposed muscle. This is sometimes referred to as a modified bare sclera technique. Unfortunately, this unprecise nomenclature can make comparing studies difficult because it is not always clear whether different authors are describing the same modification (4–6). It is also unknown whether these modifications alter the likelihood of recurrence. Depending on the amount of conjunctival closure, the modification in some cases may actually be more accurately described as a primary closure technique (4).

Previously it was thought that leaving an area of bare sclera at the limbus acted as a barrier against regrowth (23); it is now known that placement of a tissue barrier at the limbus is much more effective in preventing recurrences (7). Although rates as low as 5% have been reported with a modified bare sclera technique (4), most bare sclera series report much higher recurrence rates, usually in the range of 35% to 50% (2,5,6), and one as high as 88% (10). Indeed, one only needs to read Youngson's (24) eloquent and frank 1972 article of the unexpected and dismal results he had with bare sclera excisions in Israel to be discouraged from trying this technique. Of 174 patients, only 101 (58%) returned for follow-up, and 37 (37%) of them had recurrences in less than 7 months. Even this rate he believed was low because 61 (35% of the total) of the recurrence-free patients had been followed for 52 days or less.

Primary closure involves undermining the superior and inferior edges of the cut conjunctiva and bringing them together at the limbus to cover the defect. The only controlled study (22) of which we are aware reported a 45% recurrence rate, putting this technique's efficacy in the same poor range as a bare sclera approach. Why the recurrence rate should be so high when supposedly healthy conjunctiva is being placed as a barrier at the denuded limbus is unclear.

Pterygium Transplantation

Pterygium transplantation refers to an operation where the head of the pterygium is dissected from the cornea and buried under the conjunctiva away from the limbus so that any future growth will be "redirected." A number of people have had their names attached to this technique; the description that follows is essentially that of McReynolds (23).

The pterygium is removed from the cornea and the body is undermined (Fig. 9-2A). Scissors are used to make small radial relaxing incisions along the superior and inferior edges of the body, beginning at the limbus and proceeding for a distance corresponding to the width of the growth as it originally crossed the limbus. Further dissection is continued subconjunctivally beginning at the inferior edge of the resection and extending toward the inferior cul-de-sac to fashion a pocket into which the head will be directed. A double-armed absorbable suture (e.g., 6-0 gut) is placed through the apex of the pterygium (Fig. 9-2B). Both arms of the suture are then passed inferiorly into the subconjunctival space, and out transconjunctivally into the cul-de-sac where they are tied (Fig. 9-2C). One of the remaining ends of the suture can be used to close the inferior conjunctival edge to the underlying body of the pterygium, to decrease the risk of developing an epithelial inclusion cyst. Recurrence rates of 30% to 75% have been reported with transplantation procedures (25,26).

Placement of Free Conjunctival Autografts

In this technique, a free autograft of conjunctival tissue is used to cover the exposed sclera after the pterygium is excised. Although any portion of the bulbar conjunctiva can be used for the graft tissue, the superotemporal quadrant is recommended because it is easily accessed and heals well under the protection of the upper eyelid. Use of 6-0 silk stay sutures placed at the limbus at 12- and 6-o'clock positions aids in positioning the eye during the procedure. As originally described by Kenyon et al (7), we prefer peribulbar or retrobulbar anesthesia for maximizing both patient comfort and ease of exposure because surgical time is usually at least 1 hour in our hands. Other authors performed the surgery using a combination of topical and subconjunctival anesthesia (3,9,10). In some patients with multiple recurrent pterygia requiring major lid and fornix reconstruction, the procedure is best performed with the patient under general anesthesia (21).

After the pterygium has been excised, the area of bare sclera is measured with calipers. The dimensions of the graft required are marked on the donor site using either a surgical marking pen (our preferred method because there is no tissue damage) or light cautery spots (Fig. 9-3A). Including the marks within the excised graft helps avoid confusion and maintain proper orientation during later maneuvering. A subconjunctival injection of balanced salt solution (or anesthetic), beginning outside one's markings, will elevate the conjunctiva and aid dissection. The initial incisions are made radially along the lateral margins of the graft, which is then undermined with blunt-tipped Wescott scissors from one side to the other before the posterior edge is cut. This helps keep the thin tissue on stretch and helps prevent it from rolling on itself. The goal is to create as thin a graft as possible by dissecting the conjunctiva from the underlying Tenon's capsule. Thin grafts devoid of underlying fibrous tissue are believed to vascularize more quickly, retract less, and develop less edema postoperatively. Once the conjunctiva has been undermined between the radial margins and the posterior edge is cut, the graft is pulled forward over the cornea (epithelial side down), allowing remnants of Tenon's capsule to be removed from the undersurface. Finally, the limbal edge of the graft is cut with scissors. A margin of 2 to 3 mm of limbal conjunctiva is left to avoid any damage to the corneal limbal stem cells. The donor site heals well without covering under the protection of the upper lid (7).

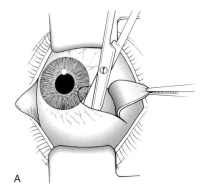
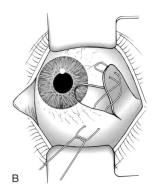
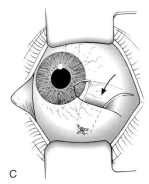

A   B   C

FIGURE 9-2.   *McReynolds procedure or subconjunctival fixation of the pterygium head. A. Formation of a subconjunctival pocket. B. A double-arm suture is passed through the apex of the pterygium and out through the inferior aspects of the previously formed subconjunctival pocket. C. Redirection of the head of the pterygium by sliding it beneath the subconjunctival pocket and tying the sutures on the external side of the conjunctiva.*

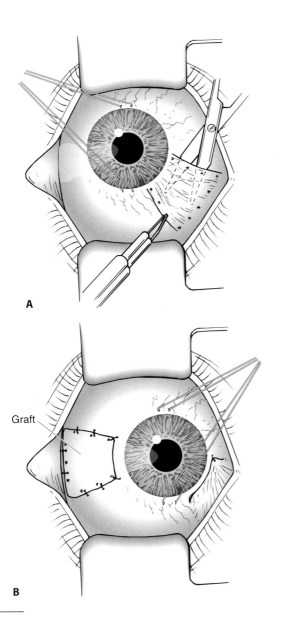

A

B

Graft

FIGURE 9-3. *Conjunctival autograft. A. Cautery or a marking pen are used to delineate the dimensions of the conjunctival transplant for excision. Two radial incisions are performed and spring-action scissors are introduced to undermine the tissue, taking care not to perforate the tissue and to make it as thin as possible. B. The conjunctival graft is placed overlying the area of previously excised pterygium, taking care to leave a 1 to 2 mm area of clear space between the limbus and the edge of the conjunctival transplant. The corner sutures are placed first and further sutures are placed to adequately secure the graft in place.*

The eye is abducted and the free conjunctival autograft is placed onto the recipient bed. Attention is given to verify that the surface epithelium is oriented upward, which the border markings will indicate. A graft placed epithelial side down will become necrotic and slough. The edge without a marking is from the limbus, and is placed along the new limbus, although if misorientation did occur it should not be a problem because stem cells are not being transferred.

As previously mentioned, the graft's primary purpose is to act as a physical barrier against regrowth of abnormal tissue. The corners of the graft are anchored to recipient episclera/sclera and conjunctiva using interrupted sutures (Fig. 9-3B). Additional interrupted sutures or a running suture are then placed between the corners, but not usually along the limbus, for added security. Some surgeons prefer using 10-0 nylon for all the sutures because it causes the least amount of tissue inflammation, which may help minimize the stimulus for recurrence. A disadvantage to nylon is that invariably some of the sutures become loose, erode, and irritate the patient. If the patient has difficulty in seeing an ophthalmologist, which may particularly be a problem in a less developed country, then the patient may be subjected to chronic irritation and possible infection. Alternatively, many surgeons use absorbable sutures, such as 8-0 polyglactin (Vicryl).

Duke-Elder cites the use of free conjunctival autografts first back to Elschnig and Speath from 1926 (15). More recently, the technique has received renewed interest after a series published in 1985 by Kenyon et al (7). They operated on 57 eyes in 54 patients. The pterygia were primary in 16 eyes and recurrent in 41 eyes. In the latter group, 14 patients had diplopia due to cicatricial involvement of the medial rectus muscle. The racial background of the majority (40/54) of patients was listed as white. Postoperative follow-up ranged from 1 to 67 months, with a mean of 24 months. There were only three recurrences reported among the 57 eyes, for a rate of 5.3%.

A discussion of the study's impressive low recurrence rate raised the question as to how many of the patients had migrated to Boston (40 patients) or Kansas City (14 patients) from locations where pterygia occur with higher frequency, and whether their residing in a less provocative climate postoperatively contributed to the low rate of recurrences (27). A number of studies since have added useful data regarding both the efficacy of the technique and the effect of study location on recurrences.

Lewallen (2) performed a randomized study on the island of St. Kitts in the Caribbean, comparing bare sclera excision versus excision with placement of a free conjunctival autograft. Almost all the pterygia were primary, and the patients were of black African race. The follow-up time ranged from 6 to 33 months, with a mean of 15 months. There were six (37%) recurrences among 16 eyes in the bare sclera group, compared to three recurrences (16%) among 19 eyes in the free autograft group. A trend was noted, but the difference was not statistically significant, owing to the small number of patients. Of note was the fact that all recurrences developed within 6 to 8 weeks of surgery, and a statistically significant association was seen between the age of a patient and the development of a recurrence. None of the patients over age 36 years (12/34) had a recurrence.

A group in Western Australia (9), where pterygia are prevalent and UV light levels are high, performed a retrospective review of 93 eyes of 85 patients who underwent free conjunctival autografting, and had results similar to those in Kenyon's study (7). The group was mainly white, with an average age of 49 years at the time of surgery. Twenty-seven eyes (29%) had had previous pterygium surgery at least once using another technique, and the mean time since surgery was 20 months (range, 6–76 months). Six recurrences (6.5%) were found, four asymptomatic and two symptomatic. Two distinct types of recurrence were described: cross graft recurrence in 3 eyes and outflanking in 3 eyes. All but one of these patients had had at least one previous pterygium excision.

Chen et al (10) reported on a prospective, double-masked randomized study comparing postoperative mitomycin C (MMC) drops to conjunctival autografting. The study was performed in Los Angeles, with 60 of 64 patients being Hispanic and only primary pterygia being included. The mean age among the autograft group was 48 years. All patients had a minimum of 6 months of follow-up, and the mean follow-up time for patients receiving MMC versus free grafts versus placebo was 12 months, 13.5 months, and 9 months, respectively. The recurrence rate after MMC (0.2 mg/mL twice daily for 5 days) was 38% (9/24), with the recurrences occurring after a mean of 5 months. Nine (39%) of 23 eyes with autografts had recurrences occurring after a mean of 4 months. Among the placebo group, which received balanced saline drops postoperatively after bare sclera excision, 15 (88%) of 17 eyes had recurrent pterygium develop after a mean of 4 months. As with Lewallen's study (7), increasing age (>50 years in their study) was associated with significantly fewer recurrences.

In 1997 a study by Prabhasawat et al (22) in Miami compared placement of amniotic membrane allografts versus primary closure versus use of free conjunctival autografts. The conjunctival autograft group included 122 eyes in 113 patients, which is the largest number reported to date. Of these, 78 eyes had primary pterygia and 44 had recurrent pterygia. The mean follow-up time for this group was 23 months, and mean age was 45 years. Racial background was not provided. The overall recurrence rate in the conjunctival autograft group was 4.9% (2.6% among primary pterygia versus 9.1% among recurrent pterygia). This was significantly better than the 14.8% overall recurrence rate for the amniotic membrane group (10.9% among primary pterygia versus 37.5% for recurrent pterygia) and the 45% recurrence rate in the primary closure group. The ages of the patients in whom recurrence developed were not statistically different from those who did not. In their discussion, the authors speculated that in addition to demographic (patient ages and study location) and ethnic differences, the amount of subepithelial fibrovascular tissue removed (surgeon technique) might be another major contributory factor that helps explain the great variation seen in recurrence rates not only between different surgical procedures but also between different groups performing the same procedure. They proposed that amniotic membrane allografts be considered an alternative to conjunctival autografts in patients with advanced and diffuse conjunctival involvement (i.e., nasal and temporal heads) or for patients in whom future glaucoma filtering is a known possibility. Practical aspects that make using amniotic membrane unappealing include logistical and technical difficulties in obtaining and preparing the tissue, and significantly increased costs to the procedure.

Other types of tissue that have been successfully used in grafting include cornea and mucous membrane (28,29). Use of autologous tissue has the advantage of avoiding a graft-versus-host immunologic reaction with possible rejection of the foreign tissue.

No vision-threatening complications have been reported after conjunctival autografting. Minor complications that occur infrequently include graft edema, corneoscleral dellen, and epithelial inclusion cysts. Corneal astigmatism, Tenon's granuloma, retraction and necrosis of the graft, and muscular disinsertion are even less frequently encountered (9,21).

Edema of the conjunctival graft may occur in the early postoperative period. It usually resolves without intervention or sequelae in 2 to 4 weeks. For severe edema one can try performing several small, vertical puncture incisions with a sharp blade followed by compression with a cotton-tip applicator in an effort to compress some of the serous fluid out of the tissue. Starck et al (21) believed that careful attention in removing excessive Tenon's tissue at the time of the harvesting of the free graft helps minimize the development of postoperative edema. Excessive elevation of the graft is sometimes due to a subconjunctival hematoma, which can form if hemostasis during surgery is inadequate. If the uneven surface is inducing formation of a dellen, puncture and drainage with pressure patching can be tried; otherwise, observation is appropriate.

Graft retraction or shrinkage can occur due to excessive residual Tenon's tissue, inadequate size, or poor graft tissue quality. The resultant effect may or may not lead to recurrence. Significant wound dehiscence can occur for these reasons, or be caused by sutures cutting through, secondary to high tension from edema or other causes. The graft can be resutured in some eyes; otherwise it may be necessary to replace the tissue. Graft necrosis is rare unless the graft has been placed epithelial side down, or the scleral bed is avascular due to prior irradiation or MMC application. In patients with avascular sclera, or corneoscleral thinning, reinforcement with a lamellas corneal or corneoscleral keratoplasty should be considered (21).

Corneoscleral dellen are treated with aggressive lubrication and sometimes patching. If patching is done, antibiotic ointment should be used concomitantly. Epithelial cysts occur 1 to 2 months after surgery, presumably due to retention and implantation of residual corneal or conjunctival epithelial cells in the conjunctival tissues. If bothersome, they are best treated by marsupialization and resection of the overlapping conjunctiva. Tenon's granulomas can occur at either the donor or the recipient site. Increased topical steroids may induce resolution of the inflammation, although in most patients the lesions are pedunculated and best treated by excision. In some patients repeated conjunctival autograft transplantation is necessary to cover the exposed tissue (21).

The above-cited studies highlight that free conjunctival autografts significantly lower the rate of recurrences compared to the rates after a bare sclera technique, primary closure, and amniotic membrane allografts, but the rate is not significantly different from those after treatment with low-dose MMC drops applied postoperatively. In a more recent comparison between intraoperative MMC application and autografting (30), the two treatments also showed no statistical difference in recurrence rates. Only one study compared the use of β-irradiation to conjunctival autografting (31). The total numbers were small and follow-up time was short; 12 eyes had bare sclera excision followed by β-irradiation and 30 eyes had a free conjunctival autograft placed. There was one recurrence (8.3%) in the irradiated group and three recurrences (3.3%) in the autograft group.

Sliding Conjunctival Flaps

A number of techniques have been described for sliding or rotating adjacent normal conjunctiva to cover the exposed sclera after pterygium excision (23,32–35). The major advantage of these approaches over free conjunctival autografts is that they are faster to perform. An additional possible benefit is that there is less disruption of vascular and lymphatic channels, which may allow for faster healing and less edema (36).

After the pterygium is excised, a limbal peritomy is continued from either the superior or inferior edge of resection for a distance equal to the amount of limbal tissue already resected. A relaxing radial incision is made at the end of the peritomy, approximately half as long as the new extension, and the bulbar conjunctiva is carefully dissected from the underlying Tenon's capsule until the flap can be slid over the intended area. The flap is secured with sutures.

We are not aware of any controlled studies comparing sliding grafts directly to free grafts. A large uncontrolled series from Queensland, Australia, reported a 3.2% recurrence rate among 222 eyes using a technique slightly different from the one just described (36). Another study from Brazil (37) found 12 recurrences among 41 eyes, to yield a 29% recurrence rate. The technique was described as a conjunctival flap rotation from the 12-o'clock position, and was also not compared to a free autograft technique.

Without studies directly comparing the two techniques, it is not possible to determine whether placement of a free graft offers a definite advantage over a sliding graft. As noted previously, there have been reports (10) where free autografts yielded recurrence rates as high as 38%. Whether this was due to an unknown variation in the surgical technique or demographic differences is unclear. Whatever the answer, it could equally explain the difference in results between the two selected sliding graft studies also. If success of the pro-cedures depends predominantly on the transplantation of completely normal conjunctiva as a barrier to the site of excision, then theoretically sliding grafts should be able to produce the same result as free grafts, *if* the transplanted conjunctiva is completely normal. In the Miami study discussed in the preceding section (22), primary closure and placement of free conjunctival autografts were among the techniques compared, with recurrence rates of 45% and 4.9%, respectively. In performing primary closure, the surgeon presumes that the abnormal tissue has been completely removed and that normal conjunctival edges are being brought together, which in essence makes primary closure a type of sliding graft technique. Based on the results from the Miami study, we speculate that a sliding graft (including primary closure) is less likely to be as successful as a free graft because it is more difficult to be sure that the surrounding conjunctiva is free of abnormal tissue.

Surgical Excision with Adjunctive Therapy

β-Irradiation

β-Irradiation has been used extensively throughout the world as an adjunctive therapy with pterygium excision since at least the early 1940s (38). It was the first adjunctive therapy to gain widespread acceptance because of its effectiveness in reducing recurrences, and its use continues in some places in the world still today.

Despite its effectiveness, β-irradiation has fallen into disfavor among many ophthalmologists because of long-term safety concerns. The most serious reported complication has been the development of scleral necrosis, which occurs in a significant minority of patients years after treatment (39,40). Additionally, lack of familiarity with how to perform the procedure, high maintenance costs and safety issues related to the radioactive equipment, and the inconvenience of some treatment regimens requiring multiple visits are other factors that make this modality less attractive.

Many variations in the administration of radiotherapy are described (39,41,42), but there are no well-controlled studies indicating the safest and most efficacious techniques and doses. They all involve applying radiation to the globe in the area of the excised pterygium, either directly by means of a strontium-90 applicator or via an external beam of radiation. A single intraoperative or postoperative treatment is used by some, whereas others apply the radiation in multiple sessions over several days or weeks. Total recommended doses of radiation exposure range from 1800 to 3000 rads (18–30 Gy), though reports clearly demonstrate the lack of consensus or uniformity of approach, with doses from 750 to 5200 rads (7.5–52.0 Gy) being used (39).

The strontium-90 applicators consist of a probe and base plate. The base plate fits onto the end of the probe and has an opening that determines the amount of active surface area from which the radiation is emitted. Shapes of the openings vary from rectilinear to circular or elliptical. Different probes have different emission rates of radioactivity, measured in rads (or Gray units) per second. The area of excision to be treated is measured. Some sources describe using an applicator that covers the entire extent of the scleral defect (41), while others place an elliptical applicator over the limbus where the excised pterygium crossed (23). The probe and base plate are cleansed with alcohol and rinsed with sterile water or saline solution before use. The applicator unit is then applied to the area of treatment for the amount of time necessary to deliver the desired amount of radiation. External-beam radiation is probably best administered by an experienced radiation therapist so that calculations and calibrations are determined accurately, and administration is performed correctly.

Recurrence rates have been quoted as low as 0.5% and as high as 83% depending on the study (43,44). MacKenzie et al (40) pointed out that the majority of these studies have been limited by either very short follow-up time or small numbers. They attempted to help clarify the issue with a retrospective study of 1102 consecutive patients who were treated with a similar regimen of β-irradiation. More than 10 years of follow-up was obtained for 585 patients, with a recurrence rate of 12%. They acknowledged a potential selection bias due to an inability to follow up approximately half the patients, which could reduce their rate to as low as 6% or increase it to as high as 42%. In either case, their reported rate was much higher than what they or many others would have expected (45). It was at considerable variance with the often-cited 1.3% recurrence rate of van den Brenk (46), who reported on 1300 cases but with only 3 months of follow-up. In final analysis, a recurrence rate of probably at least 5% to as high as 30% to 40% may be a realistic expectation, depending on such factors as technique, radiation dosage, age and race of the patient, and geographic location.

The primary complication of β-irradiation reported in the literature is scleral necrosis (39,40). Only two studies attempted to define the rate of scleral necrosis: van den Brenk (46) in 1968 reported 3 cases in 1064 patients followed for less than 1 year, and MacKenzie et al (40) found 13% having some sign of scleromalacia, with 4.5% having severe thinning. Infectious endophthalmitis and corneoscleritis are the worst sequelae of scleral necrosis, with over a dozen cases reported in the literature (39,47). One of the most extensive reports of complications is that of Tarr and Constable (39) from Perth, Australia. In addition to 51 cases of scleral ulceration, they describe corneal ulceration, endophthalmitis, glaucoma, ptosis, symblepharon, dry eye, iris atrophy, and cataractous lens changes. Among the 57 patients included, 18 (32%) described the treatment as a painful experience and 24 (42%) complained of ocular discomfort and photophobia for many years after irradiation despite protective measures and topical treatment. We believe β-irradiation should be limited only to use in practice settings where dose calculation by radiation specialists can be undertaken. Despite this, we would recommend it only if

conjunctival autografting or MMC were not able to be used as adjunctive treatment.

Mitomycin C

The effectiveness of MMC in reducing recurrences after pterygia excision was first reported in Japan in 1963 (48). The drug has been used widely in that country since (49), but it did not achieve international attention and usage until the 1990s when its beneficial effect of preventing fibroblast proliferation and scarring after glaucoma filtration surgery was recognized (50).

MMC is an antineoplastic antibiotic produced by *Streptomyces caespitosus*. It is an extremely toxic, non-cell-specific alkylating agent that selectively inhibits the synthesis of DNA and prevents cellular division, which can lead to cell death. Its cross-linking mode of action produces DNA damage similar to that of ionizing radiation, and thus MMC is referred to as being *radiomimetic*. Treated sclera may become white, or "porcelainized," due to destroyed vessels and remain so forever. Rubinfeld et al (51) hypothesized that this is due to the drug's effect on multipotential cells and the rapidly proliferating cells of vascular endothelium. In tissue cultures it is also a potent inhibitor of fibroblast proliferation (52,53).

Postoperative Application of Mitomycin C   Prior to 1994, virtually all reported experiences of adjunctive MMC for pterygia excisions involved postoperative instillation of topical solutions (3,8,10,49,51,54). Numerous concentrations and dosing schedules of the drug have been tested in an effort to determine a safe and efficacious treatment regimen. The majority of studies used concentrations ranging from 0.1 mg/mL (3) to 1.0 mg/mL (54) in dosage schedules ranging from one drop three to four times daily for 1 to 3 weeks. The report by Kunitomo and Mori (48) in 1963 described the beneficial effects of postoperative instillation of 0.4 mg/mL of MMC three times a day for 1 to 2 weeks. In the following two decades though, numerous reports from Japan described significant complications, including scleral ulceration, occurring with doses of 0.4 mg/mL applied three times a day for 1 week (49).

The realization that use of MMC can cause significant adverse effects led to numerous studies attempting to determine safe dosages for treatment. In 1988, Hayasaka et al (49) from Japan reported on 99 eyes of 80 patients with primary pterygia who were treated with either excision alone (sliding flap closure with 3 mm of bare sclera at the limbus), or excision and one of the following: 2000 rads (20 Gy) of radiation, 0.4 mg/mL of MMC three times daily for 1 week, or 0.2 mg/mL of MMC twice daily for 5 days. The follow-up time ranged from 3 to 8 years. Ten (32%) of 31 eyes in the excision-only group had recurrences, compared to 3 (15%) of 20 eyes in the radiation group, 2 (11%) of 19 eyes in the 0.4-mg/mL MMC group, and 2 (7%) of 29 eyes in the 0.2-mg/mL MMC group. Scleral ulceration occurred in 2 eyes in both the radiation and 0.4-mg/mL MMC groups, but not among the 0.2-mg/mL MMC group. The authors concluded that postoperative instillation of 0.2 mg/mL of MMC, twice a day for 5 days, was effective and safe for the treatment of primary pterygia.

Also in 1988, Singh et al (3) reported their experience using postoperative MMC drops in a largely Hispanic group of patients (36/38) in Los Angeles, California. Complete pterygium resection was performed, leaving bare sclera without any conjunctival suturing. Twenty eyes received 1.0 mg/mL of MMC drops every 6 hours for 2 weeks, 24 eyes were treated with 0.4 mg/mL of MMC, and 18 eyes received placebo drops of saline solution. One eye in the 1.0-mg/mL MMC group had a recurrence (5%) after a mean follow-up time of 20 months; there were no recurrences in the 0.4-mg/mL group after 4 months of mean follow-up, and 16 (73%) of 22 eyes in the placebo group had recurrences within a 3-month mean follow-up time (55). Apparently in the original study design, only the greater concentration (1.0 mg/mL) of MMC was to be compared to placebo, but due to significant patient discomfort from conjunctival irritation, excessive lacrimation, and punctate epithelial erosions caused by the 1.0-mg/mL solution, a decision was made to include the more dilute 0.4-mg/mL concentration (3). The authors reported no significant complications from either concentration of MMC [but with much shorter follow-up time than in Hayasaka's study (49)], and concluded that 0.4 mg/mL of MMC used every 6 hours for 14 days was a safe and effective adjunctive treatment for pterygia excisions. The lowest concentration that has been tested since then and reported to be safe and effective without any severe complications is 0.1 mg/mL (54).

Other complications reported in the Japanese literature in addition to scleral ulceration include necrotizing scleritis, globe perforation, iridocyclitis, cataract, infection, glaucoma, scleral calcification, and loss of an eye, all due to use of MMC after pterygium surgery (49,56–62). The first American report of serious complications from topical MMC used after pterygium excision was by Rubinfeld et al (51) in 1992. The report described 10 patients from several different centers who developed sight-threatening complications including severe iritis, glaucoma, and corneal and scleral necrosis and melting that were poorly responsive to medical and surgical therapy. Although some of the patients received doses as low as 0.2-mg/mL drops four times daily for 3 days, a more common element among the group was a relatively large cumulative dose due to poor compliance, with some patients using excessive numbers of drops for periods longer than instructed. Additionally, many of these patients had coexisting diseases such as Sjögren's syndrome, ocular rosacea, and ichthyosis, which may have predisposed them to developing more complications regardless of the adjunctive therapy. A limitation of the report was that a denominator for the number of cases was not included, precluding a determination of the incidence of such complications (63).

Efforts to limit inadvertent overusage of postoperative topical MMC include dispensing only the needed volume of drug solution and confiscating the bottle at the end of the course of therapy. Such efforts will probably be unnecessary in the future, given recent reports of the successful use of a single intraoperative application of MMC (see below).

Intraoperative Application of Mitomycin C   The search for effective and safe dosing and delivery of MMC has led to trials evaluating a single intraoperative application (5,6,37,64–66), much like its use in glaucoma filtering surgery. In 1995 Cardillo et al (37) published a well-designed prospective, masked study of 227 patients (mean age, 48 years) in Brazil, to compare a single intraoperative application of MMC with postoperative drops of the drug. All patients underwent surgery consisting of excision with a rotational conjunctival flap from the 12-o'clock position (sliding graft) to cover all bare sclera completely. A surgical sponge soaked with either MMC solution or placebo was placed in contact with the exposed scleral surface, with the conjunctival layer draped over the sponge for 3 minutes, followed by irrigation of 100 mL of balanced salt solution to prevent further contact of the drug with eye tissue. Patients were randomly divided into five groups: Group 1 received a single intraoperative application of 0.2 mg/mL of MMC for 3 minutes; group 2 received a single intraoperative application of 0.4 mg/mL of MMC for 3 minutes; group 3 received MMC drops, 0.2 mg/mL, three times daily for 7 days; group 4 received MMC drops, 0.4 mg/mL, three times daily for 14 days; group 5 acted as a control group and had surgery alone. After a mean follow-up time of 28 months, recurrence rates were 6.66%, 4.08%, 4.26%, 4.44%, and 29.27%, respectively. All recurrences occurred within 11 months of follow-up. The only statistical difference was between the control group and the MMC groups ($p < 0.001$). There was no statistical difference among the MMC-treated groups ($p > 0.0681$).

Their study (37) highlighted the difficulty of interpreting the variability of results between different authors. Hayasaka et al (49) compared use of 0.4 mg/mL of MMC three times daily for 1 week with 0.2 mg/mL of MMC twice daily for 5 days and found that the complication rate was higher with the 0.4-mg/mL concentration. Their conclusion and recommendation was that 0.2 mg/mL was a safe and effective concentration to use for postoperative application. Cardillo et al (37) had no significant complications in any of their treatment groups, including those who received 0.4 mg/mL three times daily for 15 days, and concluded that the variability of results of different authors suggests that factors other than dosage must be considered to judge safety. Additionally, their study was the first published one comparing intraoperative MMC with postoperative MMC, and their results showed both methods to be equally effective, regardless of the two concentrations used. The 4% to 6% recurrence rate among the treated eyes shows efficacy as good as the best reported results for free conjunctival autografting, although it would have been ideal to have included such a group for direct comparison. The 29% recurrence rate for their rotational, or sliding graft technique is difficult to interpret without comparison with bare sclera and free autograft techniques.

Manning et al (66) compared free conjunctival autografting with postoperative MMC, 0.2 mg/mL four times daily for 7 days, and intraoperative MMC, 0.4 mg/mL for 3 minutes. Recurrence rates were 22.2% (4/18), 21.1% (4/19), and 10.5% (2/19), respectively, with no statistical difference between the three groups. One patient using postoperative 0.2-mg/mL MMC drops developed thinning in an area of nonvascularized sclera, noted 4 months after surgery, which required a scleral patch graft at 18 months after surgery.

Several other studies (5,6,64,65) confirmed the efficacy and relative safety of intraoperative MMC application. Frucht-Pery et al (5) noted that although a relatively small number of patients were treated in their study to detect complications that occur at a very low rate, an intraoperative application avoided the unpleasant side effects of ocular injection, ocular pain, and punctate keratopathy reported with MMC eyedrop therapy. Additionally, no difference in the rate of epithelialization of the denuded sclera and cornea was seen between the bare sclera group and the bare sclera group treated with intraoperative MMC. Epithelialization occurred within 7 postoperative days, compared to delayed wound healing times of 3 to 4 weeks in patients previously treated with topical MMC drops for 2 weeks. The authors concluded that minimizing exposure of epithelium to MMC during application is critical for rapid healing after surgery.

As with the postoperative application of MMC, further time is needed to establish the frequency and severity of complications that may arise from the intraoperative use of MMC. In 1996 Dougherty et al (67) reported a case of corneoscleral melt in a 59-year-old man who underwent pterygium excision with intraoperative application of 0.2 mg/mL of MMC for 3 minutes, followed by a sliding conjunctival flap to cover the exposed limbus and sclera. Five weeks after the surgery, the patient had mild trauma and noted decreased vision due to a corneoscleral melt with perforation. The patient was managed with a lamellar transplant in the affected area. The melt occurred despite the fact that this patient received the lowest dose used in a series of 25 eyes using the same technique without any other complications.

Miscellaneous Adjunctive Therapies

Thiotepa is another antineoplastic agent that has been used in the past to prevent postoperative recurrences of pterygia (68). It is mentioned for historical completeness, because lack of commercial availability and its ocular side effects kept it from ever achieving widespread use. Complications include allergic conjunctivitis, conjunctival hypertrophy, and depigmentation of the eyelid skin in darkly pigmented persons.

Argon laser treatments in the early postoperative period have also been described as a means to stop recurrences (42). If evidence of regrowth occurs, laser burns of 50-μm spot size are placed in a pattern of four parallel rows at the limbus, with care taken to treat all neovascular fronds. The procedure can be repeated if necessary. We know of no studies evaluating the safety or effectiveness of this procedure.

POSTOPERATIVE MEDICATIONS AND RECURRENCE RATES OF PTERYGIA

Topical antibiotics should be used until both corneal and conjunctival epithelial defects have healed. Topical corticosteroids are also commonly used to control inflammation during postoperative healing, which presumably may act as a stimulus for recurrence, although we are unaware of any studies supporting this view. We typically employ a tapering dose over 2 to 3 months to keep the eye quiet.

Hirst et al (69) attempted to define the length of follow-up that is required to identify a recurrence in order to aid the comparison of different pterygium treatments. Survival curve analysis showed a 50% chance of recurrence in the first 120 days after surgery, and a 97% chance of recurrence within 12 months of surgery. Based on this, they suggest that a 1-year follow-up time is likely to identify a recurrence.

CONCLUSIONS REGARDING PTERYGIA TREATMENT

1. Excision leaving bare sclera is the least effective of all techniques. Most studies report recurrence rates higher than 30%, compared to rates of usually 5% to 10% for either conjunctival autografts, adjunctive β-irradiation, or adjunctive MMC.
2. Excision with a free conjunctival autograft is the safest procedure. No vision-threatening complications have been reported with autografts. Minor complications that arise infrequently include graft edema, corneoscleral dellen, and graft retraction. Graft edema and dellen are temporary problems; graft retraction or necrosis may lead to recurrence, but does not compromise globe integrity. No other procedure has been shown to be more effective than a free conjunctival autograft.
3. Adjunctive β-irradiation or MMC can cause sight-threatening complications. Extensive experience in Australia showed that β-irradiation leads to signs of scleromalacia in as many as 1 of every 10 patients, with 4.5% having severe thinning (40). MMC is currently being used widely throughout the world with good success, but it also can cause similarly serious complications as β-irradiation, although at what frequency is still unknown. It is still popular

with glaucoma filtering surgery, and it appears that a single intraoperative application of MMC may prove to be the safest and most effective manner to use in combination with pterygium excision.

RECOMMENDATIONS FOR THE MANAGEMENT OF PTERYGIA

Safety, efficacy, and patient acceptance of treatment options are the important considerations in the management of pterygia. Conjunctival autografting combined with excision is the safest technique to date, but it is also the most technically demanding and time-consuming. Rates of recurrence generally are similar for autografting as for adjunctive use of β-irradiation or MMC. We discourage the continued use of β-irradiation given the potential serious long-term risks and the availability of safer alternatives. Adjunctive MMC may prove to be acceptably safe as more long-term data are gathered. Based on the information to date, a single intraoperative application of MMC is more controlled and less likely to induce significant side effects than is postoperative topical application by a patient.

CONJUNCTIVAL INTRAEPITHELIAL NEOPLASIA

The nomenclature of conjunctival intraepithelial neoplasia (CIN) is reviewed to assist in understanding the rationale for surgical excision. Pizzarello and Jakobiec (70) first applied the concept of intraepithelial neoplasia to the conjunctiva. Dysplasia signifies an epithelial growth with a trend toward malignancy. The characteristics of dysplasia are cellular atypia and loss of polarity. *Cellular atypia* refers to individual cells seen with malignant characteristics. For example, there may be enlargement of the cell, increased nucleocytoplasmic ratio, and abnormal mitosis, as well as other findings. *Abnormal polarity* means the loss of the normal maturation sequence of the epithelial cells. There are various grades of dysplasia—mild, moderate, or severe. Anaplasia is such severe dysplasia as to be clearly malignant.

CIN indicates some grade of dysplasia without the full thickness of the epithelium being involved. Carcinoma in situ is CIN with dysplastic changes noted throughout the full thickness of the epithelium but without metastasis and no invasion beneath the epithelial basement membrane. Squamous cell carcinoma is the same as carcinoma in situ but with metastasis or extension beyond the epithelial basement membrane. Finally, *leukoplakia* is a descriptive term meaning white plaque and gives no designation as to the pathology associated with this finding.

CIN occurs in men far more frequently than women. Erie et al (71) reported 93 males and 5 females in his series whereas Fraunfelder reported a 3:1 prevalence of men to women. The age of onset tends to be late in the fifth decade. Exposure to petroleum products, cigarette smoking, and actinic exposure are believed to be factors contributing to

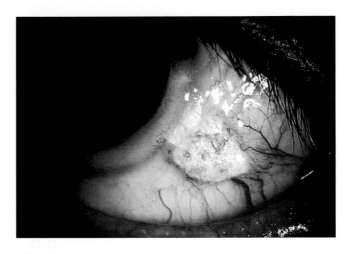

FIGURE 9-4. *Conjunctival intraepithelial neoplasia at the limbus with small extension onto the peripheral cornea.*

the development of CIN. Human papillomavirus DNA has been found in CIN tissues (72).

The clinical presentation is the development of a limbal lesion that may appear gelatinous, leukoplakic, or papillomatous with involvement of both the conjunctiva and cornea (Fig. 9-4). The corneal portion of the lesion is a thickened, gray, map-like area often with fimbriated-type finger-like projections out onto the cornea. The conjunctival portion may take any of the configurations just mentioned.

TREATMENT OF CONJUNCTIVAL INTRAEPITHELIAL NEOPLASIA

Excision plus cryotherapy is the most widely reported modality for the treatment of CIN and related disorders (73). Once the diagnosis is established by biopsy or clinical assessment, anesthetic type must be considered and controlled conveyance of the specimen to the pathologist must be arranged. The pathologists must be consulted beforehand to request their input regarding the handling of the specimen. Anesthesia could be topical or subconjunctival. Retrobulbar or peribulbar anesthesia will reduce the pain associated with the application of cryotherapy.

The area to be excised should be marked by a marking pen or by cautery. The superior edge near the limbus is a good location to begin undermining the conjunctival portion. This should be carried back posteriorly to the previously marked areas. Bulbar conjunctiva that is easily undermined is a clue that the pathology likely does not penetrate beneath the basement membrane. Once the entire conjunctival portion is undermined, it is excised. The corneal portion, if confined above Bowman's membrane, usually comes off readily with a scraping motion with a Beaver 69 blade. This scraping should begin at the area of furthest extent onto the cornea and continue in the direction of the involved limbus. Finally, a double freeze thaw of the limbus and entire margin of conjunctival resection should be accomplished. Care should be taken to elevate the conjunctival margin off of the globe so as to isolate the effect of the freezing. The scleral bed should be treated in a similar manner if there is any question of carcinoma in situ. Frozen section evaluation of the tumor margins following resection is advocated by Char (73). When excision and cryoapplication are completed, as much of the resection area as possible should be covered by approximating the conjunctiva. A small amount of bare sclera may be left but too large of an area may require a conjunctival autograft. Antibiotic ointment and a pressure patch are applied for 24 hours. Antibiotic ointment and cycloplegic as needed are then used until all of the epithelium is healed. Care must be taken to observe for infection, recurrence, and motility disturbance if the resected area extends over any muscle insertions.

Other modalities for removal include excision with topical MMC 0.02% for 10 days (74), β-irradiation with strontium 90 (75), urea (76), and immunotherapy with dinitrochlorobenzene (77).

Char (73) reported that excision with frozen section guidance and cryotherapy gives a less than 5% recurrence rate. Excision with cryotherapy of the scleral bed, conjunctival margin, and limbus gave a 4% recurrence rate at 36 months, as reported by Fraunfelder and Wingfield (78). Erie et al (71) reported a 20% recurrence rate with excision alone. Finally, Morsman (79) reported spontaneous regression of CIN following diagnostic biopsy.

REFERENCES

1. *Stedmans's medical dictionary.* 22nd ed. Baltimore: Williams & Wilkins, 1972: 1042.
2. Lewallen S. A randomized trial of conjunctival autografting for pterygium in the tropics. *Ophthalmology* 1989;96:1612–1614.
3. Singh G, Wilson MR, Foster CS. Mitomycin eye drops as treatment for pterygium. *Ophthalmology* 1988;95:813–821.
4. Anduze AL, Merritt JC. Pterygium: clinical classification and management in Virgin Islands. *Ann Ophthalmol* 1985;17:92–95.
5. Frucht-Pery J, Siganos CS, Ilsar M. Intraoperative application of topical mitomycin C for pterygium surgery. *Ophthalmology* 1996;103:674–677.
6. Mastropasqua L, Carpineto P, Ciancaglini M, Gallenga PE. Long term results of intraoperative mitomycin C in the treatment of recurrent pterygium. *Br J Ophthalmol* 1996;80:288–291.
7. Kenyon KR, Wagoner MD, Hettinger ME. Conjunctival autograft transplantation for advanced and recurrent pterygium. *Ophthalmology* 1985;92:1461–1470.
8. Rachmiel R, Leiba H, Lavartovsky S. Results of treatment with topical mitomycin C 0.02% following excision of primary pterygium. *Br J Ophthalmol* 1995;79:233–236.
9. Allan BDS, Short P, Crawford J, et al. Pterygium excision with conjunctival autografting: an effective and safe technique. *Br J Ophthalmol* 1993;77:698–701.
10. Chen PP, Ariyasu RG, Kaza V, et al. A randomized trial comparing mitomycin C and conjunctival autograft after excision of primary pterygium. *Am J Ophthalmol* 1995;120:151–160.
11. Cameron ME. *Pterygium throughout the world.* Springfield, IL: Charles C Thomas, 1965.
12. Taylor H, West S, Rosenthal F, et al. Corneal changes associated with chronic UV irradiation. *Arch Ophthalmol* 1989;107:1481.
13. Mackenzie FD, Hirst LW, Battistutta D, Green A. Risk analysis in the development of pterygia. *Ophthalmology* 1992;99:1056–1061.
14. Hect F, Shoptaugh MG. Winglets of the eye: dominant transmission of early adult pterygium of the conjunctiva. *J Med Genet* 1990;27:392.
15. Duke-Elder S. *System of ophthalmology. Diseases of the outer eye.* Vol. VIII. St. Louis: CV Mosby, 1965:573–585.
16. Detels R, Dhir SP. Pterygium: a geographical study. *Arch Ophthalmol* 1967;78:485.
17. Rasanayagam RT. The incidence and racial distribution of pterygium in West Malaysia. *Trans Ophthalmol Soc NZ* 1973;25:56.
18. Hilgers JHC. Pterygium: its incidence, heredity, and etiology. *Am J Ophthalmol* 1960;50:635.
19. Sevel D, Sealy R. Pterygia and carcinoma of the conjunctiva. *Trans Ophthalmol Soc UK* 1968;88:567.
20. Cameron ME. Histology of pterygium: an electron microscopic study. *Br J Ophthalmol* 1983;67:604–608.
21. Starck T, Kenyon KR, Serrano F. Conjunctival autograft for primary and recurrent pterygia: surgical technique and problem management. *Cornea* 1991;10:196–202.
22. Prabhasawat P, Barton K, Burkett G, Tseng SCG. Comparison of conjunctival autografts, amniotic membrane grafts, and primary closure for peterygium excision. *Ophthalmology* 1997;104:974–985.
23. King JH, Joseph AC. *An atlas of ophthalmic surgery.* 3rd ed. Philadelphia: JB Lippincott, 1981:218–229.
24. Youngson RM. Recurrence of pterygium after excision. *Br J Ophthalmol* 1972;56:120–125.
25. Jaros PA, Deluise VP. Pinguecula and pterygia. *Surv Ophthalmol* 1988;33:41.
26. Adamis AP, Starck T, Kenyon KR. The management of pterygium. *Ophthalmol Clin North Am* 1990;3:611.
27. Doughman DJ. Discussion. *Ophthalmology* 1985;92:1470.
28. Laughrea PA, Arentsen JJ. Lamellar keratoplasty for recurrent pterygium. *Ophthalmic Surg* 1986;17:106.
29. Trivedi LK, Massey DB, Rohatgi R. Management of pterygium and its recurrence by grafting with mucous membrane from the mouth. *Am J Ophthalmol* 1969;68:353.
30. Manning CA, Kloess PM, Diaz MD, Yee RW. Intraoperative mitomycin in primary pterygium excision; a prospective, randomized trial. *Ophthalmology* 1997;104:844–848.
31. Hifnawy MAM. Comparison of postoperative beta irradiation and conjunctival autograft transplantation in treatment of pterygium. *Middle East J Ophthalmol* 1997;5:19–23.
32. Stocker FW. Operation for removal of pterygium. *Arch Ophthalmol* 1942;27:925–928.
33. Aratoon V. Surgery of pterygium by conjunctival pedicle flap. *Am J Ophthalmol* 1967;63:1778–1779.
34. Wilson SE, Bourne WM. Conjunctival Z-plasty in the treatment of pterygium. *Am J Ophthalmol* 1988;106:355–357.
35. McCoombes JA, Hirst LW, Isbell GP. Sliding conjunctival flap for the treatment of primary pterygium. *Ophthalmology* 1994;101:169–173.
36. Astudillo IM, Kenyon KR, Rapoza PA. Pterygium. In: Roy FH, ed. *Master techniques in ophthalmic surgery.* Philadelphia: Williams & Wilkins, 1995:110–120.
37. Cardillo JA, Alves MR, Ambrosio LE, et al. Single intraoperative application versus postoperative mitomycin C eye drops in pterygium surgery. *Ophthalmology* 1995;102:1949–1952.
38. Leahey BD. Beta radiation in ophthalmology. *Am J Ophthalmol* 1960; 49:7–29.
39. Tarr KH, Constable IJ. Late complications of pterygium treatment. *Br J Ophthalmol* 1980;64:496–505.
40. MacKenzie FD, Hirst LW, Kynaston B, Bain C. Recurrence rate and complications after beta irradiation for pterygia. *Ophthalmology* 1991;98:1776–1781.
41. Rice TA, Michels RG, Stark WJ, eds. *Ophthalmic surgery.* 4th ed. Boston: Butterworths, 1984:73–75.
42. Insler MS, Caldwell DR, Leach DH. Pterygium. In: Brightbill FS, ed. *Corneal surgery: theory, technique, and tissue.* 2nd ed. St. Louis: Mosby-Year Book, 1993:336–338.
43. Halk GM, Ellis GS, Nowell JF. The management of pterygia: with special reference to surgery combined with beta irradiation. *Trans Am Acad Ophthalmol Otolaryngol* 1962;66:776–784.
44. Sinha A. Combined surgical and beta radiation treatment of pterygium. *Indian Pract* 1967;20:255–256.
45. Taylor HR. Discussion. *Ophthalmology* 1991;98:1781.
46. van den Brenk HAS. Results of prophylactic postoperative irradiation in 1300 cses of pterygium. *Am J Roentgenol Radium Ther Nucl Med* 1968;103:723–733.

47. Moriarty AP, Crawford GF, McAllister IL, Constable IJ. Severe corneoscleral infection. *Arch Ophthalmol* 1993;111:947–951.

48. Kunitomo N, Mori J. Studies on the pterygium. Part 4. A treatment of the pterygium by mitomycin C instillation. *Acta Soc Ophthalmol Jpn* 1963;67:601.

49. Hayasaka S, Noda S, Yamamoto Y, Setogawa T. Postoperative installation of low-dose mitomycin C in the treatment of primary pterygium. *Am J Ophthalmol* 1988;106:715–718.

50. Palmer SS. Mitomycin as adjunct chemotherapy with trabeculectomy. *Ophthalmology* 1991;98:317–321.

51. Rubinfeld RS, Pfister RR, Stein RM, et al. Serious complications of topical mitomycin C after pterygium surgery. *Ophthalmology* 1992;99:1647–1654.

52. Lee DS, Leo TC, Cortes AE, Kitada S. Effects of mithramycin, mitomycin, daunorubicin, and bleomycin on human subconjunctival fibroblast attachment and proliferation. *Invest Ophthalmol Vis Sci* 1990;31:2136–2144.

53. Yamamoto T, Varai J, Soong HK, Lichter PR. Effects of 5-fluorouracil and mitomycin C on cultured rabbit subconjunctival fibroblasts. *Ophthalmology* 1990;97:1204–1210.

54. Frucht-Pery J, Ilsar M. The use of low-dose mitomycin C for prevention of recurrent pterygium. *Ophthalmology* 1994;101:759–762.

55. Singh G, Wilson MR, Foster CS. Long-term follow-up study of mitomycin eye drops as adjunctive treatment for pterygia and its comparison with conjunctival autograft transplantation. *Cornea* 1990;9:331–334.

56. Dunn JP, Seamone CD, Ostler HB, et al. Development of scleral ulceration and calcification after pterygium excision and mitomycin therapy. *Am J Ophthalmol* 1991;112:343–344. Letter.

57. Fukamachi Y, Hikita N. Ocular complication following pterygium operation and instillation of mitomycin C. *Folia Ophthalmol Jpn* 1981;32:197–201.

58. Yamanouchi U, Takakau I, Tsuda N, et al. Scleromalacia presumably due to mitomycin C instillation after pterygium excision. *Jpn J Clin Ophthalmol* 1979;33:139–144.

59. Yamanouchi U. A case of scleral calcification due to mitomycin C instillation after pterygium operation. *Folia Ophthalmol Jpn* 1978;29:1221–1225.

60. Yamanouchi U, Mishima K. Eye lesions due to mitomycin C instillation after pterygium operation. *Folia Ophthalmol Jpn* 1967;18:854–861.

61. Singh G. Postoperative instillation of low-dose mitomycin C in the treatment of primary pterygium. *Am J Ophthalmol* 1989;107:570–571. Letter.

62. Hayasaka S, Noda S, Yamamoto Y, Setogawa T. Reply 571. To: Singh G. Postoperative installation of low-dose mitomycin C in the treatment of primary pterygium. *Am J Ophthalmol* 1989;107:570. Letter.

63. Sugar A. Who should receive mitomycin C after pterygium surgery? *Ophthalmology* 1992;99:1645–1646. Editorial.

64. Frucht-Pery J, Ilsar M, Hemo I. Single dosage of mitomycin C for prevention of recurrent pterygium: preliminary report. *Cornea* 1994;13:411–413.

65. Cano-Parra J, Diaz-Llopis M, Maldonado MJ, et al. Prospective trial of intraoperative mitomycin C in the treatment of primary pterygium. *Br J Ophthalmol* 1995;79:439–441.

66. Manning CA, Kloess PM, Diaz DM, Yee RW. Intraoperative mitomycin C in primary pterygium excision: a prospective, randomized trial. *Ophthalmology* 1997;104:844–848.

67. Dougherty PJ, Hardten DR, Lindstrom RL. Corneoscleral melt after pterygium surgery using a single intraoperative application of mitomycin C. *Cornea* 1996;15:537–540.

68. Joselson GA, Muller P. Incidence of pterygium recurrence in patients treated with thio-tepa. *Am J Ophthalmol* 1966;61:891–892.

69. Hirst LW, Allan S, Chant D. Pterygium recurrence time. *Ophthalmology* 1994;101:755–758.

70. Pizzarello LD, Jakobiec FA. Bowen's disease of the conjunctiva. A misnomer. In: Jakobiec FA, ed. *Ocular and adnexal tumors.* Birmingham, AL: Aesculapius, 1978:553–571.

71. Erie JC, Campbell RJ, Liesegang TJ. Conjunctival and corneal intraepithelial and invasive neoplasia. *Ophthalmology* 1986;93:176–183.

72. Lauer SA, Malter JS, Meier JR. Human papillomavirus type 18 in conjunctival intraepithelial neoplasia. *Am J Ophthalmol* 1990;110:23–27.

73. Char DH. *Clinical ocular oncology.* New York: Churchill Livingstone, 1989:69.

74. Frucht-Pery J, Rozenman Y. Mitomycin C therapy for corneal intraepithelial neoplasia. *Am J Ophthalmol* 1994;117:164–168.

75. Lommatzsch P. Beta-ray treatment of malignant epithelial tumors of the conjunctiva. *Am J Ophthalmol* 1976;81:198.

76. Danopoulos ED, Danopoulou IF, Liarikos SB, Merkuria KM. Effects of urea treatment in malignancies of the conjunctiva and cornea. *Ophthalmologica* 1979;178:198.

77. Ferry AP, Meltzer MA, Taub RN. Immunotherapy with dinitrochlorobenzene (DNCB) for recurrent squamous cell tumor of conjunctiva. *Trans Am Ophthalmol Soc* 1976;74:154.

78. Fraunfelder FT, Wingfield D. Management of intraepithelial conjunctival tumors and squamous cell carcinomas. *Am J Ophthalmol* 1983;95:359–363.

79. Morsman CD. Spontaneous regression of a conjunctival intraepithelial neoplastic tumor. *Arch Ophthalmol* 1989;107:1490–1491.

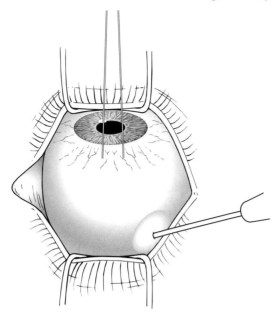

FIGURE 10-5. *Anesthetic injection. Balanced salt solution is used with a 30-gauge needle to separate the conjunctiva from Tenon's capsule. The injection site should be near the fornix so as not to perforate the eventual flap.*

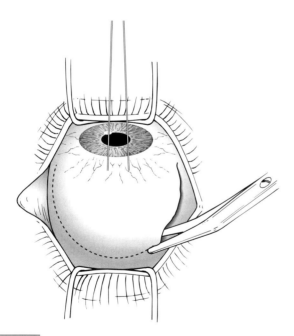

FIGURE 10-6. *Conjunctival dissection, initial incision. Scissors are used to create a large conjunctival flap superiorly, obtaining the maximal amount of tissue for the flap. One should be careful not to injure Müller's muscle.*

9. The cut edge of the superior limbal conjunctiva is secured to the site of the inferior limbus incision using 10-0 nylon sutures in a mattress and interrupted fashion. The same is done with the

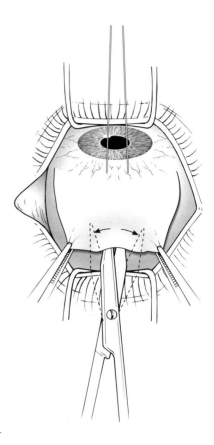

FIGURE 10-7. *Conjunctival dissection, in progress. Countertraction using smooth forceps facilitates the dissection. Blunt dissection is used, employing a closed-open technique under the conjunctiva.*

superior cut edge of the conjunctival flap to the superior limbus (Fig. 10-8).

10. If a buttonhole occurs, it should be repaired using 10-0 nylon suture on a vascular needle. Unrepaired buttonholes will serve as areas for flap retraction and exposure of the underlying cornea.

11. Antibiotic and cycloplegic drops are applied and the sutures are removed in weeks. Gradual thinning of the flap will occur over the next 6 months. The flap may become sufficiently translucent to allow anterior-segment inspection.

Scleral Flap

In general, sclera should not be used to cover perforations because it usually swells by imbibing aqueous and is poorly epithelialized. However, in certain cases, perforated ulcers at the limbus can be readily closed by swinging a flap of sclera at the limbus onto the ulcer, closing the perforation. If the hinged flap is smaller than 5 mm, it may not swell (27).

The procedure is similar to that used for dissecting a scleral flap for a trabeculectomy. If the perforation is 4 mm or smaller and within 1 mm of the limbus, it can be closed

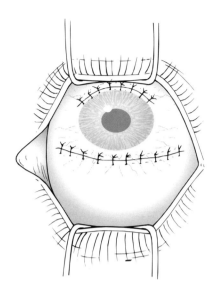

FIGURE 10-8. *Conjunctival flap in place. It is sutured with interrupted 10-0 nylon sutures.*

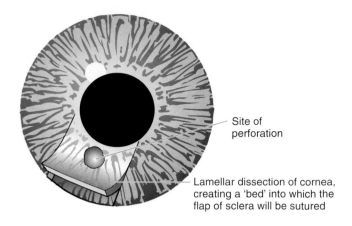

Site of perforation

Lamellar dissection of cornea, creating a 'bed' into which the flap of sclera will be sutured

FIGURE 10-10. *Preparation of corneal perforation site.*

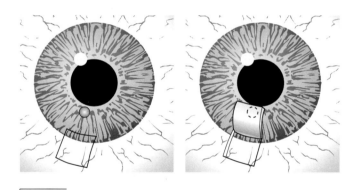

FIGURE 10-9. *Scleral flap dissection.*

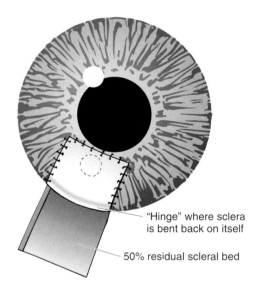

"Hinge" where sclera is bent back on itself

50% residual scleral bed

FIGURE 10-11. *Hinged scleral flap folded back into site and sutured.*

temporarily by using tissue adhesive. This will allow the anterior chamber to re-form, increasing the intraocular pressure so that scleral dissection will be facilitated (27).

Details of the procedure vary among corneal surgeons. However, the general steps of this technique are as follows (27):

1. Local anesthesia is given through lid and retrobulbar or peribulbar injections.
2. A lid speculum is placed.
3. A fornix-based conjunctival flap is made.
4. A 5 × 5mm scleral flap is then dissected from the limbus at approximately one-half thickness into clear cornea, avoiding the perforation (Fig. 10-9).
5. A lamellar bed approximately 5 × 5mm surrounding the perforation is then prepared using sharp dissection (Fig. 10-10).

6. The hinged scleral flap is then everted and sutured into the edges of the lamellar bed with 10-nylon suture (Fig. 10-11).
7. The conjunctival flap is then pulled down over the scleral defect and sutured at the limbus using interrupted 10-nylon suture.
8. Alternatively, banked sclera (preserved or otherwise) or pericardium may be used if available.

Full- or partial-thickness scleral patch can also provide efficient sealing of a persistent leak in a cystic filtration bleb (28) and closure of a perforation resulting from complications of topical mitomycin C treatment after pterygium surgery (29).

Lamellar Patch Graft

When the corneal perforation is 2 to 4mm, it can be repaired with a small lamellar or full-thickness graft. Placement of a lamellar patch graft has been successful in the treatment of descemetocele formation in a patient with a postoperative corneal dellen (30), corneal hydrops in a patient with Terrien's marginal degeneration (31), radial keratotomy complicated by sterile keratitis and corneal perforation (32), and corneal perforation after pterygium excision and topical mitomycin C therapy (33). Penetrating keratoplasty is not indicated in such circumstances because these grafts do poorly in inflamed, infected, and hypotonous eyes (34).

The general principles of this technique can be described as follows (3):

Preparation of Recipient Perforation

1. The technique and type of anesthesia to use are the surgeon's choice.
2. A lid speculum is placed.
3. The epithelium and necrotic tissue are moved for 2 to 3mm outside of the perforation site. Cyanoacrylate glue can then be applied in the usual fashion to temporarily seal the perforation.
4. After the glue has been placed, a paracentesis is made on the normal cornea. Balanced salt solution or hyaluronate is injected into the anterior chamber to restore normal depth and pressure.
5. The surgical bed is outlined, freehand or with a trephine, with edges at least 1mm outside the area of pathology in all directions.
6. Partial-thickness dissection of the normal cornea is made in the periphery of the surgical bed and all necrotic tissues are removed.

Preparation of Donor

1. A donor whole eye, either fresh, frozen, or glycerin preserved, is inflated to normal or just above normal intraocular pressure.
2. A limbal incision to 70% depth is made for insertion of the lamellar dissector.
3. A lamellar dissector is used to create a two-thirds corneal-depth lamellar dissection the entire extent of the cornea.
4. A trephine of the appropriate size, determined on prior inspection of the recipient eye, is then used to create the proper-size button for the patch graft, trephining the donor eye from epithelial side and harvesting the 70% thick donor button, which is 1mm larger in diameter than the surgical bed.

Completion of the Grafting

1. The donor button that has been created is placed over the recipient site and anchored with multiple interrupted sutures; the knots are buried.
2. A soft contact lens may be placed over the patch graft to promote re-epithelialization. Appropriate antibiotics and cycloplegic drops are administered.
3. Corneal sutures are removed 1 to 3 months after surgery.

Synthetic and Other Grafting Materials

Besides autologous and homologous conjunctiva and sclera, synthetic graft materials are also available commercially for corneoscleral surgery. Some of the common products are the Gore-Tex soft tissue patch (polytetrafluoroethylene [PTFE]), Miragel (poly[methyl acrylate-co-hydroxy-ethyl acrylate]), and Dacron (polyethylene terephthalate).

Gore-Tex has been used to patch areas with corneal ulcers, Mooren's ulcer, and necrotizing scleritis. However, there must be adequate conjunctival covering to prevent poor epithelialization, poor adhesion between the graft and surrounding tissue, and a potential infectious route (35). In some cases, the scleral reinforcement is done with polytetrafluoroethylene together with a tissue adhesive such as cyanoacrylate (21).

Research showed the long-term compatibility of Gore-Tex, Miragel, and Dacron when used as periscleral grafts in rabbits. Dacron, however, seems to be most suitable for scleral reinforcement (36).

Dehydrated human dura mater is also available commercially and can be used as a surgical patch, as can pericardium. Human donor sclera is commonly used in glaucoma surgery with a tube shunt to cover the external portion of the silicone tube and prevent its erosion through the overlying conjunctiva. Brandt (37) has reported a case of gradual melting of a scleral patch graft, which was then successfully replaced with dehydrated human dura matter. There has not been any report in the current literature on the use of dehydrated cadaveric dura mater in corneal surgery.

USE OF THERAPEUTIC SOFT CONTACT LENSES

During the last three decades, significant advancement has been made in the use of soft contact lenses for therapeutic purposes in the treatment of corneal diseases. Ophthalmologists have gained better understanding of the goals to be achieved by lens wear, the characteristics of available lenses, the indications for their use, and the complications that can occur, allowing increasingly successful use of therapeutic soft contact lens.

Goals

Various specific goals can be achieved in the treatment of ocular-surface abnormalities with soft contact lenses (38):

1. Reduction of pain
2. Mechanical protection of the ocular surface

3. Facilitation of epithelial healing and stabilization of the ocular surface
4. Maintenance of proper surface hydration

Visual improvement is often not a major therapeutic goal. However, as a result of smoothing of the refractive surface, vision may be improved in some patients.

Physiology of Soft Contact Lenses

Soft contact lenses affect the normal physiologic properties of the cornea in several ways. They induce a certain degree of anoxia, cause some amount of trauma, and change the distribution of tear film (38).

Anoxia

The degree of anoxia produced by soft contact lenses worn therapeutically is similar to that produced by routine wear for refractive purposes. However, because therapeutic lenses are often to be worn 24 hours per day, there is a greater demand on oxygen transmissibility when the eyelids are closed during sleep. The amount of oxygen dissolved in the tear film when the eyes are open is equivalent to a partial pressure of 155 mm Hg. When the eyelids are closed, the partial pressure of oxygen falls to 40 to 50 mm Hg, greatly diminishing the difference in pressure that causes oxygen to diffuse into the cornea (39). Oxygen transmission through lenses is directly related to the hydration and thickness of the lens, features that are mostly mandated by the nature of the polymer used (40). The physiologic advantage of soft, compared to hard, lenses is better direct movement of oxygen across the lens.

Mechanical Trauma

The soft contact lenses should be well fitted to allow minimal excursion. This will minimize the degree of trauma caused by the sliding of the lens over the cornea and the distortion of the epithelial cells. When the lens edges are blunter or the tear film is scanty, the trauma can aggravate. Lens-edge problems are worsened when elevation of tissue at the limbus such as with filtration blebs interferes with normal centration of the lens (39).

Tear Film Changes

In the presence of a soft contact lens, the normal layering of the tear film with the meibomian secretions interfacing with the adsorbed mucus on the epithelial cells is disorganized. The normal mixing and spreading of the tear components are also altered by the presence of a lens. Together, these changes cause increased evaporation from an eye wearing a soft lens, which may exacerbate preexisting dry eye syndromes (38).

In addition, there is relative stagnation of the tear film beneath soft lenses, causing a decrease in the usual surface flushing and cleansing that are accomplished by each blink. This may lead to occasional infections that occur with therapeutic soft lens use (38,39).

Characteristics and Types of Soft Contact Lenses

The characteristics and types of various soft contact lenses commonly used for therapeutic purposes are listed in Table 10-2. The main characteristics are the nature of the polymer, the water content, and the thickness; together, these will define the gas permeability of the lens.

Water Content and Oxygen Permeability

In a closed eye, a lens that is 40% water can be only 0.05 mm thick for sufficient oxygen to reach the corneal surface. However, a lens that is 85% water, which has decreased barrier to diffusion, could be as thick as 0.23 mm. Thus, to maximize the amount of oxygen available to the cornea, manufacturers have tried to make the lenses as thin as

Table 10-2. Common Therapeutic Soft Contact Lenses

Water Content	%	Lens Type (Manufacturers)	Polymer	Thickness (mm)
High	79	Sauflon (Visiontech)	Polymethylmethacrylate/vinyl pyrrolidone	0.22–0.45
	71	Permalens (Cooper Laboratories)	Poly (HEMA/vinyl pyrrolidone)	0.36–0.43
	58	Softcon (American Optical Corp.)	Poly (HEMA/vinyl pyrrolidone)	0.35–0.43
Medium	55	Hydrocurve II (Soft Lenses)	HEMA/diacetone acrylamide	0.06–0.07
Low	39.6	Plano T (Bausch and Lomb)	HEMA	0.17
	39	CSI (Syntex Ophthalmics)	Poly (glyceryl methacrylate/methyl methacrylate)	0.05–0.20
	38	Ultrathin 03/04 (Bausch and Lomb)	HEMA	0.035
	0	Silicone lenses	Silicone rubber	0.10–1.50

HEMA = 2-hydroxyethylmethacrylate.
Source: Modified from Thoft RA. Therapeutic soft contact lenses. In: Smolin G, Thoft RA, eds. *The cornea.* Boston: Little, Brown, 1987.

possible (38). Nevertheless, thinness must be balanced with fragility and spoilage, which are associated with both types of lenses.

Size and Base Curve

The size and base curve are important in the fitting of the therapeutic lens. The actual details of the fitting procedure are addressed elsewhere (41). In general, larger lenses tend to be more stable on the eye and may be useful in eyes with surface irregularity such as with recurrent stromal loss and subsequent healing in which the central cornea may not provide uniform support to the lens. On the other hand, a large lens will increase the area of tissue that is dependent on exchange of nutrients and may therefore exaggerate relative anoxia (38).

The base curve variation can be used to modulate the amount of lens motion and the degree of tear exchange beneath the lens. The bulk of oxygen and water exchange is across the lens and not beneath its edges, so that the size of the tear lake between the lens and the cornea is usually not directly related to the "tightness" of the lens. Theoretically, the lens should not move against the epithelial surface unless it is cushioned by a layer of tears (38).

Indications

The indications for therapeutic contact lens wear are numerous. A partial list is indicated in Table 10-3 (42–52). It is beyond the scope of this chapter to address in details each condition. However, it is very important for the ophthalmologist to choose the patients carefully. The patient must be responsible, reliable, and available for follow-up examinations. Many possible complications from therapeutic contact lens wear can occur, if patients are not seen regularly. Thus, in certain circumstances, the pathologic condition may be ideal for therapeutic lenses, but a patient's characteristics may preclude their application.

Contraindications

There are conditions in which the use of therapeutic lenses will do more harm than good. Table 10-4 lists the conditions in which therapeutic lenses are contraindicated. In general, patients with active infection, bedridden patients, immunologically incompetent patients, and patients with poor hygiene should not be fitted with a therapeutic contact lens (41). If the need for such a lens is absolute, the duration should be kept at minimal and the patient should be monitored very closely.

Experience has shown that active infectious keratitis is aggravated by contact lenses (53). Lid dysfunction may disturb adequate tear function. When tear secretion is insufficient, the lens will dry out and will irritate rather than protect the corneal epithelium. Hypoesthetic and anesthetic corneas are more prone to injuries and subsequent infection, which may not be discovered in time for adequate

treatment. Corneal hypoxia, occurring in a tightly fitted lens, may aggravate a preexisting uveitic condition (41).

Complications

There are as many possible complications from the application of therapeutic soft contact lenses as there are indications for their usage. A partial list is indicated in Table 10-5 (54–58). However, if the ophthalmologists are careful and conscious, and the patients are responsible and reliable, many of these complications can be detected early, and appropriate actions can take place before any severe damage is done.

Complications of therapeutic lenses can be divided into those secondary to the fitting of the lens and those secondary to the wearing of the lens.

Drug Delivery

In many cases, topical antibiotics must be administered in conjunction with the wearing of therapeutic soft contact lenses. There is a possible concern as to whether the presence of the contact lens will interfere with antibiotic delivery to the cornea. Research done in rabbits showed that the presence of therapeutic soft contact lens does not compromise antibiotic (aminoglycosides) delivery to the cornea (59). In addition, soft contact lenses provide significantly higher drug (chloramphenicol, gentamicin, carbenicillin) penetration than does subconjunctival therapy (60).

Monitoring of Intraocular Pressure

Patients who are wearing therapeutic soft contact lenses often still need regular measurements of their intraocular pressure. Undetected glaucoma in a patient wearing a bandage lens can be a devastating complication, resulting in extensive visual field loss. Therefore, intraocular pressure should be checked often. Whenever the lens is removed for cleaning, applanation tonometry in relatively normal corneas or pneumotonometry in irregular corneas should be performed (41).

In some patients, removing and placing a contact lens is a tremendous task. Thus, penumotonometry over the contact lens has been attempted and shown to be an effective way to estimate the intraocular pressure in patients wearing therapeutic soft contact lenses (61). In addition, Tono-Pen tonometers can be used. Mendelsohn et al (62) showed that therapeutic soft contact lenses do not have any noticeably adverse effect on the accuracy of the Pneumatonometer and Tono-Pen tonometers.

Maintenance of Contact Lenses

Prevention of microbial incubation and subsequent infection has always been a priority in contact lens users. In addition to the vast arrays of cleaning solutions, including those with enzymatic action, research indicated that microwave irradiation and ultraviolet radiation may serve as alternative

Table 10-3. Conditions That May Benefit from Therapeutic Contact Lenses

Condition	Duration	Type
Corneal dystrophies and persistent epithelial erosions	1–3 mo	High/medium water content
Traumatic corneal abrasions		
Recurrent erosion syndrome		
Recurrent corneal erosion		
Map-dot-fingerprint dystrophy		
Reis-Bucklers dystrophy		
Diabetes mellitus (neurotrophic)		
Recessive dystrophic epidermolysis bullosa (42)		
Endothelial dysfunction	As long as necessary but removed every 3 mo for cleaning	High/medium water content
Dystrophy		
Fuchs' endothelial dystrophy		
Posterior polymorphous dystrophy		
Nondystrophy		
Aphakic bullous keratopathy		
Pseudophakic bullous keratopathy		
After surgery	—	—
Complications after corneal transplantation		
Complications after trabeculectomy (43)		
After extensive epithelial debridement for corneal epithelial dystrophies		
Healing of corneal epithelial defects after vitrectomy		
Post-PRK analgesia (44)		
Infectious keratitis (infectious process has been controlled but corneal epithelial disease remains)	—	—
Herpes simplex		
Herpes zoster		
Bacterial and fungal corneal ulcers		
Superficial punctate keratopathy	—	—
Thygeson's punctate keratopathy		
Diseases of skins and lids		
Systemic diseases		
Chemical burns	As long as necessary; may use with cyanoacrylate glue	High/medium water content; large size
Recurrent epithelial erosions		
Acid		
Alkali		
Band keratopathy	—	Medium water content
Overlying epithelial erosions		
After chelation of calcium band		
Dry eye	As long as necessary	Low water content
Keratitis sicca (45)		
Sjögren's syndrome		
Other systemic diseases		
Immune disease	—	—
Super limbic keratoconjunctivitis (46)		
Cicatricial pemphigoid and erythema multiforme (47)		
Vernal keratoconjunctivitis		
Astigmatism	—	Medium/low water content
Irregular astigmatism		
Keratoconus (48)		
Piggyback (rigid lens over soft lens) (49)		
Spontaneous perforation of cornea (50)		
Trichiasis	—	—
Epithelial erosions		
Scarred cornea	—	Rigid, gas permeable soft; high/medium water content
Perforating corneal diseases (51)		
Aseptic perforation in Cockayne's syndrome (52)		

PRK = photorefractive keratectomy.
Source: Modified from Maguen E, Nesburn AB. Bandage soft contact lenses. In: Kaufman HE, Barron BA, McDonald MB, Waltman SR, eds. *The cornea*. New York: Churchill Livingstone, 1988:647–667.

Table 10-4. Contraindications to Therapeutic Lenses

Absolute contraindications
  Active infections
Relative contraindications
  Lid dysfunction
  Severely dry eyes
  Cicatricial pemphigoid
  Stevens-Johnson syndrome
  Corneal hypoesthesia
  Uveitis
  Toxic/hypersensitivity disorders
  Sterile infiltrates

Source: Modified from Maguen E, Nesburn AB. Bandage soft contact lenses. In: Kaufman HE, Barron BA, McDonald MB, Waltman SR, eds. *The cornea.* New York: Churchill Livingstone, 1988:647–667.

Table 10-5. Complications of Therapeutic Lenses

Complications secondary to therapeutic lens fitting
  Variation in lens fit
  Lens settling
  Torn or lost lens
Complications secondary to therapeutic lens wear
  Lens drying
    Nocturnal lagophthalmos
    Lagophthalmos secondary to ptosis repair or blepharoplasty
  Infection
    Microbial keratitis (bacterial, fungal, viral)
    Corneal ulceration
    Masking symptoms of infectious keratitis (54)
    Blepharitis and meibomitis
    Conjunctivitis (bacterial)
  Corneal edema (from hypoxia)
    Acute secondary to tightly fitted lens
    Chronic secondary to increased stromal thickness
  Tight lens syndrome
  Sterile corneal infiltrates and hypopyon
  Corneal neovascularization
  Superficial punctate keratopathy
  Contact lens deposits (55)
    Lipoid transparent deposits
    Proteinaceous plaque-like deposits
    Calcium deposits
  Giant papillary conjunctivitis
  Glaucoma (often preexisting)
  Pseudodendrites
  Corneal radial wrinkling
  Subepithelial corneal opacities
  Abnormalities of corneal surface
    Deficiency or abnormality of corneal wetting
    Epithelial and basement membrane hyperplasia
  Alterations in corneal curvature and sensation
  Atypical amiodarone-induced keratopathy (56)
  Increased risk of infections after corneal transplantation (57)
  Corneal immune ring (58)

Source: Modified from Maguen E, Nesburn AB. Bandage soft contact lenses. In: Kaufman HE, Barron BA, McDonald MB, Waltman SR, eds. *The cornea.* New York: Churchill Livingstone, 1988:647–667.

methods for contact lens disinfection (63,64). After exposure, there was little clinical effect on the contact lens evaluated. Also, heparin at a concentration 1000IU/mL, either included in contact lens solutions or bonded to the surface of the contact lens, decreases adherence of *Pseudomonas aeruginosa* to soft contact lenses (65).

Collagen Shield

In addition to soft and hard therapeutic contact lenses, another type of corneal bandage, the collagen shield, has become available for short-term protection of the cornea after surgery, trauma, or nontraumatic corneal surface disorders (66).

The collagen shield was first described by Aquavella et al in 1988 (67). It consists of a thin (0.0127–0.7100 mm) film of sterile non-cross-linked porcine scleral collagen. The power is plano. The shield is available in a dehydrated state. After it is applied to the anesthetized eye, it absorbs fluid from the tears and conforms to the shape of the cornea.

Collagen shields serve as short-term bandage lenses. The advantages over soft contact lenses are that they do not require fitting. Collagen shields seem to absorb medications well and if hydrated initially with antibiotics, appear to provide high sustained levels of antibiotics to the cornea for a long time. In rabbits, collagen corneal shields, compared to hydrophilic soft contact lenses, allow increased antibiotic (tobramycin) penetration into the anterior chamber (68,69).

Collagen shields can also be used in conjunction with soft therapeutic lenses. A disposable bandage soft contact lens piggybacked onto a medicated, 12-hour corneal collagen shield can promote postoperative corneal epithelial healing and provide sustained delivery of high levels of medications after corneal surgery in patients known to have poor corneal epithelial wound-healing characteristics (70).

LAMELLAR KERATOPLASTY

Von Walther first described the concept of lamellar grafting in 1840 (71). Over the years, many other corneal surgeons refined this technique. However, with the simultaneous increasing degree of success and advancement of penetrating keratoplasty, lamellar (partial-thickness) grafting has become less fashionable. Only a very small percentage of the new group of corneal surgeons trained today has had firsthand experience with this procedure. To many, this procedure is technically more difficult than penetrating keratoplasty. The indications for lamellar grafting are fewer than those for penetrating grafting. Nevertheless, there are conditions in which lamellar keratoplasty would be the ideal choice. In particular, it is an important technique for patients with destructive corneal diseases, in which the addition of corneal tissue, to build up corneal substance lost through the destructive process, is an important goal.

Currently, there are two basic techniques of lamellar grafting practiced in the United States: inlay and onlay lamellar keratoplasty.

Indications for Inlay Lamellar Keratoplasty

Superficial Stromal Pathology

Lamellar corneal grafts are used for the replacement of abnormal superficial cornea such as superficial scars. However, superficial degenerations and dystrophies such as keratoconus, Salzmann's nodular degeneration, and Reis-Bücklers corneal dystrophy can also be treated with lamellar grafting. In a recent study, corneal dystrophies were the most common indications for lamellar keratoplasty at Moorfields Eye Hospital, accounting for 28.6% of cases (72). Other indications for lamellar keratoplasty include pterygium (73), scleral and corneal ulcers, necrosis, ectasia, xanthogranuloma of the corneoscleral limbus (74,75), perforations, and melts (76). A lamellar dissection of the patient's cornea is performed to sufficient depth to remove opaque or pathologic tissue, and a partial-thickness (lamellar) donor cornea of similar thickness is sutured into the dissection bed. Therapeutic lamellar keratectomy may also be used in the management of nontuberculous *Mycobacterium* keratitis refractory to medical treatments (77,78), where corneal infiltration and infection can be removed via a freehand technique to provide a clear stromal bed.

Tectonic Purposes

Inlay lamellar grafting can also be used to add corneal substance to build up a base that is being destroyed (tectonic graft). Such destructive processes may include degenerative conditions such as pellucid degeneration, Terrien's degeneration (79), and Mooren's ulceration (80); inflammatory problems such as peripheral ulcerative keratitis, Stevens-Johnson syndrome, and rheumatoid arthritis (80); sterile "melting" of the cornea; and infectious stromal ulcers with resulting perforation. In these conditions, lamellar corneal grafting is the procedure of choice to re-establish the integrity of the globe, after antibiotic therapy has been initiated. Lamellar keratoplasty may eliminate the risk of graft rejection and rescue the risk of perforation in the event of subsequent exacerbation of the inflammatory or melting process. Lamellar grafts may then be followed by placement of a full-thickness penetrating graft for visual rehabilitation.

Indications for Onlay Lamellar Keratoplasty (Epikeratophakia)

Epikeratophakia has been developed for refractive purposes. In this procedure, no corneal stromal substance is removed (except for a small annular keratectomy in the periphery, at the site at which the onlay graft will be sutured), and the donor tissue is laid onto the bare corneal stroma of the recipient.

This surgery, still considered by many to be in an investigational stage, has been employed as a refractive technique in individuals with aphakia, myopia, keratoconus, keratoglobus, or pellucid corneal degeneration.

Commercially available lenses, freeze dried or unfrozen, are ordered with specifications to meet the refractive needs of the patient. Plus lenses can be used to correct aphakia in adults and children. Plano lenses, used as an onlay lamellar graft, can reinforce and flatten a keratoconic cornea. Minus lenses can be used to correct myopia of even a high degree, but myopic epikeratoplasty is less accurate and less stable compared with the other epikeratoplasty procedures (81).

Technique for Inlay Lamellar Keratoplasty

As with any procedure, the details of the technique, including the choice of instruments, vary with individual surgeons. However, the general principles are as follows (82). Our preferred techniques are the same as those described and illustrated for lamellar patch grafts.

Recipient Preparation

Lamellar grafting is a major surgical procedure, and thus the patient should be prepared as patients for any major ophthalmic surgery.

1. Lid separation should be performed in the usual way, making sure that the lids, lashes, and meibomian glands are isolated from the surgical field to prevent contamination. Superior and inferior rectus bridal sutures are not recommended. Instead, episcleral sutures are preferred for special stabilization of the globe.
2. Further preparation of the recipient will vary, depending on the disease entity. Patients with keratoconus or pellucid degeneration will require minimal stromal dissection. After the initial partial-thickness trephination encompassing all of the pathology, and the initiation of a stromal dissection in the periphery with a lamellar dissector, the recipient corneal lamellae can often be removed by a peeling technique, in which the edge of the corneal tissue is grasped with two forceps and is steadily, firmly pulled, allowing the separation of the lamellae. This process can be facilitated with blunt dissection, even with a dry cellulose sponge, at the interface between the tissue being removed and the cornea left behind.

   For patients who need deeper keratectomy, such as those with anterior corneal stromal scarring, automated keratectomy may be used. The quality of the dissection bed is quite good when the keractectomy is performed in this way.
3. Patients with extensive, moderately deep destruction will require extensive lamellar dissection after peripheral trephination, and the disection often must be done freehand. The trephine should encompass the geographic extent of the pathology, and the incision should be deep enough to allow the

lamellar dissection to include all of the tissue that is being actively destroyed. The interface should be kept dry. The corneal splitter or lamellar dissector is employed in such a way that the collagen fibers, as the lamellar button is being dissected from the recipient cornea, are gently dissected at the area at which the fibers join the bottom of the button. In this way, any inclination to dissect deeper into the recipient bed, and inadvertently perforate the eye, can be avoided. In addition, air can be injected into the corneal stroma to expand it to several times its normal thickness. This method is designed to facilitate dissection of the deep stroma and reduce the risk of perforation of Descemet's membrane when carrying out deep lamellar keratoplasty (83).

4. Either a vacuum or a nonvacuum trephine can be employed to accomplish the initial trephination. If the globe has been perforated, a vacuum trephine is preferred. If the vacuum cannot be accomplished, an ultrasharp, disposable trephine blade without the handle attached is preferred so that one can look through the trephine and see the centration of the blade around the pathology and can more accurately judge the depth of the trephination. Air or viscoelastic material, or both, instilled into the anterior chamber of a perforated globe can sometimes be used to produce a more firm globe, facilitating the trephination step. If the perforation is less than 3 mm, cyanoacrylate tissue adhesive can usually be used to close the perforation sufficiently to allow trephination.

5. Irregular, peripheral areas of corneal destruction, such as those seen in peripheral ulcerative keratitis, are best managed through *freehand* techniques. The freehand partial-thickness dissection can be performed with a 15-degree microsharp disposable blade to outline the area to be resected. The edge of this incision is then grasped, and the lamellar dissection of the tissue to be removed is accomplished in the manner described previously. The final step in preparing the lamellar bed, regardless of whether it has been done freehand in the periphery or with the trephine more centrally, is undermining the edge of the lamellar bed, with a Desmarres knife or a Paufique knife. This allows for the most perfect suture placement when the donor material is sutured into the lamellar bed.

Donor Preparation

1. Donor material is most easily dissected from a whole donor eyeball. An incision is made at the corneoscleral limbus, with a No. 15 Bard-Parker blade, to the approximate depth needed for the thickness of the lamellar graft (Fig. 10-12).

2. A Martinez angled corneal splitter or lamellar dissector is then used to accomplish a lamellar

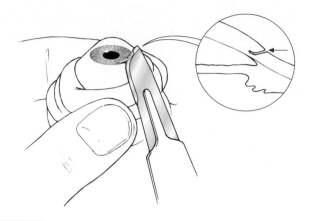

FIGURE 10-12. *Lamellar keratoplasty, donor preparation, limbal incision. A Bard-Parker blade is used to create an angled groove in the deep stroma over 90 degrees of the circumference.*

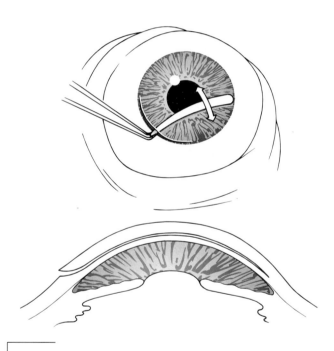

FIGURE 10-13. *Lamellar keratoplasty, donor preparation, lamellar dissection. Broad sweeping motions are used to split the lamellae by blunt dissection.*

dissection or splitting of the entire cornea of the donor eye (Fig. 10-13).

3. The trephine of the appropriate size for harvesting the donor button is then used to trephine through the entire surface of the cornea, obtaining a disk of donor material (Fig. 10-14). We generally employ a trephine size 0.25 to 0.50 mm larger than the size of the trephine used to prepare the recipient bed.

4. The edge of the donor disk is then beveled with Vannas scissors under the operating microscope, producing a watch-glass edge that because of its

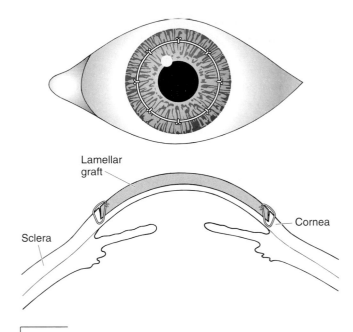

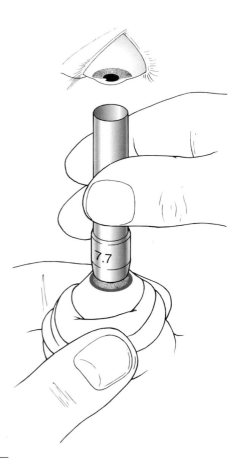

FIGURE 10-15. *Lamellar keratoplasty, lamellar graft sutured in place.*

FIGURE 10-14. *Lamellar keratoplasty, donor preparation, trephining the button. A corneal trephine is used to obtain the desired donor button; the trephination is centered by direct observation.*

thinness and shape, will fit well into the edge of the dissection bed of the recipient.

An alternative graft source is precarved lamellar corneal graft material supplied primarily for onlay epikeratophakia (Keratopatch, Allergan Medical Optics, Irvine, CA). In addition, Tayyib et al (84) and colleagues have reported the use of lathed freeze-dried corneal tissue in the treatment of corneal scarring by lamellar keratoplasty.

5. Interrupted sutures of 10-0 nylon, with buried knots, are used for securing the lamellar graft into the dissection bed (Fig. 10-15). Sutures should be well tied and tight, and the wound apposition perfect to prevent possible graft-host interface disparity problems, which can damage a successful outcome of lamellar grafting. Compression on top of the graft with a Paton spatula by the assistant is sometimes necessary to ensure that the sutures can be tightened sufficiently. In cases of lamellar grafting for keratoconus, it is sometimes necessary to decompress the globe slightly through a peripheral paracentesis wound, to sufficiently flatten the cone to allow perfect apposition of the donor edge to the recipient bed.

6. Perforations in the recipient bed pose a special problem. The perforation may be a preexisting one, as in the case of a patient who presents for the first time with a corneal ulcer that has perforated, or the perforation may be iatrogenic, inadvertently produced during the course of the lamellar dissection. The latter instance is highly undesirable and is usually avoidable. In any case, the presence of a perforation indicates that aqueous will have access to the potential space between the lamellar tissue and the recipient's cornea. Such access can result in the accumulation of large amounts of aqueous between the donor and recipient tissues, creating a pseudo anterior chamber. This undesirable situation can be obviated through the use of a mattress suture, which pulls the recipient cornea up against the back of the donor material. A 10-0 nylon double-armed mattress suture is used to clinch the recipient cornea tightly up against the back of the donor lamellar graft. This double-armed mattress stitch is full thickness to ensure a tight fit.

Technique for Onlay Lamellar Keratoplasty

There are even fewer corneal surgeons who perform onlay lamellar keratoplasty than those who do inlay keratoplasty. Nevertheless, there is no single and absolute method. However, the general steps of this technique can be described as follows (82).

Recipient Preparation

1. The epithelium is removed out to within 0.50 mm of the limbus. Epithelial removal can be facilitated through the use of 70% ethanol or 4% cocaine applied to the epithelium to be removed, taking great care not to allow these chemicals to damage the peripheral epithelium and the stem cells. A spatula is used to remove the epithelium, and great care is taken to irrigate and aspirate (with suction) all epithelium and debris from the surgical site.

2. The visual axis is marked, and a twin-blade vacuum trephine is centered over the visual axis. The trephine is used to create an incision that is 0.3 mm deep at the outer incision and 0.1 mm deep at the inner cut.

3. The tissue delimited by these incisions is then removed with Vannas scissors, creating an annular keratectomy. Again, vigorous irrigation and aspiration and cleaning of debris is critical to prevent the entrapment, eventually, of foreign material in the graft-host interface.

Donor Preparation

1. The commercially obtained donor material (Keratopatch, Allergan Medical Optics, Irvine, CA) is rehydrated for 20 minutes in balanced salt solution containing 100 microgram of gentamicin per milliliter.

2. This rehydrated donor material, ordered with the desired diameter and refractive power, is vigorously cleaned by irrigation and aspiration, and then secured onto the prepared recipient bed with 16 interrupted 10-0 nylon sutures, with the edge tucked into the annular keratectomy and the knots buried after they have been tied while the assistant compresses and flattens the cornea with a Paton spatula.

Complications of Lamellar Keratoplasty

Among the most common reasons for failure of lamellar grafts are corneal melting and sloughing of the graft (76). Other fearful complications may be inadvertent iatrogenic perforation of the recipient globe. This can be avoided by paying careful attention to the details of the technique, particularly keeping the lamellar dissection directed to the collagen fibers standing out in relief as one pulls up on the material being removed and keeping the dissection directed to the area where these fibers adjoin the material being removed.

Neovascularization of the graft-host interface is another complication. Therefore, lamellar grafting is rarely employed for patients with herpes simplex keratopathy sufficient to require grafting or with other similar disease entities that are often associated with peripheral corneal neovascularization.

Even if the graft and the graft-host wound apposition and suture tightness are perfect, peripheral stromal neovascularization will proliferate into the graft-host interface. The final result will be impaired vision, photophobia, and the creation of a high-risk penetrating graft recipient whose prospects for successful penetrating keratoplasty without transplant rejection have been substantially lowered because of neovascularization.

Formation of a pseudo anterior chamber because of an inadequately treated perforation is also a highly undesirable complication, as it will prevent healing between the graft material and the recipient bed and will produce poor vision. Foreign material in the graft interface and a poor dissection with an irregular surface in the bed of the recipient cornea will also produce poor vision.

Poor wound apposition with step formation can result in problems with re-epithelialization of the graft surface. Recurrent erosions or persistent epithelial defects may then develop.

CONCLUSIONS

The general principles, including the steps, instruments, and materials, of four different techniques of tectonic procedures—tissue adhesive application, patch grafting, use of therapeutic contact lenses, and lamellar keratoplasty—are being applied at our institution and others mentioned. However, they can be modified to be more compatible with any condition or situation. These techniques can be used to grant immediate closure of corneal perforation or to prevent complete perforation in preparation for a more definite treatment. Some of these procedures are not commonly performed by corneal surgeons and other ophthalmologists. However, all of these techniques can be very useful in specific pathologic conditions, and thus should be known as available tools in the armamentarium of ophthalmic surgeons.

REFERENCES

1. Refojo MF. Evaluation of adhesives for corneal surgery. *Arch Ophthalmol* 1968;80:645.
2. Bansal DC, Sandhu PS, Khosla AD. Clinical evaluation of cyanoacrylate glue in corneal perforations. *Indian J Ophthalmol* 1987;35:197–199.
3. Ginsberg SP, Brightbill FS. Corneal thinning and perforation. In: Brightbill FS, ed. *Corneal surgery: theory, technique, and tissue.* St. Louis: Mosby-Year Book, 1993:339–351.
4. Golubovic S, Parunovic A. Cyanoacrylate glue in the treatment of corneal ulcerations. *Fortschr Ophthalmol* 1990;87:378–381.
5. Shorr N, Cohen MS, Lessner A. Histoacryl closure of eyelid skin grafts. *Ophthalmic Plast Reconstr Surg* 1991;7:190–193.
6. Kenyon KR, Starck T, Wagoner MD. Corneal epithelial defects and noninfectious ulcerations. In: Albert DM, Jakobiec FA, eds. *Principles and practice of ophthalmology.* Philadelphia: WB Saunders, 1994:218–234.
7. Parrish CM, Chandler JW. Corneal trauma. In: Kaufman HE, Barron BA, McDonald MB, Waltman SR, eds. *The cornea.* New York: Churchill Livingstone, 1988:599–646.
8. Liesegang TJ. Bacterial and fungal keratitis. In: Kaufman HE, Barron BA, McDonald MB, Waltman SR, eds. *The cornea.* New York: Churchill Livingstone, 1988.

9. Hersh PS, Shingleton BJ, Kenyon KR. Anterior segment trauma. In: Albert DM, Jakobiec FA, eds. *Principles and practice of ophthalmology*. Philadelphia: WB Saunders, 1994:3383–3403.

10. Wagoner MD, Kenyon KR, Foster CS. Management strategies in peripheral ulcerative keratitis. *Int Ophthalmol Clin* 1986;26:147–157.

11. Gasset AR. Ocular tolerance to cyanoacrylate monomer tissue adhesive analogues. *Invest Ophthalmol* 1970;9:3.

12. Lehman RAW, West RL, Leonard F. Toxicity of alkyl 2-cyanoacrylates. *Archiv Surg* 1966;93:477.

13. Ginsberg SP, Polack FM. Cyanoacrylate tissue adhesive in occular disease. *Ophthalmic Surg* 1972;3:126.

14. Wessels IF, McNeil JI. Applicator for cyanoacrylate tissue adhesive. *Ophthalmic Surg* 1989;20:211–214.

15. Cavanaugh TB, Gottsch JD. Infectious keratitis and cyanoacrylate adhesive. *Am J Ophthalmol* 1991;11:466–472.

16. Carlson AN, Wilhelmus KR. Giant papillary conjunctivitis associated with cyanoacrylate glue. *Am J Ophthalmol* 1987;104:437–438.

17. Markowitz GD, et al. Corneal endothelial polymerization of histoacryl adhesive: a report of a new intraocular complication. *Ophthalmic Surg* 1995;26:256–258.

18. Siegal JE, Zaidman GW. Surgical removal of cyanoacrylate adhesive after accidental instillation in the anterior chamber. *Ophthalmic Surg* 1989;20:179–181.

19. Toriumi DM, et al. Histotoxicity of cyanoacrylate tissue adhesives. A comparative study. *Arch Otolaryngol Head Neck Surg* 1990;116:546–550.

20. Dean BS, Krenzelok EP. Cyanoacrylates and corneal abrasion. *J Toxicol Clin Toxicol* 1989;27:169–172.

21. Leahey AB, Gottsch JD, Stark WJ. Clinical experience with *N*-butyl cyanoacrylate (Nexacryl) tissue adhesive. *Ophthalmology* 1993;100:173–180.

22. Kim MS, Kim JH. Effects of tissue adhesive (Tisseel) on corneal wound healing in lamellar keratoplasty in rabbits. *Korean J Ophthalmol* 1989;3:14–21.

23. Henrick A, Gaster RN, Silverstone PJ. Organic tissue glue in the closure of cataract incisions. *J Cataract Refract Surg* 1987;13:551–553.

24. Mandel MA. Closure of blepharoplasty incisions with autologous fibrin glue. *Arch Ophthalmol* 1990;108:842–844.

25. Gundersen T. Conjunctival flaps in the treatment of corneal disease with reference to a new technique of application. *Arch Ophthalmol* 1958;60:880–888.

26. Raju VK. Corneal surgery. In: Duane TD, Jaeger EA, eds. *Clinical ophthalmology*. Philadelphia: Harper & Row, 1984.

27. Doughman DJ. Corneal thinnings and perforations. In: Lindquist TD, Lindstrom RL, eds. *Ophthalmic surgery*. Littleton, MA: Year Book Medical, 1990:II-C-0–II-C-14.

28. Melamed S, et al. Donor scleral graft patching for persistent filtration bleb leak. *Ophthalmic Surg* 1991;22:164–165.

29. Rubinfeld RS, et al. Serious complications of topical mitomycin-C after pterygium surgery. *Ophthalmology* 1992;99:1647–1654.

30. Insler MS, Tauber S, Packer A. Descemetocele formation in a patient with a postoperative corneal dellen. *Cornea* 1989;8:129–130.

31. Soong HK, et al. Corneal hydrops in Terrien's marginal degeneration. *Ophthalmology* 1986;93:340–343.

32. Karr DJ, Grutzmacher RD, Reeh MJ. Radial keratotomy complicated by sterile keratitis and corneal perforation. Histopathologic case report and review of complications. *Ophthalmology* 1985;92:1244–1248.

33. Fujitani A, et al. Corneoscleral ulceration and corneal perforation after pterygium excision and topical mitomycin C therapy. *Ophthalmologica* 1993;207:162–164.

34. Nobe JR. Results of penetrating keratoplasty for the treatment of corneal perforations. *Arch Ophthalmol* 1990;108:939–947.

35. Huang WJ, Hu FR, Chang SW. Clinicopathologic study of Gore-Tex patch graft in corneoscleral surgery. *Cornea* 1994;13:82–86.

36. Whitmore WG, Harrison W, Curtin BJ. Scleral reinforcement in rabbits using synthetic graft materials. *Ophthalmic Surg* 1990;21:327–330.

37. Brandt JD. Patch grafts of dehydrated cadaveric dura mater for tube-shunt glaucoma surgery. *Arch Ophthalmol* 1993;111:1436–1439.

38. Thoft RA. Therapeutic soft contact lenses. *Int Ophthalmol Clin* 1986;26:83–90.

39. Thoft RA. Therapeutic soft contact lenses. In: Smolin G, Thoft RA, eds. *The cornea: scientific foundations and clinical practice*. Boston: Little, Brown, 1987:591–604.

40. Refojo MF. Materials in bandage lenses. *Contact Intraocular Lens Med J* 1979;5:34–44.

41. Maguen E, Nesburn AB. Bandage soft contact lenses. In: Kaufman HE, Barron BA, McDonald MB, Waltman SR, eds. *The cornea*. New York: Churchill Livingstone, 1988:647–667.

42. Destro M, Wallow IH, Brightbill FS. Recessive dystrophic epidermolysis bullosa. *Arch Ophthalmol* 1987;105:1248–1252.

43. Blok MD, et al. Use of the Megasoft Bandage Lens for treatment of complications after trabeculectomy. *Am J Ophthalmol* 1990;110:264–268.

44. Arshinoff S, et al. Use of topical nonsteroidal anti-inflammatory drugs in excimer lases photorefractive keratectomy. *J Cataract Refract Surg* 1994;20(suppl):216–222.

45. Mackie IA. Contact lenses in dry eyes. *Trans Ophthalmol Soc UK* 1985;104:47–483.

46. Mondino BJ, Zaidman GW, Salamon SW. Use of pressure patching and soft contact lenses in superior limbic keratoconjunctivitis. *Arch Ophthalmol* 1982;100:1932–1938.

47. Mondino BJ. Cicatricial pemphigoid and erythema multiforme. *Ophthalmology* 1990;97:939–952.

48. Tan DT, Pullum KW, Buckley RJ. Medical applications of scleral contact lenses: a retrospective analysis of 343 cases. *Cornea* 1995;14:121–129.

49. Kok JH, van Mil C. Piggyback lenses in keratoconus. *Cornea* 1993;12:60–64.

50. Lahoud S, et al. Keratoconus with spontaneous perforation of the cornea. *Can J Ophthalmol* 1987;22:230–233.

51. Kanpolat A, Ciftci OU. The use of rigid gas permeable contact lenses in scarred corneas. *CLAO J* 1995;21:64–66.

52. Yamaguchi K, Okabe H, Tamai M. Corneal perforation in a patient with Cockayne's syndrome. *Cornea* 1991;10:79–80.

53. Brown SI, et al. Infections with the therapeutic soft lens. *Arch Ophthalmol* 1974;91:275–284.

54. Lindquist TD, Cameron JD. Unsuspected infectious keratitis in host corneal buttons. *Surv Ophthalmol* 1989;33:359–365.

55. Tripathi PC, Tripathi RC. Analysis of glycoprotein deposits on disposable soft contact lenses. *Invest Ophthalmol Vis Sci* 1992;33:121–125.

56. Rivera RP, Younge BR, Dyer JA. Atypical amiodarone-induced keratopathy in a patient wearing soft contact lenses. *CLAO J* 1989;15:219–221.

57. Varley GA, Meisler DM. Complications of penetrating keratoplasty: graft infections. *Refract Corneal Surg* 1991;7:62–66.

58. Klein P. Corneal immune ring as a complication of soft extended wear contact lens use. *Optom Vis Sci* 1991;68:853–857.

59. Matoba AY, McCulley JP. The effect of therapeutic soft contact lenses on antibiotic delivery to the cornea. *Ophthalmology* 1985;92:97–99.

60. Jain MR. Drug delivery through soft contact lenses. *Br J Ophthalmol* 1988;72:150–154.

61. Rubenstein JB, Deutsch TA. Pneumatonometry through bandage contact lenses. *Arch Ophthalmol* 1985;103:1660–1661.

62. Mendelsohn AD, et al. Comparative tonometric measurements of eye bank eyes. *Cornea* 1987;6:219–225.

63. Harris MG, et al. Microwave irradiation and soft contact lens parameters. *Optom Vis Sci* 1993;70:843–848.

64. Harris MG, et al. Effects of ultraviolet radiation on contact lens parameters. *Optom Vis Sci* 1993;70:739–742.

65. Duran JA, et al. Heparin inhibits *Pseudomonas* adherence to soft contact lenses. *Eye* 1993;7:152–154.

66. Groden LR, White W. Porcine collagen corneal shield treatment of persistent epithelial defects following penetrating keratoplasty. *CLAO J* 1990;16:95–97.

67. Aquavella JV, et al. Therapeutic applications of a collagen bandage lens: a preliminary report. *CLAO J* 1988;14:47–54.

68. O'Brien TP, et al. Use of collagen corneal shields versus soft contact lenses to enhance penetration of topical tobramycin. *J Cataract Refract Surg* 1988;14:505–507.

69. Dorigo MT, De Natale R, Miglioli S. Collagen shields delivery of netilmicin: a study of ocular pharmacokinetics. *Chemotherapy* 1995;41:1–4.

70. Palmer RM, McDonald MB. A corneal lens/shield system to promote postoperative corneal epithelial healing. *J Cataract Refract Surg* 1995;21:125–126.

71. Rycroft BW. *Corneal grafts*. London: Butterworth, 1955.

72. Morris RJ, Bates AK. Changing indications for keratoplasty. *Eye* 1989;3:455–459.

73. Laughrea PA, Arentsen JJ. Lamellar keratoplasty in the management of recurrent pterygium. *Ophthalmic Surg* 1986;17:106–108.

74. Lewis JR, et al. Juvenile xanthogranuloma of the corneoscleral limbus. *Can J Ophthalmol* 1990;25:351–354.

75. Collum LM, et al. Limbal xanthogranuloma. *J Pediatr Ophthalmol Strabismus* 1991;28:157–159.

76. The Australian Corneal Graft Registry. The Australian Corneal Graft Registry: 1990–1992 report. *Austr NZ J Ophthalmol* 1993;21(suppl):1–48.

77. Hu FR. Extensive lamellar keratectomy for treatment of nontuberculous mycobacterial keratitis. *Am J Ophthalmol* 1995;120:47–54.
78. Tseng SH, Hsiao WC. Therapeutic lamellar keratectomy in the management of nontuberculous *Mycobacterium* keratitis refractory to medical treatments. *Cornea* 1995;14:161–166.
79. Pettit T. Corneoscleral freehand lamellar keratoplasty in Terrien's marginal degeneration of the cornea—long-term results. *Refract Corneal Surg* 1991;7:28–32.
80. Bessant DA, Dart JK. Lamellar keratoplasty in the management of inflammatory corneal ulceration and perforation. *Eye* 1994;8:22–28.
81. ISORK. Statement of epikeratoplasty—The Boards of Directors of the International Society of Refractive Keratoplasty. *Refract Corneal Surg* 1989;5:33–38.
82. Foster CS. Lamellar keratoplasty. In: Albert DA, Jakobiec FA, eds. *Principles and practice of ophthalmology.* Philadelphia: WB Saunders, 1994:319–325.
83. Chau GK, et al. Deep lamellar keratoplasty on air with lyophilized tissue. *Br J Ophthalmol* 1992;76:646–650.
84. Tayyib M, et al. Lamellar keratoplasty with lyophilized tissue for treatment of corneal scarring. *Refract Corneal Surg* 1993;9:140–142.

Excimer Laser Phototherapeutic Keratectomy: Principles, Techniques, and Results

Timothy B. Cavanaugh   Paul E. Cutarelli   Andrew A. Aziz

In the past, anterior corneal pathology such as scars often required mechanical removal with superficial keratectomy or lamellar or penetrating keratoplasty. Mechanical superficial keratectomy usually involves removal of epithelium and anterior corneal pathology with a No. 64 Beaver blade. While the blade is a very effective tool for epithelial debridement, removal of subepithelial or anterior stromal lesions in this manner can result in a rough surface that provides suboptimal acuity. Mechanical debridement may also remove an opacity but leave an irregular tissue depression or "divot" which, although clear, may contribute to irregular astigmatism. Alternative treatment for a pathologic irregular corneal surface has traditionally been either hard contact lenses or partial- or full-thickness keratoplasty.

Excimer laser phototherapeutic keratectomy (PTK) is a new procedure to treat anterior corneal disease that provides superior results with less cost, risk, and morbidity. PTK removes anterior corneal pathology in a precise, controlled fashion and leaves behind a remarkably smooth stromal surface, which enhances corneal clarity and promotes uniform re-epithelialization with re-formation of basement membrane complexes even in the absence of Bowman's layer (1–3). In this fashion, the PTK-treated stromal surface not only can prevent corneal erosion but also yields the quality refractive surface necessary for good visual acuity (4–7). The excimer laser is the best corneal polishing tool developed to date. The diamond burr is sometimes used to polish the corneal surface following mechanical keratectomy with a blade but the smoothness of the resultant surface is clearly inferior to the surface achieved with excimer PTK (8). PTK has a distinct advantage over mechanical superficial keratectomy in that topically applied masking agents may be used during ablation in PTK to provide a smoothing effect in the area of pathology (4,5).

EXCIMER PHOTOABLATION OF THE CORNEA

Mechanism

The excimer laser utilizes high-energy ultraviolet light of 193 nm emitted from a decaying dimer of argon and fluoride gas laser to photoablate corneal tissue with exquisite precision on the micron order of magnitude (9,10). The term *excimer* is a combination of "excited" and "dimer," which refers to a high-energy dimerization of two normally unreactive elements, argon and fluoride. This association is achieved only with the aid of a very-high-voltage electric field forcing the two gases together (9). Because the high-energy excited dimer is inherently unstable, it rapidly decays to release the energy in the form of a photon of light. These photons are amplified and collimated to form a coherent, monochromatic laser beam (9–11). Compared with other ophthalmic lasers, the interaction of the excimer laser beam with corneal tissue is unique owing to its ability to impart extremely high levels of energy to corneal tissue while generating virtually no heat or causing optical breakdown (9–11). The photochemical reaction that occurs is termed *ablative photodecomposition*, which involves the disruption of organic molecular bonds in corneal tissue. Ultraviolet excimer laser light of 193 nm is extremely well absorbed by the covalent molecular bonds (the carbon-nitrogen linkage in peptide bonds and carbon-carbon bonds) which hold together the major macromolecules of the type I collagen and glycosaminoglycan in the corneal stroma and epithelium. The bonding energy of the macromolecular bonds for carbon-nitrogen measure about 3.0 eV while the energy of the carbon-carbon bonds is about 3.5 eV. The 6.4-eV energy emitted from the excimer beam exceeds the macromolecular bond energy and is more than ample to easily break the bonds (9). Moreover, the bond is so rapidly broken that it does not vibrate in the process of breakage, thereby avoiding the absorption of heat. The excess 2.9 to 3.4 eV of energy imparts kinetic energy to the just unbonded molecules, causing the dense molecular configuration of the solid state to convert into the low-density, gaseous or vaporized state without heat or plasma formation. When generated by laser light, this rapid bond breakage and vaporization without heat generation is termed *photoablation* (9–11) and is unique to the excimer among ophthalmic lasers. The relatively nontraumatic nature of photoablative keratectomy is primarily responsible for the subsequent relative lack of tissue-healing response in the cornea, and the preservation of the precision of the excimer laser photoablative cut. The laser is so precise that it removes only 0.25 μm of cornea per pulse within treatment zones anywhere from 0.5 to 7.0 mm.

Histopathology of Wound Healing

Knowledge of the histopathology of corneal wound healing after excimer laser photoablation is key to a full appreciation of this laser's ability to remove pathology with such precision and without a significant adverse wound-healing response. PTK results in a very clear demarcation between treated and untreated cornea at the ultrastructural level immediately after the laser procedure is completed (9). The subsequent corneal wound-healing response results in very little tissue reorganization. This is in sharp contrast to corneal incisions made with steel or diamond blades, which produce relatively irregular and diffuse tissue damage boundaries (Fig. 11-1). The tissues adjacent to the area of PTK treatment undergo minimal distortion and sustain no apparent thermal damage following 193-nm excimer laser PTK; adjacent stromal lamellae show virtually no evidence of disorganization (9).

Waring (12) divided the temporal response of corneal wound healing after surface excimer laser photoablation into three phases: acute, intermediate, and late. The acute phase occurs over 1 to 3 weeks, intermediate phase over 3 weeks to 6 months, and late phase 6 months or later. The acute-phase response after excimer laser photoablation appears to resemble the typical corneal response to epithelial removal of any etiology. Fibronectin, a glycoprotein, appears in the corneal epithelial basement membrane region during the acute corneal wound-healing phase, presumably to enhance adhesion of migrating corneal epithelial cells. These cells will both migrate and divide to fill the epithelial defect. When the corneal epithelial defect heals in 2 to 4 days, the corneal stroma is usually clear on slit-lamp examination or exhibits a slight ground-glass appearance, but no frank haze. In the 1- to 3-week period after re-epithelialization the anterior stroma is notable for marked acellularity (i.e., a reduction of keratocytes). This missing population of keratocytes restores itself gradually over the course of the acute phase, which then gives way to the intermediate phase of corneal wound

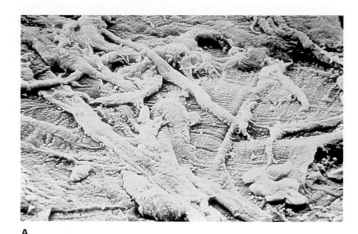

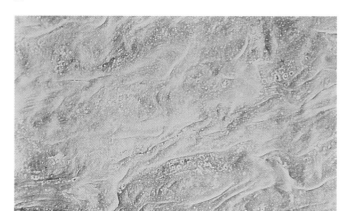

FIGURE 11-1.   *Corneal surface cut with a blade* (A) *compared to a surface cut with an excimer laser* (B).

healing. It is unclear whether the restoration of keratocyte numbers in the anterior stroma after excimer laser keratectomy is achieved exclusively by mitosis, migration, or a combination of both.

The intermediate phase of corneal wound healing after PTK is characterized by epithelial remodeling to a normal thickness. New attachment complexes, one component of which is type VII collagen anchoring fibril complex, form fibroblasts and begin to repopulate the anterior stroma and concomitantly secrete new extracellular matrix consisting of type III collagen and additional keratan sulfate proteoglycan. Clinically this may correspond to a phase of subepithelial haze formation.

The late phase of corneal healing after surface excimer laser photoablation is marked by corneal stromal remodeling. Type III and type VII stromal collagen associated with the anchoring fibril complex diminish gradually during the 18 to 24 months after photoablation. Clinically this late phase is associated with decreasing corneal haze and increased refractive stability. The duration of this phase is unknown; the potential for the late-phase corneal healing to revert to one with more intermediate-phase characteristics is debated. Late-onset corneal haze after excimer laser photoablation, although rare, may occur in a clear cornea 2 years after excimer laser treatment and anecdotally has been suggested to be precipitated by ultraviolet exposure.

BACKGROUND

In 1983, Trokel et al (10) proposed that the excimer laser could be used for precise keratectomy, either for controlled qualitative ablation of corneal pathology to restore clarity in PTK (4–7) or for quantitative modification of the corneal curvature during photorefractive keratectomy (PRK). In the United States in 1988, investigational clinical trials of PTK involving human subjects began under the close guidance of the Food and Drug Administration (FDA) and two laser manufacturers: Summit Technology (Waltham, MA) and VISX (Sunnyvale, CA). Our research site was involved in the Summit study, which consisted of 13 centers distributed across the country and a total of 249 PTK-treated eyes. All patients were over age 21 and placed into one of three treatment groups: corneal scars, irregular astigmatism, or recurrent corneal erosion. The VISX study consisted of 17 investigational sites with a total of 271 patients. It included four patient groups: corneal opacities, irregular corneal surface, superficial infectious keratitis resistant to medical therapy, and postsurgical refractive abnormalities. The clinical trial successfully proved the efficacy and safety of PTK, with both lasers receiving FDA approval in 1995.

PATIENT SELECTION

Consistent success with PTK depends on careful patient selection. Generally, candidates for PTK fall into three categories: those with corneal opacities, patients with irregular astigmatism, and those with recurrent corneal erosion. Often there is overlap between the groups (Fig. 11-2). Irregular astigmatism is not an infrequent complication of acquired corneal stromal opacity. For example, a patient with anterior lattice corneal dystrophy will have decreased acuity from the amyloid deposition as well as the irregular corneal surface induced by breakthrough of the lattice lines through Bowman's layer. This same patient will often present with bouts of pain consistent with recurrent erosion due to disruption of the normal epithelial adhesion complexes by the lattice deposits. PTK is potentially curative of all three problems.

All patients with significant surface irregularity should first try a gas-permeable contact lens and then undergo PTK if that fails. In addition, the contact lens trial can give the surgeon and patient an idea of potential visual improvement by smoothing the surface with laser. The ideal condition for PTK is an elevated anterior corneal opacity (especially stromal) in proximity to the visual axis that causes decreased visual acuity and irregular astigmatism in a myopic eye (4). The ideal patient for PTK fits the profile described in Table

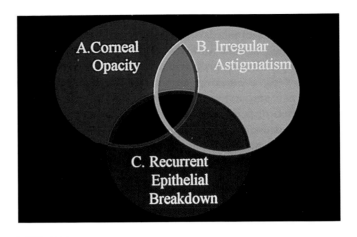

FIGURE 11-2. *Diagram depicting the overlap of indications for PTK. Corneal opacification, irregular astigmatism, and corneal erosion can often occur in the same patient.*

Table 11-1. Ideal Patient Criteria

Significant visual compromise
Pathology in anterior one-third of cornea
Elevated or flat opacity
Myopic
Under consideration for corneal transplantation
Realistic patient expectations for surgical outcome
Quiet, uninflamed eye
Recurrent erosion that does not respond to medical therapy

Table 11-2. Relative Contraindications

Pathology deeper than one-third depth
Tissue loss or depressed opacity
Thin preoperative cornea
Active ocular inflammation, e.g., uveitis
Hyperopic refractive error
Severe blepharitis
Lagophthalmos or poorly controlled dry eye
Collagen vascular diseases, e.g., rheumatoid arthritis
Immunosuppression
Unrealistic expectations for surgical outcome
Herpes simplex keratitis

11-1 and relative contraindications for PTK are listed in Table 11-2.

In general, patients should be informed about the possibility of the need for further corneal surgery such as penetrating keratoplasty should PTK fail. Treatment depth should not exceed 160 to 170μm, assuming an average central corneal thickness of 500μm. A good rule of thumb in thinner corneas is to always leave *at least* 250μm of corneal thickness after PTK; treatment deeper than that can result in instability and possibly ectasia over time. Although

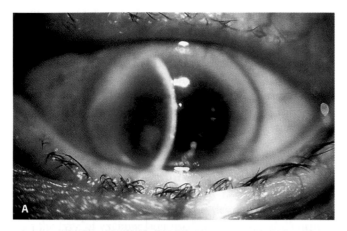

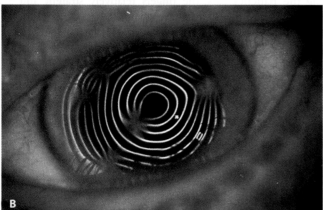

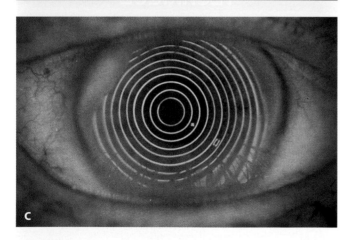

FIGURE 11-7.   *Preoperative photograph (A) showing multiple Salzmann's nodules causing both opacification and an irregular surface as demonstrated in the accompanying preoperative corneascope photograph (B). Dramatic corneal smoothing is seen on the 1-month postoperative corneascope photograph following PTK (C).*

Head Movement

Appropriate movement of the patient's head will facilitate corneal polishing maneuvers with PTK. When head movement is desired by the surgeon, he or she may initiate head movement prior to depressing the foot pedal so that the desired degree of excursion is being attained before the

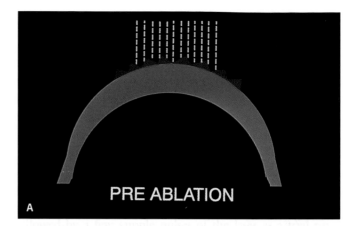

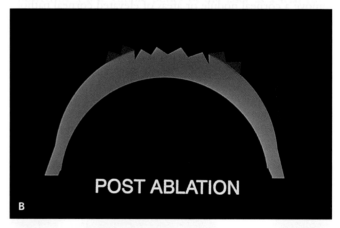

FIGURE 11-8.   A, B. *Diagrams demonstrating how the excimer laser will ablate an irregular surface deeper into the tissue without the use of a smoothing agent.*

photoablating begins. This familiarizes the patient with the concept of circular head movement while maintaining fixation on the green target light in the laser. Practice movement should always be conducted prior to the initiation of laser treatment.

Masking Agents

In recurrent erosion patients, a masking agent is rarely ever used and laser is applied directly to the affected Bowman's layer. For other patients, after mechanical removal of epithelium and any subepithelial scar tissue, the surgeon should assess the resulting corneal surface. If the surface is relatively smooth, the surgeon may then elect to proceed with PTK without a masking agent. In the vast majority of patients, however, the resultant surface is sufficiently irregular to warrant further smoothing adjuncts such as masking agents. When an excimer laser beam encounters an irregular corneal surface profile, it will ablate and remove corneal tissue but the pattern of the irregularity is preserved and etched into deeper corneal layers (4) (Fig. 11-8). Masking agents are variable-viscosity solutions of carboxymethylcellulose or similar substances that can be applied to an irregular corneal surface and act to regularize the "peaks and tics is debated. Late-onset corneal haze after excimer laser photoablation, although rare, may occur in a clear cornea 2 years after excimer laser treatment and anecdotally has been suggested to be precipitated by ultraviolet exposure.

BACKGROUND

In 1983, Trokel et al (10) proposed that the excimer laser could be used for precise keratectomy, either for controlled qualitative ablation of corneal pathology to restore clarity in PTK (4–7) or for quantitative modification of the corneal curvature during photorefractive keratectomy (PRK). In the United States in 1988, investigational clinical trials of PTK involving human subjects began under the close guidance of the Food and Drug Administration (FDA) and two laser manufacturers: Summit Technology (Waltham, MA) and VISX (Sunnyvale, CA). Our research site was involved in the Summit study, which consisted of 13 centers distributed across the country and a total of 249 PTK-treated eyes. All patients were over age 21 and placed into one of three treatment groups: corneal scars, irregular astigmatism, or recurrent corneal erosion. The VISX study consisted of 17 investigational sites with a total of 271 patients. It included four patient groups: corneal opacities, irregular corneal surface, superficial infectious keratitis resistant to medical therapy, and postsurgical refractive abnormalities. The clinical trial successfully proved the efficacy and safety of PTK, with both lasers receiving FDA approval in 1995.

PATIENT SELECTION

Consistent success with PTK depends on careful patient selection. Generally, candidates for PTK fall into three categories: those with corneal opacities, patients with irregular astigmatism, and those with recurrent corneal erosion. Often there is overlap between the groups (Fig. 11-2). Irregular astigmatism is not an infrequent complication of acquired corneal stromal opacity. For example, a patient with anterior lattice corneal dystrophy will have decreased acuity from the amyloid deposition as well as the irregular corneal surface induced by breakthrough of the lattice lines through Bowman's layer. This same patient will often present with bouts of pain consistent with recurrent erosion due to disruption of the normal epithelial adhesion complexes by the lattice deposits. PTK is potentially curative of all three problems.

All patients with significant surface irregularity should first try a gas-permeable contact lens and then undergo PTK if that fails. In addition, the contact lens trial can give the surgeon and patient an idea of potential visual improvement by smoothing the surface with laser. The ideal condition for PTK is an elevated anterior corneal opacity (especially stromal) in proximity to the visual axis that causes decreased visual acuity and irregular astigmatism in a myopic eye (4). The ideal patient for PTK fits the profile described in Table

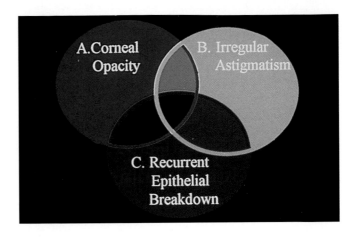

FIGURE 11-2.   *Diagram depicting the overlap of indications for PTK. Corneal opacification, irregular astigmatism, and corneal erosion can often occur in the same patient.*

Table 11-1.   Ideal Patient Criteria

Significant visual compromise
Pathology in anterior one-third of cornea
Elevated or flat opacity
Myopic
Under consideration for corneal transplantation
Realistic patient expectations for surgical outcome
Quiet, uninflamed eye
Recurrent erosion that does not respond to medical therapy

Table 11-2.   Relative Contraindications

Pathology deeper than one-third depth
Tissue loss or depressed opacity
Thin preoperative cornea
Active ocular inflammation, e.g., uveitis
Hyperopic refractive error
Severe blepharitis
Lagophthalmos or poorly controlled dry eye
Collagen vascular diseases, e.g., rheumatoid arthritis
Immunosuppression
Unrealistic expectations for surgical outcome
Herpes simplex keratitis

11-1 and relative contraindications for PTK are listed in Table 11-2.

In general, patients should be informed about the possibility of the need for further corneal surgery such as penetrating keratoplasty should PTK fail. Treatment depth should not exceed 160 to 170 μm, assuming an average central corneal thickness of 500 μm. A good rule of thumb in thinner corneas is to always leave *at least* 250 μm of corneal thickness after PTK; treatment deeper than that can result in instability and possibly ectasia over time. Although hyperopia is a relative contraindication for PTK, significant refractive shifts can be avoided with careful surgical technique. If the patient is well informed about the progression of hyperopia after surgery and is accepting of methods to treat it, such as wearing contact lenses, then hyperopic patients can be good candidates as well. Conversely, excessive ablation of peripheral corneal pathology can result in a myopic shift due to relative steepening of the central cornea induced by flattening of the periphery.

There has been some success in the treatment of herpetic corneal scars with PTK but these patients must also be well informed (13). Often herpes simplex virus (HSV) scars are flat or depressed and associated with tissue loss, so that treatment is difficult and can leave the patient with significant residual irregular astigmatism or large hyperopic shifts, or both. In addition, HSV keratitis can recur following PTK (14,15). Our recommendation is to pretreat HSV patients with oral acyclovir (400–800 mg five times a day) for 2 to 4 weeks preoperatively and for 4 to 12 weeks postoperatively on a tapering dose. This regimen is similar to what we use with penetrating keratoplasties on HSV patients and to date we have not seen any HSV recurrences with PTK.

INDICATIONS

As stated, patients for PTK typically fall into one of three categories. A wide variety of causes of corneal opacities and irregular surfaces have been described in the literature as being amenable to treatment using PTK, and these are listed in Table 11-3. The list is self-explanatory but one must remember to adhere to the patient selection criteria mentioned previously when considering each of these indications, in order to maximize positive results (16–28). We have personally had experience with PTK for each of these indications (except Meesman's dystrophy, shield ulcers, intraep-

ithelial dysplasia, and infectious crystalline keratopathy), with successful results. Although some of the listed dystrophies are stromal, PTK can fully treat the anterior varieties of these and partially treat those that extend deeper into the stroma with improvement in visual function by smoothing the corneal surface and reducing the amount of opacification. In this way, it may delay the need for keratoplasty in some patients. Painful recurrent corneal erosion or nonhealing epithelial defects have traditionally been treatment challenges and a source of considerable distress to patients. Excimer PTK has a definite role in treating a variety of epithelial adherence problems, as presented in Table 11-4. Although the mechanism for the re-establishment of epithelial basement membrane complexes with PTK is poorly understood, its remarkable effectiveness in treating recurrent corneal erosion syndrome recalcitrant to medical and standard surgical therapies has been well documented (29–34). Candidates for PTK for corneal erosion should first undergo medical therapy with lubricants, hyperosmotics, and bandage contact lenses and should proceed to PTK if this fails. In addition, surgical adjuncts such as corneal epithelial debridement with or without diamond burr polishing and stromal micropuncture have good success rates. But it is the author's strong bias that PTK is far superior to both of the aforementioned and should be considered first. Little or no scarring results from PTK in contrast to micropuncture whose very mechanism depends on the inducement of stromal scars: This procedure has no value in erosions involving the visual axis. We performed five to six PTKs on patients with recurrent erosion in whom previous micropuncture failed, and achieved a 100% cure rate. The success of PTK in the treatment of long-standing neurotrophic or similar epithelial defects is a mystery as well. It is postulated that the laser smooths the damaged Bowman's membrane or anterior stroma to provide better substrate for epithelial adherence. We strongly recommend the concurrent use of adjunctive therapy with bandage contact lenses or lateral tarsorrhaphies following PTK in this group of patients.

SURGICAL TECHNIQUE

Basic Concepts

Excimer PTK can be one of the most challenging surgical procedures to perform. A number of surgical skills are used.

Table 11-3.   Indications for PTK in Patients with Corneal Opacity or Irregular Astigmatism

Anterior corneal dystrophies (17)
    Anterior membrane dystrophy
    Reis-Buckler's dystrophy (18,19)
    Lattice dystrophy
    Granular dystrophy
    Macular dystrophy (20)
    Schnyder's crystalline dystrophy
    Meesman's dystrophy
    Recurrent dystrophies after keratoplasty (21)
Anterior corneal scars; postinfectious or posttraumatic (22,23)
Salzmann's nodular degeneration (24)
Band keratopathy
Postpterygium scars
Keratoconus apical scars (25,26)
Shield ulcers and corneal plaques in vernal (27)
Recurrent corneal intraepithelial dysplasia (28)
Infectious crystalline keratopathy (29)

Table 11-4.   Indications for PTK in Patients with Corneal Erosion/Persistent Epithelial Defect

Recurrent erosion syndrome secondary to basement membrane dystrophy (30–33)
Traumatic recurrent erosion syndrome
Idiopathic recurrent erosion syndrome
Bullous keratopathy–associated recurrent erosion (34,35)
Neurotrophic keratopathy
Nonhealing epithelial defects after keratoplasty

These include hand position, head movement, epithelial debridement, transepithelial ablation, use of masking agents, and polishing. The use of masking agents requires the most experience and is the basis for statements referring to the art of PTK. The excimer computer-controlled software can lull the surgeon into a false sense of security but unlike its PRK counterpart, the PTK technique is very surgeon dependent. Each patient is different and the surgeon must not only understand the preoperative pathology and corneal topographic profile extremely well but also be focused on the proper end point for the surgery. The surgical technique will vary with the type of corneal pathology. The three principal types of corneal pathology that dictate the surgical approach are corneal opacity, corneal stromal irregularity, and corneal epithelial adhesion abnormality (e.g., recurrent erosion syndrome) (4).

Our experience has been with the Summit Omnimed excimer laser and the description of the surgical technique reflects the suggested technique for this machine. In addition, the procedure described is one surgeon's bias and it should be noted that technique can vary not only between surgeons but also between laser systems.

Preoperative Evaluation

All new patients under consideration for PTK should have a complete ophthalmic examination including obtaining of a general medical history and review of medications being taken, to exclude any patients who fall into the contraindicated categories outlined in Table 11-2. Visual acuity with and without correction, phorometry (Phoropter) refraction, measurement of intraocular pressure (IOP), careful slit-lamp examination, and dilated fundus examination should all be performed. Irregular astigmatism and surface profile should be evaluated by keratometry, corneascopy, computerized corneal topography, or a combination of these procedures. Standard keratometry is often suboptimal owing to the limited surface area evaluated and Placido disk–type evaluations are generally superior looking for distortion in the central two or three mires. Although corneal topography provides the greatest amount of detail, the color maps can sometimes be overinterpreted by the computer's smoothing software and can be potentially misleading to the surgeon. Because of this, we always recommend comparison of the color map with the clinical appearance and the Placido disk image to aid in surgical planning. The degree of irregular astigmatism from corneal epithelial irregularity can be quite striking, with as high as 3 diopters (D) measured by Placido disk topography. Slit-lamp photographs to document preoperative clinical appearance and for comparison to postoperative photographs may be indicated. The potential for improvement in visual acuity from elimination of the irregular astigmatism or para-axial opacification is estimated by pinhole vision, potential acuity meter (PAM), and wearing of a rigid gas-permeable contact lens over refraction. Decreased visual acuity from a corneal stromal opacity is measured objectively with comparison to the patient's visual

loss tolerance and lifestyle and from these data a risk-benefit assessment is made, as one might do in the case of cataract. Photophobia and glare in the setting of anterior stromal opacity are assessed subjectively with respect to symptoms and objectively for the attendant decreased visual acuity caused by the opacity. Brightness acuity testing can be a useful adjunct to quantify the degree of degradation of visual acuity. Preoperative corneal thickness is measured by ultrasonic pachymetry and the depth of pathology can be measured by optical pachymetry (35) (Fig. 11-3). Full informed consent is obtained after the potential risks and benefits are outlined. Careful discussion of potential refractive error shifts as well as vision loss with possible later need for corneal transplantation is mandatory.

The work-up of the patient with recurrent erosion varies only slightly. The symptoms of recurrent erosion can be extremely troublesome to some patients, and proper history may reveal the significance and degree of functional impairment as well as provide clues to the exact cause. The use of a microsurgical sponge at the slit lamp may be extremely helpful in determining the presence of loosely adherent epithelium (Fig. 11-4). The sponge gently rubbed over areas

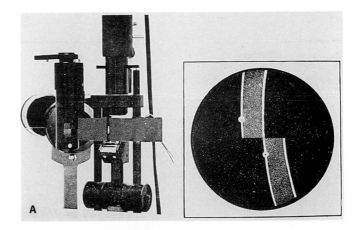

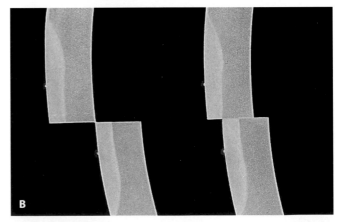

FIGURE 11-3.   A. *Optical pachymeter measuring the thickness of a normal cornea.* B. *View of a corneal scar through an optical pachymeter and judgment of the scar depth. (Courtesy of W. J. Stark, MD.)*

of suspicion will cause the loosely adherent epithelium to detach and wrinkle into folds while tightly adherent epithelium remains undisturbed. Drawings documenting the exact location of abnormal epithelial adherence during the microsurgical sponge test are recommended to act as guides during surgery.

Laser Parameters

After the excimer laser is appropriately calibrated, the surgeon may verify that the parameters of fluence, ablation diameter, repetition rate, and ablation rate are appropriate for the desired PTK treatment. The desired fluence varies with the type of excimer laser used and not with the corneal diagnosis necessitating PTK. Ablation diameter may be set by the surgeon and varied as needed throughout the session. This may be determined by the type of corneal pathology as well as the size, depth, and location of the corneal pathology. For example, the surgeon may select an ablation diameter of 6 mm for a patient with anterior basement membrane dystrophy with recurrent erosion syndrome to provide a wide treatment of the entire cornea. Conversely, for an elevated isolated scar the surgeon may use successively larger ablation diameters in order to flatten the elevated peak of the scar with PTK. Ablation and repetition rates, like fluences, are usually standardized according to the excimer laser type.

Preoperative Preparation

For most patients who have received a good education as to what to expect, no preoperative sedation is necessary. Thirty minutes preoperatively the eye is anesthetized with topical tetracaine, which is repeated every 10 minutes. All patients should be examined at the slit lamp immediately prior to being placed in the operative chair so that the surgeon has a clear view in his or her mind of the

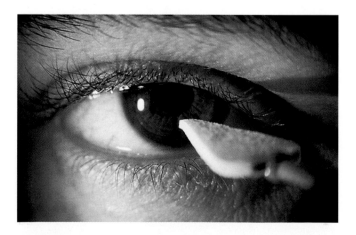

FIGURE 11-4. *Demonstration of cellulose sponge to assess adherence of corneal epithelium in recurrent erosion.*

pathology and treatment plan. The patient is then reclined supine in the operative chair and a povidone-iodine (Betadine) prepation is applied followed by placement of a wire lid speculum. An eye patch is placed over the nonoperative eye to encourage fixation only with the operative eye. The patient is then placed under the laser operating microscope and instructions are given. Visualization and familiarization with the green helium-neon (He : Ne) fixation beam in the laser is achieved and the patient is instructed to maintain this fixation throughout the procedure. The red aiming beam is focused on the central cornea and the pass-through beams are visualized on either side of the pupil. A discussion of the snapping sound and smell of the laser ensues, followed by a few sample pulses of the laser as a trial run. The surgeon should encourage the patient to relax the shoulders and neck and explain how the patient's head will be moved from side to side or around in small circles in a polishing fashion.

Epithelial Removal

Corneal epithelial removal is typically performed with a No. 64 Beaver blade or similar blade but a Paton spatula or rotating brush can be used as well. In recurrent erosion patients, all loose epithelium is removed with a cellulose sponge followed by the blade. When the No. 64 Beaver blade is used, the angle of approach should always be maintained about 45 degrees so that the blade scrapes but does not cut corneal tissue. In the treatment of opacities such as nodules, only the epithelium overlying the area of pathology needs to be removed. The edge of epithelial removal should *never* be in the visual axis however, and an additional margin of epithelium is often removed in this case. In recurrent erosion, all of the corneal epithelium that comes off easily with the sponge should be removed and the No. 64 Beaver blade is used to debride a wider margin, usually resulting in an approximately round corneal epithelial defect measuring about 7 to 9 mm. Cellulose sponges are used to remove final epithelial remnants and dry the surface for visual inspection.

In some patients, transepithelial ablation with the laser is preferable to mechanical epithelial removal. Subepithelial scar tissue should always be removed manually if possible, but in patients with significant surface irregularity caused by anterior stromal lesions it may be best to ablate directly through corneal epithelium in order to take advantage of the uncanny natural smoothing or masking ability of the epithelium. These cases can be very challenging in terms of end point determination. Transepithelial ablation should be done in a darkened room with a large-diameter ablation zone. Intact epithelium autofluoresces a light purple hue with laser beam interaction but this hue changes to a dark purple-black when ablation begins to break through the epithelial layer. Ideally, the breakthrough spots would correspond to the elevated areas of pathology visualized at the slit lamp preoperatively.

Mechanical Removal of Pathology

One error made by pioneering PTK surgeons was to remove all of the pathology with the excimer laser. While the effect can look quite dramatic, the resultant surfaces were often not as smooth as desired and excessive laser pulses were applied, resulting in thinner postoperative corneas and large hyperopic shifts (Fig. 11-5). This PTK method has been termed the *point and shoot method* and has since been abandoned for more advanced techniques (5). The currently recommended method has been referred to as the *debride and polish technique* and has proved quite effective (5) (Fig. 11-6). This technique utilizes mechanical keratectomy with the No. 64 Beaver blade in order to cleanly remove a corneal nodule or areas of elevated corneal pathology in which clear cleavage planes already exist between it and the stromal lamellae. Surprisingly dense and large areas of pathology can be removed manually, leaving a smoother underlying surface. Usually this tissue is subepithelial in nature but occasionally anterior stromal lesions also can be removed cleanly. The excimer laser with its exquisite

smoothing ability is then used as a final "polishing tool" to achieve as pristine a surface as possible (Fig. 11-7). Calcific band keratopathy should always be chelated with disodium ethylenediaminetetraacetic acid (EDTA) and scraped, leaving PTK to treat only the rough underlying exposed stroma. Finally, depressed corneal pathology where there is absence of tissue is not improved with mechanical keratectomy and should be treated with laser only.

Laser Ablation

Hand Position

The surgeon's hands are positioned with the palms covering the patient's ears, the fingers relatively straight and in contact with the patient's cheeks, and the fingertips slightly bent around the angle of the mandible. The surgeon may need to resist bending his or her fingers too much, as this may increase the patient's discomfort and cause the patient's neck to stiffen. A relaxed grip will facilitate smooth movements of the patient's head.

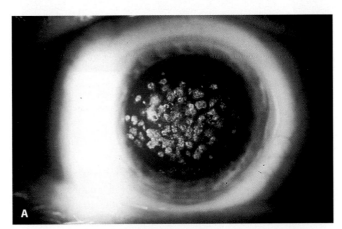

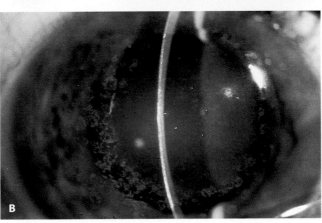

FIGURE 11-5.   A. *Preoperative photograph of a patient with anterior granular dystrophy. B. Postoperative photograph of a granular dystrophy patient treated with point and shoot PTK technique. (Courtesy of W. J. Stark, MD.)*

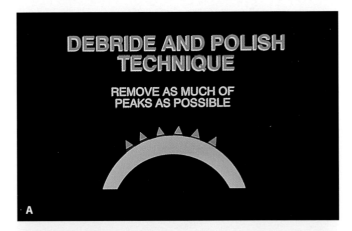

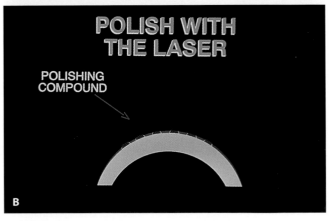

FIGURE 11-6.   A. *The debride portion of the debride and polish technique involves removal of largely elevated areas of pathology manually with a blade. B. The final polish is done with laser PTK, using a masking agent to aid in smoothing.*

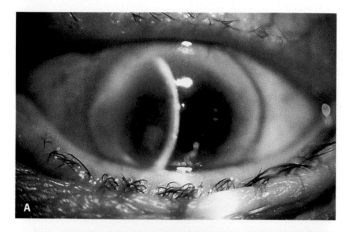

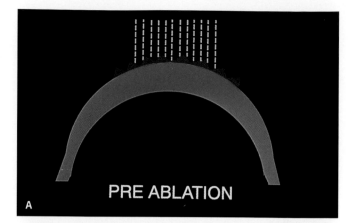

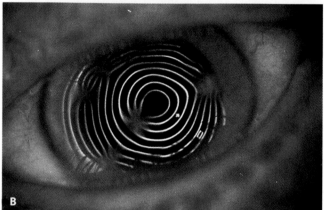

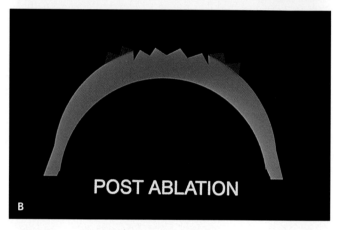

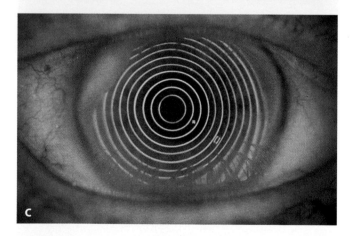

FIGURE 11-8. A, B. *Diagrams demonstrating how the excimer laser will ablate an irregular surface deeper into the tissue without the use of a smoothing agent.*

FIGURE 11-7. *Preoperative photograph (A) showing multiple Salzmann's nodules causing both opacification and an irregular surface as demonstrated in the accompanying preoperative corneascope photograph (B). Dramatic corneal smoothing is seen on the 1-month postoperative corneascope photograph following PTK (C).*

Head Movement

Appropriate movement of the patient's head will facilitate corneal polishing maneuvers with PTK. When head movement is desired by the surgeon, he or she may initiate head movement prior to depressing the foot pedal so that the desired degree of excursion is being attained before the

photoablating begins. This familiarizes the patient with the concept of circular head movement while maintaining fixation on the green target light in the laser. Practice movement should always be conducted prior to the initiation of laser treatment.

Masking Agents

In recurrent erosion patients, a masking agent is rarely ever used and laser is applied directly to the affected Bowman's layer. For other patients, after mechanical removal of epithelium and any subepithelial scar tissue, the surgeon should assess the resulting corneal surface. If the surface is relatively smooth, the surgeon may then elect to proceed with PTK without a masking agent. In the vast majority of patients, however, the resultant surface is sufficiently irregular to warrant further smoothing adjuncts such as masking agents. When an excimer laser beam encounters an irregular corneal surface profile, it will ablate and remove corneal tissue but the pattern of the irregularity is preserved and etched into deeper corneal layers (4) (Fig. 11-8). Masking agents are variable-viscosity solutions of carboxymethylcellulose or similar substances that can be applied to an irregular corneal surface and act to regularize the "peaks and valleys" so that the excimer laser beam may then encounter a fairly smooth corneal surface. The masking agent will fill the corneal tissue valleys to the level of the tissue peaks. The excimer beam can then ablate simultaneously the corneal tissue peaks and the masking agent that fills the valleys, so that the peaks are leveled but the valleys are prevented from deepening (4). The masking agents are typically used following corneal epithelial removal (Fig. 11-9).

Various masking agents have been tried over the years with varying degrees of success. These include Tears Natural II (36), polyvinyl alcohol, 1% hydroxypropyl methylcellulose (37), Healon (38), carboxymethylcellulose, and Unisol (37). The most commonly used masking agent during PTK procedures is carboxymethylcellulose. A highly viscous agent does not cover uniformly and can become clumped during ablation. A low-viscosity solution will tend to run off quickly or be knocked aside by the laser impact, thereby exposing both peaks and valleys. We prefer to use different viscosity solutions based on the task at hand. The surgical field has a triple-well container with three different concentrations of carboxymethylcellulose: 0.5% (Refresh Plus), 1.0% (Celluvisc), and 2.0% (Goniosol) (4) (Fig. 11-10). A thicker masking agent is used initially to flatten highly ele-

vated peaks. As the treatment continues and the surface gets progressively smoother, the thinner agents are employed. The carboxymethylcellulose 1% solution is the "workhorse" masking agent, as it is viscous enough to fill the corneal tissue valleys and yet remain liquid enough to flow relatively easily. The masking agent is applied with a cellulose sponge dipped into the well, acting like a paintbrush, with the excess removed with a dry sponge. Once the surgeon is happy with the smoothness of the confluent layer of masking agent, PTK commences. Short sessions of PTK ablation are interrupted by wiping the masking agent off and drying the corneal surface for close inspection. The entire process is repeated multiple times with reapplication of carboxymethylcellulose of decreasing viscosities and additional PTK until the surface is sufficiently smooth at final inspection. It is impossible to fill every valley and selectively ablate each and every corneal tissue peak, but with successive cycles of masking and photoablation, the opacity will diminish and the stromal tissue will become more regular. With experience the PTK surgeon will acquire better judgment and "touch." For a typical single PTK treatment, the surgeon will execute rapid, efficient sequences of masking agent application, sponge blotting, and excimer laser photoablation. PTK is an artistic procedure and deciding how much to mask and which concentrations to use depends on the surgeon's judgment.

Laser Treatment

The laser aiming beams should be focused on the cornea prior to application of masking agents because the viscous fluid sometimes blurs the beam image. The aiming beam should then be focused more anteriorly, to compensate for the thickness of the methylcellulose prior to commencing ablation. The laser is armed with anywhere from 25 to 100 pulses and the optical zone diameter is selected, usually 5 to 6 mm (4). With a masking agent in place, we do not

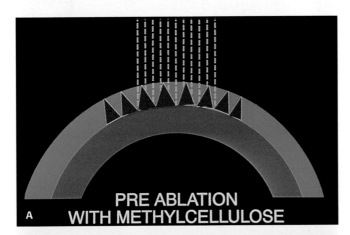

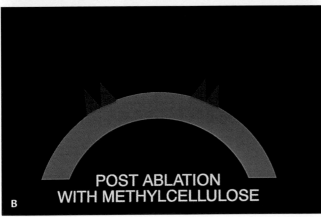

FIGURE 11-9. *A, B. Diagrams demonstrating how a masking agent can dramatically smooth an irregular corneal surface during PTK.*

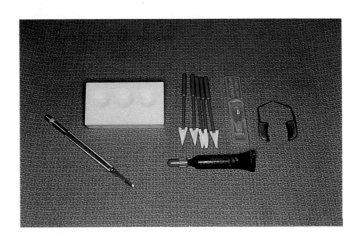

FIGURE 11-10. *Surgical field for PTK with three-well reservoir for different-viscosity masking agents, microsurgical sponges, methylcellulose, wire lid speculum, No. 64 Beaver blade, and tetracaine.*

recommend ever applying more than 100 pulses before reassessing the confluency of the methylcellulose layer and the smoothness of the underlying corneal surface and reapplying additional agent. The PTK pulses are applied while rotating the patient's head in a small circular motion to facilitate a polishing or "spray painting" technique. The entire area of corneal epithelial debridement is treated with PTK, and the surgeon ensures that the ablating spot overlaps onto the undebrided epithelium by a small amount.

After epithelial debridement and application of the appropriate masking agent in the patient with corneal surface irregularity, the surgeon must rely on both visual and audible cues termed the *sight and sound technique* as the procedure progresses (4). PTK ablation on masking agent will turn it blue-white as the excimer laser beam photoablates the carboxymethylcellulose and will be accompanied by a rapid soft audible clicking sound. When the excimer beam contacts nonprotected cornea, the fluorescence is darker blue-purple and the sound changes to a louder snapping or popping sound. The appearance of the corneal tissue valleys is that of lakes of white-blue flashes interspersed among the dark peaks of exposed corneal tissue. If the photoablation produces an all white-blue area without gaps, only the masking agent and no corneal tissue peaks are being photoablated. Ideally, the darker areas will correspond to the areas of elevation that were noted on the slit-lamp examination immediately preoperatively, signifying that the surgeon is successfully selectively ablating those areas. The force of the beam impact will move the masking agent and change the sight and sound during ablation. If the patterns seen and heard deviate from what the surgeon expects based on the pathology, the ablation should be stopped and the surface reassessed. The first set of pulses with masking agent will produce the greatest masking agent flash, the quietest pop, and the least obvious smoothing effect since the corneal tissue peaks are least broad near the apex and the most viscous masking agent is used in the early stages of the operation. As the surface is polished progressively smoother, less viscous agents are applied in less amounts, resulting in less flash, louder sound, and more rapid ablation of corneal tissue.

The optical zone diameter can be incrementally increased or decreased by the surgeon by programming the desired value with each set of 25 to 100 pulses. The choice of optical zone diameter, when to increase it, the number of pulses within a set, and the total number of sets will be determined by the surgeon with experience, and is part of the art of PTK. Again, 25 to 100 pulses per set before assessment of effect has been a good conservative benchmark for providing a demonstrable effect, yet forces frequent assessment of decreased opacification and increased smoothness while minimizing the tendency to overtreat. After one or two short treatment sessions, the surgeon should consider taking the patient to the slit lamp for a more thorough assessment of the depth of treatment and of the remaining pathology. PTK can be thought of as multiple small sur-

geries combined into one session. One should always be cognizant of the total number of pulses given and the depth achieved, given the fact that the laser ablates approximately 25 μm per pulse. The last set of pulses is usually performed at an optic zone diameter of 6 mm with wide rotational movement for a generalized polishing, nonrefractive effect.

PTK End Point

The end point of the PTK session itself requires judgment. If the opacity is clear and the cornea is smooth, the session is finished. If the opacity is clear and the cornea still only slightly rough, a final polish with carboxymethylcellulose is often used. An opacity may not be totally removable, and partial removal may be sufficient to improve the visual acuity markedly. Since drying of the cornea is not as critical as with PRK, the surgeon may move the patient to a slit lamp to judge the decrease in the opacity between sessions of PTK. The same principle applies with regard to titrating the final corneal smoothness; one should perform enough PTK to the level at which the corneal epithelium, the best smoothing agent, can provide the final restoration

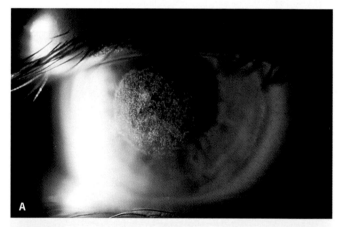

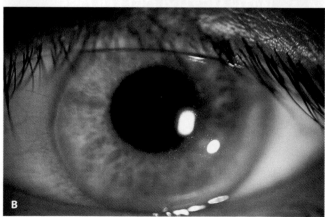

FIGURE 11-11.   A. *Significant corneal opacification causing visual loss to 20/80 in this preoperative photograph of a patient with Schnyder's crystalline dystrophy.* B. *Significant corneal clearing and improvement in vision to 20/25 in this 1-month postoperative PTK photograph.*

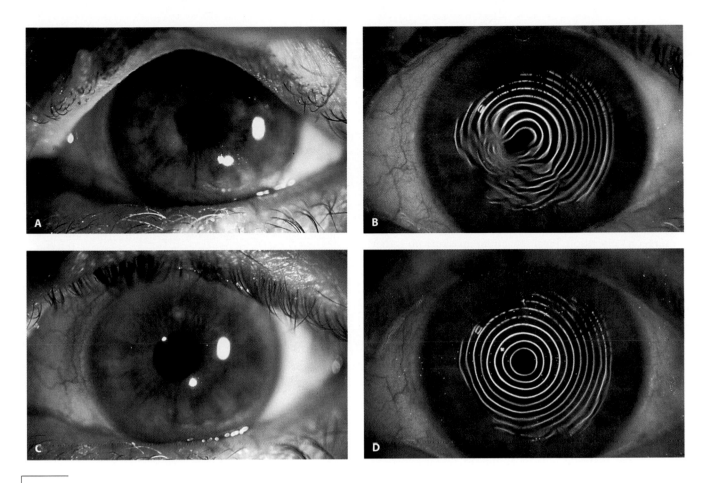

FIGURE 11-12. A. *Photograph showing preoperative view of a visually significant pericentral anterior stromal corneal scar with best-corrected acuity of 20/200. B. Preoperative corneascope shows impressive distortion of the surface profile. Following PTK there is dramatic clearing of the opacity (C) and improvement in the smoothness of the corneal surface (D) with enhanced best-corrected vision to 20/30.*

of uniformity. The principal rule of PTK is that under-treatment is better than overtreatment, an intuitively obvious concept that is easy to forget when one is actually treating the pathology. A patient whose cornea has been under-treated can return for additional treatment. With proper technique the results can be rather dramatic, as demonstrated by Figure 11-11 showing impressive clearing of Schnyder's crystalline dystrophy with PTK. Figure 11-12 demonstrates the smoothing ability of PTK as seen by the significant improvement in corneal surface profile in these corneascope photographs of a patient with a visually significant pericentral corneal scar and severe irregular astigmatism.

POSTOPERATIVE CARE

Basically, the postoperative care involves three phases:

1. Manage the epithelial defect and prevent infection.
2. Control wound healing to prevent scarring.
3. Fine-tune any refractive error.

Our postoperative regimen after PTK includes immediate administration of single drop of topical antibiotic (e.g.,

ofloxacin 0.3% or trimethoprim-polymyxin) and topical nonsteroidal agent (e.g., diclofenac 0.5%). A disposable bandage soft contact lens is placed and the fit confirmed while the patient remains supine. Typically, a loose-fitting lens with a flat base curve (9.1 or 9.3) is used to allow for tightening of the lens with hydration over the next few days. Oral pain medications such as meperidine hydrochloride 50 mg with promethazine hydrochloride 25 mg (Mepergan Fortis) or acetaminophen (Tylenol) with codeine (Tylenol No. 3) are prescribed to be taken every 4 to 6 hours as needed for pain and the patient is cautioned to minimize activity.

The patient is seen on postoperative day 1, and every 2 to 3 days until the epithelial defect heals, at which time the bandage soft contact lens is removed. Until complete re-epithelialization is apparent, the soft contact lens is not replaced at follow-up visits unless the lens is too tight or too loose and is thought to be delaying healing. The antibiotic is given four times a day along with the topical non-steroidal agent until the epithelial defect heals. Patients are instructed to use diclofenac only as needed for pain because it can delay epithelialization. In our experience, in 70% to

80% of patients re-epithelialization occurs by the third post-operative day, but this varies greatly, depending on a host of factors, not the least of which is the size of the original epithelial defect induced at the time of surgery. For patients such as those with recurrent erosion whose PTK did not extend too deeply, no topical steroid is used, as rarely do we see more than trace reticular healing haze. For patients with scars or deeper treatments, postoperative reticular haze is commonly seen; thus, a course of topical fluorometholone 0.1% (FML) is prescribed starting at four times a day and tapered according to need. In the vast majority of patients, epithelialization is completed by 1 week postoperatively; thus, the next follow-up is at 1 month. Further visits are at the surgeon's discretion. Final refractions are done no earlier than the 1-month visit, to allow for wound healing to progress; stromal remodeling, changes in epithelial thickness, and astigmatism shifts can affect the final refractive result. If a patient has significant healing haze at the 1-month visit, final refraction should definitely be delayed, as this is indicative of ongoing healing activity that will shift the refraction.

SIDE EFFECTS AND COMPLICATIONS

Refractive Shifts

The principal side effect of PTK appears to be flattening of the central cornea with resultant induced hyperopia of varying degrees (5). Proper PTK techniques with the appropriate use of masking agents and a conservative mindset can minimize the amount of induced hyperopia. If the surgeon heeds the advice given in this chapter, realizes that undertreatment is better than overtreatment, and realizes that the cornea need not be completely clear or smooth upon completion of PTK, this complication will be alleviated to a large degree.

Pain

Postoperative pain may be severe during the first 24 to 48 hours but dissipates rapidly when the epithelium heals. During the clinical trials only patching and oral pain medications were allowed postoperatively; needless to say, postoperative pain was significant. Since PTK approval, the use of postoperative bandage soft contact lenses and diclofenac 0.5% (Voltaren) has become common practice and pain has been reduced to a very tolerable level. At our center very good pain control has been achieved with the combination of bandage contact lenses and meperidine 50 mg with promethazine 25 mg (Mepergan Fortis) given orally every 4 to 6 hours, along with topical diclofenac 0.5%. Most patients complain only of burning and irritation rather than frank pain. Cycloplegics are of questionable value for control of severe pain after PTK.

Delayed Epithelialization

Although in most PTK patients re-epithelialization is complete between days 3 and 7, delayed corneal epithelial wound healing can occur after PTK. Stark et al (11) reported delayed epithelialization, requiring 3 to 4 weeks for complete healing in 2 patients with morbidity factors such as Salzman's nodular degeneration and significant alcohol intake. At our center, patients with band keratopathy (who underwent PTK with mechanical superficial keratectomy and calcium EDTA chelation) most commonly have prolonged re-epithelialization, followed by those with severe dry eye and Salzman's nodular degeneration. The routine use of bandage contact lenses has aided epithelialization in most patients but lens hydration and tightening can occur in the first few postoperative days and can delay healing due to corneal hypoxia. Adjunctive therapy such as a temporary lateral tarsorrhaphy with or without inferior punctal occlusion (silicone plug or cautery) has been extremely beneficial in recalcitrant cases.

Infection

Postoperative infection is rare but the infectious keratitis is similar to any eye with a large corneal abrasion. At our center, we experienced one pericentral staphylococcal ulcer that responded to topical ofloxacin (Ocuflox) without adverse outcome. Infections can be prevented by treating adnexal infections such as blepharitis preoperatively, using sterile operative technique, using postoperative antibiotics, and close monitoring until complete re-epithelialization is apparent. Remember that reactivation of herpes simplex keratitis can occur after PTK and appropriate preventative measures should be employed (6,7).

Stromal Haze and Scarring

Most corneas following PTK are either clear or have trace to 1+ reticular haze that is not visually significant and clears within 3 to 6 months. Prompt treatment with topical steroids can minimize the severity and course of haze. Very rarely is visually significant scarring seen as a result of PTK. More commonly, significant residual scarring may be left after PTK for scars that may have been too deep to fully ablate. In that case, penetrating keratoplasty may be indicated.

Corneal Graft Rejection

Corneal graft rejection can be induced after PTK, as reported by both Hersh et al (39) and Epstein et al (40). As with any rejection episode, prompt aggressive immunosuppressive therapy can lead to successful reversal.

Need for Subsequent Penetrating Keratoplasty

Those patients with suboptimal visual function following 3 to 6 months of full healing after PTK may benefit from either lamellar or penetrating keratoplasty. Patients treated with PTK for corneal scars should be well informed pre-operatively of the possible need for subsequent keratoplasty; thus, this should not be necessarily viewed as a complication in these patients.

OUTCOME

Our center was one of the clinical investigative centers for Summit Technology's FDA clinical PTK trial involving 249 patients with variable pathology as shown in Table 11-5. The most common diagnosis was corneal scars or irregularities followed by Salzmann's nodules and recurrent corneal erosions. Improvements in best-corrected visual acuities are presented in Tables 11-6 and 11-7. The majority of patients in the corneal opacity and irregular surface groups had substantial improvement although 18% to 22% patients also experienced loss of at least one line of vision. Most of the patients in the recurrent erosion group had no change in vision, as expected because the goal of surgery was to relieve pain from epithelial breakdown rather than to improve vision. Notably important is the fact that only 8% of this group had any loss of acuity after the procedure. Corneal cylinder reductions were seen after PTK in these patients as well, with the greatest reductions in the irregular astigmatism group, as expected since the goal of PTK in this group is corneal smoothing. The scar patients had some

reduction in cylinder with laser surface polishing while there was little if any effect on cylinder in the recurrent erosion group, as shown in Table 11-8.

The success of PTK is largely measured by improvement in best-corrected visual acuity (Table 11-9). Maloney et al (11) reported 45% of their patients had an improvement in best-corrected spectacle acuity at 12 and 24 months while 9% and 8% of treated eyes lost two or more lines of vision at 12 and 24 months, respectively. Sher et al (21) reported similar results, with 48% of their patients showing improvement in vision by two or more lines after PTK and 15% showing worsening by two or more lines. Azar et al (42) reported the average improvement in best-corrected visual acuity was 1.8 lines. Ten percent of patients lost two or more lines of best-corrected visual acuity while 45% gained two or more lines. Other studies confirmed these results (7,43).

The outcome of PTK also depends on the underlying corneal pathology. Maloney et al (41) showed that treatment

Table 11-5.

Anterior basement membrane disease	13
Band keratopathy	24
Corneal dystrophies	30
Corneal scars/Irregularities	78
Pterygium	10
Recurrent epithelial breakdown	42
Salzmann's/nodules	52
Total procedures	249

Table 11-6.

	Best Corrected Visual Acuity*		
	Improved	Unchanged	Decreased
Corneal opacity	77%	0.5%	18%
Irregular surface	70%	0.8%	22%
Epithelial breakdown	36%	46%	0.8%

* Improved or decreased represents at least one line of vision.

Table 11-7.

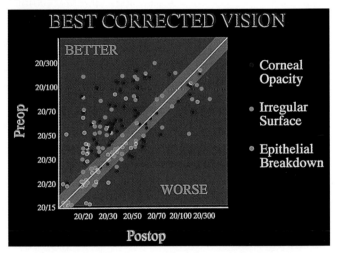

Table 11-8.   Change in Cylinder

	Preop Average	Postop Averag
Corneal opacity	−1.84 D	−1.69 D
Irregular surface	−2.33 D	−1.63 D
Epithelial breakdown	−0.98 D	−0.97 D

Table 11-9.   Changes in Best-Corrected Visual Acuity (BCVA)

Author	Improved BCVA	Loss of 2 or More Lines of BCVA
Maloney et al (42)	45%	9%
Sher et al (22)	48%	15%
Azar et al (43)	45%	10%

was most effective in eyes with hereditary corneal dystrophies, Salzmann's nodular degeneration, or corneal scars. Eyes with calcific band keratopathy appeared to improve the least. This study confirmed the results of both Chamon et al (43) and Campos et al (7). Reis-Buckler's dystrophy has also been successfully treated with PTK (17,18). Fagerholm et al (44) successfully treated all 37 patients with recurrent corneal erosions, with no further recurrences reported at 1 year. Twenty-eight of 30 patients in this study with a history of a postinfectious corneal scar also had successful treatment outcomes following PTK. Goldstein et al (22) successfully treated 2 of 3 patients with corneal scarring from trachoma. Other studies, however, did not report as much success with regard to treatment of corneal scars (7).

The visual outcome of treating corneal scars most likely depends on the stromal depth of the scar. Dausch et al (29) reported a 74% success rate in the treatment of recurrent corneal erosion with PTK. Cameron et al (26) successfully treated 3 eyes with shield ulcers and corneal plaques secondary to vernal keratoconjunctivitis. In general, patients with more superficial corneal pathology (anterior 100 μm), regardless of the underlying cause, tend to have better outcomes following PTK. Patients with deeper stromal involvement or calcific band keratopathy tend to have poorer visual outcomes (21,41,43).

Changes in refractive error are common following PTK. Postoperatively induced hyperopia is directly related to the number of stromal pulses (43,44). Maloney et al (41) reported 41% and 48% of patients with a hyperopic shift of 1 D or more at 12 and 24 months, respectively. Previous studies reported hyperopic shifts in 50% to 81% of treated eyes (21,43). This finding is not surprising since removal of central corneal tissue during PTK lessens the corneal curvature. Treatment of deeper stromal lesions can be expected to produce more postoperative hyperopia. Astigmatism may change, following PTK, with 30% to 50% of treated eyes developing an increase in astigmatism of 1 D or more (7,41). Stability of both the mean refraction and the mean best spectacle-corrected visual acuity can occur at the third postoperative month (41).

Overall, with good patient selection, the results of PTK can be outstanding. Further refinements in instrumentation and technique may serve to reduce the numbers of patients experiencing loss of best-corrected vision following PTK.

FUTURE ADVANCES

The PTK technique and understanding of the procedural nuances have come a long way since the inception of the clinical trials. Nothing can take the place of experience as the best teacher for this procedure. Future technological advances may add to experience to exponentially improve outcomes in the years to come. Second- and third-generation lasers are equipped with devices such as joy sticks and tracking systems that may improve technique and results. Both the Nidek and Chiron/Technolas excimer

lasers have joysticks that can move the excimer beam, thus obviating the need for patient head movement, and may improve the accuracy of treatment by directing the beam exactly where the surgeon points. Other laser manufacturers will provide other modalities that are beyond the scope of this chapter. Improvements in masking agents and techniques will be key to better success in patients with corneal scar and irregular astigmatism. Work has already begun in at least three clinical centers on different variations of collagen-based masking agents (45–47). A collagen polymer gel can be applied to a rough corneal surface and a hard contact lens of a predetermined curvature is placed on the gel. When the gel polymerizes to its more solid state, the contact lens is removed and the smooth curvature of the lens is transferred to the corneal surface. Since the gel is made of collagen similar to corneal collagen, it will theoretically ablate at the same rate as cornea, thereby leaving a perfectly smooth corneal surface with the same curvature as the lens. With this technique there is potential to tailor the postoperative refractive effect as well, based on the base curve of the lens selected and the resulting keratometric profile.

CONCLUSIONS

Excimer laser PTK is truly an important and powerful surgical tool in corneal surgeons' armamentarium. The precision with which the laser can polish the corneal surface is unequaled with current technology. The keys to the success of PTK are proper patient selection and conservative, meticulous surgical technique. With these keys, the surgeon can improve a patient's visual function and often prevent the need for more invasive, risky, and expensive surgical procedures such as keratoplasty.

REFERENCES

1. Fountain R, de la Cruz J, Green W, et al. Reassembly of corneal epithelial adhesion structures after excimer laser keratectomy in humans. *Arch Ophthalmol* 1994;112:967–972.
2. Fountain TR, Azar DT, de la Cruz J, et al. Reassembly of corneal epithelial adhesion structures following human excimer laser keratectomy. *Invest Ophthalmol Vis Sci* 1992;33(suppl):1106.
3. Gaster RN, Binder PS, Coalwell K, et al. Corneal surface ablation by 193 nm excimer laser and wound healing in rabbits. *Invest Ophthalmol Vis Sci* 1989;30:90–97.
4. Thompson V, Durrie DS, Cavanaugh TB. Philosophy and technique for excimer laser phototherapeutic keratectomy. *Refract Corneal Surg* 1993;9(2 suppl):81–85.
5. Durrie DS, Schumer JD, Cavanaugh TB. Phototherapeutic keratectomy: the Summit experience. In: Salz JJ, McDonnell PJ, McDonald MB, eds. *Corneal laser surgery*. St. Louis: Mosby-Year Book, 1995:227–235.
6. Talamo JH, Steinert RF, Puliafito CA. Clinical strategies for excimer laser theapeutic keratectomy. *Refract Corneal Surg* 1992;8:319–324.
7. Campos M, Nielsen S, Szerenyi K, et al. Clinical followup of phototherapeutic keratectomy for treatment of corneal opacities. *Am J Ophthalmol* 1993;115:433–440.
8. Marshall J, Trokel S, Rothery S, et al. A comparative study of corneal incisions induced by diamond and steel knives and two ultraviolet radiations from an excimer laser. *Br J Ophthalmol* 1986;70:482–500.
9. Krauss JM, Puliafito CA, Steinert RF. Laser interactions with the cornea. *Surv Ophthalmol* 1986;31:37–53.
10. Trokel SL, Srinivasan R, Braren B. Excimer laser surgery of the cornea. *Am J Ophthalmol* 1983;96:710–715.

11. Stark WJ, Chamon W, Kamp MT, et al. Clinical followup of 193nm ArF excimer laser photokeratectomy. *Ophthalmology* 1992;99:805–811.

12. Waring GO III. *Refractive keratotomy for myopia and astigmatism.* Louis: Mosby-Year Book, 1992:Chapter 19.

13. Fagerholm P, Ohman L, Orndahl M. Phototherapeutic keratectomy in herpes simplex keratitis. Clinical results in 20 patients. *Acta Ophthalmol Scand* 1994;72:457–460.

14. Pepose JS, Laycock KA, Miller JK, et al. Reactivation of latent herpes simplex virus by excimer laser photokeratectomy. *Am J Ophthalmol* 1992;114:45–50.

15. Vrabec MP, Durrie DS, Chase DS. Recurrence of herpes simplex after excimer laser keratectomy. *Am J Ophthalmol* 1992;114:96–97.

16. Orndahl M, Fagerholm P, Fitzsimmons T, Tengroth B. Treatment of corneal dystrophies with excimer laser. *Acta Ophthalmol Scand* 1994;72:235–240.

17. Lawless MA, Cohn PR, Rogers CM. Phototherapeutic keratectomy for Reis-Buckler's dystrophy. *Refract Corneal Surg* 1993;9:S96–S97.

18. McDonnell PJ, Seiler T. Phototherapeutic keratectomy with excimer laser for Reis-Buckler's dystrophy. *Refract Corneal Surg* 1992;4:306–310.

19. Droutsas DD, Tsioulias GE, Kotsiras MD, et al. Phototherapeutic keratectomy in macular corneal dystrophy with recurrent erosions. *J Refract Surg* 1996;12:S293–S294.

20. Herman SJ, Hughes WF. Recurrence of hereditary corneal dystrophy following keratoplasty. *Am J Ophthalmol* 1973;75:689–694.

21. Sher NA, Bowers RA, Zabel RW, et al. Clinical use of the 193nm excimer laser in the treatment of corneal scars. *Arch Ophthalmol* 1991;109:491–498.

22. Goldstein M, Loewenstein A, Rosner M, et al. Phototherapeutic keratectomy in the treatment of scarring from trachoma. *J Refract Corneal Surg* 1994;10:290–292.

23. Steinert RF, Puliafito CA. Excimer laser phototherapeutic keratectomy for a corneal nodule. *Refract Corneal Surg* 1990;6:352.

24. Ward MA, Artunduaga G, Thompson KP, et al. Phototherapeutic keratectomy for the treatment of nodular subepithelial corneal scars in patients with keratoconus who are contact lens intolerant. *CLAO J* 1995;21:130–132.

25. Moodaley L, Liu C, Woodward EG, et al. Excimer laser superficial keratectomy for proud nebulae in keratoconus. *Br J Ophthalmol* 1994;78:454–457.

26. Cameron JA, Antonios SR, Badr IA. Excimer laser phototherapeutic keratectomy for shield ulcers and corneal plaques in vernal keratoconjunctivitis. *J Refract Surg* 1995;11:31.

27. Dausch D, Landesz M, Schroder E. Phototherapeutic keratectomy in recurrent corneal intraepithelial dysplasia. *Arch Ophthalmol* 1994;112:22–23.

28. Eiferman RA, Forgey DR, Cook YD. Excimer laser ablation of infectious crystalline keratopathy. *Arch Ophthalmol* 1992;110:18.

29. Dausch D, Landesz M, Klein R, Schroder E. Phototherapeutic keratectomy in recurrent corneal epithelial erosion. *Refract Corneal Surg* 1993;9:419–424.

30. Ohman L, Fagerholm P, Tengroth B. Treatment of recurrent corneal erosions with the excimer laser. *Acta Ophthalmol Scand* 1994;72:461–463.

31. John ME, Van Der Karr MA, Noblitt RL, Boleyn KL. Excimer laser phototherapeutic keratectomy for treatment of recurrent corneal erosion. *J Cataract Refract Surg* 1994;20:179–182.

32. Algawi K, Goggin M, O'Keefe M. 193nm Excimer laser phototherapeutic keratectomy for recurrent corneal erosions. *Eur J Implant Refract Surg* 1995;7:11–13.

33. Thomann U, Meier-Gibbons F, Schipper I. Phototherapeutic keratectomy for bullous keratopathy. *Br J Ophthalmol* 1995;79:335–338.

34. Thomann U, Niesen U, Schipper I. Successful phototherapeutic keratectomy for recurrent erosions in bullous keratopathy. *J Refract Surg* 1996;12:S290–S292.

35. Stark WJ, Gilbert ML, Gottsch JD, Munnerlyn C. Optical pachymetry in the measurement of anterior corneal disease: an evaluative tool for phototherapeutic keratectomy. *Arch Ophthalmol* 1990;108:12–13. Letter.

36. Kornmehl EW, Steinert RF, Puliafito CA. A comparative study of masking fluids for excimer laser phototherapeutic keratectomy. *Arch Ophthalmol* 1991;109:860–863.

37. Fasano AP, Moriera H, McDonnell PJ, et al. Excimer laser smoothing of a reproducible model of anterior corneal surface irregularity. *Ophthalmology* 1991;98:1782–1785.

38. Fitzsimmons TD, Fagerholm P. Superficial keratectomy with the 193nm excimer laser: a reproducible model of corneal surface irregularities. *Acta Ophthalmol Scand* 1991;69:641–644.

39. Hersh PS, Jordan AJ, Mayers M. Corneal graft rejection episode after excimer laser phototherapeutic keratectomy. *Arch Ophthalmol* 1993;111:735–736.

40. Epstein RJ, Robin JB. Corneal graft rejection episode after excimer laser phototherapeutic keratectomy. *Arch Ophthalmol* 1994;112:157. Letter.

41. Maloney RK, Thompson V, Ghiselli BA, Durrie DS. A prospective multicenter trial of excimer laser phototherapeutic keratectomy for corneal vision loss. *Am J Ophthalmol* 1996;122:149–160.

42. Azar DT, Jain S, Woods K, et al. Phototherapeutic keratectomy: the VISX experience. In: Salz JJ, McDonnell PJ, McDonald MN, eds. *Corneal laser surgery.* St. Louis: Mosby-Year Book, 1995:213.

43. Chamon W, Azar DT, Stark IW, et al. Phototherapeutic keratectomy. *Ophthalmol Clin North Am* 1993;6:399–413.

44. Fagerholm P, Ohman L, Orndahl M. Phototherapeutic keratectomy: long-term results in 166 eyes. *Refract Corneal Surg* 1993;9:76–80.

45. Englanoff JS, Kolahdouz-Isfahani AH, Moreira H, et al. In situ collagen gel mold as an aid in excimer laser superficial keratectomy. *Ophthalmology* 1992;99:1201–1208.

46. Devore DP, Scott JB, Nordquist RE, et al. Rapidly polymerized collagen gel as a smoothing agent in excimer laser photoablation. *J Refract Surg* 1995;1:50.

47. Stevens SX, Bowyer BL, Fouraker BD, et al. Precision and accuracy of Biomask, an ablatable mask material. *Invest Ophthalmol Vis Sci* 1995;36(suppl):S709.

Corneal and Scleral Lacerations

Geoffrey J. Brent   David M. Meisler

EVALUATION

The overall goals of treating the patient with a corneal or scleral laceration include 1) preventing further injury to the eye before surgery; 2) triaging and treating associated injuries; 3) expediting preoperative evaluation and anesthesia clearance, if needed; 4) controlling infection—growing cultures and administering systemic antibiotics if indicated—and implementing tetanus prophylaxis; 5) documenting the medical record meticulously; and 6) having a comprehensive and honest discussion with the patient and family.

When one is presented with an ocular trauma patient, a quick "global assessment" of the patient's overall condition should be done before delving into a complete ocular examination. Life-threatening trauma needs to be treated before all else. Additionally, severe pain and nausea should be treated as soon as possible to minimize lid squeezing and Valsalva effects, which could lead to a loss of intraocular contents. If it is obvious that the patient has an open or unstable globe, a rigid eye shield should be secured in place until definitive eye care can be administered. The use of a plastic rather than a metal shield allows it to remain in place during most radiographic imaging studies if they are necessary.

History and Physical Examination

The mechanism of injury should be determined, to assess the likelihood of a retained intraocular or orbital foreign body and its likely composition. For medicolegal reasons the time of the injury, use of protective eye wear, and any prior treatment should be recorded. While gross disruption of the globe is obvious, one should always be suspicious for occult injury in the appropriate setting. Searching for a hidden ocular perforation is essential when dealing with "high-risk"

injuries involving sharp slender objects (such as darts, ice picks, wire, or knives) or high-speed projectiles from machinery or metal-on-metal contact, which can leave small self-sealing ocular wounds. Lacerations to the eyelids or brow area should also raise the possibility of an associated occult perforating eye injury. Relevant history and salient aspects of examination are summarized in Table 12-1.

Previous Refractive Surgery

There are few clinical data regarding the prevalence of ocular rupture in eyes that have undergone refractive surgery versus nonoperated eyes. Most data reveal that incisional refractive procedures weaken the eye and that rupture most frequently occurs at the incisional site (1,2). Traumatic ocular rupture can occur years after an incisional refractive procedure. Preliminary results of excimer laser photorefractive (PRK) and phototherapeutic (PTK) procedures suggest that PRK for up to a -10 diopter (D) correction does not significantly affect ocular integrity (1,2). The study did discover a lower bursting strength, with rupture occurring at the edge of the ablation zone with PTK of greater than 40% ablation depth, which is much deeper than that typically used clinically (1,2).

Prognosis and Patient Counseling

Effective counseling of the patient and family before surgical repair regarding the extent of the injuries and the prognosis for visual recovery is time well spent. Making sure that all involved have realistic goals and expectations eases future discussions about the need for additional surgeries, visual potential, or possible enucleation. From a medicolegal aspect, this is critical. Be honest and "guardedly optimistic" if appropriate in these discussions, but stress the fact that often the full extent of the injury cannot be discerned until

Table 12-1. History and Physical Summary of Ocular Trauma Patient

I. History
  A. Events of current injury
    1. Mechanism of injury
    2. Activity at time of injury
    3. Time elapsed since injury
    4. Use of protective equipment/eye wear
    5. Prior treatment
    6. Time since last food ingestion
  B. Past ocular history: routine, plus:
    1. Prior trauma and surgery
    2. Level of visual acuity in involved eye before injury
  C. Past medical history: routine, plus:
    1. Use of anticoagulant medications—especially over-the-counter medications which often contain aspirin
    2. Status of tetanus prophylaxis
    3. Any difficulties with prior anesthesia or surgery
II. Physical examination
  A. Visual acuity
    1. Best corrected (ideal)
    2. Pinhole
  B. External
    1. Associated life-threatening injuries—refer to appropriate personnel
    2. Associated orbital and facial injuries—possible oculoplastic, ear-nose-throat, neurosurgical, or dental consults (possibly coordinated surgery if applicable)
    3. Gross inspection of involved eye (exerting minimal pressure)
    4. Evidence of visible foreign body on adnexa, skin
  C. Motility—omit if globe is or may be lacerated
  D. Confrontational visual fields
  E. Pupils—use as dim a light as possible to minimize patient's squeezing of the lids
    1. Relative afferent pupillary defect?
    2. Distortion toward limbus?
  F. Slit-lamp examination: routine, plus:
    1. Presence of conjunctival laceration/hemorrhage—risk of underlying scleral laceration or foreign body
    2. Scleral laceration
    3. Corneal laceration or foreign body
    4. Presence of extruded intraocular contents
    5. Seidel's test if indicated
    6. Gonioscopy to look for anterior-chamber foreign body and angle damage *only* if globe is intact
    7. Note iris irregularities
    8. Iridodonesis or phakodonesis
    9. Intraocular pressure *only* if globe is intact
  G. Dilated fundus examination: routine, plus:
    1. Rule out vitreous hemorrhage, intraocular foreign body
    2. Retinal dialysis, tears, detachments, commotio
    3. Choroidal or scleral rupture
    4. Optic nerve health
    5. Depressed examination *only* if globe is intact
  H. Additional testing
  I. Ultrasound—noncontact or *gentle* pressure
  J. Imaging study—plain film, computed tomography, or magnetic resonance imaging
    1. Preoperative testing as needed

surgery, and that the primary goal is to save the eye. Restoring vision is an important but secondary goal. Advances in microsurgical techniques have improved the overall visual prognosis in penetrating ocular trauma, but for many patients the prognosis for useful vision or saving the eye may be poor. Factors at presentation that are associated with a "better" prognosis include visual ability to count fingers or better, isolated corneal lacerations (<8 mm), absence of vitreous or uveal prolapse, and absence of vitreous hemorrhage (3,4). There is a slightly better prognosis with penetrating injury due to a sharp object than with disruption of the globe due to blunt injury (3).

NONSURGICAL MANAGEMENT

Corneal injuries should be carefully examined at the slit lamp for evidence of intraocular entry. Under high magnification one should scrutinize the integrity of Descemet's membrane and look for evidence of microtrauma to the lens capsule and iris. Seidel's test should be done by painting the injured surface with fluorescein-impregnated strips to look for any leak of aqueous fluid from the anterior chamber. If no obvious leak is seen, gentle finger pressure should be applied through the upper or lower eyelid to reveal any self-sealing injury or "slow" leaks. The treatment principles for self-sealing or partial-thickness wounds are to stabilize the wound, promote healing, and prevent infection.

A simple partial-thickness corneal wound that maintains good tissue approximation may be managed medically with a broad-spectrum antibiotic ointment or drop. A cycloplegic drug will aid in patient comfort. A self-sealing puncture wound or short laceration with minimal wound gape may be treated by applying a bandage soft contact lens. For a small corneal laceration (2–3 mm) that maintains good tissue approximation with a formed anterior chamber, a bandage contact lens may be effective in splinting the wound, obviating the need for sutures. A slightly thicker soft contact lens (such as a Bausch & Lomb plano T) will provide more support for the healing cornea. The patient must be followed closely to ensure that the anterior chamber remains formed, and monitored for infection.

For wounds with a small amount of tissue loss, persistent aqueous leakage, small lacerations, or puncture, the use of cyanoacrylate tissue adhesive may be beneficial. The tissue bed must be dry and free of epithelial cells. A thin film of adhesive is applied using either a small-gauge disposable needle, a microcapillary applicator, or the broken wooden end of a sterile cotton-tipped applicator. Alternatively, a drop of adhesive can be placed in the center of a cutout piece of sterile plastic surgical drape and placed on the wound as a "patch." Following application, the adhesive should be given several minutes to dry before any further manipulation is performed. A bandage contact lens is fitted to keep the adhesive from prematurely dislodging and to minimize irritation to the tarsal conjunctiva. The adhesive will dislodge on its own as re-epithelialization occurs. While the contact lens remains in place, prophylactic antibiotic drops and a cycloplegic agent are recommended, and a topical non-steroidal anti-inflammatory drop may prove helpful for patient comfort. In poorly cooperative patients (e.g., children, demented or mentally retarded patients) or those with questioned reliability for follow-up, a definitive surgical closure would be more appropriate.

If there is evidence of intraocular penetration, even in the presence of a self-sealing wound, the patient is at an increased risk for developing endophthalmitis. These patients require close observation, and treatment with intravenous antibiotics may be considered although it is of unproven efficacy.

SURGICAL MANAGEMENT

Formation of a Surgical Therapeutic Strategy

The ophthalmologist must integrate the information gathered in the history and examination, and prepare a rational approach to repair of the traumatized ocular tissue. The goals of ocular trauma repair are to 1) restore the integrity of the globe, 2) restore the anatomy to its physiologic state, and 3) minimize current and future complications either at the initial surgery or at subsequent surgery. These goals are designed to save the eye and to restore (useful) vision. To this end, the ophthalmologist must re-form a watertight globe, remove any disrupted lens fragments or vitreous, reposition viable uvea and excise necrotic uvea, and remove any intraocular foreign body.

General anesthesia is preferred for trauma patients with a ruptured globe, since any peribulbar or retrobulbar injections would increase orbital volume, which could lead to further loss of intraocular contents. A nondepolarizing muscle relaxant such as vecuronium prevents the associated increase in intraocular pressure from contraction of the extraocular muscles, thereby decreasing the risk of expulsion of intraocular contents. Although there is still debate regarding any real benefit to the use of a nondepolarizing muscle relaxant, most anesthesiologists and ophthalmologists prefer to use one. The eye is then carefully prepped and draped, being sure not to exert any undue pressure on the globe. Exposure can be obtained by carefully inserting a lid speculum that exerts minimal pressure on the globe, or by passing 4-0 silk traction sutures through the tarsus of the upper and lower lids, or using adhesive tape Steri-Strips to retract the lids to the cheek and to the brow. All movements and manipulations of the globe should be carried out in such a way as to avoid any undue pressure on the globe, at least until a watertight closure is completed, thus reducing the risk of additional prolapse of intraocular contents.

Simple Corneal Lacerations

The traditional teaching regarding wound closure is to align the limbus and any angled aspects of the laceration first. Any pigmented lesions or scars can also be used to aid in alignment. The remaining wounds are then continually bisected by successive suture bites. This method ensures that the lateral aspects of the wound return to their original relationship, thus providing a straightforward approach to restore normal anatomic relationships and ensure a watertight closure.

A more recent suggestion is to apply some basic keratorefractive principles in the initial repair to reduce scarring in the visual axis and to minimize distortion of corneal topography. The cornea tends to flatten over any laceration or sutured wound (Fig. 12-1), and lacerations that are longer or closer to the visual axis induce greater flattening (5,6). To counteract these effects, larger compressive sutures are used to close the peripheral aspects of the corneal lacera-

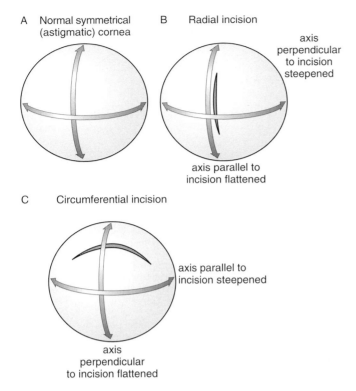

FIGURE 12-1. *Effects of radial and circumferential corneal incisions on corneal curvature.*

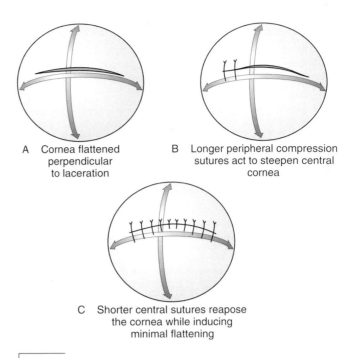

FIGURE 12-2. *Suture technique to normalize corneal curvature after laceration.*

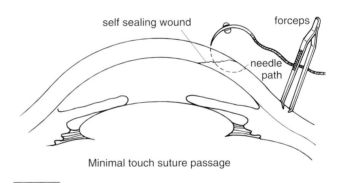

FIGURE 12-3. *"Minimal touch" suture passage avoids manipulation of wound edges and flattening of the anterior chamber in self-sealing wounds with a formed anterior chamber.*

tion that flatten the peripheral cornea and steepen the central cornea (Fig. 12-2). The central aspect of the laceration is then closed using smaller and looser suture bites to approximate the wound edges without causing excessive distortion. To aid in accurate wound closure, a temporary suture may be placed to bisect the length of the wound, to minimize lateral displacement of the wound edges during closure.

Certain "high-risk," full-thickness, self-sealing wounds involving longer lacerations (>3–4 mm), or in uncooperative patients (e.g., children, demented or mentally retarded patients) are best managed by primary surgical closure. A self-sealing wound that maintains a formed anterior chamber may be closed directly using a "minimal touch" technique. Minimal manipulation of the globe is performed to maintain the anterior chamber. Gentle fixation of the sclera at the limbus is attempted using a toothed forceps (Fig. 12-3). A one-handed technique is then used to pass the corneal sutures. The needle is directed into the cornea at a 90-degree angle, and passed through the stroma following the curve of the needle. This technique avoids manipulating the wound edge, thereby minimizing leakage of aqueous fluid and keeping the anterior chamber formed. This minimal touch technique is also advantageous when suturing near the visual axis to minimize additional iatrogenic tissue trauma from fixation forceps.

A monofilament suture of nylon or polypropylene works well in the cornea owing to its low tissue reactivity. In general, select 10-0 suture for clear cornea, and 9-0 suture near the limbus. Consider using 11-0 suture near or in the visual axis to help minimize scarring. A spatulated needle is preferred as it facilitates keeping suture passes at partial stromal thickness. Suture passes should be approximately 1.5 to 2.0 mm total in length. Slightly longer passes may be needed if the wound margin is very edematous or macerated, to ensure incorporation of healthy tissue by the suture. The suture should include approximately 85 to 95% of stromal thickness, incorporating an equal depth of tissue on each side of the wound. Sutures that are too shallow will allow the internal aspect of the wound to gape, while sutures that are too deep (full thickness) may act as a conduit for microorganisms or epithelial cells to enter the eye, and for aqueous to leak out. Suture bites should be oriented at 90 degrees with respect to the wound. Obliquely placed sutures will exert a shearing force along the length of the wound, which can lead to lateral displacement of the wound margins.

While a running suture may allow for normalization of suture tension across a wound, which may decrease induced astigmatism, unless the wound is perfectly straight it can cause lateral displacement of the wound margins, leading to an irregular closure and wound gape. Closure with a running stitch places the integrity of the entire wound on a single suture and knot, which may pose a safety risk. The use of simple interrupted sutures facilitates a more anatomic repair, as well as simplifying postoperative management of loose sutures and selected suture removal.

A simple suture exerts a zone of tissue compression along the wound that is approximately the same length of the suture. These compression zones must just overlap in order to construct a watertight repair. Longer suture bites allow a greater distance between sutures, while smaller bites require more closely spaced sutures. Excessive overlap of compression zones can lead to excessive scarring and tissue flattening.

Suture knots should be tied with either three-one-one or two-one-one throws, and the loose ends cut short with Fine stitch scissors or a 15-degree (super-sharp) blade. The knots should then be buried away from the visual axis, and the cut suture ends should be directed away from the corneal surface to facilitate future suture removal.

The architecture of a beveled corneal laceration or incision provides it with a self-sealing mechanism (the basis for shelved cataract incisions, Fig. 12-4). A full-thickness, perpendicularly oriented laceration or incision is prone to leak because any pressure (interior or exterior) will serve to unapproximate the wound edges. Therefore, all perpendicular aspects of the laceration should be repaired first to allow a more rapid watertight closure, facilitating re-formation of the anterior chamber. Passage of temporary sutures may be needed to form a watertight closure, allowing the anterior chamber to be re-formed. These may then be replaced with better-situated permanent sutures.

It is often difficult to obtain a watertight closure with stellate corneal lacerations, especially when they involve tissue avulsion. When there is no tissue loss and the apices are well formed, simple suture closure with the aid of bridging sutures may be helpful. With tissue loss, or apices that approximate poorly, the purse-string technique proposed by Eisner (7) may provide adequate closure (Fig. 12-5). A diamond blade set at half stromal thickness is used to make a small incision in the normal cornea between the base and apex of each pedicle. A continuous 10-0 nylon suture is then passed from incision to incision in a purse-string fashion and tied. The knot is then buried. If there is persistent leakage from the wound, tissue adhesive and a bandage soft contact lens may be used. A conjunctival flap will not stop a persistent corneal wound leak, and it will obscure the view of the anterior chamber, making follow-up more difficult.

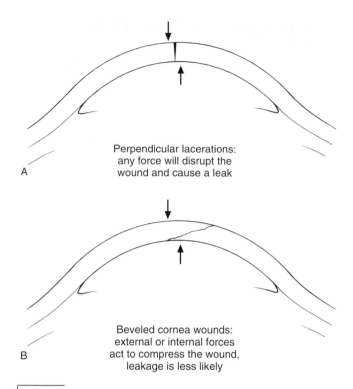

FIGURE 12-4. *A full-thickness perpendicular laceration is unstable. Surgically reapproximate these areas first to help maintain a formed anterior chamber. A beveled laceration tends to be self-sealing, and can be closed last.*

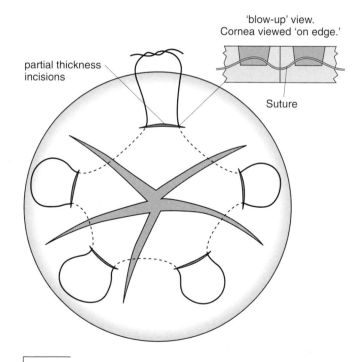

FIGURE 12-5. *Stellate laceration repair. Partial-thickness incisions are made in each facet using a guarded (diamond) blade. A deep stromal continuous suture is passed. Additional interrupted sutures are placed to achieve a watertight closure.*

Additionally, conjunctival flaps are visually and cosmetically inferior to direct surgical repair.

If an avulsed piece of corneal tissue is present, it should be sutured back into place. Start by securing the apices of the avulsed tissue, then add any additional sutures as needed to reapproximate the wound.

A flat or shallow anterior chamber will need to be reformed with either balanced salt solution, an air bubble, or a viscoelastic substance. Try balanced salt solution or air first; if either adequately maintains the chamber, the ophthalmologist can avoid using a viscoelastic substance that can complicate matters by mimicking vitreous, making tissue and suture manipulation more difficult, and require removal from the eye to prevent intraocular pressure spikes. The chamber may be re-formed either through the original wound or through a separate limbus-based paracentesis port positioned 90 degrees away. Although often difficult to perform due to hypotony, a separate paracentesis is advantageous as it can be made self-sealing and it avoids any further manipulation of the wound margin. A diamond blade rather than a metal blade may facilitate creation of the paracentesis. All wounds should be checked for watertight closure using a dry cellulose sponge.

Dealing with Iris Prolapse

Patients with larger and more peripheral corneal lacerations or flattening of the anterior chamber are prone to iris incarceration in the wound or iris prolapse. To minimize postoperative complications such as refractive problems secondary to excess light scatter, peripheral anterior synechiae formation, and cosmetic appearance from a missing iris, prolapsed tissue should be repositioned, and the repaired wound should be free of incarcerated tissue. In general, tissue exposed for less than 24 to 36 hours is probably safe to reposition if it appears healthy. However, prolapsed iris tissue that is obviously necrotic, macerated, or contaminated should be excised rather than accepting the increased risk of infection and inflammation associated with repositioning the tissue. If any sign of surface epithelialization exists, it is better to excise the tissue rather than risk introducing epithelial cells into the anterior chamber. To excise prolapsed tissue, gently grasp the edge of the exposed iris with smooth forceps, exerting minimal traction, and cut the tissue flush with the cornea using Vannas or Castroviejo scissors. Try to preserve as much viable-appearing iris tissue as possible to facilitate reconstruction of the iris diaphragm.

In cases with minimal iris prolapse or incarceration and a formed anterior chamber, pharmacologic manipulation of the iris may suffice. A dilating agent (intraocular epinephrine 1:10,000) may free iris trapped in the central aspect of a corneal laceration. Conversely, a miotic agent (acetylcholine or carbachol) may free iris entrapped in the peripheral aspect of a corneal laceration.

If the anterior chamber is at least partially formed, further deepening the chamber with intraocular saline solution or a viscoelastic substance may relieve the incarceration. Inject-

ing a viscoelastic agent between the iris and the peripheral cornea can also be used to push or "steamroll" the iris out of the wound. If the iris still will not release, an instrument such as a cyclodialysis or iris spatula or a blunt irrigating cannula may be used to sweep the iris from the wound. While avoiding the corneal endothelium and the lens, try to "tease" the iris from the wound. Working from the center toward the periphery will minimize tension on the iris root, thereby reducing the risk of creating an iridodialysis cleft or tearing the iris root, which can cause additional bleeding (8).

With a flat anterior chamber the wound must be closed so that the chamber can be re-formed. It may be necessary to place shallow temporary suture bites to avoid impaling iris tissue while allowing a watertight closure so that the anterior chamber can be re-formed (Fig. 12-6). Through a paracentesis site, injected viscoelastic substance or mechanical iris sweep will separate the incarcerated iris from the posterior aspect of the wound. The temporary sutures can then be replaced with deeper, more appropriate sutures.

Before excising prolapsed peripheral iris, or in lacerations near the limbus, carefully inspect the involved uveal tissue

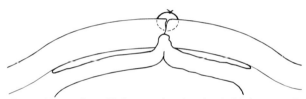

Corneal laceration with flat anterior chamber to iris incarcerated in wound. Shallow suture bites passed to reform the anterior chamber and avoid capturing the iris

A

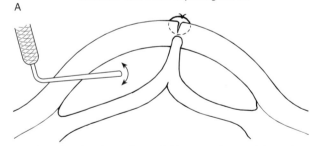

Anterior chamber reformed. Iris sweep inserted through paracentesis site and iris is pulled free from posterior aspect of wound. Viscoelastic may also be used

B

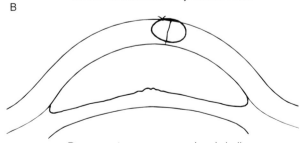

Deeper sutures are passed and shallow temporary sutures are removed. There is no iris incarcerated in wound

C

FIGURE 12-6. *Repair of corneal laceration with iris incarceration using temporary shallow corneal sutures.*

to make sure that the ciliary body is not involved, as any unnecessary manipulation can cause bleeding. If significant iris bleeding is encountered during surgical repair, a viscoelastic substance can be used as a tamponade. If the globe is watertight, gentle pressure may be applied to the globe, or infusion pressure may be increased if an infusion line is in use. Additionally, intraocular epinephrine 1:10,000 can be injected for its vasoconstrictive effect. A surgical peripheral iridectomy should be performed in an area where peripheral iris incarceration was relieved to minimize the risk of peripheral anterior synechiae formation.

Associated Iris Trauma

An iris laceration is repaired to maintain a tight iris diaphragm, which will decrease the risk of peripheral anterior synechiae and iris-corneal adhesions. Restoring the pupil shape is important for refractive and cosmetic reasons. Repair of the iris defect can be accomplished primarily or secondarily. At the primary surgery a 10-0 polypropylene suture on a vascular needle can be used to close the iris defect. Keep the cut suture ends short to avoid contact with nearby tissues. Alternatively the iris laceration may be repaired using the McCannel suture technique (8) (Fig. 12-7). A similar technique can be used to repair an area of iridodialysis.

Anterior-Segment Trauma with Associated Lens Damage

Once a projectile or foreign body breaches the cornea, there is little to prevent it from disrupting the crystalline lens as well. A thorough preoperative and intraoperative evaluation of the lens is essential but often difficult owing to poor visibility caused by corneal edema and anterior-chamber blood or fibrin. Depending on the type and extent of the corneal wound, a thorough evaluation may best be accomplished before wound closure. In eyes with poor pupillary dilation it may be necessary to use a Graether collar button or cyclodialysis spatula to push or retract the iris, enabling the lens to be thoroughly inspected. A fibrinous anterior-chamber reaction that deposits across an intact anterior lens capsule may obscure the lens or appear as a dense cataract (9), or after restoration of the anterior chamber, adequate visibility of the lens may not be achieved secondary to corneal edema; in these instances, it would be better to wait and let the eye quiet down, re-evaluate, and possibly do a secondary cataract extraction if indicated. Further, a small breach of the lens capsule (such as after a penetrating injury from a wire or a small in-and-out projectile) may seal spontaneously and only cause a localized opacity of the lens that is not visually significant, and may be safely observed.

In patients with a dense cataract and an adequate view after repair of the corneal laceration, a primary lensectomy may be carried out. This will allow easier follow-up examination of the fundus, prevent additional phacogenic inflam-

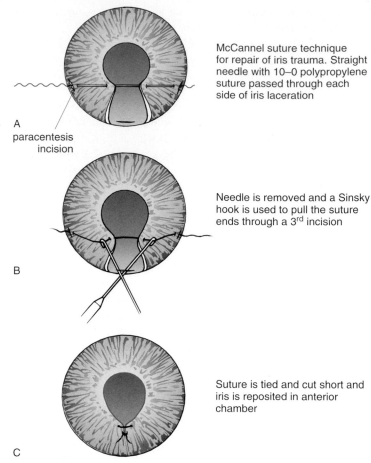

McCannel suture technique for repair of iris trauma. Straight needle with 10–0 polypropylene suture passed through each side of iris laceration

A   paracentesis incision

Needle is removed and a Sinsky hook is used to pull the suture ends through a 3rd incision

B

Suture is tied and cut short and iris is reposited in anterior chamber

C

FIGURE 12-7.   *Repair of iris trauma with sector defect. Do not make the pupil "too small," or fundus examination will be difficult.*

mation, and may avoid a second ocular surgery. The use of flexible iris hooks inserted through multiple paracentesis incisions may aid in exposure if there is poor pupillary dilation. If there appears to be minimal capsular disruption, good zonular support, and an intact posterior capsule, a standard extracapsular or phacoemulsification technique may be used. A limbal- or temporal-based incision is constructed and surgery is carried out according to standard technique. The surgeon should be vigilant for significant amounts of zonular dehiscence and be prepared to convert his or her technique for lens delivery if necessary. In patients with extensive zonular dehiscence an intracapsular cataract extraction technique should be considered.

If the lens is subluxated, severely disrupted, or dislocated, with vitreous prolapse into the anterior chamber, then vitrectomy instrumentation should be used to perform a lensectomy and vitrectomy. If possible, use of a limbal-based entrance may allow preservation of the posterior capsule and may minimize the chance of lens fragments sinking into the vitreous. Every attempt should be make to preserve as much posterior capsule as possible so that a posterior-chamber lens may be placed either in the bag, or in the sulcus primarily or at a second surgery. The vitrectomy cutting instrument and irrigation are introduced through the limbus or the pars plana, depending on the surgeon's preference or the type of injury. The cutting instrument is used to remove vitreous and liberated lens material from the anterior chamber. An anterior capsular rent can be trimmed and if possible converted to a capsulotomy, or perhaps a continuous-tear capsulorrhexis. The remaining lens material may be removed using aspiration and cutting. Very hard nuclear material may need to be removed by nuclear expression or phacoemulsification. If necessary, a thorough anterior vitrectomy is performed. The anterior chamber is carefully evaluated to ensure that there is no vitreous remaining that could become incarcerated in the wound, leading to postoperative vitreous traction, inflammation, retinal traction, or a "vitreous wick" causing a wound leak and increasing the risk of infection.

The insertion of an intraocular lens at the primary surgery remains controversial. A primary lens implant could save the patient from secondary surgery, yet the selection of the proper lens power, anatomic placement, and the risk of implanting a prosthetic device in a potentially contaminated wound are of great concern. A secondary implantation has the advantage of more reliable calculation of intraocular lens power based on actual keratometry readings, and operating on a quiet eye which may facilitate proper lens placement. In eyes with an adequate view through the cornea after repair, with no gross wound contamination or evidence of infection, with anterior or posterior capsular support, and with no evidence of significant posterior-pole trauma, a primary intraocular lens implantation may be a reasonable choice (10–12). Lens-power determination can be sufficiently accurate by using keratometry and axial-length measurements of the fellow healthy eye (10,11). Even if the determination were inaccurate, it could be reasoned that it would be better to be 4- or 5-D ametropic than aphakic. Children in the amblyogenic age range can benefit from a faster visual rehabilitation time, and it may be possible to avoid the difficulties of fitting a contact lens in an eye with corneal scarring or sutures. If adequate capsular support is present, an intraocular lens should be placed in the bag or in the sulcus. Without an intact capsule, a transsclerally sutured posterior-chamber lens could be placed, or an anterior-chamber lens could be used. Because of concerns of long-term tolerance and increased anterior-segment complications in a traumatized eye, it may be best to avoid an anterior-chamber lens in a younger patient. The patient will likely need to wear a contact lens to neutralize irregular astigmatism resulting from the corneal laceration.

Corneoscleral Lacerations

A localized peritomy is made to improve visibility of the wound being repaired. Avoid excessive manipulation of the globe or extensive exploration until all visible wounds are closed. If the wound edges are significantly separated, closure is facilitated by regrasping the needle after passage through the first wound edge. Small well-delineated corneoscleral lacerations or small isolated scleral lacerations from sharp penetrating injury may be primarily repaired and may not require extensive exploration. Large lacerations and lacerations associated with severe blunt trauma require exploration of all quadrants of the globe to look for occult injury. Smaller scleral lacerations may be repaired using nonabsorbable 8-0 nylon or silk suture or absorbable 7-0 polyglactin (Vicryl). For larger corneoscleral lacerations it is best to start by approximating the limbus using nonabsorbable 8-0 or 9-0 nylon suture (silk is also appropriate, but may cause more inflammation if used at the corneal limbus). Proceed posteriorly with the repair using simple interrupted sutures, and closing the wound as it becomes exposed ["zippered" closure (8)]. In lacerations that extend far posteriorly, the use of a half-round needle will make suture passes easier when working in a deep "hole." If exposure of the posterior aspect of the wound is difficult because of orbital tissue prolapse, a small malleable retractor or a pediatric nasal speculum can be used to improve visibility, taking care not to exert any pressure on the globe.

Prolapsed vitreous should be engaged with a dry cellulose sponge, then cut flush with the wound using fine scissors; alternatively the vitreous cutting device may be used. Care should be taken to minimize any unnecessary traction on the vitreous. Prolapsed uveal tissue should be repositioned before wound closure. Ideally, there should be no vitreous or uveal tissue incarcerated in the surgically closed wound. Every attempt is made to preserve any prolapsed uveal tissue. Repositioning of prolapsed uveal tissue may be facilitated by having an assistant gently push the prolapsed tissue back into the wound using a smooth flat spatula as the surgeon passes the sutures. The wound edges may also be gently raised with a forceps while passing suture bites, to keep uveal tissue from being impaled by the suture needle. Uveal tissue is handled with extra care as it can bleed easily and profusely. If it is necessary for uveal tissue to be removed, precauterizing will help to control bleeding. Wounds with extensive uveal prolapse have a worse visual prognosis (3). Viscoelastic substances should not be injected in the subretinal space to reposition uveal tissue because they are poorly absorbed and may lead to excessive inflammation and increase the risk of retinal detachment.

Once all visible wounds are closed, a 360-degree peritomy is made, and all four quadrants are opened, through Tenon's capsule, and explored. Placement of one or more bridle sutures of 4-0 silk under an extraocular muscle or tendon, or through the limbus may be useful to rotate the globe to aid in exploration. Particular attention is directed to the anatomically thinnest area of the sclera, which is posterior to the insertions of the extraocular muscles, to inspect for occult scleral rupture (13). If lacerations extend through or under extraocular muscles, an assistant can gently retract the muscle using a muscle hook to aid in exposure. If more exposure is needed, the muscle tendon can be secured using a double-armed polyglactin (Vicryl) suture with a spatulated needle, then severed from its insertion and reattached after the laceration is repaired.

It may not be possible to surgically close a scleral wound that extends far posteriorly, near the optic nerve. Prolapsed vitreous and uveal tissue will also be more difficult to manage in far posterior lacerations. In these cases, it is better to leave the posterior aspect of the wound open rather than cause additional damage and further tissue prolapse that would occur with the extreme globe manipulation required to expose and attempt closure of the laceration. An isolated posterior scleral laceration or rupture from blunt trauma, projectile injury, or a perforating wound of the globe may occur without associated corneal injury. This should be suspected with the appropriate history, and may demonstrate decreased visual acuity, focal subconjunctival hemorrhage and chemosis, conjunctival laceration, uveal "show" under the conjunctiva, decreased intraocular pressure, hyphema, vitreous hemorrhage, pupillary irregularity, or a shallow or deep anterior chamber (8). These injuries are repaired just as anterior scleral lacerations, by using a 360-degree peritomy with exploration of all four quadrants and wound closure as the wounds are uncovered. An isolated far posterior (near the nerve) scleral wound, such as seen with penetrating trauma of the globe, may best be managed without primary surgical closure. This avoids the extreme manipulation of the globe that would be necessary for closure and that could lead to further vitreous and uveal prolapse. In these cases the orbital tissue will serve to tamponade the wound as it heals.

Corneoscleral Lacerations with Associated Tissue Loss

Every attempt should be made to find and reposition any avulsed corneal or scleral tissue. Injuries involving loss of a small tissue area may be closed using tight sutures, although this can lead to significant amounts of tissue distortion and wound tension, which may impede healing and complicate visual rehabilitation. If possible, tissue adhesive may aid in their closure. Avulsion of larger tissue areas requires replacement with either fresh or preserved donor corneal or scleral tissue. It is best to remove frankly necrotic or infected-appearing tissue before placing a graft. Devitalized or irregular margins are then trimmed using scissors or a sharp blade to form a smooth circular recipient bed. Care should be taken to avoid further injury to underlying uveal tissue. Alternatively a partial-thickness trephination may be performed and the remaining tissue removed with scissors or a sharp blade as in a penetrating keratoplasty. Trephination of an open, unpressurized globe may be technically more difficult to perform; however, the trephine blade may be inked (as with corneal markers for radial keratotomy) and used as a marker to define a distinct border to cut along, and will make fitting a watertight patch easier. Depending on the wound architecture, either partial-thickness (lamellar) or full-thickness graft tissue may be used.

A full-thickness or penetrating graft requires a recipient bed with a well-defined rim of healthy tissue to suture to. The patch is cut approximately 0.5 mm larger than the recipient bed and secured into place using simple interrupted sutures: 10-0 nylon for a corneal patch, 8-0 nylon or silk for sclera. Start by placing four cardinal sutures at the 3-, 6-, 9-, and 12-o'clock positions to secure and align the graft and make watertight closure easier. The anterior chamber can then be re-formed and the wound integrity checked.

A lamellar graft is indicated for areas of tissue loss that have irregular margins or margins with macerated or previously thinned stromal tissue. To begin, a partial-thickness incision is made around the wound using a trephine or a sharp blade. A partial-thickness recipient bed is then formed. The lamellar graft is fashioned slightly larger and with approximately the same thickness as the recipient bed; if the recipient bed was trephined, the patch may be trephined 0.5 mm larger, and if the recipient bed is irregular, then the patch can be fashioned by hand. The patch is then laid into place and secured using 10-0 nylon simple interrupted sutures. The sutures should exit from the donor material at approximately 90% to 95% thickness and enter the deepest portion of the recipient shelf. The knots are trimmed short and buried as for a regular corneal suture.

Penetrating keratoplasty is rarely performed for repair of acute trauma. Graft survival is guarded due to the added inflammation associated with acute trauma (14–16). For acute repair a patch graft may be used until a full-thickness keratoplasty can be performed secondarily. In the setting of extensive tissue loss, a penetrating keratoplasty may be appropriate.

Irreparable Tissue Injury

With extensive tissue loss or severe disruption of the globe with loss of intraocular contents, primary surgical repair may be impractical. Every attempt should be made to restore the integrity of the globe and allow the patient and family time to accept the necessity of a secondary enucleation. If primary repair is not possible and primary enucleation has been discussed and consented to preoperatively, it should be done at the initial surgery. This will save the patient the time and risk of a second surgery under general anesthesia, and reduce the risk of sympathetic ophthalmia.

REFERENCES

1. Vinger PF, Mieler WF, Oestreicher JH, Easterbrook M. Ruptured globes following radial and hexagonal keratotomy surgery. *Arch Ophthalmol* 1996;114:129–134.
2. Campos M, Lee M, McDonnell PJ. Ocular integrity after refractive surgery: effects of photorefractive keratectomy, phototherapeutic keratectomy, and radial keratotomy. *Ophthalmic Surg* 1992;23:598–602.
3. Barr CC. Prognostic factors in corneoscleral lacerations. *Arch Ophthalmol* 1983;101:919–924.

4. Adhikary HP, Taylor P, Fitzmaurice DJ. Prognosis of perforating eye injury. *Br J Ophthalmol* 1976;60:737–739.

5. Rowsey JJ, Hays JC. Refractive reconstruction for acute eye injuries. *Ophthalmic Surg* 1984;15:569–574.

6. Rowsey JJ. Ten caveats in keratorefractive surgery. *Ophthalmology* 1983;90:148–155.

7. Eisner G. *Eye surgery: an introduction to operative techniques.* New York: Springer, 1986.

8. Hersh PS, Zagelbaum BM, Kenyon KR, Shingleton BJ. Surgical management of anterior segment trauma. In: Tasmer W, ed. *Duane's clinical ophthalmology.* New York: Lippincott-Raven, 1995:1–19.

9. Muga R, Maul E. The management of lens damage in perforating corneal lacerations. *Br J Ophthalmol* 1978;62:784–787.

10. Lamkin JC, Azar DT, Mead MD, Volpe NJ. Simultaneous corneal laceration repair, cataract removal, and posterior chamber intraocular lens implantation. *Am J Ophthalmol* 1992;113:626–631.

11. Anwar M, Bleik JH, von Noorden GK, et al. Posterior chamber lens implantation for primary repair of corneal lacerations and traumatic cataracts in children. *J Pediatr Ophthalmol Strabismus* 1994;31:157–161.

12. Chan TK, Mackintosh G, Yeoh R, Lim ASM. Primary posterior chamber IOL implantation in penetrating ocular trauma. *Int Ophthalmol* 1993;17:137–141.

13. Cherry PMH. Indirect traumatic rupture of the globe. *Arch Ophthalmol* 1978;96:252–256.

14. Kenyon KR, Starch T, Hersh PS. Penetrating keratoplasty and anterior segment reconstruction for severe ocular trauma. *Ophthalmology* 1992;99:396–402.

15. Shingleton BJ, Hersh PS, Kenyon KR, eds. *Eye trauma.* St. Louis: Mosby-Year Book, 1991.

16. Webster RG. Corneal trauma; physical agents. In: Smolin G, Thoft RA, eds. *The cornea.* 3rd ed. Boston: Little, Brown, 1994:605–617.

Management of Recurrent Corneal Erosions

DAVID R. HARDTEN   TIMOTHY J. EHLEN

Hansen first described recurrent corneal erosions in 1872 (1). He accurately described many characteristics of the disease, including the observation that many patients had a history of antecedent corneal trauma. In 1874, another German physician, Von Arlt, first used the term *recurrent erosion* to describe the same condition the term refers to today (2).

Recurrent corneal erosions are characterized by acute attacks of sudden pain, frequently with waking in the morning or after several hours of sleep. The patient will have a history of similar episodes with symptom-free intervening periods of various length in between episodes. Obvious epithelial irregularities and defects may be all that is seen on slit-lamp examination, or subtle epithelial edema and irregular epithelium may be all that is noted. Whatever the appearance, the patient's symptoms are frequently out of proportion to the clinical findings.

Recurrent erosions commonly occur in eyes that have suffered trauma, usually with a sharp or abrading injury. Recurrent erosions also occur without preceding trauma in patients with an underlying epithelial, basement membrane, or anterior stromal dystrophy.

Recurrent erosions can be a difficult and frustrating problem for patients and the treating physicians. Most patients seem to do well with initial conservative measures, such as lubrication, patching, or bandage contact lenses. Some patients may require surgical therapy. Anterior stromal puncture, superficial keratectomy, phototherapeutic keratectomy, and neodymium:yttrium-aluminum-garnet (Nd:YAG) anterior stromal treatment are all options for the more difficult and recalcitrant cases.

ETIOLOGY

Recurrent erosion syndrome may follow minor corneal trauma. It can occur days to years following the initial injury.

The correlation between the trauma and subsequent recurrent erosion has been noted since the first descriptions of the syndrome (1,2). The trauma is most often minor. Sharp injuries such as those caused by a fingernail, paper edge, or tree leaf may be more likely to predispose a patient to recurrent erosions (3). One study noted that recurrent erosions are five times more likely if the initial abrasion is caused by a fingernail, paper, or plant than by other harder, sharper objects (4). It has also been noted that recurrent erosions seldom follow foreign body removal or wounds that involve Bowman's membrane (3–6).

Nontraumatic causes of recurrent erosion also occur. Many of the epithelial, basement membrane, and anterior stromal dystrophies predispose a patient to recurrent erosions. Anterior basement membrane dystrophy is the most frequently seen dystrophy, and has been estimated to be present in more than 70% of patients with recurrent erosion over the age of 50 (7). Up to 54% of anterior basement membrane dystrophy patients have had symptoms of recurrent erosion (8). Another report indicated that up to 26% of all recurrent erosion patients have identifiable map lines (9). These map lines, which represent abnormal thickened areas of anterior basement membrane, are often quite subtle, and the incidence may be higher than 26% because they may be missed on slit-lamp examination (Fig. 13-1). Historically, Reis-Buckler's dystrophy and Cogan's microcystic dystrophy have been extensively studied and have been used as models for comparing the pathology found in posttraumatic recurrent erosions (3,10). Lattice and granular stromal dystrophies have also been associated with particularly recalcitrant nontraumatic recurrent erosion (11).

Other forms of nontraumatic corneal insult have been linked to recurrent erosions. Previous herpes simplex and herpes zoster infections of the cornea are known to be associated with subsequent recurrent erosion syndrome. Previous bacterial or fungal infections, neurotrophic ulcers, and

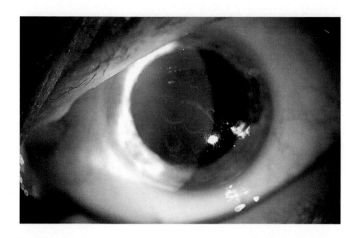

FIGURE 13-1. *Geographic maplike lines of thickened anterior basement membrane material in a patient with anterior basement membrane dystrophy.*

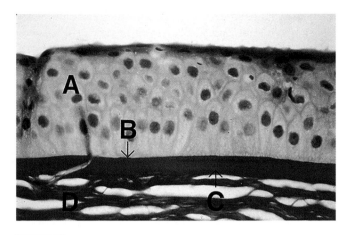

FIGURE 13-2. *Photomicrograph of normal cornea. A = epithelium; B = basement membrane; C = Bowman's layer; D = stroma. (Courtesy of J. Douglas Cameron, MD, Minneapolis, MN.)*

chemical or thermal burns may lead to recurrent erosions (12). Local abnormalities such as severe blepharitis and systemic illnesses also may predispose a patient to recurrent erosions. Diabetes mellitus patients have been found to have a primary abnormality of the epithelial–basement membrane adhesion complex, resulting in poorly attached epithelium (11,13). Graft-versus-host disease, keratoconjunctivitis sicca, Sjögren syndrome, underlying collagen-vascular disease, contact lens wear, Stevens-Johnson syndrome, and ocular cicatricial pemphigoid also may alter the integrity of the epithelium and the epithelial–basement membrane complexes, predisposing a patient to recurrent erosions (14).

HISTOPATHOLOGY

The anterior cornea consists of an epithelial layer, a basement membrane layer, the fibrous Bowman's layer, and stroma.

The normal corneal epithelium is five or six cell layers thick. Epithelial cells in the basal layer are more cuboidal in shape than the more squamous, flatter superficial cells. The basal layer of epithelial cells is firmly attached to the underlying tissue, the basement membrane, by well-defined attachment complexes. The interface of the basal epithelial cell and the anterior corneal stroma consists of several layers: basal epithelial cell membrane, hemidesmosomes and tonofibrils, lamina lucida, lamina densa, and the relatively fibrous Bowman's layer (11). Basement membranes are known to support and provide a boundary for cells and to influence cell size, shape, and orientation. Basement membranes are composed of proteoglycans and glycosaminoglycans. The major components of the human corneal epithelium basement membrane are laminin, type IV collagen, and fibronectin (11,15). Basement membrane substrates are secreted from the basal epithelial cells (Fig. 13-2).

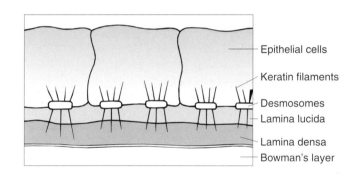

Epithelial cells

Keratin filaments

Desmosomes

Lamina lucida

Lamina densa

Bowman's layer

FIGURE 13-3. *High-magnification schematic of a hemidesmosome complex. Labeled elements of the diagram include hemidesmosome plaque, epithelial cell membrane, superficial basement membrane, and tonofibrils.*

Corneal epithelium is normally firmly attached to Bowman's layer and the underlying stroma by an epithelial–basement membrane complex. The pivotal structure of this complex is the hemidesmosome. Hemidesmosomes are button-like plaques of epithelial cell membrane–basement membrane contact that firmly anchor the cell to the underlying tissue. Intermediate filaments connect the hemidesmosome to the intracellular matrix, and also extend extracellularly through basement membrane into Bowman's layer. Healthy basal epithelial cells and normal basement membrane are necessary for this anchoring attachment to occur (16,17) (Fig. 13-3).

Several ultrastructural abnormalities in both the basement membrane and the epithelial cells have been identified in recurrent erosion syndrome. Thickened and multilaminar basement membranes, and basement membrane discontinuities have been described by several authors (12,18–20). It is believed that thickened basement membrane may be due to poorly regulated membrane production, while multilaminar membranes may be due to membrane reduplication, as seen in anterior basement membrane dystrophy.

Investigators recently showed that in areas where normal basement membrane is present in patients with recurrent erosion, epithelial cells are attached to it in a normal manner (15). It has also been shown that although basement membrane is present and identifiable in the presence of recurrent erosion, it is seen in a variable and inconsistent pattern (15). Immunostaining techniques showed that decreased amounts of the main basement membrane substrates (i.e., collagen type IV, fibronectin, and laminin) closely correlate with areas of loose epithelium in recurrent erosion syndrome (6,11). These recent findings suggest that abnormal amounts or abnormal histologic patterns of basement membrane material interfere with efforts to solidly adhere epithelium to underlying tissue.

Abnormalities in the epithelial cells from affected corneal epithelium in recurrent erosion were described recently (6). Multinucleate giant epithelial cells and binucleate cells have been identified in the loose epithelium of eyes with recurrent erosion. The intricate details of the relationship between abnormal basement membrane and abnormal epithelial cells in recurrent erosion are not yet known.

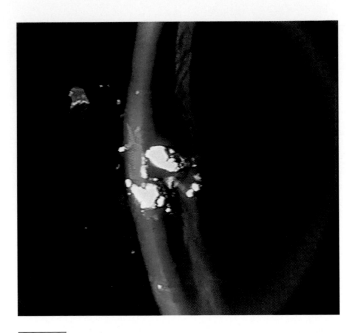

FIGURE 13-4.   *Patient with recurrent erosion due to anterior basement membrane dystrophy. Irregular edges of the epithelium are seen at the edge of the epithelial defect.*

MEDICAL MANAGEMENT

The goal of treating recurrent erosions is to provide the most favorable environment to encourage epithelial growth, migration, and adhesion to the underlying corneal structures. Initial medical therapy is undertaken in most patients because this is usually successful in curing the patient (12). Educating and providing the patient with insight into the etiology and course of the problem is equally important.

Initial management of an acute recurrent erosion consists of antibiotic ointment and pressure patching until the patient becomes asymptomatic. Alternatively, topical lubricating drops or ointments alone can be utilized, as some patients are more comfortable without patching.

An acute erosion may have frankly loose epithelium (Fig. 13-4). In these cases, debridement of this tissue may be helpful prior to patching or other therapy. Removing this tissue allows for fresh epithelium to migrate in, which may have the advantage of being more closely approximated to the underlying Bowman's layer. This also prevents the loose edges from being traumatized by eyelid action, which may be quite painful for the patient. After debridement, the physician may use topical antibiotics and lubricants or patching.

When the symptoms subside, applying an ointment at bedtime may provide adequate lubrication to prevent a recurrence upon waking in the morning. Nighttime lubrication with ointment should be continued for 6 to 12 months after the patient recovers from the acute episode. In addition, teaching the patient how to open the eyelid in a nontraumatic way in the morning may be helpful. Pulling on the upper lid above the tarsal plate to physically remove it from the corneal surface prior to opening the eye in the morning may help to carefully separate the lid from the cornea, thus preventing erosions. The most common difficulty with this technique is remembering to perform the maneuver prior to opening the eye.

Hyperosmotic topical lubricating ointments also can be used at bedtime. These have an added benefit of providing a hyperosmolar environment that is not only lubricating, but also dehydrates the epithelium (11,12,21). The result is that the epithelium is more closely approximated to Bowman's layer with less intervening fluid. A more rapid reattachment of the epithelium occurs in this environment. A 5% sodium chloride ointment (Muro 128, Bausch & Lomb, Tampa, FL; Adsorbanac, Alcon, Fort Worth, TX; AK-NaCl, Akorn, Abita Springs, LA) or a 40% glucose ointment (Glucose-40, Ciba Vision, Duluth, GA) can be used to create this hyperosmolar environment.

Investigators have looked into topical hyperosmotic colloidal suspensions, which may even cause more dehydration as compared to hypertonic sodium chloride ointments (21,22). Using a topical colloidal dextran polysaccharide solution (Dehydrex, Holles Laboratories, Cohasset, MA), patients who did not respond to previous therapy (including patching, lubricants, and hypertonic saline ointments) had marked and lasting effect of increased visual acuity and decreased recurrence of symptoms (21).

BANDAGE CONTACT LENS

When medical management fails to promote epithelial adhesion and relieve the patient's symptoms, the use of a soft contact lens can be quite helpful (23–25). Any loose epithelial tissue should be debrided prior to application, since this tissue may interfere with regrowth of new epithelium and may provide a nidus for infection (25).

Soft contact lenses promote healing by protecting the poorly adherent and the new epithelial tissue from the trauma induced by the movement of the eyelids (11). Formation of new basement membrane and attachment complexes may require up to 2 to 3 months, and the bandage lens may be helpful during this healing period (12).

While the contact lens is in place, daily use of prophylactic antibiotics may be considered, at least until the epithelium is healed. The contact lens, although meant to protect the cornea, inherently alters the local microenvironment. One of the more important effects is introducing an increased risk for microbial infection. Other problems with bandage contact lens wear include contact lens intolerance, reduced oxygen tension at the corneal surface, increasing epithelial and stromal edema, peripheral neovascularization, and giant papillary conjunctivitis (24,25).

Some patients may find long-term symptomatic relief in daily-wear or extended-wear lenses. If daily-wear lenses are used, use of nonpreserved lubricants is helpful during the day, and lubricating ointments should be used at night. Because of the inconvenience and risks associated with contact lens wear, the patient and physician often prefer alternative therapies.

ANTERIOR STROMAL PUNCTURE

It has long been noted that recurrent corneal erosions rarely occur following trauma when a breach of Bowman's layer has occurred. Superficial lacerations of the cornea heal with a significantly smaller chance of subsequent recurrent erosion syndrome. Recurrent erosion syndrome also rarely follows removal of a foreign body. These observations eventually led to the idea of artificially creating breaches of Bowman's membrane, hoping for a similar decrease in the incidence of subsequent recurrent erosions. The procedure referred to as *anterior stromal puncture* is one method of creating these violations of Bowman's layer (5).

Recent studies showed that at sites of anterior stromal puncture, there is a proliferation of subepithelial fibrotic connective tissue. Immunohistochemical staining showed that at the puncture sites, laminin, fibronectin, and type IV collagen are all locally present where the epithelium is firmly attached. It appears that only a breach of Bowman's layer, exposure to stroma, or both, results in the production, excretion, and organization of these proteins (6,15).

Anterior stromal puncture is reserved for patients who do not respond to conservative medical therapy. Several studies demonstrated favorable results with this technique and variations of the basic technique or instrumentation have also been described with similar results (5,26). The procedure is quick, done in the office at the slit lamp, relatively safe, and inexpensive and involves a short recovery period for the patient.

The procedure begins with the application of topical anesthesia. A drop of fluorescein solution prior to beginning the punctures allows for a brighter visualization of the areas that have been punctured.

The choice of needle or instrument used to perform the punctures relies somewhat on the surgeon's preference. Different puncturing instruments have been described. A straight, 20-gauge needle can be used, but because of the inconsistent depth of punctures and the potential for full-thickness corneal perforation, most surgeons no longer use a straight needle. The tip of the needle can be bent to prevent inadvertent deep punctures. The needle shaft can also be bent to allow better positioning of the hand during the procedure. A bend similar to that of a cystotome used for the capsulotomy at the time of cataract surgery is optimal. The result is an instrument with a built-in depth gauge, leading to a consistent stromal penetration depth and less risk of corneal perforation, as well as allowing better visualization of the treated area (Fig. 13-5).

The needle is applied to the corneal surface with enough force to enter the anterior stroma through Bowman's layer. Indentation of the cornea is probably not necessary if a sharp needle is used and excessive indentation can lead to an increase in corneal edema. The punctures are applied over areas of loose or sloughing epithelium. The entire area of the erosion should be covered with punctures 0.5 to 1.0 mm apart. The visual axis is avoided to prevent scarring in the visual axis, which can lead to decreased vision and glare from light scattering (5,26) (Fig. 13-6).

At the conclusion of the procedure a drop of cycloplegic such as 1% cyclopentolate can be applied and antibiotic ointment such as erythromycin is applied and the eye is typically patched. The patient is seen the following day to evaluate the healing of the corneal epithelium and to examine for possible infection. Antibiotic ointment is continued until complete re-epithelialization occurs. The patient should

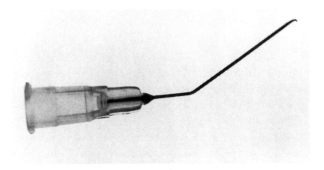

FIGURE 13-5. *Anterior stromal puncture needle. Note the bend at the base of the shaft, allowing for a comfortable hand position, and the bend at the tip of the needle allowing for consistent depth of corneal penetration. (Reprinted with permission from Rubinfeld RE, Laibson PR, Cohen EJ, et al. Anterior stromal puncture for recurrent erosion: further experience and new instrumentation. Ophthalmic Surg 1990;21:318–326. Figure 1.)*

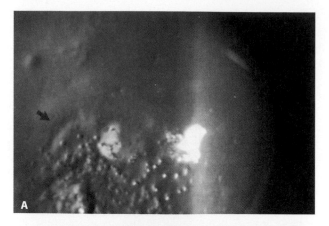

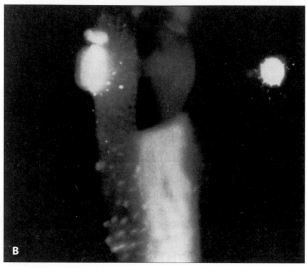

FIGURE 13-6.   *Anterior stromal puncture scars.* A. *Retro-illumination slit-lamp photograph taken immediately after anterior stromal puncture.* B. *Slit-lamp photograph demonstrating corneal scarring at sites of deep stromal penetration during anterior stromal puncture. (Reprinted with permission from Rubinfeld RE, Laibson PR, Cohen EJ, et al. Anterior stromal puncture for recurrent erosion: further experience and new instrumentation. Ophthalmic Surg 1990;21:318–326. Figures 5 and 6.)*

continue applying a plain lubricating or a hypertonic ointment at bedtime for 6 months to 1 year or more depending on the nature, severity, and longevity of the preoperative erosions. Should the erosions recur, second and third trials of anterior stromal puncture can be beneficial. However, alternative therapies such as phototherapeutic keratectomy with the excimer laser may be more useful if recurrence occurs or the disease involves an area within 2.5 mm of the visual axis.

Several authors documented the success of treating recurrent erosions with anterior stromal puncture. In a trial by Rubinfeld et al (26) in 1990, a total of 25 patients with recurrent erosions resistant to cure by conservative therapy underwent a single trial of anterior stromal puncture. In a follow-up period ranging from 2 to 30 months, only one

recurrent erosion was reported. Other clinicians reported anterior stromal puncture success rates of 70% to 90% in treating recurrent erosions in patients with erosions that were previously resistant to medical therapy (6,27).

SUPERFICIAL EPITHELIAL KERATECTOMY

Another effective form of surgical intervention in recurrent erosion patients is superficial epithelial keratectomy. Superficial epithelial keratectomy, like anterior stromal puncture, is not a first-line treatment but is usually reserved for erosions that persist despite medical therapy. The procedure was originally described as a treatment for recurrent erosion associated with excessive aberrant epithelial basement membrane, such as may be seen with anterior corneal dystrophies (27). This is an extremely useful technique for managing recurrent erosions in these patients.

Superficial keratectomy is most easily performed under an operating microscope. A relatively simple microscope in the office can be used. Topical anesthesia such as proparacaine is applied immediately prior to the procedure. Topical nonsteroidal anti-inflammatory agents such as diclofenac may also be used to help reduce postoperative pain (28). A lid speculum is applied. The region to be debrided is identified by the surgeon, and the loosely adherent epithelium is gently scraped away with a PRK Spatula, Tooke knife, or No. 64 Beaver blade (Fig. 13-7). Excessive lubrication should be avoided to allow easy removal of the epithelium. Drying the corneal surface allows any remaining clumps of epithelium or abnormal basement membrane material to be visualized more easily. These regions are polished with a dry cellulose sponge in a circular manner to make certain there is no remaining epithelium or anterior basement membrane material. In patients with anterior basement membrane dystrophy, care must be taken to remove all abnormal material, even in areas that may not have had documented erosions. A dry cellulose sponge will help to identify other loose areas of epithelium, which will be removed when polished with the sponge. Care must be taken to leave at least 0.5 mm of epithelium adjacent to the limbus to allow these stem cells to survive and repopulate the cornea with epithelial cells. If an edge of the thickened anterior membrane is elevated, a jeweler's forceps may be used to peel these sheets from Bowman's layer, but this should be followed by polishing with the sponge once again. At the conclusion of the procedure, there should be a fully exposed and clean Bowman's layer in the region of debridement.

Pain can vary significantly from patient to patient. The typical patient is initially quite comfortable, until the effect of the topical anesthetic wears off. At the conclusion of the procedure, the cornea is lubricated with antibiotic ointment and a pressure patch may be applied. The patient should keep the patch on for 24 hours, until returning to clinic the next day.

Alternatively, the patient may be more comfortable with the eye left unpatched and a bandage soft contact lens placed

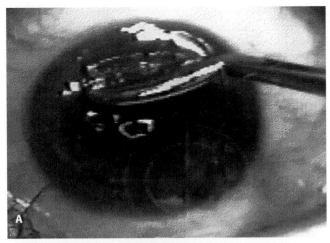

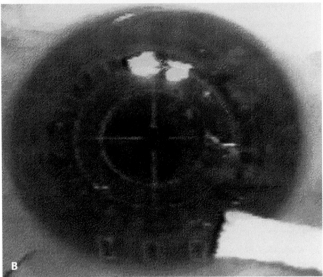

FIGURE 13-7.   *Photograph of superficial keratectomy procedure.* A. *A hockey-stick blade is used to sweep across the cornea to remove epithelium.* B. *Remaining epithelium is removed with a cellulose sponge after most of the epithelium was removed with a blade.*

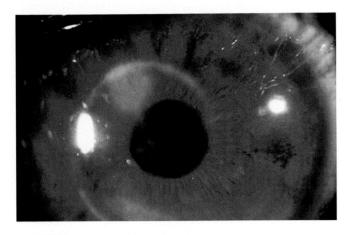

FIGURE 13-8.   *Inflammatory infiltrates in a patient following superficial keratectomy and excimer laser treatment. This patient was treated with a bandage contact lens and topical nonsteroidal agents. No topical steroids were used. The patient responded well with resolution of the infiltrates when topical steroids were instituted.*

on it. If a contact lens is used, topical antibiotic, topical steroid, and topical nonsteroidal anti-inflammatory drugs are quite helpful in controlling pain and preventing infectious keratitis. If a topical nonsteroidal agent is used for postoperative discomfort, it is important that it be used as seldom as necessary to control pain. When topical nonsteroidal anti-inflammatory medicines are used, they are typically applied four times the first day, three times the second day, and twice the third day. This is usually adequate to control pain. Topical steroids should be concomitantly used with the nonsteroidal agent to prevent inflammatory infiltrates (28,29) (Fig. 13-8). Copious topical nonpreserved lubrication should be used to assist in postoperative comfort. The patient should be followed closely until complete epithelialization occurs, which depends on the size of the area debrided.

The size of the area to be debrided depends on the pathology in the individual patient. If only a small region of the cornea is affected and the remainder of the cornea is perfectly normal, then a shorter postoperative recovery period and less postoperative pain are encountered if only the affected area is debrided. Determining that a certain region of a cornea is normal is sometimes very difficult. Often, microscopic pathology is difficult to fully correlate with clinical findings in the presence of a dystrophy such as anterior basement membrane dystrophy. For this reason, some surgeons elect to debride the entire corneal surface if any epithelium appears to be abnormal in the setting of diseases such as anterior basement membrane dystrophy. In this case, one must be careful to avoid the peripheral 0.5 or 1.0 mm of the cornea to ensure maintaining limbal integrity. This allows the peripheral epithelial stem cells to rapidly re-epithelialize the surface. Complete epithelial debridement has the advantage of treating any areas that may have unrecognized pathology, thereby potentially avoiding a future erosion. The normal epithelium will usually be much more adherent when an attempt is made to remove it with the dry cellulose sponge. It must be remembered that the postoperative course and length of recovery may be a day or two longer, and there may be more discomfort with a larger epithelial defect.

Buxton and Fox (27) reported an 85% success rate of relieving patients from symptoms of recurrent erosions that were resistant to medical therapy. In most patients, visual acuity improved after complete corneal epithelialization occurred.

DIAMOND BURR KERATECTOMY

The use of a diamond burr has been advocated to assist in removal of epithelium and anterior basement membrane material in certain situations. Some surgeons find it useful to remove large nodules of epithelium that are not easily managed with the standard superficial keratectomy techniques (30). The diamond burr has also been recommended for use in the perilimbal region of the cornea, approximately 0.5 to 1.0 mm from the limbus, where a near-complete superficial keratectomy is indicated, as for anterior basement membrane dystrophy (27). The postoperative care of a patient in whom a diamond burr was used to assist with epithelial and anterior basement membrane removal is identical to the postoperative care for patients who have undergone the above-described superficial keratectomy.

PHOTOTHERAPEUTIC KERATECTOMY

The argon-fluorine 193-nm excimer laser emits ultraviolet light that can remove fractions of a micron of corneal tissue in a short period of time without causing damage to adjacent tissues. The excimer laser has gained enormous popularity since its first application in human corneas in 1988. The most common current application is photorefractive keratectomy for correcting myopic refractive errors (30–32). The excimer laser also has several therapeutic applications in treating anterior corneal pathology. It can be used to smooth irregular corneal surfaces and remove visually impairing, superficial scarring from the anterior 100 to 150 μm of the cornea. Anterior corneal dystrophies, traumatic scars, infectious scars, and Salzmann's nodular degeneration are some of the pathologies amenable to treatment with phototherapeutic keratectomy (30–36). Recurrent erosions that are refractory to other treatment modalities have also been treated by phototherapeutic keratectomy (30,36–42).

The excimer laser is now accessible to ophthalmologists, with several 193-nm excimer lasers now being produced. Several studies reported on the capabilities of phototherapeutic keratectomy with the excimer laser for managing recurrent erosion syndrome (30,36–42). The excimer laser is also capable of treating any anterior corneal surface irregularities or scarring that may be related to the recurrent erosion. In some patients the excimer laser may provide an alternative to lamellar or penetrating keratoplasty.

Phototherapeutic keratectomy in patients from whom significant amounts of corneal tissue are removed may flatten the cornea. In some patients with preexisting myopic refractive errors, this may be beneficial, yet in patients who are already hyperopic this may be a disadvantage (37). The amount of tissue removed for most patients with recurrent erosion only minimally changes the refractive error.

Patients undergoing phototherapeutic keratectomy for recurrent erosions should have a complete ophthalmologic examination. Of particular importance is the visual acuity with and without best correction, a detailed slit-lamp examination, and a dilated-fundus examination. A drawing of the location and depth of pathology with respect to other landmarks is helpful. Additional important procedures include pachymetry of the affected region, computerized topographic analysis of the cornea, and keratometry.

One eye at a time is operated on, waiting until complete epithelialization and recovery of vision before the second eye is operated on. The more severely affected eye is treated first. Topical anesthetic is instilled into the eye. A drop of topical nonsteroidal anti-inflammatory drug such as diclofenac may be useful in reducing postoperative pain (28,29). A drop of topical antibiotic or steroid may also be instilled. The nonoperative eye is taped closed, which helps the patient to fixate on the fixation target. The eyelid margins are prepped with a 50% solution of povidone-iodine, and a lid speculum is placed. The patient is centered under the operating microscope, and appropriately positioned so that the iris plane is perpendicular to the laser beam. The patient is asked to fixate on the operating microscope fixation target. An inability of the patient to hold fixation is not crucial to phototherapeutic keratectomy for recurrent erosions because the treatment is not always centered over the pupil (30).

A 7.0- or 8.0-mm optical zone marker can be used to mark the visual axis in areas where centration is important. The region to be debrided is identified by the surgeon, and the loosely adherent epithelium is gently scraped away with a Tooke knife or No. 64 Beaver blade. Excessive lubrication should be avoided to allow easy removal of the epithelium. Drying the corneal surface allows any remaining clumps of epithelium or abnormal basement membrane material to be visualized more easily. These regions are polished with a dry cellulose sponge in a circular manner to make certain there is no remaining epithelium or anterior basement membrane material. In patients with anterior basement membrane dystrophy, care must be taken to remove all abnormal material, even in areas that may not have had documented erosions. A dry cellulose sponge will help to identify other loose areas of epithelium, and they will be removed when polished with the sponge. Care must be taken to leave at least 0.5 mm of epithelium adjacent to the limbus, to allow these stem cells to survive and repopulate the cornea with epithelial cells.

If an edge of the thickened anterior basement membrane is elevated, a jeweler's forceps may be used to peel these sheets from Bowman's layer but this should be followed by polishing with the sponge once again. There should be fully exposed and clean Bowman's layer in the region of debridement. The presence of an irregular surface prior to photoablation will result in an irregular postoperative surface unless care is taken to protect low-lying areas and expose elevated areas. Methylcellulose can be used as a modulating agent to smooth and protect the valleys while exposing the peaks if there is significant irregularity (30,36). In patients with minimal surface irregularities, the surface should be relatively dry prior to the beginning of ablation. The patient is asked to fixate on the fixation target, centration is rechecked, and photoablation can proceed.

In the typical eye with anterior basement membrane dystrophy without subepithelial scarring, the corneal surface is relatively smooth after the mechanical superficial keratectomy. In these eyes, the goal should be to remove 5 µm of tissue from all affected areas of the cornea. If the pathology is limited to the central 6 mm of the cornea, the laser can be set in the phototherapeutic keratectomy mode for a treatment depth of 5 µm (only 20 pulses), and the foot pedal depressed to perform the treatment. If the pathology extends over the entire cornea, as is often the case, then the laser is set for a depth of 30 µm, and the eye is moved under the laser during the treatment to obtain even application of laser energy throughout the cornea, ablating to a depth of about 5 µm in each area of the cornea (Fig. 13-9). It is important that all areas that had epithelium removed be treated with the laser to allow better adhesion.

At the conclusion of the procedure, a drop of mild steroid, a nonsteroidal anti-inflammatory drug, a topical antibiotic, and a bandage contact lens are applied. The contact lens is used until re-epithelialization occurs. Postoperative comfort may be supplemented with oral analgesics. Topical antibiotics should be used three to four times daily until complete epithelialization occurs, at which point they can be discontinued. The steroids are used four to six times daily and tapered slowly over 1 to 6 months, depending on the depth of ablation.

Nonsteroidal anti-inflammatory drops can be used to reduce postoperative pain, but excessive use may result in delayed epithelial healing or sterile infiltrates. Concomitant topical steroids may help to reduce or prevent the sterile infiltrates associated with nonsteroidal anti-inflammatory use (28,29). Nonsteroidal agents are used, at most, four times the first day, three times the second day, and twice the third day. It is important to continue frequent lubrication with a hypertonic ointment for up to 1 year after phototherapeutic keratectomy for recurrent erosion, to prevent an early recurrence of the erosion.

Talley et al (37) reported a series of 12 eyes (11 patients) that underwent phototherapeutic keratectomy for recurrent erosions. In all 12 eyes medical therapy had failed to prevent recurrent erosions; in 9, at least one trial of superficial keratectomy had failed and in 1, previous superficial keratectomy and anterior stromal puncture procedures had failed. Eleven of these 12 eyes had no recurrence of recurrent erosion symptoms in a follow-up period of 4 to 24 months after phototherapeutic keratectomy, and all had best-corrected visual acuity equal to or better than the preoperative visual acuity. Only 1 of the 12 eyes experienced a recurrent erosion, but this erosion occurred outside the treated area.

Phototherapeutic keratectomy is an effective treatment for recurrent erosions, involves rapid visual recovery, and is flexible, with the potential for treating a number of other anterior corneal pathologic conditions. When conservative therapy fails, the patient may be treated with phototherapeutic keratectomy before anterior stromal puncture, especially when very large areas are affected or when the visual axis is involved. Superficial keratectomy is still extremely effective, and less expensive than phototherapeutic keratectomy, and therefore may become the first surgical procedure for many patients, though phototherapeutic keratectomy is an excellent alternative when superficial keratectomy fails. Phototherapeutic keratectomy is especially useful in patients with scarring, patients with identifiable underlying anterior corneal pathology, or when anisometropia could be reduced with central corneal flattening.

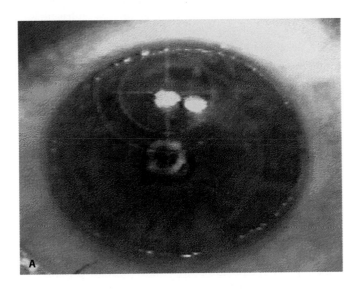

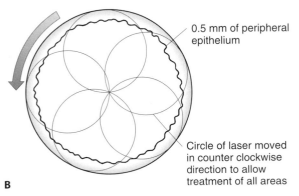

0.5 mm of peripheral epithelium

Circle of laser moved in counter clockwise direction to allow treatment of all areas

FIGURE 13-9. *Phototherapeutic keratectomy of recurrent erosion. A. Photograph of the starting position of the circle of laser energy. Note how the outer circle of the reticle overlaps peripheral intact epithelium to ensure treatment of the entire cornea, which has been debrided of epithelium. B. Circle of laser energy moved in a counterclockwise direction to allow treatment of all areas.*

Nd:YAG ANTERIOR STROMAL PUNCTURE

The Nd:YAG laser is useful in several settings in ophthalmology, but perhaps the most recent application is as a device to perform anterior stromal puncture in a precise, nontraumatic, and reproducible manner (43). This procedure can be easily performed in any office equipped with a Nd:YAG laser, and requires only topical anesthetic. No long-term study is available, but early anecdotal evidence suggests promising results.

The patient is anesthetized with topical anesthetic, and is positioned at the laser. Topical antibiotics may be applied. The epithelium in the affected area is debrided using cellulose sponges and the area to be treated should have a smooth, shiny appearance indicating that all epithelium is removed. The aiming beam is carefully focused just in front of the basement membrane zone, and several 1.8- to 2.2-mJ shots are fired. It is important to realize that more punctures will have to be performed than with conventional anterior stromal puncture because of their markedly smaller size. The laser punctures are spaced approximately 0.2 mm apart. Audible snapping may be heard as the laser shock wave hits the cornea.

Immediate postoperative care includes a combination steroid-antibiotic ointment and pressure patching. Topical antibiotics should be continued, and the patient followed daily until re-epithelialization occurs. After the defect is healed, the antibiotic is discontinued and a lubricating ointment is used at bedtime for up to 1 year.

Complications are primarily the result of poor aim. If the laser is focused too deeply in the cornea, a bubble can form within the stroma. This bubble dissipates over ensuing weeks to leave a small gray scar. This scar is reportedly smaller than a conventional anterior stromal puncture scar. Another potential complication is any effect the shock wave may have on the endothelium. One animal study demonstrated focal endothelial and Descemet's membrane damage in 2% of animals undergoing Nd:YAG anterior stromal puncture (43).

CHEMICAL CAUTERY

Chemical cautery has also been advocated for the treatment of recurrent erosions. Like contemporary surgical treatment used today, it was reserved for recurrent erosion that responded poorly to lubrication. Reports of cure rates of up to 90% have been published (3).

As with phototherapeutic keratectomy and other therapeutic procedures for recurrent erosions, an important step in successful treatment of recurrent erosions is removal of all affected epithelium prior to application of the chemical. Several chemical preparations have been used, but the most common has been 2% chlorine water. Trichloroacetic acid 10% and iodine are some other preparations that have been successful (3,11).

COMPLICATIONS

All the procedures described have potential complications. The risk of infection is quite low, while scarring and haze formation are seen regularly after some procedures, but are rarely visually significant.

Increased risk of infection occurs any time the corneal epithelium is altered. Patients with recurrent erosions are at risk of infectious keratitis even without surgical intervention. Debridement of loose or sloughed tissue and the judicious use of antibiotics may reduce the incidence of infection. However, the most important measures to minimize the risk of infection and corneal scarring are careful clinical observation and patient education. In the event that an infectious keratitis is suspected, appropriate cultures should be promptly obtained and antibiotic therapy begun.

Subepithelial scar and haze formation can occur after anterior stromal puncture, superficial keratectomy, phototherapeutic keratectomy, and the Nd:YAG anterior stromal puncture procedures, but it is also a result of long-standing, untreated recurrent erosions, as well as the underlying pathologic condition leading to the recurrent erosions. Scar and haze can be very unpleasant and dissatisfying to the patient, resulting in photophobia, glare, and decreased visual acuity. Scar and haze are due to new collagen formation in the affected area of the cornea. They can occur at any level from the subepithelial to the posterior stromal regions, in response to inflammatory destruction of the normal tissue. Corneal haze following all excimer laser ablations decreases gradually over the first year or two after treatment. Topical steroids are used to decrease the local inflammatory response and also are important to decrease the formation of corneal haze and sterile infiltrates associated with topical nonsteroidal anti-inflammatory medicines (28–30,44,45).

The postoperative care recommended with each therapeutic modality is designed to minimize these complications. Such care is considered an integral step in all of the described procedures, and is important if the surgeon is to obtain the best possible results. Careful postoperative observation is the single most important measure toward preventing complications and minimizing them should they occur.

CONCLUSIONS

Recurrent erosions have significant clinical morbidity for the patient. Incapacitating effects associated with an erosion include epiphora, pain, photophobia, and decreased visual acuity. Recurrent erosions can be a difficult and challenging clinical problem for both patient and ophthalmologist.

Although most recurrent erosions are successfully treated with adequate artificial lubrication, some patients do not respond well to this treatment. Bandage contact lenses, anterior stromal puncture, superficial epithelial keratectomy, diamond burr keratectomy, chemical cautery, and phototherapeutic keratectomy are all effective treatments for recurrent erosions in the appropriate clinical settings. In deciding which treatment is best for an individual patient, the physician should take into consideration the severity and longevity of the recurrent erosions, any underlying pathology associated with the erosions, and the patient's compliance with medical regimens.

REFERENCES

1. Hansen E. Om den intermitterende keratitis vesicularis neuralgia af traumatisk opindelse. *Hospitals Tidende* 1872;51:201–203.

2. Von Arlt F. Ueber die verletzungen des Arges in Gericht-sarztilicher beziehung. *Wien Medizen/Wachenscher* 1874;23:447–449.

3. Chandler PA. Recurrent erosion of the cornea. *Am J Ophthalmol* 1945;28:355–363.

4. Weene LE. Recurrent corneal erosion after trauma: a statistical study. *Ann Ophthalmol* 1985;17:521.

5. McLean EN, MacRae SM, Rich LF. Recurrent erosion treatment by anterior stromal puncture. *Ophthalmology* 1986;93:784–788.

6. Hsu JKW, Rubinfeld RS, Bary P, Jester JV. Anterior stromal puncture: immunohistochemical studies in human corneas. *Arch Ophthalmol* 1993;111:1057–1063.

7. Basic clinical and science course section No. 8. External disease and cornea. San Francisco, CA: American Academy of Ophthalmology, 1995:181–183.

8. Trobe JD, Laibson PR. Dystrophic changes in anterior cornea. *Arch Ophthalmol* 1972;87:378–382.

9. Brown NA, Bron AJ. Recurrent erosion of the cornea. *Br J Ophthalmol* 1976;60:84–86.

10. Fogle JA, Kenyon KR, Stark WJ, Green WR. Defective epithelial adhesion in anterior corneal dystrophies. *Am J Ophthalmol* 1975;79:925–940.

11. Wood TO. Recurrent erosion. *Trans Am Ophthalmol Soc* 1984;82:850–898.

12. Kenyon KR. Recurrent corneal erosion. *Int Ophthalmol Clin* 1978;19:169–195.

13. Albert DM, Jakobiec FA. *Principles and practice of ophthalmology—clinical practice.* Vol. 1. Philadelphia: WB Saunders, 1984:218–234.

14. Aitken DA, Beirouty ZA, Lee WR. Ultrastructural study of the corneal epithelium in the recurrent erosion syndrome. *Br J Ophthalmol* 1995;79:282–289.

15. Alberts B. *Molecular biology of the cell.* 2nd ed. New York: Garland, 1989:798–820.

16. Sugrue SP, Hay ED. The identification of extracellular matrix (ECM) binding sites on the basal surface of embryonic corneal epithelium and the effect of ECM binding on epithelial collagen production. *J Cell Biol* 1986;102:1907–1916.

17. Schultz PO, Van Dorn DL, Peters MA, et al. Diabetic keratopathy. *Trans Am Ophthalmol Soc* 1981;79:180–199.

18. Kenyon KR, Hannimen LA, Gibson IK, et al. Clinico-pathological correlations of epithelial basement membrane morphology in human corneal erosion. *Invest Ophthalmol Vis Sci* 1981;20(suppl):39.

19. Alvarado J, Murphy C, Juster R. Age related changes in basement membrane of the human corneal epithelium. *Invest Ophthalmol Vis Sci* 1983;24:1015–1028.

20. Foulks GN. Treatment of recurrent corneal erosion and corneal edema with topical osmotic colloidal solution. *Ophthalmology* 1981;88:801–803.

21. Lamberts DW, Foulks GN, Holly FT. Effect of colloidal isoosmotic solutions on edema and epithelialization of denuded rabbit cornea in vivo. *Invest Ophthalmol Vis Sci* 1978;277(suppl).

22. Dohlman CH, Boruchoff SA, Mobilia EF. Complications in use of soft contact lenses in corneal disease. *Arch Ophthalmol* 1973;90:367–371.

23. Mobilia EF, Foster CS. The management of recurrent erosions with ultrathin lenses. *Contact Intraoc Lens Med J* 1978;4:25–29.

24. Langston R, Machemer CJ, Norman CW. Soft lens therapy for recurrent erosion syndrome. *Ann Ophthalmol* 1978;10:875–878.

25. Thoft RA, Mobilia EF. Complications with therapeutic extended wear soft contact lenses. *Int Ophthalmol Clinic* 1981;21:197–208.

26. Rubinfeld RE, Laibson PR, Cohen EJ, et al. Anterior stromal puncture for recurrent erosion: further experience and new instrumentation. *Ophthalmic Surg* 1990;21:318–326.

27. Buxton JN, Fox ML. Superficial epithelial keratectomy in the treatment of epithelial basement membrane dystrophy. *Arch Ophthalmol* 1983;101:392–395.

28. Sher NA, Frantz JM, Talley A, et al. Topical diclofenac in the treatment of ocular pain after excimer photorefractive keratectomy. *Refract Corneal Surg* 1993;9:425–436.

29. Teal P, Breslin C, Arshinoff S, Edmison D. Corneal subepithelial infiltrates following excimer laser photorefractive keratectomy. *J Cataract Refract Surg* 1995;21:516–518.

30. Harden DR, Lindstrom RL. Excimer laser photorefractive and phototherapeutic keratectomy. In: Lindquist TM, Lindstrom RL, eds. *Ophthalmic surgery.* St. Louis: Mosby, 1995:II-J0–II-J34.

31. Sher NA, Chen V, Bowers RA. The use of the 193-nm excimer laser for photorefractive keratectomy in sighted eyes: a multi-center study. *Arch Ophthalmol* 1991;109:1525–1530.

32. Talley AR, Hardten DR, Sher NA, et al. Results one year after using the 193-nm excimer laser for photorefractive keratectomy in mild to moderate myopia. *Am J Ophthalmol* 1994;118:304–311.

33. Campos M, Nielson S, Szerenyi K, et al. Clinical follow-up of phototherapeutic keratectomy for treatment of corneal opacities. *Am J Ophthalmol* 1993;115:433–440.

34. Fagerholm P, Fitzsimmons TD, Omdahl M, et al. Phototherapeutic keratectomy: long-term results in 166 eyes. *Refract Corneal Surg* 1993;9(suppl):S76–S81.

35. Sher NA, Bowers RA, Zabel RW, et al. Clinical use of the 19-nm excimer laser in the treatment of corneal scars. *Arch Ophthalmol* 1991;109:491–498.

36. Rapuano CJ, Laibson PR. Excimer laser photokeratectomy. *CLAO J* 1993;190:235–240.

37. Talley A, Sher NA, Doughman DJ, et al. Phototherapeutic keratectomy for the treatment of recurrent corneal erosion syndrome. *Trans Acad New Orleans Ophthalmol Sci* 1995;42:113–119.

38. Hersh PS, Sinak A, Garrana R, Mayers M. Phototherapeutic keratectomy: strategies and results in 12 eyes. *Refract Corneal Surg* 1993;9(suppl):S90–S95.

39. Hahn TW, Sah WJ, Kim JH. Phototherapeutic keratectomy in nine eyes with superficial corneal diseases. *Refract Corneal Surg* 1993;9(suppl):S115–S117.

40. Forster W, Grewe S, Atzler U, et al. Phototherapeutic keratectomy in corneal diseases. *Refract Corneal Surg* 1993;9(suppl):S85–S90.

41. Dausch D, Landesz M, Klein R, Schroder E. Phototherapeutic keratectomy in recurrent corneal epithelial erosion. *Refract Corneal Surg* 1993;9(suppl):419–424.

42. Gartry D, Muir MK, Marshall J. Excimer laser treatment of corneal surface pathology: a laboratory and clinical study. *Br J Ophthalmol* 1991;75:258–269.

43. Geggel HS. Successful treatment of recurrent corneal erosion with Nd:YAG anterior stromal puncture. *Am J Ophthalmol* 1990;10:404–407.

44. Tuft SJ, Zabel RW, Marshall J. Corneal repair following keratectomy: a comparison between conventional surgery and laser photoablation. *Invest Ophthalmol Vis Sci* 1989;30:1769–1777.

45. Wu WC, Stark WJ, Green WR. Corneal wound healing after 193-nm excimer laser keratectomy. *Arch Ophthalmol* 1991;109:1426–1432.

Chapter

14

Traumatic Cataract with Other Anterior-Segment Injury

GLENN C. COCKERHAM   PETER A. RAPOZA   KENNETH R. KENYON

Cataracts associated with trauma present unique diagnostic and treatment challenges in anterior-segment surgery. The reported incidence of lenticular damage in ocular trauma series from the United States and other countries varies widely from 7% to 54% (1–6). Traumatic cataract was present in 43% (88/205) of eyes injured by a sharp object (7), and in 47% of eyes with perforating injuries and retained intraocular foreign bodies (8). Trauma accounts for approximately one-half of lens dislocations or subluxations (9). Ocular trauma frequently occurs in younger individuals, with the potential threat of amblyopia further complicating decision making. Traumatic cataract is often associated with other ocular injuries, including corneoscleral lacerations, hyphema, angle recession, iris tears or dialysis, and vitreous hemorrhage (10–12). In a study of 1004 cases of traumatic cataract, only 17% manifested as uncomplicated cataract alone, without other ocular damage (13). Sequelae of such anterior-segment trauma can include endophthalmitis, corneal scarring, irregular astigmatism, peripheral anterior synechiae (PAS), anterior-chamber membranes, glaucoma, cystoid macular edema (CME), epiretinal membrane, retinal detachment, amblyopia, and strabismus (14).

PATHOPHYSIOLOGY

Both blunt force– and sharp-object–induced injuries cause cataractous changes. Sharp object–induced injuries that violate the lens capsule lead to rapid cataract formation in the area of injury. The eventual extent of the lens opacity may depend on the size of the capsular defects. Concussive forces may be directly transmitted to the lens as a coup injury. The lens capsule may rupture posteriorly (in its thinnest area) or anteriorly. A contrecoup injury may arise from disruption by a shock wave at fluid interfaces, including the anterior or posterior lens capsule (15). An unrecog-nized capsular tear at the lens equator may also occur from equatorial expansion of the eye secondary to an axial compressive force (11,15). The extent of ocular damage is likely proportional to the amount of force applied. Lens epithelium proliferates in an attempt to seal the wound (16).

Traumatic cataract can also occur in the presence of an intact lens capsule (Fig. 14-1). Concussive damage to the lens epithelium may directly injure the adenosine tri-phosphate–dependent sodium-potassium ion pump, allowing an influx of sodium and water into the lens substance, with cortical hydration and opacification (10). Ultrastructural studies showed rapid epithelial deterioration after either blunt force– or sharp-object–induced injury, with changes of adjacent cortical fibers, which may explain the frequent occurrence of posterior subcapsular cataracts after trauma (17). A common pathway for traumatic cataract appears to be lens hydration, as ultrastructural analysis of posterior subcapsular cataracts demonstrated grossly swollen cortical fibers in the area of opacification (16). The resultant change in refractive index between normal cortex and swollen cortex may account for the lens opacity and reduced vision (Fig. 14-2). Computed tomography (CT) studies of traumatic cataract demonstrated a consistently increased water content (10,18). The hydrated cortex becomes flocculent and in the presence of a capsular dehiscence, may be liberated into the anterior chamber. The entire lens may swell and opacify, with eventual rupture. If left undisturbed, the cortex will resorb in some patients, especially in younger patients, with eventual formation of Soemmering's ring. A tough, thin membranous cataract may form, with fibrous metaplasia of the lens epithelium.

Intraocular foreign bodies can induce cataract formation through penetration or perforation of the lens. Reactive metals can cause additional lens damage: For example, iron is the most frequent constituent of metallic foreign bodies,

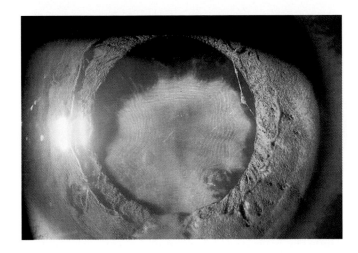

FIGURE 14-1. *Typical rosette cataract due to blunt trauma.*

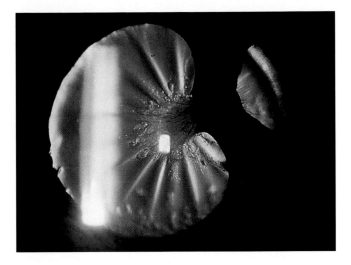

FIGURE 14-3. *Retroillumination highlights a traumatic cataract and iridodialysis.*

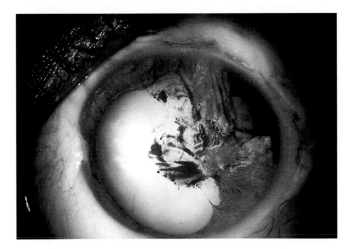

FIGURE 14-2. *Mature cataract and severe iridodialysis following blunt trauma from a racquet ball.*

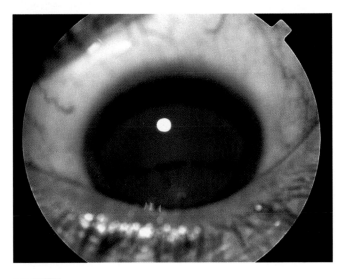

FIGURE 14-4. *Zonular disruption, lens subluxation, and disinsertion of the vitreous base induced by blunt trauma.*

and can lead to siderosis, with brown deposits in the lens epithelium (19). Siderosis can affect other intraocular epithelial tissues, causing iris heterochromia and atonicity, retinal degeneration, and open-angle glaucoma. Iron-containing foreign bodies contained within the lens can remain inert (20). Foreign bodies from copper or one of its alloys (brass or bronze) usually occur with wire injuries or cartridge explosions (19). Generally, intraocular foreign bodies of copper are extremely inflammatory, especially if the copper content exceeds 85%, but can remain inert if embedded in the lens. Chalcosis, or copper toxicity, can lead to deposition of copper particles on basement membranes. Clinical features of chalcosis include deposition of copper particles on the peripheral part of Descemet's membrane; a green, sluggish iris; a green or brown "sunflower" anterior capsular cataract; and metallic particles along retinal vessels or in the macula (19).

Other clinical consequences of lenticular trauma are well recognized. Zonular damage can occur at the time of injury, with subluxation or dislocation (luxation) of the lens (Figs. 14-3 and 14-4). The lens can dislocate posteriorly into the vitreous or anteriorly into the anterior chamber, the latter potentially involving lens-endothelial touch and corneal edema. Free lens protein, presumably sequestered from the immune system by an intact lens capsule in normal circumstances, can incite intense (phacotoxic) inflammation. Phacolytic glaucoma can occur from blockage of the aqueous outflow system by macrophages engorged with lens material. An injured lens can grossly enlarge, become tumescent, and produce a pupillary block, with resultant phacomorphic glaucoma. Lens injury after sharp trauma is strongly associated with endophthalmitis (7).

EVALUATION

A logical, stepwise approach to ocular trauma patients is essential to document the site and severity of injury, as well as to record pertinent negative findings. This is especially true for acute injuries, as the evaluation will form the basis for therapeutic decisions and has medicolegal significance as well. The initial examination may afford the only opportunity to inspect the posterior structures, before corneal edema, cataract, or hemorrhage ensues.

Important historical points for acute trauma include the time of the most recent oral intake, tetanus status, drug allergies, general health (including sickle-cell status or other hematologic abnormalities), medications, and previous anesthetic and surgical history. Best-corrected and uncorrected visual acuity prior to the injury, and past ocular history including glaucoma, previous injuries, ocular medications, previous eye surgery, and any conditions predisposing to lens subluxation (such as syphilis, Marfan's syndrome, and homocystinuria) are recorded. Prior cataract surgery, especially by an intracapsular or extracapsular technique with a large limbal incision, can predispose to wound rupture even years later. Similarly, previous radial keratotomy incisions can remain permanently weak (21).

The events surrounding the injury should be reconstructed. The time of injury, type and magnitude of force applied, and any protective devices or eye wear used can alert the examiner to potential occult injuries and guide further testing. Globe rupture, optic nerve damage, and orbital fractures must be suspected with significant blunt trauma. Known perforating injury or a history suggestive of high-velocity metal particles (e.g., grinding or hammering metal on metal) should raise suspicion of an intraocular foreign body (20,21).

In instances of traumatic cataract after contusion without perforating injury or symptomatic hemorrhage or inflammation, patients may present weeks or months after the time of injury. Fluctuating vision may be a symptom of a subluxated lens, while decreased vision may be attributable to a progressive cataract or a dislocated lens (11).

Ocular trauma patients can be difficult to evaluate in the acute setting because of age, associated injuries, anxiety, and intoxication or other mental impairment. Initial consideration must be given to prevention of further damage or injury. If a ruptured globe is suspected, no external pressure should be applied, to avoid extrusion of intraocular contents. Likewise, no topical medications should be administered until globe rupture has been definitively ruled out. A protective metal eye shield should be utilized immediately. A lid or regional nerve block may be necessary to overcome eyelid spasm and thereby facilitate ocular examination. Antiemetics are useful in nauseated patients.

Documentation of visual function is important to establish a baseline and for medicolegal considerations. Initial uncorrected and (if possible) best-corrected visual acuities are determined or at least verified personally by the ophthalmologist. Near vision with a reading card is usually sufficient (with appropriate reading, add lens for presbyopic patients). If possible, distance visual acuity, including pinhole acuity, should also be measured. A vision of no light perception should be verified with a bright light source (e.g., indirect ophthalmoscope) and witnessed by other examiners, as this finding is of great significance for surgical decision making. Pupillary testing for an afferent defect and appropriate visual field testing should also be performed.

For adequate inspection of the anterior segment, slit-lamp biomicroscopy should be carefully performed. Conjunctival lacerations, chemosis and subconjunctival hemorrhage, or uveal pigment may indicate occult globe injury. The presence and location of any corneal lacerations are noted, and they are tested for leakage with 2% fluorescein. The anterior chamber is inspected for signs of inflammation, vitreous, lens fragments, and blood. Deepening of the chamber is suggestive of globe rupture with vitreous loss, whereas shallowing can be caused by lens swelling or a retained foreign body. If no evidence of globe rupture is found, then visualization of the chamber angle with gonioscopy is important to rule out iridodialysis, angle recession, and foreign body or lens fragments.

The size and shape of the pupil are noted. A peaked pupil can indicate vitreous in the anterior chamber, or iris prolapse through a scleral wound. Retroillumination may detect iris perforations, suggesting accompanying lens damage. Iridolenticular adhesions indicate prior trauma or inflammation.

Examination of the lens is conducted before and after pupil dilatation. The position of the lens relative to the iris is noted, and the presence and location of lens luxation (dislocation) or subluxation are noted. Iridodonesis, a tremulous, shimmering movement of the iris overlying an unstable lens, indicates zonular dehiscence. Sectoral vitreous prolapse into the anterior chamber also evidences zonular rupture. A Vossius' pigment ring indicates that the lens has sustained significant blunt concussive force. The integrity of the anterior and posterior capsule is carefully determined with the narrow slit beam, as the status of the posterior capsule is especially important for surgical planning. The presence of flocculent gray material is evidence of a breach in the capsule with hydration of the cortex. Lens clarity is determined with direct and indirect illumination, noting any nuclear sclerosis, opacities, sectoral defects, or foreign bodies. Fibrin may coat the lens and simulate lenticular opacification. The ocular examination is completed by dilated examination of the vitreous, retina, and optic nerve and measurement of intraocular pressure. In instances where applanation tonometry is not possible, tactile estimation of intraocular pressure may be very useful.

Ultrasound is helpful to image intraocular structure when visualization is poor owing to the presence of blood, fibrin, or corneal opacity. A foreign body can be detected and localized. CT is useful to evaluate the bony orbit, extraocular muscles, and optic nerve and is capable of distinguishing a traumatic cataract from a normal lens. In a study of 69 eyes with acute orbital trauma, many with opaque media, clinically cataractous lenses had statistically significantly lower attenuation values by CT than did normal lenses in the uninvolved fellow eye, with this effect attributed to increased intralenticular fluid (10). CT of a traumatic cataract 3 months after a penetrating lens injury occurred showed a hyperdense rim surrounding a hypodense center, the latter due to increased fluid content (18). CT can also localize a retained metallic foreign body, whereas magnetic resonance imaging (MRI) is contraindicated if metallic foreign bodies are present or suspected, because of potential displacement of the object by the magnetic force.

MANAGEMENT

The optimal management of a traumatic cataract and anterior-segment injury is determined on an individual basis. Important factors to consider include vision and visual potential, the patient's age, the location of the opacification, the status of the lens capsule and zonules, and the presence and degree of lens-induced glaucoma, as well as the various concomitant injuries of the ocular anterior and posterior segments. Indeed, some traumatic cataracts will remain visually insignificant. Pieramici et al (22) followed five patients with lens capsule disruption and peripheral opacification from foreign body injury; the cataracts did not progress and all patients maintained at least 20/40 vision. Paracentral lens opacities can be managed by pharmacologic pupil constriction to reduce glare and blur. Thus, the indications for surgical intervention include a visually significant cataract; lens-induced glaucoma; uncontrollable lens-, blood-, or vitreous-induced inflammation; and significant zonular disruption with subluxation.

Pediatric Traumatic Cataract

The management of traumatic cataract in children requires special consideration. The surgical goal is to obtain clear ocular media, especially in young children at risk for deprivation amblyopia, although lens removal can be delayed if no definite capsule rupture is noted on initial examination or the lens is not visualized because of blood or fibrin in the anterior chamber (23). Indications for surgery in children include a large capsular tear, visual acuity less than 20/70 or loss of central fixation despite patching of the uninjured eye, or development of strabismus (23). Endocapsular aspiration of the cataract is usually combined with discission of the posterior capsule and a limited anterior vitrectomy (23,24). A peripheral iridectomy can be performed. Postoperative topical and systemic steroids and cycloplegic agents are required to suppress inflammation and prevent the formation of synechiae.

Prompt optical correction of unilateral surgical aphakia, combined with occlusion therapy, is necessary for children under the age of 7, but the best approach remains controversial. Results with spectacle correction are poor (23,25). Contact lenses are often used, but the disadvantages of extended contact lens wear are many, including the associated expense, parent frustration with lens care and lost lenses, difficulty with fit after corneal injury, and the obvious multiple socioeconomic factors (26,27). Epikeratophakia, or placement of a prelathed lenticule of donor corneal tissue onto a host corneal bed, has demonstrated good results in patients with contact lens intolerance or corneal lacerations, but the current limited availability of appropriately prepared lenticules is a major problem (28–30).

Correction of traumatic unilateral aphakia by placement of an anterior-chamber, iris-clip, iridocapsular, or posterior-chamber intraocular lens (IOL) has been reported (23–27, 31–34). We currently favor only the use of posterior-chamber IOLs in children, usually with capsular or scleral suture fixation, given the availability of excellent IOLs, sutures, and techniques for this specific situation. Suggested indications for IOL implantation in aphakic pediatric patients include a coexisting corneal injury complicating contact lens fitting and age younger than 7, because of difficulties with contact lens wear in this age group (27,34). IOLs have been implanted in children as young as 1 year (31,34) but are most commonly utilized after the ages of 2 to 3 years. Lens power can be calculated from keratometry and axial-length measurements, or an adult lens power can be implanted to accommodate anticipated growth and changes in refraction. Heparin-coated IOLs have been recommended to lessen the incidence of inflammatory precipitates (27). The posterior capsule may be discissed at surgery, or afterward with a yttrium-aluminum-garnet (YAG) laser.

Lens Removal

In adult patients under the age of 40, traumatic cataracts can be aspirated by an endocapsular technique with automated or manual irrigation-aspiration, in the presence of adequate zonular support. A limited vitrectomy can be performed if vitreous has prolapsed through a zonular rupture. In older patients with less than 60 degrees of zonular dehiscence, phacoemulsification or extracapsular cataract extraction can be attempted (35). For extracapsular extraction, nucleus removal by an irrigating lens loop is safer than nuclear expression. The surgeon must always be prepared to convert to lensectomy or cryoextraction, if unrecognized zonular instability is discovered. Lensectomy or cryoextraction, frequently including anterior vitrectomy, is indicated for an unstable lens. If a lens loses all zonular support during surgery and submerges into the vitreous, a viscoelastic agent should be immediately placed behind it to prevent further posterior movement. If the lens can be stabilized anteriorly, then the wound is enlarged to at least 10 mm, and the lens or lens fragment is removed with a lens loop, and an anterior vitrectomy performed. If such retrieval of the lens is not readily possible, a pars plana lensectomy can be performed primarily or as a secondary procedure. We strongly discourage the use of copious intravitreal irrigation to attempt to "refloat" the dislocated lens, as the likelihood of a posterior-segment complication is unacceptably high, whereas removal by a vitreoretinal approach is very successful and may be combined with posterior-chamber IOL fixation.

Membranous cataracts often occur with adhesions to the pupil or vitreous face. Although some membranes may be amenable to YAG laser disruption, removal of the dense fibrous cataract and scar tissue usually requires sharp dissection and excision with intraocular scissors or use of an automated vitreous cutter. As the scar tissue is often vascularized and prone to bleed, endodiathermy must be available intraoperatively. Manipulation of posterior adhesions to the vitreous face can cause vitreous loss.

Lens Dislocation or Subluxation

Traumatically dislocated lenses may be displaced into the anterior chamber or into the vitreous or extrude through a corneal or scleral wound outside of the eye. Indications for surgery of traumatic ectopia lentis include dislocation into the anterior chamber with corneal touch, mature cataract, lens-induced uveitis or glaucoma, visual aberration, and increasing lens subluxation (9). A lens with an intact capsule dislocated posteriorly into the vitreous may be well tolerated and require no surgical treatment. If removal is necessary, a bimanual vitrectomy technique is preferred, as the ability to grasp and manipulate the unstable lens is enhanced. A dislocated lens in the anterior chamber is contained by pupillary constriction, then removed by lens aspiration, phacoemulsification, or intracapsular extraction. As previously discussed, the appropriate surgical procedure for removal of a subluxated lens depends on the degree of subluxation and remaining zonular support, the patient's age and the status of the vitreous. In younger patients (<40 years), endocapsular aspiration of the cataract can be performed with either manual or automated irrigation-aspiration, provided there is sufficient zonular support or subluxation of less than one-half the lens diameter, and limited vitreous prolapse into the anterior chamber. If vitreous is present in the anterior chamber, zonular loss exceeds 90 degrees, or the lens is subluxed more than one-half the diameter, then pars plana lensectomy and vitrectomy are recommended. In patients older than 40, aspiration is generally unsuccessful because of increased density of the lens nucleus, necessitating an extracapsular or phacoemulsification technique if the vitreous face is intact and zonular support is adequate. With anterior vitreous prolapse and inadequate zonular support, an anterior vitrectomy may be performed, followed by an intracapsular extraction. If the lens is extremely unstable, without zonular support, then pars plana vitrectomy and lensectomy are indicated (35).

Anterior Vitrectomy

Vitreous that has become fibrotic following incarceration in a corneoscleral wound should be excised. All prolapsed vitreous should be removed from the anterior chamber, as a limited anterior vitrectomy facilitates iris reconstruction and IOL insertion or transscleral fixation. An automated vitrector with minimal irrigation is used to remove vitreous atraumatically and to lyse iridovitreal and other adhesions. No irrigation is necessary if an open-sky technique is used. Isolated vitreous strands may be removed with a cellulose sponge (e.g., Weck-cel) and Vannas or Westcott scissors. At the conclusion of vitrectomy, the anterior chamber should be free of vitreous strands and the iris should assume its normal anatomic plane.

Goniosynechialysis

Lysis of PAS may improve aqueous outflow and reduce the incidence or severity of postoperative glaucoma. It also frees incarcerated iris tissue for reconstructive iridoplasty. A blunt instrument is used to separate iris from the periphery of the cornea. In open-sky techniques, a cellulose sponge is preferred. If an area of synechiae cannot be liberated, it can be excised after radial cuts are made in the iris along either side of it. Bleeding can be managed by a viscoelastic agent, by irrigation with 1:10,000 epinephrine, or in open-sky surgery, by either application of a thrombin-soaked cellulose sponge or direct cauterization with bipolar underwater diathermy.

Removal of Anterior-Segment Membranes

Posttraumatic fibrovascular or thin Descemet-like membranes often form over the anterior part of the iris, the angle, and the posterior area of the cornea. Removal of these membranes is indicated to prevent further fibrosis, synechial formation, iris retraction, and endothelial loss. A dry cellulose sponge can be used to identify the cleavage plane between membrane and normal tissue. Fine tissue forceps are used to grasp the edge and gently peel off the membrane.

Intraocular Lens Placement

For many years, anterior-chamber IOLs were preferred for visual rehabilitation in aphakia, and remain useful today for primary or secondary implantation predominantly in nontraumatized eyes of older patients who do not have adequate capsular support for a sulcus-fixated posterior-chamber IOL. Improvements in lens quality and design have gradually evolved over the past two decades. Rigid one-piece Choyce-style anterior-chamber IOLs were abandoned because of manufacturing and design problems, as well as a frequent association with the uveitis, glaucoma, hyphema

(UGH) syndrome (36). Leiske-style, closed-loop, semiflexible anterior-chamber IOLs were discontinued because of the frequent occurrence of corneal edema (pseudophakic bullous keratopathy) and CME. Criteria for an acceptable anterior-chamber IOL include a well-polished, one-piece, all-polymethylmethacrylate (PMMA), flexible, open-loop lens with Choyce-type broad haptics (37,38). Flexible, open-loop anterior-chamber IOLs, such as the Kelman Omnifit and similar designs, do not appear to have the multiple complications seen with previous generations of lenses (39).

Anterior-chamber IOLs have been used as secondary implants after the removal of traumatic cataracts in adults, usually for intolerance of contact lenses or aphakic spectacles (40,41). Although anterior-chamber IOLs have been implanted after traumatic cataract in children, they are best reserved for use in nontraumatized eyes of elderly patients. Relative contraindications to their usage include PAS, glaucoma, angle recession, a large sector iridectomy, and corneal compromise (42).

Placement of a posterior-chamber IOL into the capsular bag by standard techniques is the preferred method for implantation, provided enough zonular support exists for lens stability. In situations of suboptimal posterior capsular support, ciliary sulcus placement of a large-diameter-optic (6.5–7.0-mm), posterior-chamber IOL without suture fixation may be effective. In a series of eyes with at least six clock hours of peripheral zonular support, all sulcus-fixated posterior-chamber IOLs remained centered after a mean follow-up of 10.5 months (43). Iris suture fixation may be readily employed in an open-sky technique. Short (2-inch) double-armed 10-0 polypropylene (Prolene) sutures with BV100-4 vascular needles (Ethicon) are girth-hitched through positioning holes in a one-piece, all-PMMA lens, are brought through the undersurface of the mid-peripheral region of the iris, and are then secured as mattress sutures on the anterior part of the iris.

Transscleral fixation through the ciliary sulcus with suspensory sutures allows placement of a posterior-chamber IOL into the nodal point of the eye, despite inadequate capsular support. Nonabsorbable suture material, usually 10-0 polypropylene, is preferred, as pathologic studies demonstrated that haptic placement in uncomplicated cases may be outside the ciliary sulcus, and that no appreciable fibrosis around the haptics occurs by 6 months (44). The ideal location for transscleral passage has been shown in cadaver eyes to be 0.83 mm posterior to the posterior surgical limbus in the vertical meridian and 0.46 mm in the horizontal meridian (45). Thus, while the eye remains pressurized, triangular, limbus-based, half-thickness scleral flaps are fashioned at the 10-o'clock and 4-o'clock meridians (for righthanded surgeons), avoiding the horizontal ciliary vessels. Other meridians may be used, depending on the surgeon's preference, as long as the haptics are situated 180 degrees apart. After lens removal, and anterior vitrectomy if indicated, the wound is enlarged. A one-piece, all-PMMA

lens with haptic eyelets is placed on the surgical field. A modified C-loop haptic with a total diameter of 11.5 to 12.5 mm is preferred, to conform to the mean diameter of 11.15 mm of the ciliary ring (46). In cases without penetrating keratoplasty, a 13.3-mm-long needle with 10-0 polypropylene (CIF-4, Ethicon) is tied or girth-hitched to the IOL haptics and passed through the scleral incision and across the anterior chamber closely behind the iris in order to exit through the bed of the scleral flap. Alternatively, a 25-gauge retrobulbar needle can be similarly passed through the limbal incision, across the anterior chamber, under the iris, to exit through the ciliary sulcus. The suture can then be threaded through the needle lumen and exit through the limbal incision, where it is affixed to the IOL (47). If the cornea is removed and an open-sky approach is employed, the posterior-chamber IOL is easily sutured to the iris by utilizing 2-inch 10-0 polypropylene sutures with BV100 needles (Ethicon), which are girth-hitched to the positioning holes on the IOL optic and passed through the midperipheral part of the iris.

Modifications of transscleral fixation include creation of one flap superiorly and two adjacent flaps inferiorly, to allow three-point IOL fixation, as described by Rapoza (48) (Figs. 14-5 to 14-14). Polypropylene suture on a CIF-4 needle can be used for transscleral fixation inferiorly, with iris fixation performed by using polypropylene on double-armed BV100-4 needles passed superiorly through a limbal incision (49). Polypropylene suture on an STC-6 needle

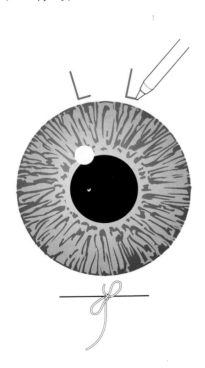

FIGURE 14-5. *Prepare scleral tunnel incision, remove lens material and prolapsed vitreous. Inject viscoelastic to protect corneal endothelium and stabilize vitreous. Prepare partial thickness sclerotomies at 5:30 and 7:30.*

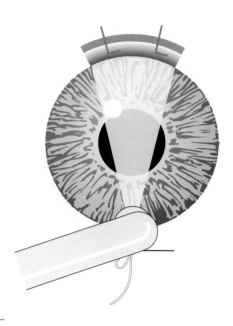

FIGURE 14-6.   *Transilluminate ciliary sulcus to ensure secure placement of IOL haptices.*

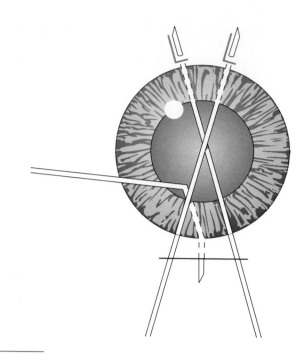

FIGURE 14-7.   *Pass pre-bent 25-gauge hypodermic needles through the sclerotomies to serve as suture introducers.*

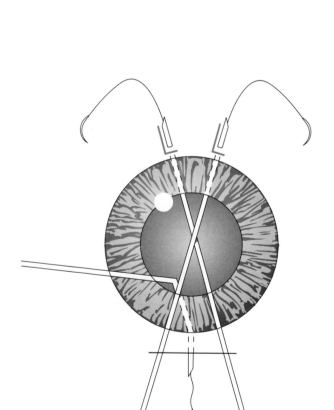

FIGURE 14-8.   *Pass 10-0 prolene suture through hypodermic needles. (Note: each needle and suture are passed one at a time.)*

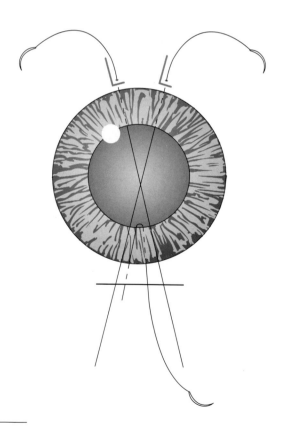

FIGURE 14-9.   *Remove hypodermic needles. Externalize suture ends.*

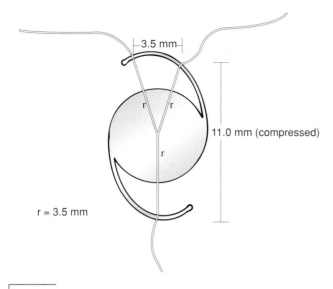

FIGURE 14-10.   *Fixate sutures to haptics.*

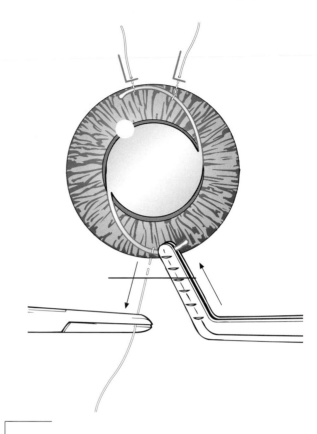

FIGURE 14-12.   *Implant superior haptic into the ciliary sulcus.*

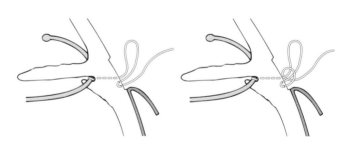

FIGURE 14-13.   *Anchor prolene sutures to scleral bed.*

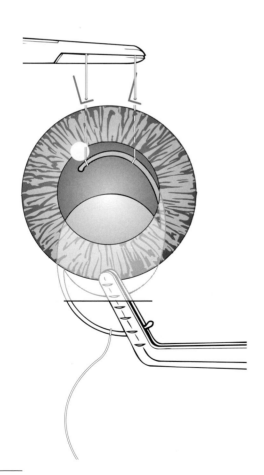

FIGURE 14-11.   *Introduce inferior haptic into the ciliary sulcus.*

(Ethicon) can be used (50). Suture material can be secured to an IOL by placement of either a girth hitch or a knot.

Iridodialysis Repair

Traumatic iridodialysis can cause diplopia and glare and be cosmetically disfiguring. Repair in a closed system can be accomplished by placing a 10-0 polypropylene suture with a double-armed CIF-4 needle (Ethicon). A limbal peritomy is performed parallel to the edge of the dialysis and a stab paracentesis placed 180 degrees away from the dialysis. The straight needle is passed through the paracentesis site, through the peripheral edge of dehisced iris, and through the globe to exit 0.5 mm posterior to the posterior surgical

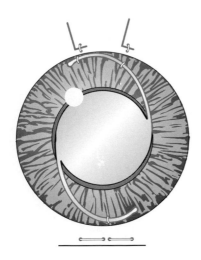

FIGURE 14-14. *Remove viscoelastic and any remaining vitreous anterior to the IOL. Close limbal wound and conjunctiva.*

limbus. The second needle is passed through the same paracentesis wound, engaging iris 1.0 to 1.5 mm adjacent to the first suture and exiting the globe in the same coronal plane as the first needle. Additional sutures can be appropriately used for repair of a large dialysis. The knots are rotated and buried, and the conjunctiva replaced. This technique is best suited for a pseudophakic eye (51,52).

Iridoplasty

Iridoplasty is accomplished after removal of all iris adhesions, membranes, and scar tissue, and after completion of lens removal, anterior vitrectomy, and IOL implantation. The goals of iris reconstruction are 1) restoration of a tight iris diaphragm to lessen the risk of future synechial formation, 2) improvement in corneal transplant survival by prevention of iridocorneal adhesions and glaucoma, 3) formation of a stable iris platform for IOL support, and 4) restoration of a functional pupil to prevent or reduce glare and to improve appearance (14). Closure of any iris defects is performed with interrupted sutures of either 10-0 nylon or polypropylene. This is readily accomplished in the open-sky situation of penetrating keratoplasty. In the closed eye setting, modifications of the McCannell suturing technique are employed, utilizing the CIF-4 needle with 10-0 polypropylene suture, which is passed through the peripheral region of the cornea to engage both iris edges, and then exited out the other side through the peripheral region of the cornea. The needle is cut off and the suture ends are retrieved and externalized with an iris hook through an adjacent limbal incision. The suture is tied externally and slipped into the anterior chamber.

RESULTS

The results obtained by medical or surgical management of traumatic cataract depend on the visual potential of the injured eye as a consequence of multiple factors. Corneal scarring or edema, irregular astigmatism, glaucoma, vitreous hemorrhage, CME, epiretinal membrane, retinal detachment, and amblyopia can all limit visual outcome. Differences in therapy, surgical techniques, and age groups make comparisons of visual results difficult among series of pediatric traumatic cataracts. In general, the younger the patient at the time of injury and the longer the interval between cataract development and surgery, the greater the risk of amblyopia (2,26). The end result of untreated traumatic cataract in young children is dismal. Of 26 patients under age 6 with traumatic cataracts reported in 1961, some treated by lens removal and some by lens resorption, only 1 patient, managed with spectacle correction and occlusion therapy, obtained vision of 20/40 or better (53). Aphakic contacts lenses are a therapeutic advance, but results have been poor in children under the age of 7, despite occlusion therapy (25). Aspiration of lens material combined with the wearing of spectacles or contact lens allowed vision of 20/40 or better in 41% of patients with traumatic cataracts; however, some of these patients were adults (54). In a group of children with corneal lacerations and traumatic cataract treated with corneal repair and lens aspiration, followed by contact lens correction and patching, 20/40 vision was achieved in 27% (27). Vision of 20/40 or better was recorded in 77% of children over age 6 with traumatic cataract managed with lens aspiration plus contact lens wear and occlusion therapy (2).

Four (25%) of 12 children with surgical aphakia after unilateral traumatic cataract obtained 20/50 or better vision with epikeratophakia (28). Epikeratophakia grafts were successful in 5 of 6 children under age 3 years and 3 months with corneal lacerations and traumatic cataracts; vision in these 5 patients ranged from 20/30 to 20/80 (30).

Several large series analyzed results of unilateral traumatic cataract corrected surgically with a variety of IOLs. Hiles (31) reported that 54 (60%) of 90 children achieved a best-corrected visual acuity of 20/40 or better with either an anterior-chamber, iris-suture, or posterior-chamber IOL. In a study of 584 eyes, in children and adults, Fyodorov et al (13) reported 90% with 20/50 or better vision with a sputnik-style lens. In a study by Blumenthal et al (33), 71% of 36 pediatric patients obtained 20/40 or better vision with an iris, iridocapsular, or posterior-chamber IOL. Hemo and Ben Ezra (24) found 20/40 or better vision in 77% of children with primary IOL implantation and 69% with secondary IOL implantation, using either an anterior-chamber or posterior-chamber IOL. In a series by Gupta et al of younger children, age 3 to 11 years, 45% obtained 20/40 or better vision with either an anterior-chamber (4) or posterior-chamber IOL (18,26). Anwar et al (27) found that 11 (73%) of 15 children age 3 to 8 years managed with aspiration, posterior-capsule discission, and anterior vitrectomy and placement of a posterior-chamber IOL achieved a visual acuity of 20/40 or better. Aggressive occlusion therapy is required in children under the age of 7 or 8.

After anterior-segment reconstruction, including penetrating keratoplasty, in 39 severely injured adult eyes, visual acuity improved in 31 (79%). Visual acuity improved from 20/100 or better in 10% of eyes preoperatively to 49% postoperatively. The majority of patients with PAS preoperatively (80%) had no recurrence after goniosynechialysis (14). Doren et al (55) similarly performed penetrating keratoplasty, with anterior-segment reconstruction as needed, on 41 adult and pediatric eyes with traumatic corneal scars. Three patients required cataract extraction. The authors reported a final visual acuity of 20/100 or better in 30 (74%) of their patients.

COMPLICATIONS

General anesthesia is usually required for cataract surgery or trauma repair in children, with the remote risk of death or neurologic impairment. Visual impairment from optic nerve injury, globe perforation, or retrobulbar hemorrhage can occur with retrobulbar anesthetic injection. Complications of trauma repair and cataract surgery include corneal decompensation due to endothelial damage or stripping of Descemet's membrane, hemorrhage, glaucoma, CME, retinal tear or detachment, infection, and sympathetic ophthalmia.

There are several complications related to specific techniques or devices. Although the risk is lower with a flexible, open-loop anterior-chamber IOL than with earlier models, corneal decompensation and pseudophakic bullous keratopathy may still develop with anterior-chamber IOLs. Glaucoma may occur from formation of PAS, from pupillary block, or from the UGH syndrome. Other complications found with anterior-chamber IOLs include lens malposition and fibrinous membrane formation. A higher incidence of CME has been noted in eyes with vitreous prolapse and anterior vitrectomy (42,56).

Ciliary body hemorrhage can occur during passage of a needle during transscleral suture fixation of a posterior-chamber IOL. Dislocation or tilt of a posterior-chamber IOL can occur in instances where there is less capsular support than anticipated for sulcus fixation (57). Dislocation or tilt of a posterior-chamber IOL can also occur after transscleral suture fixation if a knot slips, or the suture is inadvertently cut externally (58). Tilt, decentration, rotation, or "propellering" of a lens may occur after two-point suture fixation. Solomon et al (59) noted erosion of a polypropylene suture through a half-thickness scleral flap in 22 (73%) of 30 eyes from 1 to 12 months after surgery, although this has not been our personal experience. *Hemophilus influenzae* endophthalmitis occurred in a patient with an exposed

suture 5 months after transscleral suture fixation of a posterior-chamber IOL (60).

CONCLUSIONS

Traumatic cataract remains a potentially blinding condition. Eye trauma is especially problematic in children with an immature visual system because of the threat of deprivation amblyopia. The prognosis for unilateral traumatic cataract in children has improved significantly with prompt removal of the opaque lens, aggressive occlusion therapy, and correction of aphakia by wearing of a contact lens, epikeratophakia, or implantation of an IOL. A posterior-chamber IOL, anchored by either capsular support or transscleral suture fixation, is the preferred and recommended approach in both children and adults. Although associated anterior-segment injuries may limit final visual outcome, a thorough and meticulous reconstruction of the anterior segment may restore useful vision in even severely injured eyes.

REFERENCES

1. Insler MS, Helm CJ. Traumatic cataract management in penetrating ocular injury. *CLAO J* 1989;15:78–81.
2. Jain IS, Bansal SL, Dhir SP, et al. Prognosis in traumatic cataract surgery. *J Pediatr Ophthalmol Strabismus* 1979;16:301–305.
3. De Juan E, Sternberg P, Michels RG. Penetrating ocular injuries: types of injuries and visual results. *Ophthalmology* 1983;90:1318–1322.
4. Muga R, Maul E. The management of lens damage in perforating corneal lacerations. *Br J Ophthalmol* 1978;62:784–787.
5. Eagling EM. Perforating injuries of the eye. *Br J Ophthalmol* 1976;60:732–736.
6. Pieramici DJ, MacCumber MW, Humayun MU, et al. Open globe injury: update on types of injuries and visual results. *Ophthalmology* 1996;103:1798–1803.
7. Thompson WS, Rubsamen PE, Flynn HW, et al. Endophthalmitis after penetrating trauma: risk factors and visual acuity outcomes. *Ophthalmology* 1995;102:1696–1701.
8. Williams DF, Mieler WF, Abrams GW, Lewis H. Results and prognostic factors in penetrating ocular injuries with retained intraocular foreign bodies. *Ophthalmology* 1988;95:911–916.
9. Jaffe NS, Jaffe MS, Jaffe GF. Lens displacement. In: Jaffe NS, Jaffe MS, Jaffe GF, eds. *Cataract surgery and its complications.* St. Louis: CV Mosby, 1990:303–316.
10. Boorstein JM, Titelbaum DS, Patel Y, et al. CT diagnosis of unsuspected traumatic cataracts in patients with complicated eye injuries: significance of attenuation value of the lens. *AJR Am J Roentgnol* 1995;164:181–184.
11. Irvine JA, Smith RE. Lens injuries. In: Shingleton BJ, Hersh PS, Kenyon KR, eds. *Eye trauma.* St. Louis: Mosby-Year Book, 1991:126–135.
12. Cowden JW. Anterior segment trauma. In: Spoor TC, Nesi FA, eds. *Management of ocular, orbital, and adnexal trauma.* New York: Raven, 1988:21–49.
13. Fyodorov SN, Egorova EV, Zubareva LN. One thousand four cases of traumatic cataract surgery with implantation of an intraocular lens. *Am Intraocular Implant Soc J* 1981;7:147–153.
14. Kenyon KR, Starck T, Hersh PS. Penetrating keratoplasty and anterior segment reconstruction for severe ocular trauma. *Ophthalmology* 1992;99:396–402.
15. Wolter JR. Coup-contrecoup mechanism of ocular injuries. *Am J Ophthalmol* 1963;56:785–795.
16. Fagerholm PP, Philipson BT. Human traumatic cataract: a quantitative microradiographic and electron microscopic study. *Acta Ophthalmol* 1979;57:20–32.
17. Rafferty NS, Goossens W, March WF. Ultrastructure of human traumatic cataract. *Am J Ophthalmol* 1974;78:985–995.
18. Segev Y, Goldstein M, Lazar M, Reider-Groswasser I. CT appearance of a traumatic cataract. *AJNR Am J Neuroradiol* 1995;16:1174–1175.
19. De Bustros S. Posterior segment intraocular foreign bodies. In: Shingleton BJ, Hersh PS, Kenyon KR, eds. *Eye trauma.* St. Louis: Mosby-Year Book, 1991:226–237.

20. Smiddy WE, Stark WJ. Anterior segment intraocular foreign bodies. In: Shingleton BJ, Hersh PS, Kenyon KR, eds. *Eye trauma*. St. Louis: Mosby-Year Book, 1991:169–174.

21. Hamill WB. Clinical evaluation. In: Shingleton BJ, Hersh PS, Kenyon KR, eds. *Eye trauma*. St. Louis: Mosby-Year Book, 1991:3–24.

22. Pieramici DJ, Capone A, Rubsamen PE, Roseman RL. Lens preservation after intraocular foreign body injuries. *Ophthalmology* 1996;103:1563–1567.

23. Hiles DA, Wallar PH, Biglan AW. The surgery and results following traumatic cataracts in children. *J Pediatr Ophthalmol* 1976;13:319–325.

24. Hemo Y, BenEzra D. Traumatic cataracts in young children. *Ophthalmic Pediatr Genet* 1987;8:203–207.

25. Binkhorst CD, Gobin MH. Pseudophakia after lens injury in children. *Ophthalmologica* 1967;154:81–87.

26. Gupta AK, Grover AK, Gurha N. Traumatic cataract surgery with intraocular lens implantation in children. *J Pediatr Ophthalmol Strabismus* 1992;29:73–78.

27. Anwar M, Bleik JH, von Noorden GK, et al. Posterior chamber lens implantation for primary repair of corneal lacerations and traumatic cataracts in children. *J Pediatr Ophthalmol Strabismus* 1994;31:157–161.

28. Morgan KS, Stephenson GS, McDonald MB, Kaufman HE. Epikeratophakia in children. *Ophthalmology* 1984;91:780–784.

29. Morgan KS, Marvelli TL, Ellis GS, Arffa RC. Epikeratophakia in children with traumatic cataracts. *J Pediatr Ophthalmol Strabismus* 1986;23:108–114.

30. Morgan KS, Stephenson GS. Epikeratophakia in children with corneal lacerations. *J Pediatr Ophthalmol Strabismus* 1985;22:105–108.

31. Hiles DA. Intraocular lens implantation in children with monocular cataracts: 1974–1983. *Ophthalmology* 1984;91:1231–1237.

32. Binkhorst DC, Gobin MH, Leonard PAM. Post-traumatic artificial lens implants (pseudophakoi) in children. *Br J Ophthalmol* 1969;53:518–529.

33. Blumenthal M, Yalon M, Treister G, Hashomer T. Intraocular lens implantation in traumatic cataract in children. *Am Intraocular Implant Soc J* 1983;9:40–41.

34. Bienfait MF, Pameijer JH, Blecourt-Devilee M. Intraocular lens implantation in children with unilateral traumatic cataract. *Int Ophthalmol* 1990;14:271–276.

35. Koch DD, Emory JM. Subluxated lens: intracapsular aspiration. In: Heilman K, Paton D, eds. *Atlas of ophthalmic surgery: techniques—complications*. Vol 2. New York: Thieme Medical, 1987:4.66–4.70.

36. Smith PW, Wong SK, Stark WJ, et al. Complications of semiflexible, closed-loop anterior chamber intraocular lenses. *Arch Ophthalmol* 1987;105:52–57.

37. Auffarth GU, Wesendahl TA, Brown SJ, Apple DJ. Are there acceptable anterior chamber intraocular lenses for clinical use in the 1990s? An analysis of 4104 explanted anterior chamber intraocular lenses. *Ophthalmology* 1994;101:1913–1922.

38. Auffarth GU, Brown SJ, Wesendahl TA, Apple DJ. Clinical use for AC IOLs. *Ophthalmology* 1995;102:857–859. Letter.

39. Weene LE. Flexible open-loop anterior chamber intraocular lens implants. *Ophthalmology* 1993;100:1636–1639.

40. Leatherbarrow B, Trevett A, Tullo AB. Secondary lens implantation: incidence, indications and complications. *Eye* 1988;2:370–375.

41. Hayward JM, Noble BA, George N. Secondary intraocular lens implantation: eight year experience. *Eye* 1990;4:548–556.

42. Lyle WA, Jin J. Secondary intraocular lens implantation: anterior chamber Vs posterior chamber lenses. *Ophthalmic Surg* 1993;24:375–381.

43. Smiddy WE, Avery R. Posterior chamber IOL implantation with suboptimal posterior capsular support. *Ophthalmic Surg* 1991;22:16–19.

44. Lubniewski AJ, Holland EJ, Van Meter WS, et al. Histologic study of eyes with transsclerally sutured posterior chamber intraocular lenses. *Am J Ophthalmol* 1990;110:237–243.

45. Duffey RJ, Holland EJ, Agapitos PJ, Lindstrom RL. Anatomic study of transsclerally sutured intraocular lens implantation. *Am J Ophthalmol* 1989;108:300–309.

46. Apple DJ, Price FW, Gwin T, et al. Sutured retropupillary posterior chamber intraocular lenses for exchange or secondary implantation: The 12th annual Binkhorst lecture, 1988. *Ophthalmology* 1989;96:1241–1247.

47. Spigelman AV, Lindstrom RL, Nichols BD, et al. Implantation of a posterior chamber lens without capsular support during penetrating keratoplasty or as a secondary lens implant. *Ophthalmic Surg* 1988;19:396–398.

48. Rapoza PA. Posterior chamber intraocular lenses-sclera-fixated. In: Brightbill FS, ed. *Corneal surgery: theory, technique, and tissue*. 2nd ed. St. Louis: Mosby, 1993:171–176.

49. Stark WJ, Goodman G, Goodman D, Gottsch J. Posterior chamber intraocular lens implantation in the absence of posterior capsular support. *Ophthalmic Surg* 1988;19:240–243.

50. Mittelviefhaus H. A modified technique of transscleral suture fixation of posterior chamber lenses. *Ophthalmic Surg* 1992;23:496–498.

51. Nunziata BR. Repair of iridodialysis using a 17-millimeter straight needle. *Ophthalmic Surg* 1993;24:627–629.

52. Kaufman SC, Insler MS. Surgical repair of a traumatic iridodialysis. *Ophthalmic Surg Lasers* 1996;27:963–966.

53. McKinna AJ. Results of treatment of traumatic cataract in children. *Am J Ophthalmol* 1961;52:43–53.

54. Ryan SJ, Von Noorden GK. Further observations on the aspiration technique in cataract surgery. *Am J Ophthalmol* 1971;71:626–630.

55. Doren GS, Cohen EJ, Brady SE, et al. Penetrating keratoplasty after ocular trauma. *Am J Ophthalmol* 1990;110:408–411.

56. Wong SK, Koch DD, Emory JM. Secondary intraocular lens implantation. *J Cataract Refract Surg* 1987;13:17–20.

57. Hahn TW, Kim MS, Kim JH. Secondary intraocular lens implantation in aphakia. *J Cataract Refract Surg* 1992;18:174–179.

58. Hu BV, Shin DH, Gibbs KA, Hong YJ. Implantation of posterior chamber lens in the absence of capsular and zonular support. *Arch Ophthalmol* 1988;106:416–420.

59. Solomon K, Gussler JR, Gussler C, Van Meter WS. Incidence and management of complications of transsclerally sutured posterior chamber lenses. *J Cataract Refract Surg* 1993;19:488–493.

60. Heilskov T, Joondeph BC, Olsen KR, Blankenship GW. Late endophthalmitis after transscleral fixation of a posterior chamber intraocular lens. *Arch Ophthalmol* 1989;107:1427. Letter.

15

Refractive Surgery— Incisional Radial Keratotomy

John W. Cowden   Thomas P. Cowden

HISTORY

Radial keratotomy (RK), a surgical procedure for the reduction or elimination of myopia, was developed by S. N. Fyodorov of the USSR and introduced into the United States in 1978 by Leo Bores. At that time the operation consisted of 16 partial-thickness radial incisions of the anterior part of the cornea that caused central flattening, thus decreasing the corneal curvature and degree of myopia. The first operation to flatten the cornea and correct the astigmatism was reported by Snellen in the German literature in 1869. Bates reported a similar procedure in the United States in 1894. In 1953 Sato described the technique of incising the cornea internally and externally to cause a flattening of the curvature. Although this procedure reduced myopia, it was technically difficult and caused damage to the corneal endothelium, eventually leading to the development of bullous keratopathy. Since 1980 thousands of articles have been written on all aspects of RK. There have been glowing reports on its effectiveness and safety (1,2). There have also been reports of serious complications, such as perforation during surgery resulting in cataracts, endophthalmitis, and the loss of the eye. There have been drawn-out legal proceedings regarding alleged antitrust violations, arguments regarding experimental versus investigational status, concern about its effectiveness and safety, and reports of complications, new instrumentation, and the psychological, sociological, and economic impacts. RK was the forerunner of modern refractive corneal surgery, and as such, will continue to find its place along with a variety of procedures that have been or will be developed to modify the corneal surface to improve the uncorrected vision of the eye (3,4).

PRINCIPLES OF RADIAL KERATOTOMY

RK is an incisional procedure of the cornea that steepens the peripheral aspect causing a compensatory flattening of the center, thus reducing myopia. The incised peripheral region of the cornea is steepened by the intraocular pressure acting to push the weakened area outward, which reduces the central corneal curvature (Figs. 15-1 and 15-2). If the procedure is done properly, the procedure can be varied to control the effect, thus resulting in the desired correction [emmetropia ± 1.00 diopter (D)] in 80% or more of the eyes, as reported in the National Eye Institute's Prospective Evaluation of Radial Keratotomy (PERK) study, which assessed the efficacy, safety, predictability, and stability of RK (5,6).

Surgical variables that influence the desired effect are 1) the diameter of the central optical zone, 2) the number of radial incisions, 3) the depth of the incision, and 4) the length of the incision. The surgeon must select the values for these surgical parameters that will provide the best result. The diameter of the optical zone can be varied between 3.0 and 5.5 mm, with the smaller optical zone providing the greatest amount of correction. However, this is not directly correlated. The number of radial incisions selected also helps to determine the amount of correction. Thus, four radial incisions will achieve more than 75% of the effect achieved with eight incisions (7,8). Superficial incisions or shallow incisions result in a loss of correction; thus, the deeper the incision, the greater the degree of central flattening. Longer corneal incisions tend to cause a greater central flattening.

Two patient variables must be considered when selecting the surgical technique and the values for the parameters: 1) the degree of myopia and 2) age. With increasing degrees

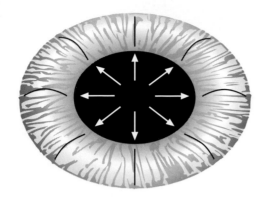

FIGURE 15-1. *Peripheral radial incisions cause a relative steepening of the peripheral cornea and compensatory central flattening. (Adapted from slides by S. N. Fyodorov, MD.)*

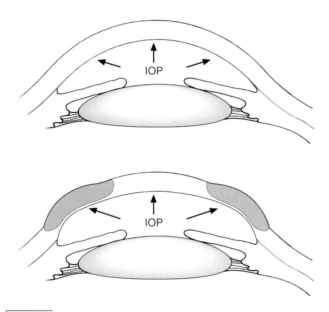

FIGURE 15-2. *(Top) Cross section of normal cornea showing even corneal curvature. (Bottom) Cross section of cornea showing peripheral steepening due to intraocular pressure (IOP) causing bulging of weakened peripheral cornea with compensatory central flattening. (Adapted from slides by S. N. Fyodorov, MD.)*

of myopia, smaller optical zones, more incisions, and deeper incisions are needed to achieve the largest amount of correction (9). The patient's age is a significant factor. The older the patient, the greater the effect achieved; thus, an identical surgical technique will have a greater effect in a 40 year old than a 20 year old. There is a 1½% to 2% greater effect for each year. A 40-year-old person would have 30% to 40% more correction than a 20-year-old person would. A number of other patient variables have been identified as possibly affecting the results but have not been statistically proved. These include corneal curvature, diameter, and thickness; intraocular pressure; and ocular rigidity.

Three methods of incising the cornea have been effective. The American technique, introduced in the United States by Leo Bores, requires centrifugally placed incisions of the cornea from the optical zone toward the periphery (4,10,11). The Russian technique, which starts at the periphery and incises the cornea toward the optical zone centripetally, results in a deeper and smoother incision but is associated with some difficulties in control (12–15). A combination of the American and Russian techniques, using a specially designed diamond knife, has been devised and is presently the method utilized by most RK surgeons (11,16–21). Lindstrom (22) determined that the length of the incision could be decreased from 11 mm to 7 mm (mini-RK) with a loss of less than 8% in effect but providing an increased margin of safety and corneal stability. An additional principle that should be considered is staging. By doing four-incision RK followed later by two- to four-incision RK, one can achieve a greater amount of correction than when doing the same total number of incisions at one time. Additional accuracy can be achieved with less chance of overcorrection (23).

PATIENT SELECTION AND PREOPERATIVE WORK-UP

Not all myopic patients are candidates for RK. New techniques such as excimer-laser photorefractive keratotomy (PRK), automated lamellar keratectomy (ALK), and laser-assisted in-situ keratomileusis (LASIK) have shown promise for correcting moderate to high levels of myopia, leaving RK as the procedure of choice for low levels of myopia. Therefore, the refractive surgeon must be familiar with all of the procedures and offer the appropriate technique to the qualified patient.

Most importantly, RK is elective, and because the operation is performed on a structurally normal eye, the patient must fully understand the risks and benefits of the procedure. Most myopes who request refractive surgery are well educated and participate actively in seeking information about the results and consequences of surgery. Patients are drawn to refractive procedures primarily to improve their uncorrected vision, cosmetic appearance, or job performance or for convenience (16,24). Thus, the ophthalmologist's role is not as traditionally thought, to correct blindness, but rather is the more humbling role of improving the quality of a patient's visual function. Therefore, the physician's responsibility of informed consent requires that the patient be familiar with the minor complications, such as overcorrection, undercorrection, and irregular astigmatism, as well as accept the possible morbidity of rare, but serious, vision-threatening complications. Prior to the procedure, each concern, preconceived or unrealistic expectation, question, and needs of the patient must be addressed, and nonsurgical options explored, because only the fully informed patient can decide if the benefits outweigh the risks.

Contraindications for RK exist. Patients who have unrealistic expectations or who cannot fully understand and accept the possible complications should not be treated by RK. Candidates less than 21 years old are excluded because they have exaggerated wound healing, there may be more pronounced progressive hyperopic drift over their lifetime, and myopia may progress. A patient's refraction should be stable, within 0.5 D, over a 2-year period prior to RK. This requires ruling out corneal warpage as the cause of an unstable refraction. Rigid gas-permeable and prolonged soft contact lens wear, lid pathology, and aggressive rubbing can cause refractive variability, and must be addressed prior to refractive surgery. Patients should not wear a rigid gas-permeable contact lens for 3 weeks or a soft contact lens for 3 days prior to refractions (8). Other corneal conditions such as keratoconus and irregular astigmatism are not likely to be corrected with RK, and may worsen following the procedure. Collagen vascular disease, severely dry eyes, and uncontrolled diabetes mellitus are relative contraindications because they are associated with a poor healing response. Ocular inflammation including blepharoconjunctivitis and keratoconjunctivitis should be controlled prior to surgery. Herpes simplex keratitis may be reactivated and patients with a history of this should be excluded (25). Other causes of induced myopia such as nuclear cataract, diabetic lens changes, or a posterior staphyloma must be investigated and excluded.

A variety of mechanisms for screening patients prior to a formal preoperative work-up are available. Prior to presenting for refractive surgery, most patients have knowledge gained through the media, Internet, optometrists, friends, physicians, or other individuals. However, a repetitive education process involving published and presented material should be instituted. Topics should include myopia, astigmatism, the basic anatomy of the eye, the clinical evaluation process, the surgical procedure, postoperative care and precautions, benefits, predictability of results, risks and complications, alternatives to RK, patient selection criteria, glossary and definition of terms, history and development of RK. Illustrations and photographs should be provided. Commonly asked questions, the clinic's address and telephone number, and the physician's training and experience and references should be given prior to the actual clinical evaluation. This process can screen out inappropriate candidates.

The formal preoperative work-up begins with obtaining a thorough history, including social, family, ocular, medical, and surgical components. Age, gender, occupation, interest, associated medical problems that might influence wound healing such as rheumatoid arthritis or diabetes, corneal or anterior-segment diseases, and contact lens history must be noted. A knowledge of current medications, including ocular antiglaucoma agents that can enhance regression of the procedure effect (26), and topical or systemic steroids that can alter wound healing, as well as allergies is critical. Preoperative pachymetry values in eight radial zones centrally, paracentrally, and peripherally as well as keratometry

readings should be recorded. Retinoscopy and computerized corneal topography can be used to help rule out early keratoconus or asymmetric astigmatism. A stable manifest and cycloplegic refraction over 2 years is imperative for predictable results. The best-corrected visual acuity, presbyopic correction, intraocular pressure, pupil size and irregularities, and side of the dominant eye must be recorded. The examination must include an evaluation of the lids and adnexa to rule out lesions inducing astigmatism, and inflammation. The tear film and function are assessed to rule out dry eye. A complete corneal, anterior-segment, and fundus examination concludes the work-up.

SURGICAL TECHNIQUES

Four techniques are described: Lindstrom, Casebeer, Thornton, and Nordan. Various refractive surgeons have utilized individual modifications of each of these techniques.

The Lindstrom Technique

Topical 0.5% proparacaine hydrochloride is administered one drop every 1 to 5 minutes times three. The patient is asked to fixate on the light filament of the operating microscope. The center of the visual axis is marked with a blunt 30-gauge cannula or Sinskey hook just inferior to the opposite end of the filament reflex as viewed with the surgeon's dominant eye (Fig. 15-3). A central optical zone marker of the appropriate size is centered over the mark, and an indentation made in the epithelium. An 8-mm mark is then placed concentrically around the first mark. A corneal pachymetry reading is taken temporally adjacent to the

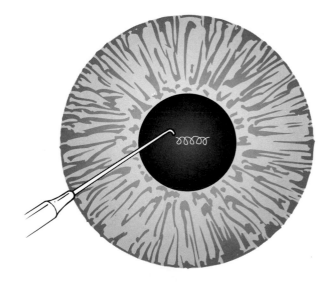

FIGURE 15-3. *Marking the visual axis; surgeon fixates with the right eye while a mark is made with a small blunt tipped instrument (Sinskey hook or 30-gauge canula), just inferior to the left side of the coaxial light reflex of the microscope.*

central optical zone marker, and the diamond micrometer knife is set at 110% of the temporal paracentral pachymeter reading.

For the American technique (centrifugal incisions), the central-most portion of the knife is placed at the optical zone ring and plunged directly into the cornea until the footplates are firmly positioned. Following a short pause, a continuous incision is made peripherally while the globe is fixated with forceps or a Thornton's ring. A slightly moistened cornea is preferable. A bimanual cutting technique is done using opposing forces by pulling the fixation forceps and the knife in opposite directions at the same time. The blade is kept perpendicular to the cornea surface while this incision is made. The blade is inserted at the inner portion of the optical zone ring and the incision extended until the footplates cross the peripheral zone circle (Fig. 15-4).

For the Russian technique (peripheral to central cutting), the knife is set just outside the 8-mm zone marker and extended centrally until the central optical zone ring is cut. A small central rotation of the knife at the end of the incision is done to undercut the deeper stroma (Fig. 15-5).

The third technique, known as the double-pass technique, is a combination of the American and Russian incisions using a specially designed knife known as the Duotrac or Genesis blade. This blade is designed with a shortened interior cutting edge on the vertical facet that is sharpened only to 200 to 250μ from the tip, preventing penetration of the central optical zone and thus avoiding inadvertent incision into the clear optical zone and also providing a uniform deepened incision (Fig. 15-6).

For four-incision RK, the first three incisions can be made with the dominant hand and are most commonly placed at 10:30, 7:30, and 1:30 positions, with the 4:30 incision made with the other hand. There will be no scars visible in the palpebral aperture, thus producing less glare at night. For eight-incision RK, the incisions should be made in an opposing fashion in order to reduce the amount of astigmatism and inadvertent perforation. The sequence of the incisions should be such that the last incision is in the inferior temporal portion where the cornea is often the thinnest and microperforation is most likely to occur (Figs. 15-7 and 15-8) (9,22).

The Casebeer Technique

Charles Casebeer developed a systematic approach to radial and astigmatic keratotomy which he made into a comprehensive course utilizing nomograms, a course manual, tapes, equipment manufactured by Chiron Intraoptics, diamond blades manufactured by Magnum Diamond Corporation, and the ultrasonic pachymeter manufactured by Sonogauge. His system is described in his manual, *A Comprehensive System of Refractive Surgery* (19). A number of authors reported postoperative visual acuity of 20/40 or better in 95% to 99% of the patients (24).

Casebeer's surgical technique, performed after his detailed preoperative evaluation is completed, is as follows: Topical lidocaine 4% (Xylocaine) drops are given three times before the patient enters the operating room and immediately before surgical preparation, which is similar to that used for cataract surgery. Following placement of the lid speculum,

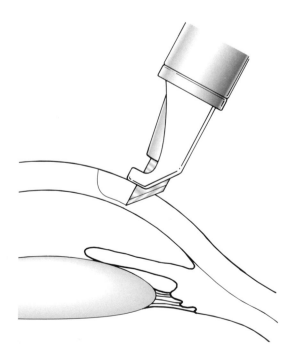
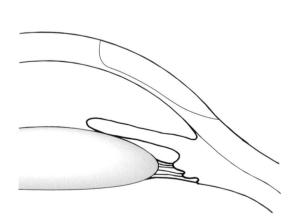

FIGURE 15-4. *Back cutting diamond knife blade making centrifugal radial incision (American technique).*

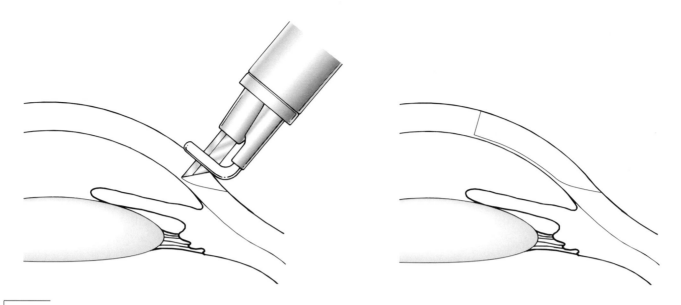

FIGURE 15-5.   *Front cutting diamond knife blade making centripedal radial incision (Russian technique).*

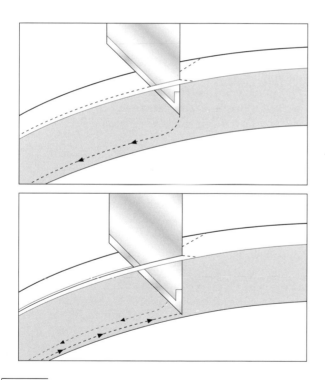

FIGURE 15-6.   *Double-edged knife blade making combined radial incision (Casebeer technique).*

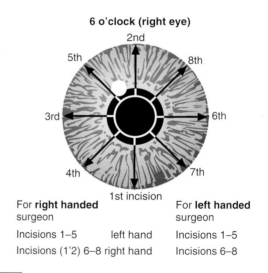

FIGURE 15-7.   *Incisional sequence right eye. (Adapted from R. Lindstrom, MD.)*

the patient is instructed to look at the light or fixation device. Ultrasonic pachymetry is performed only once at a position 1.5 mm temporal to the light reflex while the patient is fixating. Once the patient has achieved fixation, the optical zone marker appropriate for the myopic correction according to the incisional nomogram is centered by

placing the pointer of the marker 1 mm inferior and to the opposite end of the coaxial light reflex from the operating microscope as viewed by the surgeon's fixating eye. Marking of the visual axis is not required. If astigmatic correction is to be performed, the arcuate marker is placed outside of the spherical optical zone at the 7-mm optical zone of astigmatism. Finally, an 8-mm optical zone marker is placed concentrically around the inner optical zone or zones. Astigmatic cuts are made prior to radial cuts. The Duotrac system blade is utilized for radial incisions; usually there is no need for fixation of the globe. However, if the patient is unable to maintain fixation, the eye is stabilized with forceps

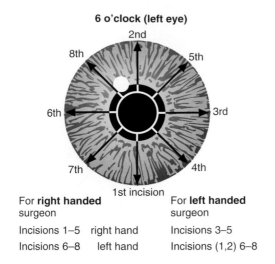

6 o'clock (left eye)

For **right handed**
surgeon

Incisions 1–5   right hand

Incisions 6–8   left hand

For **left handed**
surgeon

Incisions 3–5

Incisions (1,2) 6–8

FIGURE 15-8.   *Incisional sequence left eye. (Adapted from R. Lindstrom, MD.)*

or a clamp at the limbus opposite to the incision that is being made. Excessive pressure on the globe is to be avoided. The incision is started at the outer edge of the central optical zone and extended peripherally to the 8-mm mark, utilizing enough pressure to slightly distort the cornea. Once the blade touches the 8-mm ring, the incision is stopped, and then without removing the blade, reversed toward the center optical zone by applanating the cornea but not indenting it. This results in deepening of the initial incision. At the end of the incision, the blade will stop automatically as it runs into the uncut tissue at the central optical axis. No irrigation or manipulation of the wound is performed. A broad-spectrum antibiotic is instilled into the eye and patching is not required.

The Thornton Technique

The Thornton RK technique is different from those of Casebeer and Lindstrom, which used the Russian technique originally. Thornton uses the American method developed by Leo Bores, incising from the edge of the optical zone outward but stopping short of the limbus, best described as "limbal sparing." The Thornton RK technique uses the American method as follows (27):

1. Deep topical anesthesia is achieved by administering proparacaine inferiorly and then superiorly while the patient is supine. After preparation with povidone-iodine (Betadine) and placement of the eyelid speculum, a drop of 4% lidocaine is instilled.
2. The visual axis is marked using Thornton's technique of having the patient fixate on a previously marked dot on the center of the microscope lens, with the microscope light turned off but the room lights on. This method does not depend on a reflection or decentration of a coaxial light reflex.

3. The preselected low profile marker is used to outline the optical zone.
4. A Thornton fixation ring is used to stabilize the eye with light pressure while the incisions are made.
5. The preset diamond blade is inserted to its full depth at the edge of the optical zone mark and drawn slowly to just before the limbus.
6. Each additional incision is made similar to the first while light pressure is reapplied with the fixation ring. The peripheral incision can be deepened if indicated according to Thornton's nomogram.
7. When the incisions are completed, they are inspected for length and depth using the Thornton incision spreading forceps, and irrigated to remove any blood or debris.
8. An additional drop of anesthetic along with any antibiotic drop is instilled and the eye is patched.

A full description of the Thornton technique can be found in his book (27).

The Nordan Technique

The Nordan/Maxwell RK method is based on Fred Kremer's original American-style technique and includes several important features (28).

The nomogram takes into account the patient's refractive error, gender, intraocular pressure, and corneal thickness. It does not include preoperative keratometry and measurement of corneal diameter.

Pachymetry is performed under the microscope at the edge of the optical zone mark.

The American technique is used on all new cases. The goal is a depth of 85% of the corneal thickness at the central aspect of the incision. Therefore, a back-cutting blade is increased 5% to 10% deeper than the corneal thickness measurement. The blade is advanced when there is a 5% difference in pachymetry readings (about 0.04mm), which usually entails one change in blade length per case for the superior or superior-nasal incisions. A diamond blade width of 120 to 150μ (at the 0.5-mm length) works equally well in clinical practice.

Nordan believes that a consistently accurate *achieved* incision depth is the key to accurate, stable incisions. This is best accomplished by a single pass of a blade, which has a single corneal-stromal relationship and results in the thinnest scar. He strongly disagrees with the double-pass concept for RK incisions, because a front-cutting blade will cut deeper than a back-cutting blade the same length. Therefore, a double-pass technique can never be as accurate as a single-pass technique, since the blade is achieving about 70% depth on the first pass and a questionable depth on the forward second pass. An achieved depth of 85% to 90% of corneal thickness is important for consistency. It is interesting to consider that a back-cutting blade, which is set 10% longer than the cornea is thick, achieves an incision depth to 85%

to 90% of the corneal thickness. This 15% to 20% difference between blade length and achieved incision depth is due to the give of the cornea under pressure from the blade (i.e., the small but significant resistance offered to the penetration of the diamond blade) and the tendency of the back-cutting blade to "water ski" out of the cornea during the incision.

Bias

Bias is the percentage that must be added to the corneal pachymetry measurement to determine which blade length will achieve the desired result. This bias can be positive or negative and is determined by the diamond blade construction and direction of incision. For example, assume a corneal measurement of 0.60 mm. In order for a quality back-cutting diamond blade to obtain a 90% incision, the blade depth chosen might be 0.60 + 0.06, or 0.66 mm. The 0.06 refers to a +10% bias with a blade length of 110% of the pachymetry measurements.

For a front-cutting (vertical) blade to obtain the same 90% incision depth, a −5% bias might be necessary. The blade length would be 0.60 mm − 0.05(0.60), or 0.57 mm. Front-cutting diamond blades usually create a corneal incision that is about 5% less deep than the length of the blade. Therefore, a front-cutting blade will produce a corneal incision about 15% deeper than a back-cutting blade of the same length, which equals 0.09 mm with an initial blade setting of 0.60 mm.

A front-cutting blade offers the advantage of improved viability for the surgeon and a perpendicular incision at the optical zone limit; however, the drawbacks of a front-cutting blade are that it distorts the optical zone line during a radial incision and, more importantly, can easily *cut through the patient's visual axis during inadvertent eye movement*. For this reason, front-cutting blades should be used for astigmatic keratotomy and redeepening of RK incisions but not for the primary RK incisions. The safety of the American (center to periphery) technique for RK incisions is undeniable and greater depth can always be achieved by increasing blade length.

Achieved corneal incision depths of more than 95% of corned thickness can lead to a greater effect but also *corneal instability* and fluctuating vision. Achieved corneal incision depths of less than 75% can lead to severe undercorrection or even *total regression* of a reasonable result after several weeks or months.

Marking the Visual Axis

Most surgeons prefer to mark the visual axis in order to accurately center the optical zone. This is done by asking the patient to fixate on the light filament within the operating microscope, providing it is a coaxial illumination system. The surgeon, using his or her dominant eye and closing the nondominant eye, views the patient's cornea through the microscope. Then, with a fine blunt instrument,

such as a 3-gauge cannula tip or a Sinskey hook, an indentation in the cornea is placed on the opposite side, just inferior to the light filament reflex. Thus, a surgeon viewing with the right eye would make the mark on the left inferior edge of the filament. The optical zone marker is then centered over the epithelial indentation, located in the visual axis and pressed onto the cornea, and an indentation of the desired diameter is made in the epithelium. Some surgeons prefer to use a radial incision marker consisting of four to eight radial blades to indent the epithelium, to act as a guide for making the radial incisions.

Postoperative Management

Irrigation of the incisions is not required. An antibiotic-steroid solution is placed on the cornea along with one or two drops of a nonsteroidal anti-inflammatory agent, before and after the procedure, which significantly decreases postoperative pain. Postoperative examinations are necessary at 1 week and 3 months, unless enhancements are anticipated, in which case more frequent visits are necessary.

COMPLICATIONS

Experience, attention to detail, improved technique, and new instrumentation have all contributed to the low rate of complications from RK. The incidence of the more common complications including overcorrection and undercorrection can be reduced if the surgeon does not exceed the reasonable limits of correction possible with RK. The majority of severe complications are associated with surgeons who avoid the experience and teachings of others. In several large studies, overall complication rates of up to 8% were estimated (29,30). In the PERK study, at 1 year, 10% of the patients were dissatisfied with the procedure (31). However, at 5 years, 80% of the patients had a good to excellent outcome based on the visual function score, using both refraction and uncorrected visual acuity (32), and at 10 years, the uncorrected vision in 85% of the patients was 20/40 or better (6). Although most complications from RK resolve with time, knowledge of and treatment for these complications should be fully understood prior to performing this popular procedure. They can be divided into intraoperative, early postoperative, late postoperative, and severe/vision-threatening complications (Table 15-1).

Intraoperative Complications

The frequency of the majority of complications involving anesthesia has been reduced by using topical techniques. Although rare, toxicity and cross-reactivity to topical anesthetics occur (33). The use of retrobulbar anesthesia, during the early development of RK, produced several complications including globe perforations, subconjunctival hemorrhages leading to corneal blood staining, retrobulbar hemorrhages, and optic nerve damage. Therefore, it has

Table 15-1. Complications of Radial Keratotomy

Intraoperative
  Anesthesia related
    Allergy
    Globe perforations
    Optic nerve damage
    Retrobulbar hemorrhage
    Subconjunctival hemorrhage
    Toxicity
  Planning/technique errors
    Corneal microperforation
    Corneal macroperforation (requiring sutures)
    Inaccurate optical zone marking, number of incisions,
      meridian marking
    Inadequate depth of incisions
    Inadequate instrumentation
    Intersecting incisions
    Invasion of optical zone
    Involvement of limbus
    Lens capsule perforation
    Wound debris
Early postoperative
  Subjective
    Fluctuating vision
    Anisometropia/aniseikonia
    Diplopia
    Distortion of image
    Glare, flare, sunburst, photophobia
    Pain
  Optical
    Astigmatism: induced, residual, irregular
    Overcorrection
    Premature presbyopia
    Regression of effect
    Undercorrection

  Corneal
    Anterior basement membrane changes
    Delayed wound healing
    Edema
    Endothelial cell loss
    Epithelial defects
    Recurrent erosions
    Wound leak
  Orbit
    Ptosis
    Strabismus
Late postoperative
  Optical
    Progressive hyperopia
    Reduced best-corrected visual acuity
  Corneal
    Epithelial iron deposits
    Epithelial inclusion cysts
    Loss of ability to wear contact lens
    Recurrent erosions
    Scarring
    Vascularization
Serious/vision threatening
  Cataracts
  Endophthalmitis
  Glaucoma
  Inflammation/iritis
  Keratitis: bacterial, fungal, herpes simplex virus, sterile
  Retinal detachment
  Stromal melt
  Traumatic rupture

generally been replaced by less invasive, topical methods (34,35).

Perforations of the cornea may result in shallowing of the anterior chamber, leading to the development of peripheral anterior synechiae, glaucoma, or cataract, and can predispose the eye to endophthalmitis (Fig. 15-9). Microperforations, those not leading to a shallow chamber, and shallow cuts are usually due to incorrect setting of the blades or improper technique. Rates of microperforations of between 5% to 37% have been reported (30,36,37). The rates have been reduced to 0% to 2% with the use of diamond knives and ultrasonic pachymetry (38). Microperforations can occur occasionally. Therefore, it is imperative that when the surgeon identifies aqueous at any point, the incision be stopped, to avoid extending a self-sealing perforation into a large full-thickness incision into the anterior chamber (Fig. 15-10). Macroperforations, those leading to a shallowing of the anterior chamber, are reported at rates of between 1% and 13% (29,39). Usually 10-0 nylon sutures are required to re-form the anterior chamber and there may be an increased

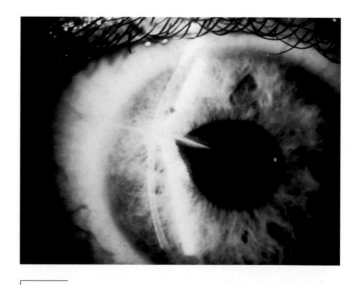

FIGURE 15-9. *Slit-lamp photo of anterior synechiae secondary to perforated radial keratotomy (RK) incision.*

risk of severe complications (Fig. 15-11). Endophthalmitis, epithelial downgrowth, scarring, endothelial cell loss, iris adhesions to the cornea, asymmetric astigmatism, decreased globe integrity, persistent iritis with resultant cystoid macular edema, cataracts, and secondary inflammatory glaucoma have occurred with entrance into the anterior chamber (33,40–44). Attention to details such as blade depth, irregularities of the knife footplates, perpendicular positioning of the blade, corneal thickness, and corneal hydration will reduce the incidence of RK becoming an intraocular procedure.

Technique errors leading to errant incisions, either incorrect number, incorrect meridian, intersecting incisions, incisions across the limbus, curvilinear incisions, or deviations into the optical zone, can be reduced by carefully planning

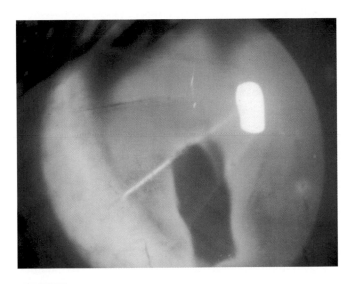

FIGURE 15-10.   *Cobalt blue photo showing aqueous leak from perforating radial keratotomy (RK) incision.*

the surgical procedure prior to entering the operating room (Fig. 15-12). Improper incisions can result in instability of the cornea, healing difficulties, epithelial inclusion cysts, stromal melt, and vascularization of the incisions (17,33,44). Visual complaints of glare, ghost images, starbursts, and monocular diplopia are more common with improper incision techniques and decentered optical zones (39,45).

Early Postoperative Complications

Subjective symptoms of pain lasting from 24 to 72 hours are common after RK. During the PERK study, patients experienced more intense pain when their eyes were patched postoperatively. Experience has shown that the use of oral analgesics, narcotics, or sedatives can reduce the severity of the postoperative pain (31,46). Patient satisfaction has improved with the postoperative use of a topical nonsteroidal agent such as diclofenac (Voltaren) or ketorolac tromethamine (Acular). Some patients benefit from wearing a bandage soft contact lens; however, this may increase the risk of postoperative corneal edema (33).

Photophobia, glare, and sunbursts may occur 1 to 2 weeks postoperatively and persist for months, as seen in 40% of the patients in the PERK study (31). Causes include persistent epithelial defects, inflammation, iridocyclitis, and epithelial edema. These symptoms are less severe when fewer incisions and larger optical zones are used, and are limited when topical nonsteroidal anti-inflammatory medications, artificial tears, and topical steroids are administered (33).

Diurnal fluctuation of vision, ranging from 0.50 to 4.25 D, occurs in approximately 80% of eyes following RK (31,47,48). It is likely due to incomplete healing and corneal edema near the radial incisions, causing increased central flattening. The effect is more pronounced early in the morning, when corneal edema may exist owing to

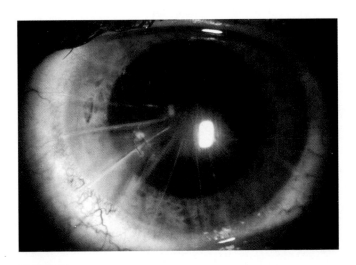

FIGURE 15-11.   *Photo of sutured RK incision (same case as Fig. 15-10).*

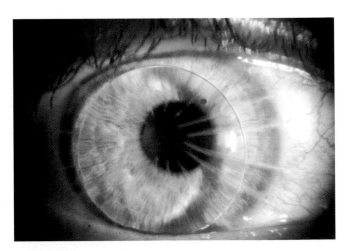

FIGURE 15-12.   *RK incisions extending into central optical zone.*

overnight closure of the lids. In the majority of patients, diurnal fluctuation resolves after 4 to 8 weeks, once the wound has stabilized. Factors that may destabilize the wound such as eye rubbing, chronic postoperative contact lens wear, and an increased intraocular pressure may prolong visual fluctuations, even for many years following the surgery (49,50).

Diminished night vision is due to pupillary dilation incorporating the refractive component of the steeper peripheral cornea (33). The more irritating monocular diplopia and multiple ghost images are common in patients in whom small optical zones and many incisions were used, resulting in irregular astigmatism and abnormal corneal topography (45).

Early postoperative non-vision-threatening refractive complications include regression, undercorrection, overcorrection, progression, and induced regular or irregular astigmatism, anisometropia, and presbyopia. Regression of effect is usually due to early wound healing and varies among patients. Because this wound-healing response is unpredictable in individual patients, undercorrection is often the goal of the procedure; it can be modulated with enhancement procedures (33). Significant undercorrection occurs more frequently with attempts at correcting higher myopia. The PERK study found that vision in 26% of the patients was undercorrected more than −0.5 D at 10 years after the surgery (6). High degrees of preoperative myopia, shallow incisions, low intraocular pressures postoperatively, thin corneas, miscalculation, and aggressive wound healing may contribute to undercorrection (48,51). Undercorrection is also more common in young female patients. Correction with spectacles or contact lenses and enhancement procedures such as adding incisions, reincising shallow incisions, shortening the optical zone, and excimer phototherapeutic keratectomy are successful in treating undercorrection (24,51,52). Postoperative steroids can enhance the effect of the initial surgery by modifying wound healing (53).

Overcorrection, as defined in the PERK study, is hyperopia greater than +1.00 D (32). Reported rates range from 0.8% to 36.0% (29,33). Current nomograms include age as a major factor in correction of myopic error. Thus, the overcorrection rate is now significantly lower than the 36% seen in the PERK study patients who were not grouped by age (17). Other circumstances causing overcorrection include temporary central flattening due to postoperative edema, incorrect surgery such as too small of an optical zone, overresponse to surgery, and progressive hyperopia (54). The primary treatment is prevention, such as planning undercorrection for the initial procedure and employing enhancement techniques later if necessary. Medical and surgical treatment options include wearing spectacles or contact lenses, administering topical antiglaucoma medications (epinephrine or pilocarpine) to augment regression of the effect, and reopening and scraping out fibrous tissue or epithelial cysts from the wounds with subsequent suturing to reverse the effect (26,55). A pursestring suture, or multiple interrupted sutures can be used to reverse overcorrected radial incisions (9).

Residual astigmatism, induced astigmatism, and irregular astigmatism commonly occur following RK. Although most surgeons do not attempt to correct astigmatism of less than 0.75 D, residual astigmatism may persist after RK with or without concomitant astigmatic keratotomy. The PERK study did not include patients with more than 1.50 D of preoperative astigmatism, but found at 5 years that 15% of the eyes developed 1 D or more of refractive astigmatism (32). This induced astigmatism can be regular or irregular. Although patients may tolerate up to 1 D of regular induced astigmatism, larger amounts, more common with 8- to 16-incision surgery, enhancement procedures, and perforations, can limit uncorrected visual acuity or cause monocular diplopia (56). Careful preoperative evaluation to exclude patients with corneal warpage from contact lens wear or with corneal pathology, including keratoconus, may prevent postoperative visual loss due to irregular astigmatism. Induced irregular astigmatism can also occur if fewer incisions are made than planned, if they are more shallow than required, if the incisions are asymmetric around the visual axis, if the optical zone is decentered, or if astigmatic and radial incisions cross. Significant complication such as epithelial plugs, stromal melt, and secondary infective keratitis are due to the wound gape and poor healing that occur when astigmatic and RK incisions cross (17). If incisions do intersect, interrupted 10-0 nylon sutures should be placed to reduce wound gape and reapproximate the corneal architecture. Although in the majority of patients, induced astigmatism resolves with time, careful corneal topography and photokeratoscopy should be used to determine the extent and resolution of the irregularity in order to determine the need for treatment. Treatment depends on the etiology and may include the wearing of rigid contact lenses, placement of subsequent incisions based on corneal topography, or lamellar or penetrating keratoplasty (57).

Simultaneous bilateral RK may reduce the incidence of transient anisometropia in moderate to high myopes, while increasing the chance of devastating complications such as bilateral bacterial keratitis (54). To reduce this risk, one can perform unilateral RK and unilateral contact lens or spectacles can be worn until the second eye undergoes RK.

Late Postoperative Period

Other complications that may have long-term consequences and variable visual morbidity include contact lens intolerance, epithelial basement membrane disorders, epithelial inclusion cysts, foreign bodies in the grooves, stellate epithelial iron lines, vascularization of incisions, hypertrophic incision scars, diminished corneal strength, and endothelial cell loss (58) (Figs. 15-13 and 15-14). Any incision into Bowman's membrane can cause redundant basement membrane (59), recurrent erosion syndrome (48), subepithelial fibrosis (60), and rust-colored epithelial inclusion cysts,

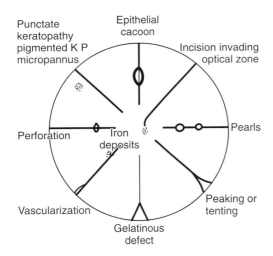

FIGURE 15-13. *Diagrammatic examples of corneal pathology due to radial keratotomy (RK) incisions.*

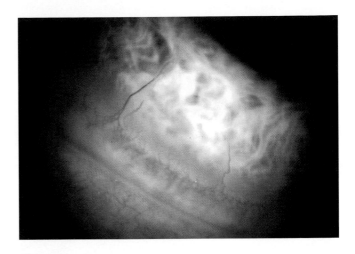

FIGURE 15-15. *Neovascularization or RK incisions associated with soft contact lens wear.*

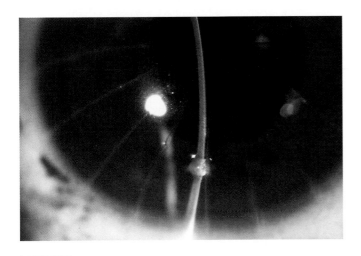

FIGURE 15-14. *Epithelial cyst in RK incisional scar.*

which were present in 7% of PERK patients at 1 year (48). Although less common with modern mini-RK incisions, which do not extend to the limbus, corneal vascularization of the radial wounds occurs when contact lens wear, crossed incisions, or postoperative inflammation or infection complicate RK (61) (Fig. 15-15).

Most long-term studies reported the occurrence of progressive hyperopia (6,37,49). This is defined as a shift in spectacle correction of more than 1.00 D hyperopic due to continued flattening of the central cornea after RK (6). In the PERK study 22% of the eyes at 5 years and 43% of the eyes by 10 years manifested changes of progressive hyperopia (32). Other more recent studies reported similar progressive hyperopic rates of between 17% and 54% (6,62–65). This effect seems to be more dramatic when smaller optical zones, multiple enhancement procedures, increasing

numbers of incisions, or incisions extending to the limbus were used. Treatment is similar to that for overcorrection. Other surgical options included hyperopic epikeratoplasty, and lamellar or penetrating keratoplasty for severe progressive hyperopia (57,66). Mini-RK, the procedure in which the peripheral 2.0 to 2.5 mm of cornea is spared by shorter corneal incisions, showed promising results in reducing the rate of progressive hyperopia as well as postoperative overcorrection (22,67).

A decrease in best-corrected visual acuity is a significant complication, especially when operating on physiologically normal eyes except for the myopia. Much dialogue regarding the ethics of this issue has been offered over the 50-year history of RK. The PERK study found that 24 (3%) of 793 eyes lost two or more lines of best-corrected visual acuity at 10 years (6). Marmer (29) found that only 0.9% of more than 63,000 cases of RK surveyed resulted in a decrease in best-corrected visual acuity. The American Academy of Ophthalmology Assessment of Radial Keratotomy reported that about 1% of patients may expect to have a decrease in best-corrected visual acuity following RK (68). The possibility of a decrease in best-corrected visual acuity, although rare, is thus real and must be included in the complete informed consent process for the refractive procedure.

Noncorneal postoperative complications such as esotropia and blepharoptosis have been reported following RK. Patients who possess reduced fusional amplitudes, which had been compensated for by their preoperative myopia, can develop postoperative esotropia due to an increased need for accommodation and reduced fusional divergence amplitudes once their vision has been overcorrected to a mild hyperopic state (69). Inadvertently disinserting the levator aponeurosis while placing the lid speculum during surgery is thought to result in the observed cases of ptosis following RK (70).

Serious/Vision-Threatening Complications

More unusual but nevertheless devastating complications of RK can result in permanent visual loss. The PERK study followed 793 eyes for 10 years and only 2 eyes suffered a potential sight-threatening complication (bacterial keratitis), both of which were treated and returned to 20/20 vision (6). In a 5-year period, Bates et al (71) found no vision-threatening complications or loss of best-corrected visual acuity in 300 eyes. Other studies confirmed the rarity of severe complications, even following macroperforations, which were managed appropriately with sutures (38).

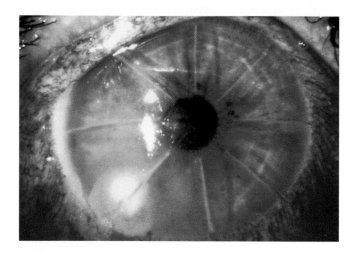

FIGURE 15-16.   *Delayed keratitis in RK incision 40 month post op.*

Vision-threatening complications include retinal detachment; endophthalmitis; bacterial, fungal, and herpes simplex keratitis; delayed sterile keratitis; stromal melt; cataract formation; secondary glaucoma; epithelial downgrowth; traumatic globe rupture; and delayed wound healing. Retinal tears leading to retinal detachment may follow globe perforation and decompression with subsequent ciliary spasm, or may result after the use of miotics in the early postoperative period (72,73). *Staphylococcus epidermidis*, causing endophthalmitis, was cultured from 3 eyes, each following an incision perforation (37,73). Early infectious keratitis reportedly has been caused by *Staphylococcus aureus*, *S. epidermidis*, *Streptococcus pneumoniae*, diphtheroids, *Pseudomonas* species, *Serratia marcescens*, and *Mycobacterium chelonei* (37,54,74–77). *Candida* and *Aspergillus* organisms can cause fungal keratitis along the radial incision in the early postoperative period (78,79). Delayed keratitis, mostly related to contact lens wear, occurred 40 months after surgery (80) (Fig. 15-16). Responsible bacteria include *S. epidermidis*, *Propionibacterium acnes*, *Pseudomonas aeruginosa*, *M. chelonei*, *Enterobacter gergoviae*, and *Serratia liquefaciens* (75,80,81). The trauma to the cornea during refractive surgery may reactivate herpes simplex keratitis, and therefore the procedure should not be undertaken in patients with a history of herpetic keratitis (25,33). Patients with dry eye, rheumatoid arthritis, or other collagen vascular diseases are not good candidates for incisional keratotomy because of the increased risk of stromal melt. Crossed incisions also increase the risk of subsequent stromal melting (17). Cataract formation occurred following prolonged steroid use after RK, and after large macroperforation violated the lens capsule (73,82).

Table 15-2.   Outcomes (4,6,22,24,32,46,62,64)

Study	No. of Eyes	Technique	Follow-up	Unaided VA			Complications
				20/40	20/25+	±1D	
Arrowsmith (62)	123	A	5 yr	75%	—	53%	15% ↓ VA ≥ 2 lines 22% Hyperopic shift
Samelson (4)	134	A	5 yr	62%	—	56%	30% ↓ VA ≥ 2 lines 15% Hyperopic shift
Dietz (64)	675	R	5 yr	88%	—	76%	3% ↓ VA ≥ 2 lines 31% Hyperopic shift
PERK, Waring (32)	757	A	5 yr	88%	60%	66%	3% ↓ VA ≥ 2 lines 22% Hyperopic shift
PERK, Waring (6)	693	A	10 yr	85%	53%	60%	3% ↓ VA ≥ 2 lines 43% Hyperopic shift
Casebeer technique, Waring (46)	557	C	6 mo	95%	—	89%	4% perforation
Casebeer technique, Werblin (24)	205	C	1 yr	99%	86%	—	
Lindstrom technique, mini-RK (22)	100	M	6 mo	94%(100%)	72%(76%)	92%(98%)	2% Microperforation (8% Reoperation)

A = American technique; R = Russian technique; C = Casebeer technique; M = mini-RK; VA = visual acuity.

Mild postoperative iridocyclitis was observed in eyes with perioperative microperforations, and postoperative epithelial defects (83). Synechial formation, caused by shallowing of the anterior chamber during perforations, and topical steroid use may result in secondary glaucoma (42). Binder (84) reported a case of epithelial downgrowth occurring 4 months after RK; cryotherapy was required. Although there have been many cases of blunt trauma to globes following incisional keratotomy, without rupture of the incisions, severe trauma can result in perforations in the weakened radial incisions long after surgery (85). Therefore, patients must be aware of the risk of blunt trauma and use protective eye wear accordingly.

OUTCOMES

Numerous studies have reported the results of variou authors' series of cases using the different techniques. However, most are flawed by changes in the surgical techniques, insufficient follow-up time and lack of follow-up patient numbers.

The best designed prospective study was the National Eye Institute, Prospective Evaluation of Radial Keratotomy (PERK) study. Its limitation was also an asset: only one type of RK technique was studied in a rigidly controlled patient population with excellent follow-up for 10 years.

A comparison of 5 different long-term studies using different techniques is shown in Table 15-2.

REFERENCES

1. Shepard DD. Radial keratotomy: analysis of efficacy and predictability in 1058 consecutive cases. Part I: efficacy. *J Cataract Refract Surg* 1986;12:632–643.
2. Shepard DD. Radial keratotomy: analysis of efficacy and predictability in 1058 consecutive cases. Part II: predictability. *J Cataract Refract Surg* 1987;13:32–34.
3. Cowden JW. Endothelial changes following radial keratotomy. In: Schacher RA, Schacher L, eds. *Refractive keratoplasty*. Denison, TX: LAL Publishing, 1983:351–359.
4. Cowden JW. Current status of radial keratotomy. *Ophthalmol Clin North Am* 1990;3:679–686.
5. AAO Anonymous. Radial keratotomy for myopia. *Ophthalmology* 1993;100:1103–1115.
6. Waring GO, Lynn JJ, McDonnell PJ, the PERK study group. Results of the Prospective Evaluation of Radial Keratotomy (PERK) study 10 years after surgery. *Arch Ophtholmol* 1994;112:1298–1308.
7. Spigelman AV, Williams PA, Lindstrom RL. Further studies of four incision radial keratotomy. *Refract Corneal Surg* 1989;5:292–295.
8. Spigelman AV, Williams PA, Nichols BD, et al. Four-incision radial keratotomy. *J Cataract Refract Surg* 1988;14:125–128.
9. Linquist TD, Williams PA, Lindstrom RL. Surgical treatment of overcorrection following radial keratotomy: evaluation of clinical effectiveness. *Ophthalmic Surg* 1991;22:12–15.
10. Hoffman RF. *Radial keratotomy surgical techniques*. Thorofare, NJ: Slack, 1986.
11. Lane S. Radial keratotomy surgical techniques. In: Krachmer JH, Mannis MJ, Holland EJ, eds. *Cornea*. Vol. III. St. Louis: Mosby-Year Book, 1997:2059–2082.
12. Ellis W. Surgical techniques. In: *Keratotomy surgery for myopia, hypermyopia, and astigmatism*. El Cerrito, CA: Eye Center of Northern California Medical Textbook Division, 1991:163–200.
13. Ellis W. *A textbook of radial keratotomy and astigmatic surgery*. Irvine, CA: Keith C. Terry & Associates, Medical Textbook Division, 1986:77–146.
14. Fyodorov SN. Methods of radial keratotomy. In: Schacher RA, Levy NS, Schacher L, eds. *Radial keratotomy*. Denison, TX: LAL Publishing, 1980:35–66.
15. Salz IJ. Radial keratotomy. In: Thompson FB, ed. *Myopia surgery*. New York: Macmillan, 1990:31–65.
16. Assil KK, Kassoff J, Schanzlin DJ, Quantock AJ. A combined incision technique of radial keratotomy: a comparison of centripetal and centrifugal incision techniques in human donor eyes. *Ophthalmology* 1994;101:746–754.
17. Assil KK, Schanzlin DJ. *Radial and astigmatic keratotomy*. Thorofare, NJ: Slack, 1994.
18. Assil KK. Radial keratotomy: the combined technique. *Int Ophthalmol Clin* 1994;34:55–77.
19. Casebeer JC. *A comprehensive system of refractive surgery*. 1994 course syllabus.
20. Lindstrom RL, Lindquist TD. *Radial keratotomy*. Vol. II. St. Louis: Mosby-Year Book, 1995:1–25.
21. Percival S, Piers B, Vyas AV. Radial keratotomy for myopia from 5.00 to 13.00 diopters two years after surgery. *J Refract Surg* 1996;12:86–90.
22. Lindstrom RL. Minimal invasive radial keratotomy and mini RK. *J Cataract Refract Surg* 1995;21:27–34.
23. Cowden JW, Lynn MJ, Waring GO. Repeated radial keratotomy in the Prospective Evaluation of Radial Keratotomy study. *Am J Ophthalmol* 1987;103:423–431.
24. Werblin TP, Stafford EM. The Casebeer system for predictable keratorefractive surgery. *Ophthalmology* 1993;100:1095–1102.
25. Haruta Y, et al. Recurrent herpes simplex virus type I corneal lesions after radial keratotomy in the rabbit. *Arch Ophthalmol* 1987;105:692–694.
26. Busin M, Suasez H, Bieber S, et al. Overcorrected visual acuity improved by antiglaucoma medication after radial keratotomy. *Am J Ophthalmol* 1985;101:374–375.
27. Thornton SP. *Radial and astigmatic keratotomy—the American system of precise predictable refractive surgery*. Thorofare, NJ: Slack, 1994.
28. Nordan LT. *Correcting myopia and astigmatism, radial keratotomy—the American way, the Nordan Maxwell approach*. Westmont, IL: American Surgical Instruments, 1992.
29. Marmer RH. A study of radial keratotomy complications. *Ann Ophthalmol* 1987;19:409–411.
30. Rowsey JJ, Balyeat HD. Radial keratotomy: preliminary report of complications. *Ophthalmic Surg* 1982;13:27–35.
31. Baurque LB, et al. Reported satisfaction, fluctuation of vision, and glare among patients one year after surgery in the Prospective Evaluation of Radial Keratotomy (PERK) study. *Arch Ophthalmol* 1986;104:356–363.
32. Waring GO, Lynn MJ, Nizam A, et al. Results of the Prospective Evaluation of Radial Keratotomy (PERK) study five years after surgery. The PERK study group. *Ophthalmology* 1991;98:1164–1176.
33. Stevens SX, Young SA, Polack PJ, et al. Complications of radial keratotomy. In: Krachmer JH, Mannis MJ, Holland EJ, eds. *Cornea*. Vol. III. St. Louis: Mosby-Year Book, 1997:2101–2116.
34. Cross WD, Head WJ. Complications of radial keratotomy: an overview. In: Sanders D, Hofmann RF, Salz J, eds. *Refractive corneal surgery*. Thorofare, NJ: Slack, 1986:349–399.
35. Rapizzi A, Prosdcino G, Gorla C, Martinuzzi A. Blood staining of the cornea following radial keratotomy. *J Refract Surg* 1991;7:188–189.
36. Cowden JW, Bores LD. A clinical investigation of the surgical correction of myopia by the method of Fyodorov. *Ophthalmology* 1981;88:737–741.
37. Dietz MR, Sanders DR, Marks RG. Radial keratotomy: an overview of the Kansas City study. *Ophthalmology* 1984;91:467–478.
38. Leroux les Jardins S, Bertrand I, Massin M. Intraoperative and early postoperative complications in 466 radial keratotomies. *J Refract Corneal Surg* 1992;8:215–216.
39. Rowsey JJ, Balyeat HD. Preliminary results and complications of radial keratotomy. *Am J Ophthalmol* 1982;93:433–455.
40. Carter J, Bruce A, Basson MD, et al. Cystoid macular edema following corneal-relaxing incisions. *Arch Ophthalmol* 1987;105:70–72.
41. Gelender H, Gelber EC. Cataract following radial keratotomy. *Arch Ophthalmol* 1983;101:1229–1231.
42. Hersh PS, Kalevar V, Kenyon KR. Penetrating keratoplasty for severe complications of radial keratotomy. *Cornea* 1987;10:170–174.
43. Schachar RA. Indications, techniques, and complications of radial keratotomy. *Int Ophthalmol Clin* 1983;23:119–128.
44. Zamora RL, Goldberg MA, Pepose JS. Presumed epithelial cyst in the anterior chamber following refractive keratotomy. *Refract Corneal Surg* 1994;10:652–655.
45. Waring GO, et al. Three year results of the Prospective Evaluation of Radial Keratotomy (PERK) study. *Ophthalmology* 1987;94:1339–1354.
46. Waring GO. *Refractive keratotomy for myopia and astigmatism*. St. Louis: Mosby, 1992.
47. Schanzlin DJ, et al. Diurnal change in refraction, corneal curvature, visual acuity, and intraocular pressure after radial keratotomy in the PERK study. *Ophthalmology* 1986;93:167–175.

48. Waring GO, et al. Results of the Prospective Evaluation of Radial Keratotomy (PERK) study one year after surgery. *Ophthalmology* 1985;92:177–197.

49. McDonnell PJ, Nizam A, Waring GO. Morning to evening change in refraction, corneal curvature, and visual acuity 11 years after radial keratotomy in the Prospective Evaluation of Radial Keratotomy study. The PERK study group. *Ophthalmology* 1996;103:233–239.

50. Nizam A, Waring GO, Lynn MJ, et al. Stability of refraction and visual acuity during 5 years in eyes with simple myopia. The PERK study group. *Refract Corneal Surg* 1992;8:439–447.

51. Frangie JP, et al. Excimer laser keratectomy after radial keratotomy. *Am J Ophthalmol* 1993;115:634–639.

52. Hoffman RF, Starling JC, Masler W. Contact lens fitting after radial keratotomy: one year results. *J Refract Surg* 1986;2:155–163.

53. Rowsey JJ, et al. Predicting the results of radial keratotomy. *Ophthalmology* 1983;90:642–654.

54. Duffey RJ. Bilateral *Serratia marcescens* keratitis following simutaneous bilateral radial keratotomy. *Am J Ophthalmol* 1995;119:233–236.

55. John ME. High hyperopia after radial keratotomy. *J Cataract Refract Surg* 1993;19:446–447.

56. Arrowsmith PN, Saunders DR, Marks RG. Visual, refractive, and keratometric results of radial keratotomy. *Arch Ophthalmol* 1983;101:873.

57. Binder PS, Charlton KH. Surgical procedures performed after refractive surgery. *Refract Corneal Surg* 1992;8:61–74.

58. Davis RM, et al. Corneal iron lines after radial keratotomy. *J Refract Surg* 1988;2:174–178.

59. Nelson JD, et al. Map-finger-dot changes in the corneal epithelial basement membrane following radial keratotomy. *Ophthalmology* 1985;92:199–204.

60. Gieser J, Sugar A. Radial keratotomy and corneal scarring. *Arch Ophthalmol* 1992;119:1527–1528.

61. Duffey RJ. Postoperative complications of radial keratotomy. In: Krachmer JH, Mannis MJ, Holland EJ, eds. *Cornea*. Vol. III. St. Louis: Mosby-Year Book, 1997:2117–2142.

62. Arrowsmith PN, Marks RG. Four-year update on predictability of radial keratotomy. *J Refract Surg* 1988;4:37–45.

63. Deitz MR, Sanders DR, Raanan MG. Progressive hyperopia in radial keratotomy. *Ophthalmology* 1986;93:1284–1288.

64. Dietz MR, et al. Long term (5 to 12 year) follow-up of metal blade radial keratotomy procedures. *Arch Ophthalmol* 1994;112:614–620.

65. Salz JJ, et al. Ten years' experience with a conservative approach to radial keratotomy. *Refract Corneal Surg* 1991;7:12–22.

66. Thornton SP, et al. Management of hyperopic shift after radial keratotomy. *Refract Corneal Surg* 1992;8:325–330.

67. Thornton SP, et al. Options on mini-radial keratotomy. *Refract Corneal Surg* 1993;9:476–479.

68. Waring GO. Ophthalmic procedures assessment—radial keratotomy for myopia. *Ophthalmology* 1988;95:671–687.

69. John ME, Howard C. Esotropia following radial keratotomy. *J Cataract Refract Surg* 1991;17:246–247.

70. Lindberg JV, et al. Ptosis following radial keratotomy: performed using a ridged eyelid speculum. *Ophthalmology* 1986;93:1509–1512.

71. Bates AK, Morgan SJ, Steele AD. Radial keratotomy: a review of 300 cases. *Br J Ophthalmol* 1992;76:586–589.

72. Feldman RM, et al. Retinal detachment following radial and astigmatic keratotomy. *Refract Corneal Surg* 1991;7:252–253.

73. O'Day DM, Feman SS, Elliott JH. Visual impairment following radial keratotomy: a cluster of cases. *Ophthalmology* 1986;93:319–326.

74. Cottingham AJ, et al. Bacterial corneal ulcers following keratorefractive surgery: a retrospective study of 14,163 procedures. Presented at the Ocular Microbiology and Immunology Group meeting, San Francisco, September 28, 1986.

75. Mataba AY, et al. Bacterial keratitis after radial keratotomy. *Ophthalmology* 1989;96:1171–1175.

76. Robin JB, et al. *Mycobacterium chelonei* keratitis after radial keratotomy. *Am J Ophthalmol* 1986;102:72–79.

77. Wilhelmus KR, Hamburg S. Bacterial keratitis following radial keratotomy. *Cornea* 1983;2:143–146.

78. Heidemann DG, Dunn SP, Watts JC. Aspergillus keratitis after radial keratotomy. *Am J Ophthalmol* 1995;120:254–256.

79. Maskin SL, Alfonso E. Fungal keratitis after radial keratotomy. *Am J Ophthalmol* 1992;114:369–370.

80. Mandelbaum S, et al. Late development of ulcerative keratitis in radial keratotomy scars. *Arch Ophthalmol* 1986;104:1156–1160.

81. Shivitz IA, Arrowsmith PN. Delayed keratitis after radial keratotomy. *Arch Ophthalmol* 1986;104:1153–1155.

82. Baldone JA, Franklin RM. Cataract following radial keratotomy. *Ann Ophthalmol* 1983;15:416–418.

83. Starling J, Hofmann R. Case report: anterior uveitis and transient hyperopia following radial keratotomy. *J Refract Surg* 1986;2:96–98.

84. Binder PS. Presumed epithelial ingrowth following radial keratotomy. *CLAO J* 1986;12:247–250.

85. Simons KB, Linsalata RP, Zaragosa AM. Ruptured globe secondary to blunt trauma following radial keratotomy. *J Refract Surg* 1988;4:132–135.

Astigmatic Keratotomy

C. J. Anderson

Naturally occurring astigmatism is greater than 0.50 diopters (D) in 44% of the population and greater or equal to 1.50 D in 8.44% of the general population (1). Regular astigmatism is present when two distinct focal points occur on the retina, corresponding to the steep and flat axes of the cornea (Fig. 16-1A). Irregular astigmatism occurs when an uneven corneal surface causes multiple retinal images. Astigmatism is classified as hyperopic, myopic, and compound, depending on whether the spherical equivalent is plus, minus, or neutral. Astigmatism can be hereditary or can be caused by trauma, surgery, contact lens wear, or eyelid pathology. Most cases of regular stable astigmatism are amenable to refractive surgery with the exception of astigmatism due to temporary causes such as contact lens wear or eyelid (chalazia) pathology. The treatment for temporary astigmatism is the withdrawal of the source of the astigmatism. This chapter covers the incisional surgical management of regular, naturally occurring and post–cataract surgery astigmatism.

PATIENT SELECTION

The most common symptoms of uncorrected astigmatism include blurring of vision, ghosting of images, monocular diplobia, and asthenopia. Most patients complain that they cannot see clearly at any distance. Symptomatic astigmatic refractive errors are most frequently corrected with spectacles and contact lenses although some patients are contact lens or spectacle intolerant. Other patients who are not intolerant of contact lenses or spectacles desire better uncorrected visual acuity for lifestyle enhancement, occupational requirements, or cosmetic reasons. The surgeon must identify the motivations and occupational history in all patients requesting refractive surgery.

A key responsibility of the surgeon is to discuss with each patient a realistic goal for visual improvement after refrac-

tive surgery. The goal is to achieve better uncorrected vision and functional improvement. It should be clear to patients that the surgeon cannot guarantee a specific level of uncorrected vision (e.g., 20/20) or a level of vision comparable to that achieved with spectacles or contact lenses. Furthermore, some patients have adjusted to their amount and axis of astigmatism and will find that a surgically induced change may be a difficult adjustment. Patients in the presbyopic age range are told that reading glasses may still be required after surgery. The surgeon is wise to counsel patients who have unrealistic expectations against having refractive surgery, to avoid disappointment with postsurgical results.

A history of stable refractive error is another prerequisite to refractive surgery. For this reason, patients should be at least 18 years old. Current refraction is always compared to spectacles and ophthalmic records. Also, patients who have had cataract surgery should have stable refraction without suture influence before refractive surgery is performed. A history of unstable diabetes or pregnancy might result in unstable refractions that would counterindicate refractive surgery.

The surgeon should perform a thorough ophthalmic examination on all refractive surgery candidates. The examination includes assessments of uncorrected, best-corrected, and near vision. Technicians and the physician perform manifest and cycloplegic refraction along with tonometry, keratometry, slit-lamp biomicroscopy, and retinal examination. The goal is to rule out other ocular diseases such as cataract or glaucoma and to measure the astigmatic error for surgical planning. The surgeon should carefully examine the cornea for evidence of trauma, dystrophy (keratoconus), and degeneration that might be the cause of astigmatic error. Corneal computerized topography is an adjunctive test that graphically illustrates the amount and axis of astigmatism and helps to rule out subtle corneal disease such as

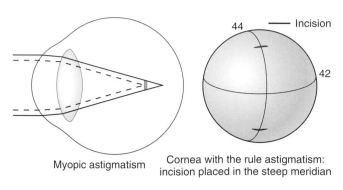

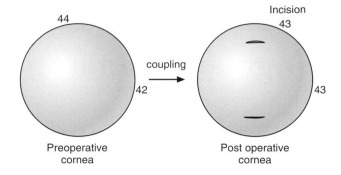

A

B

FIGURE 16-1.   A. *Astigmatic eye.* B. *Astigmatic incisions are placed in the steep corneal meridian to correct astigmatism.*

FIGURE 16-2.   *Coupling means that an incision across the steep meridian (axis) will flatten this meridian and steepen the meridian 90 degrees away.*

subclinical keratoconus or irregular astigmatism. If the refraction, keratometry, and computerized topography results do not agree, the surgeon must recheck the results and look for lenticular-induced astigmatism.

The patient should then go through a comprehensive informed consent process that might include viewing a video, receiving staff counseling, reading written material, and taking quizzes as well as signing a consent form. The surgeon should also discuss common side effects including foreign body sensation, glare, and fluctuating vision; complications such as infection, trauma, overcorrection, undercorrection; and irregular astigmatism and its implications; reoperations; and answers to all questions. The surgeon should have a feeling of understanding and rapport with his or her patient.

SURGICAL PLANNING

The surgeon devises a surgical plan for the correction of astigmatism for each individual patient based on history, examination, topography, and goals. Certain well-defined principles will assist the surgeon in the plan. First, the surgeon always places astigmatic incisions on the steep or plus axis of astigmatism in order to flatten this meridian (2). For example, the surgeon would make superior and inferior incisions perpendicular to the plus cylinder axis at 90 degrees for astigmatism with the rule (see Fig. 16-1B). A plus cylinder refraction automatically identifies the correct axis and therefore is most useful in surgery.

Another important principle is that an incision that flattens the steep meridian will have an effect to steepen the meridian 90 degrees away. This relationship is defined as coupling (3). If the coupling ratio is 1, there will be an equal amount of flattening in the incised meridian as there is steepening in the opposite orthogonal meridian (Fig. 16-2). A ratio of more than 1 will produce more flattening in the incised meridian than steepening in the nonincised meridian and a ratio of less than 1 will result in the opposite. The amount of coupling is determined by characteristics of the incision such as length and curvature. Short transverse inci-

Table 16-1.   Astigmatism Alone*

Correction (D)	T Marker Size (mm)	Optical Zone (mm)
0.75	2.5	7.00
1.12	3.0	7.00
1.25	2.5	6.00
1.67	3.0	6.00
2.00	2.5	5.00
2.25	3.0	5.00
2.50	2.5	4.75
2.75	3.0	4.75
3.00	2.5	4.50
3.50	3.0	4.50

*   Do not use with addition or modification of radial incisions.
Primary and enhancement procedures.
System exception: Pachymetry at most temporal and/or superior incision site.
System diamond blade set to pachymetry value.
A total or two (2) transverse incisions on the axis of the positive cylinder.
One transverse incision on each side of the cornea.

sions have a high coupling ratio, resulting in more flattening of the steep meridian. Longer transverse incisions may have a coupling of less than 1, whereas arcuate incisions tend to have a more equal coupling ratio. Sometimes more or less coupling is desirable depending on whether the surgeon wants an overall flattening effect on the cornea. For example, choosing an astigmatic incision with a coupling ratio higher than 1 would have an overall effect of flattening the entire cornea, causing a reduction of myopia or increasing hyperopia, depending on the baseline refractive error.

A third principle is that an incision placed closer to the visual axis has a greater effect on correcting astigmatism than does an equal-length incision placed farther from the optical zone (Fig. 16-3 and Table 16-1) (2). One approach is to make an equal-length transverse incision called a T incision at varying distance from the visual axis, depending on the degree of astigmatism to be corrected. However, incisions closer than 5 mm may cause overcorrections or irregular

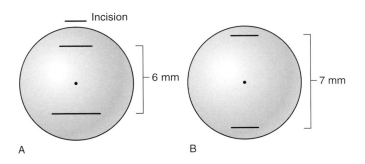

FIGURE 16-3.   *Equal-length incisions have a greater effect at a smaller optical zone (A) than a larger optical zone (B).*

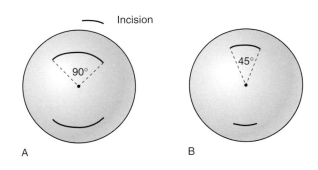

FIGURE 16-4.   *Longer incisions at the same optical zone (A) have a greater effect than do shorter incisions (B).*

Table 16-2.   Lindstrom/Casebeer Arc "T" Astigmatic Nomogram[a]

	Age				
	18–25	26–35	36–49	50–80	>80
1.0	30° × 2[b]	30° × 2[b]	30° × 2[b]	30° × 1	30° × 1
1.5	30° × 2[b]	30° × 2[b]	30° × 2[b]	30° × 2[b]	30° × 1
2.0	45° × 2[c]	45° × 2[c]	45° × 2[c]	30° × 2[b]	30° × 2[b]
2.5	60° × 2	45° × 2[c]	45° × 2[c]	30° × 2[b]	30° × 2[b]
3.0	60° × 2	60° × 2	45° × 2[c]	45° × 2[c]	30° × 2[b]
3.5	75° × 2	60° × 2	60° × 2	45° × 2[c]	30° × 2[b]
4.0	75° × 2	75° × 2	60° × 2	60° × 2	45° × 2[c]
4.5	75° × 2	75° × 2	60° × 2	60° × 2	45° × 2[c]
5.0	—	75° × 2	75° × 2	60° × 2	45° × 2[c]
5.5	—	—	75° × 2	75° × 2	45° × 2[c]
6.0	—	—	—	75° × 2	60° × 2
6.5	—	—	—	75° × 2	60° × 2
7.0	—	—	—	—	60° × 2

[a]   Pachymetry measurement taken 1.5 mm temporal to central visual axis.
Arcs must never exceed 90 degrees.
Two (2) symmetric arcs should be used unless corneal topography dictates otherwise.
Add 50 μm to pachymetry value when setting the arc "T" diamond blade, to overcome compressibility.
[b]   For enhancement only, 30° × 2 = 45° × 1.
[c]   For enhancement only, 45° × 2 = 75° × 1.

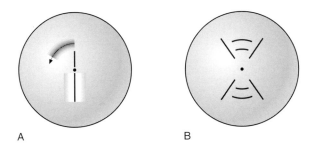

FIGURE 16-5.   A. *Radial incisions have a flattening effect that diminishes farther away from the incisions.* B. *Transverse incisions combined with radial incisions have a more flattening effect than do transverse incisions alone.*

The effect of a second incision is reduced by 25% of the effect obtained with the first incision (2).

Sometimes it is desirable to place radial incisions to correct astigmatic errors. Radial incisions placed in the steep meridian will also flatten the cornea and astigmatism. The maximal effect of a radial incision is over the incised cornea, with the effect decreasing the farther the distance from the incision (Fig. 16-5A) (5). For example, the surgeon may correct a refractive error of −1.25 + 1.50 X90 by placing two radial incisions at the 90-degree axis. Furthermore, transverse incisions have a greater refractive effect if combined with radial incisions in the same meridian. The procedure using multiple transverse incisions combined with radial incisions is called *trapezoidal keratotomy* (Ruiz procedure). It is a less popular, unpredictable operation for correcting high degrees of astigmatism (6). Likewise, if the surgeon uses transverse incisions along with radial incisions, combined radial and astigmatic keratotomy, there is usually greater surgical effect on the astigmatism than if the same incision was made without the radial incisions (Fig. 16-5B and Table 16-3). When the surgeon combines radial with tangential incisions, an important principle is not to cross or intersect the incisions, to avoid problems including irregular astigmatism, edge lift, and perforations (Fig. 16-6).

astigmatism. A more recently popularized technique is making an arcuate incision of increasing length at the same optical zone to correct increasing amounts of astigmatism (Table 16-2 and Fig. 16-4) (3,4). For example, an arcuate incision of 45 degrees corrects more astigmatism than one of 30 degrees but less astigmatism than one at 60 degrees at the same 7-mm optical zone. The surgeon can make arcuate incisions closer to the visual axis at the 6-mm zone or multiple incisions at different optical zones, though most of the effect is from the incision closest to the optical zone.

Table 16-3.   Astigmatism with Myopia*

Correction (D)	T Marker Size	Optical Zone (mm)
1.00	2.5	7.00
1.25	3.0	7.00
1.50	2.5	6.00
2.00	3.0	6.00
2.25	2.5	5.75
2.62	3.0	5.75
3.00	2.5	5.50
3.50	3.0	5.50
4.00	2.5	5.25
4.50	3.0	5.25
5.00	2.5	5.00
5.50	3.0	5.00
5.75	2.5	4.50
6.00	3.0	4.50

* Use in conjunction with the addition or modification of radial incisions.
Primary and enhancement procedures.
Pachymetry 1.5 mm temporal to central optical axis.
System diamond blade set to pachymetry value.
A total of two (2) transverse incisions on the axis of the positive cylinder.
One transverse incision on each side of the cornea.

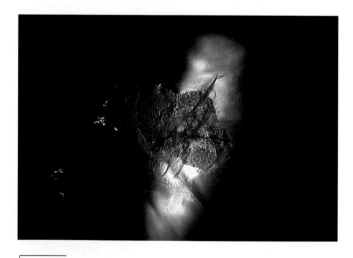

FIGURE 16-6.   *Corneal perforation at the site of intersecting radial and transverse incisions, requiring corneal glue.*

There are two other considerations in the surgical plan. One is that incisions have a greater effect the older the patient's age is. Many nomograms adjust for the effect of age. For example, a 30-year-old patient would generally have half the refractive effect from the same incision as an 80-year-old patient would. The second consideration is that the deeper the incision, the greater the effect. Incisions about 90% of the corneal depth are necessary to have maximum effect, whereas incisions of 50% or less depth may have little refractive effect (Fig. 16-7).

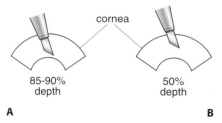

FIGURE 16-7.   A. *The depth of the incisions should be through 85% to 90% of the corneal thickness.* B. *Shallow incisions usually cause undercorrection.*

Using these basic principles and nomograms, the surgeon derives the surgical plan. It is very helpful for the surgeon to track his or her own results and develop a personalized nomogram for astigmatic surgery.

SURGICAL TECHNIQUE

Primary Procedure

The surgeon performs the surgical procedure according to the surgical plan. Adequate preparation and equipment including a clean operating environment and an operating microscope are essential. The most commonly used instruments include optical zone markers, usually 5, 6, and 7 mm; radial markers, usually four and eight incisions; transverse markers (2.5 and 3 mm) or arcuate markers measured in degrees; and a Sinsky hook. An astigmatic dial or a reticle in the operating microscope is useful in finding the correct axis of astigmatism. The surgeon begins by measuring the corneal thickness with the pachymeter and using the micronscope to measure the extension of the diamond blade (Fig. 16-8). Diamond blades used for correcting astigmatism have a front-cutting blade and a calibrated micron handle and come in a number of different configurations, for example, square or angled. The operating staff prepares and sterilizes the instruments before the patient enters the operating room.

The staff prepares patients simultaneously in another room and obtains a brief medical history, allergy history, and vital signs. The patient signs a formal informed consent form. Nurses give an oral sedative such as diazepam (Valium) depending on the patient's state of anxiety, and several sets of topical anesthetic approximately 15 minutes before surgery. It is rarely necessary to administer a retrobulbar or general anesthetic, with the possible exception of patients with severe nystagmus or uncooperative patients.

In the operating room the patient lies in a prone position under the operating microscope. The surgeon asks the patient to fixate on the light filament or a central fixation device on the operating microscope, and marks the center of the pupil or visual axis with a Sinsky hook and makes the appropriate optical zone mark by indenting the cornea or placing dye on the marker (Figs. 16-9 and 16-10). The surgeon must identify the axis of astigmatism as precisely as

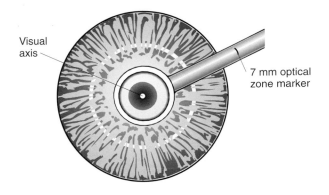

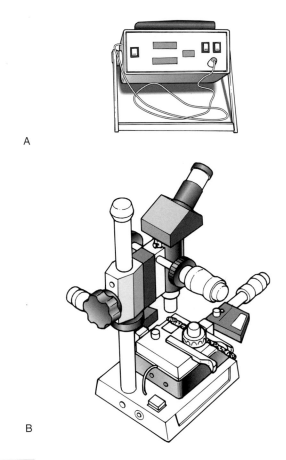

FIGURE 16-8. A. *Corneal pachymeter.* B. *Microscope (Micronscope II, Chiron Vision, Irvine, CA).*

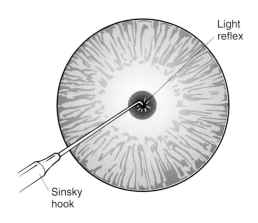

FIGURE 16-9. *The center of the pupil or visual axis is marked with a Sinsky hook.*

FIGURE 16-10. *The optical zone marker is used to measure the distance from the center of the pupil to the incision site.*

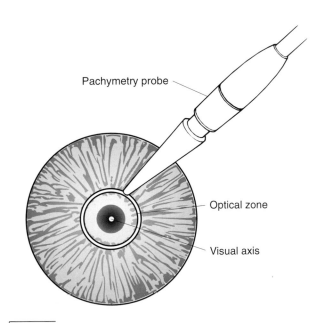

FIGURE 16-11. *The reticle in the microscope, or a handheld astigmatic dial, is used to identify the axis of astigmatism.*

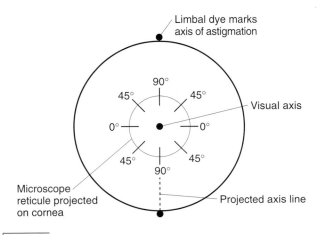

FIGURE 16-12. *A radial keratotomy marker can determine the length of the arcuate incision in degrees.*

possible. It is helpful to identify a landmark at the limbus such as a vessel or nevus, or alternatively the surgeon can mark the 6- and 12-o'clock limbi preoperatively at the slit lamp with a gentian violet dye or a small scratch. Marking at the slit lamp with the patient upright avoids the possibility of cyclotorsion in the prone position. The surgeon lines up a reticle in the microscope or a handheld astigmatic

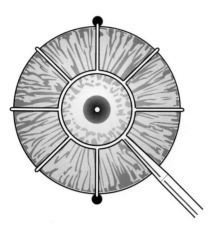
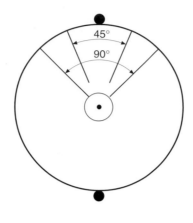

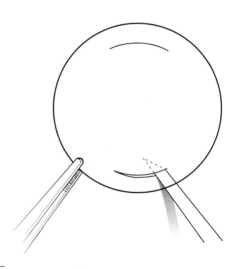

FIGURE 16-13.   *Corneal thickness is measured by pachymetry over the incision site.*

dial with the limbal marks so the 90-degree axis of the dial lines up with the 6- and 12-o'clock limbal marks, and marks the patient's axis of astigmatism with a line or a radial mark (Fig. 16-11). I like to use one of the radial lines of a standard 8, 12, or 16 radial keratotomy (RK) incision marker to mark the axis because then this marker also determines the length in degrees of the arcuate incision. For example, the distance between two radial marks on an 8 RK marker is 90 degrees and as a 16 RK marker it is 45 degrees. Therefore, if the surgeon uses one radial of the 16 RK marker to mark the axis, then an incision the length of adjacent radial marks would give an arcuate incision of 45 degrees (Fig. 16-12). The surgeon can alternatively purchase special markers for varying degrees or lengths of either arcuate or transverse incisions. Transverse incisions are made with straight marks, usually 2.5 or 3 mm in length.

Corneal pachymetry measurements are taken over the area of the incision (Fig. 16-13). The diamond blade is set for 100% of the thinnest pachymetry value, either with a separate microscope called the microscope, designed to measure the distance from the footplate of the blade to the tip, or with the micrometer handle on the diamond blade. Some surgeons measure only the central part of the cornea with pachymetry and then add 50 μm to the blade to compensate for the thicker peripheral area of the cornea where the astigmatic incisions are made.

The surgeon fixates the globe with forceps and the front-cutting diamond penetrates the cornea and seats deeply at the edge of the mark. The surgeon makes the desired incision by following the prepared marks carefully, viewing the tip of the blade (Fig. 16-14). For longer arcuate incisions of more than 45 degrees, the surgeon curves the incision by developing a slight roll of the fingers. The surgeon repeats the procedure for paired arcuate incisions on the opposite side of the astigmatic axis. When the surgeon makes radial incisions to correct myopia, he or she makes the astigmatic incisions first and places the radial incisions either adjacent to or such that they skip over the astigmatic incisions. The surgeon should be viewing the front edge of the blade on a semidry cornea, watching for any aqueous leakage that would indicate a perforation. The incision must be stopped in the event of microperforation, to avoid a larger macro-

FIGURE 16-14.   *Corneal incisions are made with a knife set at 100% of the pachymetry value at the incision site.*

perforation that could lead to anterior-chamber collapse or persistent aqueous leak requiring sutures. No further irrigation or manipulation of the incisions is necessary unless obvious debris is seen in them.

Antibiotic drops are then applied and the patient is sent home with an antibiotic or antibiotic-steroid combination to be used about 1 week during the time the epithelium is healing. Instructions are given to avoid getting dust, dirt, and water in the eyes for 2 weeks. Sunglasses are advised to help with glare and the patients are given pain and sleeping medication. Follow-up appointments are arranged for 1 day, 1 week, 1 month, and then as necessary for the first year.

Enhancements

Reoperations for either residual astigmatism or newly induced astigmatism are not performed for several months after the initial surgery until the refractive error and corneal topography have stabilized. If the incisions look shallow at the slit lamp, the surgeon should recheck the pachymetry measurement and blade extension and deepen them. Alter-

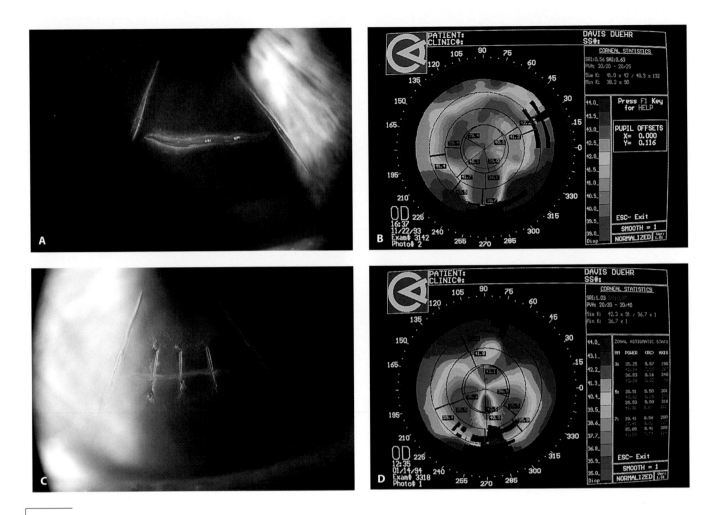

FIGURE 16-15.   *Poorly healed inferior astigmatic scar (A) resulting in abnormal corneal flattening and overcorrection (B). Treatment consisted of debridement of the scar and suturing of the incision with 10-0 polypropylene (Prolene) (C), with reversal of the overcorrection (D).*

natively, the surgeon can either lengthen the initial incision or add additional incisions at a smaller optical zone. If the astigmatism in properly healed incisions is at a different axis than the original, either there is an overcorrection or an error in axis identification of the cylinder. In this case, the surgeon uses the same technique with careful identification of the correct axis and possibly with a more conservative surgical plan, to avoid overcorrection in the opposite 90-degree meridian. Radial incisions made in the first procedure should not intersect with these recent incisions and therefore the astigmatic incision may have to skip over radial incisions.

Keratotomy in Cataract Surgery

Many surgeons use a variety of techniques for astigmatism correction in cataract surgery. One commonly used technique is to plan the cataract incision to intersect the axis of the patient's astigmatism. Depending on the length and location of the cataract incision from the limbus, the surgeon induces flattening of the steep meridian (7). For greater amounts of astigmatism, the surgeon makes corneal incisions

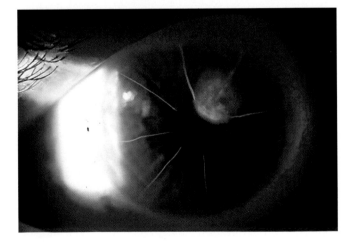

FIGURE 16-16.   *Corneal infiltrate at the incision site.*

at the time of cataract surgery or postoperatively using the standard technique for astigmatic keratotomy. The nomogram should be conservative, taking the generally older age of the patient into consideration. If the surgeon uses astigmatic keratotomy simultaneously with cataract surgery and the patient receives peribulbar, retrobulbar, or general anesthesia, the technique is more difficult because the inability of the patient to fixate may cause globe rotation. A qualitative or quantitative keratometry or intraoperative topography may be useful in this situation to identify the correct axis of astigmatism. With the use of topical or conjunctival anesthesia for cataract surgery, the surgeon avoids these difficulties and can use the standard technique.

COMPLICATIONS

Intraoperative complications include microperforations and macroperforations. A microperforation is defined as a small leak of aqueous that is self-sealing. There is no specific retreatment with the exception of more observation and antibiotics. A larger macroperforation results in continuous leak of aqueous or anterior-chamber collapse. The surgeon treats this by either placing a bandage contact lens or suturing the incisions.

The most frequent postoperative complications in astigmatic surgery are overcorrection and undercorrection. Undercorrection usually occurs either because of improper marking of the visual axis so the astigmatic incision does not bisect the axis of astigmatism or because the incisions are made too shallow. An improperly located axis of astigmatism also leads to a shift in the axis of the astigmatism. The surgeon treats undercorrection by a repeat operation, either making the incision deep enough or making a new incision at the proper axis or at a smaller optical zone.

Overcorrection usually occurs because of errors in marking or making the incision at the proper optical zone. Another cause is making the incision longer than is intended according to the nomogram. There is also the possibility, due to biologic variability or poor healing, that the incisions are correct but the patient overresponded. Many poorly healed incisions appear to have wide scars and epithelial plugs (Fig. 16-15). Sometimes the treatment of choice is to clean out the incisions and suture them closed.

Another rare complication is irregular astigmatism, defined as an irregular corneal surface that causes a reduction in best-corrected spectacle visual acuity. Also, keratometry and corneal topography demonstrate irregular astigmatism. A rigid contact lens usually improves vision better than spectacles and is an additional diagnostic and therapeutic aid.

Incisional keratitis presents in the early postoperative course as an edematous "fluffy" incision, with the patient complaining of pain, glare, and photophobia. The surgeon manages keratitis with antibiotic-steroid drops and observation. If obvious infiltrate develops, the surgeon can irrigate the incision with antibiotic solution and administer intensive antibiotics, similar to the treatment of corneal ulceration (Fig. 16-16).

Other complaints such as foreign body sensation and dry eyes are common. One relatively common finding is corneal iron lines, probably related to changes in the tear film. Occasionally, corneal dellen or corneal vascularization occurs postoperatively.

OUTCOMES

There is no large controlled study of astigmatic keratotomy similar to the Prospective Evaluation of Radial Keratotomy (PERK) study of radial keratotomy (8). One study showed a variable range of astigmatic shift using a variety of surgical procedures, with the greatest shift being with the trapezoidal keratotomy and lesser shift with transverse incisions alone. All procedures suffered from a variable degree of accuracy (9). Two recent studies that included eyes that had both radial and astigmatic incisions reported excellent results, even with beginning surgeons (10,11). Astigmatic surgery can also be effective in conjunction with cataract surgery (12–14).

CONCLUSIONS

Astigmatic keratotomy, whether primary or associated with radial keratotomy or cataract surgery, is a simple, low-cost, and effective procedure. The procedure will likely survive for the foreseeable future, even in the era of increasingly sophisticated technology such as the excimer laser.

REFERENCES

1. Guyton DL. Prescribing cylinders: the problem of distortion. *Surv Ophthalmol* 1977;22:177–188.
2. Rowsey JJ. Ten caveats in keratorefractive surgery. *Ophthalmology* 1983;90:148–155.
3. Thornton SP. Astigmatic keratotomy: a review of the basic concepts with case reports. *J Cataract Refract Surg* 1990;16:430–435.
4. Agapitos PJ, Lindstrom RL. Astigmatic keratotomy. *Ophthalmol Clin North Am* 1992;5:709–715.
5. Duffey RJ, Jain VN, Tchah H. Paired arcuate keratotomy. A surgical approach to mixed and myopic astigmatism. *Arch Ophthalmol* 1988;106:1130–1135.
6. Ibrahim O, Hussein HA, El-Sahn MF, et al. Trapezoidal keratotomy for the correction of naturally occurring astigmatism. *Arch Ophthalmol* 1991;109:1374–1381.
7. Axt JC, McCaffery JM. Reduction of postoperative against the rule astigmatism by lateral incision technique. *J Cataract Refract Surg* 1993;19:380–386.
8. Waring GO, Lynn MJ, McDonnell PJ. Results of the Prospective Evaluation of Radial Keratotomy (PERK) study 10 years after surgery. *Arch Ophthalmol* 1994;112:1298–1307.
9. Agapitos PJ, Linstrom RJ, Williams PA, et al. Analysis of astigmatic keratotomy. *J Cataract Refract Surg* 1989;15:13–18.
10. Werblin TP, Stafford GM. The Casebeer system for predictable keratorefractive surgery. *Ophthalmology* 1993;100:1095–1102.
11. Friedberg ML, Imperia PS, Elander R, et al. Results of radial and astigmatic keratotomy by beginning refractive surgeons. *Ophthalmology* 1993;100:746–751.
12. Shepard JR. Correction of preexisting astigmatism at the time of small incision cataract surgery. *J Cataract Refract Surg* 1989;15:55–57.
13. Davidson JA. Transverse astigmatic keratotomy combined with phacoemulsification and intraocular lens implantation. *J Cataract Refract Surg* 1989;15:38–44.
14. Osher RH. Transverse astigmatic keratotomy combined with cataract surgery. *Ophthalmol Clin North Am* 1992;5:717–725.

Technique for Myopic Photorefractive Keratectomy

ROGER F. STEINERT

Most of the important elements of the technique for photorefractive keratectomy (PRK) for the correction of myopia are similar, regardless of the specific laser employed. In this chapter, I discuss the common elements in preoperative evaluation, preparation of the patient, removal of the epithelium, stromal ablation, immediate postoperative treatment, postoperative medications, management of common complications, and outcomes.

PREOPERATIVE EVALUATION

A comprehensive ophthalmic examination, including dilated indirect ophthalmoscopy, is mandatory. Prior to instillation of any drops that may disturb the corneal surface, including applanation tension, a careful manifest refraction with defogging is performed. Many myopic patients wear spectacles or contact lenses with excessive minus power.

Two special evaluations are needed in addition to a conventional comprehensive examination. Videokeratography with computer-assisted topographic analysis provides information that may be important initially or later in the healing course. Preoperatively, the topographic analysis discloses irregular astigmatism, most commonly forme fruste keratoconus, that may lead to a poor result despite excellent technique and normal postoperative healing. Preoperative topographic analysis also discloses any disparity between the refractive astigmatism and the corneal cylinder, possibly due to lenticular astigmatism, posterior staphyloma, or inaccurate refraction. Postoperatively, the preoperative topographic analysis provides the baseline against which postoperative results are measured. Increasingly sophisticated topographic software allows highly useful analyses of induced change.

A cycloplegic refraction should be performed at the time of the dilated fundus examination. Excessive accommodation is more commonly a problem in younger patients, but even patients over the age of 40 sometimes demonstrate a marked disparity between a manifest refraction and a cycloplegic refraction.

The most important element in the preoperative evaluation is the determination that refractive surgery in general, and PRK in particular, is appropriate for the individual patient. For the physician, this assessment is a combination of an analysis of the objective data and of the patient's understanding of the procedure and expectations of outcome. For the patient, a fully informed decision requires the transfer of larger amounts of information about refractive errors, the treatment modality, the risks and benefits of the proposed treatment, and the alternatives. In addition, however, the patient needs perspective, which will be guided both by the physician and the office staff and by any individuals known to the patient who have previously undergone PRK.

PREPARATION OF THE PATIENT

Considerable variation exists among treatment centers regarding specific details of the preoperative preparation of the patient. The general trend, however, is toward minimization of preoperative manipulations. Traditional preparation for ophthalmic microsurgery often includes antiseptic cleansing of the skin around the eyes, administration of antibiotic solutions to the ocular surface, and a sterile surgical drape. Most practitioners have found that these steps are not necessary for PRK.

Some surgeons administer miotic drops such as pilocarpine 2% approximately ½ hour preoperatively, to minimize the size of the entrance pupil. The goal is to achieve increased ease of centration of the PRK ablation zone. The patient has the additional advantage of some reduction in photophobia from the microscope's illumination lights. Disadvantages of pharmacologic miosis include inducing brow ache from stimulation of the iris sphincter and ciliary muscles, a postoperative sense of darkness, and the statistically small but real possibility of a miotic-induced peripheral retinal break, particularly in a myopic population. Surgeons frequently believe that mild miosis is helpful early in their experience, but increasingly omit this step as experience is gained.

Some patients desire systemic sedation to lessen their anxiety at the time of treatment, while other patients strongly wish to avoid any alteration in their level of awareness. Many surgeons offer an oral antianxiety medication and allow the patient to choose. A commonly used drug is diazepam (Valium), 5 to 10 mg depending on body weight, approximately 30 minutes prior to the laser procedure. All patients should have a companion to assist the patient in returning home after the treatment. If a systemic antianxiety drug is dispensed, however, it is especially mandatory that the presence of a companion be verified prior to administration of the drug.

REMOVAL OF THE EPITHELIUM

Techniques for removal of the epithelium to expose the underlying stroma can be grouped into three categories: mechanical, chemically assisted, and laser.

Mechanical De-epithelialization

The most straightforward means of removing epithelium, employed in most of the early investigations, utilizes a purely mechanical debridement of the epithelium with a sterile blade or spatula-type device. To avoid excessive de-epithelialization, an optical zone marker is centered over the optical axis and a forceful mark placed. Typically, a 7.0-mm optical zone marker is employed for a 6.0-mm PRK. In addition to providing a visual guideline for the margin of the de-epithelialization, the optical zone marker physically transects the epithelium. If the initial debridement is performed at the edge of the optical zone and the blade is swept in a circular fashion just inside the optical zone marker, the epithelium will peel off up to, but not across, the mark. Most surgeons will debride the periphery first and then an island of central epithelium at the end. In this manner, excessive dehydration of the critical central area is avoided during the slow peripheral de-epithelialization (1). Several blunt and semiblunt reusable surgical instruments have been designed for debridement. An alternative is a disposable surgical blade such as the No. 64 Beaver blade, with care taken to tilt the blade at a low angle to avoid any cutting of the stroma (Fig. 17-1). After the debridement, the clumps of epithelium are removed from the surgical field.

The base of the exposed Bowman's layer is "polished" with a cellulose surgical spear. The spear can be minimally moistened, but not saturated, with a medium-viscosity artificial tear agent such as ½% carboxymethylcellulose (Refresh

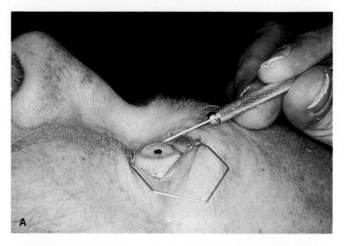

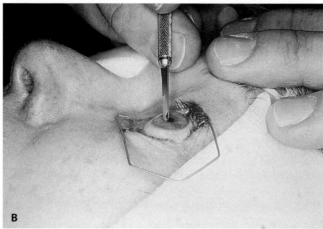

FIGURE 17-1.   A. *When de-epithelialization is performed by debridement with a surgical blade, the blade is rotated to a flat angle to avoid the potential for lacerating Bowman's layer. B. A sharp blade at an acute angle is more likely to nick Bowman's layer and should be avoided.*

Plus, Allergan, Irvine, CA) (Fig. 17-2). The goal is to ensure full removal of any residual nests of epithelial cells and create a maximally smooth surface. The artificial tear moisture may help by "filling in" any depressed areas, similar to the application of masking fluids in phototherapeutic keratectomy. The surface should appear dry and not frankly moistened before the laser treatment is started, as any residual moisture will absorb laser energy and reduce the optical effect of the PRK.

A recent variant of mechanical debridement involves the use of a rotating brushlike device that has a diameter matching the desired PRK treatment zone. These disposable brushes are typically powered by a conventional consumer battery-operated electric toothbrush handle (2).

Chemically Assisted De-epithelialization

The epithelium may be loosened by disrupting cells through the application of several toxic agents (3). Direct application

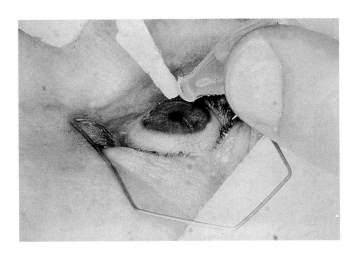

FIGURE 17-2. *After mechanical de-epithelialization, the base is cleaned with a cellulose surgical spear lightly moistened by a medium-viscosity nonpreserved artificial tear agent.*

of drops is inadvisable, because of the spread of the toxic fluid to the peripheral epithelium and limbal germinal epithelium which are critical in re-establishing the epithelium after PRK. The distribution of the agent can be controlled by using a soaked pledget of sterile filter paper shaped in an appropriately sized disk, such as approximately 7.0 mm in diameter. After only several minutes of application, the underlying epithelium is notably more easily removed. Topical anesthetic agents such as proparacaine and tetracaine are the most commonly used agents, although other topical anesthetics such as lidocaine (Xylocaine) and even liquid cocaine and toxic antibiotics such as aminoglycosides have been used.

The potential effect of these agents on the underlying stroma is unknown, however. Any pharmacologic agent that disrupts epithelium will, by definition, enter at least the anterior stroma, and quite possibly rapidly penetrate full thickness down to endothelium and even the anterior chamber. Whether or not these agents have any effect on postoperative inflammatory cells and the keratocytes is unknown. These effects could be potentially harmful or beneficial, and careful investigations are needed to evaluate these effects.

Transepithelial Ablation

The excimer laser itself can ablate through epithelium (4,5). Typically, a planar ablation with an optical zone equal to, or slightly larger than, the optical ablation is programmed. If the room lights and optical microscope illumination are turned off, the epithelium can be observed to fluoresce with a readily seen cobalt blue color. The underlying stroma does not fluoresce. When the laser ablation begins to break through the epithelium, islands of black (nonfluorescent) tissue will be seen to expand with each pulse as more

epithelium is fully denuded. The most common area of initial penetration is the superior region, although considerable individual variation occurs. Epithelium is usually thickest either centrally or inferiorly.

If the laser is used to fully ablate all epithelium, then it is unnecessary to manipulate the base of the ablation zone before proceeding with optical PRK of the stroma, other than to dry any residual moisture if present. Because some stroma will have been removed with the final pulses of transepithelial ablation, most surgeons employing this technique reduce the programmed amount of optical correction by 0.50 to 0.75 diopter (D). The precise amount of direction varies depending on the specific technique and equipment employed, and the surgeon employing this technique should check with colleagues to determine their experience, as well as carefully monitor his or her own results and personally modify the predictive nomogram.

An alternative technique that does not require modification of the PRK nomogram uses the laser to ablate most of the epithelium, but stops near or at the exact point of first perforation of the epithelium. With the Summit Apex system operating at 180 mJ/cm^2 and 10 Hz, normal epithelial perforation rarely occurs with fewer than 145 pulses, and more typically perforation is first seen between 160 and 180 pulses. One strategy is to program 150 pulses in the phototherapeutic (PTK) mode with a 6.0-mm optical zone, and then mechanically wipe off the remaining basal remnants. A slightly different approach, one that I currently employ, is to program 200 pulses, and simply stop as soon as I begin to see perforation of the epithelium as judged by the disappearance of fluorescence. The base is then wiped or dried of residual cell remnants and moisture.

To clean the base of the epithelial ablation zone, a dry cellulose surgical spear is usually adequate. A dull or sharp blade can be used as an additional aid, acting almost as a "squeegee" to wipe off any basal elements. Unlike mechanical epithelial debridement, no thick cell elements will remain, and the maneuver is not forceful. The goal is to remove residual moisture and the basal laminar fragments.

STROMAL ABLATION

Each laser requires a specific input of parameters and, in many cases, offers the surgeon several choices in specific ablation parameters.

Refractive Goal

For most ophthalmic excimer lasers, the surgeon inputs the desired refractive goal in diopters. Particularly for corrections above 4 D, the surgeon must know whether the laser algorithm corrects for vertex distance or whether a vertex distance correction should be calculated manually, in order to shift the spectacle correction to the corneal plane. If a soft contact lens power is used to determine the refractive goal, then no vertex correction is needed. A hard contact lens power should never be used, because hard contact lens power is determined by the base curve of the hard contact lens in addition to any optical power on the anterior contact lens surface.

Most surgeons use a "dry" manifest refraction performed with a defogging technique to determine the amount of myopia to be corrected. In addition, however, a cycloplegic refraction is mandatory preoperatively to eliminate the potential for latent accommodation, a common finding in myopic patients wearing spectacles. In addition, a patient undergoing evaluation for PRK often has a heightened degree of anxiety and is more prone to accommodation even with careful defogging refraction techniques. The cycloplegic refraction itself may not accurately represent the patient's true refractive status, however. The most common source of error in the cycloplegic refraction is the inclusion of the aspheric peripheral and midperipheral cornea in the optics being refracted, as well as the potential for a shift in position of the lens-iris diaphragm. Schallhorn et al (7) proposed improving the utility of cycloplegic refractions by placing a 3- to 4-mm aperture in the phorometer (Phoroptor) or trial frame during the cycloplegic refraction, thereby eliminating at least some of the aspheric peripheral corneal optical aberrancy.

Multizone Ablation

Some surgeons hypothesized that regression after PRK may be due, at least in part, to the abrupt transition from the treated zone to the untreated zone (6). The basic refractive algorithm assumes a spherical correction, but this is imposed on an increasingly aspheric peripheral cornea. To achieve a more gradual peripheral transition, a "multizone" ablation can be performed. The concept is similar to flattening the peripheral base curves of a contact lens.

In a laser system where the operator can select different optical zone sizes, a peripheral multizone ablation can be performed manually. For example, for a 6-D correction, the laser is first programmed for a 4-D correction with a 4.0-mm optical zone, followed by a 1.0-D correction with a 5.0-mm optical zone, and an additional 1.0-D correction with a 6.0-mm optical zone. Sequential ablations also create a "multipass" treated surface, as discussed below. Laser devices may be programmed to offer the surgeon the ability to preprogram a "single-pass" multizone contour, which can be readily created through a modification of the algorithms controlling the rate of opening of the aperture in a large-area ablation system or the scanning pattern of a smaller-beam system.

Clinicians have experienced good outcomes after multizone ablations. Little work has been done, however, to prove the advantage of this technique. Large trials prospectively randomizing patients between single-zone and multizone ablations will be needed to determine whether any benefit occurs after multizone ablation.

Multipass Ablation

Several surgeons reported an improvement in their results when the final ablation was the sum of two or more sequential ablations on the same site at the same session (6). This is often combined with a multizone ablation, as noted already. Multipass ablation can be programmed as an optional technique in some devices.

The advantage of multipass ablation may be in reducing the irregularities due to inhomogeneities in the laser beam, as well as perhaps an averaging of other biologic variables. Clinical benefit from a multipass technique needs to be verified through a large prospective randomized trial.

Centration

Centration of the ablation over the visual axis is critical in avoiding optical distortions postoperatively (8). Decentered ablations will result in irregular astigmatism, multiplopia, and the perception of glare and halos (9).

The surgeon must take particular care to center the ablation over the entrance pupil. Because the corneal dome is approximately 4mm in front of the iris plane, it is not adequate to rely simply on the patient viewing a central fixation light in the laser system. The laser system must provide some external centration reference so that the surgeon can determine the placement of the optical zone on the cornea. Meticulous attention to the manufacturer's recommended technique for centration is critical to the success of the procedure (Fig. 17-3).

High-speed eye tracking systems have been incorporated out of necessity into the small-spot scanning laser systems. Precise registration of each laser spot relative to the other is necessary to achieve a smooth and predictable ablation. An additional benefit may be the ability to maintain centration if eye movement occurs. The surgeon cannot be lulled into a false sense of confidence with an eye tracking device, however (10). The eye tracker will follow the beam location initially established by the surgeon; if the optical zone is initially decentered, the tracking device will maintain the same decentration throughout the procedure! For lasers with large-area ablation systems, any advantage of an automated eye tracking system over surgeon-controlled centration has yet to be established.

Central Island Prevention

Some manufacturers have specific recommendations for "pretreatment" of a small central zone, to reduce or eliminate the incidence of a central steep area generally referred to as a *central island*. One of the many theories of central island formation is that the accumulation of excess moisture centrally reduces the laser beam intensity (11,12). If so, interrupting the laser ablation to dry the central area with a cellulose surgical spear may be helpful.

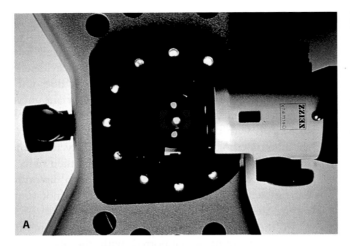
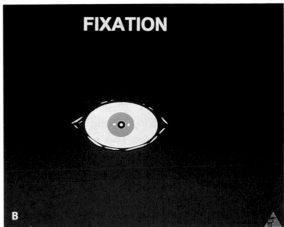
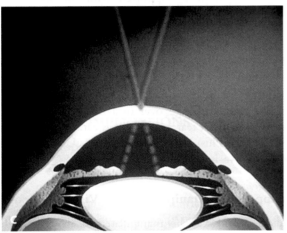
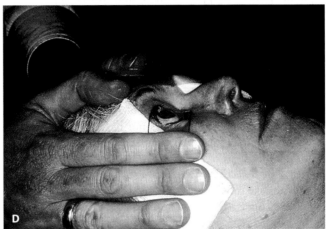

FIGURE 17-3. A. *In the Summit Technology Apex system, the patient fixates on a green, coaxial aiming light that is surrounded by a red illuminated circle.* B. *The surgeon focuses a dual external helium-neon (He-Ne) laser beam on the corneal apex, directly over the visible reflection of the green fixation light.* C. *The divergent He-Ne beams strike the edge of the pupillary sphincter at 3- and 9-o'clock positions.* D. *The surgeon stabilizes the patient's head with his or her hands. Note the surgical gauze pad taped to the temporal region of the head to absorb moisture that would otherwise run into the patient's ear, causing distraction. The untreated eye is protected with a gauze eye pad of an occlusive shield.*

Another approach that is currently gaining popularity is to "pretreat" a central area of about 2.5 to 3.0 mm in diameter, either as a separate step before the principal ablation or as a modification of the laser algorithm.

The efficacy of these techniques has not been proved and remains anecdotal.

POSTOPERATIVE MEDICATION

Many variations on postoperative management exist, dependent on both surgical preference and specific experience with a particular laser system. The postoperative regimen continues to evolve with increased experience, and the reader must remain up-to-date on current medication regimens. This section offers my personal approach at the time of writing.

Immediate Postoperative Medications

At the conclusion of the ablation, three drops of diclofenac (Voltaren) are applied, followed by one drop of ofloxacin (Ocuflox) and fluorometholone 0.1% (FML, Fluor-Op, E-flone). A bandage contact lens is applied. My current preference is the extremely thin and generally well-tolerated ProTek bandage soft contact lens (Ciba) with a 8.9-mm base curve. The lens is applied with sterile technique, utilizing two cellulose surgical spears. The patient then utilizes the ofloxacin and fluorometholone four times daily until re-epithelialization occurs, typically 2 days after transepithelial ablation and 3 to 4 days after manual debridement. The patient is checked daily until re-epithelialization occurs. The diclofenac drops are used as needed for pain but no more than every 4 hours on the first day postoperatively (13,14).

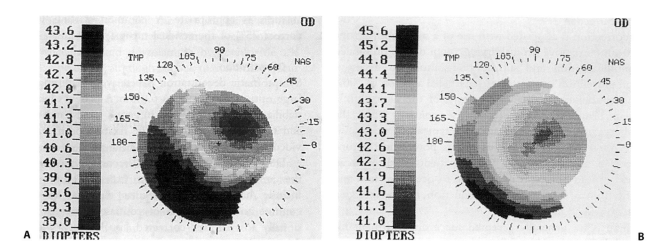

FIGURE 17-5.   A. *Severe decentration is evident on topographic analysis. The patient's vision was 20/25 and he complained of severe glare and multiplopia.* B. *After retreatment, topographic analysis shows extension of the flattened ablation zone into more of the visual axis. Although incompletely treated, the patient reported approximately 90% resolution of his visual disturbances.*

Table 17-1.   Published Outcomes After Photorefractive Keratectomy for Low to Moderate Myopia with a 6.0-mm Optical Zone

	Pop and Aras (6)	Schallhorn et al (7)	McCarty et al (36)	Shah and Hersh (37)
Follow-up (mo)	6	12	12	6
Range of myopia (D)	−1.0 to −6.0	−2.0 to −5.5	−8.8 to −5.25	−1.5 to −6.0
No. of patients	145	30	274	45
Laser system	VISX	Summit	VISX	Summit
Uncorrected visual acuity (%)				
≥20/20	NR	100	47	62
≥20/25	89.4	100	NR	NR
≥20/40	97.9	100	87	100
Predictability (%)				
±0.5 D	84.8	70	NR	62.2
±1.0 D	95.5	93	87	84.4

NR = not reported.

for myopia will not result in improvement of visual acuity in the presence of long-standing amblyopia, nor will visual acuity improve in the presence of myopic macular degeneration. Psychological or social expectations may be unspoken and yet may be major motivations in a patient seeking refractive surgery. Elimination of the use of spectacles will not resolve unrealistic patient expectations.

OUTCOMES

The typical outcomes after myopic PRK continue to improve. Results in published series lag behind current results, as techniques and technology continue to evolve rapidly. Table 17-1 summarizes the findings of several series published in 1995 and 1996 with a 6.0-mm optical zone, but note the procedures were performed in 1993 and 1994.

REFERENCES

1. Campos M, Trokel SL, McDonnell PJ. Surface morphology following photorefractive keratectomy. *Ophthalmic Surg* 1993;24:822–825.
2. Pallikaris IG, Karoutis AD, Lydataki SE, Siganos DS. Rotating brush for fast removal of corneal epithelium. *J Refract Corneal Surg* 1994;10:439–442.
3. Campos M, Raman S, Lee M, McDonnell PJ. Keratocyte loss after different methods of deepithelialization. *Ophthalmology* 1994;101:890–894.
4. Alio JL, Ismael MM, Artola A. Laser epithelium removal before photorefractive keratectomy. *Refract Corneal Surg* 1993;9:395.
5. Gimbel HV, DeBroff BM, Beldavs RA, et al. Comparison of laser and manual removal of corneal epithelium for photorefractive keratectomy. *J Refract Surg* 1995;11:36–41.
6. Pop M, Aras M. Multizone/multipass photorefractive keratectomy: 6 month results. *J Cataract Refract Surg* 1995;21:633–643.
7. Schallhorn SC, Blanton CL, Kaupp SE, et al. Preliminary results of photorefractive keratectomy in active-duty United States Navy personnel. *Ophthalmology* 1996;103:5–22.
8. Schwartz-Goldstein BH, Hersh PS. Corneal topography of phase III excimer laser photorefractive keratectomy: optical zone centration analysis. *Ophthalmology* 1995;102:951–962.

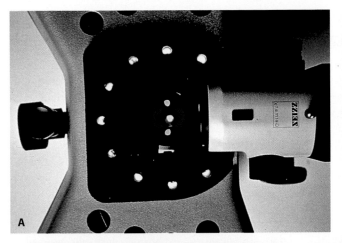
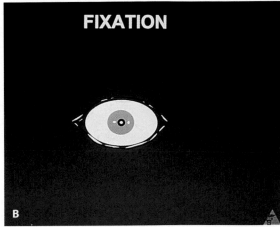
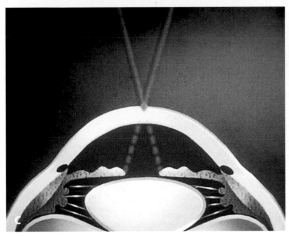
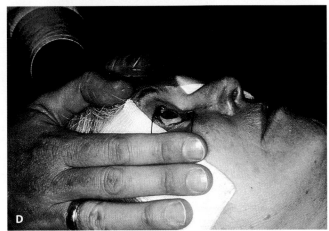

FIGURE 17-3.   *A. In the Summit Technology Apex system, the patient fixates on a green, coaxial aiming light that is surrounded by a red illuminated circle. B. The surgeon focuses a dual external helium-neon (He-Ne) laser beam on the corneal apex, directly over the visible reflection of the green fixation light. C. The divergent He-Ne beams strike the edge of the pupillary sphincter at 3- and 9-o'clock positions. D. The surgeon stabilizes the patient's head with his or her hands. Note the surgical gauze pad taped to the temporal region of the head to absorb moisture that would otherwise run into the patient's ear, causing distraction. The untreated eye is protected with a gauze eye pad of an occlusive shield.*

Another approach that is currently gaining popularity is to "pretreat" a central area of about 2.5 to 3.0 mm in diameter, either as a separate step before the principal ablation or as a modification of the laser algorithm.

The efficacy of these techniques has not been proved and remains anecdotal.

POSTOPERATIVE MEDICATION

Many variations on postoperative management exist, dependent on both surgical preference and specific experience with a particular laser system. The postoperative regimen continues to evolve with increased experience, and the reader must remain up-to-date on current medication regimens. This section offers my personal approach at the time of writing.

Immediate Postoperative Medications

At the conclusion of the ablation, three drops of diclofenac (Voltaren) are applied, followed by one drop of ofloxacin (Ocuflox) and fluorometholone 0.1% (FML, Fluor-Op, E-flone). A bandage contact lens is applied. My current preference is the extremely thin and generally well-tolerated ProTek bandage soft contact lens (Ciba) with a 8.9-mm base curve. The lens is applied with sterile technique, utilizing two cellulose surgical spears. The patient then utilizes the ofloxacin and fluorometholone four times daily until re-epithelialization occurs, typically 2 days after transepithelial ablation and 3 to 4 days after manual debridement. The patient is checked daily until re-epithelialization occurs. The diclofenac drops are used as needed for pain but no more than every 4 hours on the first day postoperatively (13,14).

Because nonsteroidal anti-inflammatory drugs (NSAIDs) delay re-epithelialization, persistent use of the diclofenac drops is discouraged unless the drop is clearly resulting in reduction in discomfort. In any case, the diclofenac drops are taken from the patient after 24 hours and discarded.

Additional measures may be needed for postoperative comfort. For pain control, I prefer the meperedine-promethazine combination 25 mg (50 mg/25 mg; Mepergan Fortis) as much as every 4 hours. This is a highly effective, narcotic, systemic pain-relieving agent, and also has sedative properties. A patient with discomfort ideally keeps the eye closed and sleeps. A cold compress applied to the closed eyelid also yields significant pain relief, as well as helps to reduce any lid inflammation or edema. An ice cube in a sealed plastic pouch wrapped with a thin towel applied gently to the eyelid is highly effective. Systemic NSAIDs may also provide some relief, but this is usually less effective than the above-mentioned measures.

Some patients will experience a distinct foreign body sensation under the eyelid, often perceived by the patient as the edge of the bandage soft contact lens. This is usually deceptive, although the contact lens should be inspected to make sure that it is centered and does not have any damage to the edge or foreign material trapped under it. In the absence of definite signs of contact lens–induced hypoxia or a poor-fitting or defective lens, removal of the contact lens is usually a mistake and results in even more pain. Manipulation of the contact lens until re-epithelialization occurs should be avoided. If a specific indication for lens removal or exchange occurs, use of a topical anesthetic is mandatory to control the intense pain that will result. A foreign body sensation under the upper eyelid is usually due to the corneal epithelial defect rather than the contact lens, despite the perception of a superior location of a foreign body. If the patient has discomfort with lid movement, then the eyelid should be closed over the contact lens, either with a pressure patch or by eyelid taping. The contact lens is retained.

Verma et al (15) suggested that topical anesthetics may be employed acutely after PRK with excellent pain relief but no significant toxicity. This observation must be confirmed in large trials.

If the patient is intolerant to the contact lens or the lens is lost, an alternative is pressure patching (16). The patient must be carefully instructed about the technique for appropriate pressure patching, as an incomplete patch will risk damage to the epithelium. If patching is used, the medication regimen can remain unchanged or a combination antibiotic-steroid ointment [such as tobramycin-dexamethasone (Tobradex)] can be employed four times daily.

After Re-epithelialization

When re-epithelialization occurs, the soft contact lens is gently removed by sliding it to the side, to avoid dislodging the freshly healed and fragile epithelium. The lens is discarded and the use of antibiotics discontinued.

Routine use of fluorometholone postoperatively is highly controversial. Gartry et al (17,18) provided evidence that routine use of topical steroids postoperatively does not yield better results, but many clinicians disagree or are uncertain. My current practice is to restrict the use of topical steroids to patients with corrections of 3.1 D or higher. In that case, the fluorometholone is used four times daily for 1 month, three times daily for the second month, and then twice daily for 2 weeks, once daily for 2 weeks, and then discontinued. Patients with corrections of 3.0 D or less do not routinely receive steroids.

In the first days after re-epithelialization, the freshly healed epithelium is supported with the use of highly viscous nonpreserved artificial tear drops such as carboxymethylcellulose 1% (Celluvisc). After several days, any surface discomfort will generally be resolved and the epithelium becomes smoother. Visual acuity rapidly improves. At that point, the highly viscous artificial tear agent can become more troublesome than helpful. I generally suggest that the patient change over to a moderate-viscosity nonpreserved artificial tear agent such as carboxymethylcellulose ½% (Refresh Plus). This is used as needed, and discontinued when the eye is comfortable.

Postoperative Manipulation of Visual Outcomes

Topical steroids can be manipulated in an effort to influence the postoperative refractive status or the development of haze or both. As of this date, no clinical study has definitively proved the efficacy of these approaches, yet many clinicians believe that some benefit may occur from these manipulations (19-21). For a patient with an unusual amount of haze that may be visually significant, and for patients with regression of the initial correction into the myopic range, an intense course of topical steroids may be helpful (22). In general, I believe in an aggressive steroid regimen if any intervention is to be undertaken at all. In most cases, prednisolone acetate 1% (Pred Forte) is prescribed for use every 2 hours for 2 weeks while awake and then four times daily for a second 2 weeks, with the patient re-evaluated at 1 month. If no favorable effect has occurred, the steroids are discontinued. If there is reduction in the amount of regression or haze, then a slow tapering of the topical steroids is performed over as much as 3 or 4 months.

Conversely, if a patient's vision is overcorrected and the patient shows little tendency for typical regression, then routine steroids are either tapered more rapidly or abruptly discontinued. This can trigger some increased healing and regression to reduce or eliminate hyperopia.

Corneal scraping procedures, to debride the epithelium under topical anesthesia, have been advocated for both residual hyperopia and myopia or scar formation. In the case of hyperopia, the goal is to stimulate wound healing and regression. The de-epithelialization is performed with a sterile surgical blade and no steroids are applied postoperatively. One small series failed to document a major regression, although an average of approximately 0.5 D of regression did occur after 1 year following debridement for hyperopia (23).

In the case of excessive regression, often accompanied by some degree of excess haze, debridement performed relatively early may succeed in "stripping" new collagen deposition from the base of the ablation zone and eliminating the opacity. In this case, very aggressive steroid treatment similar to the protocol described for steroid treatment of regression is employed. For this treatment to be successful, it must be employed relatively early in the course of the scar formation, or the scar will be impossible to manually debride. An alternative is to allow full and stable healing, usually at least 6 months after the initial PRK, and then perform a reablation, the amount of which is calculated for the residual myopia, and also remove superficial scar tissue (24–27).

COMPLICATIONS

Early Postoperative Complications

Delayed Re-epithelialization
Epithelium normally closes over the treated area within 3 to 4 days. After transepithelial ablation with an optical zone no larger than the ablation zone (typically 6.0 mm), re-epithelialization occurring within 48 hours is common. Typically, a cluster of superficial punctate keratitis or a linear ridge with a pseudodendrite appearance is common.

Delay of re-epithelialization is usually attributable to one or more of the following: exposure, toxicity from topical medication, external disease such as blepharitis or keratitis sicca, and collagen-vascular disease.

Treatment of delayed re-epithelialization begins with addressing the underlying disorder. In addition, the current unsuccessful regimen must be changed. Options for enhancing re-epithelialization include use of a pressure patch, taping of the lids, application of a bandage soft contact lens, and a temporary tarsorrhaphy. Any regimen, if unsuccessful, should be modified. Failure to progressively re-epithelialize under a bandage soft contact lens suggests a tight lens syndrome, and changing the treatment to patching or lid taping may be helpful. Conversely, a persistent epithelial defect with patching or lid taping usually responds to a bandage soft contact lens. Lid suturing to create a temporary tarsorrhaphy is usually the ultimate treatment, withheld as the treatment of last resort, but is usually ultimately successful when less aggressive treatment fails.

When a persistent epithelial defect resists treatment of any underlying disorders and all common treatment regimens, the surgeon must be suspicious of topical anesthetic abuse. Patients after PRK frequently experience some degree of discomfort, and often become aware that the physician has access to a "magic drop" of topical anesthetic. The patient may obtain a bottle of topical anesthetic without observation, and apply it repeatedly postoperatively, with devastating toxicity to the epithelium. In the presence of a persistent epithelial defect, particularly extending longer than 1 week and with the appearance of grayness or necrosis, hospitalization to eliminate the possibility of self-administered anesthetic should be considered.

Keratitis
The appearance of localized infiltrates in the early postoperative period is usually associated with application of a bandage soft contact lens and nonsteroidal agents in the absence of an antibiotic active against gram-positive organisms and the absence of a topical steroid (28–31). It is impossible to definitely assess the infectious or sterile nature of an infiltrate, and therefore any infiltrate should be cultured and treated presumptively for infection. Many surgeons believe that use of concomitant steroids with nonsteroidal agents and a bandage contact lens, especially with an antibiotic active against gram-positive organisms, markedly reduces, if not virtually completely eliminates, the appearance of sterile infiltrates. No large series has yet confirmed this clinical impression, however.

Infectious keratitis, when it occurs, often appears on day 2 or 3 postoperatively. This is a rare event, occurring at a rate of only 0.1% or less. Most cultures will reveal only gram-positive organisms such as *Staphylococcus* and *Streptococcus*, although a more aggressive gram-negative organism cannot be excluded on clinical examination. Risk factors for an infiltrate include blepharitis, tear film pathology, and the use of a bandage soft contact lens. Antibiotic prophylaxis may reduce the risk of infectious keratitis, but it cannot be completely eliminated.

Any deep stromal infiltrate must be cultured, and a localized "pinhead" superficial infiltrate not covered by epithelium also must be assumed to be infectious, requiring appropriate cultures and antibiotic therapy.

Elevated Intraocular Pressure
Elevated intraocular pressure is usually secondary to topical steroid application. Intraocular pressure must be measured at examinations beginning the first postoperative month, when the epithelium is secure, in order to diagnose elevations. In the presence of a healthy optic disk, elevated intraocular pressure to a level of less than 30 mm Hg is usually well tolerated for several weeks or even months. Pressures above 30 mm Hg or any preexisting damage to the optic nerve head may require initiation of pressure-reducing medication.

The first step of therapy is to immediately discontinue steroid therapy, or change to a steroid less likely to induce pressure elevation [rimexolone (Vexol) or fluorometholone]. If steroids must be continued, or the pressure does not return to adequate levels with an alteration in steroids, then initiation of pressure-reducing medication is appropriate. In the absence of asthma or contraindicating cardiovascular disease, β-blockers are typically the first agent of choice. Topical apraclonidine (Iopidine) is often well tolerated and highly successful, and dorzolamide hydrochloride 2% (Trusopt) may be useful, although surface toxicity may occur and must be carefully monitored.

Late Postoperative Complications

Central Islands and Peninsulas

Central islands, or circumscribed areas of central steepening in the presence of overall flattening after PRK, are evident on topography 1 month postoperatively (11,12). A peninsula is an extension of the peripheral corneal curvature, steeper than the ablated zone, toward the center. A peninsula may be peripheral or extend into the center. The origin is usually located inferiorly. The natural history is that most islands resolve by 6 postoperative months.

Prevention of central islands requires careful following of manufacturer's recommendations. These include "anti-island" ablation treatments and, at least in some patients, interrupting PRK several times to dry the central stroma with a cellulose surgical sponge.

Figure 17-4 demonstrates the typical appearance of a central island and its spontaneous resolution. Although histopathologic documentation of the healing of central islands remains unavailable, a common hypothesis is that the central island represents unablated stromal tissue. The "healing" consists of a thickening of the epithelium in the midperiphery surrounding the island, which gradually envelops and covers the island. To expand on the "island" metaphor, the "sea of epithelium" rises and covers the island; the stromal island does not "sink" into the ocean.

In general, before one considers retreatment, it is prudent to wait at least 6 months to observe the healing pattern in patients with symptomatic central islands or peninsulas. Some topographically evident central islands do not cause visual symptoms, and these islands should be ignored. Patients with symptomatic central islands and peninsulas will experience some combination of the following: mild loss of best-corrected visual acuity, multiplopia, "ghost images," halos and glare, and increased astigmatism. When these symptoms are present and unchanging after 6 months, and the topography and refractive status is stable, then treatment should be considered.

Two treatment options have been advocated. In the first, the central epithelium is removed with a blade, exposing the central stromal island. The peak of the island is then treated either with a PRK algorithm whose optical zone is set to the diameter of the island and whose dioptric correction matches the height of the island, or with a phototherapeutic keratectomy (PTK) algorithm, again with the diameter set to the width of the island and with the number of pulses calculated to create the dioptric flattening needed. In either case, the dioptric correction is based on the height of the island as detected by early topography, usually the 1-month topographic analysis. By 3 to 6 months, the island may

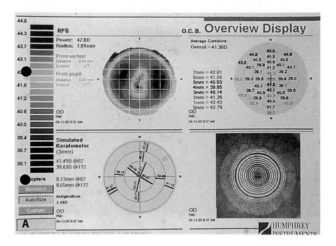

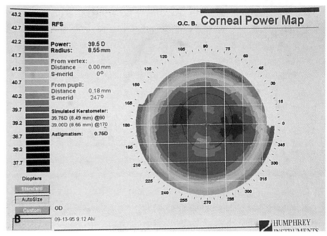

FIGURE 17-4. A. A large central island is evident 1 month postoperatively. Vision was 20/25 with "ghost images". B. At 3 months, the island has nearly resolved. Vision was 20/15 without any multiplopia.

appear to be less elevated owing to partial hyperplasia of the surrounding epithelium, and therefore retreatment will be incomplete.

An alternative treatment technique is to retain the epithelium and use phototherapeutic keratectomy disk ablation equal to the largest diameter of the island. The first area of stroma to be exposed should be at the peak of the island. This can be visualized as the "breakthrough" of the cobalt blue–colored fluorescence that occurs with ablation of the epithelium, a fluorescence readily visualized when the room lights and operating microscope lights are shut off. The ablation through the epithelium will progressively expose the island, while the thicker peripheral epithelium will shield the surrounding stroma. When the central dark nonfluorescent stromal island reaches the size of the topographic island at 1 month, the island ablation is complete.

In either of these techniques, after removal of the island, aggressive topical steroids should be utilized to discourage any central scarring, until stable healing and refractive status are achieved.

Overcorrection

Overcorrection is associated with use of a small optical zone (<6.0 mm); excessive stromal drying, often due to prolonged de-epithelialization and surface preparation; an excessive "island prevention" program; transepithelial ablation of 100% of the epithelium without adjustment of the algorithm; a gaussian beam that is more intense centrally than the periphery; or an incorrect refraction, typically a noncycloplegic refraction with excessive minus power due to unrecognized accommodation. Older patients with reduced corneal wound healing may be prone to overcorrection and benefit from a small (e.g., 5%) reduction in the intended correction (24,32,33).

There is no generally accepted successful treatment for residual hyperopia. Hopefully, a hyperopic PRK or some other hyperopic refractive procedure will be helpful for these patients.

Anecdotal endorsement of two strategies has arisen, although these have not been demonstrated to succeed in a larger series. The first approach is to debride the central epithelium, in an effort to stimulate irritation of the underlying stroma and subsequent healing of the stroma and epithelium with reduction in central flattening. No topical steroids are used postoperatively. One small clinical trial failed to show any large reproducible benefit from this procedure, however (23). Alternatively, a soft contact lens is used chronically and persistently postoperatively, resulting in a reduction of central flattening either due to the irritation stimulated by the contact lens or due to some degree of hyperplasia of the epithelium caused by the protection of the overlying contact lens which vaults the ablation zone.

Undercorrection/Regression

Initial undercorrection may be due to an overly moist or wet cornea, reducing the transmission of energy to the intended stromal ablation zone; an excessively "flat" beam contour; or refraction error. In some but not all patients, regression is accompanied by haze. Haze is attributed to deposition of disorganized new collagen in the ablation zone.

Retreatment of undercorrected myopia is less predictable than the initial PRK (24–27). Generally, reduction of the intended correction by at least 0.5 D is prudent pending further experience. Intense topical steroids are used postoperatively to reduce the likelihood of an aggressive healing response after the retreatment. For the very small number of patients in whom an optically significant scar aggressively re-forms after two sets of treatments, further retreatments are unadvisable.

Retreatment is usually considered after a minimum of 6 months' healing, with documentation of stable refraction and topography. If the optical zone is smaller than 6.0 mm, reablation to a full 6.0-mm optical zone is performed (27). Scar tissue should be removed with repeat ablation if it does not easily become dislodged with scraping. Because of the potential for overcorrection, undercorrection at the repeat ablation is appropriate. A common starting value is to correct 75% of the residual myopia.

Decentration

Symptomatic decentration is best avoided through use of a large optical zone, such as 6.0 mm. A patient's head must be stabilized, typically by the surgeon's hands, and the patient and surgeon must monitor the fixation-beam pattern provided by the manufacturer.

Decentration generally will become symptomatic when the amount of decentration exceeds 1 mm. Symptoms include halos, glare, monocular diplopia, loss of image contrast and overall loss of contrast sensitivity, and occasionally loss of best-corrected visual acuity with extreme decentrations.

Definitive treatment of symptomatic decentration requires further excimer laser ablation (34). In one approach, the epithelium is retained over the topographically flattened zone to act as a mask. The epithelium is debrided mechanically outside of the ablation zone, in an area that appears to be steep on topography. A ridge at the border of the treatment zone is usually exposed. The ridge is ablated as needed with a small–optical-zone PTK. A PRK is then performed in the undercorrected area with the optical power guided by the topography. The already flattened treatment zone is protected by the preexisting epithelium and, if necessary, the application of high-viscosity artificial tear fluids. Figure 17-5 depicts improvement in the centration of the ablated area after following the above-described protocol. The patient's symptoms of halos, glare, and multiplopia are rated as "90% improved" by the patient after the retreatment.

Alternatively, a decentration may be addressed by a second ablation that is decentered 180 degrees away from the first ablation site (35).

Steroid-Induced Cataract

The surgeon must be mindful of the potential for inducing cataract through prolonged topical steroid administration. The use of strong penetrating steroids should be restricted to treatment of regression or haze that requires such agents, and the total dosage should be monitored, with a change over to nonpenetrating weaker steroids as soon as possible. Steroid-induced cataracts are best avoided, of course, if no topical steroids are needed on a routine basis postoperatively.

The Unexpectedly Disappointed Patient

Patients unhappy with the quality of their postoperative vision without any evident cause should first be examined for evidence of visually significant residual irregular astigmatism. The best test for irregular astigmatism is a refraction with a diagnostic hard contact lens.

In the absence of symptomatic residual irregular astigmatism, the unexpected disappointment is most often the result of unreasonable preoperative expectations. In particular, it is important for any patient to understand that PRK

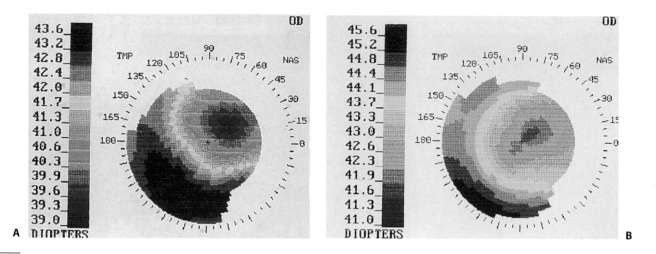

FIGURE 17-5.   A. *Severe decentration is evident on topographic analysis. The patient's vision was 20/25 and he complained of severe glare and multiplopia. B. After retreatment, topographic analysis shows extension of the flattened ablation zone into more of the visual axis. Although incompletely treated, the patient reported approximately 90% resolution of his visual disturbances.*

Table 17-1.   Published Outcomes After Photorefractive Keratectomy for Low to Moderate Myopia with a 6.0-mm Optical Zone

	Pop and Aras (6)	Schallhorn et al (7)	McCarty et al (36)	Shah and Hersh (37)
Follow-up (mo)	6	12	12	6
Range of myopia (D)	−1.0 to −6.0	−2.0 to −5.5	−8.8 to −5.25	−1.5 to −6.0
No. of patients	145	30	274	45
Laser system	VISX	Summit	VISX	Summit
Uncorrected visual acuity (%)				
≥20/20	NR	100	47	62
≥20/25	89.4	100	NR	NR
≥20/40	97.9	100	87	100
Predictability (%)				
±0.5 D	84.8	70	NR	62.2
±1.0 D	95.5	93	87	84.4

NR = not reported.

for myopia will not result in improvement of visual acuity in the presence of long-standing amblyopia, nor will visual acuity improve in the presence of myopic macular degeneration. Psychological or social expectations may be unspoken and yet may be major motivations in a patient seeking refractive surgery. Elimination of the use of spectacles will not resolve unrealistic patient expectations.

OUTCOMES

The typical outcomes after myopic PRK continue to improve. Results in published series lag behind current results, as techniques and technology continue to evolve rapidly. Table 17-1 summarizes the findings of several series published in 1995 and 1996 with a 6.0-mm optical zone, but note the procedures were performed in 1993 and 1994.

REFERENCES

1. Campos M, Trokel SL, McDonnell PJ. Surface morphology following photorefractive keratectomy. *Ophthalmic Surg* 1993;24:822–825.
2. Pallikaris IG, Karoutis AD, Lydataki SE, Siganos DS. Rotating brush for fast removal of corneal epithelium. *J Refract Corneal Surg* 1994;10:439–442.
3. Campos M, Raman S, Lee M, McDonnell PJ. Keratocyte loss after different methods of deepithelialization. *Ophthalmology* 1994;101:890–894.
4. Alio JL, Ismael MM, Artola A. Laser epithelium removal before photorefractive keratectomy. *Refract Corneal Surg* 1993;9:395.
5. Gimbel HV, DeBroff BM, Beldavs RA, et al. Comparison of laser and manual removal of corneal epithelium for photorefractive keratectomy. *J Refract Surg* 1995;11:36–41.
6. Pop M, Aras M. Multizone/multipass photorefractive keratectomy: 6 month results. *J Cataract Refract Surg* 1995;21:633–643.
7. Schallhorn SC, Blanton CL, Kaupp SE, et al. Preliminary results of photorefractive keratectomy in active-duty United States Navy personnel. *Ophthalmology* 1996;103:5–22.
8. Schwartz-Goldstein BH, Hersh PS. Corneal topography of phase III excimer laser photorefractive keratectomy: optical zone centration analysis. *Ophthalmology* 1995;102:951–962.

9. Seiler T, Holschbach A, Derse M, et al. Complications of myopic photore-fractive keratectomy with the excimer laser. *Ophthalmology* 1994;101:153–160.

10. Terrel J, Bechara SJ, Nesburn A, et al. The effect of globe fixation on ablation zone centration in photorefractive keratectomy. *Am J Ophthalmol* 1995;119:612–619.

11. Lin DT. Corneal topographic analysis after excimer photorefractive keratectomy. *Ophthalmology* 1994;101:1432–1439.

12. Colin J, Cochener B, Gallinaro C. Central steep islands immediately following excimer photorefractive keratectomy for myopia. *Refract Corneal Surg* 1993;9:395–396. Letter.

13. Stein R, Stein HA, Cheskes A, Symons S. Photorefractive keratectomy and postoperative pain. *Am J Ophthalmol* 1994;117:403–405.

14. Sher NA, Frantz JM, Talley A, et al. Topical diclofenac in the treatment of ocular pain after excimer laser photorefactive keratectomy. *Refract Corneal Surg* 1993;9:425–436.

15. Verma S, Corbett MC, Marshall J, Hamilton AMP. Pain control after PRK: do topical anesthetics have a role? *Ophthalmology* 1995;102(suppl):102. Abstract.

16. Demers PE, Thompson P, Bernier RG, et al. Effect of occlusive pressure patching on the rate of epithelial wound healing after photorefractive keratectomy. *J Cataract Refract Surg* 1996;22:59–62.

17. Gartry DS, Kerr Muir M, Marshall J. The effect of topical corticosteroids on refraction and corneal haze following excimer laser treatment of myopia: an update. A prospective, randomised, double-masked study. *Eye* 1993;7:584–590.

18. O'Brart DP, Lohmann CP, Klonos G, et al. The effects of topical corticosteroids and plasmin inhibitors on refractive outcome, haze, and visual performance after photorefractive keratectomy: a prospective, randomized observer-masked study. *Ophthalmology* 1994;101:1565–1574.

19. Carones F, Brancato R, Venturi E, et al. Efficacy of corticosteroids in reversing regression after myopic photorefractive keratectomy. *Refract Corneal Surg* 1993;9(suppl):52–56.

20. Fitzsimmons TD, Fagerholm P, Tengroth B. Steroid treatment of myopic regression: acute refractive and topographic changes in photorefractive patients. *Cornea* 1993;12:358–361.

21. Tengroth B, Epstein D, Fagerholm P, et al. Excimer laser photorefractive keratectomy for myopia: clinical results in sighted eyes. *Ophthalmology* 1993;100:739–745.

22. Durrie DS, Lesher MP, Cavanaugh TB. Classification of variable clinical response after photorefractive keratectomy for myopia. *J Refract Surg* 1995;11:341–347.

23. Gauthier CA, Fagerholm P, Epstein D, et al. Failure of mechanical epithelial removal to reverse persistent hyperopia after photorefractive keratectomy. *J Refract Surg* 1996;12:601–606.

24. Epstein D, Tengroth B, Fagerholm P, Hamberg-Nystrom H. Excimer retreatment of regression after photorefractive keratectomy. *Am J Ophthalmol* 1994;117:456–461.

25. Seiler T, Derse M, Pham T. Repeated excimer laser treatment after photorefractive keratectomy. *Arch Ophthalmol* 1992;110:1230.

26. Matta CS, Piebanga LW, Deitz MR, Tauber J. Excimer retreatment for myopic photorefractive keratectomy failures: six-to-18-month follow-up. *Ophthalmology* 1996;103:444–451.

27. Kalski RS, Sutton G, Lawless MA, Rogers C. Multiple excimer laser retreatments for scarring and myopic regression following photorefractive keratectomy. *J Cataract Refract Surg* 1996;22:752–754.

28. Sher NA, Krueger RR, Teal P, et al. Role of topical corticosteroids and nonsteroidal antiinflammatory drugs in the etiology of stromal infiltrates after excimer laser photorefractive keratectomy. *J Refract Corneal Surg* 1994;10:587–588.

29. Sampath R, Ridgway AE, Leatherbarrow B. Bacterial keratitis following excimer laser photorefractive keratectomy: a case report. *Eye* 1994;8(Pt 4):481–482.

30. Lavery FL. Photorefractive keratectomy in 472 eyes. *Refract Corneal Surg* 1993;9:98–100.

31. Faschinger C, Faulborn J, Gauser K. Infektiose horn-hautgescnure-einmal mit endophthalmitis nach PRK mit einmal-kontaktlinse. *Klin Monatsbl Augenheilkd* 1995;206:96–102.

32. Seiler T, Wollensak J. Myopic photorefractive keratectomy with the excimer laser, one year follow-up. *Ophthalmology* 1991;98:1156–1163.

33. Dutt S, Steinert RF, Raizman MB, et al. One-year results of excimer laser photorefractive keratectomy for low to moderate myopia. *Arch Ophthalmol* 1994;112:1427–1436.

34. Lim-Bon-Siong R, Williams JM, Steinert RF, Pepose JS. Retreatment of decentered excimer photorefractive keratectomy ablations. *Am J Ophthalmol* 1997;123:122–124.

35. Seiler T, Schmidt-Petersen H, Wollensak J. Complications after myopic photorefractive keratectomy primarily with the Summit excimer laser. In: Salz JJ, ed. *Corneal laser surgery*. St Louis: Mosby-Year Book, 1995: 131–142.

36. McCarty CA, Aldred GF, Taylor HR, the Melbourne Excimer Laser Group. Comparison of results of excimer laser correction of all degrees of myopia at 12 months postoperatively. *Am J Ophthalmol* 1996;121:372–383.

37. Shah SI, Hersh PS. Photorefractive keratectomy for myopia with a 6mm beam diameter. *J Refract Surg* 1996;12:341–346.

Refractive Surgery: Basic Techniques for Astigmatism

STEVE JOHNSON

Astigmatism is an anomaly of refraction that was first addressed by Sir Isaac Newton in 1727 (1). Since that time, the correction of astigmatism has provided a great challenge. Often in conjunction with myopia or hyperopia, naturally occurring astigmatism is usually of low-enough magnitude that optical devices including spectacles and gas-permeable contact lenses provide adequate refractive correction. However, astigmatism that occurs after surgery such as large-incision extracapsular cataract surgery or keratoplasty can prove to be too great for such optical devices. Developments in managing wound construction and wound closure have attempted to reduce postoperative astigmatic error, yet residual astigmatism is not uncommon. Surgical correction of astigmatism may be required to reduce the ametropia.

Since the reintroduction of incisional techniques by Fyodorov et al (2), surgical correction for astigmatism has not been limited only to postoperative complications. Multiple incisional techniques have been explored to correct naturally occurring regular astigmatism.

In 1983 Trokel et al (3) proposed the use of the 193-nm argon-fluoride (ArF) excimer laser as a new tool for refractive surgeons. Using excimer laser to create large-area ablations, Marshall et al (4) demonstrated the ability to change the refractive state of the cornea. This ablative process, called *photorefractive keratectomy* (PRK), is used to reshape the cornea. Use of PRK to flatten the central part of the cornea in an attempt to reduce myopia has proved to be effective (5–7). To date two excimer laser companies, Summit (Waltham, MA) and VISX (Sunnyvale, CA), have received approval from the Food and Drug Administration (FDA) for use in correcting low and moderate myopia.

Treatment of astigmatism using excimer laser technology exists as only a partially chartered frontier. Differing ablation concepts and methods have been and are continually being explored. Broad-beam lasers have been used in con-

junction with diaphragms, masks, and apertures to reduce astigmatism (8–10). Along with continued refinement in broad-beam laser use, new technology incorporating scanning-beam lasers is being developed. Only early postoperative data on astigmatism reduction are available for some laser techniques. With limited long-term published results available, comparing differing laser techniques for astigmatic correction is difficult.

This chapter reviews the introductory principles of optics, keratometry, and incisional surgery to aid in the understanding of excimer laser use for the correction of astigmatism. An overview of the presently used laser procedures and published follow-up results may help the clinician analyze the efficacy and safety of this new refractive tool.

OPTICS AND ASTIGMATISM

For clinicians and refractive surgeons to understand how changes in the anterior surface of the cornea can affect the myopic, hyperopic, and astigmatic state of the eye, knowledge of optics and refraction is important. Myopia and hyperopia require corrective lenses with concave and convex surfaces, respectively. The refracting power of concave and convex surfaces focuses light to a point (Fig. 18-1). Concave and convex surfaces are considered spherical surfaces if they have the same curvature and thus the same refracting power in all meridians. Realistically, the cornea has a slightly aspheric anterior surface that is steeper centrally than peripherally. However, to understand the refractive powers of the cornea, it is easier to consider the anterior surface of the cornea as a spherical convex surface.

Elementary optics explain that in the plano refractive state the cornea has a spherical convex surface focusing light to a point on the retina. A myopic refractive error has a focus point anterior to the retina. Attempts to bring the

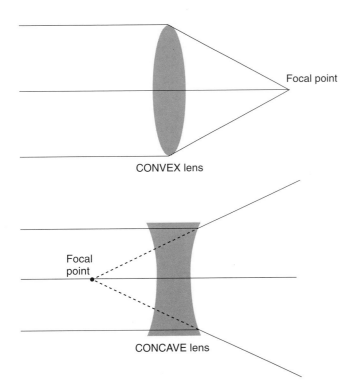

FIGURE 18-1.   *Concave and convex lenses.*

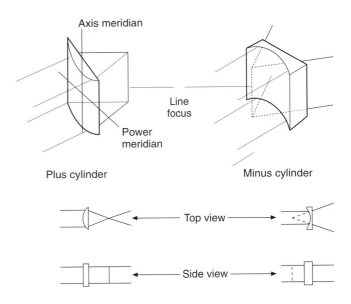

FIGURE 18-2.   *Plano cylindrical lens.*

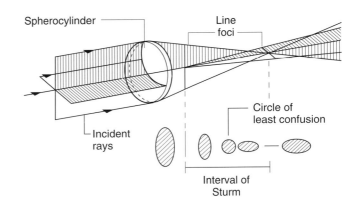

FIGURE 18-3.   *Conoid of Sturm.*

focus point of a myopic eye onto the retina will require, in theory, either moving the retina anteriorly or decreasing the convex vergence power of the anterior corneal surface so that the focus point moves posteriorly.

When astigmatism is considered, the optics are slightly more difficult. Contrary to a spherical surface that has the same curvature in all meridians, an astigmatic lens has a curvature that is greatest in one meridian and least in a meridian 90 degrees away. Because an astigmatic surface is not equal in all meridians, it cannot focus light to a point, but rather focuses it to a line. The name *astigmatic* means "not point-like."

An example of an astigmatic lens is a cylindrical lens. A cylindrical lens has a focal line rather than a focal point. A specific type of regular cylindrical lens called a *plano cylindrical lens* has two primary meridians (Fig. 18-2). One primary meridian is parallel to the flat plano surface and is called the *axis meridian*. Light rays parallel to this axis are not refracted. The second primary meridian, called the *power meridian*, is perpendicular to the axis meridian. Light rays parallel to the power meridian are refracted to a focal line parallel to the axis meridian.

When astigmatism is present as part of the refractive error of the eye, the astigmatic error primarily occurs in the anterior corneal surface. This astigmatic corneal surface is not just a plano cylindrical surface, but rather a spherocylindrical surface, otherwise, called a *toric surface.*

Two plano cylinders with axis meridians oriented 90 degrees apart could be considered spherocylindrical; however, a spherocylindrical lens can simply be thought of as a combination of a spherical lens and a cylindrical lens. A spherocylindrical lens focuses light not to a point, but instead to two focal lines. Between these two focal lines, there is a circle of least confusion where light is focused with least distortion (Fig. 18-3). A refractionist attempting to refract a spherocylindrical lens refers to this circle of least confusion as the *spherical equivalent.*

Refractive surgeons always use the spherical equivalent when computing what refractive error must be corrected to get to the best overall focus of the spherocylindrical lens in question. Through calculation of the spherical equivalent, the average spherical power of all meridians is appreciated.

If one primary axis of the spherocylindrical corneal surface is greater than the second primary axis, then residual cylindrical power can be considered. Correcting for spherical equivalent with an appropriate convex or concave lens, using either spectacles or contact lenses, is usually not difficult. If residual cylindrical power is present, that too can often be corrected with toric lenses.

There are several clinical methods to assess and quantify residual cylindrical power and axis of a toric corneal surface. Basic keratometric techniques are able to provide accurate measurements of the central 3 to 4 mm of the cornea, specifically the dioptric power and axis orientation of the two primary axes (Fig. 18-4). When regular astigmatism is present with primary lens axes approximately 90 degrees apart, this common measuring technique is often clinically sufficient.

However, as the breadth of knowledge and experience increased with respect to attempts at surgically reducing spherical refractive errors, so did the need to develop other techniques to assess both central and midperipheral keratometric values. Hence, keratoscopy and photokeratoscopy gained significant favor among clinicians, specifically anterior-segment surgeons attempting to quantify residual astigmatism following cataract surgery, penetrating keratoplasty, and early refractive surgical procedures. Similar to basic keratometric techniques, keratoscopy uses reflected corneal images (Fig. 18-5). Keratoscopy can use a single ring or multiple rings to assess astigmatic error. Circular rings when reflected on a spherical surface will reflect circular images, whereas the same circular rings reflected off toric surfaces will reflect elliptical or oval images. When multiple-ring keratoscopes are used, both the individual ring configuration and the spatial relationship of each ring with other reflected rings are important clues for understanding corneal curvature. Meridians where reflected rings are spaced very close together have greater steepness and thus greater power than

do meridians where reflected rings are spaced farther apart. With regular toric surfaces, individual rings are oval, indicating one primary axis has a greater steepness and curvature than does the axis 90 degrees away. Common examples often used to describe a toric surface are the back surface of a spoon, ladle, or a cross section of a ring doughnut.

Clinically, refractive surgeons usually want to identify the steeper axis and attempt to decrease or flatten its curvature. For this reason, a useful example of a toric surface is a football lying on its side. There are two distinct curvatures, one stretching from tip to tip of the ball and the other going around the middle of the ball where the laces are holding the cover together (Fig. 18-6A). The curvature from tip to tip is flat compared to the curvature 90 degrees away across the laces. To flatten the steeper curvature one could consider loosening the laces (Fig. 18-6B).

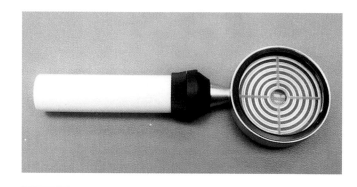

FIGURE 18-5. *Hand-held keratoscope.*

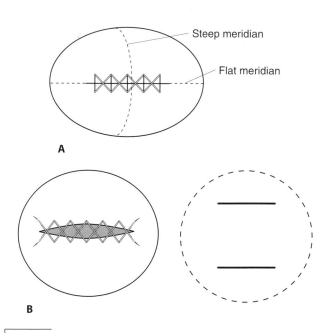

FIGURE 18-6. *Toric surface. A. Football lying on its side, demonstrating curvature stretching from tip to tip. B. Curvature around the middle of the ball, where the laces are holding the cover together.*

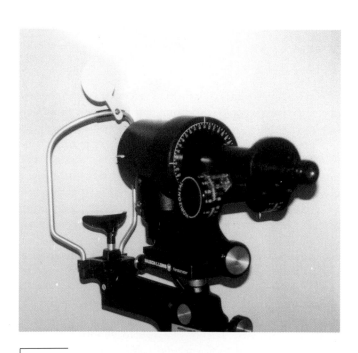

FIGURE 18-4. *Bausch-Lomb keratometer.*

This philosophy is used when correcting astigmatic surfaces with incisional surgery. Detecting football-shaped keratoscopic rings and loosening the "laces" of the steep axis with relaxing incisions across the steep meridian helps surgeons flatten and round out keratoscopically reflected rings.

New technology that combines computer-assisted video imaging and data analysis to measure the curvature of the anterior corneal surface has been developed and referred to as *computerized video keratography* (CVK) (11) (Fig. 18-7). Using placido-based topography systems and interpolating information between specific data points, clinicians have developed a three-dimensional understanding of the quality and quantity of a corneal surface. With this technique, topographic changes after refractive procedures can be evaluated. CVK has become an indispensable tool for measuring not only corneal surfaces with regular astigmatic errors, but also other corneal surface irregularities. With CVK, regular astigmatism often presents itself as a figure-eight configuration lined up along the steepest axis (Fig. 18-8). CVK uses not

only configurations but also color-coded maps to help the clinician interpret the data.

Many refractive surgeons use CVK in preoperative refractive surgery evaluations to help detect naturally occurring astigmatism (Fig. 18-8) and the axis of greater curvature as well as to detect areas of irregular curvature, such as an increased inferior steepness seen in a patient with early keratoconus. CVK is also helpful to evaluate astigmatic error induced by corneal transplantation or various refractive surgical procedures. After procedures used to correct myopia, a central uniform flattening is appreciated on CVK. After correction of astigmatism, meridianal flattening is seen. Postoperatively, corneas that have undergone surface ablation with an excimer laser must re-epithelialize. During this period of re-epithelialization, as well as the rest of the healing phase, corneal surface irregularities can be present. Surface irregularities can lead to irregular astigmatism and potentially a reduction in best-corrected vision. CVK is extremely helpful in not only identifying surface irregularities, but also quantitating with a numerical value the amount of irregularity. With these surface irregularity values, serial CVKs can be used to assess the healing process (Fig. 18-9).

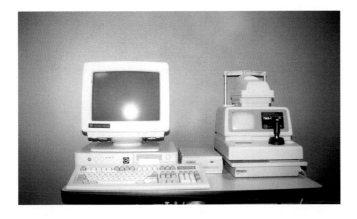

FIGURE 18-7.   *Tomey computerized video keratoscope.*

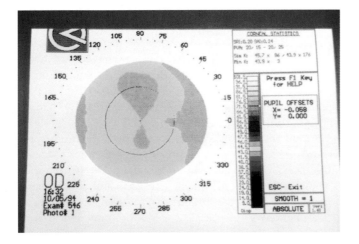

FIGURE 18-8.   *Example of regular astigmatism with the characteristic figure-eight pattern seen on computerized video keratography.*

SURGICAL REDUCTION OF ASTIGMATISM AND INCISIONAL KERATOTOMY

As mentioned earlier, most ametropic errors can be corrected with spectacles or contact lenses. Because of intolerance or personal preference, a fraction of the population has chosen to reduce their dependency on an optical device through surgical correction. Attempts to surgically correct low to moderate myopia with present refractive surgical procedures such as radial keratotomy and PRK have been relatively successful (12).

However, surgical procedures to decrease astigmatic error for the most part have been those that like radial keratotomy involve relaxation of corneal fibers through deep corneal incisions.

As noted by Jose Barraquer (13), a pioneer in refractive surgery for over 40 years, present refractive surgical techniques can be classified into three types of procedures.

1. Procedures that involve relaxation of the corneal fibers such as incisions of the Sato type improved by Fyodorov. Included in this group are radial keratotomy, which is used for the reduction of low or moderate myopia, and operations to reduce astigmatism, such as T and L incisions, Ruiz trapezoidal incisions, arcuate incisions, and Troutman relaxing incisions.
2. Procedures that involve a modification of corneal thickness by subtraction of tissue, with examples including automated lamellar keratectomy (ALK) and photoablative keratectomy [photorefractive keratectomy (PRK), photoastigmatic refractive

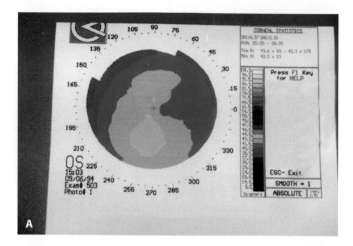

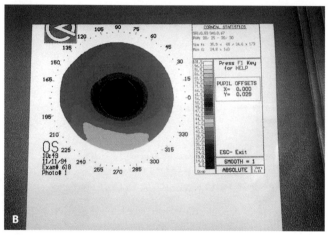

FIGURE 18-9.   *Toric ablation with the excimer laser. Preoperative (A) and postoperative (B) computerized video keratography.*

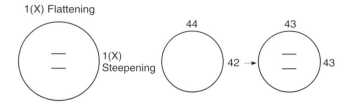

FIGURE 18-10.   *A schematic depiction of the effect on spherical equivalent of transverse incisions. Transverse incisions flatten the steeper meridian an equivalent amount as they steepen the flatter meridian, resulting in no change in spherical equivalent ($+1.00 - 2.00 \times 180 \rightarrow plano$).*

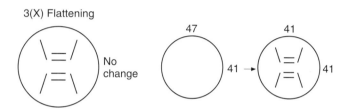

FIGURE 18-11.   *If a perfect result is achieved when performing trapezoidal astigmatic keratotomy, one should be left with only the spherical component of the refraction when expressed in a minus cylinder form. Plano $-6.00 \times 180 \rightarrow plano$.*

keratectomy (PARK), and laser-assisted in situ keratomileusis (LASIK)].

3. Procedures that involve a modification of corneal thickness by addition of tissue. Epikeratophakia and placement of intracorneal lenticules are included in this group.

In reviewing Barraquer's classifications, one can appreciate the conceptual difference between new photorefractive methods such as PRK and PARK, and the more time-tested incisional keratotomy methods used in radial keratotomy and astigmatic keratotomy.

To date, incisional keratotomy has been the primary surgical procedure performed to reduce astigmatism. Since 1885 when Schiøtz reported using full-thickness incisional therapy to treat astigmatism, full- and partial-thickness corneal incisions have been used to relax corneal fibers (14). Following the pioneering work of Sato (15–17) in the 1940s and early 1950s, Fyodorov and Durner (2) in 1981 reintroduced corneal incisional surgery as a surgical modality to reduce myopia and astigmatism. Since that time multiple techniques and surgical patterns have been explored. The most common patterns include transverse T, trapezoidal, and arcuate keratotomies. The primary plan for each of these types of keratotomies is to relax the corneal fibers across the steep corneal meridian.

Relaxation of these fibers would flatten the steep meridian. Coupled with flattening of the steep meridian, the curvature of the original flat meridian may be affected.

Lindstrom et al (18) reported that with transverse T paired incisions there is a net effect so that for X amount of flattening in the steep meridian, there is X amount of steepening in the flatter meridian 90 degrees away (Fig. 18-10). Because of this one-to-one coupling effect, transverse incisions do not change the spherical equivalent. In comparison, trapezoidal incisions differ in that they produce $3X$ amount of flattening in the steep meridian and no change in the flat meridian (Fig. 18-11).

Within the last few years the majority of incisional procedures used to reduce astigmatism involved either a straight transverse T or arcuate keratotomy. Lindstrom (19) reported a comparison study of straight transverse and arcuate keratotomies. Based on the Lindstrom nomogram, straight transverse incisions were placed at a 5- or 7-mm optical zone and were all 3 mm in length, while arcuate incisions varied from 45 to 90 degrees and were always placed at a 7-mm optical zone. In the straight transverse keratotomy group, 24 eyes with a mean preoperative refractive cylinder of 4.35 ± 2.35 diopters (D) had a reduction to 2.88 ± 2.71 D at 6-

to 18-month follow-up. Two eyes in this group had an increase in astigmatism between 1.25 and 2.00 D. The arcuate transverse keratotomy group, 22 eyes, had a mean preoperative refractive cylinder of 4.75 ± 2.78 D and mean postoperative refractive cylinder of 2.33 ± 2.27 D at 6- to 18-month follow-up.

Recently Price and the Arc-T Study Group (20), in an attempt to evaluate the predictability of astigmatism reduction using specifically the Lindstrom nomogram, reported results for 160 eyes with a mean preoperative refractive cylinder of 2.8 ± 1.2 D (Table 18-1). At 1-month follow-up the postoperative refractive cylinder for 144 eyes was 1.2 ± 0.8 D.

Concentrating on the fact that astigmatic corrections involved both dioptric change as well as axis variance, the authors performed vector analysis using the Holladay, Cravy, Koch (HCK) vector analysis method (21). The HCK change in cylinder for these 144 eyes was 2.3 ± 1.4 D. The authors used multiple regression analysis to conclude that certain factors have important predictive values for astigmatic keratotomy. Their analysis showed greater astigmatic change with an increased number of incisions, increased incision length, and increased age of the patient and in male patients.

Utilizing either straight or arcuate keratotomies can provide satisfactory astigmatic surgical correction; however, results can be variable, with significant undercorrections, overcorrections, and long-term refractive instability (19). Undercorrection can occasionally be managed with

Table 18-1. Descriptive Statistics for 1-Month Postoperative Results

	n	Mean ± SD	Min	Max
Preoperative refractive cyl (D)	160	2.8 ± 1.2	1.0	6.5
Postoperative refractive cyl (D)	144	1.2 ± 0.8	0.0	5.0
Absolute change in cyl (D)	144	1.6 ± 1.1	−0.5	4.8
HCK change in cyl	144	2.3 ± 1.4	0.1	6.7

Cylinder	Preoperative, No. (%)	Postoperative, No. (%)
<0.5	0	11 (8)
0.5–0.99	0	45 (31)
1.0–1.49	14 (9)	48 (33)
1.5–1.99	23 (14)	16 (11)
2.0–2.99	63 (39)	17 (12)
3.0–3.99	33 (21)	4 (3)
4.0–4.99	13 (8)	2 (1)
5.0–6.5	14 (9)	1 (1)

Min = minimum; Max = maximum; cyl = cylinder; D = diopter; HCK = Holladay, Cravy, and Koch (21).
Source: Price FW, Grene RB, Marks RG, Gonzales JS, the Arc-T Study Group. Astigmatism Reduction Clinical Trial: a multicenter perspective evaluation of the predictability of arcuate keratotomy. *Arch Ophthalmol* 1995;113:279.

enhancements while overcorrection may require compression sutures placed across astigmatic keratotomies. With regards to surgical correction of astigmatism, variable results with incisional surgery allowed for other avenues to be explored and developed.

Through use of ultraviolet-range, 193-nm excimer light, precise excisions or ablations can be performed on the cornea. Corneal tissue is removed when pulsed exposure of excimer light breaks molecular bonds. Understanding that a specific amount of corneal tissue would be removed with each individual pulsed exposure of excimer light, one can calculate the excisions or ablations to a specific depth of the cornea.

Through original work by Trokel et al (3) in 1983, smooth surface corneal ablations were achieved with significant accuracy and minimal damage to the surrounding tissue.

With this knowledge, investigators developed procedures whereby uniform, concentric surface ablations with ablated depths greater centrally than peripherally reduced myopia.

Surface ablation to correct myopia is called *photorefractive keratectomy* (PRK). Significant studies and data concerning PRK and its efficacy are covered more extensively in the preceding chapter.

EVOLUTION OF PHOTOASTIGMATIC REFRACTIVE KERATECTOMY

With early appreciation for the excimer laser's precision, direction was taken to use the excimer laser as a fancy light blade to make excisions much as a diamond or steel blade would make incisions. Hypothetically, linear excisions would function much the same as the corneal incisions of radial or astigmatic keratotomy through relaxation of corneal fibers. Seiler et al (22) performed pioneering work with excimer laser linear corneal T excisions. Published in 1988, their study was designed to create astigmatic refractive changes in nonastigmatic blind eyes. The study also attempted to reduce astigmatic error in contact lens–intolerant, severely astigmatic sighted eyes. In the first group, eight nonsighted eyes from eight patients, paired transverse T excisions were placed at a 6.0-mm optical zone to induce astigmatism. Corneal ablations were made using a broad homogeneous excimer beam masked by a premanufactured polymethylmethacrylate (PMMA) block covered with foil. The mask had a transverse slit 4.5 mm long and 150 mm wide. Because with corneal ablation, tissue is actually removed, Seiler et al referred to the transverse slits as *excisions*, as compared to incisions made by steel and diamond blades (Fig. 18-12).

Similar in theory to the relaxation of corneal fibers with astigmatic keratotomy, the paired T excisions were placed to induce flattening in the corneal meridian perpendicular to the excisions as well as a coupled steepening in the corneal meridian parallel to the excision.

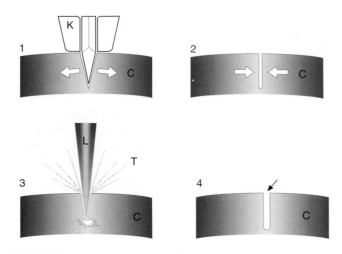

FIGURE 18-12.   *Comparison of cutting action of diamond knife and excimer laser. 1. An incision into the cornea (C) with a diamond knife (K) splits (arrows) the tissues. 2. The resulting incision is very narrow. 3. The excimer laser (L) on the other hand actually removes corneal tissue (T) and creates a trough in the cornea (C). 4. The laser does not create an incision but actually produces an excision of tissue (arrow) as seen in the result (compare 4 with 2).*

In the study, each eye showed the expected flattening in the perpendicular axis and steepening in the parallel axis, with total induced astigmatic change involving the coupling of these two effects on corneal curvature. With a minimum of 3 months of follow-up, clinical data from the eight patients showed that the mean total keratometric change was 2.49 D, with a range of 1.32 to 4.16 D.

In the second group, which included five sighted eyes in 4 patients, preoperative astigmatic errors ranged from 3.5 to 6.5 D. T excisions were placed perpendicular to the steep corneal meridian, with a clear optical zone of 6.0 mm. Excision depths estimated by slit-lamp micrographs ranged from 80% to 95% of the total corneal thickness. Results in this group showed that the mean total keratometric change was 3.15 D, with a range of 1.86 to 4.06 D.

Interestingly, unlike incisional astigmatic keratotomy where the coupling effect usually shows a greater or similar flattening effect on the meridian perpendicular to the incision than the steepening effect 90 degrees away from the incision, T excisions in all 13 eyes resulted in a mean flattening of 1.16 D and a mean steepening of 1.58 D. This moderate coupling difference suggests that though the overall directional change in corneal curvature for incisional and excisional techniques may be the same, the exact mechanism by which that change occurs may be different.

Seiler, Waring, and colleagues (23) attributed the failure of excimer laser excisional keratotomy to 1) excisional V-shaped cuts rather than the thin linear cuts by conventional diamond knives; 2) differences in the amount of wound healing between incised and ablated corneal tissue; and 3) greater expense with laser excisional procedures compared to incisional techniques.

SURGICAL REDUCTION OF ASTIGMATISM AND BROAD-BEAM EXCIMER LASER

Excimer laser technology then evolved to a surface ablative technique (4). PRK was used to reduce myopia by sculpting and reducing the anterior corneal curvature. Many early PRK studies limited patients to those with low astigmatism such as 1.0 D or less, concentrating primarily on the safety and efficacy of PRK for surgically correcting spherical myopia (24–26).

A circular beam of varying diameter can be used to remove more tissue centrally than peripherally, thus flattening the central lenticular power of the cornea. After the advent of PRK, McDonnell et al (27) attempted to create toric surface ablations to correct cylindrical error. With a broad-beam excimer laser source and an expanding rectangle-shaped slit, cylindrical changes could be carved into the cornea.

These cylindrical changes would have no refractive change parallel to the slit opening; however, they would have a flattening effect produced in the meridian in which the slit was expanded. Referring back to basic optics, if a plano cylindrical lens is ablated into the cornea, there would be an axis through which no refractive change would occur. Perpendicular to that axis, light rays would be refracted to a focal line. Different curvatures of that plano cylindrical lens would produce different dioptric power changes. By expanding a slit while exposing the slit to a broad-beam excimer laster source, the surgeon would ablate corneal tissue in the shape of a rectangular trough.

This rectangular trough similar to a cylindrical lens would have an axis parallel to the long axis of the slit. The long axis of the slit was termed the *mechanical axis*. Theoretically if one is trying to correct for regular (with the rule) astigmatism with greater corneal steepness at the 90-degree meridian, the mechanical axis or long axis of the slit would be aligned parallel to the 180-degree meridian. With this alignment the flattening effect of the induced cylindrical change would be in the 90-degree axis.

After initial encouraging results with creating toric ablations on PMMA blocks and rabbit corneas using the expanding slit technique, in 1991 McDonnell et al (8) published results on the first human eyes to have toric ablations (Fig. 18-13). These four patients were all contact lens intolerant; one patient had naturally occurring high astigmatism, two patients had postoperative astigmatic error from penetrating keratoplasty, and one patient had astigmatism secondary to a corneal scar following corneal ulcer infection.

These four eyes were fixated with a vacuum suction ring. Spherical and cylindrical refractive errors were placed into minus cylindrical form, with the mechanical axis of the slit oriented in the same axis as the minus cylinder. This orientation of the slit axis would produce flattening in the most steep meridian 90 degrees away from that axis. A computer controlled the separation of the slit depending on the amount of cylindrical correction intended.

In three of the four patients, full cylindrical refractive corrections were sought while in the one postgrafting patient with a preoperative cylindrical error of 12, surgical correction of only 6 D was planned.

Results showed the achieved correction ranged from 63% to 100% of that intended, with a mean (± standard deviation) for the four eyes of 83 ± 17%.

The prerefractive and postrefractive cylindrical axis showed a shift ranging from 0 to 11 degrees with a mean shift of 7 ± 5 degrees. Though complications such as residual regular and irregular astigmatism, mild superficial corneal haze, and reactivation of herpes simplex epithelial keratitis (in one patient) occurred, the procedure appeared to be quite safe and effective. Multiple subsequent studies were done using a computer-controlled expanding slit and iris

diaphragm to correct for astigmatism and myopia, respectively. When PRK was performed to correct myopia and astigmatic corrections were also intended, this procedure was coined *photoastigmatic refractive keratectomy* (PARK).

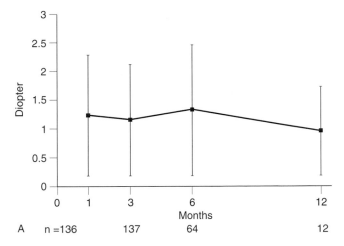

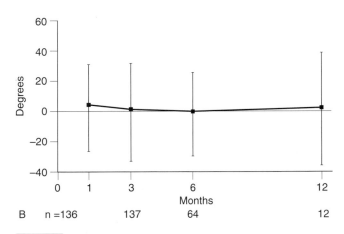

FIGURE 18-15. A. *Surgically induced astigmatism for photoastigmatic refractive keratectomy (PARK) cylindrical correction determined by vector analysis.* B. *Angle of error for PARK cylindrical correction determined by vector analysis.*

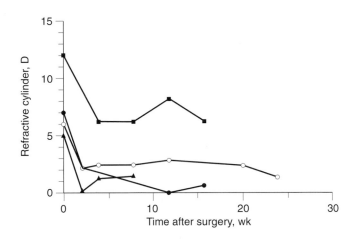

FIGURE 18-13. *Plot of refractive cylindrical error before and after toric excimer laser ablation.* Squares *represent patient 1;* closed circles, *patient 2;* triangles, *patient 3; and* open circles, *patient 4. Patient 1 had 6 D of attempted correction of refractive cylinder that measured 12 D; all other patients had attempted correction of all cylinders.*

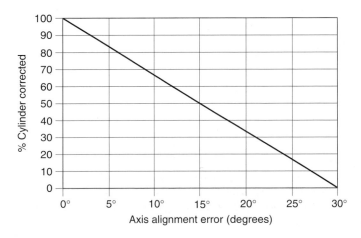

FIGURE 18-14. *Cylinder axis alignment.*

Table 18-2.   Summary of Selected Published Studies Using Broad-Beam ArF (193-nm) Excimer Laser and Expanding Slit/Iris Diaphragm to Correct Myopic Astigmatism

Study (yr)	Laser	Preoperative Refractive Data	Findings
McDonnell PJ, et al (8) (1991)	VISX (Twenty-Twenty Sunnyvale, CA)	N = 4 Intended range of cylinder correction (5.5 to 6.75 D)	First published data of toric ablations on human subjects. The achieved correction ranged from 63% to 100% of that intended, with a mean ($\pm$ SD) for the 4 eyes of 83% $\pm$ 17%. All patients experienced a shift of the spherical equivalent toward hyperopia. Follow-up revealed a shift in axis ranging from 0 to 11 degrees with a mean shift of 7 $\pm$ 5 degrees.
Taylor HR, et al (28) (1993)	VISX (Twenty-Twenty)	N = 54 Mean cylindrical refraction preoperatively -1.39 ± 1.33 D Mean spherical equivalent preoperatively (approximation by interpreting published graph) 4.0 D	3-month follow-up showed a mean postoperative cylindrical refraction of -0.61 ± 0.53 D, significant to the p level (0.0002). 6-month mean spherical equivalent was 0.29 $\pm$ 0.73 D. Vector analysis using method discussed by Alpins (29) assessed "angle error" at 6 mo to be -1.1 ± 23.9 degrees. At 6 postoperative mo, 19 (95%) of the 20 patients had uncorrected visual acuity of 6/12 (20/40) or better, with 6 patients losing one line of best-corrected vision and 2 patients losing 2 lines.
Pender PM, et al (30) (1994)	VISX (Twenty-Twenty)	N = 8 Preoperative mean astigmatic error, 1.28 D (range, 0.75 to 2.25 D) Preoperative mean spherical refractive error, -4.06 D (range, -2.00 to 7.00 D)	Mean postoperative residual cylinder for all 8 cases was 0.46 D, with 3 eyes having residual cylinder 0.75 D or greater and one eye showing no change in magnitude of cylinder postoperatively. Overall improvement showed 25% of patients achieving 20/20 or better uncorrected visual acuity, 62.5% achieving 20/40 or better uncorrected acuity, and 100% achieving 20/50 or better uncorrected visual acuity. In 2 cases there was one line loss in best-corrected visual acuity from 20/20 to 20/25. The importance of error in axis alignment resulting in undercorrection was discussed and a graph displays percentage of cylinder corrected plotted against axis alignment error (Fig. 18-14).
Taylor HR, et al (31) (1994)	VISX (Twenty-Twenty)	N = 139 for 3-mo data N = 65 for 6-mo data Mean spherical equivalent was divided into 3 groups: I N = 59 < -5.00 D II N = 59 -5.00 to -10 D III N = 21 > -10.00 D Range of astigmatic error, ≤ -6.00 D	3-mo data showed mean and standard deviation spherical equivalent for the 3 groups to be: I -0.34 ± 1.06 D II -0.55 ± 1.27 D III -1.83 ± -1.72 D Though there were less patients in the 6-mo follow-up (N = 65), there was definite regression in mean spherical equivalent for group III to -3.96 ± 2.08 D. Using vector analysis (29), overall mean surgically induced astigmatism was 1.15 D at 3 mo and 1.32 D at 6 mo with a mean angle of error of 1.55 degrees at 3 mo and 0.16 degree at 6 mo (Fig. 18-15).
Spigelman AV, et al (32) (1994)	VISX (Twenty-Twenty)	N = 70 for 6-mo follow-up N = 12 for 12-mo follow-up Mean preoperative sphere for 70 patients, -4.96 D Mean preoperative cylinder for 70 patients, -1.52 D	Results in 70 patients at 6-mo follow-up showed a mean postoperative sphere of -0.14 D and mean postoperative cylinder of -0.54 D. 1-yr data for 12 of the 70 patients with mean preoperative sphere and cylinder was -3.85 D and -1.19 D, respectively. Postoperative mean for the 12 patients showed a mean postoperative sphere and cylinder of -0.05 D and -0.59 D, respectively. At 6 mo, 71% had 20/40 or better uncorrected visual acuity and 83% of the 1-yr follow-up group had 20/40 or better uncorrected visual acuity. At 1 yr 2 patients had lost one line of best-corrected visual acuity. Sequential vs elliptical technique was discussed with concerns about sequential technique creating transition zones.
Kim YJ, et al (33) (1994)	VISX (Twenty-Twenty)	N = 168 Mean preoperative astigmatism, 1.51 $\pm$ 0.81 D (range, 0.50 to 4.25 D) Mean spherical refractive error, -7.27 ± 2.66 D (range, -2.50 to -17.25 D)	Mean postoperative astigmatism was 0.70 $\pm$ 0.58 D at 3 mo and 0.67 $\pm$ 0.60 D at 6 mo. Vector analysis using Holladay, Cravy, and Koch rectangular coordinates (21) showed that at 3 mo, 72% and at 6 mo, 65.2% were within $\pm$ 0.50 D of intended astigmatic correction. Vector analysis also showed that postoperative axis was less than 10 degrees off preoperative intended axis in 60.1% of patients. Discussion about the practical problem of exact axis alignment and which axis to use if axis determined by manifest refraction and that by cycloplegic refraction differ. Also, question concerning when axis differences are determined by topography.

Table 18-2.   *Continued*

Study (yr)	Laser	Preoperative Refractive Data	Findings
Snibson GR, et al (34) (1995)	VISX (Twenty-Twenty)	Total N = 76 Mean preoperative spherical equivalents divided into 3 groups: I N = 30 −3.55 ± 0.94 D II N = 39 −6.55 ± 1.23 D III N = 7 −14.18 ± 2.49 D Range of astigmatic error, ≤6 D	1-yr results show postoperative mean spherical equivalents for the 3 groups to be: I −0.59 ± 0.61 D II −1.09 ± 1.07 D III −2.61 ± 1.92 D After 1 yr 72% of eyes were within 1 D of planned refraction and 87% within 2 D. Vector analysis (29) demonstrated a −1.07 ± 29.47-degree (mean ± SD) angle of error for these eyes with 1 D or more of astigmatism. 83% ± 33% of the intended magnitude of the cylindrical correction was achieved at 12 mo. At 12 mo, 9 patients (6%) experienced a reduction in best-corrected visual acuity of 2 or more Snellen lines with 2 patients having best-corrected visual acuity less than 20/40. Authors noted persistent loss of best-corrected visual acuity to be largely (but not entirely) attributable to residual corneal opacity. 29 patients underwent retreatment of one eye within 12 mo of the initial procedure.
Alio JL, et al (35) (1995)	VISX (Twenty-Twenty)	N = 46 Mean preoperative spherical refraction, −0.25 ± 0.25 D (range, −0.50 to 0 D) Mean preoperative cylindrical refraction, −2.50 ± 0.70 D (range, −1.50 to −4.00 D)	Mean residual manifest cylindrical correction was −0.50 ± 0.20 D at 12 mo. In all eyes, the axis of residual cylinder was ±5 degrees of the preoperative astigmatic axis. At 12 mo 8 eyes had lost one line of best-corrected visual acuity. Mean uncorrected preoperative visual acuity was 20/100 and mean uncorrected postoperative visual acuity was 20/25.

SD = standard deviation.

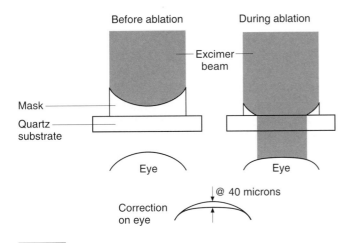

FIGURE 18-16.   *Shape transfer with the Erodible Mask.*

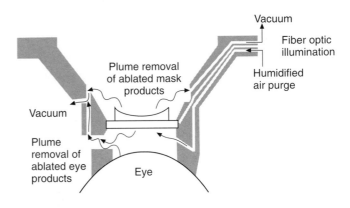

FIGURE 18-17.   *Eye cup holding the Erodible Mask.*

Table 18-2 provides a summary of studies using expanding slit procedures (8,28–35).

During that similar period in time (between 1992–1996), use of broad-beam excimer laser and expanding slit was not the only technique developed and evaluated for the correction of astigmatism.

Other techniques involving broad-beam laser ablation used either an erodible mask (9) or oval apertures (10). Use of an erodible mask to create an ablation surface without steps was developed in an attempt to correct both myopia and astigmatism. Hypothetically the erodible mask technique could create almost any new anterior corneal curvature. The Erodible Mask consists of a PMMA button mounted on a quartz plate transparent to the 193-nm radiation (Fig. 18-16). A plastic shell surrounds both the PMMA button and the quartz plate. The plastic shell, when placed onto the cornea, functions like a suction ring, with a space between the shell and the cornea allowing for a vacuum and a humidified controlled environment (Fig. 18-17). Initially the technique involved mask-corneal contact, with the surgeon manually holding and aligning the mask into position. Later procedures also incorporated a fixed stand on the laser machine to hold the mask in place.

The PMMA mask has a similar ablation rate as that of corneal stroma. The mask can be created into any specific shape. With a broad laser beam the entire mask can be exposed to the laser whereby as soon as the thinnest area of the mask is ablated, the corneal stroma is ablated. With regards to correcting regular astigmatism and in theory flattening the steep corneal meridian, a mask creating a cylindrical correction with the axis 90 degrees away from the steep meridian could be used.

In a study by Brancato et al (36), scanning electron microscopy of PMMA plates ablated using the Erodible Mask (Fig. 18-18) demonstrated smoother surfaces compared to PMMA plates ablated using the conventional diaphragm technique, where microsteps due to diaphragm movements were seen.

In that same study, Brancato et al (36) showed early clinical results using the erodible mask technique to correct

myopic astigmatism in four human eyes. After 3 months of follow-up, these patients who had preoperative myopia ranging from -2.00 to $-10.00\,\mathrm{D}$ were all within $\pm1.00\,\mathrm{D}$ of the intended spherical correction. Preoperative astigmatism ranged from -1.50 to $-2.50\,\mathrm{D}$, with only one eye at 3 months showing complete correction and the other three eyes being undercorrected.

Table 18-3 provides a summary of studies using the laser and the Erodible Mask (9,36–42).

To date, most toric ablation research has involved a broad-beam excimer laser technique. As described already, the two most common techniques involved either an expanding slit or an ablatable mask placed in front of a broad homogeneous beam. Within the last several years, conceptually differing techniques in lasering systems have been developed.

With a 193-nm ArF excimer laser as the ablative source, scanning rather than constant broad-beam laser exposure has been used to correct myopia and myopic astigmatism.

SCANNING EXCIMER LASER SYSTEMS

Scanning motors (galvanometers) similar to those used for laser light shows are utilized in scanning excimer laser systems, except they are faster and smaller. A computer controls the galvanometer to place the beam in a manner that will ablate the steep meridian and make it flatter. In some situations this treatment area will have a rectangular shape when only astigmatism is corrected whereas an oval or elliptical shape can be created when myopic and astigmatic corrections are attempted.

Certain high-speed systems provide feedback on the actual scanning position and the computer compares this to the command position to verify the beam location. This feedback system is an attempt to improve treatment accuracy. A small beam of variable size is used to ablate a given toric pattern in the cornea. The theory behind the primary procedural techniques using the scanning beam to correct regular myopic astigmatism is the same as that for the broad-beam system.

The steepest corneal meridian can be flattened by ablating a cylindrical correction with the cylindrical axis aligned 90 degrees away from the steepest meridian. With the patient's refractive error computed in minus cylinder form, the axis of attempted cylindrical ablation is placed along that same minus cylinder axis. Spherical corrections can coincide with astigmatic corrections, with overlapping treatment zones to help create smooth ablative surfaces.

One excimer laser model made by Technolas is the Keracor 116. The Keracor 116 is a broad-beam laser that has the capability to operate in a scanning mode for the astigmatic portion of the treatment, but then switches back to the broad-beam expanding-iris-diaphragm mode to perform the spherical portion of the treatment. The Keracor 116 is a hybrid of broad-beam and scanning lasers (Laswell LA, personal communication, 1996).

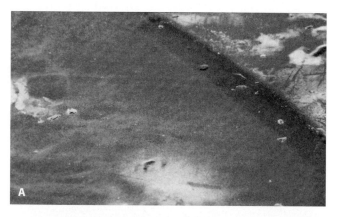

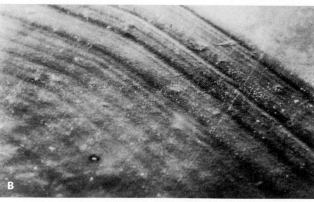

FIGURE 18-18.   *A. A PMMA plate ablated using an erodible mask. Note the smoothness of the surface, and the presence of a "step" in the margin of the ablation zone. B. A PMMA plate ablated using the conventional diaphragm technique. Note the presence of several steps due to diaphragm movements. [Reproduced with permission from Brancato R, Carones F, Trabucchi G, et al. The erodible mask in photorefractive keratectomy for myopia and astigmatism. Refract Corneal Surg 1993;9(suppl):S127.]*

Table 18-3.   Summary of Selected Studies Using Broad-Beam ArF Excimer (193-nm) Laser and an Erodible Mask to Correct Myopic Astigmatism

Study (yr)	Laser	Preoperative Data	Findings
Gordon M, et al (9) (1992)	Summit (Summit Technology, Waltham, MA)	N = 5 Mean preoperative sphere, −2.15 D (range, −0.50 to −3.50 D) Mean preoperative cylinder, −2.7 D (range, −2.00 to −4.00 D)	2-mo follow-up results showed mean sphere of +2.25 ± 0.91 D above desired correction and mean postoperative cylindrical correction of −0.85 D.
Brancato R, et al (36) (1993)	Summit	N = 4 Preoperative myopia (range, −2.00 D to −10.00 D) Preoperative astigmatism (range, −1.50 to 2.50 D)	Results at 3 mo showed preoperative myopia had been corrected to ±1.00 D of intended correction for all 4 eyes. Only 1 eye had complete astigmatic correction, with the other 3 eyes having astigmatic undercorrection. Findings also included smoother ablated PMMA surfaces when comparing erodible mask technique to diaphragm technique, using scanning electron microscopy.
Hersh PS, et al (37) (1994)	Summit (Omnimed)	Toric group N = 10 Preoperative myopia, < −6.50 D Preoperative refractive astigmatism, 1.48 D Preoperative keratometric astigmatism, 1.99 D	Follow-up period not documented. Postoperative refractive astigmatism was decreased to 0.86 D while postoperative keratometric astigmatism decreased to only 1.96 D. Potential causes of astigmatic undercorrection were noted, such as consequence of toric ablation algorithm, miscentration of ablation, misalignment of cylindrical axis, and/or meridianal effects of wound healing (8,38).
Cherry PMH, et al (39) (1994)	Summit (Omnimed)	Group I: Preoperative spherical component 5.75 D or less Preoperative keratometric astigmatism mean, 2.26 D (N = 9) Preoperative refractive astigmatism mean, 2.17 D (N = 16) Group II: Preoperative spherical component, −6.00 D or more Preoperative keratometric astigmatism, 2.07 D (N = 13) Preoperative refractive astigmatism, 2.52 D (N = 18)	3-mo follow-up for group I showed mean keratometric astigmatism of 2.66 D and a mean refractive astigmatism of 1.21 D. Mean refractive astigmatism was reduced from 2.17 to 1.21 D while mean keratometric astigmatism interestingly increased from 2.26 to 2.66 D. 3-mo follow-up for group II showed mean refractive astigmatism reduced from 2.52 to 1.23 D. However, this group II, like group I, had an increase in mean keratometric astigmatism from 2.07 to 2.59 D. The authors submitted one possible explanation for this difference between refractive and keratometric findings—that potential irregular haze may cause several microareas of differing keratometric findings.
Gomez de Liano MZ, et al (40) (1995)	Summit (Excimed UV 200 LA)	N = 229 Preoperative mean spherical equivalent, −4.35 ± 2.15 D Preoperative mean astigmatic error, −2.28 ± 1.25 D	3-mo follow-up for 110 eyes showed a mean postoperative spherical equivalent +0.73 ± 0.75 D and mean postoperative correction of −1.68 ± 0.79 D. 1-yr follow-up for 53 eyes showed a mean postoperative spherical equivalent of +0.52 ± 0.88 D and mean postoperative astigmatic correction of −1.40 ± 0.78 D. Pertinent finding was loss of spectacle corrected visual acuity, with 18% having lost lines of best-corrected vision. Breaking down that 18%, the authors noted 62% of that group of eyes lost one line, 19% lost 2 lines, and 19% lost 3 lines.
Niles C, et al (41) (1996)	Summit (Omnimed)	N = 25 Preoperative mean sphere, −7.46 D (range, −3.25 D to −13.50 D) Preoperative mean cylinder, 2.31 D (range, 1.25 to 6.25 D)	6-mo follow-up showed a mean postoperative sphere of −0.71 D and a mean postoperative cylindrical correction of 0.69 D. Authors noted greater than expected undercorrection and overcorrection of the myopic component while astigmatic correction was more predictable. The mean astigmatism correction at 6 mo was 73.1%. Because of some difficulties encountered during treatment, authors offered a possible suggestion of sequential treatment using an erodible mask for astigmatic correction and the routine PRK treatment for residual myopia.

Table 18-3.   *Continued*

Study (yr)	Laser	Preoperative Data	Findings
Brancato R, et al (42) (1996)	Summit (Excimed UV 200)	N = 21 Attempted myopic correction: mean, −7.07 D (range, −1.50 to −10.00 D) Attempted astigmatic correction: mean, −2.43 D (range, −1.50 to −4.00 D)	At 6-mo after treatment mean spherical correction was +0.18 D (range, −2.50 to +3.50 D) and mean cylinder correction was −1.25 D (range, −2.00 to −0.50 D). Ten eyes (48%) were within ±1.00 D of intended astigmatic correction, with 11 eyes (52%) showing an undercorrection of greater than 1.00 D. The authors calculated the overall percentage of the magnitude of astigmatism corrected at 6 mo to be 35.5%. None of the eyes lost spectacle-corrected visual acuity lines 6 or 12 mo after surgery.

PMMA = polymethylmethacrylate; PRK = photorefractive keratectomy.

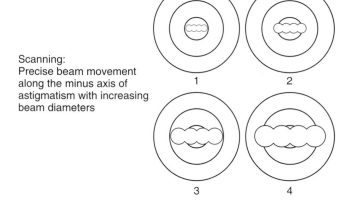

Scanning:
Precise beam movement along the minus axis of astigmatism with increasing beam diameters

FIGURE 18-19.   *Excimer laser correction of astigmatism using the scanning technology of Keracor 116.*

The Keracor 116 uses a two-phase treatment approach that consists of a separate treatment to correct the cylinder component of the refractive error followed by treatment to correct the spherical component of the refractive error.

Once the desired spherocylindrical refractive correction is programmed into the laser's computer, the treatment begins with the astigmatic portion of the correction. The current algorithm employs an elliptical treatment zone of 4.0 × 12.0 mm. The laser commences its treatment by "marching" back and forth along the meridian of the minus cylinder axis (the flatter corneal meridian) using a very narrow circular beam whose width is controlled by the iris diaphragm in the optical pathway of the laser (Fig. 18-19). With each pass across the cornea, the iris diaphragm opens slightly more until the full astigmatic correction has been delivered.

The long axis of the beam (12.0 mm) is the cylinder axis, while the shorter dimension (4.0 mm) is where the minus

cylinder power is generated by the ablation. When completed, there is a rounded rectangular or elliptical zone that now has the cylindrical correction.

Following the cylinder correction, the laser reverts to the circular expanding-iris-diaphragm mode to apply the spherical portion of the treatment using a multizone treatment algorithm. Thus, the spherical correction is overlaid on top of the cylindrical correction. The goal of performing the procedure in this order is to smooth out any edge irregularities created by the cylinder correction; the wobbling scanning mirrors employed to direct the laser beam create a "polishing" effect on the corneal surface, which helps to minimize the step effects that would otherwise result from the use of an expanding iris diaphragm with discrete step sizes and fixed bending mirrors.

Two Chiron Vision phase II studies of PRK correction for myopia and astigmatism using the Keracor 116 laser have been conducted, and unpublished 6-month results became available (Laswell LA, personal communication, 1996). Both studies involved corrections for astigmatism ranging from 1.0 to 5.0 D of cylinder, with the spherical intended correction divided into low myopia ranging from −1.5 to −6.0 D and moderate myopia ranging from −6.12 to −10.0 D. With use of the scanning technology to correct astigmatic error, cylinder deviation from the intended correction as determined by vector analysis was within 1.0 D for 73% of the eyes in the low-myopia group and for 85% of the eyes in the moderate-myopia group. Table 18-4 provides the mean preoperative and postoperative spherical and cylindrical powers for both low and moderate myopia with astigmatism.

As described earlier, the Technolas Keracor 116 is a hybrid laser incorporating both broad-beam iris-diaphragm spherical correction and a scanning technique for correction of astigmatism. At the present time, multiple new true scanning lasers are being developed whereby the laser beam is scanned across the cornea to correct spherical and astigmatic refractive errors.

Table 18-4. Results of Phase II Clinical Studies of PRK for Myopic Astigmatism Treatment with the Chiron Technolas Keracor 116 Excimer Laser*

Parameter/Finding	Low Myopia with Astigmatism (1.5–6.0 D sphere with 1.0–5.0 D of cylinder)	Moderate Myopia with Astigmatism (6.12–10.0 D sphere with 1.0–5.0 D of cylinder)
Mean age (SD), range	43.3 (7.8), 22.2–60.0 yr	39.7 (9.2), 19.4–60.3 yr
Mean preop sphere power (cycloplegic), range	−3.77 D (1.28), −6.00 to −1.50 D (N = 125)	−7.61 D (1.23), −10.0 to −4.75 D (N = 133)
Mean preop cylinder power (cycloplegic), range	−1.83 D (0.85), −1.00 to −4.75 D	−1.68 D (0.69), −1.00 to −4.50 D
Postop mean cycloplegic deviation from intended spherical correction, range	−0.02 D (0.80), −2.00 to +2.21 D (N = 89)	0.18 D (1.18), −4.50 to +3.41 D (N = 124)
% Within ±1.0 D of intended spherical correction	82%	72%
% Overcorrected by >1.0 D	8%	18%
% Undercorrected by >1.0 D	10%	10%
Mean spherical cycloplegic refraction, range	−0.07 D (0.78), −2.00 to +2.00 D (N = 89)	−0.38 D (1.15), −5.00 to +2.25 D (N = 124)
Mean cylinder cycloplegic refraction, range	−0.72 D (0.61), −2.50 to plano (N = 89)	−0.57 D (0.47), −2.00 to plano (N = 124)
Cylinder deviation from intended correction by vector analysis	±1.0 D = 73% ±0.50 D = 53% (N = 89)	±1.0 D = 85% ±0.50 D = 55% (N = 124)
Uncorrected acuity at 6 mo postop		
20/40 or better	88% (N = 91)	79% (N = 126)
20/20 or better	46%	30%
Change in best-corrected acuity at 6 mo		
Loss of >2 lines	1% (N = 104)	2% (N = 126)
Loss of 2 lines	4%	2%
Increase of 3 lines	2%	1%
Increase of 2 lines	13%	3%

* All follow-up data are from 6-month postoperative examinations.
SD = standard deviation.

Specific scanning mechanisms differ among several of these newer lasers. Unique delivery systems exist with capabilities of delivering either a scanning slit or scanning spot. Advantages and disadvantages of these new laser systems with respect to operating time, eye-tracking requirements, and ability to treat regular astigmatism need to be evaluated further.

Beyond the physics and engineering of scanning beam laser, the computer technology and derived algorithms that direct the scanning beam are key elements. Changing the computer program and algorithm, differently shaped treatment areas and treatment pattern sequences can be derived. This flexibility without having to change laser hardware may prove quite valuable.

COMBINED PHOTOREFRACTIVE KERATECTOMY AND ASTIGMATIC KERATOTOMY

Astigmatic keratotomy may be combined with PRK or LASIK to correct myopic astigmatism.

Ring et al (43) utilized transverse keratotomy combined with spherical PRK for compound myopic astigmatism in their study of 40 eyes. Following the popular nomograms of Thorton and Lindstrom (Fig. 18-20), arcuate incisions were made in an attempt to decrease the astigmatic error. In conjunction with arcuate keratotomies, PRK myopic correction was attempted using a Summit Omnimed laser. Six-month data showed correction of the mean spherical equivalent from −6.82 preoperatively to −0.01 D postoperatively.

The range of preoperative spherical correction was −1.5 to −13.50 D, with a mean of −5.99 D. The mean preoperative cylindrical correction of −1.73 D was corrected to a mean residual astigmatism of −0.32 D. Seventy-five percent of the patients achieved uncorrected visual acuity of 20/40 or better. When transverse keratotomy is combined with PRK, Ring et al suggested a time interval between keratotomy and PRK if astigmatism was 2.00 D or greater. Coupling effects and stability of the cornea were considered.

Astigmatism is not always regular. Steep and flat corneal meridians may be separated by an angle other than 90 degrees. A symmetric corneal curvature and a specific meridian may be present. Varying astigmatic axis or dioptric power, or both, across a corneal surface lead to irregular astigmatism. Any or all of these astigmatic variables can develop clinically secondary to a specific corneal pathology

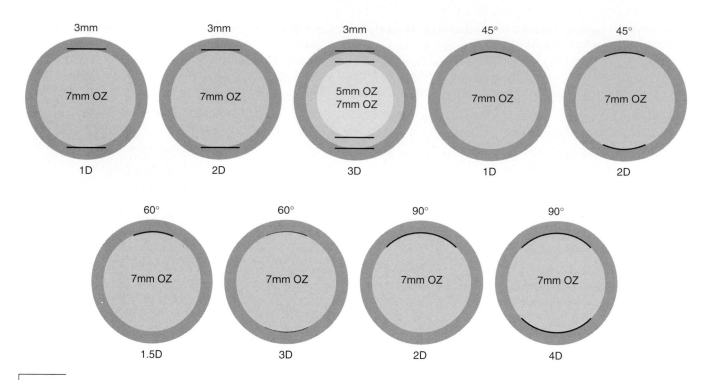

FIGURE 18-20.   *Lindstrom nomogram for astigmatic keratotomy nomogram modifiers:*

1. *Zone: 7 mm for arcuate keratotomy, 7 mm and 5 mm for straight keratotomy.*
2. *Knife setting: 100% of thinnest paracentral pachometry at zone mark in the meridian of astigmatism.*
3. *Over/under age 30: Increase or decrease efficacy 2% per year e.g.,*
    Age 20 = 80% of age 30
    Age 55 = 150% of age 30
    Age 80 = 200% of age 30
4. *While mild overall corneal flattening may occur, assume a coupling ratio of 1 : 1.*
5. *The procedure may be combined with a four-incision or eight-incision radial keratotomy, although radial and transverse incisions should not touch.*
6. *Assume a range of effect of ±2.00 D when planning surgery.*

OZ = optical zone.

such as with corneal scar, pterygium, basement membrane dystrophy, and keratoconus; however, a common presentation is in the postsurgical patient. Following such procedures as cataract extraction, penetrating keratoplasty, radial keratotomy, and automated lamellar keratectomy, residual astigmatism is not always regular.

PHOTOASTIGMATIC REFRACTIVE KERATECTOMY AND KERATOPLASTY

With respect to penetrating keratoplasty, suture position and tension, graft-donor alignment, and wound healing can all lead to visually disabling astigmatism. Use of postkeratoplasty relaxing incisions or wedge resections to correct astigmatism has been described (44). Corneal excimer ablations to correct postkeratoplasty astigmatism was described by Campos et al (45), who used expanding slit technology to perform strictly cylindrical correction on 12 postkeratoplasty eyes that were contact lens and spectacle intolerant.

The mean preoperative refractive cylinder was 7.0 ± 3.6 D and postoperatively the mean value was 4.3 ± 2.9 D, with the follow-up time ranging from 6 to 14 months. Limited postoperative complications with respect to corneal graft clarity, re-epithelialization, corneal haze, pain, and infection were observed; however, one patient with a history of herpes simplex keratitis developed a recurrence 10 months after laser treatment that later resulted in graft rejection.

In a more recent study, Nordan et al (46) performed both spherical and toric ablations for residual myopic astigmatism following keratoplasty. This small group of five eyes had a mean preoperative refraction of −7.40 ± 4.37 D sphere and +3.05 ± 1.47 D cylinder. Following spherical and toric ablation with iris diaphragm and expanding slit apertures, the refraction was −3.35 ± 3.04 D sphere and +1.30 ± 0.62 D cylinder.

Though preliminary, the results noted in these two studies (45,46) may provide some hope for corneal transplant surgeons who are always looking for means to prevent or treat postkeratoplasty ametropia.

REFERENCES

1. Duke-Elder S. *The practice of refraction.* St. Louis: CV Mosby, 1949:91.
2. Fyodorov SN, Durner VV. Surgical correction of complicated myopic astigmatism by means of dissection of circular ligament of cornea. *Ann Ophthalmol* 1981;13:115–118.
3. Trokel SL, Srinivason R, Braren B. Excimer laser surgery of the cornea. *Am J Ophthalmol* 1983;96:710–715.
4. Marshall J, Trokel S, Rothery S, Krueger RR. Photoablative reprofiling of the cornea using an excimer laser photorefractive keratectomy. *Lasers Ophthalmol* 1986;1:21–48.
5. Gartry DS, Kerr Muir MG, Marshall J. Excimer laser photorefractive keratectomy: 18 month follow up. *Ophthalmology* 1992;99:1209–1219.
6. Snibson GR, Carson CA, Aldred GF, Taylor HR, for the Melbourne Excimer Laser Group. One-year evaluation of excimer laser photorefractive keratectomy for myopia and myopic astigmatism. *Arch Ophthalmol* 1995;113:994–1000.
7. Tengroth B, Epstein D, Fagerholm P, et al. Excimer laser photorefractive keratectomy for myopia: clinical results in sighted eyes. *Ophthalmology* 1993;100:739–745.
8. McDonnell PJ, Moreira H, Clapham TN, D'Arcy J, Munnerlyn CR. Photorefractive keratectomy for astigmatism: initial clinical results. *Arch Ophthalmol* 1991;109:1370–1373.
9. Gordon M, Brint SF, Durrie DS, Seiler T, et al. Photorefractive keratectomy (PRK) at 193nm using an erodible mask. *SPIE Proc* 1992;1644(II):11–19.
10. Forster W, Beck R, Borrmann A, Busse H. Correcting myopic astigmatism with an areal 193nm excimer laser ablation. *J Cataract Refract Surg* 1995;21:278–281.
11. Gormley DJ, Gersten M, Koplin RS, Lubkin V. Corneal modeling. *Cornea* 1988;7:30–35.
12. Binders PS. Excimer laser photoablation and radial keratotomy for the correction of myopia. *Refract Corneal Surg* 1994;10:443–464.
13. Boyd BF. *Highlights of ophthalmology refractive surgery with the masters.* Vol. 2. Coral Gables, FL: Highlights of Ophthalmology, 1987:4–5.
14. Schiøtz HA. Ein Fall von hochgradigem Horn hautastigmatismus nach Staarextraction. Besserung auf operativem Wege. *Arch Augenheilk* 1885;15:178–181.
15. Sato T. Treatment of conical cornea by incision of Descement's membrane. *Acta Soc Ophthalmol Jpn* 1939;43:541.
16. Sato T, Shibata H, Akiyama K. Anterior and posterior half-corneal incisions for myopia, results in human eyes. *Acta Soc Ophthalmol Jpn* 1952;56:1137–1140 (In Japanese).
17. Sato T, Akiyama K, Shibata H. A new surgical approach to myopia. *Am J Ophthalmol* 1953;36:823–829.
18. Lindstrom RL, Lindquist TD. The surgical correction of postoperative astigmatism. *Cornea* 1988;7:138–148.
19. Lindstrom RL. The surgical correction of astigmatism: a clinician's perspective. *Refract Corneal Surg* 1990;6:441–454.
20. Price FW, Grene RB, Marks RG, Gonzales JS, the Arc-T Study Group. Astigmatism Reduction Clinical Trial: a multicenter perspective evaluation of the predictability of arcuate keratotomy. *Arch Ophthalmol* 1995;113:277–282.
21. Holladay JT, Cravy TV, Koch DD. Calculating the surgically induced refractive change following ocular surgery. *J Cataract Refract Surg* 1992;18:429–443.
22. Seiler T, Bende T, Wollensack J, Trokel S. Excimer laser keratectomy for correction of astigmatism. *Am J Ophthalmol* 1988;105:117–124.
23. Waring GO III, Seiler T, Fantes FE, Hanna KD. *Refractive keratotomy for myopia and astigmatism.* St. Louis: Mosby-Year Book, 1992:718.
24. McDonald MB, Liu JC, Byrd TJ, et al. Central photorefractive keratectomy for myopia: partially sighted and normally sighted eyes. *Ophthalmology* 1991;98:1327–1337.
25. Maguire LJ, Zabel RW, Parker P, Lindstrom RL. Topography and ray tracing analysis of patients with excellent visual acuity three months after excimer laser photorefractive keratectomy for myopia. *Refract Corneal Surg* 1991;7:122–128.
26. Lindstrom RL, Sher NA, Chen V, et al. Use of 193-nanometer nm excimer laser for myopic photorefractive keratectomy in sighted eyes: a multicenter study. *Trans Am Ophthalmol Soc* 1991;89:155–182.
27. McDonnell PJ, Moreira H, Garbus J, et al. Photorefractive keratectomy to create toric ablations for correction of astigmatism. *Arch Ophthalmol* 1991;109:710–713.
28. Taylor HR, Guest CS, Kelly P, Alpins NA, for the Excimer Laser and Research Group. Comparison of excimer laser treatment of astigmatism and myopia. *Arch Ophthalmol* 1993;111:1621–1626.
29. Alpins NA. A new method of analyzing vectors for planning and understanding changes in astigmatism. *J Cataract Refract Surg* 1993;19:524–533.
30. Pender PM, Excimer Laser Study Group. Photorefractive keratectomy for myopic astigmatism: phase II A of the Federal Drug Administration study (12–18 month follow up). *J Cataract Refract Surg* 1994;20(suppl):262–264.
31. Taylor HR, Kelly P, Alpins N. Excimer laser correction of myopic astigmatism. *J Cataract Refract Surg* 1994;20(suppl):243–251.
32. Sigelman AV, Albert WC, Cozean CH, et al. Treatment of myopic astigmatism with the 193nm excimer laser utilizing aperture elements. *J Cataract Refract Surg* 1994;20(suppl):258–261.
33. Kim YJ, Sohn J, Tchan H, Lee CO. Photoastigmatic refractive keratectomy in 168 eyes: six month results. *J Cataract Refract Surg* 1994;20:387–391.
34. Snibson GR, Carson CA, Aldred GF, Taylor HR, for the Melbourne Excimer Laser Group. One-year evaluation of excimer laser photorefractive keratectomy for myopia and myopic astigmatism. *Arch Ophthalmol* 1995;113:994–1000.
35. Alio JL, Artola A, Ayala MJ, Claramonte P. Correcting simple myopic astigmatism with the excimer laser. *J Cataract Refract Surg* 1995;21:512–515.
36. Brancato R, Carones F, Trabucchi G, et al. The erodible mask in photorefractive keratectomy for myopia and astigmatism. *Refract Corneal Surg* 1993;9(suppl):S125–S133.
37. Hersh PS, Patel R. Correction of myopia and astigmatism using an ablatable mask. *J Refract Corneal Surg* 1994;10(suppl):S250–S254.
38. Shieh E, Moreira H, D'Arcy JD, et al. Quantitative analysis of wound healing after cylindrical and spherical excimer laser ablations. *Ophthalmology* 1992;99:1050–1055.
39. Cherry PMH, Tutton MK, Bell A, et al. Treatment of myopic astigmatism with photorefractive keratectomy using an erodible mask. *J Refract Corneal Surg* 1994;10(suppl):S239–S245.
40. Gomez de Liano MZ, Jimenez-Alfaro I, Carreras I, et al. The Spanish User Group. Photorefractive keratectomy for myopic astigmatism using the emphasis erodible mask. *J Refract Corneal Surg* 1995;11:S343–S348.
41. Niles C, Culp B, Teal P. Excimer laser photorefractive keratectomy using an erodible mask to treat myopic astigmatism. *J Cataract Refract Surg* 1996;22:436–440.
42. Brancato R, Carones F, Venturi E, et al. Refractive keratectomy for compound myopic astigmatism with an eye cup erodible mask delivery system. *J Refract Surg* 1996;12:501–510.
43. Ring CP, Hadden OB, Morris AT. Transverse keratotomy combined with spherical photorefractive keratectomy for compound myopic astigmatism. *J Refract Corneal Surg* 1994;10:S217–S221.
44. Krachmer JH, Fenzl RE. Surgical correction of high postkeratoplasty astigmatism: relaxing incisions versus wedge resections. *Arch Ophthalmol* 1980;98:1400–1402.
45. Campos M, Hertzog L, Garbus J, et al. Photorefractive keratectomy for severe postkeratoplasty astigmatism. *Am J Ophthalmol* 1992;114:425–436.
46. Nordan LT, Binder PS, Kassar BS, Heitzmann J. Photorefractive keratectomy to treat myopia and astigmatism after radial keratotomy and penetrating keratoplasty. *J Cataract Refract Surg* 1995;21:268–273.

Lamellar Keratoplasty and Laser In Situ Keratomileusis

C. A. SWINGER

PRINCIPLES

Radial keratotomy (RK) for low to moderate myopia, although providing good clinical results and immediate visual recovery, has been associated with long-term instability in some patients, exhibiting a shift toward hyperopia. Currently, it is most often reserved for low levels (1–4 D) of myopia. Surface ultraviolet photorefractive keratectomy (PRK) is increasingly being performed on candidates who might have undergone RK in the past. The clinical results with PRK for correction of low to moderate myopia have been very good. Disadvantages of the technique, however, are a prolonged wound-healing response and slower visual rehabilitation; the need in some patients for corticosteroids for several months, which may be associated with intraocular complications; and a rapid decline in both safety and efficacy, as evidenced by a higher incidence of haze and regression, at higher levels of correction. An alternative form of surgery, lamellar refractive keratoplasty (LRK), for correction of both myopia and hyperopia, has been performed for many years and is undergoing an increasingly rapid evolution.

Conceived and developed by José I. Barraquer of Bogotá, Colombia, lamellar refractive surgery was for years performed by only a small group of elite surgeons around the world. LRK has distinct biologic and clinical advantages over surface PRK, such as preservation of both epithelial and Bowman's layers; a markedly reduced inflammatory and wound-healing response, which reduces haze, scarring, and regression; a rapid visual recovery; reduced intraocular complications, such as glaucoma and cataract, which sometimes result from prolonged corticosteroid use; and an easier postoperative management. Improvements in microkeratome technology and the substitution of laser precision for the tissue modification step have spawned a revolution in this

area, creating intense worldwide interest and application of lamellar surgery for correction of all ametropias (1–54). This chapter introduces the lamellar refractive techniques, emphasizing those most commonly performed.

HISTORY

More than three decades ago, Barraquer began developing the LRK techniques of keratophakia and keratomileusis (4,5). Barraquer first reported clinical results with autoplastic myopic keratomileusis (MKM) in 1964 (4). It was more than a decade later, however, when refractive surgery began to grow beyond the domain of its innovator. In 1977, Troutman and Swinger introduced LRK for hyperopia into the United States and in 1978 Swinger began performing keratomileusis for myopia (54). These techniques demanded mastery of the complicated cryolathe for their performance, which severely limited their dissemination. The cryolathe freeze process caused significant tissue damage and delayed visual recovery. The development of epikeratoplasty by Werblin and Kaufman (23) provided a technically simplified procedure and reduced costs when lyophilized lenticules were made commercially available, but epikeratoplasty was marked by inaccuracy and delayed visual recovery (37).

Modern lamellar refractive surgery began expanding in earnest when Swinger and Krumeich developed the concepts, techniques, and instrumentation for performing LRK without freezing or lyophilization, embodied in the Barraquer-Krumeich-Swinger (BKS) refractive set, providing great simplification and rapid visual recovery (51). Ruiz carried on the nonfreeze concept by pioneering lamellar stromectomy, described long ago by Krawicz (27), where the optical resection was performed on a keratectomized bed, as opposed to on a resected lamellar disk as had been done until then, using an automated microkeratome (43,44). The procedure was called *keratomileusis in situ* (KMIS), and it is also known as *automated lamellar keratoplasty* (ALK).

Mechanical microkeratomes provide limited accuracy with respect to tissue resection depths. They are satisfactory for the creation of a flap, as the exact dimensions may vary slightly without affecting the accuracy of the procedure. However, they have been less than satisfactory when creating the second, or optical, resections in BKS keratomileusis or KMIS, where errors measured in microns can result in significant residual refractive error (2,9,11,16,18,20,22,30). For this reason, ultraviolet laser ablation was investigated for the tissue modification step, and it is now used ubiquitously (46).

Peyman et al (41) first proposed using laser energy to shape keratectomized corneal tissue and Krwawicz (27) and later Pureskin (42) first presented the concept of surgery under a corneal flap. Pallikaris et al (38–40) performed a lenticular variant of KMIS under a corneal flap, using an excimer laser rather than a microkeratome for the optical cut, and called the procedure *LASIK*, an acronym for *laser in situ keratomileusis*. Buratto et al (13,14) first performed excimer laser ablation on a resected anterior cap, or excimer laser keratomileusis. A free anterior lamellar cap was obtained with the BKS microkeratome and its stromal surface ablated. Disadvantages with this approach are an inability to use a hinged flap, and a keratectomy of considerable thickness is necessary, which may be associated with some postoperative instability. Also, if the first resection was unexpectedly thin, it may be inadequate to accommodate the desired depth and diameter of ablation. Therefore, the preferred approach, now used universally, is to use a hinged flap method and ablate the stromal bed.

TECHNIQUES

Theory

LRK modifies refraction through lamellar interaction on the cornea. Technically, even PRK falls into this category, though for convenience sake it is referred to simply as PRK. LRK is then used to include all procedures that remove or add tissue or alloplastic materials across the central cornea, sparing Bowman's layer, for refractive purposes. Of such procedures, whether autoplastic, homoplastic, or alloplastic, most, such as keratophakia, keratomileusis, epikeratoplasty, and LASIK, are lenticular procedures, and they may be called forms of lenticular lamellar keratoplasty (LLK). Others, such as KMIS and hyperopic lamellar keratotomy (HLK), are forms of LRK but not LLK, as they do not add or remove lenticular-shaped material.

All lamellar refractive procedures with the exception of HLK and high-refractive-index keratophakia alter, in theory, only the anterior corneal curvature. In a procedure such as HLK (and RK), both corneal surfaces have a new shape following surgery. An exception to this is experimental alloplastic keratophakia using a high-refractive-index

material (29). Here there is minimal change in anterior corneal curvature but some change in posterior curvature. In this case, refractive change is effected not by changing the anterior corneal curvature but by inserting a high-refractive-index lens of appropriate shape into a stromal pocket.

The fundamental equation relating anterior corneal curvature to corneal refractive power in diopters (D) is:

$$\text{Anterior corneal refractive power (D)} = 376/\text{radius of curvature (mm)}$$

Current surgical procedures that correct myopia decrease the anterior corneal refractive power, and this is effected by increasing the radius of curvature of the cornea, thus flattening the cornea. One can calculate the necessary final radius of anterior corneal curvature for an eye from the above equation by simply subtracting the patient's spectacle refraction, referred to the corneal vertex, from the initial mean corneal refractive power (keratometry). Such calculations are the modified basis of nomograms made available at training courses, and they are employed in laser algorithms. For correction of hyperopia the radius of curvature must be reduced and the cornea steepened. On the other hand, although one can calculate the needed final radius of curvature for a hyperopic eye to be treated by HLK, there has been no mathematic basis developed for the HLK weakening procedure, and surgical parameters were developed empirically, by investigation.

Lamellar surgery may be accomplished in several ways. As pioneered by Barraquer, Swinger, Krumeich, and Buratto, keratomileusis for myopia (Fig. 19-1) begins with a complete lamellar keratectomy on the patient's cornea. The resected disk is modified with a cryolathe (Barraquer), BKS device (Barraquer, Krumeich and Swinger), or photoablation (Buratto) by resecting stromal tissue primarily in the center. Replacing the modified cap onto the bed results in a compensatory flattening of the central cornea. In hyperopic keratomileusis, tissue is resected primarily in the periphery of the disk.

In keratophakia, a convex corneal tissue or alloplastic lens, such as a hydrogel, is placed into the interface following a lamellar keratectomy with a microkeratome (Fig. 19-2). When high-refractive-index lenses of polysulfone were used in experimental keratophakia, they were usually placed after manual dissection of a deep lamellar pocket, without incising through Bowman's layer. The use of alloplastic materials imposes a number of challenges such as biocompatibility, permeability to oxygen and nutrients, refractive index considerations, and pressure necrosis of adjacent cornea (35).

In epikeratoplasty (Fig. 19-3), a shallow, peripheral 360-degree trough is created through de-epithelialized cornea. A homoplastic plano, myopic, or hyperopic tissue lens is placed atop Bowman's membrane of the recipient and sutured into the trough. Following surgery, the cornea has two Bowman's layers.

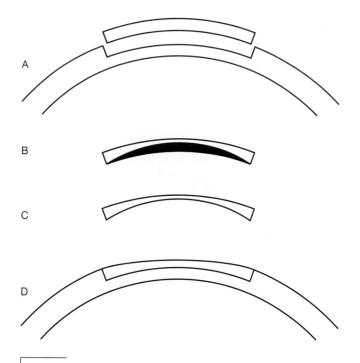

FIGURE 19-1. *Myopic keratomileusis. A. Lamellar keratectomy created with a microkeratome. B. Stromal tissue removed, more so centrally (shaded area). C. Refractive lenticule with divergent power. D. Flattened cornea upon replacement of the cap.*

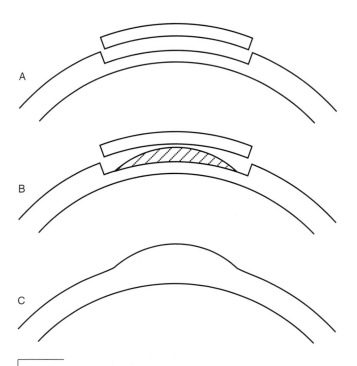

FIGURE 19-2. *Keratophakia (for hyperopia and aphakia). A. Lamellar keratectomy created with a microkeratome. B. Stromal or alloplastic lens placed (striped) on the bed. C. Steepened and thickened central cornea upon replacement of the cap.*

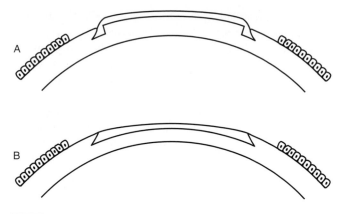

FIGURE 19-3. *Myopic epikeratophakia. A. Peripheral groove created in peripheral de-epithelialized cornea. B. Flattened cornea upon placement of a donor lenticule, thicker in the periphery and thinner in the center, atop the cornea and into the groove.*

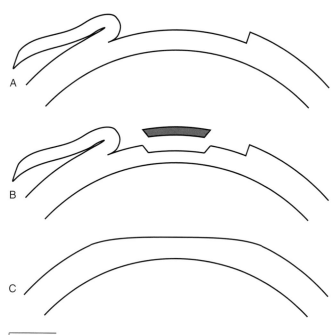

FIGURE 19-4. *Keratomileusis in situ. A. Lamellar flap created with a microkeratome. B. A second microkeratome resection, on the bed, removes a parallel-faced disk of tissue. C. Flattened central cornea upon replacement of the flap.*

In KMIS, or myopic ALK, an incomplete corneal lamellar flap is created, usually with an automated microkeratome. Next, a lamellar disk of tissue, smaller in diameter than the flap but concentric with it, is resected from the bed with a second pass of the microkeratome and discarded (Fig. 19-4). The flap is then replaced. In HLK, or hyperopic ALK (Fig. 19-5), a deep lamellar flap is created with a single pass of the microkeratome. The intraocular pressure (IOP), displacing the thin posterior corneal layer anteriorly, produces an ectasia of the cornea, resulting in corneal steepening and

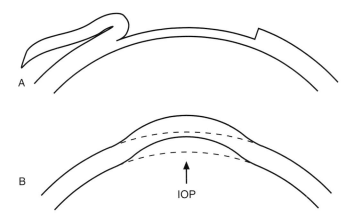

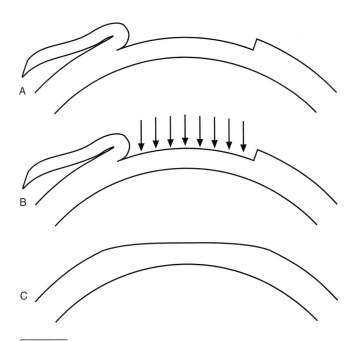

FIGURE 19-5. *Hyperopic lamellar keratotomy. A. Lamellar flap, approximately 70% of the corneal thickness, created with a microkeratome. B. Intraocular pressure (IOP) displaces the thin posterior layer and overlying flap anteriorly, causing central corneal steepening. The original corneal shape is shown with dashed lines.*

FIGURE 19-6. *Myopic LASIK. A. Lamellar flap created with a microkeratome. B. Laser energy delivered more so to the central cornea to remove a positive meniscus lens from the stromal bed. C. Flattened central cornea following replacement of the cap.*

correction of hyperopia. The amount of ectasia and correction is directly related to the depth and inversely related to the diameter of the keratectomy. For keratectomies less than about 60% of the corneal thickness, minimal ectasia and effect result, whereas for keratectomies of 80% or more, uncontrolled ectasia may result in a keratoconus-like condition. There is a practical limit to how small the keratectomy may be made, limiting the correction to +4 to +5 D. KMIS and HLK are frequently referred to as automated lamellar keratoplasty, or ALK. However, the microkeratome need not be automated to perform these techniques, and the term is not medically precise.

In LASIK (Fig. 19-6), lenticular lamellar ablation is performed on a keratectomized bed using laser photoablation. The shape of the tissue ablated is similar to that for surface PRK, though sometimes with smaller ablation diameter. LASIK, like surface PRK and unlike other forms of LRK, can correct myopia, hyperopia, astigmatism, and combinations thereof.

PATIENT SELECTION

Indications

The primary medical indication for LRK is high anisometropia that cannot be corrected by contact lens wear. Since it is well established that best-corrected acuity often improves following LRK for moderate to high myopia, it is also indicated in patients with subnormal vision to improve best-corrected acuity. Most patients, however, seek surgery for improvement of their uncorrected vision for various occupational, professional, or personal reasons.

Patients should have reached the legal age of consent, usually 18 years, and their refractive error should have stabilized, as evidenced by a 0.5-D change or less in both the

spherical and astigmatic components of the refraction during the previous year. All forms of LRK, except LASIK, are limited to the correction of spherical refractive errors only. Thus, patients with significant astigmatism must either be treated with LASIK or have their procedure combined with an astigmatic keratotomy procedure, either simultaneously or secondarily.

LRK is also indicated in patients who have previously undergone surgery such as RK, PRK, penetrating keratoplasty, or even LRK, and who are dissatisfied because of a residual refractive error. I have used homoplastic keratomileusis, whereby a refractive donor cap replaces the resected anterior cap from the patient's eye, to correct up to 28 D of myopia and to rehabilitate patients with anterior corneal scars and refractive error, whereby both may be eliminated simultaneously (52). Homoplastic keratomileusis can also be used following RK to correct secondary hyperopia and to remove glare-producing incisions from the pupillary zone (49). One should wait up to 2 years, however, to ensure that the radial incisions are well healed. HLK following RK should not be employed as a first line of treatment, as severe ectasia may result in a cornea already weakened by radial incisions. Other methods such as the Grene lasso, a reversible suture technique, and surface PRK have been applied successfully to eyes overcorrected by RK and should be attempted first.

Although being investigated for up to 30 D of myopia using various ablation profiles and multizonal patterns, autoplastic myopic LRK, including LASIK, is best reserved for myopia between −6 to −15 D until results conclusively demonstrate safety and efficacy for higher corrections. Homoplastic keratomileusis may sometimes be used to obtain higher corrections. For hyperopes, it is my experience that corneas steepened to a mean power of 60 to 62 D or more may have significant loss of visual acuity, and hyperopic procedures should be limited to corneal power and refractive correction combinations that respect this limit. In the future, very high refractive errors may be treated with phakic intraocular lens implant surgery. HLK is best reserved for hyperopia in the range of +1 to +4 D, although this technique has been replaced by hyperopic LASIK to a great extent, which is being investigated in hyperopes to up to +8 D or more.

Until recently, LRK had been reserved for myopia greater than 6 D. With the advent of laser technology, however, myopic and hyperopic LASIK techniques are being investigated for refractive errors as low as 1 D. However, the baseline surgical complications, even in expert hands, may be higher in the technically more complex LASIK procedure than in RK or PRK. Although LASIK does offer advantages to the patient, its application in patients with low levels of myopia is currently being investigated and needs fuller evaluation of safety and efficacy, comparing the complication rates and acuity results to RK and PRK, before being applied on a widespread basis. Ultimately, each surgeon performing refractive procedures needs to critically evaluate his or her own capabilities and results to determine the range of application for each procedure.

Table 19-1 provides a summary of the clinical applications of LRK techniques, used currently and in the past.

Contraindications

One should not perform refractive surgery without good reason on patients whose refractive error is unstable. Lamellar refractive procedures for myopia, including LASIK, are better reserved for myopic errors of less than −12 to −15 D. For errors above this range, the procedure is considered investigational and applied by experienced LRK surgeons, and the results can be unsatisfactory, exhibiting regression or accompanied by subjective complaints if small ablation zones are used. The exact cutoff point may depend on a number of factors such as visual acuity, pachymetry results, keratometry values, and the laser used, with its associated physical characteristics and ablation profile.

Eyes with active external infectious or inflammatory disease processes are to be avoided, as are thin corneas that would need to be excessively thinned by the proposed procedure. Corneas with neovascularization or pannus that would be transected by the microkeratome and corneas with significant endothelial dystrophy (cell count < 1500) are best avoided, although KMIS may be less traumatic to the endothelium than a broad-beam LASIK procedure. Corneas with basement membrane dystrophy or a history of recurrent erosion may be better treated with surface PRK rather

Table 19-1.   Clinical Applications of Lamellar Refractive Surgery

Autoplastic keratomileusis [cryolathe, Barraquer-Krumeich-Swinger (BKS) procedure]
Myopia, 6–15 D
Hyperopia, 4–10 D
Homoplastic keratomileusis
Myopia, 6–30 D
Hyperopia, 4–12 D
Keratophakia
With lamellar keratectomy—stromal or hydrogel inlay
Hyperopia, 6–20 D
With pocket dissection—polysulfone inlay
Myopia, 6–30 D
Aphakia, 6–20 D
Epikeratoplasty
Myopia, 6–30 D
Hyperopia, 6–20 D
Keratomileusis in situ
Myopia, 6–30 D
Hyperopic lamellar keratotomy
Hyperopia, 1–6 D
LASIK
Myopia, 1–30 D
Hyperopia, 1–6 D
Toric, 1–6 D

than LRK to stabilize the anterior corneal surface postoperatively. Flat corneas (<41 D) may be associated with a free cap following the keratectomy. Though surgery is not contraindicated for such corneas, the surgeon may elect to operate on challenging cases after moderate experience is gained. LASIK is best avoided in eyes with a history of herpetic keratitis. Scarred corneas (though homoplastic keratomileusis may be used in some) including eyes with keratoconus, except in an investigational setting, are best treated by experienced LRK surgeons, as should challenging cases such as eyes previously treated by RK or PKP, as studies in such eyes are few. Eyes with stable forme fruste keratoconus with a normal corneal thickness in a patient 30 to 35 years or older may be considered.

Eyes with a very small palpebral fissure, eyes with external pathology such as conjunctival adhesions or lesions, deeply set eyes, or eyes with an abnormal orbital configuration may present problems during the keratectomy and should be avoided.

Surgery should not be performed on patients who are pregnant, who have autoimmune disease or diseases, or who are taking medications that can adversely affect wound healing. Also, patients with severely dry eyes, significant glaucoma, a history of herpes zoster ophthlamicus (for LASIK), and eyes with treatable retinal pathology that could lead to detachment should be avoided. Eyes with retinal tears or holes may undergo surgery after treatment and clearance by the retinal surgeon specialist. Eyes with retinal vascular disease, systemic vascular disease, or significant glaucomatous cupping are best avoided because posterior-pole complications may develop owing to the necessary elevation of IOP for up to several minutes during the procedure. Refractive surgery of any type should be applied not at all or most cautiously to patients with good vision in only one eye. Finally, the surgeon must assess the expectations of the patient and ensure that they are realistic, and that the patient accepts that there are no guarantees and always the possibility of complications. If not, one should defer surgery.

INSTRUMENTATION

Microkeratome Set

Many microkeratomes are now commercially available, and they may vary significantly. This section describes the salient features of the commonly used microkeratomes.

Microkeratome Head and Motor

Current LRK procedures require a lamellar keratectomy performed with a microkeratome. These units are also useful for therapeutic lamellar keratoplasty. The classic Barraquer and BKS microkeratomes consist of a detachable head that uses a commercial stainless-steel razor blade. The head is mechanically connected to and powered by a high-speed (12,000–14,000 rpm) direct-current motor, though variant models may be turbine driven and operate at even higher speeds. The motor is typically in the body of the handle and held in the surgeon's hand.

The head of the microkeratome has two sections, which may be hinged. Separation allows for placement of the stainless-steel blade, which extends beyond the head proper and presents the cutting edge. The blade should be used for only one procedure, examined carefully under the microscope to ensure it is free from defects before use, and handled with great care during insertion to avoid damage. A stop attachment or means of limiting the keratectomy so as to provide an incomplete flap rather than a complete cap is provided. The cutting blade is preceded by a flat plate that applanates the spherical cornea during the keratectomy such that a lamellar resection of constant thickness is made possible. Recently, disposable microkeratome heads were developed. There have been no studies, however, demonstrating their safety and efficacy. Each microkeratome model has its own sterilization requirements.

Most surgeons no longer use these manually driven microkeratomes but use instead automated microkeratomes. The first was developed by Ruiz and is called the Automatic Corneal Shaper (ACS) (Chiron Vision, Claremont, CA) (Fig. 19-7). It is propelled by a series of external gears. Other companies subsequently developed other means and models such as the Universal Keratome (Phoenix Keratek, Scottsdale, AZ), for example. The ACS uses an inclined blade that oscillates somewhat more slowly (7500 rpm) than many

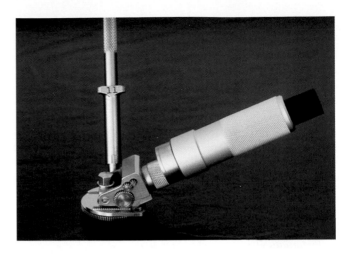

FIGURE 19-7. *Automated microkeratome and suction ring (Automatic Corneal Shaper).*

microkeratomes, whereas the Universal Keratome has a specially designed blade without inclination. Both devices use only a single adjustable suction ring, the former in three pieces, adjustable with respect to the cornea, to vary the diameter of the resection. Another automated microkeratome (Storz GMBH, Heidelberg, Germany) uses a circular rotating blade rather than the linear oscillating blade used in most units. Automated microkeratomes pass across the cornea at constant speed and would be expected to provide a more consistent surface quality, especially for beginning LRK surgeons.

In addition to microkeratomes using metal blades, a sapphire-blade microkeratome with a 0-degree incline (Schwind, Kleinostheim, Germany) and a water-jet microkeratome have been developed (Medjet, Inc., Edison, NJ). The BKS microkeratome has been upgraded to an automated version that is available not only with steel blades, but also with sapphire and diamond blades. Gem blades increase surface quality and may provide greater precision and reproducibility, as they are very sharp and may be used for hundreds of procedures.

Microkeratome performance is dependent on many factors such as careful maintenance, which is critical; blade type, sharpness, and angle; motor speed and vibration; suction ring design; speed of translation; exposure of the eye; IOP; suction; centration; and technique.

Base (Depth, Thickness) Plates

Most microkeratomes have a series of interchangeable base plates that allow one to vary the depth of the keratectomy in small increments, such as 50 μm. The plate is inserted into the head of the microkeratome. The thicker the plate inserted, the less the gap between the head's applanation plate and the blade edge, reducing the thickness of the resection. Plates are labeled according to the resection depth expected. For example, a 160 plate should provide a resection thickness of 160 μm. For LASIK, primarily 130- and

160-μm plates are used. Flaps thinner than 130 μm are difficult to handle and tend to wrinkle but seat well, and flaps thicker than 160 μm necessitate ablation deeper into the stroma, where the ablation rate may differ or endothelial damage may ensue. Plates up to 200 μm are sometimes used, however, for very low corrections.

Blades often vary in dimension, and a special optical microscope may be used to measure the gap and confirm that it is as required. Additional shim plates may be inserted into the ACS to bring the gap to within 5% of that required to improve accuracy. Some units may allow only a single resection depth for LASIK and may not be usable for other applications.

Pneumatic Fixation (Suction) Ring(s)

Microkeratomes come with one adjustable or a set of perilimbal suction rings that vary in height, attach to the globe by suction, and allow for variable corneal protrusion through their central aperture (see Fig. 19-7). They deliver suction to the globe via tubing from the control unit's vacuum pump and serve to fixate the globe, to vary the diameter of the keratectomy, and to guide the microkeratome during the resection. As the ring height above the limbus increases, corneal protrusion and applanation are reduced, and the diameter of the resection is smaller. As LASIK has become the procedure of choice, only a single, low ring is necessary, one allowing a large-diameter resection, so that the flap will not be inadvertently ablated while accommodating large ablation diameters for hyperopic or toric corrections.

Applanation Lens(es)

To estimate the resection diameter prior to the actual cut, an applanation lens with a circular reticle of known diameter on its lower surface is used for comparison with the applanated corneal reflex (Fig. 19-8). A lens with appropriate reticle, depending on the diameter required (usually 8.5 mm for LASIK), is chosen and inserted into the suction ring. The lens may be clamped into the ring (ACS) or held down firmly against the ring during use for accurate measurement. The upper surface of the acrylic lens is a magnifier, and its flat lower surface lies in the plane of the cutting blade, thereby allowing prediction of the diameter that will be obtained. The cornea must be dry during use to prevent errors from a fluid meniscus. Should the measured diameter be incorrect, the ring is changed or adjusted upward or downward until the necessary diameter is applanated. In LASIK, the largest possible diameter is usually desired.

Applanation Tonometer

A smooth, regular keratectomy of desired diameter is best ensured when the IOP is elevated to 65 mm Hg or higher. A conical applanation tonometer with a circular reticle on its lower surface that corresponds to an IOP of 65 mm Hg is used to confirm this (Fig. 19-9). The upper convex surface acts as a magnifier. The lower surface is allowed to rest on the dry corneal dome and applanates the cornea a given amount, depending on the IOP. The area of the applanation reflex is compared to the area of the reticle. If the IOP is 65 mm Hg, the reflex will match the reticle. If the pressure is more than 65 mm Hg, the reflex is smaller. If the IOP is less, the reflex is larger.

Low IOP while the suction ring in place is frequently caused by conjunctival chemosis resulting from ring placement. Chemosis may be manually reduced by compressive posterior stroking with a dull instrument or by withdrawal of any fluid with a very fine needle. In rare cases, a retrobulbar injection of normal saline solution (not anesthetic, which would interfere with patient fixation in LASIK), or a peritomy, with application of the ring to the sclera may help. If the IOP remains inadequate, it is best to abort the procedure because a thin, small, or irregular flap may be obtained, which could lead to an eccentric ablation or result in ablation of the flap.

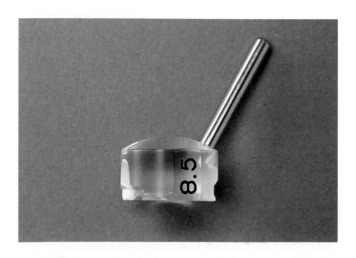

FIGURE 19-8.   *Barraquer applanation lens.*

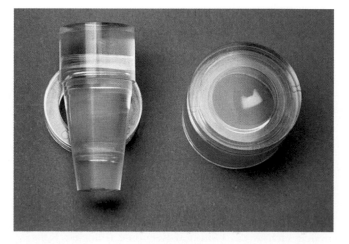

FIGURE 19-9.   *Barraquer applanation tonometer.*

Control Unit

The control unit provides a source of direct current for operation of the microkeratome and has a suction pump to provide a vacuum for the suction ring. It usually has foot pedals for independent operation of these two functions. The microkeratome advance pedal may have two positions, one for forward and one for reverse translation (ACS).

Miscellaneous

Most units include assorted tools and wrenches to assist in setup, and may come with an antidesiccation chamber in case a free cap is obtained, a reference marker, and a spatula. An optical scope to measure the cutting gap is optional.

Ultrasonic Pachymeter

Pachymetry is a very important part of LRK, both before and during surgery. An ultrasonic unit should be used, and it is advantageous that it be able to take very thin readings, so that the flap can be measured directly.

Computer

Although a computer is used during LASIK for laser input, nomograms are invariably used for the remainder of LRK procedures. Nomograms provide the surgeon with the diameters and depths of resections and base plates, if applicable, to be used to achieve the desired refractive correction.

Laser

LASIK requires a laser capable of tissue ablation. To date, all studies have employed ultraviolet (UV)-wavelength photoablation lasers, either excimer or solid state. Any UV laser can be used, and in the future infrared lasers, such as the erbium : yttrium–aluminum–garnet (YAG), may also find application. The laser's microscope should have a working distance of at least 5 inches to accommodate the microkeratome. A laser with low fluence or a small spot reduces the acoustic shock waves at the endothelial level and may increase safety. Most, though not all, lasers are capable of correcting astigmatism. A laser with an active eye tracker could potentially add safety to the procedure, as the patient's fixation during LASIK may be impaired.

PREOPERATIVE EVALUATION

Soft contact lens wearers should remove their lenses at least 2 weeks prior to the baseline examination, and gas-permeable and hard [polymethyl methacrylate (PMMA)]-lens wearers should remove their lenses for 3 weeks. With rigid-lens wearers, stability of the refraction should be documented by two refractions at least 1 week apart where the spherical and astigmatic components demonstrate stability within 0.25 D.

A complete history is obtained and ophthalmologic examination is performed and includes uncorrected and best-corrected distance and near visual acuities and a dilated retinal examination, as myopic refractive patients may exhibit retinal pathology. Any pathology in the posterior pole, such as macular degeneration, lacquer cracks, and Fuchs' spot, should be documented. Other tests to be performed include a cycloplegic refraction to accurately determine the refractive error. Many surgeons base the surgery on the manifest refraction for myopic procedures, while others use the cycloplegic refraction. The cycloplegic refraction will ensure that the patient was not accommodating. If a significant discrepancy exists between the manifest and cycloplegic refractions, the manifest refraction should be rechecked. For high corrections, it is important to measure the vertex distance of the refraction to properly assess the refractive error. The cycloplegic refraction is important for hyperopic corrections, and surgery is often based on the cycloplegic refraction. If the visual acuity is subnormal, one should determine the etiology, and one may consider laser interferometry or potential acuity measurements to determine the visual potential, to properly inform the patient of the postoperative prognosis.

Keratometry is useful to determine any regular or irregular astigmatism or keratoconus. Computerized videokeratography is useful to determine any corneal irregularities or asymmetries, which may be the only sign of early keratoconus, to assist in the placement of astigmatic incisions, and to follow any irregularities thought to have been induced by contact lens wear.

The palpebral aperture should be checked and found to be of sufficient size to accommodate the suction ring. The lids should be checked for signs of blepharitis or infection. Conjunctival adhesions or other abnormalities should be noted, as these can interfere with suction ring placement. Tonometry is important to detect glaucoma. Patients with borderline high or elevated IOP may exhibit an enhanced response to HLK or even postoperative instability.

Pachometry is very important in LRK, as the depth of the tissue resection in some procedures and the minimal requisite thickness (approximately 250 μm) of the posterior corneal layer postoperatively, to maintain stability, are related to the initial corneal thickness. In cases of high correction, a reduced ablation diameter or multizonal ablation is being evaluated. If the pachometry value is less than 450 μm, approximately, LRK is usually not performed. If the pachometry value is less than 525 μm, a 130- rather than 160-μm flap should be considered.

An axial length measurement is useful in investigational studies attempting to document postoperative stability. Endothelial cell counts may be evaluated before performing LASIK on patients who have had prior surgery, such as penetrating keratoplasty, in whom the endothelial cell count may be reduced, and when evaluating new laser technologies.

Lastly, and most importantly, during the informed-consent process the patient should be given detailed information regarding the risks and benefits, other available modalities of correction, and the typical postoperative course, both short term and long term. The patient should be informed of the relative percentages of success, the time course of visual recovery, the nature and incidence of common complications, the possible effects of postoperative presbyopia, the possibility that surgery may be aborted due to an inadequate keratectomy or laser failure, and the fact that optical aids or enhancement surgery may be needed following surgery, along with their timing.

SURGICAL PROCEDURES

In this section, the techniques of LASIK, the procedure most commonly performed, KMIS, and HLK are described. In most countries, laser technology is available and KMIS and HLK have been replaced by LASIK.

In the United States, LRK is usually performed unilaterally, allowing the obvious advantages of safety and normal function of the fellow eye until the surgical eye is rehabilitated. If the surgery was uncomplicated and the postoperative corneal topography is satisfactory, one may anticipate a full recovery of vision and perform surgery on the second eye within days to weeks. Unilateral surgery does have disadvantages, however, such as inconvenience and added costs. There is increasing interest in performing simultaneous bilateral surgery, especially with LASIK, and the surgeon's experience along with the patient's desires and needs will determine the most suitable course of action for each patient.

All LRK procedures are performed as outpatient surgery, usually with the patient under topical anesthesia. Though the procedures are ostensibly easy to perform, the surgeon and staff must be well trained and practiced in these techniques. It is best that the surgeon have considerable corneal experience with techniques such as radial and astigmatic keratotomy and lamellar and penetrating keratoplasty to perform LRK well. Enhancement and combined surgery, along with management of complications, demand these capabilities.

Laser In Situ Keratomileusis

In LASIK a microkeratome creates a superficial, nasally hinged lamellar flap, approximately 130 to 160 μm thick and 8 to 10 mm in diameter. Initially, the keratectomy was a complete resection of a free lamellar cap. A hinged flap is now used routinely, because it provides advantages such as prevention of loss or inversion, less trauma, easier alignment, shorter procedure time, and preservation of some of the corneal anterior nerve net. The distal 1 mm of the resection, approximately, is left incomplete, leaving the lamellar flap fixated by a tag of tissue. This flap is reflected over the nasal aspect of the globe to allow access to the stromal bed for the second step, laser ablation. The flap is then replaced.

The hinged flap technique increases the safety of the sutureless technique, while the thinner anterior resection contributes to increased corneal stability postoperatively. A potential disadvantage of ablating the stromal bed, however, is that laser energy is delivered deeper into the corneal tissue than it is with surface PRK. However, this has not been associated with levels of endothelial cell loss to cause concern if surgery maintains at least 250 μm of tissue in the posterior layers. Each manufacturer's laser, commercially or individually developed, should be individually shown to be safe in this respect, as each laser differs in beam dynamics, repetition rate, and energy density.

Experience has shown that LASIK algorithms may differ from those used for surface PRK, and they are still undergoing development. Further, each laser model is characterized by its own variance between these two algorithms, and they must be independently determined by investigation. One reason for this variance is the lower ablation rate of the deeper stroma due to a higher level of hydration. Increased hydration most likely plays a role in the genesis of central islands, also seen following LASIK.

Because broad laser beams, associated with greater acoustic shock, are known to produce central islands, in both PRK and LASIK, a scanning spot laser with low fluence may be advantageous, as scanning spot lasers are not associated with central islands. With broad-beam lasers, the surgeon must be aware of the possibility of central islands when optic zones larger than 5.0 mm are used and of the possibility of visual symptoms when optic zones smaller than 6.0 mm are used. As the refractive correction increases, the ablation zone may need to be made smaller in diameter to limit the depth of the ablation. This may result in visual symptoms in darkened environments or reduced contrast sensitivity if corrections too high are attempted. A method to maximize ablation diameter and minimize ablation depth is to use multizonal ablation, whereby the total correction is partitioned into two, three, or even many zones of varying diameter. Prospective studies, however, need to be done to conclusively demonstrate the advantages and disadvantages of new approaches such as this in this rapidly developing procedure. It is important to remember that the results obtained with one laser may not apply to others, as lasers vary in beam profile, edge treatment, and so on.

Preoperative

Lamellar surgery should be performed in as clean an environment as possible, to minimize foreign bodies in the interface. Care must be taken to avoid any contact of instruments with cloth or fiber products, to minimize foreign bodies. During surgery the surgeon must avoid contact of the intrastromal area with any instrument that has had contact with the epithelium, to prevent seeding into the interface. The surgeon should use powderless or no gloves. Before LASIK, it is essential that the laser room and laser be prepared, the laser calibrated, and the patient's data entered into the laser's computer. If an astigmatic correction is to be performed, the axis is marked on the eye with the patient in the upright position. The axis is verified with the patient in the supine position and adjustments made if necessary. It is critical that the microkeratome be fully and accurately assembled and tested for performance before the procedure is started. This includes checking and inserting the blade and ensuring that the correct depth plate (usually 160 µm) is fully inserted, checking the blade gap with an optical scope if available and applicable, checking the stopper to prevent a free cap, and ensuring in a "dry run" that the head passes smoothly forward and back through the ring to be used.

The lids may be scrubbed if indicated but care must be taken not to chemically insult the conjunctiva. Oral or intravenous sedation or both may be used to allay anxiety. Topical antibiotics are often used prior to surgery, and sometimes a nonsteroidal anti-inflammatory agent is given. To center the suction ring more easily, which is critical, it is best not to dilate the pupil. Miotics should not be used as they may displace the pupil, cause conjunctival edema, or lower IOP, all of which interfere with the keratectomy. Topical anesthesia is obtained with several drops of 0.5% proparacaine hydrochloride, for example. Topical anesthetics are best given shortly before the keratectomy and in conservative doses, as they are toxic to the epithelium. A traumatized epithelium either from overdosage of anesthetic or from being anesthetized too long preoperatively can result in an epithelial defect from the keratectomy or delayed visual recovery.

The usual surgical preparation is carried out and care is taken that chemical agents do not enter the eye, which could cause conjunctival chemosis and poor suction ring adherence. The fellow eye is best covered with an opaque shield. The patient's head is aligned beneath the laser's surgical microscope.

Corneal Flap

The cul-de-sac and fornices may be well irrigated to remove secretions, and the eye is draped to prevent exposure of the lashes, which could interfere with microkeratome passage. The bulbar conjunctiva may be further anesthetized, if desired, by application of an anesthetic-moistened surgical spear. A speculum is placed to provide a wide clearance for passage of the microkeratome, and central pachymetry is performed. Pachymetry is always performed without the suction ring on the eye, as quickly as possible after any resection, and without the addition of fluids, which can hydrate the cornea and give false readings.

Surgery begins by using a dye-coated marker to imprint the reference marks on the corneal epithelium. A marker commonly used has two concentric circles, one large (10 mm) and one small (3.5 mm), that assist in centering the suction ring with the pupil, and a pararadial line that will later assist in repositioning the flap.

Suction Ring

The surgeon next places the perilimbal suction ring in proper orientation, depending on the unit, and centers it well, using the epithelial marks as a guide, before applying suction. If access to the globe is not adequate while the ring is in place, the speculum may be depressed slightly to further expose the globe, or in rare cases a retrobulbar injection of saline solution may be used to further proptose the globe. The diameter of the proposed resection, typically 8 to 10 mm, is confirmed by inserting the applanation lens with an appropriate-diameter reticle into the ring and comparing the applanated corneal reflex to the reticle. The cornea must be dry during use of the applanation lens and tonometer, or faulty readings will be obtained. To adjust the resection diameter, the ring is rotated on a thread (ACR) while on the eye, being adjusted up or down until the desired diameter is applanated. Currently, most microkeratomes use a single LASIK ring that is not adjustable. The surgeon should confirm that the vacuum gauge of the unit reads at its maximal value (typically in the range of 22–28 mmHg) as determined earlier by digital occlusion of the ring aperture with the suction on. This indicates maximal potential, and the intraoperative reading, if less, may indicate less than adequate ring fixation, which could result in an irregular keratectomy. The reason should be sought and rectified.

Usually, for LASK, the largest available diameter is preferred to prevent inadvertent laser ablation of the flap, accommodate large-diameter ablations for hyperopic and toric corrections, and provide flexibility should the flap have been somewhat decentered. For good success, hyperopic and, with some lasers, toric LASIK procedures necessitate a larger ablation diameter than does myopic LASIK. The maximal depth of the ablation is in the periphery in hyperopic corrections, and the ablation profile must then be returned back to the peripheral surface, necessitating a peripheral blend zone, to allow for good wound coaptation and anterior corneal contour. For toric ablations, some lasers provide a significant taper along one of the axes to assist wound healing.

Tonometry

The weight of the applanation tonometer is allowed to rest on the dry corneal dome. If the IOP is 65 mmHg or higher, the diameter of the applanated area will be equal to or less than that enclosed by the reticle on the lower surface of the tonometer, which corresponds to a pressure of 65 mmHg. If the IOP is inadequate, chemosis should be sought and treated and, as a last resort, a retrobulbar injection of 3 to 4 mL of normal saline solution or a 360-degree peritomy, to allow ring application directly to the sclera, should be considered. If the IOP is still not adequate, the procedure should be aborted. The surgeon should not leave the suction applied to the globe for longer than approximately 3 minutes at any one time, to avoid complications in the posterior pole.

Keratectomy

After the parameters of diameters and IOP have been satisfied, the cornea is moistened with balanced salt solution and the microkeratome is inserted carefully and gently into the ring. The microkeratome is advanced by stepping on the foot pedal, if automated, or by manually passing it across the cornea. It is then reversed in similar fashion, being careful not to tear the delicate flap. Microkeratomes are typically passed from the temporal side of the cornea toward the nasal side and are then withdrawn, automatically or manually, in the opposite direction, leaving a hinged flap. The surgeon performs the keratectomy using the low magnification of the laser's microscope.

The microkeratome base plate used in creating the flap should provide a cut approximately 160 μm thick. For low corrections in LASIK, thicker flaps can be considered to facilitate handling. It is most important to ensure that the microkeratome is not used without a base plate (if the unit uses a base plate) as the anterior chamber may be inadvertently entered, with catastrophic results.

If the initial corneal thickness minus the sum of the planned ablation depth plus the 160 μm is higher than 250 μm, approximately, a 130-μm flap is created to maintain adequate tissue (250 μm) in the posterior layer postoperatively. Some surgeons, as a rule of thumb, use 50% of the initial corneal thickness as the minimal postoperative thickness to be maintained. It is important in LASIK to maintain an adequate layer of posterior corneal tissue, which if too thin may result in instability or ectasia. It also provides a margin of safety against endothelial damage secondary to laser-induced acoustic shock waves.

Surgeons differ with respect to desired hinge size. Larger hinges add stability and ease realignment, especially for inexperienced surgeons, whereas smaller hinges lessen the possibility of ablation of the flap. Large-diameter flaps may allow both advantages.

The suction ring is removed and the hinged flap is carefully reflected nasally using a thin cannula. The flap and stromal bed are examined for any irregularities in thickness, shape, or surface quality. Pachymetry is used to determine flap or central corneal thickness, allowing calculation of flap thickness. Should the flap be inadequately resected, grossly decentered, or obviously incompatible with a good clinical result, it is immediately replaced and surgery aborted. Surgery may be repeated at the same depth after several months. If the flap is resected completely in the form of a free cap, the surgeon may place it into a sealed antidesiccation chamber to prevent dehydration and loss during the next step of the procedure of leave it in the microkeratome head to minimize handling. Free caps, which have a low incidence, may result in corneas with a small diameter, if the IOP is low or if the stop is not set appropriately. With free caps, it is important that the surgeon not confuse the epithelial and stromal sides of the cap and that it be replaced correctly.

Laser Ablation

The cul-de-sacs are dried to remove any fluid. Depending on which, if any, eye tracker is used, the tracker may be engaged with the flap in position while the patient is instructed to fixate on the laser's fixation target. When this is confirmed, the flap is carefully reflected nasally onto the limbus with a fine instrument such as a cyclodialysis spatula and ablation is performed. When an eye tracker is not used, some surgeons complete the ablation with the suction ring in place but with the vacuum disengaged. This allows the surgeon to facilitate centration, as the patient's fixation during LASIK is impaired, partly by the reduced optical quality of the keratectomized bed and partly by the retinal hypoxia caused by the high IOP during the keratectomy.

The dry stromal lamellar bed is exposed to the laser beam such that the desired dioptric correction is imposed. Should a technical problem arise with the laser, the flap is replaced and kept moist until the laser is again ready. During LASIK, unlike KMIS, a lenticular-shaped resection is created, as in surface PRK. The surgeon, using midrange magnification, monitors the helium-neon beams, if available, to ensure continued fixation and, with large ablation diameters as in hyperopia, or with only moderately sized flaps, may cover the flap with a spatula to prevent it from being ablated. Otherwise, one may induce irregular astigmatism or even perforate the flap. Depending on the laser used, significant hydration may appear centrally as ablation proceeds; such hydration is caused in part by a broad beam, and by laser-induced acoustic shock waves acting on the deeper stroma, which has a higher degree of hydration. When this occurs, surgeons may pause the ablation and use a spatula or cannula from time to time to mechanically express the fluid from the central cornea.

Reconstruction

The flap and bed are examined for any foreign bodies, which may be removed with a moist cellulose microsurgical sponge (Merocel), being careful not to deposit further foreign bodies. Some surgeons irrigate the bed at this point to remove any debris or epithelial cells. On the other hand, others irrigate the bed under the flap, after it has been replaced. The stromal side of the flap is made wet with balanced salt solution. It is replaced atop the bed by inserting an instrument such as a cyclodialysis under the flap at the hinge, and in smooth, complete motion it is carefully reflected back onto the bed. A narrow-gauge cannula may be inserted under the flap and filtered balanced salt solution used to irrigate the interface.

The flap is carefully allowed to set into place as the surgeon, using the previously placed linear reference mark, ensures that it is properly aligned and seated without wrinkles or folds and that it is concentric with the edge of the keratectomy. Flap replacement is a very important step to minimize irregular astigmatism postoperatively and demands full attention. The delicate flap must never be grasped with a sharp forceps, as edge damage can occur and cause postoperative sequelae. A moist cellulose microsurgical sponge is used to help seat the flap with a gentle motion, and it is left unsutured. The presence of striae, however, is an indication that the flap is not aligned properly, and it should be lifted and realigned. The gutter around the flap may be dried with the sponge, but the epithelium should be kept moist to prevent a postoperative epithelial defect. The flap may be allowed to air dry for up to 5 minutes.

Flap adherence is demonstrated by depressing the adjacent cornea with a smooth forceps such that striae are induced and seen to radiate into the area of the flap, affecting the entire circumference, without causing edge elevation (striae test). Topical medications such as an antibiotic, a corticosteroid, non-steroidal antiinflammatory drop, and viscous tears are instilled and the speculum carefully removed without dislodging the flap. Ointments should not be used after lamellar surgery, as they can cloud the interface. The lids are moved over the flap to demonstrate that they do not displace it (blink test). Free caps can usually be left unsutured if the striae and blink tests demonstrate adherence. In this case the lids are carefully taped together to prevent displacement, and bandage lenses and patches are avoided. If not adherent, the cap is sutured with an 8-bite antitorsion suture. The eye is covered with a shield and the patient requested to avoid manipulating the shield and eye. Some surgeons check the patient after a short period to ensure good flap position prior to discharge. The patient is instructed to return for evaluation the following day.

Keratomileusis In Situ (or Myopic ALK)

In KMIS, the microkeratome creates a superficial, nasally hinged lamellar flap, 130 to 160 μm thick and 7.50 to 8.00 mm in diameter, and the flap is reflected over the nasal part of the globe to allow access for the second, refractive, resection. The microkeratome makes a second resection within the confines of the flap and the tissue is discarded. The flap is then replaced.

Preoperative
The preoperative preparations and examinations are the same as those described for LASIK.

Corneal Flap
The creation of the corneal flap is as described for LASIK with the exception that clinical studies in the past used smaller flaps, 7.25 to 7.50 mm in diameter. Recently, suction rights that allow larger-diameter flaps were designed for LASIK surgery. In principle, such rings and larger-diameter flaps could be used for KMIS also, though data are not available.

Refractive Modification Step
Suction Ring   The microkeratome is prepared for the second resection by inserting the base plate indicated by the

nomogram. The gap can be measured and adjusted with shim plates if necessary. The suction ring is again placed on the eye in the imprinted groove made by the first resection, centered with the 10-mm circular imprint, and adjusted upward to provide the smaller resection diameter dictated by the nomogram. It is important to note that it is very difficult to center the suction ring in a new position for this second, critical cut. It is most important, therefore, that the first application was well centered. If it was decentered, the optical resection will likely be decentered, and this could lead to visual symptoms postoperatively. An applanation lens with a reticle of appropriate diameter is used to ensure the resection diameter, which typically ranges between 3.5 and 5.0 mm. The diameter and depth of this second resection determine the refractive correction.

Tonometry
The applanation tonometer confirms that the IOP is at least 65 mm Hg. If not, measures are taken as described earlier for LASIK.

Keratectomy
The second microkeratome resection is performed concentric to and within the confines of the first. This second resection produces a lamellar depression of constant central thickness (that is, not lenticular) and peripheral taper in the stromal bed. Repeat central pachymetry allows calculation of this resection thickness.

Reconstruction

The flap is then replaced as described for LASIK and irrigation carried out under the flap to remove any epithelial cells or debris. The edge of the flap is dried with a cellulose sponge while the central corneal epithelium is kept moist with a drop of balanced salt solution. The striae and blink tests are performed as already described. A nonsteroidal anti-inflammatory drop may be applied along with topical antibiotic and corticosteroid, and the eye covered with a protective shield. The postoperative care is described later.

HYPEROPIC LAMELLAR KERATOTOMY (OR HYPEROPIC ALK)

HLK is performed similarly to the initial steps of LASIK and KMIS, already described. A nomogram indicating a range of hyperopic corrections provides the required diameter of resection. It is critical that the corneal thickness be accurately measured preoperatively and confirmed intraoperatively. The depth of the resection is calculated to be 70% of the measured corneal thickness in previously unoperated eyes and 60% in eyes that have undergone RK, as there is greater instability in a weakened cornea. The surgeon chooses a base plate that will provide the necessary depth. The gap is measured and shims added, if necessary, to bring the gap to within ±5% of the calculated value.

Microkeratomes will more often make thinner rather than thicker cuts due to reduced ring adherence to the globe, inadequate IOP, poor blade quality, and so on. In some eyes with steep corneas or in eyes where the IOP induced by the ring is very high, resection thickness may be slightly increased compared to the expected value.

After the suction ring is applied, it is adjusted, using the applanation lens whose reticle corresponds to the diameter of resection indicated by the nomogram, until the desired diameter (typically 5.6–6.6 mm) is applanated. The microkeratome is inserted into the ring, and the resection is completed as a hinged flap. The bed is examined and the flap replaced. The bed and flap are left wet before the flap is replaced. The flap is left unsutured after adequate adherence is demonstrated with the striae and blink tests. An 8-bite antitorsion suture may be used if needed.

POSTOPERATIVE CARE

The postoperative course of LRK is straightforward. At surgery a shield is placed, and when there is free cap the lids are also taped. Pain is usually minimal, except for some foreign body sensation for 1 to 2 days, and is easily controlled with a mild pain reliever. An epithelial defect is unusual when the patient is examined on the first postoperative day. If present, a bandage lens and nonsteroidal anti-inflammatory drugs may be used. The eye should not be patched, however, to avoid displacing the cap. The uncorrected acuity is checked and is often 20/40 or better. The flap should be in place without striae, folds, or displacement, and the interface should be without significant haze or edema. Small debris may be noted in the interface, but is usually of no consequence and need not be removed. If the flap is displaced or has wrinkles or folds, it must be repositioned. Should a free cap be found lost, or displaced and shrunken, a homoplastic cap can be used to reconstruct the cornea, after irrigation and debridement of the bed to remove any epithelium. The surgeon must be experienced with homoplastic lamellar surgery, however. Following LASIK or KMIS, some surgeons will simply allow the stromal bed to epithelialize over in such cases. The smoother the bed, the less haze and scarring might be expected. Should the result be unsatisfactory, further laser or homoplastic surgery may be performed. Following HLK, however, the cornea must be reconstructed to maintain the integrity of the thinned cornea.

Patients may return to normal activity as soon as is convenient, and a few special precautions including emphasizing that the eye should not be rubbed, squeezed, or manipulated for 1 to 2 weeks if not longer, need to be taken. A shield may be used at night for 7 to 10 days and protective sunglasses used during the day, to reduce glare and to prevent inadvertent rubbing or foreign bodies. Patients should be advised that their near vision may be impaired and that they may have some glare at night in the early postoperative period. The eye is usually treated with a topical antibiotic and corticosteroid for 5 to 7 days, along with viscous lubricating drops for several days. Ointments should not be used. The role of corticosteroids in LASIK surgery has not been fully evaluated. In my experience, the intrastromal wound-healing process is usually minimal but, if significant, the eye may be treated with steroids for a longer period. Regression is more often due to epithelial hyperplasia or possibly from the IOP acting on the thinned posterior layer. Neither situation would be expected to be ameliorated with steroids. The patient is usually next seen in 1 to 2 weeks, and at 1, 3, 6, and 12 months postoperatively.

Any sutures are removed in approximately 1 week. In the early postoperative period the surgeon must observe for epithelialization of the interface, which typically manifests after 7 to 10 days. If it appears to be significant—being central, causing irregular astigmatism, visual symptoms, or visual loss—it must be debrided. This can be done by lifting the flap and gently debriding the flap and bed, or by inserting a bent irrigating cannula or dulled needle to remove it with irrigation.

Visual recovery is rapid following LRK, and patients usually have a dramatic improvement in their uncorrected vision on the first day. Typically by 4 to 6 weeks one will have an accurate estimate of the final refraction and uncorrected and best-corrected acuities, although higher myopes can still show significant regression thereafter. At the 1-month visit, if undercorrection and unsatisfactory uncorrected acuity exist, the patient may be told that enhancement surgery will be needed.

Although LASIK adds the step of a lamellar keratectomy across the visual axis to the laser ablation of PRK, visual rehabilitation is typically more rapid than following surface PRK, because of the presence of Bowman's membrane and a reduced would-healing response. Also, postoperative pain is greatly reduced compared to surface PRK. The postoperative management of LRK is less than for PRK, where patients must be closely monitored for possible steroid-induced glaucoma, haze, and regression.

Enhancement surgery following LASIK can usually be performed after the third month. In lower myopes, the refraction may not have changed much between the first- and third-month visits, and the patient may then be treated. Usually, this is accomplished by lifting the flap and performing a second ablation to correct the residual refractive error (34). The surgeon must carefully identify the edge of the flap and use an instrument such as a Suarez spreader to carefully separate the layers, held together primarily in the periphery. In high myopes, regression may continue 6 months or longer. The refractive error should be followed and allowed to stabilize before retreatment. In the interim, soft or disposable lenses may be fit, though sometimes with difficulty because of the flat central cornea. Rigid lenses are best avoided during the first 4 to 6 postoperative months, as they may induce significant regression in some patients.

Three months after KMIS, enhancement surgery is usually performed for residual myopia or astigmatism with a keratotomy procedure, although I have also used surface PRK with good results. Treatment of secondary hyperopia is more of a challenge. One may consider a transepithelial hyperopic surface PRK, to avoid dislodging the flap with manual removal, or intrastromal ablation, but these approaches have not been studied. Hyperopic ablations require larger ablation diameters for best results. If the initial flap was of relatively small diameter or decentered somewhat, this approach may be made more challenging. The weakened cornea following HLK is also a challenge with respect to enhancement surgery. Astigmatic keratotomy may reduce astigmatism, but the application of enhancement procedures in this group of patients has not been evaluated.

COMPLICATIONS

Considering the complexity of LRK, the reported complications, although varied, usually do not compromise visual acuity in the majority of patients. The known complications of LRK are given in Table 19-2. Nevertheless, LRK is very demanding with respect to surgical skill and attention to details. The learning curve is quite steep and cannot be avoided. Complication rates as high as 25% have been reported for beginning LRK surgeons, but, with practice and persistent dedication, rates should eventually be lower than 5%. Complications are in large part related to the keratectomy, by far the most difficult and critical part of the procedure, and flap or cap management. One should be very familiar with the possible complications of LRK and either be in a position to treat them, should they occur, or have on hand an experienced lamellar surgeon to whom complications may be referred.

Intraoperative

Intraoperative complications are usually related to the keratectomy. These include a flap that is of wrong diameter, too thin or too thick, free, irregular, or only partially completed. Careful attention to all the details of the steps in creating the flap, such as determining the diameter and pressure, should prevent most of these complications. One should be aware that flat corneas, less than 41 D, have a tendency to produce free caps, and the stop of the microkeratome might be adjusted to account for this. However, there is always the possibility of an imperfect blade or microkeratome jam or failure during the cut. If the flap is inadequate or one is in doubt, it may be prudent to replace the flap and perform surgery again after 3 months, as either LASIK or surface PRK if the surgeon believes a problem with the keratectomy may occur again. If the bed is irregular, its modification could result in irregular astigmatism postoperatively, as the flap-bed relationship will have been disturbed. There usually are no sequelae after replacement of flaps or caps.

Table 19-2. Complications of Keratomileusis In Situ, Hyperopic Lamellar Keratotomy, and LASIK

Intraoperative
 Microkeratome related
  Incomplete resection, microkeratome failure
  Eccentric resection
  Resection too thin or too thick
  Irregular resection and/or surface
  Free cap
  Perforation into eye
  Traumatized flap
 Laser ablation
  Corneal perforation
  Laser failure
Postoperative
 Optical
  Subjective symptoms
  Reduction of best-corrected vision
  Inaccuracy—undercorrection, overcorrection
  Regular astigmatism
  Irregular astigmatism
  Regression of effect
 Conjunctiva/cornea
  Lost or displaced cap
  Irregularly seated flap/cap
  Subconjunctival hemorrhage
  Epithelial defect, erosion
  Filamentary keratitis
  Refractile deposits in interface
  Foreign bodies in interface
  Epithelium in interface
  Necrosis of Bowman's membrane
  Stromal melt
  Keratitis—inflammatory, infectious
  Haze of scarring of interface
  Ectasia
  Central island
  Endothelial cell loss
 Intraocular
  Fuchs' spot
  Retinal vessel occlusion—branch vessel, central retinal artery

Corneal perforation during surgery occurs only rarely, and its incidence should be reduced with improvements in technique and instrumentation. It can result in expulsion of the ocular contents with catastrophic consequences. It is avoided by ensuring that an adequate depth plate is fully inserted into the microkeratome before use. Because two microkeratome resections are performed in KMIS, there is greater potential risk, as the microkeratome depth plate must be changed in the middle of the procedure, usually by the surgical assistant. Should the laser ablation perforate the cornea, the aqueous would attenuate the beam and prevent further damage.

Decentration of the laser ablation or second resection may result in visual symptoms as the pupil dilates over the untreated area, or from induced irregular astigmatism. This can be minimized by attention to centration during the procedure. There are several novel approaches for correcting this difficult problem, such as repeat ablation in an asymmetric fashion and asymmetric surface PTK, and I am working with customized irregular ablation using topographic data and small-spot scanning. Regardless of the magnitude of the problem I have found that, ultimately, symptoms can be eliminated in many patients by a deep lamellar keratoplasty with the microkeratome, with subsequent refractive surgery as indicated. In almost all patients, penetrating keratoplasty is avoidable.

Postoperative

Patients may experience a variety of symptoms following LRK. These include glare, halos, and multiple images, which are especially associated with small or decentered resections, and a reduction in contrast sensitivity or night vision. In a multicenter study of KMIS, 29% of patients experienced light sensitivity, 62% night glare, and 40% day glare (47). Occasionally, following KMIS, patients may experience their vision as less than desirable and revert to contact lens wear, despite excellent acuity. These symptoms are in large part caused by small or eccentric optic zones, large pupils, and irregular astigmatism. In some patients following LASIK, the symptoms may be reduced by a second procedure using a larger ablation diameter, if there is some residual refractive error. Although the second resection in KMIS is significantly smaller than the ablation zone typically used in LASIK, the effective optic zone, determined by videokeratography postoperatively, is increased in KMIS and reduced in LASIK, compared to what might be expected. This is because of the geometry of the area modified, which in KMIS results in an effective increase as the Bowman's membrane bends over the edge of the trough. In LASIK, there is a smooth and tapered-edge contour that may fail to alter the overlying Bowman's membrane effectively at the zonal margin.

On the first day or two following surgery, an epithelial defect may be seen. Also, as the flap is not as securely held down by an epithelial cover as it soon will be, a free cap or dislocated flap may be seen. Or, one may observe folds, wrinkles, or striae in the flap. These should be repaired early as described previously.

Infection is an infrequent complication of LRK, but does occur. Meticulous care of instrumentation and good technique should minimize infection. When it occurs, it is more likely to be at the interface. One should treat any infection aggressively with broad-spectrum antibiotics. If necessary, the flap may be removed to allow access to the bed for diagnosis or treatment. The bed can be left to heal and the cornea repaired later with further surgery as indicated.

More common complications of concern are epithelialization of the interface and irregular astigmatism. Epithelium may gain access to the interface by seeding during the microkeratome pass, by ingrowth from the periphery, or by direct spread from a transected radial incision. Small patches of epithelium in the peripheral interface are of little or no concern. However, if the epithelium is more centrally located and decreases vision either directly or by producing irregular astigmatism, it should be debrided. Larger patches of epithelium (2–3 mm) may result in melting of the overlying stroma, and should be removed early. If in doubt, the surgeon can closely follow the patient, observing the refraction, acuity, topography, and slit-lamp appearance. With experience, it is rather clear when to intervene. This is done by reflection of the flap and careful, sharp mechanical debridement of the bed and flap. The condition should be treated early to avoid permanent mild opacification of the stroma and, if so treated, rarely results in a reduction of visual acuity. If the flap has become irregular because of a melt, it will sometimes regularize by epithelial fill-in. In other cases, the surgeon must decide whether to replace the flap with a cap of homoplastic lamellar tissue or simply let the bed epithelialize over and manage the eye thereafter as one would an eye that has undergone surface PRK.

The major concern with LRK is irregular astigmatism. Although some slight irregularity is common, it causes a reduction in visual acuity in only a small percentage of patients. Reductions in acuity are significantly higher with KMIS than with LASIK, where the laser creates the crucial optical cut with submicron accuracy, unlike the microkeratome. Nevertheless, if the ablation in LASIK is decentered, visual loss secondary to irregular astigmatism may result. Newer lasers with eye trackers may reduce such problems. Reported series of KMIS noted an incidence of up to 14% visual loss attributable to irregular astigmatism (1,2,9,30,47). When visual loss occurs, it is usually mild, occurs at finer levels of acuity, and is at most of several lines. Subjective symptoms, however, caused by an irregular refracting surface may be more bothersome to the patient than a small loss of acuity. As the best-corrected acuity is frequently increased after LRK for myopia, owing to elimination of image minification, some patients without an improvement in acuity may harbor minor corneal irregularities that cause visual symptoms. Most patients with severe, irregular astigmatism may be treated by flap adjustment or replacement, if indicated, or by a deep lamellar keratoplasty to restore the cornea to its normal thickness and to regularize the anterior contour. Refractive surgery can then be repeated at a later date. In the future, such patients may be treated with a customized ablation using a small-spot laser.

More long-term postoperative complications are overcorrection, undercorrection, and induced astigmatism. Undercorrection may manifest early or result from regression, especially in higher myopes. The causes of inaccuracy are many, and include errors in planning and instrumentation setup, defective surgical technique, microkeratome or laser algorithm inaccuracy, hydration and dehydration factors, and epithelial modulation of the final result. The accuracy of LASIK in particular has been improving significantly with dedicated investigation.

Residual refractive errors can be treated with enhancement surgery. In the interim, the patient can be fit with a disposable contact lens to improve performance. As described earlier, undercorrections following LASIK can be treated by lifting the flap and ablating a second time. Following LASIK the flap can be lifted as late as 1 year and further laser ablation applied (34). When re-treating with the laser, one may need to augment the desired correction somewhat, because the ablation rate of the bed may be slightly reduced by the wound-healing process. One may also perform surface PRK, which brings with it a prolonged postoperative course, or RK. If RK is used, one must ensure that accurate pachymetry is performed to avoid perforation of the cornea with an altered thickness profile.

Secondary hyperopia is more challenging to correct. Some surgeons have used holmium laser thermal keratoplasty successfully, hyperopic surface PRK, or a hyperopic ablation on the bed following lifting of the flap. Younger patients with accommodation may adapt to the situation, or after the second eye is operated on, a slight overcorrection in the first eye may not be as bothersome. Because the standard deviation increases as higher corrections are attempted, it may be best to err on the side of undercorrection and treat undercorrections with a second ablation rather than risk overcorrection.

There is typically some regression following LRK, including LASIK. The regression appears greater as the attempted correction increases, and high myopes can have regressions of 4 D or more in the first 6 months following surgery. However, one must pay careful attention to the pachymetry values, as the cause of the regression in the first place may be a mild ectasia of a too-thinned posterior corneal layer. Further ablation will worsen such a situation and should be avoided. Another cause of regression is epithelial hyperplasia. I have seen a relatively sudden regression of several diopters, often in one eye, develop after several years. The cause was diagnosed as epithelial hyperplasia, and it was treated by mechanical debridement of the central epithelium, with recovery of the initial result and lack of recurrence over the intermediate term. In rare cases, there may be haze and scar formation in the interface in aggressive healers, though this is of much lower incidence than after surface PRK. Such patients may be re-treated by ablation, preferably early after stabilization with steroids, to remove the new collagen.

After LASIK, as after surface PRK, central islands may be encountered frequently when broad-beam lasers have been used, and may result in visual symptoms, undercorrection, and visual loss. Some surgeons and laser manufacturers have developed central pretreatment protocols to reduce the incidence of central islands. Central islands may resolve to a lesser extent following LASIK than following surface PRK. Newer lasers using scanning beam technology appear to have eliminated this complication. Should a central island be of clinical significance, it may be treated by lifting the flap

and performing a small-diameter (2–3-mm) ablation at the island site.

The most disastrous complications following LRK are central retinal artery occlusion (only one known case, following myopic keratomileusis in which a retrobulbar injection was used), corneal perforation during the keratectomy, and infection. A central retinal artery occlusion may result from vasospasm or hemorrhage, if a retrobulbar injection is used. Currently, retrobulbar injection is used only if the IOP cannot be elevated adequately or inadequate physical access to the eye requires such as injection to proptose the eye.

OUTCOME

Although LRK has been performed for many years, there are, unfortunately, few published reports on KMIS and HLK despite many surgeons' having performed these techniques (1,2,9,15,18,22,24,47). However, there is a large body of scientific data now accumulating for LASIK, the procedure of choice. Studies to date demonstrated the superiority of LASIK over mechanical LRK with respect to subjective symptomatology, surgical accuracy, ability to treat astigmatism, and visual results for both myopia and low hyperopia. When evaluating these procedures and reading the literature, it is important for the reader to distinguish studies with and those without enhancement surgery, to properly ascertain the effects of the primary procedure alone.

Refractive Correction

The mean refractive change in a given series obviously depends on patient selection. Keratometry and topography often underestimate the refractive correction after myopic procedures but not hyperopic procedures. In a study of HLK for up to +5 D of hyperopia, 79% of the eyes were within −1.0 to +0.87 D of the intended correction (24).

Although refractive corrections well over 20 D have been reported following KMIS and LASIK, eyes with large corrections may have small optic zones, postoperative instability, or subjective symptoms. Very high corrections should be limited to patients with thick corneas and perhaps with reduced acuity. In general, many surgeons currently agree that the upper limit of myopic correction safely and reproducibly attainable with LRK, whether performed by KMIS or LASIK, is approximately 12 to 15 D, although some studies showed good success with higher corrections.

With respect to surgical accuracy, mean percentage corrections after LRK are frequently close to 100%, but inaccuracy remains apparent with nonlaser techniques, as evidenced by the standard deviations reported, which typically range from 20% to 30%, and the percentages of cases lying outside given refractive intervals. Studies of KMIS show 35% to 53% of eyes within ±1 D of the desired correction (15,22), and one study needed an eventual enhancement rate of 48% (15). Another series, with an enhancement rate of 77%, showed 76% of eyes within ±1 D of the intended correction (30). In the U.S. ALK study of KMIS in 1124 myopes, following enhancements the vision in 75% of eyes with up to 6 D of myopia was 20/40 or better uncorrected, decreasing to 66% in the −6 to −10 D group and 51% in the −10 to −20 D group (47). For 370 HLK procedures, 71% of eyes that were +1 to +4 D preoperatively had 20/40 or better uncorrected vision postoperatively, with 73% within ±1.50 D of the intended correction (47). The accuracy of the KMIS and HLK procedure is probably on the order of ±2 D.

Although many factors may contribute to an inaccuracy of KMIS and HLK, such as contact of tissue with air and fluid, complex instrumentation, and wound healing, it is the intrinsic inaccuracy of the microkeratome that is the major cause. KMIS has been plagued by undercorrection, primarily from the inability of the metal blade to cut as deeply as predicted in a given patient. In one study, 57% of the eyes had greater than 1 D of myopia with a mean residual myopia of −1.86 D (22). There is little question that LASIK can provide superior accuracy, although published LASIK studies were carried out while surgical algorithms were still being developed. Also, results may vary depending on the laser used. Early studies showed that up to 74% of eyes with up to 20 D of myopia are correctable to within ±1.0 D (28).

Astigmatism

Lamellar refractive surgery can induce both regular and irregular astigmatism, although the incidence of induced regular astigmatism appears to be low with good technique. Studies showed a mean increase of 0.4 to 0.5 D in regular astigmatism following KMIS (15,22). Following LASIK in one series, 8% of eyes reportedly had an induced cylinder of greater than 1 D (33). Common causes of regular and irregular astigmatism are an irregular keratectomy, irregular flap healing, eccentricity of the ablation, ablation of the flap, or epithelialization. Regular astigmatism may be treated after 3 months with a second ablation or keratotomy procedure.

A study of combined KMIS and arcuate keratotomy in the bed showed the ability to correct mild astigmatism, but the mean correction was only 29%, which is less efficacious than arcuate keratotomy performed alone (31). Whereas regular astigmatism is usually of little concern following KMIS, irregular astigmatism is of concern. One may find persistent irregular astigmatism in a small percentage of eyes following KMIS. Minor irregularities are discernible from the topography of many eyes following mechanical LRK and may cause a reduction in best-corrected visual acuity or a reduction in contrast sensitivity. Experience has shown that the risks of irregular astigmatism may be greater following mechanical surgery than LASIK, although one LASIK study reported an incidence of 6% (33).

Visual Results

Because there is little wound-healing response in the central cornea, visual recovery is rapid after all forms of LRK, especially LASIK, with patients frequently seeing 20/40 or better on the first postoperative day.

In a study of HLK for up to +5 D of hyperopia, 76% of eyes achieved 20/40 or better uncorrected acuity (24). However, 13% of the eyes lost one to three lines of best-corrected acuity.

Uncorrected acuity following KMIS is often unsatisfactory without enhancement. Studies showed 21% to 58% of eyes with 20/40 acuity or better before enhancement (15,22,47) and one study 86% 20/40 vision or better after enhancement, with a 77% enhancement rate (30). Following LASIK, 36% to 60% of eyes had 20/20 vision or better and 50% to 81% had 20/40 vision or better prior to enhancement (10,28).

It has been well documented that best-corrected visual acuity may improve following LRK when performed on eyes with subnormal vision. For example, a study of cryolathe keratomileusis showed an improvement in best-corrected acuity in more than 60% of the eyes (48). Usually, 20/20 or better preoperative vision will be regained postoperatively following LRK, especially LASIK, though in a small percentage of patients the vision may be reduced. In general, if the surgery was uncomplicated, one can expect the vision to return to its preoperative level. The major causes of minor reduction in visual acuity following LRK are irregular astigmatism and scarring following debridement of the interface for treatment of epithelialization. Following KMIS, 5% to 14% of eyes lose two to five lines of best-corrected acuity (15,22), and following LASIK the reported incidence is in the range of 3.6% to 21.0%, the latter being in a U.S. phase I study (12).

Stability

Stability of the refractive correction following LRK is usually attained early, although 15% of eyes or more may exhibit a regression of 0.50 D or more in the first year. During the first year after LASIK, up to a mean of 1.50 D of regression has been seen. Typically, when new-generation lasers without an initial hyperopic overshoot are used to correct myopia, the correction appears stable within 1 to 2 months, although there may be some slight adjustment over the first 6 months. The correction after KMIS also stabilizes quickly, though it is slightly more variable in this respect than LASIK. In one study of KMIS there was mean loss of correction of 2 D between 1 and 12 months (15).

Studies of long-term results are only available for cryolathe myopic keratomileusis. Barraquer (8) reported an average loss of correction of 15.42% during the first year. When based on refraction, the mean loss was 0.45 D between years 1 and 9 when compared to the control fellow eye. It thus appears that long-term stability is good following LRK. Therefore, one may reasonably expect good long-term stability following KMIS and LASIK, as the resected anterior cap is thinner than that following cryolathe myopic keratomileusis, and results in lessened ability of the anteriorly directed force from the flattened Bowman's membrane and the IOP to displace the greater mass of the posterior bed.

FUTURE HORIZONS

Corneal Sculpting

New technologies and approaches are being developed to determine corneal shape and thickness profiles, and older ones have expanded their capabilities. Soon, such devices may be used in either real time or at surgery to allow more accurate results. Also, topographic data will be input or coupled to the new small-spot laser technologies to allow true corneal sculpting. I recently evaluated an investigational software program of the LightBlade laser (Novatec Laser Systems, Carlsbad, CA) and found that it allows immediate ablation of any shape that has been input into the laser's computer. The coupling of refined topographic analysis and very-small-spot scanning lasers opens new possibilities for individualized ablation patterns and complex algorithms to maximize the effectiveness of laser ablation procedures.

Laser Keratome

Coworkers and I developed a new solid-state laser, using both UV and transmissive wavelengths, and described the first experimental use of a laser keratome (LightBlade) (52). Using a penetrating wavelength the laser is able to produce a lamellar keratectomy of any desired shape by focusing the laser's transmissive wavelength appropriately. Others subsequently used such an approach (36). This approach, which is still experimental, could eventually lead to a keratomileusis procedure performed only by laser, thereby avoiding mechanical microkeratomes and their limitations. The refractive ablation could be performed either with the penetrating wavelength, resulting in a keratomileusis procedure whereby the flap is never lifted, eliminating some complications such as epithelialization, or with the UV wavelength following reflection of the cap.

Intrastromal Ablation

Another approach to keratomileusis-like procedures is intrastromal ablation, whereby a penetrating wavelength is focused in the anterior corneal stroma to ablate a tissue lens by laser photodisruption (52). The shape of the ablation cavity is designed such that the desired deformation of the anterior corneal curvature results on collapse of the cavity.

Using animal eyes, coworkers and I demonstrated the ability to precisely create cavities with the desired degree of

spacing or overlap, and achieved up to 15 D of refractive change. Electron micrographic studies showed little collateral damage. Other investigators confirmed the ability of intrastromal lasers to ablate cavities that result in changes in anterior corneal curvature, although unpredictably. Experience has shown, however, that deformation of a primate cornea with Bowman's membrane is difficult. In one human study using a neodymium : yttrium-lithium fluoride (Nd : YLF) picosecond laser, significant corneal thinning up to $119\,\mu m$ was found, although the result was only 2 D of myopic correction (32). There were no complications.

The novelty of this approach is exciting, as the anterior cornea is left undisturbed and a mechanical microkeratome is not needed. Intrastromal ablation would be a painless procedure with rapid visual recovery and possibly reduced complications. Concerns remain over the effect of the shock waves produced on various aspects of the eye, especially the endothelium, although studies to date demonstrated no endothelial damage if the cavities are kept in the anterior stroma. Another approach is to outline the intrastromal tissue lens with the laser and then remove the lens in toto through a peripherally created incision. The major challenges are obtaining significant refractive correction and accuracy.

CONCLUSIONS

Lamellar refractive surgery has undergone a long period of development. Interest and innovation are increasingly being brought to this surgical approach, to attempt to refine its applications and improve its safety and accuracy. Although several approaches currently exist, further clinical investigation will be necessary to determine which techniques are most efficacious and applicable in a given setting. It has become increasingly clear, however, that lasers will play an important role in the future of LRK, either in the form of LASIK, which has already demonstrated its superiority, or in the form of new approaches as laser technology undergoes further evolution and refinement. LASIK currently provides relatively high corrections while avoiding the long-term instability of RK, the surface wound-healing processes of surface PRK, and the inaccuracy of mechanical KMIS. Thus, LASIK appears to be the procedure of choice for correcting most refractive errors, especially those above 6 D.

REFERENCES

1. American Academy of Ophthalmology. Automated lamellar keratoplasty. *Ophthalmology* 1996;103:703–704.
2. Arenas-Archila E, Sanchez-Thorin JC, Naranjo-Uribe JP, Hernandez-Lozano A. Myopic keratomileusis in situ: a preliminary report. *J Cataract Refract Surg* 1991;17:424–435.
3. Barker BA, Swinger CA. Keratophakia and keratomileusis. *Int Ophthalmol Clin* 1988;28:126–133.
4. Barraquer JI. Keratomileusis for the correction of myopia. *Arch Soc Am Oftalmol Optom* 1964;5:27–48.
5. Barraquer JI. Special methods in corneal surgery. In: King JH Jr, McTigue JW, eds. *The cornea.* Washington, DC: Butterworths, 1965:593–604.
6. Barraquer JI. Keratomileusis for myopia and aphakia. *Ophthalmology* 1981;88:701–708.

7. Barraquer JI. Keratomileusis for the correction of myopia. *Arch Soc Am Oftalmol Optom* 1982;16:221–232.

8. Barraquer JI. Long term results of myopic keratomileusis—1982. *Arch Soc Am Oftalmol Optom* 1983;19:137–148.

9. Bas AM, Nano HD Jr. In situ myopic keratomileusis results in 30 eyes at 15 months. *Refract Corneal Surg* 1991;7:223–231.

10. Bas AM, Onnis R. Excimer laser in situ keratomileusis for myopia. *J Refract Surg* 1995;11:S229–S233.

11. Bosc JM, Montard M, Delbosc B, et al. Non-freeze myopic keratomileusis. Retrospective study of 27 consecutive operations. *J Fr Ophtalmol* 1990;13:10–16.

12. Brint SF, Ostrick DM, Fisher C, et al. Six-month results of the multicenter phase I study of excimer laser myopic keratomileusis. *J Cataract Refract Surg* 1994;20:610–615.

13. Buratto L, Ferrari M. Excimer laser intrastromal keratomileusis: case reports. *J Cataract Refract Surg* 1992;18:37–41.

14. Buratto L, Ferrari M, Genisi C. Myopic keratomileusis with the excimer laser: one-year follow up. *Refract Corneal Surg* 1993;9:12–19.

15. Casebeer JC, Ruiz L, Slade S. *Lamellar refractive surgery*. Thorofare, NJ: Slack, 1996:138.

16. Durand L, Burillon C, Resal R. Refractive surgery and the non-freeze BKS set. Reliability of our Lyon methods. *Bull Soc Ophtalmol Fr* 1990;90:441–443.

17. Fiander DC, Tayfour F. Excimer laser in situ keratomileusis in 124 myopic eyes. *J Refract Surg* 1995;11:S234–S238.

18. Gomes M. Keratomileusis in situ using manual dissection of corneal flap for high myopia. *J Refract Corneal Surg* 1994;10(suppl):S255–S257.

19. Guell JL, Muller A. Laser in situ keratomileusis (LASIK) for myopia from −7 to −18 diopters. *J Refract Surg* 1996;12:222–228.

20. Hagen KB, Kim EK, Waring GO. Comparison of excimer laser and microkeratome myopic keratomileusis in human cadaver eyes. *Refract Corneal Surg* 1993;9:36–41.

21. Helmy SA, Salah A, Badawy TT, Sidky AN. Photorefractive keratectomy and laser in situ keratomileusis for myopia between 6.00 and 10.00 diopters. *J Refract Surg* 1996;12:417–421.

22. Ibrahim O, Waring GO, Salah T, El Maghraby A. Automated in situ keratomileusis for myopia. *J Refract Surg* 1995;11:431–441.

23. Kaufman HE. The correction of aphakia. *Am J Ophthalmol* 1980;89:1–10.

24. Kezirian GM, Gremillion CM. Automated lamellar keratoplasty for the correction of hyperopia. *J Cataract Refract Surg* 1995;21:386–392.

25. Kim HM, Jung HR. Laser assisted in situ keratomileusis for high myopia. *Ophthalmic Surg Lasers* 1996;27:S508–S511.

26. Kornmehl EW, Swinger CA, Pugh W, et al. Corneascope evaluation of myopic keratomileusis. *Invest Ophthalmol Vis Sci* 1985;26(suppl):203. ARVO abstracts.

27. Krwawicz T. Experimental operations of partial lamellar excision of corneal stroma for the correction of myopia. *Klin Oczna* 1963;33:574–579.

28. Kremer FB, Dufek M. Excimer laser in situ keratomileusis. *J Refract Surg* 1995;11:S244–S247.

29. Lindstrom RL, Lane SS. Polysulfone intracorneal lenses. In: Sanders DR, Hofmann RF, Sal JJ, eds. *Refractive corneal surgery*. Thorofare, NJ: Slack, 1986:549–563.

30. Lyle WA, Jin GJ. Initial results of automated lamellar keratoplasty for correction of myopia: one year follow-up. *J Cataract Refract Surg* 1996;22:31–43.

31. Manche EE, Maloney RK. Astigmatic keratotomy combined with myopic keratomileusis in situ for compound myopic astigmatism. *Am J Ophthalmol* 1996;122:18–28.

32. Marchi V, Gualano Z, Zumbo G, Marchi S. Intrastromal photorefractive keratectomy for myopia by Nd:YLF picosecond laser. *J Refract Surg* 1996;12:S284–S287.

33. Marinho A, Pinto MC, Pinto R, et al. LASIK for high myopia: one year experience. *Ophthalmic Surg Lasers* 1996;27:S517–S520.

34. Martines E, John ME. The Martines enhancement technique for correcting residual myopia following laser assisted in situ keratomileusis. *Ophthalmic Surg Lasers* 1996;21:S512–S516.

35. Mc Carey BE. Alloplastic refractive keratoplasty. In: Sanders DR, Hofmann RF, Sal JJ, eds. *Refractive corneal surgery*. Thorofare, NJ: Slack, 1986:529–548.

36. Mitsutoshi I, Quantock AJ, Malhan S, et al. Picosecond laser in situ keratomileusis with a 1053-mm Nd:YLF laser. *J Refract Surg* 1996;12:721–728.

37. Neumann AC, McCarty G, Sanders DR. Delayed regression of effect in myopic epikeratophakia vs myopic keratomileusis for high myopia. *Refract Corneal Surg* 1989;5:161–166.

38. Pallikaris I, Papatzanaki ME, Georgiadis A, Frenschock O. A comparative study of neuronal regeneration following corneal wounds induced by an argon fluoride excimer laser and mechanical methods. *Lasers Light Ophthalmol* 1990;3:89–95.

39. Pallikaris IG, Papatzanaki ME, Siganos DS, Tsilimbaris MK. A corneal flap technique for laser in situ keratomileusis. Human studies. *Arch Ophthalmol* 1991;109:1699–1702.

40. Pallikaris IG, Papatzanaki ME, Stathi EZ, et al. Laser in situ keratomileusis. *Lasers Surg Med* 1990;10:463–468.

41. Peyman GA, Badaro RM, Khoobehi B. Corneal ablation in rabbits using an infrared (2.9 microns) erbium:YAG laser. *Ophthalmology* 1989;96:1160–1169.

42. Pureskin N. Weakening ocular refraction by means of partial stromectomy of the cornea under experimental conditions. *Vestn Oftalmol* 1967;8:1–7.

43. Ruiz L. Presented at the American Academy of Ophthalmology, Dallas, TX, 1986.

44. Ruiz L, Rowsey J. In situ keratomileusis. *Invest Ophthalmol Vis Sci* 1988;29(suppl):392.

45. Salah T, Waring GO III, El Maghraby A, et al. Excimer laser in situ keratomileusis under a corneal flap for myopia of 2 to 20 diopters. *Am J Ophthalmol* 1996;121:143–155.

46. Seiler T, Kahle G, Kriegerowski M. Excimer laser (193 nm) myopic keratomileusis in sighted and blind human eyes. *Refract Corneal Surg* 1990;6:165–173.

47. Slade SG. Overview of lamellar refractive surgery. In: Machat JJ, ed. *Excimer laser refractive surgery*. Thorofare, NJ: Slack, 1996:270–281.

48. Swinger CA, Barker BA. Prospective evaluation of myopic keratomileusis. *Ophthalmology* 1984;91:785–792.

49. Swinger CA, Barker BA. Myopic keratomileusis following radial keratotomy. *J Refract Surg* 1985;1:53–55.

50. Swinger CA, Barraquer JI. Keratophakia and keratomileusis: clinical results. *Ophthalmology* 1981;88:709–715.

51. Swinger CA, Krumeich J, Cassiday D. Planar lamellar refractive keratoplasty. *J Refract Surg* 1986;2:17–24.

52. Swinger CA, Lai ST. Solid state photoablative decomposition—the Novatec laser. In: Salz JJ, McDonnell PJ, McDonald MB, eds. *Corneal laser surgery*. St. Louis: Mosby, 1995:261–267.

53. Swinger CA, Villasenor RA. Homoplastic keratomileusis for the correction of myopia. *J Refract Surg* 1985;1:219–223.

54. Troutman RC, Swinger CA. Refractive keratoplasty—keratophakia and keratomileusis. *Trans Am Ophthalmol Soc* 1978;76:329–339.

Surgical Pathology of the Cornea

JAYNE S. WEISS   RICHARD M. AHUJA

NORMAL CORNEAL HISTOLOGY

The cornea forms the anterior one-sixth of the human eye. The cornea's anatomy is intrinsically linked to its major functions of protection and refraction of light. The cornea must be transparent to maintain optical clarity and function and concurrently provide strength for the protection of intraocular contents (1). The corneal surface also must be smooth for proper interaction with the tear film because the tear-air interface is a key refracting surface, and the tear film conveys oxygen to the cornea.

The cornea measures 10.6 mm vertically, 11.7 mm horizontally, and 11.7 mm in diameter. Its thickness is approximately 1.2 mm peripherally and 0.5 to 0.6 mm centrally (2). The cornea is composed of the following five layers: epithelium, Bowman's layer, stroma, Descemet's membrane, and endothelium.

The corneal epithelium consists of a stratified squamous nonkeratinized layer that is organized to provide a smooth, transparent, optical surface for the eye's major refracting surface. Its central thickness is 50 to 60 μm. It is composed of five to seven layers: three to four layers of squamous cells, one to three layers of wing cells, and a single layer of basal cells. At the corneoscleral junction the epithelium thickens to ten or more cell layers, becoming contiguous with the bulbar conjunctiva. Neurons, melanocytes, and modified macrophages are also present in the epithelial layer of the cornea. A high density of unmyelinated sensory nerve endings, about 300 to 400 times that of the epidermis, penetrate the epithelial squamous cells (3).

The corneal epithelium cytoskeleton is composed primarily of three proteins: intermediate filaments, microtubules, and actin filaments. The filaments are linked to form an elaborate web of cytoskeletal meshwork that affects both epithelial shape and metabolism.

The most superficial squamous cell layer of the corneal epithelium is two to three cells thick. The cells are flat and contain organelles designed primarily for protein synthesis such as Golgi cisternae and Golgi-associated vesicles with horizontal nuclei internally (4). The most flattened apical cells have unique membrane specializations including microvilli 1 μm long and microplicae, which are apical membrane ridgelike folds that may help to increase metabolite absorption and stabilize the tear film (5). The laterally located tight junctions or zonulae occludens prevent the penetration of microorganisms and help to keep the stroma dehydrated by blocking the entrance of fluids and metabolites.

Scanning electron microscope examination of these surfaces demonstrates that apical cells scatter electrons variably. Cells that scatter electrons to a greater degree are termed *light cells*. The light cells have a higher density of surface microvilli and microplicae, which help to retain the tear film (6). The dark cells may represent older cells that desquamate into the tear film.

The middle layer of cells of the corneal epithelium are referred to as *wing cells* because of their multisided shape with a convex anterior surface and concave posterior surface. Their lateral borders have numerous interdigitations and desmosomes that attach to neighboring cells. The cytoplasmic faces of the membranes at the desmosome are associated with dense plaques and intermediate filaments of keratin or cytokeratin (7).

The corneal epithelial basal cell layer is composed of a single layer of tall columnar cells along the basement membrane. These cells have few cytoplasmic organelles and fewer desmosomal attachments than do the wing cells. Hemidesmosomes extend from the cell cytoskeleton through the basement membrane to the anchoring fibril network. The hemidesmosome has a cytoplasmic plaque to which the keratin filaments insert. The lateral borders of the basal cells interdigitate and are attached by desmosomes along the basement membrane (2).

Complete turnover of the corneal epithelium occurs approximately every 5 to 7 days (8). Mitotic activity occurs at the basal cell layer after which cells migrate toward terminal differentiation and anteriorly until they desquamate at the apical surface of the epithelium. Although studies indicated no regional variation in mitotic rates over the cornea, there is evidence to support the statement that basal cells of the limbal region at the periphery of the cornea are probably the stem cells of the corneal epithelium (9).

The epithelial basement membrane is periodic acid–Schiff (PAS) positive and is strongly adherent to the underlying Bowman's layer. The basement membrane forms a scaffold on which the epithelium rests. Its surface components play a role in the migration and adhesion of epithelial cells during wound healing (10).

Bowman's layer (Fig. 20-1) is a complex of fine, randomly oriented collagen fibrils that lies between the epithelial basement membrane and the highly organized stroma. Its thickness measures between 8 and 10 μm. Bowman's layer has type VII collagen–containing anchoring fibrils that are attached to the lamina densa of the epithelial basement membrane and to anchoring plaques in the fibrillar stroma (11). The components of Bowman's layer are theorized to be produced by stromal keratocytes and epithelial cells.

The corneal stroma forms about 90% of the corneal thickness and consists of collagen fibrils between 20 and 30 nm that are arranged within 200 to 250 stacked lamellae that run parallel to the stromal surface. Within each lamella the fibrils are packed in parallel arrays. The fibrils contain mostly type I collagen and are in the same direction in a given lamella but at right angles to fibrils in neighboring lamellae. Fewer amounts of type III and some type IV collagen are also present. The transparency of the corneal stroma is produced by the small, uniform diameter of the stromal fibrils and their close, regular packing, which minimizes light scatter through the cornea (Fig. 20-2) (12).

The collagen fibers are embedded in glycosaminoglycans (GAGs), which hold the collagen fibrils in an orderly array. The GAGs are sugars in which repeating disaccharide units form a long polymer chain. Keratin sulfate and chondroitin sulfate are found in the corneal stroma. The GAGs are aligned between the collagen fibrils and hold the fibrils at a fixed distance of 30 to 60 nm.

Many theories have been proposed to explain the control of the diameters of the collagen fibrils. Fibrillogenesis experiments in vitro showed that the relative proportion of type V collagen helps determine the orderly spacing of collagen fibrils (13,14). Type VI collagen filaments are also present between collagen fibrils and also play a role in maintaining the proper fibril separation needed for corneal transparency (15).

Flattened fibroblasts, termed *keratocytes*, lie in between adjacent lamellae and synthesize the extracellular matrix of the stroma. These keratocytes can migrate to an area of a wound site. Polymorphonuclear leukocytes, plasma cells, and lymphocytes are also present in stroma.

Descemet's membrane is the PAS-positive basement membrane of the corneal endothelium and lies on the posterior surface of the stroma. This thick basal lamina is synthesized by corneal endothelium and is composed of type IV and type VII collagen, fibronectin, laminin, heparin sulfate, and dermatan sulfate proteoglycans (16,17).

Descemet's membrane is composed of an anterior and a posterior layer. The anterior portion is 3 μm thick with a

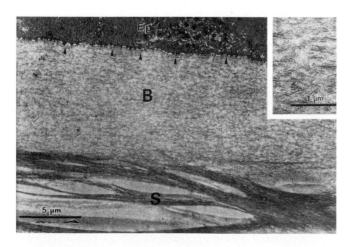

FIGURE 20-1.   *Transmission electron micrograph of a cross section of the human cornea through Bowman's layer (B). The anterior surface of Bowman's layer has an irregular profile (arrowheads) reflecting the basal contour of the epithelium (Ep). S = stroma. (×6300.) (Reproduced by permission from Komai Y, Ushiki I.* Invest Ophthalmol Vis Sci *1981;32:2244–2258.)*

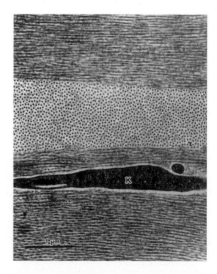

FIGURE 20-2.   *Collagen fibrils in the cornea have a uniform diameter and are arranged in the same direction within the lamellae with interspersed keratocytes (k). (Reproduced by permission from Komai Y, Ushiki I.* Invest Ophthalmol Vis Sci *1981;32:2244–2258.)*

vertical banded pattern and is laid down in utero. The posterior portion is a 10-μm-thick nonbanded layer that can thicken with aging. Descemet's membrane prevents penetration of leukocytes and blood vessels into stroma but does not prevent transmission of water and smaller molecules.

When breaks occur in Descemet's membrane, it retracts and coils toward the stroma. Endothelial cells migrate over the damaged site and secrete a new basement membrane (Fig. 20-3). This secondarily secreted tissue appears as a gray sheet on the posterior surface of the cornea termed a *retrocorneal membrane* or *posterior collagenous layer*.

The corneal endothelium rests on Descemet's membrane and consists of a single layer of flattened, polygonal, closely apposed cells with five to seven sides (18). Each hexagonal cell is about 5 μm thick and 20 μm in diameter with a surface area of 250 μm². In the young adult, cell density varies between 2000 and 4000 cells/mm² (19). Although a critical number of endothelial cells are needed to maintain corneal deturgescence, cells can enlarge to maintain functional ability and preserve corneal clarity. Scanning electron microscopy of the apical endothelial cells surface shows short microvilli, lateral interdigitating processes, pitlike openings of pinocytic vesicles, and flat bulges on the posterior layer caused by round nuclei (20,21).

Endothelial cells also contain numerous intracellular organelles such as a large oval nucleus with prominent nucleoli, numerous mitochondria, prominent Golgi bodies, and elaborate endoplasmic reticulum. The presence of these intracellular organelles reflects a high level of metabolic activity with the endothelial cells.

The corneal endothelium maintains corneal deturgescence by balancing fluid movement across the cellular layers via a pump-leak system. With use of an active transport pump the endothelium can transport fluid against normal hydrostatic pressure. In a normal state the stromal hydration is 78% and stromal thickness is 0.50 mm. There are approximately 3.0×10^6 pump sites per cell and the number can decrease both with age and with disease states (22).

The endothelial cells are joined together laterally by focal tight junctions that aid in forming a barrier to aqueous humor, and gap junctions that aid in cell-to-cell communication (23). Gap junctions also allow the penetration of small molecules and electrolytes between endothelial cells, creating a leaky barrier to aqueous humor. These connections are very important, as the major function of the endothelium is the regulation of corneal stromal water content. Cytoplasmic processes also extend from the basal aspect of the endothelial cells into Descemet's membrane (24).

NORMAL WOUND HEALING

The three corneal layers—epithelium, stroma, and endothelium—heal by tissue repair not regeneration. Surgical scars that have extensions into the stroma are opaque because of the disordered array of collagen fibers and also have less tensile strength than does normal cornea. The three layers of the cornea differ in the wound-healing response.

The corneal epithelium, a five- to seven-layer stratified squamous epithelium, is a self-renewing structure with complete turnover occurring in 5 to 7 days. It can be regenerated by limbal basal cells, which have a higher mitotic index than do the cells of the central epithelium (25). The healing rate in corneal epithelial wounds is rapid and there is relatively minimal to no scarring. Epithelial injuries heal by migration, mitosis, and differentiation of newly formed basal cells (26). In full-thickness defects, an epithelial sheet of polygonal cells migrates over the denuded stroma within the first hour after injury. The earliest sliding cells are wing cells followed by the basal cells. The defect is covered by a sliding of the newly formed cells that involves a complex process of repeated cellular adhesion and lysis (27). In limbal wounds, healing occurs by migration of conjunctival epithelium or proliferation of the remaining corneal epithelial cells.

Fibronectin and laminin are released initially (28–30). Fibronectin is a high-molecular-weight plasma and extracellular matrix glycoprotein that deposits with fibrin on denuded corneal basement membrane soon after the epithelium is initially injured, and slowly regresses after wound repair is completed. Fibronectin with fibrinogen forms the initial meshwork facilitating fibroblast invasion and attachment to collagen (31). Laminin is present in corneal basement membrane and functions as an attachment glycoprotein for epithelial cells (28).

Polymorphonuclear neutrophils migrate to the site of injury within 1 to 5 hours after the injury occurs, and help remove remnants of injured cells.

Configurational changes in the cell cytoskeleton with lysis of intracellular desmosomal attachments occur in basal epithelial cells at the edge of the injury. Filopodia are

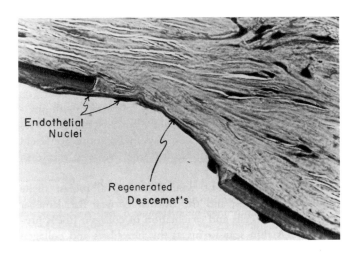

FIGURE 20-3. *Descemet's membrane is partially regenerated in this specimen 2.5 years after surgery, with flattened endothelial cell nuclei. (H & E, ×595.) (Reproduced by permission from Flaxel JT, Swan KC. Arch Ophthalmol 1969;81:653–659.)*

Endothelial Nuclei

Regenerated Descemet's

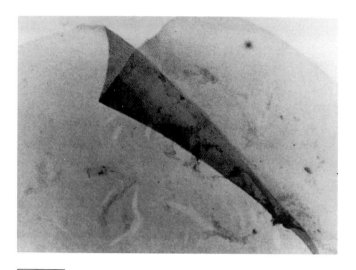

FIGURE 20-8.   *Folded Descemet's membrane after intraocular surgery. (Reprinted with permission from Zeiter HJ, Zeiter JT. J Am Intraocular Implant Soc 1983;9:36–39.)*

staining pigmented cells may be present where Descemet's membrane turns away from the stroma. Hassall-Henle warts are present, with marked flattening of endothelial cell nuclei over the summit of the warts (89). In an eye with Descemet's membrane detachment secondary to injection of sodium hyaluronate, light microscopy reveals a normal corneal epithelium and Bowman's layer, with Descemet's membrane and endothelium detached by a lightly staining material.

Electron microscopy of the same eye demonstrates an anatomically intact endothelium and stripped Descemet's membrane. Numerous electron-dense globules of a fine granular material are present in the space between the membrane and the stroma. A monolayer of endothelial cells of 2.5 μm is present on the anterior surface of Descemet's membrane, with the cells appearing degenerated with multimembranous inclusions. The most posterior lamellae of the stroma appears abnormal because of the less-dense network of collagen (95).

Fibrous ingrowth was found after 22% of adult and 10% of congenital cataract extractions complicated by Descemet's membrane detachments (94). Of these eyes, 60% with fibrous ingrowth had detached fragments of Descemet's membrane. The amount of corneal edema and opacity depends on the size of the detachment. Minor detachments have a minor impact on vision, whereas extensive detachments of Descemet's membrane can lead to bullous keratopathy (87,96). The detached Descemet's membrane may curl back into place or the denuded area of stroma may be covered by newly formed Descemet's membrane. If this does not occur, iris may also adhere to the denuded portion of stroma, forming anterior synechiae.

Sharp Injuries

Perforating surgical injuries or wounds are usually limbal or perilimbal in location and have clean, sharply defined edges on pathologic examination. Wounds with a radius of curvature shorter than that of the cornea pucker or remain open, whereas linear wounds longer than the radius of curvature tend toward self-approximation (69). In deeper lacerations, the iris, lens, or ciliary body can be incarcerated in the wound.

In penetrating keratoplasty wounds, the stromal margins heal similarly to full-thickness incisions of the cornea. However, most of the fibroblasts are provided by recipient cornea. After perforating injuries the cornea begins the healing process in the first few hours. Epithelial downgrowth or fibrous ingrowth can complicate wound healing.

Retrocorneal Membranes and Epithelial Downgrowth

Retrocorneal membranes can occur after surgical perforating trauma. Epithelial downgrowth, fibrous ingrowth, endothelial proliferation, and retrocorneal melanin pigmentation (RCP) can produce membranous opacities behind the cornea. These membranes may appear as fine gray lines on the posterior corneal surface (Fig. 20-9).

Epithelial Downgrowth

Epithelial downgrowth carries a poor prognosis for vision. This relatively rare complication of surgical injury occurs at rates of 0.6% for all traumatic and surgical perforating injuries, up to 0.2% after cataract surgery, and 0.27% after penetrating keratoplasty (98–103).

Under normal circumstances, epithelium may grow into the depth of the corneal stromal wound, but as healing progresses, the epithelium is displaced to its proper level, preventing entry into the anterior chamber. However, if there is delayed wound closure, a poorly apposed wound, wound dehiscence, or incarceration of epithelial tissue in the surgical wound, the epithelium may continue to grow into the anterior chamber.

Epithelial downgrowth does not occur simply because access to the anterior chamber is present. Other factors are also necessary (104). The absence of contact inhibition by healthy corneal endothelium may allow for epithelium to enter the anterior chamber (105,106). Presence of a smooth surface such as a lens capsule or fibrin may aid the movement of the epithelial cells (107). Growth factors released in inflamed eyes owing to loss of the blood-ocular barrier may promote epithelial proliferation (108,109).

The histopathologic finding of nonkeratinized stratified squamous epithelium on the posterior surface of the cornea or over the iris is diagnostic (101). The epithelium is several layers thick when it covers well-vascularized surfaces, with nutrition provided by uveal tissue and aqueous humor (110).

vertical banded pattern and is laid down in utero. The posterior portion is a 10-μm-thick nonbanded layer that can thicken with aging. Descemet's membrane prevents penetration of leukocytes and blood vessels into stroma but does not prevent transmission of water and smaller molecules.

When breaks occur in Descemet's membrane, it retracts and coils toward the stroma. Endothelial cells migrate over the damaged site and secrete a new basement membrane (Fig. 20-3). This secondarily secreted tissue appears as a gray sheet on the posterior surface of the cornea termed a *retrocorneal membrane* or *posterior collagenous layer*.

The corneal endothelium rests on Descemet's membrane and consists of a single layer of flattened, polygonal, closely apposed cells with five to seven sides (18). Each hexagonal cell is about 5 μm thick and 20 μm in diameter with a surface area of 250 μm². In the young adult, cell density varies between 2000 and 4000 cells/mm² (19). Although a critical number of endothelial cells are needed to maintain corneal deturgescence, cells can enlarge to maintain functional ability and preserve corneal clarity. Scanning electron microscopy of the apical endothelial cells surface shows short microvilli, lateral interdigitating processes, pitlike openings of pinocytic vesicles, and flat bulges on the posterior layer caused by round nuclei (20,21).

Endothelial cells also contain numerous intracellular organelles such as a large oval nucleus with prominent nucleoli, numerous mitochondria, prominent Golgi bodies, and elaborate endoplasmic reticulum. The presence of these intracellular organelles reflects a high level of metabolic activity with the endothelial cells.

The corneal endothelium maintains corneal deturgescence by balancing fluid movement across the cellular layers via a pump-leak system. With use of an active transport pump the endothelium can transport fluid against normal hydrostatic pressure. In a normal state the stromal hydration is 78% and stromal thickness is 0.50 mm. There are approximately 3.0×10^6 pump sites per cell and the number can decrease both with age and with disease states (22).

The endothelial cells are joined together laterally by focal tight junctions that aid in forming a barrier to aqueous humor, and gap junctions that aid in cell-to-cell communication (23). Gap junctions also allow the penetration of small molecules and electrolytes between endothelial cells, creating a leaky barrier to aqueous humor. These connections are very important, as the major function of the endothelium is the regulation of corneal stromal water content. Cytoplasmic processes also extend from the basal aspect of the endothelial cells into Descemet's membrane (24).

NORMAL WOUND HEALING

The three corneal layers—epithelium, stroma, and endothelium—heal by tissue repair not regeneration. Surgical scars that have extensions into the stroma are opaque because of the disordered array of collagen fibers and also have less tensile strength than does normal cornea. The three layers of the cornea differ in the wound-healing response.

The corneal epithelium, a five- to seven-layer stratified squamous epithelium, is a self-renewing structure with complete turnover occurring in 5 to 7 days. It can be regenerated by limbal basal cells, which have a higher mitotic index than do the cells of the central epithelium (25). The healing rate in corneal epithelial wounds is rapid and there is relatively minimal to no scarring. Epithelial injuries heal by migration, mitosis, and differentiation of newly formed basal cells (26). In full-thickness defects, an epithelial sheet of polygonal cells migrates over the denuded stroma within the first hour after injury. The earliest sliding cells are wing cells followed by the basal cells. The defect is covered by a sliding of the newly formed cells that involves a complex process of repeated cellular adhesion and lysis (27). In limbal wounds, healing occurs by migration of conjunctival epithelium or proliferation of the remaining corneal epithelial cells.

Fibronectin and laminin are released initially (28–30). Fibronectin is a high-molecular-weight plasma and extracellular matrix glycoprotein that deposits with fibrin on denuded corneal basement membrane soon after the epithelium is initially injured, and slowly regresses after wound repair is completed. Fibronectin with fibrinogen forms the initial meshwork facilitating fibroblast invasion and attachment to collagen (31). Laminin is present in corneal basement membrane and functions as an attachment glycoprotein for epithelial cells (28).

Polymorphonuclear neutrophils migrate to the site of injury within 1 to 5 hours after the injury occurs, and help remove remnants of injured cells.

Configurational changes in the cell cytoskeleton with lysis of intracellular desmosomal attachments occur in basal epithelial cells at the edge of the injury. Filopodia are

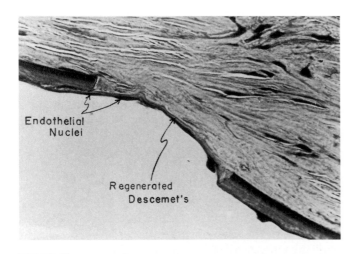

FIGURE 20-3. *Descemet's membrane is partially regenerated in this specimen 2.5 years after surgery, with flattened endothelial cell nuclei. (H & E, ×595.) (Reproduced by permission from Flaxel JT, Swan KC. Arch Ophthalmol 1969;81:653–659.)*

Endothelial Nuclei

Regenerated Descemet's

extended and a monolayer of basal cells migrates onto the surface of the epithelial wound within 6 hours after injury (26). Migration is an active process during which there is a continuous formation and destruction of cellular adhesions to extracellular matrix proteins. Mitosis occurs to form new epithelial cells to replace the forward migrating cells and to restore epithelial thickness. Superficial epithelial cells then terminally differentiate and re-form intermediate filaments that are specific to the cornea. Endothelial growth factor, fibroblast growth factor, and transforming growth factor stimulate mitosis and migration in the process of corneal epithelial wound healing (32,33).

The corneal stroma heals at a much slower rate than the epithelium and other connective tissues. Following perforating lacerations of the cornea, healing begins to occur as early as 1 day after injury but may proceed for many months or years. Initially there is a release of soluble and cellular factors, after which epithelium migrates to form a fibrin plug in the posterior aspect of the wound which persists from 10 days to years (26). A diffuse gray haze with faint edema due to swelling in the middle or periphery of the stroma develops slowly in the first hour after injury.

Keratocytes near the wound edge are phagocytosed and proteoglycans are lost. Nearby stromal keratocytes and monocytes activate and transform into fibroblast-like cells and migrate to fill the wound (Fig. 20-4) (34,35). Although, in animals the wound fills with fibrin, initiating the contractile phase of stromal wound healing, there is little fibrin present in human stromal wounds (26,34,36). Proteoglycans including keratin and chondroitin and dermatan sulfate accumulate within the wound in animals (37). The fibroblasts secrete a soluble procollagen that polymerizes at the surface to form true collagen.

Collagen types I, III, V, and VI are synthesized and stress fibers containing f-actin, nonmuscle myosin, and α-actinin develop (34,38). Tensile strength is derived from the collagen fibrils—the length and organization of collagen within the fibrils and the covalent-noncovalent interactions in and between the fibrils (39). Remodeling occurs in the scar tissue over years with changes in transparency, but the scar may never reach the tensile strength of uninjured tissue. The injured Bowman's layer does not regenerate and does not adversely affect anterior corneal surface wound healing.

In rabbit corneal endothelial cells, scanning confocal microscopy reveals a high mitotic rate after wounding. Three days after an injury occurs, the posterior fibrin plug of the corneal wound is covered by fibroblast-like cells and newly divided endothelial cells (40). These transformed endothelial cells produce a new Descemet's membrane, which is regenerated over weeks (41).

The corneal endothelial monolayer in humans loses its capacity to mitose to replace lost or injured cells in an adult. Unlike animal endothelium, which heals through mitosis of endothelial cells, endothelial healing in humans is normally amitotic (42). Because of the limited mitotic response, repair occurs primarily by migration of neighboring cells to cover

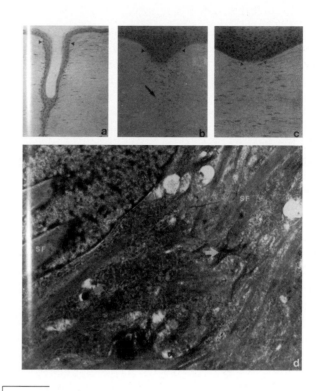

FIGURE 20-4.   *Light microscopy of a cat corneal wound at 3 (a), 14 (b), and 30 (c) days. Transmission electron microscopy of corneal wound-healing fibroblasts at 14 days (d). The wound is initially covered by corneal epithelium forming an epithelial plug (a), which is later replaced by fibrotic tissue (b) (arrowheads). During the precontractile phase of wound healing, the wound appears to increase in size (a, b, arrowheads). From days 14 to 30, corneal wounds show a decrease in wound gape, suggesting wound contraction (b, c, arrowheads) with a concomitant decrease in the number of fibroblasts. Fibroblasts after radial keratotomy surgery show prominent stress fiber bundles (SF) throughout the cell. (a, ×125; b, ×160; c and d, ×1500.) (Reproduced by permission from Garana RM, Petroll WM, Chen WT, et al. Radial keratotomy II: the role of the myofibroblast in corneal wound contraction. Invest Ophthalmol Vis Sci 1982;33:3271–3282.)*

the wound, with enlargement and flattening of these cells (43). Studies have described the repair of large endothelial defects to involve cell translocation to cover the wound gap. This translocation response involves migration, with individual cells moving to the wound by breaking contacts with neighboring cells, and spreading, with the entire confluent monolayer adjacent to the wound moving as a whole to cover the wound (44).

In the late phases of wound healing, fibroblast tissue cellularity decreases, and the normal corneal flat, lamellar arrangement of cells and orientation of collagen fibrils predominate. A thin scar forms as the fibroblasts and collagen fibrils are reorganized. The contraction of myofibroblasts and decrease of cellularity cause a shrinkage of the wound. Light microscopy reveals that the healed wound has a different orientation of collagen fibers than does the surrounding corneal lamellae (45).

WOUND HEALING WITH
AND WITHOUT SUTURES

The placement of corneal sutures leads to a variety of histopathologic changes in the cornea. Suture placement has an important effect on corneal wound healing and corneal curvature. The healing of unsutured corneal wounds is slower than that of sutured wounds (46–50).

There are major differences in structural healing between sutured and unsutured corneal wounds (Fig. 20-5) (51–53). Unsutured wounds may gape more because of retraction of stromal lamellar collagen fibers in Bowman's layer, which may be abnormally increased by eyelid or intraocular pressure. Epithelial plug formation occurs in unsutured corneal wounds, compared to the permanent distortion of normal lamellar structure from incarceration of Bowman's layer in sutured wounds. If the orientation of fibroblasts is parallel to the sutured wound, subsequent collagen fiber deposition is also parallel to the wound. This results in ineffective wound closure and repair. In unsutured wounds epithelial contact inhibition may delay stromal repair. Unsutured corneal wounds also invoke less inflammatory response than do sutured wounds. Insufficient keratocyte activation may delay the repair process.

Therefore, suture placement accelerates wound repair by increasing wound apposition and maintenance of normal collagen structure (51). In keratotomy or unsutured wounds, fibroblast orientation parallel to the epithelial plug correlates with an ineffective scar tissue organization parallel to the wound. However, in sutured wounds the initial fibroblast orientation parallel to the wound eventually results in pseudolamellar or transverse scar tissue organization (51,53–57). A biphasic fibroblast reaction with cell orientation changing directions characterizes the repair process in both sutured and unsutured wound healing. This may result from contact guidance (alignment along tissue structures), chemotaxis (alignment over a chemical gradient), and stress distribution (alignment along stress forces) (58).

Based on electron microscopic analysis, the early phases of unsutured wound healing are associated with complete elimination of the epithelial plug, with a transverse fibroblast orientation over the entire wound depth. In early sutured wounds, there is a lack of scar tissue organization. Fibroblast orientation is sagittal to the wound (59).

In later stages of wound healing, there is a decline in the approximation toward lamellar restoration in the unsutured wound. The initially disorganized sutured wounds demonstrate a recovery of lamellar organization across the wound progressing from anterior to posterior. Because pseudolamellar repair results in maintenance of tensile strength across the wound, the ineffective remodeling in unsutured wounds may lead to a progressive weakening of the wound and more corneal flattening. This correlates to the progressive hyperopia noted in as many as 30% of patients after radial keratotomy surgery (60).

Both continuous and interrupted sutures are used in penetrating keratoplasty. In animal studies, histopathology shows a greater inflammatory response in the corneal stroma and a faster rate of wound healing with interrupted sutures than with continuous sutures. Though wounds closed with continuous sutures heal more slowly, they provide a greater impedance to the growth of vessels (61).

For repair of ocular surgical wounds the sutures most commonly used are silk, nylon, and polyester sutures such as Mersilene. Silk suture produces a greater inflammatory response in tissue and buries poorly, and therefore is rarely used to repair corneal wounds (62). Monofilament nylon has prolonged tensile strength and induces minimal inflammation in tissue. It also hydrolyzes and biodegrades in vivo, with free ends coming to the surface, creating a foreign body reaction and a nidus for vascularization (63–65). Hydrolysis of polyamide structures such as nylon suture is mediated by lysosomal enzymes and causes less erosion in the cornea and conjunctiva than in uveal tissue (65). Polypropylene (Prolene) suture is not hydrolyzable and does not biodegrade, and therefore is the preferred suture for iris fixation. It has a stronger tensile strength than nylon, and produces more tissue compression than nylon (62).

Mersilene, a polyester suture, is not biodegradable and may provide better long-term wound stability than nylon (66). For keratoplasty Mersilene is used alone or in combination with nylon. Its advantages in corneal grafts are its nonbiodegradability and lower rate of inflammation when free of foreign body adherence (67,68).

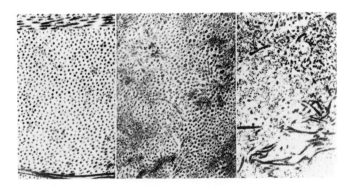

FIGURE 20-5. *Scanning electron microscopy of an unwounded area* (left), *a sutured wound* (center), *and an unsutured wound* (right) *within the same monkey eye 2.5 months after surgery. The sutured wound area shows compact collagen fiber deposition. The unsutured wound area demonstrates irregular and less-compact fiber deposition. Fine or coarse granular, electron-dense depositions are visible between fibrils in sutured and unsutured wounds. (×36,000.) (Reproduced by permission from Melles GRJ, Binder PS. A comparison of wound healing in sutured and unsutured corneal wounds.* Arch Ophthalmol *1990;108:1460–1469.)*

CORNEAL NEOVASCULARIZATION

Corneal neovascularization (CNV) can occur in a number of pathologic states and is characterized by new vessel loops

extending from the limbus into adjacent deep or superficial corneal stroma. Neovascularization represents a part of the normal repair response to inflammation and is seen with edema, cellular infiltration, and tissue necrosis (69). It occurs in response to a variety of pathologic conditions: infections, trauma, burns, exposure to toxins, graft rejection, metabolic disorders, vasculitides, and anoxia from contact lens wear and nutritional deficiencies. Changes in pH, liberation of various enzymes from inflammatory cells, and alterations in the oxidative process can stimulate growth of new vessels.

CNV may also interfere with the differentiation of migrating conjunctival epithelium during healing of corneal epithelial defects. Vascularization may result in recurrent erosions, low-grade inflammation, and lipid deposition.

Nonspecific inflammatory insults can induce CNV. Polymorphonuclear neutrophils (PMN) and lymphocytes may stimulate vascularization of the cornea (70). Stimulated lymphocytes may cause immunologic mediated CNV found in immune reactions such as corneal graft rejection and herpes simplex virus (HSV) keratitis (71). Lymphocytic infiltration induces the release of diffusible factors capable of initiating directional vessel growth in the normally avascular cornea.

Interleukin (IL)-2 is one of the soluble mediators released by the stimulated lymphocytes. IL-1 and IL-2 cause acute inflammation composed of stromal PMN infiltration. IL-1 is also found in the setting of CNV with a significant infiltration of PMNs (72). Other lymphocyte-secreted mediators such as prostaglandins also induce angiogenesis (73).

CNV may cause increased exposure to mediators of inflammation via the patent blood vessels, resulting in allograft rejection. In corneas with extensive neovascularization the rate of graft rejection is as high as 65% (74).

Many methods of treatment of CNV including cryotherapy, β-irradiation, creation of corneal scars, corticosteroid injections, laser photocoagulation, and photothrombosis have been investigated (75,76). Potential complications include delayed corneal wound healing, infections, cataract formation, corneal ulceration, corneal opacification, and revascularization of the cornea.

CNV can be treated with argon laser photocoagulation. The argon beam penetrates the cornea with low absorption and high efficiency in order to coagulate stromal vessels. One day after argon laser treatment, light microscopy showed coagulative necrosis, inflammatory cells, and engorged blood vessels (77,78). Compared to control samples, there was a reduction in inflammatory cells and blood vessels, with an increase in fibroblastic proliferation and ghost vessels.

Yellow-dye laser as compared to argon blue green laser has a higher absorption by oxyhemoglobin and reduced hemoglobin. Transmission electron microscopy of corneas treated with a 577-nm yellow-dye laser showed damaged endothelial cells lining the stromal vessels. The stroma demonstrated a disorganized array of collagen fibrils, edema, extravasated erythrocytes, and a perivascular inflammatory

cell infiltrate (79). Control corneas demonstrated smooth, contoured stromal blood vessels, with normal endothelial cells with a uniform pattern of stromal collagen fibrils and no inflammatory cells (77). Histopathology showed intracorneal hemorrhages in 21% of corneas treated by yellow-dye laser, but these generally resolved within 2 weeks. None of the laser-treated corneas showed any damage to the deep stroma or the endothelium.

The treatment of CNV by photothrombosis involves vascular occlusion mediated by aggregating platelets that respond to photochemically induced endothelial damage. Studies have used argon laser irradiation with intravenous injection of photosensitizing dye such as rose bengal to permanently occlude the new vessels. Examination of treated corneas revealed involution of occluded corneal vessels 1 week after treatment, with improvement in corneal clarity and surface smoothness (Fig. 20-6). Fluorescein angiography

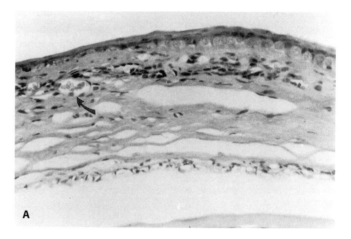

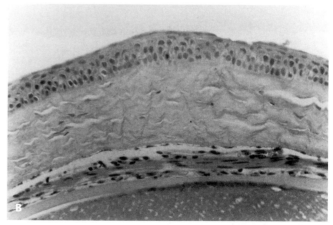

FIGURE 20-6. A. *Histologic section of a control cornea with neovascularization reveals mature vessels* (arrow) *and moderate mononuclear infiltrate. (H & E, ×80.) B. Following photodynamic therapy after injection of DHE, there is a decrease in stromal cellularity and neovascularization with normal underlying iris and mild vascularization of the lens. (H & E, ×80.) (Reproduced by permission from Epstein RJ, Harris DM. Photodynamic therapy for corneal neovascularization.* Cornea *1991;10:424–432.)*

also confirmed occlusion, with no further recanalization of the vessels in a 4-month study period (80).

Pretreatment of CNV with photothrombosis improves corneal graft survival with 75% of pretreated corneas remaining clear, while only 12.5% of untreated corneas remained clear. However, occlusion of the new vessels may be temporary; histologic examination revealed subsequent regrowth or recanalization of corneal blood vessels. Permanent occlusion can occur, but photothrombosis can help to prevent vascular invasion into the graft tissue (81). More studies and modification of delivery methods are needed to make photothrombosis clinically applicable.

Photodynamic therapy (PDT) has also been used to induce regression of CNV. PDT is generally administered through fiberoptics following injection of a photosensitizing dye such as dihematoporphyrin ether (DHE). PDT is thought to generate singlet oxygen radicals, which are cytotoxic to vessels that supply them. Histopathologic studies demonstrated attenuated vessels in the area of the injection site. Centrally there is a decrease in the number of keratocytes within the stroma with no damage to underlying endothelium. Peripherally, inflammatory cells are also present in association with attenuated blood vessels. PDT with DHE significantly reduces the area of CNV but does not completely eliminate it (82).

SURGICAL CORNEAL TRAUMA

Surgical injury to the cornea may be blunt or sharp. Blunt surgical trauma includes corneal epithelial abrasions and Descemet's membrane tears. Sharp injuries include penetrating and perforating wounds.

Corneal Epithelial Abrasions

Surgical trauma and topical medications used postoperatively, including steroids, antiglaucoma medications, and antibiotics, can damage the corneal epithelium (Fig. 20-7). There is a complex structural attachment of epithelium to stroma. The epithelial basement membrane is strongly adherent to the underlying Bowman's layer and is anchored by hemidesmosomes with the lamina lucida containing laminin and bullous pemphigoid antigen, below which lies the lamina densa (83,84). When tangential force is applied, the epithelial cells separate from their attachments at the junction between the bullous pemphigoid layer and laminin (85).

A superficial epithelial abrasion occurs when the surface and polygonal cell layers are traumatized without disruption of the basal cell layer or its basement membrane attachment. This type of abrasion heals by migration of adjacent polygonal epithelial cells (69).

Full-thickness wounds of the corneal epithelium heal by migration, mitoses, and differentiation. If the basement membrane is disrupted, the re-epithelialization can occur prior to the formation of adhesion complexes. Firm adhe-

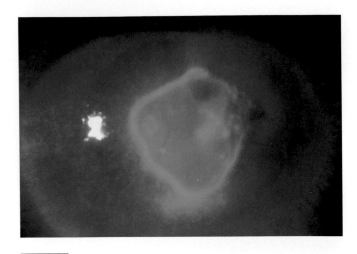

FIGURE 20-7. *Traumatic corneal epithelial abrasion (fluorescein stain). (Courtesy of R. M. Ahuja.)*

sion to Bowman's membrane may not develop for several weeks if the basement membrane needs to be regenerated (86). The lack of firm adhesions to Bowman's membrane can lead to recurrent erosions.

Limbal corneal injury repair occurs from migration of epithelium from the conjunctival epithelium. Conjunctival flaps are used to cover nonhealing corneal epithelial defects. If conjunctival vessel ingrowth has not occurred, the conjunctival epithelium loses its goblet cells and assumes the appearance of normal corneal epithelium after weeks (69). Conjunctival flaps are used because epithelial healing in corneal and conjunctival tissue is very similar. However, whereas the cornea forms only fibroblastic tissue, the conjunctiva, because of its vascularity, forms granulation tissue (45).

Tears of Descemet's Membrane

Descemet's membrane detachments may result from intraocular surgery. Cataract extraction with or without intraocular lens (IOL) placement, penetrating keratoplasty, iridectomy, and cyclodialysis can cause stripping of Descemet's membrane (87–94). A retrospective review revealed a history of prior intraocular surgery in 80% of patients, with the most frequent procedure being cataract extraction, in 52% (95). Descemet's membrane can be stripped by implantation of an IOL; use of dull instruments such as knife, keratome, or scissors or phacoemulsification hand pieces; vigorous irrigation and aspiration; and injection of intraocular solutions such as sodium hyaluronate (94–96). Some patients may have an inherent anatomic predisposition to Descemet's tears (91,97).

Light microscopy of Descemet's tears following IOL placement reveals thinning of the corneal epithelium with the edge of the broken Descemet's membrane folded upon itself, forming a cystlike space (Fig. 20-8). Non-iron-

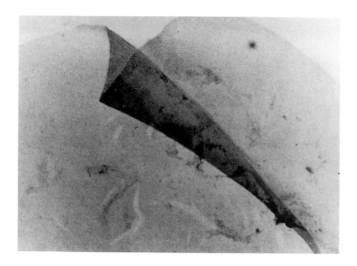

FIGURE 20-8. *Folded Descemet's membrane after intraocular surgery. (Reprinted with permission from Zeiter HJ, Zeiter JT. J Am Intraocular Implant Soc 1983;9:36–39.)*

staining pigmented cells may be present where Descemet's membrane turns away from the stroma. Hassall-Henle warts are present, with marked flattening of endothelial cell nuclei over the summit of the warts (89). In an eye with Descemet's membrane detachment secondary to injection of sodium hyaluronate, light microscopy reveals a normal corneal epithelium and Bowman's layer, with Descemet's membrane and endothelium detached by a lightly staining material.

Electron microscopy of the same eye demonstrates an anatomically intact endothelium and stripped Descemet's membrane. Numerous electron-dense globules of a fine granular material are present in the space between the membrane and the stroma. A monolayer of endothelial cells of 2.5 μm is present on the anterior surface of Descemet's membrane, with the cells appearing degenerated with multimembranous inclusions. The most posterior lamellae of the stroma appears abnormal because of the less-dense network of collagen (95).

Fibrous ingrowth was found after 22% of adult and 10% of congenital cataract extractions complicated by Descemet's membrane detachments (94). Of these eyes, 60% with fibrous ingrowth had detached fragments of Descemet's membrane. The amount of corneal edema and opacity depends on the size of the detachment. Minor detachments have a minor impact on vision, whereas extensive detachments of Descemet's membrane can lead to bullous keratopathy (87,96). The detached Descemet's membrane may curl back into place or the denuded area of stroma may be covered by newly formed Descemet's membrane. If this does not occur, iris may also adhere to the denuded portion of stroma, forming anterior synechiae.

Sharp Injuries

Perforating surgical injuries or wounds are usually limbal or perilimbal in location and have clean, sharply defined edges on pathologic examination. Wounds with a radius of curvature shorter than that of the cornea pucker or remain open, whereas linear wounds longer than the radius of curvature tend toward self-approximation (69). In deeper lacerations, the iris, lens, or ciliary body can be incarcerated in the wound.

In penetrating keratoplasty wounds, the stromal margins heal similarly to full-thickness incisions of the cornea. However, most of the fibroblasts are provided by recipient cornea. After perforating injuries the cornea begins the healing process in the first few hours. Epithelial downgrowth or fibrous ingrowth can complicate wound healing.

Retrocorneal Membranes and Epithelial Downgrowth

Retrocorneal membranes can occur after surgical perforating trauma. Epithelial downgrowth, fibrous ingrowth, endothelial proliferation, and retrocorneal melanin pigmentation (RCP) can produce membranous opacities behind the cornea. These membranes may appear as fine gray lines on the posterior corneal surface (Fig. 20-9).

Epithelial Downgrowth

Epithelial downgrowth carries a poor prognosis for vision. This relatively rare complication of surgical injury occurs at rates of 0.6% for all traumatic and surgical perforating injuries, up to 0.2% after cataract surgery, and 0.27% after penetrating keratoplasty (98–103).

Under normal circumstances, epithelium may grow into the depth of the corneal stromal wound, but as healing progresses, the epithelium is displaced to its proper level, preventing entry into the anterior chamber. However, if there is delayed wound closure, a poorly apposed wound, wound dehiscence, or incarceration of epithelial tissue in the surgical wound, the epithelium may continue to grow into the anterior chamber.

Epithelial downgrowth does not occur simply because access to the anterior chamber is present. Other factors are also necessary (104). The absence of contact inhibition by healthy corneal endothelium may allow for epithelium to enter the anterior chamber (105,106). Presence of a smooth surface such as a lens capsule or fibrin may aid the movement of the epithelial cells (107). Growth factors released in inflamed eyes owing to loss of the blood-ocular barrier may promote epithelial proliferation (108,109).

The histopathologic finding of nonkeratinized stratified squamous epithelium on the posterior surface of the cornea or over the iris is diagnostic (101). The epithelium is several layers thick when it covers well-vascularized surfaces, with nutrition provided by uveal tissue and aqueous humor (110).

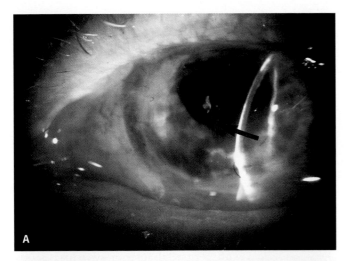

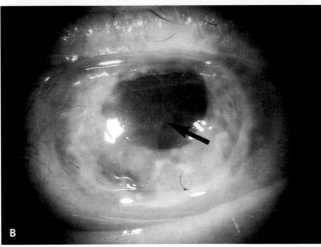

FIGURE 20-9. *A. A fine white line (arrow) is noted on the posterior cornea of a patient with keratoplasty. B. Seven months later, florid progression of epithelial downgrowth (arrow) is seen posterior to the corneal endothelium, with corneal decompensation. (H & E, ×40.) (Courtesy of J. S. Weiss.)*

Unlike endothelium, which is normally a monolayer, the epithelium is composed of more than one layer of cells and can therefore be differentiated from endothelium by hematoxylin and eosin stain (111).

Three types of cells are seen on cytopathologic examination: a flattened, rectangular surface cell; a rounded, basal cell; and the goblet cells with large vacuoles (111). Electron microscopic studies reveal wide intracellular borders, numerous surface microvilli, and prominent tonofilaments at the leading edge of the membrane. The prominent edge of the epithelial downgrowth noted on slit-lamp examination correlates to an increased epithelial cell thickness noted on histopathologic examination (99). The underlying endothelium is mostly degenerated or has undergone epithelial metaplasia (112–114). The trabecular meshwork appears dis-

organized and frequently results in intractable glaucoma (112).

Fibrous Ingrowth

Fibrous ingrowth is a rare complication of intraocular surgery and leads to the formation of a retrocorneal membrane as a result of fibrous proliferation and in-vasion of connective tissue into the anterior chamber. Histopathologic confirmation is infrequently obtained, as these eyes retain function and are not likely to be enucleated.

Henderson (115) first described fibrous ingrowth as a proliferation of subconjunctival connective tissue that invades the anterior chamber as a result of poorly healed cataract wounds, with incarcerated iris or lens acting as a bridge for the connective tissue ingrowth. Normally, endothelium bridges the inner aspect of the wound within 2 weeks after surgery, which confines fibroblast migration to the stromal defect alone. However, vitreous incarceration interferes with this normal wound healing. The frequency of fibrous ingrowth after cataract surgery with vitreous incarceration is reported to be 84%. Fibrous ingrowth was found in 36% of eyes enucleated owing to complications after cataract surgery and 15% of eyes enucleated after complications from glaucoma surgery (116–118). Fibrous ingrowth occurred in 50% to 80% of penetrating keratoplasty eyes (116).

There may be multiple causes of fibrous ingrowth. Hemorrhage in the anterior chamber may serve as a scaffold for fibrous proliferation. Inflammation in the anterior chamber can cause fibrous metaplasia of endothelial cells. Malposition of wound edges may cause persistent irritation and slow healing, allowing for fibrous ingrowth. Traumatic surgical perforating wounds causing rupture of Descemet's membrane may also lead to fibrous proliferation from metaplasia of stromal keratocytes or transformed endothelial cells (116,119).

Histopathologically, fibrous downgrowth is a multilayered sheet of fibroblast-like cells covering the posterior corneal surface (Fig. 20-10). The number of cell layers and thickness vary in different areas of the cornea. The multilaminar structure is composed primarily of collagen fibrils in addition to banded, fibrillar, and fibrocellular cells (120).

An abnormally increased response of the typical fibroblastic repair in surgical wound healing can lead to fibrous ingrowth (118). This may originate from either subepithelial connective tissue, corneal or limbal stromal fibroblasts, or metaplastic endothelium (116,119,121,122). Normal stromal wound healing requires cells that migrate from the limbus and transformation of existing stromal cells into keratocytes and then into fibroblasts which deposit new collagen. These stromal fibroblasts may be a source of the fibroplasia (123). Normally, endothelial cells convert into fibroblasts, which can regenerate Descemet's membrane, but the endothelial cells can undergo fibrous metaplasia because

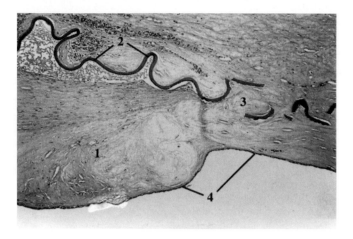

FIGURE 20-10. *A mass of dense connective tissue (1) rets on the posterior surface of Descemet's membrane (2), which is folded. The fibrosis communicates with the corneal stroma via breaks in Descemet's membrane at the site of the surgical wound (3). A thin layer of epithelial ingrowth (4) is seen on the posterior surface of the fibrous ingrowth. (PAS, ×25.) (Reproduced by permission from Lee SY, Rapuano CJ. Retrocorneal membranes. In: Krachmer JH, Mannis ML, Holland EJ, eds. Cornea: surgery of the cornea and conjunctiva. Vol. 3. St. Louis: Mosby-Year Book, 1996:1709–1717. Courtesy of Ralph Engle Jr, MD.)*

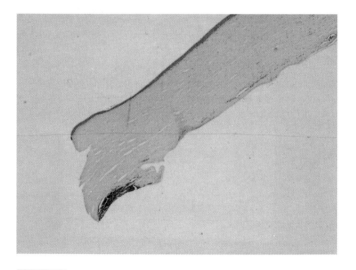

FIGURE 20-11. *Retrocorneal pigment noted after prior penetrating trauma. (H & E, ×40.) (Courtesy of J. S. Weiss.)*

they are mesodermally derived cells, as are fibroblasts (69,116).

Retrocorneal Melanin Pigmentation

RCP usually results from surgical penetrating trauma (Fig. 20-11). Histopathologic examination of 200 eyes with RCP revealed four cell types: iris stromal melanocytes, iris pigment epithelial cells, corneal endothelial cells with phagocytosed pigment granules, and pigmented macrophages (124).

Ninety-five percent of these eyes with RCP had a history of accidental or surgical trauma.

The iris stromal melanocytes form a golden-colored plaque on the endothelial surface with either a monolayer of dendritic-shaped cells or a multilayer of spindle-shaped cells, as seen by scanning electron microscopy. The melanin granules of iris melanocytes are smaller than iris pigment epithelial cells. Scanning electron microscopy shows melanocytes in anterior iris synechiae, enmeshed within fibrous or cellular strands connected to the retrocorneal surface by small fibrils.

Iris pigment epithelial cells are darker and plumper with sharp outlines. Transmission electron microscopy shows rounder melanin granules that are more variable in size. These cells also replace corneal endothelial cells and are always associated with peripheral anterior synechiae or iris incarceration in postsurgical corneal wounds.

Corneal endothelial cells that have engulfed pigment clumps form a more scattered pattern or a Krukenberg spindle. Transmission electron microscopy shows melanin granules to be in endothelial cells with a larger and more varied appearance than other types of melanin granules.

Pigmented macrophages are thick and round, densely pigmented cells with less contact to the posterior corneal surface. Transmission electron microscopy shows pseudopodia, secondary lysosomes with pigment granules, and the absence of a basement membrane. These cells are seen in combination with other cell types, especially endothelial cells with phagocytosed pigment granules, and are less specific to the release of pigment granules by the iris.

Endothelial Downgrowth

Corneal endothelial migration and proliferation in the anterior chamber can occur as a result of surgical trauma. Herbert (125) first described a "glass membrane" in eyes with chronic iridocyclitis. Donaldson and Smith (126) coined the term *tubular-appearing structure* in association with vitreous incarceration in corneal surgical wounds. Such membranes may represent a growth of endothelium onto zonular fibers (127).

In human endothelial wound healing, mitotic cell divisions are seen under unusual or pathologic conditions and indicate an abnormal proliferation of the cells (128,129). Proliferation of endothelium is a rare process after intraocular surgery (130). However, an abnormal response can occur and cause excess production of Descemet's membrane by the transformed endothelial cells, producing a fibrous tissue that is incorporated into Descemet's membrane and creating a thickened multilaminar Descemet's membrane (131). Corneal endothelium can abnormally proliferate in the anterior chamber and cover all free surfaces. Tubular structures are formed when endothelium proliferates along zonular fibers or vitreous strands adherent to a corneal wound (Fig. 20-12) (126). Histopathology of the fibers shows a solid cylinder with a connective tissue core covered by an elaborated Descemet's membrane–like material with

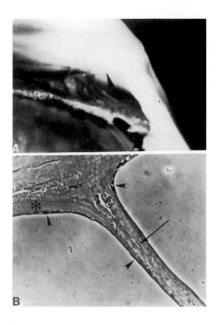

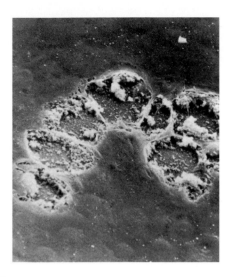

FIGURE 20-12.   *Phase-contrast photomicrograph of the inner aspect of a cataract wound, with thin, irregularly spaced endothelial cells (arrowheads) lining Descemet's membrane (asterisk) and vitreous strand (arrow). (Para-thenylenediamine, ×320.) (Reproduced by permission from McDonnell PJ, Cruz ZC, Green WR. Vitreous incarceration complicating cataract surgery. Ophthalmology 1986;93:247–253.)*

FIGURE 20-13.   *Scanning electron micrograph of human corneal endothelium following touch to the intraocular lens (dipped in balanced salt solution) for 15 seconds. The anterior membranes of cells have been torn off. (×600.) (Reproduced by permission from Kaufman HE, Katz JI. Endothelial damage from intraocular lens insertion.* Invest Ophthalmol Vis Sci *1976;15:996–1000.)*

PAS and von Giesen staining identical to that of Descemet's membrane. These may develop years after the original surgery. Corneal endothelial cell overgrowth of the angle occurs in association with peripheral anterior synechiae, with membranes covering the trabecular meshwork containing fibrillar structures, and glaucoma results (132).

Descemet's membrane may be regenerated by endothelial cells after vitreous incarceration in corneal surgical wounds, as early as 4 months postoperatively (118). Histopathology reveals spindle-shaped fibroblastic cells and collagen fibrils in the vitreous strands or Descemet's membrane surrounding vitreous, causing glassy tubes. Vitreous prevents the normal endothelial wound-healing process, allowing fibroblastic cellular proliferation with endothelial cell migration onto the vitreous strand and descemetization of the vitreous surface. Wolter and Fechner (133) described the histopathology of a glassy tube extending from the ciliary body to the vitreous as corneal endothelium and a secondary Descemet's membrane surrounding a core of vitreous. Sheetlike glassy membranes can also cover the iris and all other anterior-chamber structures (131).

INTRAOCULAR LENS PLACEMENT

Recent advances in cataract surgery techniques and IOL implants have helped to greatly reduce the nature and frequency of complications from cataract surgery, and modern IOL implantation overall carries a very low rate of compli-

cations. However, corneal complications still occur in association with IOL insertion.

Pseudophakic bullous keratopathy (PBK) is a serious complication of IOL implantation. Despite advances in the understanding of potential corneal complications and improvements in surgical techniques and IOLs, corneal endothelial damage still occurs (Fig. 20-13). In a recent literature review of 27 studies on complications following cataract surgery, the incidence of PBK varied from 0% to 3.0% after phacoemulsification, from 0% to 6% after extracapsular cataract extraction (ECCE), and from 0% to 0.1% after phacoemulsification or ECCE (134). In cohort studies, the proportion of eyes with PBK following phacoemulsification or ECCE was similar. A majority of cases involving psuedophakic corneal decompensation and bullous keratopathy result from long-term complications secondary to implantation of older IOLS that are no longer used. However, eyes with corneal decompensation are at increased risk for infection and secondary corneal ulceration.

Specular microscopic studies showed that in eyes that developed corneal edema after IOL implantation, there was a higher mean preoperative coefficient of variation of cell area, polymegathism (135). The eyes with greater preoperative polymegathism were more vulnerable to surgical trauma and had less functional reserve than did normal corneas. Pathologically, a marked variation in cell size represents a defect in cell morphology that may result in diminished functional ability. The larger cells may not interdigitate well with small cells, creating an ineffective structural barrier of endothelium and resulting in compromised function and corneal edema. At present no definitive answer has arisen to explain the role of corneal endothelial cell density and the postoperative development of corneal edema.

Edema is defined as the accumulation of fluid in the keratocytic extracellular space. Although 500 cells/mm² is usually considered a critical number for maintenance of corneal deturgescence, corneal edema can occur from a critical reduction of endothelial cell function.

The five histopathologic features of corneal edema are a deposition of collagen between the epithelium and Bowman's layer, a degenerative pannus, a loss of the clefts between stromal lamellae, deposition of basement membrane material within the epithelium with appearance of sub-epithelial bullae, and hydropic degeneration where the cytoplasm of the epithelial cells appears washed out (136).

Healthy corneas have a regular arrangement and distribution of different collagen types to help maintain a stable shape and clarity. Changes in collagen composition can alter the regular arrangement of stromal fibrils and lamellae, leading to a loss of clarity. Transmission electron microscopy studies of corneas from eyes with severe PBK associated with an anterior-chamber IOL showed the presence of collagen types I and III, possibly secondary to a transformation of corneal endothelial cells into fibroblasts, which secrete a scar tissue containing types I and III collagen fibrils in response to chronic stimulation by the anterior-chamber IOL. Type IV collagen was also produced in higher amounts in eyes with posterior-chamber IOLs, probably due to endothelial cell stimulation by IOL implantation. There was absence of type VI collagen in the posterior-chamber IOL group, which may have caused a disorganization of the orderly type I collagen fibril array and regularity of the interfibrillar space, leading to diminished corneal clarity (137).

Corneal decompensation due to long-term IOL contact occurs with less frequency because of the common use of posterior-chamber IOLs. Iris-supported IOLs are associated with the greatest rate of postoperative corneal edema. In a study comparing rigid anterior-chamber IOLs and posterior-chamber IOLs, at 5-year follow-up there was a 20% greater decrease of endothelial cell density of the central cornea in the anterior-chamber IOL group (138). A review of 13 studies in which 8515 iris fixation IOLs were implanted, the rate of corneal decompensation was 3.2 ± 4.3% (139). In another review of 3047 ECCE procedures with up to 10 years of follow-up, the rates of endothelial cell loss were 0.4% with no IOL, 5.0% with anterior-chamber IOLs, 3.6% with iris fixation IOLs, and 0.06% with posterior-chamber IOLs (140).

Endothelial cell loss and cell damage are greatest in the superior aspect of the cornea. Histology of the cornea immediately after cataract surgery shows that the endothelial cells lose their hexagonal shape and uniform size as they try to cover the defects of lost or damaged cells. The endothelial cells in the superior and central regions of the cornea show similar structural changes while the inferior corneal endothelial cells do not. The cells under normal

wound healing return to normal configuration within 3 months postoperatively. The corneal thickness returns to normal sooner because the endothelial pump regains normal function sooner (141,142).

Placement of IOLs can also lead to a progressive loss of endothelial cells. A 10-year postoperative analysis of patients who underwent cataract extraction with IOL implantation showed a 2.5% annual rate of corneal endothelial cell loss, which was 2.5 to 8.0 times the rate in healthy, age-matched, unoperated eyes (143). Fifty percent of the study patients had an ECCE with placement of a transiridectomy clip lens, 30% had an intracapsular cataract extraction with placement of an iris fixation lens, and 20% had an ECCE with placement of a posterior-chamber IOL. The lens type used did not affect the rate of endothelial cell loss, but eyes with corneal guttata continued to lose cells at twice the rate as other postoperative eyes. It is theorized that because of similar rates of cell loss between intracapsular and extracapsular extraction, the presence of the IOL may not be the cause of the cell loss (144). Cell loss may be due to other factors such as vitreous contact, chronic inflammation, toxic effects of intraoperative solutions, or changes in aqueous humor secondary to lack of a crystalline lens.

Contact between the IOL and the corneal endothelium can lead to endothelial cell damage and progressive loss. Specular microscopy shows loss of endothelial cells after IOL placement (145). Scanning electron microscopy demonstrates endothelial cell damage occurring from direct contact between the surface of the IOL and corneal endothelium, resulting in clinical endothelial cell loss (146).

PENETRATING KERATOPLASTY

The most frequent histopathologic finding in failed corneal grafts is the retrocorneal fibrous membrane (147) (Fig. 20-14, see also Fig. 20-11), which is found in 58% of corneal buttons removed for graft failure (148). Retrocorneal membranes are also common in functional grafts.

Postmortem examination of 30 eyes that had undergone prior penetrating keratoplasties revealed 26 of the grafts to be clear. Sixteen eyes had localized retrocorneal fibrous tissue posterior to the wound site (149). Overriding wound margins were frequent, with incarceration of Descemet's membrane in 22, incarceration of Bowman's membrane in 11, and incarceration of both structures in 9. Iris was incarcerated in the wound in 14 and vitreous was incarcerated in 8.

Sixty-one percent of the eyes that had undergone intracapsular cataract extraction had iris and vitreous incarceration. Of the eyes that had undergone ECCE, 18% had iris incarceration and none had vitreous incarceration. Twenty percent of specimens had retrocorneal pigmentation, the majority with iris incarceration.

Tissue incarceration in the corneal wound may predispose to wound-healing abnormalities (150,151). Wound

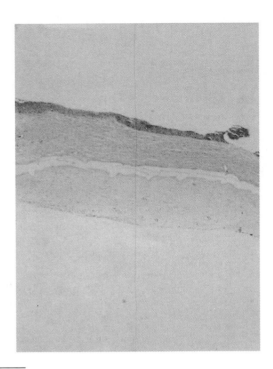

FIGURE 20-14. *Stromal downgrowth posterior to a failed graft. (H & E, ×100.) (Courtesy of J. S. Weiss.)*

margins heal similarly to other full-thickness incisions, with fibroblasts migrating from the adjacent stroma.

After re-epithelialization of the transplant, specular microscopy reveals abnormal cells that are irregular, large, nucleate or spindle-shaped up to 6 months postoperatively (152). Donor epithelium may disappear between 10 days (153) and 6 months (154).

Graft endothelial cells are maintained but are lost at a greater than normal rate during the life of the transplant. Specular microscopy reveals that endothelial cell density decreases 7.8% between 3 and 5 years after keratoplasty. At 1 and 3 years after surgery there is a significant relationship between the risk of graft failure and endothelial cell density. Endothelial failure accounts for 30% of graft failures but graft rejection is the most common cause of failure, causing 34% (155).

Confocal microscopy has been used in rabbits to diagnose graft rejection. Vessels with leukocyte infiltrates are observed at the capillary terminals and there is a reduction of stromal keratocyte density in the region of the infiltrate. Cellular infiltration in the stroma is also noted on histopathologic examination (156). Electron microscopic examination reveals lymphocytic invasion in the epithelium, stroma, and endothelium during the rejection episode (157).

Lymphocytes may travel through vascular channels to penetrate the anterior chamber through the graft-host interface. Consequently, poorly healed or aligned wounds may be at higher risk for rejection (158–160). Likewise, corneal vascularization also predisposes to rejection (161–163). Presence of Langerhans' cells that are immunocompetent

increases the risk of rejection for an oversized graft approaching limbus (164). Prior inflammation may increase the presence of immunocompetent cells and is associated with an increased risk of graft rejection.

Graft rejection may be classified by the specific location of the graft that is being attacked. Epithelial rejection causes a disorganization of cells in the area of the rejection line, which contains polymorphonuclear leukocytes with lymphocytes and blast cells (165).

During stromal rejection, monocytes, lymphocytes, plasma cells, and fibroblasts destroy the basement membrane. Immunoblast-like cells may be present in the area of the rejection, with disruption of the stromal lamellae and presence of new blood vessels. There may be extravasation of lymphocytes and plasma cells (166,167).

Endothelial graft rejection begins with endothelial cell destruction near the host-graft junction. The rejected endothelial cells lose their cell junctions and become elongated or rounded (168,169). Fibroblasts are also noted in areas of posterior collagenous layers (119,170).

RADIAL KERATOTOMY

Histopathologic examination of radial keratotomy wounds reveals changes that are similar to those in other unsutured corneal wounds. In normal wound healing, the epithelial plug regresses by 14 days when the fibroblasts have become fibrocytes. Myofibroblasts and scar tissue are oriented parallel (171) to the wound, resulting in wound closure (53) and wound stabilization by 6 months (52).

Analysis of corneal autopsy specimens from patients who previously underwent radial keratotomy revealed three separate adjacent morphologic zones of healing. The superficial duplicated basement membrane complex covers a zone resembling Bowman's membrane and a deeper zone with collagen parallel to the plugs. The orientation of the scar tissue is transverse at the base of the epithelial plug and sagittal in the deeper wound (171).

Histopathologic examination demonstrated prolonged intraincisional retention of epithelial cysts (52) from 3 to 47 months (172–174) after radial keratotomy (Fig. 20-15). In patients who required penetrating keratoplasty 5 to 6 months following radial keratotomy, histopathologic examination revealed incisional gaping and epithelial plugs up to 15 cell layers in depth and 11 cell layers in width (175).

Complete wound healing can take up to 66 months after radial keratotomy (174). Prolonged changes in wound healing are also confirmed by lectin-binding patterns, which differ 11 months and 66 months after radial keratotomy.

Wound depth may also affect healing. Incisions transversing more than 80% of the stromal depth may result in endothelial cell rupture. Tangential incisions can heal quicker than corresponding semiradial incisions, possibly because of their shallower depth (176).

Scar organization determines the ultimate recovery of tensile strength. Delayed corneal wound healing is the most

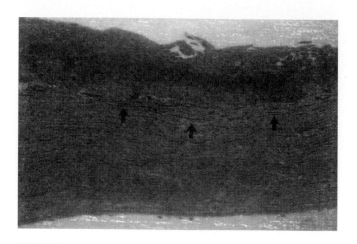

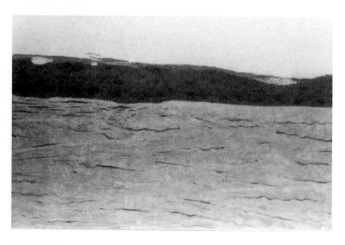

FIGURE 20-15.   *Human keratotomy wounds containing epithelial plugs at 46% (left), 18% (center), and 7% (right) stromal depths. The area with the transverse scar tissue organization directly underneath the base of the plug is indicated by an* arrowhead; *deeper wound regions show disorganization of cells and extracellular matrix. (Mallory's azure II–methylene blue with basic fuchsin counterstains, ×750.) (Reproduced by permission from Melles GRJ, Binder PS, Moore MN, Anderson A. Epithelial-stromal interactions in human keratotomy wound healing.* Arch Ophthalmol *1995;113:1124–1130.)*

FIGURE 20-16.   *Light micrograph of ablated cornea 4 months after photorefractive keratectomy, illustrating the smooth ablation into the stroma. (Toluidine blue and basic fuchsin, original magnification ×67.) (Reproduced by permission from Beuerman RW, McDonald MB, Shofner RS, et al.* Arch Ophthalmol *1994;112:1103–1110.)*

PHOTOREFRACTIVE KERATECTOMY

The pathologic changes that occur in the cornea following excimer laser photorefractive (PRK) or phototherapeutic (PTK) keratectomy mimic those changes ordinarily found after corneal wound healing. The time course of wound healing after PRK in monkeys is similar to that found after simple superficial keratectomy (184–195). Regardless of the preciseness of actual PRK treatment, the accuracy of the final refraction depends on the individual's capacity for stromal regeneration (184–193).

Soon after the initial ablation, a slide of epithelial cells is detected (184), followed by cellular division and migration (196–198). At 4 weeks, light microscopy reveals a thickened epithelium with columnar basal cells, which are noted to have larger dimensions than those in the untreated adjacent tissue (193). Scanning electron microscopy at 4 weeks demonstrates normal-appearing epithelial cells (193). At 12 weeks, the amount of epithelial thickening noted at the ablation edge is proportional to the depth of the ablation or the amount of myopia treatment (185,199). By 3 to 6 months, histology reveals normal epithelium (187,188,193,200) (Fig. 20-16). Specular microscopy confirms this finding in humans 6 months after PRK (200). By 4 to 18 months after PRK in monkeys, the basal laminae are almost totally regenerated although they appear more undulated (185).

The stability of the epithelial resurfacing requires accurate re-establishment of the epithelial adhesions to the underlying stroma. By day 7, an anchoring fibril zone is noted with small gaps at the edge of the ablated zone (190). Hemidesmosomes are present in normal number and distribution at 4 weeks (193) or are decreased in number (185). At the same time, tonofilaments are not very prominent but

common histopathologic finding in keratotomy wounds and explains subsequent refractive instability (57). Incomplete wound healing may result in progressive wound gape, corneal flattening, and hyperopia. Binder and Charlton (177) examined (51,176) corneal specimens removed after prior radial or astigmatic keratotomy and found wound-healing abnormalities that correlated with symptoms of decreased visual acuity, glare, undercorrection, and overcorrection.

There may also be an increased predisposition for a fully healed keratotomy wound to rupture if increased incisional stress concentration is caused by the presence of an epithelial plug in that incision (178). Rupture of a radial keratotomy incision from blunt ocular trauma can occur up to 10 years after the original surgery (179).

Retained epithelial plugs may result in corneal surface irregularities, subclinical recurrent erosions, and a predisposition to subsequent ulceration (180). Histopathologic examination of keratotomy sites in patients with bacterial keratitis who subsequently required keratoplasty revealed delayed corneal wound healing (181).

Because unpredictable wound healing causes unpredictable refractive results, other methods of refractive correction have been explored. Intrastromal rings composed of polymethylmethacrylate have been implanted in the peripheral cornea to flatten the corneal curvature and decrease myopia (182). Eight months after ring explantation, histopathologic examination of the human cornea demonstrated slight collagen compression and keratocyte loss where the ring had been (183).

become well established by 6 months. In human corneas that underwent prior PTK but were subsequently removed at the time of penetrating keratoplasty, normal anchoring fibrils were noted in only 8% of basal epithelial cells at 6 months and 35% at 15 months. The hemidesmosome population ranged from 35% to 37% during the same period of time. In fact, there was an almost linear increase in the percentage of basal cells noted to have anchoring fibrils proportional to the increased duration of wound healing. Although these findings were observed in abnormal corneas (201), they are confirmed by findings in monkeys where the basement membrane demonstrated focal areas of thickening, fragmentation, and absence as long as 18 months after PRK (184,202–204).

Destruction of Bowman's layer and the concomitant associated stromal changes are a major determinant of refractive results of PRK. Serial confocal microscopy in rabbits demonstrates maximal keratocyte loss between 24 and 48 hours, with an increase in spindle-shaped fibroblasts noted by 7 days. Deeper ablations demonstrate a longer duration of keratocyte loss and later appearance of fibroblasts (205). At 3 weeks, subepithelial fibroblasts are noted to have three times the density of normal keratocytes but this resolves by 9 months after PRK (188). At 4 weeks, light microscopy reveals vacuolization of the anterior stroma (193) with a high degree of resolution by 6 months. Deeper ablation shows more profound disturbances (Fig. 20-17).

In the monkey, keratocyte density peaked at 4 months but returned to normal at 12 months (185). Confocal microscopy in rabbits demonstrates at 1 month a densely reflective material between the anterior stroma and the epithelium which could correlate to stromal haze (206).

There is a positive correlation between the amount of new collagen deposited in the anterior stroma and the depth of the ablation or the amount of myopia treated (199). By specular microscopic study at 3 and 12 months following PRK in humans, the corneal endothelium appears to sustain no change (207).

Histopathologic and immunohistochemical changes including an accumulation of newly synthesized type 3 collagen and increased amounts of keratin sulfate are noted as late as 18 months after PRK (190).

These changes may correlate with the corneal haze. The haze appears to become maximal in amount from 4 to 6 months after PRK and then diminishes (184,208–210). In patients whose epithelium was removed after excessive myopic regression after PRK, the epithelium stained positively for hyaluronic acid, which seemed to correlate clinically with the higher amounts of stromal haze (211). Haze formation (see Fig. 21-16) may be related to the deposition of extracellular matrix in the subepithelial stroma (185,204,212–214) and stromal fibroblast hyperplasia (205,215,216). In monkeys, persistent haze at 12 months correlates with electron-lucent spaces in the subepithelial zone and these extracellular accumulations may cause the stromal opacity. New collagen deposition increases with deeper ablations, which would support the increased regression noted with corrections of higher degrees of myopia. Epithelial hyperplasia may contribute to myopic regression. Repeat PRK with the excimer laser was performed in monkeys 3 months after the initial PRK. Wound-healing changes appeared more pronounced and persistent than those after the initial PRK. Three months after the second PRK there was increased subepithelial haze, epithelial hyperplasia, increased subepithelial fibroblasts, and some disorganization of newly produced extracellular matrix (213). As late as 15 months after the second PRK, there was persistent basal vacuolization, focal basement membrane disruption, and organized subepithelial fibrous tissue.

REFERENCES

1. Kuwabara T. Current concepts in anatomy and histology of the cornea. *Contact Intraocular Lens Med J* 1978;4:101–113.
2. Snell RS, Lamp MA, eds. *Clinical anatomy of the eye.* Boston: Blackwell Science, 1989:119–136.
3. Rozsa AJ, Beuerman RW. Density and organization of free nerve endings in the corneal epithelium of the rabbit. *Pain* 1982;14:105–120.
4. Gipson IK, Sugrue SP. Cell biology of the corneal epithelium. In: Albert DM, Jakobiec FA, eds. *Principles and practice of ophthalmology.* Basic sciences. Philadelphia: WB Saunders, 1994:3–16.
5. Nichols BA, Chiappino ML, Dawson CR. Demonstration of the mucous layer of the tear film by electron microscopy. *Invest Ophthalmol Vis Sci* 1985;25:464–473.
6. Pfister RR. The normal and abnormal human corneal epithelial surface: a scanning electron microscopic study. *Invest Ophthalmol Vis Sci* 1977;16:614–622.
7. Schwarz MA, Owaribe K, Kartenbeck J, Franke WW. Desmosomes and hemidesmosomes: constitutive molecular components. *Annu Rev Cell Biol* 1990;6:461–491.
8. Hana C, O'Brien JE. Cell production and management in the epithelial layer of the cornea. *Arch Ophthalmol* 1960;64:536–540.
9. Lavker RM, Dong G, Chen SZ, et al. Relative proliferative rates of limbal and corneal epithelia: implications of corneal epithelial migration, circadian rhythm, and suprabasally located DNA synthesizing keratinocytes. *Invest Ophthalmol Vis Sci* 1991;32:1864–1875.
10. Waring GO. Corneal structure and pathophysiology. In: Leibowitz HM, ed. *Corneal disorders: clinical diagnosis and management.* Philadelphia: WB Saunders, 1984:3–56.
11. Schittny JC, Timpl R, Engel J. High resolution immunoelectron microscopic localization of functional domains of laminin, collagen, and heparin sulfate

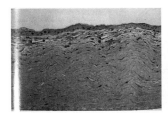
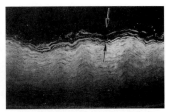

FIGURE 20-17. *Subepithelial scar formation after excimer laser keratectomy in a rabbit. Left. Epithelial irregularity is overlying diffuse, moderate to marked subepithelial hypercellular scar tissue formation. (H & E, ×190.) Right. Fluorescence microscopy demonstrates hypofluorescence in the area of the subepithelial scar formation with interdigitations between the stroma (fluorescent material) and new scar tissue in the wound bed. (×200.) (Reproduced by permission from Talamo J, Gollamudi S, Green WR, et al. Arch Ophthalmol 1991;109:1141–1146.)*

proteoglycan in epithelial basement membrane of mouse cornea reveals different topological orientations. *J Cell Biol* 1988;107:1599–1610.

12. Maurice DM. The structure and transparency of the corneal stroma. *J Physiol* 1957;136:263–268.

13. Linsenmayer TF, Fitch JM, Birk DE. Heterotypic collagen fibrils and stabilizing collagens. Controlling elements in corneal morphogenesis? *Ann NY Acad Sci* 1990;580:143–160.

14. Birk DE, Fitch JM, Babiarz JP, et al. Collagen fibrillogenesis in vitro: interaction of types I and V collagen regulates fibril diameter. *J Cell Sci* 1990;95:649–657.

15. Cho H, Covington HI, Cintron C. Immuno localization of type VI collagen in development and healing of rabbit cornea. *Invest Ophthalmol Vis Sci* 1990;31:1096–1202.

16. Yue BY, Baum JL, Silbert JE. Synthesis of glycosaminoglycans by cultures of normal corneal endothelial and stromal cells. *Invest Ophthalmol Vis Sci* 1978;17:523–527.

17. Sawada H, Konomi H, Hirosawa K. Characterization of the collagen in the hexagonal lattice of Descemet's membrane: its relation to type VIII collagen. *J Cell Biol* 1990;110:219–227.

18. Rao GN, Lohman LE, Aquavella JV. Cell size-shape relationship in corneal endothelium. *Invest Ophthalmol Vis Sci* 1982;22:271–274.

19. Hiles DA, Biglan AW, Fetherolf EC. Central corneal endothelial cell counts in children. *Am Intraocular Implant Soc J* 1979;5:292–300.

20. Davanger M, Olsen EG. The corneal endothelial cell interface. *Acta Ophthalmol* 1985;63:443–448.

21. Sherrard ES, Ng YL. The other side of the corneal endothelium. *Cornea* 1990;9:48–54.

22. Geroski DH, Edelhauser HF. Quantitation of Na/K ATPase pump sites in the rabbit corneal endothelium. *Invest Ophthalmol Vis Sci* 1984;25:1056–1060.

23. Rae JL, Lewno AW, Cooper K, Gates P. Dye and electrical coupling between cells of the rabbit corneal endothelium. *Curr Eye Res* 1989;8:859–869.

24. Iwamoto T, Smelser GK. Electron microscopy of the human corneal endothelium with reference to transport mechanisms. *Invest Ophthalmol* 1965;4:270–276.

25. Schemer A, Galvin S, Sun TT. Differentiation: related expression of a major 64K corneal keratin in vivo and in culture suggests limbal location of corneal epithelial stem cells. *J Cell Biol* 1996;103:49–62.

26. Schultz G. Modulation of corneal wound healing. In: Krachmer JH, Mannis MJ, Holland EJ, eds. *Cornea: fundamentals of cornea and external disease.* Vol. 1. St. Louis: Mosby-Year Book, 1996:183–198.

27. Jeanblatt MM, Neufeld AH. A final culture of corneal epithelial wound closure. *Invest Ophthalmol Vis Sci* 1986;27:8–13.

28. Burrill PH, Bernadini J, Kleinman HK, Kretchmer N. Effect of serum fibronectin and laminin on adhesion of rabbit intestinal epithelial cells in culture. *J Supramol Struct Cell Biochem* 1981;16:385–392.

29. Fujikawa LS, Foster CS, Harriet HJ, et al. Fibronectin in healing rabbit corneal wounds. *Lab Invest* 1981;45:120–129.

30. Fujikawa LS, Foster CS, Gipson IK, Colvin RB. Basement membrane components in healing rabbit corneal epithelial wounds: immunofluorescence and ultrastructural studies. *J Cell Biol* 1984;98:128–138.

31. Phan TM, Foster CX, Wasson PJ, et al. Role of fibronectin and fibrinogen in healing of corneal epithelial scrape wounds. *Invest Ophthalmol Vis Sci* 1989;30:377–385.

32. Frati L, Daniele S, Delogu A, Covelli I. Selective binding of epidermal growth factor and its specific effects on the epithelial cells of the cornea. *Exp Eye Res* 1972;14:135–141.

33. Khaw PT, Schultz GS, Mackay SLD, et al. Detection of transforming growth factor alpha messenger RNA and protein in human corneal epithelial cells. *Invest Ophthalmol Vis Sci* 1992;33:3302–3306.

34. Garana RM, Petroll WM, Chen WT, et al. Radial keratotomy II: the role of the myofibroblast in corneal wound contraction. *Invest Ophthalmol Vis Sci* 1992;33:3271–3282.

35. Skalli O, Schurch W, Seemayer T, et al. Myofibroblasts from diverse pathologic conditions are heterogeneous in their content of actin isoforms and intermediate filament protein. *Lab Invest* 1989;60:275–285.

36. Jester J, Steel D, Salz J, et al. Radial keratotomy in non-human primate eyes. *Am J Ophthalmol* 1981;92:153–157.

37. McDermott ML. Stromal wound healing. In: Brightbill FS, ed. *Corneal surgery.* 2nd ed. Chicago: Mosby-Year Book, 1993:44–51.

38. Luttrull JK, Smith RE, Jester JV. In vitro contractility of avascular corneal wounds in rabbit eyes. *Invest Ophthalmol Vis Sci* 1985;26:1449–1452.

39. Davian PF, Gallary EJ. Connective tissue remodeling in corneal and scleral wounds. *Invest Ophthalmol Vis Sci* 1986;27:1478–1484.

40. Ichuima H, Jester JV, Petroll WM, Cavanaugh HD. Laser and tandem scanning confocal microscopic studies of the rabbit corneal wound healing. *Scanning* 1994;16:263–268.

41. Jaffee NS, Jaffee MS, Jaffee GF. *Cataract surgery and its complications.* St. Louis: CV Mosby, 1990:21–34.

42. Van Horn DL, Sendele DD, Seidman S, Buco PJ. Regenerative capacity of the corneal endothelium in the rabbit and rat. *Invest Ophthalmol Vis Sci* 1977;16:597–613.

43. Sherrard ES. The corneal endothelium in vivo: its response to mild trauma. *Exp Eye Res* 1976;22:347–357.

44. Joyce ND, Meklin B, Neufeld AH. In vitro pharmacologic separation of corneal endothelial migration and spreading responses. *Invest Ophthalmol Vis Sci* 1990;31:1816–1826.

45. Yanoff M, Fine BS, eds. *Ocular pathology: a text and atlas.* 3rd ed. Philadelphia: JB Lippincott, 1989.

46. Lang GK, Green WR, Maumenee AE. Clinicopathologic studies of keratoplasty eyes obtained post mortem. *Am J Ophthalmol* 1986;101:28–40.

47. Swan KC, Morrison JC. Corneal wound healing after penetrating keratoplasty. *Trans Pan Coast Otol Ophthalmol Soc* 1985;66:99–109.

48. Morrison JC, Swan KC. Full thickness lamellar keratoplasty: a histologic study in human eyes. *Ophthalmology* 1982;89:715–719.

49. Luttrull JK, Luttrull JK, Smith RE, Jester JV. In vitro contraction of avascular corneal wounds in rabbit eyes. *Invest Ophthalmol Vis Sci* 1985;26:1449–1452.

50. Coldwell KA, Binder PS. High voltage electron microscopic analysis of wound healing after human radial keratotomy. *Invest Ophthalmol Vis Sci* 1988;29(suppl):280–287.

51. Melles GRJ, Binder PS. A comparison of wound healing in sutured and unsutured corneal wounds. *Arch Ophthalmol* 1990;108:1460–1469.

52. Binder PS, Wickham MG, Zabala EY, Ackers PH. *Corneal anatomy and wound healing.* In: *Symposium on medical and surgical disease of the cornea. Transactions of the New Orleans Academy of Ophthalmology.* St. Louis: CV Mosby, 1980:1–35.

53. Binder PS. What we have learned about corneal wound healing from refractive surgery. *Refract Corneal Surg* 1989;5:98–120.

54. Cintron C, Szamier RB, Hassinger LC, Kublin CL. Scanning electron microscopy of rabbit corneal scars. *Invest Ophthalmol Vis Sci* 1982;23:50–63.

55. Cintron C, Hassinger LC, Kublin CL, Cannon DJ. Biochemical and ultrastructural changes in collagen during corneal wound healing. *Ultrastruct Res* 1978;65:13–22.

56. Davison PF, Gallbavy EJ. Connective tissue remodeling in corneal and scleral wounds. *Invest Ophthalmol Vis Sci* 1986;27:478–484.

57. Jester JV, Villasenor RAM, Schanzlin DJ, Cavanagh HD. Variations in corneal wound healing after radial keratotomy: possible insights into mechanisms of clinical complications and refractive effects. *Cornea* 1992;11:191–199.

58. Melles GRJ, Binder PS, Anderson JA. Variation in healing throughout the depth of long-term, unsutured, corneal wounds in human autopsy specimens and monkeys. *Arch Ophthalmol* 1994;112:100–109.

59. Troutman RC. Microsurgery of the anterior segment of the eye. In: Spencer WH, ed. *The cornea. Optics and surgery.* Vol. 2. St. Louis: CV Mosby, 1977:263–273.

60. Melles GRJ, Binder PS, Beekhaus WH. Scar tissue orientation in unsutured and sutured corneal wound healing. *Br J Ophthalmol* 1995;79:760–765.

61. McCulley JP, Eliason JA. A comparison of interrupted and continuous suturing in keratoplasty. *Invest Ophthalmol Vis Sci* 1978;17(suppl):120–125.

62. Leibowitz HM, Waring GO. Operative procedures in penetrating keratoplasty. In: Leibowitz HM, ed. *Corneal disorders: clinical diagnosis and management.* Philadelphia: WB Saunders, 1984:589–629.

63. Acheson JF, Lyons CJ. Ocular morbidity due to monofilament nylon corneal surfaces. *Eye* 1991;5:106–112.

64. Balyeat HD, Davis RM, Rowsey J. Nylon suture toxicity after cataract surgery. *Ophthalmology* 1988;95:1509–1514.

65. Haysaka S, Ishiguro S, Shiono T, et al. A scanning EM study of nylon degradation by ocular tissue extracts. *Am J Ophthalmol* 1982;93:111–117.

66. Drews RC. Astigmatism after cataract surgery: nylon versus Mersilene. *J Cataract Refract Surg* 1995;21:70–72.

67. Freuh BE, Brown SI, Feldman ST. 11-0 Mersilene as running suture for penetrating keratoplasty. *Am J Ophthalmol* 1992;113:406–411.

68. Frucht-Perry J. Mersilene sutures for corneal surgery. *Ophthalmol Surg* 1995;26:117–120.

69. Spencer WH. Cornea. In: Spencer WH, ed. *Ophthalmic pathology: an atlas and textbook.* Vol. 1. 4th ed. Philadelphia: WB Saunders, 1996:157–333.

70. Fromer CH, Klintworth GK. An evaluation of the role of leukocytes in the pathogenesis of experimentally induced corneal vascularization: III. Studies related to the vasoproliferative capability of polymorphonuclear leukocytes. *Am J Pathol* 1996;82:157–170.

71. Epstein RJ, Stulting RD. Corneal neovascularization induced by stimulated lymphocytes in inbred mice. *Inves Ophthal Vis Sci* 1987;28:1505–1513.

72. Ben Ezra D, Hemo I, Maftzir G. In vivo antigenic activity of interleukins. *Arch Ophthalmol* 1990;108:573–576.

73. Ben Ezra D. Neovasculogenic ability of prostaglandins, growth factors and synthetic chemoattractants. *Am J Ophthalmol* 1978;86:455–461.

74. Khodadoust AA. The allograft rejection reaction: the leading cause of late failure of corneal graft rejection. *Ciba Found Symp* 1973;15:151–164.

75. Cherry PMH, Faulkner JD, Shaver RP, et al. Argon laser treatment of CNV. *Ann Ophthalmol* 1973;5:911–920.

76. Michaelson IC. Effect of cortisone upon corneal vascularization induced experimentally. *Arch Ophthalmol* 1952;47:459–464.

77. Reed JW, Fromer C, Klintworth GK. Induced corneal vascularization. Remission with argon laser therapy. *Arch Ophthalmol* 1975;93:1017–1019.

78. Nirankari VS, Dandera L, Rodrigues MM. Laser photocoagulation of experimental corneal stromal vascularization—efficacy and histopathology. *Ophthalmology* 1994;100:111–118.

79. Hemady RK, Baer JC, Foster CS. Biomicroscopic and histopathologic observation after corneal laser photocoagulation in a rabbit model of CNV. *Cornea* 1993;12:185–190.

80. Huang AJW, Watson BD, Hernandez E, Tseng SCG. Photothrombosis of corneal neovascularization by intravenous rose bengal and argon laser irradiation. *Arch Ophthalmol* 1988;106:680–685.

81. Corrent G, Roussel TJ, Scheffer CG, Watson BD. Promotion of graft survival by photothrombotic occlusion of corneal vascularization. *Arch Ophthalmol* 1989;107:1501–1506.

82. Epstein RJ, Harris DM. Photodynamic therapy for corneal neovascularization. *Cornea* 1991;10:424–432.

83. Hamill B. Corneal injury. In: Krachmer JH, Mannis MJ, Holland EJ, eds. *Cornea: fundamentals of cornea and external disease.* Vol. 1. St. Louis: Mosby-Year Book, 1996:1403–1422.

84. Fujikawa LS, Foster CS, Gipson IK, Colvin RB. Basement membrane component in healing rabbit corneal epithelial wounds: immunofluorescence and ultrastructural studies. *J Cell Biol* 1984;98:128–138.

85. Parrish CM, Chandler JW. Corneal trauma. In: Kaufman HE, ed. *The cornea.* New York: Churchill Livingstone, 1988.

86. Khodadoust AA, Silverstein AM, Kenyon KR, Dowling JJ. Adhesion of regenerating corneal epithelium: the role of the basement membrane. *Am J Ophthalmol* 1968;65:339–348.

87. Sugar HS. Prognosis in stripping of Descemet's membrane in cataract extraction. *Am J Ophthalmol* 1967;63:140–143.

88. Goodman DF, Stark WJ, Gottich J. Complication of cataract extraction and intraocular lens implantation. *Ophthalmic Surg* 1989;20:132–140.

89. Makey TA, Keates RH. Detachment of Descemet's membrane and insertion of intraocular lens. *Ophthalmic Surg* 1980;11:492–494.

90. Sparks GM. Descemetopexy. Surgical reattachment of stripped Descemet's membrane. *Arch Ophthalmol* 1967;78:31–34.

91. Samuel B. Detachment of Descemet's membrane. *Trans Am Ophthalmol Soc* 1928;26:427–437.

92. Lang GK, Green WR, Maumenee AE. Clinicopathological studies of keratoplasty eyes obtained post mortem. *Am J Ophthalmol* 1986;101:26–40.

93. Brown SI, Dohlman CH, Boruchoff SA. Dislocation of Descemet's membrane during keratoplasty. *Am J Ophthalmol* 1973;76:51–53.

94. Bettman JW. Pathology of complications of intraocular surgery. *Am J Ophthalmol* 1969;68:1037–1050.

95. Pieramici D, Bree WR, Stark WJ. Stripping of Descemet's membrane: a clinicopathologic correlation. *Ophthalmic Surg* 1994;25:226–231.

96. Sugar A. Surgical trauma—pseudophakia and aphakic corneal edema. In: Krachmer JH, Mannis ML, Holland EJ, eds. *Cornea and external disease: clinical diagnosis and management.* Vol. 2. St. Louis: Mosby-Year Book, 1996:1423–1435.

97. Reese AB. Discussion of Scheie HG. Stripping of Descemet's membrane in cataract extraction. *Trans Am Ophthalmol Soc* 1964;62:131–138.

98. Theobald GD, Haas JS. Epithelial invasion of the anterior chamber following cataract extraction. *Trans Am Acad Ophthalmol Otol* 1948;52:470–479.

99. Weiner MJ, Trentcoste J, Pon DM, Albert DM. Epithelial downgrowth: a 30 year clinicopathological review. *Br J Ophthalmol* 1989;73:6–11.

100. Otradover J, Zicha Z. Epithelial invasion of the anterior chamber after cataract extraction. *Cesk Oftalmol* 1960;16:131–142.

101. Bernardino VB, Kim JC, Smith TR. Epithelialization of the anterior chamber after cataract extraction. *Arch Ophthalmol* 1969;82:742–750.

102. Sugar A, Meyer RF, Hood CI. Epithelial downgrowth following penetrating keratoplasty in the aphake. *Arch Ophthalmol* 1977;95:464–467.

103. Feder RS, Krachmer JH. The diagnosis of epithelial downgrowth after keratoplasty. *Am J Ophthalmol* 1985;99:697–703.

104. Lee SY, Rapuano CJ. Retrocorneal membrane in the cornea. In: Krachmer JH, Mannis MJ, Holland EJ, eds. *Cornea. Fundamentals of the cornea and external disease.* Vol. 2. St. Louis: Mosby-Year Book, 1996:1709–1717.

105. Davenger M, Olsen EG. Experimental epithelial ingrowth. Epithelial/endothelial interaction through a corneal perforation studied in organ culture. *Acta Ophthalmol* 1985;63:443–448.

106. Cameron JD, Flaxman BA, Yanoff M. In vitro studies of corneal wound healing: epithelial/endothelial interactions. *Invest Ophthalmol Vis Sci* 1974;13:575–579.

107. Bruner WE, Green WR, Stark WJ. A case of epithelial ingrowth primarily involving the lens capsule. *Ophthalmic Surg* 1986;17:483–485.

108. Pack A, Tso MOM, Yul B. Cellular deposits on intraocular lenses. *Acta Ophthalmol Suppl (Copenh)* 1985;170:54–57.

109. Smith DR, Sommerville GM, Shew M. An experimental model of epithelialization of the anterior chamber. *Can J Ophthalmol* 1967;2:158–162.

110. Lytle RA, Simmons RJ. Epithelial and fibrous proliferation. In: Albert DM, Jakobiec FA, eds. *Principles and practice of ophthalmology.* Vol. 3. Philadelphia: WB Saunders, 1994:1479–1485.

111. Engel HM, Green WR, Michaels RG, et al. Diagnostic vitrectomy. *Retina* 1981;1:121–149.

112. Zavala EY, Binder PS. The pathologic findings of epithelial ingrowth. *Arch Ophthalmol* 1980;98:2007–2014.

113. Yamaguchi T, Polack FM, Valenti J. Electron microscopy study of epithelial downgrowth after penetrating keratoplasty. *Br J Ophthalmol* 1981;65:374–382.

114. Burris TE, Rowsey JJ, Nordquist RE. Model of epithelial downgrowth: scanning and transmission electron microscopy of corneal epithelialization. *Cornea* 1985;4:249–255.

115. Henderson T. A histological study of the normal healing of wounds after cataract extraction. *Ophthalmic Rev* 1907;26:107–113.

116. Waring GO, Laibson RR, Rodriques MM. Clinical and pathologic alterations of Descemet's membrane: with emphasis on endothelial metaplasia. *Surv Ophthalmol* 1974;18:325–368.

117. McDonnell PJ, de la Cruz ZC, Green WR. Vitreous incarceration complicating cataract surgery. *Ophthalmology* 1986;93:247–253.

118. Allen JC. Epithelial and stromal ingrowth. *Am J Ophthalmol* 1968;68:179–182.

119. Waring GO, Bourne WM, Edelhauser HF, Kenyon KR. The corneal endothelium: normal and pathologic structure and function. *Ophthalmology* 1982;89:532–590.

120. Waring GO. Posterior collagenous layer of the cornea: ultrastructural classification of abnormal collagenous tissue posterior to Descemet's membrane in 30 cases. *Arch Ophthalmol* 1982;100:122–134.

121. Swan KC. Fibroblastic ingrowth following cataract extraction. *Arch Ophthalmol* 1973;89:445–449.

122. Rodriques MM, Waring GO, Laibson PR, Weinreb S. Endothelial alterations in congenital corneal dystrophies. *Am J Ophthalmol* 1975;80:678–689.

123. Weimar VL. The sources of fibroblasts in corneal wound repair. *Arch Ophthalmol* 1958;60:93–109.

124. Kampik A, Patrinely JR, Green WR. Morphologic and clinical features of retrocorneal melanin pigmentation and pigmented pupillary membranes: review of 225 cases. *Surv Ophthalmol* 1982;27:161–180.

125. Herbert H. Glass membrane formation in chronic iridocyclitis. *Trans Ophthalmol Soc UK* 1927;47:155–164.

126. Donaldson DD, Smith TR. Descemet's membrane tubes. *Trans Am Ophthalmol Soc* 1966;64:89–109.

127. Wolter JR. Descemet's membrane tubes on the zonular fibers of the lens. *J Pediatr Ophthalmol* 1969;6:153–156.

128. Binder RF, Binder HF. Regenerative processes in the endothelium of cornea. *Arch Ophthalmol* 1957;57:11–13.

129. Cogan DG. Applied anatomy and physiology of the cornea. *Trans Am Acad Ophthalmol Otol* 1951;55:229–259.

130. Rowsey JJ, Gaylor JR. Intraocular lens disasters: peripheral anterior synechiae. *Ophthalmology* 1980;87:646–664.

131. Smith SG, Lindstrom RL, eds. *Intraocular lens: complications and management.* Thorofare, NJ: Slack, 1988:1–43.

132. Harris M, Tso AY, Kaba FW, et al. Corneal endothelial overgrowth of angle and its evidence of myoblastic differentiation in 3 cases. *Ophthalmology* 1984;91:1154–1160.

133. Wolter JR, Fechner PU. Glass membranes on the anterior iris surface. *Am J Ophthalmol* 1962;53:235–243.

134. Powe NR, Schein DD, Gieser SC, et al. Synthesis of the literature on visual acuity and complications following cataract extraction with intraocular lens implantation. *Arch Ophthalmol* 1994;112:239–252.

135. Rao GN, Aquavella JV, Goldberg SH, Beck SL. PBK: relationship to preoperative corneal endothelial status. *Ophthalmology* 1984;91:1135–1140.

Evolution and Current Status of Cataract Surgery

Henry M. Clayman

HISTORY

Cataract has been an affliction since time immemorial and it is natural that mankind would have sought a remedy. The earliest documentations of cataract surgery are derived from the Assyrian code of Hammaurabi and ancient Hindu medicine, specifically the teachings of Susrata. The exact dates of Susrata's work are debatable but have been estimated as emanating 2000 years ago. The Susrata technique was termed *couching* and involved displacement of the crystalline lens into the posterior chamber, thus clearing the visual axis. In this technique the sclera was perforated with a sharp instrument, after which a blunt instrument was inserted through the scleral incision and the cataractous lens was displaced posteriorly. Though techniques varied, couching was practiced into this century by native healers in India.

Duke-Elder (1) cited an ancient technique that surely was a harbinger of contemporary surgery. He noted that the Arabian surgeon Ammar (996–1020) operated on a soft cataract by inserting an intralenticular hollow tube and aspirating the cataractous material. However, it is Jacques Daviel (1696–1762) of France who may be considered the founder of modern cataract surgery. In 1748 Daviel described his technique of cataract surgery in which the cataractous lens was extracted from the eye, directly from its natural position behind the iris. The Daviel technique was not a modified couching procedure by which the cataract was displaced anteriorly into the anterior chamber and then removed; it was in fact a planned extracapsular extraction (ECCE).

Intracapsular cataract extraction (ICCE), in which the crystalline lens is extracted in entirety, was first practiced about 250 years ago, almost concurrent with the Daviel technique. In these early techniques the lens was literally squeezed out of the eye by digital pressure on the limbus or sclera after the appropriate limbal incision was made. Instruments were later used to apply suitable pressure, perhaps the best-known maneuver being the *Smith Indian technique* wherein pressure was applied by a muscle hook at the inferior limbus and the cataract was expelled through a superior incision. ICCE was also performed with spoons and forceps, the former being inserted behind the cataract, which was then lifted out of the eye. Forceps extractions involved grasping the anterior lens capsule and with gentle traction either sliding or tumbling the cataract out of the eye, a technique that persisted into the 1960s. Inherent in these early cataract techniques was the risk of both vitreous loss and capsule rupture. The profession therefore sought other techniques in the hope of facilitating a safer operation. Several surgeons devised techniques using a suction cup to fixate the anterior capsule and these ran the gamut from a simple suction cup to an electrically controlled device called an *erisiphake* (2). Diathermy was also proposed.

The seminal event in ICCE instrumentation was the introduction of cryoextraction by Krwawicz of Poland in 1961 (3). Krwawicz devised a nickel-plated, copper ball-tip applicator which he called a *cryoextractor*. This instrument had no inherent refrigerant capabilities and was chilled, prior to intraoperative use, by immersion into a thermos flask containing a mixture of dry ice and methyl alcohol. Kelman, influenced by neurosurgical applications of tissue freezing and unaware of Krwawicz's prechilled cryoextractor, independently introduced cryoextraction in the United States using liquid nitrogen as the refrigerant. The cryoextraction technique, infrequently used in the United States nowadays, is described in the next chapter. At this point in the discussion, note should be made of an important pharmacologic observation reported by J. Barraquer in 1957. In an attempt to dissolve an extensive hyphema, Barraquer

71. Epstein RJ, Stulting RD. Corneal neovascularization induced by stimulated lymphocytes in inbred mice. *Inves Ophthal Vis Sci* 1987;28:1505–1513.

72. Ben Ezra D, Hemo I, Maftzir G. In vivo antigenic activity of interleukins. *Arch Ophthalmol* 1990;108:573–576.

73. Ben Ezra D. Neovasculogenic ability of prostaglandins, growth factors and synthetic chemoattractants. *Am J Ophthalmol* 1978;86:455–461.

74. Khodadoust AA. The allograft rejection reaction: the leading cause of late failure of corneal graft rejection. *Ciba Found Symp* 1973;15:151–164.

75. Cherry PMH, Faulkner JD, Shaver RP, et al. Argon laser treatment of CNV. *Ann Ophthalmol* 1973;5:911–920.

76. Michaelson IC. Effect of cortisone upon corneal vascularization induced experimentally. *Arch Ophthalmol* 1952;47:459–464.

77. Reed JW, Fromer C, Klintworth GK. Induced corneal vascularization. Remission with argon laser therapy. *Arch Ophthalmol* 1975;93:1017–1019.

78. Nirankari VS, Dandera L, Rodrigues MM. Laser photocoagulation of experimental corneal stromal vascularization—efficacy and histopathology. *Ophthalmology* 1994;100:111–118.

79. Hemady RK, Baer JC, Foster CS. Biomicroscopic and histopathologic observation after corneal laser photocoagulation in a rabbit model of CNV. *Cornea* 1993;12:185–190.

80. Huang AJW, Watson BD, Hernandez E, Tseng SCG. Photothrombosis of corneal neovascularization by intravenous rose bengal and argon laser irradiation. *Arch Ophthalmol* 1988;106:680–685.

81. Corrent G, Roussel TJ, Scheffer CG, Watson BD. Promotion of graft survival by photothrombotic occlusion of corneal vascularization. *Arch Ophthalmol* 1989;107:1501–1506.

82. Epstein RJ, Harris DM. Photodynamic therapy for corneal neovascularization. *Cornea* 1991;10:424–432.

83. Hamill B. Corneal injury. In: Krachmer JH, Mannis MJ, Holland EJ, eds. *Cornea: fundamentals of cornea and external disease.* Vol. 1. St. Louis: Mosby-Year Book, 1996:1403–1422.

84. Fujikawa LS, Foster CS, Gipson IK, Colvin RB. Basement membrane component in healing rabbit corneal epithelial wounds: immunofluorescence and ultrastructural studies. *J Cell Biol* 1984;98:128–138.

85. Parrish CM, Chandler JW. Corneal trauma. In: Kaufman HE, ed. *The cornea.* New York: Churchill Livingstone, 1988.

86. Khodadust AA, Silverstein AM, Kenyon KR, Dowling JJ. Adhesion of regenerating corneal epithelium: the role of the basement membrane. *Am J Ophthalmol* 1968;65:339–348.

87. Sugar HS. Prognosis in stripping of Descemet's membrane in cataract extraction. *Am J Ophthalmol* 1967;63:140–143.

88. Goodman DF, Stark WJ, Gottich J. Complication of cataract extraction and intraocular lens implantation. *Ophthalmic Surg* 1989;20:132–140.

89. Makey TA, Keates RH. Detachment of Descemet's membrane and insertion of intraocular lens. *Ophthalmic Surg* 1980;11:492–494.

90. Sparks GM. Descemetopexy. Surgical reattachment of stripped Descemet's membrane. *Arch Ophthalmol* 1967;78:31–34.

91. Samuel B. Detachment of Descemet's membrane. *Trans Am Ophthalmol Soc* 1928;26:427–437.

92. Lang GK, Green WR, Maumenee AE. Clinicopathological studies of keratoplasty eyes obtained post mortem. *Am J Ophthalmol* 1986;101:26–40.

93. Brown SI, Dohlman CH, Boruchoff SA. Dislocation of Descemet's membrane during keratoplasty. *Am J Ophthalmol* 1973;76:51–53.

94. Bettman JW. Pathology of complications of intraocular surgery. *Am J Ophthalmol* 1969;68:1037–1050.

95. Pieramici D, Bree WR, Stark WJ. Stripping of Descemet's membrane: a clinicopathologic correlation. *Ophthalmic Surg* 1994;25:226–231.

96. Sugar A. Surgical trauma—pseudophakia and aphakic corneal edema. In: Krachmer JH, Mannis ML, Holland EJ, eds. *Cornea and external disease: clinical diagnosis and management.* Vol. 2. St. Louis: Mosby-Year Book, 1996:1423–1435.

97. Reese AB. Discussion of Scheie HG. Stripping of Descemet's membrane in cataract extraction. *Trans Am Ophthalmol Soc* 1964;62:131–138.

98. Theobald GD, Haas JS. Epithelial invasion of the anterior chamber following cataract extraction. *Trans Am Acad Ophthalmol Otol* 1948;52:470–479.

99. Weiner MJ, Trentcoste J, Pon DM, Albert DM. Epithelial downgrowth: a 30 year clinicopathological review. *Br J Ophthalmol* 1989;73:6–11.

100. Otradover J, Zicha Z. Epithelial invasion of the anterior chamber after cataract extraction. *Cesk Oftalmol* 1960;16:131–142.

101. Bernardino VB, Kim JC, Smith TR. Epithelialization of the anterior chamber after cataract extraction. *Arch Ophthalmol* 1969;82:742–750.

102. Sugar A, Meyer RF, Hood CI. Epithelial downgrowth following penetrating keratoplasty in the aphake. *Arch Ophthalmol* 1977;95:464–467.

103. Feder RS, Krachmer JH. The diagnosis of epithelial downgrowth after keratoplasty. *Am J Ophthalmol* 1985;99:697–703.

104. Lee SY, Rapuano CJ. Retrocorneal membrane in the cornea. In: Krachmer JH, Mannis MJ, Holland EJ, eds. *Cornea. Fundamentals of the cornea and external disease.* Vol. 2. St. Louis: Mosby-Year Book, 1996:1709–1717.

105. Davenger M, Olsen EG. Experimental epithelial ingrowth. Epithelial/endothelial interaction through a corneal perforation studied in organ culture. *Acta Ophthalmol* 1985;63:443–448.

106. Cameron JD, Flaxman BA, Yanoff M. In vitro studies of corneal wound healing: epithelial/endothelial interactions. *Invest Ophthalmol Vis Sci* 1974;13:575–579.

107. Bruner WE, Green WR, Stark WJ. A case of epithelial ingrowth primarily involving the lens capsule. *Ophthalmic Surg* 1986;17:483–485.

108. Pack A, Tso MOM, Yul B. Cellular deposits on intraocular lenses. *Acta Ophthalmol Suppl (Copenh)* 1985;170:54–57.

109. Smith DR, Sommerville GM, Shew M. An experimental model of epithelialization of the anterior chamber. *Can J Ophthalmol* 1967;2:158–162.

110. Lytle RA, Simmons RJ. Epithelial and fibrous proliferation. In: Albert DM, Jakobiec FA, eds. *Principles and practice of ophthalmology.* Vol. 3. Philadelphia: WB Saunders, 1994:1479–1485.

111. Engel HM, Green WR, Michaels RG, et al. Diagnostic vitrectomy. *Retina* 1981;1:121–149.

112. Zavala EY, Binder PS. The pathologic findings of epithelial ingrowth. *Arch Ophthalmol* 1980;98:2007–2014.

113. Yamaguchi T, Polack FM, Valenti J. Electron microscopy study of epithelial downgrowth after penetrating keratoplasty. *Br J Ophthalmol* 1981;65:374–382.

114. Burris TE, Rowsey JJ, Nordquist RE. Model of epithelial downgrowth: scanning and transmission electron microscopy of corneal epithelialization. *Cornea* 1985;4:249–255.

115. Henderson T. A histological study of the normal healing of wounds after cataract extraction. *Ophthalmic Rev* 1907;26:107–113.

116. Waring GO, Laibson RR, Rodriques MM. Clinical and pathologic alterations of Descemet's membrane: with emphasis on endothelial metaplasia. *Surv Ophthalmol* 1974;18:325–368.

117. McDonnell PJ, de la Cruz ZC, Green WR. Vitreous incarceration complicating cataract surgery. *Ophthalmology* 1986;93:247–253.

118. Allen JC. Epithelial and stromal ingrowth. *Am J Ophthalmol* 1968;68:179–182.

119. Waring GO, Bourne WM, Edelhauser HF, Kenyon KR. The corneal endothelium: normal and pathologic structure and function. *Ophthalmology* 1982;89:532–590.

120. Waring GO. Posterior collagenous layer of the cornea: ultrastructural classification of abnormal collagenous tissue posterior to Descemet's membrane in 30 cases. *Arch Ophthalmol* 1982;100:122–134.

121. Swan KC. Fibroblastic ingrowth following cataract extraction. *Arch Ophthalmol* 1973;89:445–449.

122. Rodriques MM, Waring GO, Laibson PR, Weinreb S. Endothelial alterations in congenital corneal dystrophies. *Am J Ophthalmol* 1975;80:678–689.

123. Weimar VL. The sources of fibroblasts in corneal wound repair. *Arch Ophthalmol* 1958;60:93–109.

124. Kampik A, Patrinely JR, Green WR. Morphologic and clinical features of retrocorneal melanin pigmentation and pigmented pupillary membranes: review of 225 cases. *Surv Ophthalmol* 1982;27:161–180.

125. Herbert H. Glass membrane formation in chronic iridocyclitis. *Trans Ophthalmol Soc UK* 1927;47:155–164.

126. Donaldson DD, Smith TR. Descemet's membrane tubes. *Trans Am Ophthalmol Soc* 1966;64:89–109.

127. Wolter JR. Descemet's membrane tubes on the zonular fibers of the lens. *J Pediatr Ophthalmol* 1969;6:153–156.

128. Binder RF, Binder HF. Regenerative processes in the endothelium of cornea. *Arch Ophthalmol* 1957;57:11–13.

129. Cogan DG. Applied anatomy and physiology of the cornea. *Trans Am Acad Ophthalmol Otol* 1951;55:229–259.

130. Rowsey JJ, Gaylor JR. Intraocular lens disasters: peripheral anterior synechiae. *Ophthalmology* 1980;87:646–664.

131. Smith SG, Lindstrom RL, eds. *Intraocular lens: complications and management.* Thorofare, NJ: Slack, 1988:1–43.

132. Harris M, Tso AY, Kaba FW, et al. Corneal endothelial overgrowth of angle and its evidence of myoblastic differentiation in 3 cases. *Ophthalmology* 1984;91:1154–1160.

133. Wolter JR, Fechner PU. Glass membranes on the anterior iris surface. *Am J Ophthalmol* 1962;53:235–243.

134. Powe NR, Schein DD, Gieser SC, et al. Synthesis of the literature on visual acuity and complications following cataract extraction with intraocular lens implantation. *Arch Ophthalmol* 1994;112:239–252.

135. Rao GN, Aquavella JV, Goldberg SH, Beck SL. PBK: relationship to preoperative corneal endothelial status. *Ophthalmology* 1984;91:1135–1140.

136. Joyce NC. Cell biology of the corneal endothelium. In: Albert DM, Jakobiec FA, eds. *Principles and practice of ophthalmology*. Basic sciences. Philadelphia: WB Saunders, 1994:17–37.

137. Delaique O, Arbeille B, Rossazza C, et al. Quantitative analysis of immunogold labelings of collagen type I, III, IV and VI in healthy and pathological human cornea. *Graefes Arch Clin Exp Ophthalmol* 1995;233:331–338.

138. Numa A, Nakamura J, Tahashima M, Kani K. Long term corneal evaluation. *Jpn J Ophthalmol* 1983;37:78–87.

139. Drews RC. Symposium of complication of modern surgical procedures: inflammatory response, endophthalmitis, corneal dystrophy, glaucoma, retinal detachment, dislocation, refractive error, lens removal and enucleation. *Ophthalmology* 1978;85:164–175.

140. Chambless WE. Incidence of anterior and posterior segment complications in over 3000 cases of extracapsular cataract extractions, intact and open capsules. *Am Intraocular Implant Soc J* 1985;11:146–148.

141. Schultz RD, Glasser DB, Matsuda M, et al. Response of corneal endothelium to cataract surgery. *Arch Ophthalmol* 1986;104:1164–1169.

142. Yee R, Geroski D, Matsuda M. Cellular migration and morphology in corneal endothelial wound repair. *Invest Ophthalmol Vis Sci* 1985;26:1191–1201.

143. Bourne WM, Nelson LR, Hodge DO. Continued endothelial cell loss after lens implantation. *Ophthalmology* 1994;101:1014–1023.

144. Oxford Cataract Treatment and Evaluation Team (OCTET). Long-term corneal endothelial cell loss with cataract surgery: results of a randomized controlled trial. *Arch Ophthalmol* 1986;104:1170–1175.

145. Bourne WN, Kaufman HE. Endothelial damage associated with intraocular lenses. *Am J Ophthalmol* 1976;81:482–485.

146. Kaufman HE, Katz JI. Endothelial damage from intraocular lens insertion. *Invest Ophthalmol Vis Sci* 1976;15:996–1000.

147. Kurz GH, D'Amico RA. Histopathology of corneal graft failures. *Am J Ophthalmol* 1968;66:184–199.

148. Hales RH, Spencer WH. Unsuccessful penetrating keratoplasties. *Arch Ophthalmol* 1963;70:805–810.

149. Lang GK, Green WR, Maumenee AE. Clinicopathologic studies of keratoplasty eyes obtained postmortem. *Am J Ophthalmol* 1986;101:28–40.

150. Morrison JC, Swan KC. Bowman's layer in penetrating keratoplasties of the human eye. *Arch Ophthalmol* 1962;100:1835–1838.

151. Morrison JC, Swan KC. Descemet's membrane in penetrating keratoplasties on the human eye. *Arch Ophthalmol* 1983;101:1927–1929.

152. Tsubota K, Mashima Y, Murata H, et al. Corneal epithelium following penetrating keratoplasty. *Br J Ophthalmol* 1995;79:257–260.

153. Dohlman CH. On the fate of the corneal graft. *Acta Ophthalmol* 1975;35:286–302.

154. Silverstein AM, Rossman AM, Leon AS. Survival of donor epithelium in experimental corneal xenografts after penetrating keratoplasty. *Am J Ophthalmol* 1970;69:448–453.

155. Bourne WM, Hodge DO, Nelson LR. Corneal endothelium five years after transplantation. *Am J Ophthalmol* 1994;118:185–196.

156. Cohen RA, Chew SJ, Gebhardt BM, et al. Confocal microscopy of corneal graft rejection. *Cornea* 1995;4:467–472.

157. Forstot DL, Blackwell WL, Jaffee NS, et al. Effect of intraocular lens implantation of corneal endothelium. *Trans Am Acad Ophthalmol Otol* 1977;83:195–203.

158. Smolin G, Beswell R. Corneal graft rejection associated with anterior iris adhesion. Case report. *Ophthalmology* 1978;10:1603–1604.

159. Tragakis MP, Brown SI. The significance on anterior synechiae after corneal transplantation. *Am J Ophthalmol* 1973;74:532–533.

160. Maguire MG, Stark WJ, Gottsch JD, et al. Risk factors for corneal graft failure and rejection in the collaborative corneal transplantation study. *Ophthalmology* 1994;101:1536–1547.

161. Arentsen JJ. Corneal transplant allograft rejection: possible predisposing factors. *Trans Am Ophthalmol Soc* 1983;81:361–402.

162. Batchelor JR, Carey TA, Werb A, et al. HLA matching and corneal grafting. *Lancet* 1976;7959:551–554.

163. Voker-Dieben HJ, D'Amora J, Kokvan Alphen CC. Hierarchy of prognostic factors for corneal allograft survival. *Aust N Z J Ophthalmol* 1987;15:11–18.

164. Gilette TE, Chandler JW, Greiner JV. Langerhans cells of the ocular surface. *Ophthalmology* 1982;89:700–710.

165. Kanai A, Polack FM. Ultramicroscopic alteration in corneal epithelium in corneal grafts. *Am J Ophthalmol* 1971;72:119–126.

166. Pouliquen LF, Sourdille GJ, Offret G. *Les greffes de la cornee*. Paris: Masson, 1948.

167. Polack FM. The corneal graft reaction. An immunological pathological and clinical perspective. In: Steinberg GH, Guy F, Nussenblatt RB, eds. *Immunology of the eye*. Workshop I Immunol Abstracts. Special supplement. 1980.

168. Polack FM. Histopathologic and histochemical alteration in the early stages of corneal graft rejection. *J Exp Med* 1962;116:8709–8718.

169. Renard GF, Moncourirer P. The action of sensitized lymphocytes of the corneal endothelium of rabbits. *Graefes Arch Clin Exp Ophthalmol* 1997;203:201.

170. Galin MA, Lin LL, Fetherolf EC, et al. Time analysis of corneal endothelial cell density after cataract extraction. *Am J Ophthalmol* 1979;88:93–96.

171. Melles GRJ, Binder PS, Moore MN, Anderson JA. Epithelial-stromal interactions in human keratotomy wound healing. *Arch Ophthalmol* 1995;113:1124–1130.

172. Yamaguchi T, Tamak K, Kaufman HE, et al. Histologic study of a pair of human corneas after anterior radial keratotomy. *Am J Ophthalmol* 1985;100:281–292.

173. Jester JV, Villasenor RZ, Miyashiro J. Epithelial inclusion cysts following radial keratotomy. *Arch Ophthalmol* 1983;101:611–615.

174. Binder PS, Nayak SK, Deg JK, et al. An ultrastructural and histochemical study of long term wound healing after radial keratotomy. *Am J Ophthalmol* 1987;103:432–440.

175. Deg JK, Zavala EY, Binder PS. Delayed corneal wound healing following radial keratotomy. *Ophthalmology* 1985;92:734–748.

176. Deg JK, Binder PS. Wound healing after astigmatic keratotomy in human eyes. *Ophthalmology* 1987;94:1290–1298.

177. Binder PS, Charlton KH. Surgical procedures performed after refractive surgery. *Refract Corneal Surg* 1992;8:61–74.

178. Bryant MR, Szerenyi K, Schmotzer H, McDonnell PJ. Corneal tensile strength in fully healed radial keratotomy wounds. *Invest Ophthalmol Vis Sci* 1994;35:3022–3031.

179. McDermott ML, Wilkinson WS, Ukel DV, et al. Corneoscleral rupture ten years after radial keratotomy. *Am J Ophthalmol* 1990;110:575–577.

180. Matoba AY, Torres J, Wilhelmus KR, et al. Bacterial keratitis after radial keratotomy. *Ophthalmology* 1989;96:1171–1175.

181. Geggel HS. Delayed sterile keratitis following radial keratotomy requiring corneal transplantation for visual rehabilitation. *Refract Corneal Surg* 1990;6:55–58.

182. Assil KK, Barrett AM, Fouraker BD, Schanzlin DJ. One-year results of the intrastromal corneal ring in nonfunctional human eyes. *Arch Ophthalmol* 1995;113:159–167.

183. Quantock AJ, Kincaid MD, Schanzlin DJ. Stromal healing following explantation of an ICR (intrastromal corneal ring) from a nonfunctional human eye. *Arch Ophthalmol* 1993;113:208–209.

184. Tuft SJ, Gartry DS, Rawe IM, Meedk KM. Perspective: photorefractive keratectomy: implications of corneal wound healing. *Br J Ophthalmol* 1993;77:243–247.

185. Beuerman RW, McDonald MB, Shofner RS, et al. Quantitative histological studies of primate corneas after excimer laser photorefractive keratectomy. *Arch Ophthalmol* 1994;112:1103–1110.

186. Taylor DM, L'Esperance RA Jr, Del Pero RA, et al. Human excimer laser lamellar keratectomy. *Ophthalmology* 1989;96:654–664.

187. Del Pero RA, Gigstad JE, Roberts AD, et al. A refractive and histopathologic study of excimer laser keratectomy in primates. *Am J Ophthalmol* 1990;109:419–429.

188. Fantes FE, Hanna KD, Waring GO III, et al. Wound healing after excimer laser keratomileusis (photorefractive keratectomy) in monkeys. *Arch Ophthalmol* 1990;108:665–675.

189. Malley DS, Steineert RF, Puliafito CA, Dobi ET. Immunofluorescence study of corneal wound healing after excimer laser anterior keratectomy in the monkey eye. *Arch Ophthalmol* 1990;108:1316–1322.

190. Sundar Raj N, Geiss MJ III, Fantes F, et al. Healing of excimer laser ablated monkey corneas. *Arch Ophthalmol* 1990;108:1604–1610.

191. Kahle G, Stadter H, Seiler T, Wollensak J. Gas chromatographic and mass spectroscopic analysis of excimer and erbium:yttrium aluminum garnet laser ablated human cornea. *Invest Ophthalmol Vis Sci* 1992;33:2180–2184.

192. Van Setten GB, Koch JW, Tervo K, et al. Expression of tenascin and fibronectin in the rabbit cornea after excimer laser surgery. *Graefes Arch Clin Exp Ophthalmol* 1992;230:178–183.

193. Marshall J, Trokel SL, Rothery S, Krueger RR. Long term healing of the central cornea after photorefractive keratectomy using an excimer laser. *Ophthalmology* 1988;95:1411–1421.

194. Hirst LW, Kenyon KR, Fogle JA, et al. Comparative studies of corneal surface injury in the monkey and rabbit. *Arch Ophthalmol* 1981;99:1066–1073.

195. Kenyon KR. Morphology and the pathologic responses of the cornea to disease. In: Smolin G, Thoft RA, eds. *The cornea: scientific foundations and clinical practice.* 2nd ed. Boston: Little, Brown, 1983:63–98.

196. Thoft RA, Friend J. The X, Y, Z hypothesis of corneal epithelial maintenance. *Invest Ophthalmol Vis Sci* 1983;24:1442–1443.

197. Ebato B, Friend J, Thoft R. Comparison of limbal and peripheral human corneal epithelium in tissue cultures. *Invest Ophthalmol Vis Sci* 1988;29:1533–1537.

198. Cotsarelis G, Cheng SZ, Dong G, et al. Existence of slow cycling limbal epithelial basal cells that can be preferentially stimulated to proliferate: implications on epithelial stem cells. *Cell* 1989;57:210–219.

199. Shieh E, Moreira H, D'Arch J, et al. Quantitative analysis of wound healing after cylindrical and spherical excimer laser ablations. *Ophthalmology* 1992;99:1050–1055.

200. Amano S, Shimizu K, Tsubota K. Specular microscopic evaluation of the corneal epithelium after excimer laser photorefractive keratectomy. *Am J Ophthalmol* 1994;117:381–384.

201. Fountain TR, de la Cruz ZC, Green WR, et al. Reassembly of corneal epithelial adhesion structures after excimer laser keratectomy in humans. *Arch Ophthalmol* 1994;112:967–972.

202. Khodadoust AA, Silverstein AM, Kenyon KR, Dowling JE. Adhesion of regenerating corneal epithelium. The role of basement membrane. *Am J Ophthalmol* 1968;65:339–348.

203. Gipson IK, Spurr-Michaud S, Tisdale A, Keough M. Reassembly of the anchoring structures of the corneal epithelium during wound repair in the rabbit. *Invest Ophthalmol Vis Sci* 1989;30:424–434.

204. Hanna KD, Pouliquen YM, Savoldelli M, et al. Corneal wound healing in monkeys 18 months after excimer laser photorefractive keratectomy. *Refract Corneal Surg* 1990;6:340–345.

205. Chew SJ, Beuerman RW, Kaufman HE, McDonald MD. In vivo confocal microscopy of corneal wound healing after excimer laser photorefractive keratectomy. *CLAO J* 1995;21:273–280.

206. Essepian JP, Rajpal RK, Azar DT, et al. The use of confocal microscopy in evaluating corneal wound healing after excimer laser keratectomy. *Scanning* 1994;16:300–304.

207. Carones F, Brancato R, Venturi E, Morico A. The corneal endothelium after myopic excimer laser photorefractive keratectomy. *Arch Ophthalmol* 1994;112:920–924.

208. Gartry DS, Kerr Muir MG, Marshall J. Photorefractive keratectomy with an argon fluoride excimer laser: a clinical study. *Refract Corneal Surg* 1991;7:420–435.

209. Gartry DS, Kerr-Muir MG, Marshall JJ. Excimer laser photorefractive keratectomy: 18 month follow-up. *Ophthalmology* 1992;99:1202–1219.

210. Gartry DS, Kerr-Muir MG, Lohmann CP, Marshall J. The effect of topical corticosteroid on refractive outcome and corneal haze after photorefractive keratectomy. *Arch Ophthalmol* 1992;110:944–952.

211. Fagerholm P, Hamberg-Nystrom H, Tengroth B. Wound healing and myopic regression following photorefractive keratectomy. *Acta Ophthalmol* 1994;72:229–234.

212. Lohmann C, Gartry D, Muir MK, et al. "Haze" in photorefractive keratectomy: its origins and consequences. *Laser Light Ophthalmol* 1991;4:15–34.

213. Hanna KD, Pouliquen YM, Waring GO, et al. Corneal wound healing in monkeys after repeated excimer laser photorefractive keratectomy. *Arch Ophthalmol* 1992;110:1286–1291.

214. Alleman N, Chamon W, Silverman RH, et al. High-frequency ultrasound quantitative analysis of corneal scarring following excimer laser keratectomy. *Arch Ophthalmol* 1993;111:968–973.

215. Trokel SI, Srinivisan R, Braen B. Excimer laser surgery of the cornea. *Am J Ophthalmol* 1983;96:710–715.

216. McDonald MB, Frantz JM, Klyce SD, et al. One year refractive results of central photorefractive keratectomy for myopia in the nonhuman primate cornea. *Arch Ophthalmol* 1990;108:40–47.

Evolution and Current Status of Cataract Surgery

Henry M. Clayman

HISTORY

Cataract has been an affliction since time immemorial and it is natural that mankind would have sought a remedy. The earliest documentations of cataract surgery are derived from the Assyrian code of Hammaurabi and ancient Hindu medicine, specifically the teachings of Susrata. The exact dates of Susrata's work are debatable but have been estimated as emanating 2000 years ago. The Susrata technique was termed *couching* and involved displacement of the crystalline lens into the posterior chamber, thus clearing the visual axis. In this technique the sclera was perforated with a sharp instrument, after which a blunt instrument was inserted through the scleral incision and the cataractous lens was displaced posteriorly. Though techniques varied, couching was practiced into this century by native healers in India.

Duke-Elder (1) cited an ancient technique that surely was a harbinger of contemporary surgery. He noted that the Arabian surgeon Ammar (996–1020) operated on a soft cataract by inserting an intralenticular hollow tube and aspirating the cataractous material. However, it is Jacques Daviel (1696–1762) of France who may be considered the founder of modern cataract surgery. In 1748 Daviel described his technique of cataract surgery in which the cataractous lens was extracted from the eye, directly from its natural position behind the iris. The Daviel technique was not a modified couching procedure by which the cataract was displaced anteriorly into the anterior chamber and then removed; it was in fact a planned extracapsular extraction (ECCE).

Intracapsular cataract extraction (ICCE), in which the crystalline lens is extracted in entirety, was first practiced about 250 years ago, almost concurrent with the Daviel technique. In these early techniques the lens was literally squeezed out of the eye by digital pressure on the limbus

or sclera after the appropriate limbal incision was made. Instruments were later used to apply suitable pressure, perhaps the best-known maneuver being the *Smith Indian technique* wherein pressure was applied by a muscle hook at the inferior limbus and the cataract was expelled through a superior incision. ICCE was also performed with spoons and forceps, the former being inserted behind the cataract, which was then lifted out of the eye. Forceps extractions involved grasping the anterior lens capsule and with gentle traction either sliding or tumbling the cataract out of the eye, a technique that persisted into the 1960s. Inherent in these early cataract techniques was the risk of both vitreous loss and capsule rupture. The profession therefore sought other techniques in the hope of facilitating a safer operation. Several surgeons devised techniques using a suction cup to fixate the anterior capsule and these ran the gamut from a simple suction cup to an electrically controlled device called an *erisiphake* (2). Diathermy was also proposed.

The seminal event in ICCE instrumentation was the introduction of cryoextraction by Krwawicz of Poland in 1961 (3). Krwawicz devised a nickel-plated, copper ball-tip applicator which he called a *cryoextractor*. This instrument had no inherent refrigerant capabilities and was chilled, prior to intraoperative use, by immersion into a thermos flask containing a mixture of dry ice and methyl alcohol. Kelman, influenced by neurosurgical applications of tissue freezing and unaware of Krwawicz's prechilled cryoextractor, independently introduced cryoextraction in the United States using liquid nitrogen as the refrigerant. The cryoextraction technique, infrequently used in the United States nowadays, is described in the next chapter. At this point in the discussion, note should be made of an important pharmacologic observation reported by J. Barraquer in 1957. In an attempt to dissolve an extensive hyphema, Barraquer introduced α-chymotrypsin into the eye. The next day he observed that the patient's crystalline lens had subluxed and made the correct deduction that here was a safe means to lyse zonules, which heretofore had been managed by mechanical means when necessary (4).

ADVENT OF PHACOEMULSIFICATION

When one considers the current state of cataract surgery, the predominant technique is ECCE or one of its variants, which includes phacoemulsification. Intraocular lenses (IOLs) evolved in parallel, but coincidentally fueled the further development of cataract surgery. Though the history of IOLs is discussed in a subsequent chapter, the point germane to the current status of cataract surgery is the pioneer IOL surgeons' search for the optimum location to fixate an IOL. Following the introduction of Binkhorst's iridocapsular IOL, which was inserted in conjunction with an ECCE (5), ophthalmologists slowly became persuaded that an intact posterior capsule conferred ocular advantages beyond a vehicle for IOL fixation (6). Specifically, the incidences of cystoid macular edema and retinal detachment were less (7,8). As the era of modern ECCE dawned, Kelman independently developed phacoemulsification in an attempt to remove the cataractous lens through a small incision and conceptualized this project in 1961 (9). Kelman's work became a small-incision ECCE technique which nicely matched the direction that IOL development and insertion were moving. However, the combination was not instant and had to await further evolution of IOL design and materials, improvement in phacoemulsification equipment (10), the introduction of viscoelastic agents and advances in phacoemulsification technique (Fig. 21-1). Moreover, Kelman's efforts were met with considerable skepticism, if not hostility, by some of his colleagues. At the 1974 annual meeting of the American Academy of Ophthalmology, DeVoe, in discussing phacoemulsification, stated, "It is not, and probably will not become a universal replacement for the conventional procedure. . . ." (11).

Kelman's original technique involved a 1- to 2-mm limbal incision and introduction of a Kelman irrigating cystotome through this incision (12). Irrigation was necessary to maintain the anterior chamber during the anterior capsulectomy maneuver because this era antedated the availability of viscoelastic agents. A *Xmas tree* anterior capsulectomy was performed and the underlying nucleus was next engaged with the tip of the irrigating cystotome. An attempt was made to prolapse the nucleus into the anterior chamber, which often was a challenging maneuver and, in my view, one of the impediments to the wider adoption of phacoemulsification by the profession at that time (Fig. 21-2).

Assuming that the nucleus had been prolapsed into the anterior chamber, the next step was to enlarge the original incision to 3 mm and insert the phacoemulsification handpiece, whose modalities comprised irrigation, aspiration, and ultrasound. The nucleus was then emulsified in the ultrasound

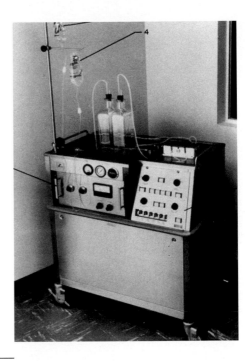

FIGURE 21-1.   *Original Kelman phacoemulsification equipment. (Courtesy of Charles D. Kelman, MD.)*

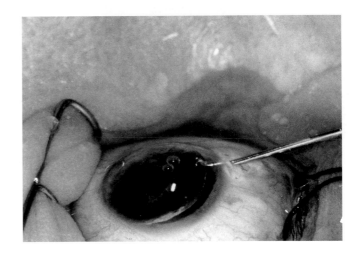

FIGURE 21-2.   *Nucleus prolapsed into the anterior chamber.*

mode, which also provided continuous irrigation and aspiration (Fig. 21-3). On completion of this phase of the operation, the ultrasonic handpiece was withdrawn from the eye and replaced with the irrigation-aspiration handpiece. The cortical remnants were aspirated from the eye with simultaneous irrigation to maintain the anterior chamber and define tissue planes. On conclusion of irrigation and aspiration, a posterior capsular opacity was sometimes noted, frequently amenable to removal by a burr that was attached to the cystotome handpiece. The surgeon then either enlarged the incision for IOL insertion or sutured the 3-mm incision if the patient was to be left aphakic. At this time most surgeons were

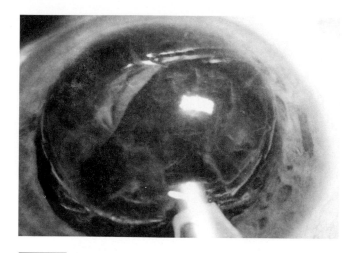

FIGURE 21-3.   *Ultrasonic probe emulsifying the nucleus in the anterior chamber.*

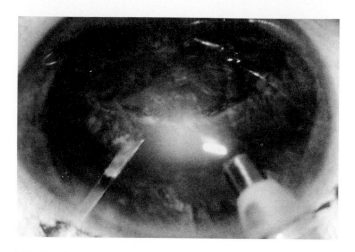

FIGURE 21-5.   *Nucleus secured by the nucleus rotator as a prelude to phacoemulsification of the superior pole.*

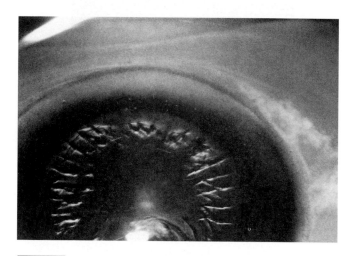

FIGURE 21-4.   *Can-opener anterior capsulectomy.*

still performing a peripheral iridectomy as part of the initial procedure and some were performing a primary discission of the posterior capsule. The latter was done because the neodymium:yttrium-aluminum-garnet (Nd:YAG) laser had not yet been introduced for ophthalmic use, so when a visually significant secondary cataract developed, a subsequent discission would be required, which would necessitate a second invasive procedure.

Kratz (13) and Little (14) devised a two-handed phacoemulsification technique in an attempt to overcome the difficulties sometimes encountered with the nuclear prolapse maneuver. The anterior capsulectomy was modified to the *can-opener* format (Fig. 21-4), though the irrigation-aspiration phases of the Kelman technique were unchanged. In the Kratz version, an additional limbal incision of about 1 mm was made at the 2-o'clock position (for a right-handed surgeon) to allow the subsequent introduction of a spatula-like second instrument. With the Kratz and Little

techniques, no attempt was made to prolapse the nucleus into the anterior chamber following anterior capsulectomy. Instead the nucleus was sculpted using the ultrasound mode, such that a ledge was left at the inferior third of the nucleus. At this point the second instrument was introduced and placed against the vertical portion of the inferior nuclear ledge while the ultrasonic handpiece was withdrawn to the level of the superior iris whereupon irrigation was terminated. For this maneuver, Kratz inserted the second instrument through the 2-o'clock incision while Little used the original incision. As a result, the anterior chamber shallowed slowly but not uniformly because the forward movement of the inferior nucleus was impeded by the instrument placed at the inferior ledge. As a consequence, the superior pole of the nucleus became exposed at the superior pupillary margin where it was secured by the tip of the ultrasonic handpiece. Irrigation was then initiated and rapidly reformed the anterior chamber, leaving the superior nuclear pole engaged at the superior iris plane, hence the term *iris plane phacoemulsification.* The second instrument, held in the surgeon's left hand, was then used to secure the lateral edge of the nucleus as the superior pole was emulsified (Fig. 21-5). The nucleus was then rotated by this instrument to the ultrasonic tip such that successive portions of the nuclear periphery were emulsified. The residual central portion usually presented into the anterior chamber spontaneously, where it was held against the ultrasonic tip by the second instrument as emulsification was completed.

IMPACT OF POSTERIOR-CHAMBER INTRAOCULAR LENSES ON SURGICAL TECHNIQUE

As the Kratz and Little techniques evolved, so did IOL surgery, specifically the introduction of the Shearing posterior-chamber IOL that is placed in the ciliary sulcus

(15). This single-plane IOL was in synchrony with phacoemulsification techniques and ciliary sulcus placement was usually amenable to placement under air since viscoelastic agents were not yet available (Fig. 21-6). As more Shearing IOLs were implanted (16), surgeons had the opportunity to evaluate the postoperative results and noted various types of malpositions that were attributed to ciliary sulcus fixation. These included nonfixation wherein the IOL moved from side to side with ocular movement, the so-called *windshield wiper syndrome* (17), but the most common malposition was the *sunrise syndrome* (18) in which the optic was displaced superiorly by inadvertent placement of one loop in the capsular bag or cul-de-sac, usually the inferior, and the other in the ciliary sulcus. Even if the optic was rotated, it was still displaced away from the loop in the bag, which was overcompressed in comparison to the sulcus-placed loop. Apart from innovations in IOL design, the desirability of in-the-bag fixation slowly became apparent. The problem was while the inferior loop could usually be correctly positioned in the bag, in the absence of viscoelastic substances, placement of the superior loop could be capricious. When viscoelastic agents finally became available, the surgeon was able to reinflate the capsular bag and form the anterior chamber, thus defining the anatomy and tissue planes of the anterior segment with a medium that would not significantly dissipate during subsequent IOL insertion.

With the wider adoption of in-the-bag placement, the profession discerned another potential problem, namely, radial tears in the anterior capsule during nuclear phacoemulsification or IOL placement. In an attempt to overcome this problem, capsulorrhexis was proposed (19). This is a technique in which the anterior capsulectomy is performed by tearing the anterior capsule in a continuous circular motion. The result is a capsulectomy margin with a smooth edge, in contradistinction to the multiple serrations of the can-opener technique. The next problem was how to

get access to the nucleus in the presence of a circular tear because the margins of the anterior capsule were an impediment to exposure of the superior pole of the nucleus, a requisite for execution of the two-handed phacoemulsification technique. Furthermore, even if the nucleus was exposed, subsequent manipulations during phacoemulsification could tear the margin of the anterior capsule. It also should be added that there has been a tendency to make the circular tear of a smaller diameter to better fixate foldable IOLs and this has compounded the problem of nuclear access. As a result, a number of techniques have been devised to phacoemulsify the nucleus in-the-bag, following capsulorrhexis. The common theme in all these methods was to divide the nucleus into smaller fragments as a prelude to phacoemulsification (20,21); hence, the name *divide and conquer* was attributed to one of these techniques (22).

If laser phacoemulsification were currently available, in-the-bag phacoemulsification procedures might be simplified, but at the time of writing such devices were still investigational (23). To advance the topic even further, what if the capsular bag could be evacuated through a puncture wound and then refilled with a substance to mimic the action of the crystalline lens and possibly retain accommodation. Futuristic as this may seem, the technique has been named *phacoersatz* and is the topic of active research (24). One of the problems of contemporary extracapsular cataract surgery is the incidence of capsular opacification. Originally this was treated with a discission but since the advent of the Nd:YAG laser, a noninvasive procedure has been available. This modality and viscoelastic substances merit some additional discussion.

VISCOELASTIC SUBSTANCES

Viscoelastic agents are an integral part of contemporary cataract surgery, but as with other elements of the current scene were a fortuitous development that blended nicely with the ascendancy of phacoemulsification and IOL surgery. The benchmark viscoelastic substance is hyaluronic acid, which is present in significant concentrations in the vitreous. Its use as an adjunct to retinal detachment surgery was attempted in the 1960s, and in 1967 Laboratoires Chibret of France manufactured a product called *Etamucine* which is a bovine-derived hyaluronic product. Balazs et al (25) began the investigation of hyaluronic acid extracted from human umbilical cord and later combined this with hyaluronic acid derived from rooster comb, a source that yields substantial quantities of a high polymer hyaluronic acid. Healon, a viscoelastic predicated on the work of Balazs et al, was eventually marketed by Pharmacia of Sweden. Miller and Stegmann (26) reported on the use of a 1% sodium hyaluronate solution in conjunction with anterior-segment surgery in 1980 and, in the same year, Soll et al (27) advocated chondroitin sulfate derived from shark as an intraoperative corneal protectant. A product combining

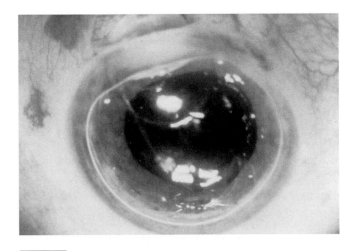

FIGURE 21-6. *Insertion of posterior-chamber IOL under air.*

sodium chondroitin sulfate and sodium hyaluronate is marketed as Viscoat, and methylcellulose, as suggested by Fechner in 1978 (28), is available as Ocucoat, which is 2% hydroxypropylmethylcellulose.

It is interesting to reflect on how a substance, conceptualized as a vitreous substitute, was insidiously adopted by surgeons performing anterior-segment surgery (29). The initial impetus was protection of the corneal endothelium during IOL insertion (30). In the beginning of the 1980s, iris-clip IOLs, in conjunction with an ECCE, were still inserted in 50% of cataract patients (31). These IOLs were of two planes (i.e., the posterior loops were offset from the back surface of the IOL) and there was a tendency for the incision to gape during IOL insertion. This time frame antedated the introduction of viscoelastic agents; therefore, air was routinely used to form the anterior chamber as a prelude to IOL insertion. Unfortunately, in many patients the air escaped as these two-plane IOLs were introduced through the incision, resulting in contact between the corneal endothelium and the IOL optic. This was believed to cause postoperative keratopathy, and therefore viscoelastic substances were originally adopted by surgeons for their protective qualities (Fig. 21-7). As the prevailing surgical technique evolved to ECCE and then phacoemulsification with in-the-bag IOL placement, the need to definitively delineate tissue planes produced the almost universal adoption of viscoelastic substances for intraoperative use. These products have made the difficult routine simple and the only caveat beyond their cost is their propensity to raise the intraocular pressure if they are left in the eye postoperatively (32), which is why they are generally evacuated from the eye at the conclusion of the procedure. Viscoelastic substances represent an example of the serendipity involved in so many aspects of contemporary cataract surgery, where a vitreous substitute now facilitates the cataract surgeon.

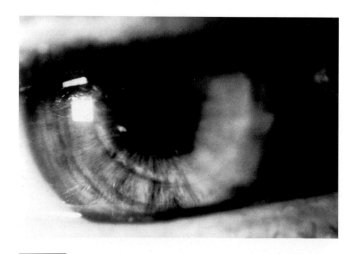

FIGURE 21-7.   *Keratopathy in patient with Worst Medallion iris-fixated IOL in situ.*

Nd:YAG LASER

Though the history of ophthalmic lasers is beyond the scope of this text, the emergence of the Nd:YAG laser as an ophthalmic tool is pertinent to the current status of cataract surgery. The Nd:YAG laser's ability to perform a noninvasive posterior capsulotomy is predicated on photodisruption whereby a pulsed, high-energy, ionizing laser beam effects tissue breakdown. The pivotal words are *high energy* and this became possible with McClung and Hellwarth's introduction of Q-switching in 1967 (33). Krasnov (34) described the use of a Q-switched ruby laser for goniotomy in 1972 and Gaasterland, working in the United States, performed the photodisruption of a pupillary membrane with a Q-switched ruby laser in 1979 (35). The main problems with the ruby laser were the relatively large focal spot size (175 μm), the necessity to cool the ruby laser element for several minutes between applications, and the very high energies that were required.

Fankhauser and Aron-Rosa introduced the Nd:YAG laser to ophthalmology, prior use having been for industrial purposes. In 1981 Fankhauser et al (36) described the use of the Nd:YAG laser for anterior ocular segment interventions, whereas a year earlier Aron-Rosa et al (37) reported on 20 IOL recipients who had a Nd:YAG posterior capsulotomy performed from 4 weeks to 8 months postoperatively. The emergence of the Q-switched Nd:YAG laser coincided well with the evolution to extracapsular techniques and avoided an invasive discission in the management of posterior capsular opacities. To be sure there were complications peculiar to lens implantation, such as inadvertent laser markings of the IOL (38), commonly called *dings*, which were demonstrated in experimental studies by Clayman et al (39). Moreover, spontaneous late enlargement of the posterior capsulotomy was sometimes observed with IOL dislocation (40) and the incidence of both retinal detachment and cystoid macular edema probably slightly increased following a Nd:YAG posterior capsulectomy (41). Nevertheless the Nd:YAG laser is an essential component of the contemporary ophthalmologist's armamentarium and its use has been expanded to the management of pupillary membranes and anterior IOL opacities (42) (Fig. 21-8). If one assumes that the long-term incidence of posterior capsular opacification following extracapsular surgery is in double digits, albeit under 50%, then it is hard to imagine providing modern patient care without this modality. Yet this is another case of serendipity because the Nd:YAG laser was a product of laser evolution, not IOL or cataract surgical techniques, that fortunately interfaced with the direction that cataract surgery was taking.

EPILOGUE

Another evolutionary step is being played out. At the time of writing approximately 90% of cataract surgeries in the United States were performed by phacoemulsification, and

and enlarge it to place an IOL? Why not devise an IOL that could be inserted through the original phacoemulsification incision? In response to this idea, foldable IOLs and their various insertion devices were introduced and these modalities currently comprise more than 50% of IOL sales in the United States. If we were to revisit this matter in a few years, foldable IOLs might well dominate the IOL market if the pricing were compatible with the economic trends impacting ophthalmology.

REFERENCES

1. Duke-Elder S. *System of ophthalmology.* St. Louis: CV Mosby, 1969:250.
2. Barraquer J, Boberg-Ans J. Cataract surgery. *Br J Ophthalmol* 1959;43:69–77.
3. Krwawicz T. Intracapsular extraction of intumescent cataract by application of low temperature. *Br J Ophthalmol* 1961;45:279–283.
4. Barraquer J. Enzymatic zonulolysis. *Proc R Soc Med* 1959;52:973–981.
5. Binkhorst CD, Kats A, Leonard PAM. Extracapsular pseudophakia. Results in 100 two-loop iridocapsular lens implantations. *Am J Ophthalmol* 1972;73: 625–636.
6. Binkhorst CD. The iridocapsular (two-loop) lens and the iris-clip (four loop) lens in pseudophakia. *Trans Am Acad Ophthalmol Otolaryngol* 1973;77:589–617.
7. Binkhorst CD, Kats A, Tjan TT, Loones LH. Retinal accidents in pseudophakia—intracapsular vs extracapsular surgery. *Trans Am Acad Ophthalmol Otolaryngol* 1976;81:120–127.
8. Binkhorst CD. Corneal and retinal complications after cataract extraction. *Ophthalmology* 1980;87:609–617.
9. Kelman CD. Phacoemulsification and aspiration: a new technique of cataract removal. *Am J Ophthalmol* 1967;64:23–25.
10. Kelman CD. History of emulsification and aspiration of senile cataracts. *Trans Am Acad Ophthalmol Otolaryngol* 1974;78:OP5–OP13.
11. DeVoe AG. Symposium: phacoemulsification. Introduction. *Trans Am Acad Ophthalmol Otolaryngol* 1974;78:OP3–OP4.
12. Kelman CD. The Kelman phacoemulsification procedure. In: Emery JM, Little JH, eds. *Phacoemulsification and aspiration of cataracts.* St. Louis: CV Mosby, 1979:172–174.
13. Kratz RP. The Kelman phacoemulsification procedure. In: Emery JM, Little JH, eds. *Phacoemulsification and aspiration of cataracts.* St. Louis: CV Mosby, 1979:191–192.
14. Little JH. Technique of phacoemulsification. In: Emery JM, Little JH, eds. *Phacoemulsification and aspiration of cataracts.* St. Louis: CV Mosby, 1979:193–196.
15. Shearing SP. A practical posterior chamber lens. *Contact Intraocular Lens Med J* 1978;4:114–119.
16. Kratz RP, Mazzocco T, Davidson B, Colvard DM. The Shearing intraocular lens: a report of 1000 cases. *Am Intraocular Implant Soc J* 1981;7:55–57.
17. Böke WRF, Krüger HCA. Causes and management of posterior chamber lens displacement. *Am Intraocular Implant Soc J* 1985;11:179–184.
18. Smith SG, Lindstrom RL. Malpositioned posterior chamber lenses: etiology, prevention and management. *Am Intraocular Implant Soc J* 1985;11:584–591.
19. Gimbel HV, Neuhan T. Development, advantages and methods of the continuous circular capsulorrhexis technique. *J Cataract Refract Surg* 1990;16:31–37.
20. Sheperd JR. In situ fracture. *J Cataract Refract Surg* 1990;16:436–440.
21. Fine IH. The chip and flip phacoemulsification. Technique. *J Cataract Refract Surg* 1991;17:366–371.
22. Gimbel HV. Divide and conquer nucleofractis phacoemulsification: developments and variations. *J Cataract Refract Surg* 1991;17:281–291.
23. Bath PE. Laserphaco: an introduction and review. *Ophthalmic Laser Ther* 1988/89;3:75–82.
24. Haefliger E, Parel JM. Accommodation of an endocapsular silicone lens (phacoersatz) in the aging rhesus monkey. *J Refract Corneal Surg* 1994;10:550–555.
25. Balazs EA, Freeman MI, Klöti R, et al. Hyaluronic acid and replacement of vitreous and aqueous humor. *Mod Probl Ophthalmol* 1972;10:3–21.
26. Miller D, Stegmann R. Use of Na-hyaluronate in anterior segment eye surgery. *Am Intraocular Implant Soc J* 1980;6:13–15.
27. Soll DB, Harrison SE, Arturi SC, Clinch T. Evaluation and protection of the corneal endothelium. *Am Intraocular Implant Soc J* 1980;6:239–242.
28. Fechner PU. Methyl-cellulose in lens implantation. *Am Intraocular Implant Soc J* 1978;3:180–181.

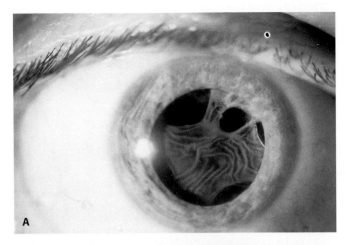

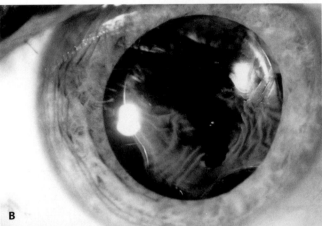

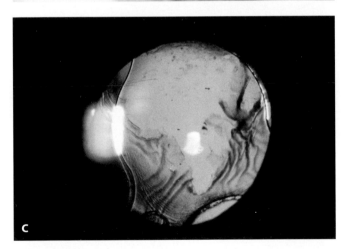

FIGURE 21-8. A. *Remnant of anterior capsule adherent to the anterior IOL surface.* B. *Same eye after lysis of the membrane with a Nd : YAG laser.* C. *Retroillumination of same eye.*

the balance by a planned ECCE, with ICCE rarely used. Nearly all patients received posterior-chamber IOLs, with anterior-chamber IOLs reserved for special situations. Given the ascendancy of phacoemulsification, the profession asked of itself, Why take the 3-mm phacoemulsification incision

29. Page LG, Balazs EA. Use of sodium hyaluronate (Healon) in human anterior segment surgery. *Ophthalmology* 1980;87:699–705.

30. Sugar J, Mitchelson J, Kraff M. Endothelial trauma and cell loss from intraocular lens insertion. *Arch Ophthalmol* 1978;96:449–450.

31. Clayman HM. The trend in intraocular lens implantation. *Am Intraocular Implant Soc J* 1980;6:15.

32. Binkhorst CD. Inflammation and intraocular pressure after the use of Healon® in intraocular surgery. *Am Intraocular Implant Soc J* 1980;6:340–341.

33. McClung FJ, Hellwarth RW. Giant optical pulsating from ruby. *J Appl Physiol* 1967;33:828–831.

34. Krasnov MM. Laser puncture of the anterior chamber angle in glaucoma. *Vestn Oftalmol* 1972;3:27–31.

35. Steinert RF, Puliafito CA. *The Nd : YAG laser in ophthalmology.* Philadelphia: WB Saunders, 1985:8.

36. Fankhauser F, Roussel P, Steffen J, et al. Clinical studies on the efficiency of a high power laser irradiation upon some structures of the anterior segment of the eye. *Int Ophthalmol* 1981;3:129–139.

37. Aron-Rosa D, Aron J, Greisemann J, Thyzel R. Use of the neodymium-yag laser to open the posterior capsule after lens implant surgery. A preliminary report. *Am Intraocular Implant Soc J* 1980;6:352–354.

38. Dickerson DE, Gilmore JE, Gross J. The Abraham lens with the neodymium-YAG laser. *Am Intraocular Implant Soc J* 1983;9:438–440.

39. Clayman HM, Karrenberg FC, Parel JM. Intraocular lens damage from the neodymium : YAG laser. *Ann Ophthalmol* 1984;16:551–556.

40. Clayman HM, Jaffe NS. Spontaneous enlargement of neodymium : YAG posterior capsulotomy in aphakic and pseudophakic eyes. *J Cataract Refract Surg* 1988;14:667–669.

41. Grevens CM, Sanders RJ, Brown GC, et al. Pseudophakic retinal detachments: anatomic and visual results. *Ophthalmology* 1992;99:257–262.

42. Gandha SB, Brown RH, Katz LJ, Lynch MG. Neodymium : YAG membranectomy for pupillary membranes on posterior chamber intraocular lenses. *Ophthalmology* 1995;102:1846–1852.

Anesthesia for Cataract Surgery

PASCAL D. IMESCH

ANATOMIC, PHYSIOLOGIC, AND PHARMACOLOGIC CONCEPTS

The goal of every anesthesia is to allow surgery without pain under optimal conditions. For the eye and the eyelids in cataract surgery, this means anesthesia of the globe, conjunctiva, and partly the lids, as well as paralysis of the eye muscles and lid akinesia. Additionally, stable choroidal and retinal blood flow and a regulated intraocular pressure are desired. To understand the possible options for optimal anesthesia during cataract surgery, one must understand a few anatomic, physiologic, and pharmacologic concepts. The goal of this introduction is not to provide detailed insight into orbital anatomy, physiology, and pharmacology but to stress the basic concepts pertaining to anesthesia for cataract surgery.

Anatomy

Sensory Innervation

Sensory innervation to the eye and upper lid is carried by the first branch of the trigeminal nerve. Only a part of the lower lid is innervated by the second branch of the trigeminal nerve, the maxillary nerve. The maxillary nerve enters the orbit through the inferior orbital fissure outside the annulus of Zinn and takes its course along the orbital floor where it may be prone to trauma from a needle scratching along the orbital floor. The first branch of the trigeminal nerve, the ophthalmic nerve, splits into three subportions. One of them, the nasociliary nerve, enters the orbit inside the annulus of Zinn and passes through the muscle cone, whereas the other two branches, the frontal and lacrimal nerves, enter the orbit through the superior orbital fissure outside the muscle cone. By a strictly intraconal injection

of anesthetic, the frontal and lacrimal nerves are not anesthetized, leaving some sensibility to the conjunctiva and the lids. Table 22-1 shows the sensory innervation of different ocular structures by these different nerves (1).

Motor Innervation

The ocular muscles are innervated by the trochlear nerve (IV), the abducens nerve (VI), and the oculomotor nerve (III), which also carries proprioceptive and parasympathetic fibers that pass through the ciliary ganglion. All nerves are innervated multifocally by small nerve branches entering their respective muscles along their posterior and anterior parts (1). The oculomotor and the abducens nerves enter the orbit inside the annulus of Zinn and can be affected by intraconally injected agents (2). The oculomotor nerve splits into a superior part innervating the superior rectus and the levator palpebrae muscle while the inferior portion divides into even more branches innervating the medial rectus, the inferior rectus, and the inferior oblique muscle. The presynaptic parasympathetic fibers mentioned before arise from the Edinger-Westphal nucleus and separate from the inferior portion of the oculomotor nerve to enter the ciliary ganglion.

The trochlear nerve enters the orbit through the superior oblique orbital fissure outside the muscle cone together with the two sensory nerves, the frontal nerve and the lacrimal nerve, and passes over the levator palpebrae muscle to innervate the superior oblique muscle. This explains isolated activity of the superior oblique muscle after an isolated retrobulbar anesthesia.

The orbicular muscle of the eyelids is innervated by the facial nerve, which splits into multiple branches at the level of the parotid gland and innervates the orbicular muscle via multiple fine branches crossing over the lateral orbital rim

Table 22-1.   Sensory Innervation Areas of Different Portions of the First Branch of the Trigeminal Nerve

Nerve	Innervation
Frontal	Medial two-thirds of conjunctival skin
Lacrimal	Lateral third of conjunctival skin
Nasociliary	Medial canthus, caruncle, canaliculi, lacrimal sac
	Cornea, perilimbal conjunctiva, iris, ciliary body, optic nerve sheath (through the ciliary ganglion)

Table 22-2.   Motor Innervation of Ocular Muscles and Eyelids

Nerve	Innervation
Oculomotor (III)	Superior, medial, and lateral rectus muscles; levator palpebrae muscle
	Ciliary muscle, iris sphincter muscle (parasympathetic branches synapsing in the ciliary ganglion)
Abducens (VI)	Lateral rectus muscle
Trochlear (IV)	Superior oblique muscle
Facial	Orbicular muscle

into the muscle. A summary of the innervation of different ocular structures is shown in Table 22-2.

The Orbit

Topography, Connective Tissue, and Fat   The medial orbital wall is roughly in a sagittal plane forming a 45-degree angle with the lateral wall. The inferior wall rises to the apex at an angle of approximately 10 degrees. The volume of the orbit is approximately $30 \, cm^3$. The depth of the orbit from the inferior orbital rim to the apex ranges from 42 to 54 mm (3). The globe is centered in the anterior part of the orbit and therefore is located temporally to the orbital apex. The anatomic axis of the orbit diverges by 23 degrees from the visual axis in primary gaze position, which lies in the sagittal plane.

The separation of the orbital compartments into an intraconal and extraconal space is overly simplified, although it is still valid as a basic concept. The orbit is compartmentalized by a framework of partly discontinuous connective tissue septa (4,5) that form different connections in different locations within the orbit, leading to a complex system of partly communicating orbital compartments. In general, these septa are more developed in the anterior part of the orbit than in the retrobulbar region and toward the apex where the intermuscular septa are partly missing in the inferotemporal and superotemporal quadrants. There are structural differences between the intraconal and extraconal fat compartments, although the less mobile extraconal fat lobules communicate with the more fusiform and mobile

intraconal fat lobules through gaps in the septa between the rectus muscles (6).

The ocular muscles are embedded in this framework of orbital septa and are in close proximity to the orbital walls. Only the medial rectus muscle is separated from the orbital wall by a fat compartment. This compartment communicates with superior and inferior compartments and ultimately with the orbital apex.

Optic Nerve and Ciliary Ganglion   The optic nerve leaves the globe 3 mm to the nasal side of its posterior pole. The intraorbital portion of the optic nerve measures 3 cm and takes a winding course to pass the space of 2.5 cm between the posterior pole and the optic foramen (7). This excessive length of the optic nerve allows free eye movements without tearing the optical nerve fibers in extreme gaze positions.

The cerebrospinal fluid communicates freely with the subdural space around the optic nerve. The dura fuses anteriorly with the sclera and posteriorly with the periorbita around the optic foramen.

The ciliary ganglion is located temporal to the optic nerve inside the muscle cone 7 to 10 mm anterior to the orbital apex (1,8). Sensory fibers from various ocular structures pass through the ciliary ganglion from the short posterior ciliary nerves to reach the nasociliary branch of the ophthalmic nerve. Preganglionic parasympathetic fibers from the Edinger-Westphal nucleus synapse in the ciliary ganglion and the postganglionic fibers innervate the ciliary muscle and the iris by way of the short posterior ciliary nerves. Additionally postganglionic sympathetic fibers from the superior cervical ganglion pass through the ciliary ganglion to innervate ocular blood vessels via the short posterior ciliary nerves.

Orbital Blood Supply   Because the orbit forms a cone, the space is narrower toward the apex and delicate orbital structures are more tightly packed in the posterior portion of the orbit. In the anterior and middle regions of the orbit, however, the inferotemporal, the superotemporal, and the extremely medial compartments are relatively avascular.

The ophthalmic artery enters the orbit inferonasal to the optic nerve (9). It then runs around the optic nerve, crosses it superiorly, or inferiorly in a minority of cases, and runs under the superior oblique muscle toward the medial part of the orbit (10).

The large principal orbital "superior ophthalmic" vein is located in the superior medial quadrant running along the medial border of the superior rectus muscle. It enters the muscle cone and passes through it within a septum of connective tissue to exit the intraconal space laterally and the orbit through the superior orbital fissure (11). The superior medial quadrant and the lateral part of the orbital apex have the highest concentration of large vessels.

The vortex veins run from the equator of the globe posteriorly and one of them is in close proximity with the lateral border of the inferior rectus muscle (12,13).

Because of the large variability of the venous and even arterial blood supply to the orbit, it is safest to avoid the superior medial quadrant and the orbital septa close to the rectus muscles entirely. The inferotemporal, the superotemporal, and the extremely nasal orbital adipose compartments, however, are relatively free of delicate vascular structures, especially in the anterior and middle regions of the orbit.

Physiology

Intraocular Pressure

Intraocular pressure is influenced by different factors such as aqueous humor production, the osmotic pressure difference between the aqueous humor and the blood plasma, the choroidal blood volume, and most importantly for ocular anesthesia, the extrinsic pressure to the globe. This pressure obviously increases during the administration of anesthetic into the confined orbital space. The pressure depends on the site of injection (i.e., intraconal or extraconal) and the speed of injection (3,14–16). Pressure equilibration between the extraconal and intraconal compartments takes about 5 minutes (17).

Age also plays a role in the time course and amount of increased intraocular pressure by increased extrinsic pressure. In older patients the more rigid sclera may resist extrinsic pressure more than the soft sclera of younger people, which will transmit extrinsic pressure changes more quickly to the intraocular compartment.

The aqueous outflow is influenced by the capacity of the outflow path, the difference between intraocular and venous pressures, as well as the viscosity of the aqueous humor (18). From these factors the intraocular pressure can readily and immediately be influenced by application of additional extrinsic pressure. A decrease in intraocular pression therefore can be accelerated by ocular compression, with a rate of approximately 5 mm Hg within the first 5 minutes and much slower thereafter (16). A concern of increased intraocular pressure induced by oculopression is the potential to induce ischemia (19–22). To date there are no documented reports in the literature of an ischemic insult (23). Evidence, however, exists of transient ischemic abnormalities documented by fluorescein angiography and electroretinography (24–26). A controlled amount of oculopression may increase the margin of safety before accidentally inducing ischemic damage prior to surgery.

Pharmacology

Local Anesthetics

The oldest amide-linked local anesthetic introduced in the 1950s is lidocaine hydrochloride. Because of its very good tissue-penetrating properties and its effectiveness even for topical anesthesia, it has long been considered the anesthetic of choice (27). A disadvantage is its relatively short duration of action due to its inherent vasodilating properties. These can be diminished and the duration of action prolonged by approximately 75% by adding epinephrine.

Mepivacaine hydrochloride is similar to lidocaine but has less vasodilating activity and therefore a duration of action that is about 50% longer than that of lidocaine hydrochloride. This duration can also be prolonged with the addition of epinephrine. Contrary to lidocaine hydrochloride, however, it is not effective topically.

There are additional drugs that are modifications of either lidocaine or mepivacaine hydrochloride with essentially longer-duration properties.

Bupivacaine hydrochloride has higher lipid solubility and therefore a long duration of action. One disadvantage is its slow tissue penetration and therefore its slow onset of anesthesia. Low concentrations (0.25%, 0.50%) suffice for sensory anesthesia whereas higher concentrations (0.75%) are required for a motor block. This can result in a prolonged diplopia more than 24 hours after surgery.

Another modification is the popular (28,29) drug etidocaine hydrochloride. It has a faster onset of anesthesia than bupivacaine hydrochloride with a similar duration of action. Patients may also experience prolonged diplopia beyond 24 hours.

In ophthalmology, using mixtures of drugs with different properties for local anesthesia is a common practice (30). The effects of a drug of long duration such as bupivacaine hydrochloride combined with a drug with a fast onset and good tissue-penetrating properties such as lidocaine hydrochloride provide good and quick satisfactory anesthesia as well as excellent postoperative prolonged analgesia (31). Additionally it is reported that warming the anesthetic to 37°C will render the local anesthesia less painful (32,33).

Topical Anesthetics

Because of its increased corneal epithelial–penetrating properties most topical anesthetics are ester-linked chemicals, with cocaine being its most prominent member. Other agents include amethocaine, proparacaine, lignocaine, oxybuprocaine, and benoxinate. All these compounds produce corneal toxicity if used over a prolonged period of time, with cocaine causing the greatest problem (34). Also, corneal wound healing may be decreased (35,36).

As mentioned earlier, lidocaine can also be used as a topical anesthetic, with less corneal toxicity than cocaine and even proparacaine (34,37,38). Also bupivacaine in high concentrations (0.75%) can be used for a prolonged topical anesthesia (39).

Adjuvants

Epinephrine causes blood vessel constriction and therefore decreases the systemic distribution of a locally injected drug (40) and increases the duration of action (41,42). The final concentration should be no more than 5 µg/mL and the total amount injected should not exceed 0.2 mg (43).

For regional orbital anesthesia, the use of epinephrine is controversial because orbital vasoconstriction can lead to irreversible ischemic damage to ocular structures (35, 44,45).

Hyaluronidase is an enzyme known to break down collagen and therefore allows locally injected anesthetics to more readily penetrate tissues (46). Because the injected anesthetic will diffuse easier and faster throughout the orbit (47), large amounts of anesthetic can be injected without a drastic local increase in tissue pressure (44,48–52). In contrast, omission of hyaluronidase from the anesthetic solution may result in high intraocular pressure during surgery (53). The use of hyaluronidase may reduce the complications during surgery (46). Multiple dilutions of the enzyme have been used and there is no study documenting the optimal dosage (54).

GENERAL ANESTHESIA VERSUS LOCAL ANESTHESIA

In the beginning of this century, local anesthesia techniques for ocular surgery were highly favored over general anesthesia. With the onset of new and safer general anesthesia this trend changed in the 1950s and 1960s (55), to reverse again to local anesthesia techniques in our era (56–58).

The decision about whether to perform surgery under general or local anesthesia is multifactorial and is based not only on the patient's medical condition but also on other factors, with the most important being patient cooperation.

There are only a few stringent indications for general anesthesia. These include patients who are completely uncontrollable such as small children and people who are, for a multitude of reasons, unable to cooperate during surgery. Additionally, people who object to local anesthesia and people who have contraindications to local anesthesia will have to undergo general anesthesia.

There is a concern that general anesthesia is associated with a greater risk of complications than is any form of local anesthesia (59). However, no differences have been found in the rate of cognitive dysfunction in elderly patients after general or local anesthesia (60). Other studies examining mortality showed no significant difference between local versus general anesthesia for cataract surgery (61). The patient population in these studies, however, was carefully selected and placed in appropriate anesthesia groups showing a low risk of cataract surgery in general.

In contrast, unplanned hospital admissions were increased after cataract surgery with general anesthesia compared to surgery with local anesthesia (62). The risks of general anesthesia increase not with age but with the number of additional diseases (63). Patients with an underlying disorder indicating a higher risk for general anesthesia will benefit from local anesthesia. Patient selection and the correct indication for either local or general anesthesia are obviously crucial (64).

Postoperative analgesia has been reported to be better after local anesthesia (65) than general anesthesia. However, the advantage of local anesthesia is not only better postoperative analgesia and increased safety for patients with preexisting diseases, but also independence from a large staff of anesthesiologists and time as well as cost savings (66).

When deciding for local anesthesia, however, one must also consider psychological factors. Detailed information provided to the patient about the surgery and the patient's confidence in the surgeon are much more effective factors in calming the patient and increasing the chances for a successful surgery than are sedative drugs (67). During surgery, however, unnecessarily repeated questions about pain or discomfort will lead to the contrary effect and frighten the patient (68). The personality and charisma of a cataract surgeon are therefore important variables influencing the patient's confidence and collaboration during surgery and should be considered when deciding on general or local anesthesia (35). Simply compensating for a lack of communication skills and a missing human touch by increasing the use of sedative drugs will worsen the surgical outcome (55,56,69,70).

All these factors support the concept that patient cooperation is the major determinant when deciding on local or general anesthesia, if the choice is not diminished by contraindications for either form of anesthesia. Uncooperative or uncontrollable patients as well as their surgeon will benefit from general anesthesia whereas in most other cases local anesthesia is advantageous.

REGIONAL ANESTHESIA

There exists a multitude of fine variance between different regional anesthesia techniques, which are often combined to have the desired effect. As outlined earlier, the common goal is to anesthetize the sensitive ocular nerves and to paralyze the ocular and facial lid muscles. Additionally the anesthesia itself should be as painless to administer as possible, ensure low pressure in the orbit and the globe, as well as avoid local and systemic complications (71).

Retrobulbar Anesthesia

In recent surveys 59% of all surgeons preferred a retrobulbar block; 40% of them additionally chose a facial nerve block.

The basic description of this technique is from Atkinson, written in 1955 (72).

Basically a needle is inserted through the skin of the lower lid or the conjunctiva above the orbital rim in the inferotemporal quadrant in a sagittal plane. The bevel of the needle should be toward the globe, to minimize the risk of scleral engagement with the needle tip (73,74). As the needle tip presumably has reached the equator, the needle is directed upward and inward and pushed into the retrobulbar muscle cone. Often increased resistance will be felt when reaching the connective tissue forming the muscle cone and resistance will rapidly decrease when the needle has penetrated the cone. Anesthetic is injected along the path and in the muscle cone, where the bulk of the anesthetic is delivered (72). Avoidance of large pivotal or slicing needle movements is important to prevent injury to orbital vessels (75).

Variations of this technique concern the gaze of the patient, the entry location of the needle, the amount and type of anesthetic injected in different places while directing the needle into the muscle cone, the number of injections and needles, as well as the shape and size of the needle itself.

Gaze

Atkinson (72) described an upward and inward gaze. This technique has been challenged and called obsolete by some showing that in this gaze the needle may be very close to the optic nerve, the ophthalmic artery, and the superior ophthalmic vein and that the macular area is more exposed to injury (7,76,77). This observation was based on documentation of the needle position by computed tomography on one cadaver with its gaze position fixed by sutures. As important as this experimental result may be, in a clinical setting others found no significant difference in central nervous system spread of anesthetic in patients with an upward and inward versus a straight gaze in primary position (78). Today other gaze positions are predominant. When the needle reaches the muscle cone from an injection site located temporoinferiorly, the optic nerve is safest when the patient is looking out and down, which moves the optic nerve away from the needle (76,77,79). This position may be awkward for the patient as he or she watches the needle approach the eye. Therefore, a more comfortable and reasonable gaze may be down and in or the primary gaze position straight ahead (7).

Entry Location of the Needle

Instead of entering the peribulbar space through the skin of the lower eyelid, the needle can be inserted through the conjunctiva (74). Easy and good topical anesthesia of the conjunctiva can be achieved with anesthetic drops or a cotton-tipped applicator soaked in full-strength local anesthetic held to the conjunctiva, making the approach less painful. Orientation of the needle tangential to the globe may also be easier. Even in a case of a scleral engagement with the needle tip, the angle between the needle and a tangential plane to the globe will be smaller than when the needle is moved toward the sclera through the skin of the lower eyelid. This renders a possible perforation less probable with a conjunctival approach.

Anesthetic Agents

An overview of the feature of the main anesthetic agents was provided earlier. For retrobulbar anesthesia, 1% lido-

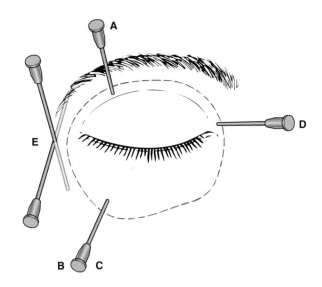

FIGURE 22-1. *Schematic of the possible injection sites for a superotemporal peribulbar injection (A), for an inferotemporal peribulbar or a retrobulbar injection (B, C), for an extremely medial peribulbar injection (D), and for a Van Lindt facial block (E).*

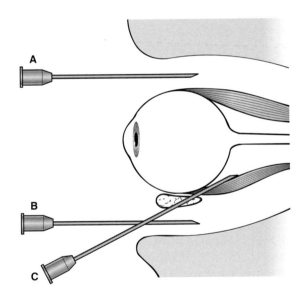

FIGURE 22-2. *Schematic in a sagittal view of the needle position in a superotemporal peribulbar block (A), an inferotemporal peribulbar block (B), and a retrobulbar block (C). The bevel of the needle is directed toward the globe. The angle in a retrobulbar injection is shallow and the needle may easily deliver anesthetic into the inferior rectus muscle.*

caine, 0.75% bupivacaine, and 2% mepivacaine, with or without 1:200,000 epinephrine and hyaluronidase, are the most commonly used (5,74). For surgery lasting longer than 90 minutes, long-acting agents such as bupivacaine and etidocaine in high-enough concentrations are the anesthetic of choice. The use of hyaluronidase (e.g., 7.5 units/mL) is generally recommended (45,51,53,80,81).

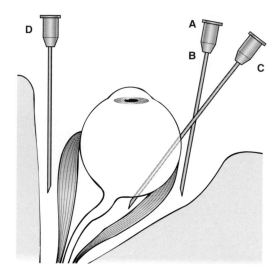

FIGURE 22-3.   *Schematic in a horizontal view of the needle position in a superotemporal or an inferotemporal peribulbar block (A, B), a retrobulbar block (C), and an extremely medial peribulbar block (D). The optic nerve moves away from the needle in an outward and downward gaze but approaches the needle in an upward and inward gaze.*

Number of Injections

Multiple injections are a modification of the basic retrobular approach, but represent more a combination of retrobular anesthesia and one or more additional peribulbar injections.

To avoid the globe, multiple injections in a safe place have been advocated over one "high-risk" injection by the strictly peribulbar anesthesia technique. Since the blood supply to the orbit is highly variable, even an injection in relatively avascular areas harbors the risk of perforating an orbital vessel. The risk increases with the number of injections (82,83). Additionally, all retrobulbar or intraconal anesthesia techniques, respectively, include at least one injection into the intraconal space, hence the name. Weighing all the risks, it may be safest to limit the administration of anesthetics to as few injections into the orbit as necessary to achieve a satisfactory anesthesia with a retrobulbar technique. It may also comfort the patient and increase his or her confidence in the surgeon to receive one injection instead of having to undergo a lengthy procedure with multiple needle switching.

The basic concept of multiple injections is to anesthetize the region around the orbital septum, with the first injection sometimes including diluted anesthetics (84). Then anesthetic is injected into the retrobulbar space. To provide lid akinesia, anesthetic is also injected into variable preseptal locations upon withdrawal of the needle. If akinesia is not complete, more anesthetic is selectively injected into the peribulbar space around the muscle not completely paralyzed. This mostly happens via a superotemporal or an

extremely nasal injection directing the needle more superiorly or inferiorly as needed.

Hustead described up to five injections using four needles. With the first two injections with the same needle, he entered through the skin of the lateral part of the lower eyelid and delivered the first dose to the peribulbar space at a depth of 20 mm. Upon withdrawing the needle, he also injected anesthetic in the region of the anterior orbital septum. With the third and fourth injections he reached the retro-orbital space and the preseptal area again upon withdrawing the needle. If akinesia was not complete, he performed a nasal injection medial to the caruncle into the medial superior or medial inferior quadrant. Anesthetic injected into this medial fat compartment will distribute easily to the orbital apex. To ensure complete akinesia he sometimes performed a fifth superior temporal peribulbar injection through the skin of the upper eyelid (5). This additional superior temporal injection may be necessary if spread of the anesthetic agent to the superior rectus muscle is impaired by thick connective tissue around the superior ophthalmic vein (11). There are additional slight variations to this technique used by others (5,64,73), always pertaining to the same principle of anesthetizing the nasociliary sensory nerve and the motor nerves by an intraconal injection of anesthetic and by completing the block by additional direct peribulbar injections into the superotemporal quadrant or into the superonasal and inferonasal quadrants, respectively, by an extremely medial approach.

By the use of hyaluronidase, spread of the anesthetic agent anterior to the orbital septum and within the orbit is facilitated. This helps to anesthetize the fine nerve branches innervating the orbicular muscle and renders an additional facial block unnecessary (16,74,85).

Needle

Eleven percent of optic nerves can easily be perforated with needles measuring 38 mm in length (8). There is interindividual variability because of the different lengths of the orbits. To keep a safe distance from the optic nerve and the large vessels at the apex of the orbit, it has been suggested that the needle length should not exceed 31 mm. This advice has been widely accepted (8).

A recent study using ultrasonographic localization of the needle showed that needles of this length end up between 0.2 and 3.3 mm behind the globe. This shows the extreme proximity of the needle to the posterior sclera and demands extra prudence and careful evaluation of the indication for retrobulbar anesthesia in myopic eyes (86). Needles without cutting edges and a blunt rounded tip are thought to push vessels out of the way instead of cutting into them (5,87–90). Additionally globe penetration may be more difficult with a blunt-ended needle (91–93) although it is not prevented completely (94,95). Other reports considered blunt-ended needles not as safe as sharp needles (91,95). Blunt-ended needles may need more force to be pushed through tissues, causing less tactile control (86). Sharp needles have also been reported to be less painful than blunt-ended needles (82,91,96,97). Additionally some physicians favor needles with a bent or curved design. Needles are bent in midhalf (5) or curved (83) to form a 10- to 30-degree angle, to better mold the needle shape to the orbital floor and to make sure the needle tip lies freely within the muscle cone without attachment to one of the surrounding eye muscles, particularly the inferior rectus muscle.

Peribulbar Anesthesia

From 1985 to 1993 the popularity of peribulbar anesthesia has increased from 4% to 35% of American Society of Cataract and Refractive Surgery (ASCRS) surgeons using it (98).

Strictly peribulbar anesthesia is used to prevent the risk of injury to the optic nerve or the ophthalmic vein and artery located in the retrobulbar cone.

With the needle directed in close proximity to the orbital walls, the distance to the globe is maximized and a potential scleral perforation is made more difficult (5). However, perforations have been reported using a peribulbar technique (90,94,95,99–103). Up to 10 mL of anesthetic is injected into the orbit outside the cone into the peribulbar space (89,104). Needles are usually shorter than 31 mm since they do not have to reach the retrobulbar cone.

The techniques of injection correspond to those for additional injections in a multiple injection approach described in the section on retrobulbar anesthesia. At least two injections are usually performed inferotemporally and superotemporally or superonasally, injecting 1 to 5 mL each time into the respective peribulbar fat pads. Since these fat compartments communicate with each other but are separated by a framework of connective tissue septa, the use of hyaluronidase will facilitate the even distribution of anesthetic within the orbit and is highly recommended with peribulbar anesthesia (105,106).

The rate of unsuccessful complete akinesia with exclusively peribulbar anesthesia varies among reports from 5% to 50% (45,89,104). Since the anesthetic agent has to diffuse throughout the orbit to reach the nerves in demand, the onset of anesthesia is generally slower than with a retrobulbar injection (45,82,107). An additional disadvantage is that more anesthetic has to be injected (83), leading to a higher extrinsic pressure to the globe (3) and to a more pronounced degree of conjunctival chemosis (107–109).

While anesthesia may not be as complete with a strictly peribulbar technique than with a combined peribulbar-retrobulbar technique, serious complications such as retrobulbar hemorrhage, optic nerve injury, and globe perforation may be reduced, which explains the growing popularity of this form of regional anesthesia (110).

Sub-Tenon's Anesthesia

This form of anesthesia has gained popularity since 1990 (111), although it was described for the first time in 1956 (112). Sub-Tenon's space is in communication with the subdural retrobulbar space (5,113). Since Tenon's fascia reaches up to the perilimbal conjunctiva, sub-Tenon's space can be accessed from there. This is the easiest and safest access to the retrobulbar space.

With this technique the conjunctiva is anesthetized topically first. Then sub-Tenon's space is dissected surgically at a distance of 2 to 3 mm behind the limbus (13,114,115). Greenbaum (115) made a point that by careful coagulation of the conjunctiva at this location, the underlying Tenon's capsule fuses with the conjunctiva, allowing easy dissection of both layers and access to sub-Tenon's space. Although dissection more posterior to the limbus is possible, it is more complicated requiring dissection through the conjunctiva, Tenon's capsule, and the intermuscular septum. Through a very small opening (0.5 mm), a blunt-ended curved cannula is inserted into sub-Tenon's space and directed into the retrobulbar cone (116). Greenbaum (115) used a polyethylene cannula with a flat bottom while Stevens (117) described a curved metal cannula. If the opening in the conjunctiva is tight enough to prevent retrograde flow of liquid, the anesthetic agent is injected briskly into the retrobulbar space. The force of quickly injected liquid will mechanically further dissect sub-Tenon's space, allowing fast, precise, and safe distribution of the anesthetic agent. One milliliter to 5 mL of anesthetic has been used. The effect of the anesthesia is immediate. Akinesia, however, takes 5 minutes to develop. This technique also seems to be safer with regard to the extrinsic extraocular pressure generated. No significant intraocular pressure increase is noted after sub-Tenon's anesthesia when compared with retrobulbar or peribulbar anesthesia.

On the other hand, a vortex vein could potentially be injured, with a risk for orbital hemorrhage (13). There are also reports of incomplete anesthesia requiring additional injections (118). However, compared to blind approaches with sharp needles, this technique appears very safe and promising without the drawbacks of topical anesthesia. Since sub-Tenon's anesthesia has been more widely adopted just recently, we will certainly see more uses for it in the future.

Facial Block

Retrobulbar anesthesia usually does not provide akinesia of the eyelids because the branch of the facial nerve innervating the orbicular muscle is located anterior to the orbital septum where anesthetic does not spread from the retrobulbar cone. Peribulbar anesthesia is more complete in this regard by spreading more anesthetic forward around the terminal branches of the facial nerve and around the orbicular muscle. Greenbaum (64) stated that in sub-Tenon's block, the need for lid akinesia is obviated, because the patient feels neither pain nor has any remaining vision. He or she therefore has no need to close the eyes (64). Again patient cooperation appears as a crucial factor in local anesthesia.

Most surgeons will probably agree that facial blocks may still be required in certain situations and with certain patients. The possible techniques are the Van Lindt block, the O'Brien block, and the Atkinson block, with the Van Lindt block being the oldest and probably the most widely used.

In the Van Lindt block a needle is inserted at the temporal orbital margin into the skin and the subdermal connective tissue is infiltrated, directing the needle upward toward the eyebrow and, after the needle is withdrawn slightly, it is directed downward toward the lower orbital rim (119). This anesthetizes the terminal facial nerve branches when crossing the temporal orbital rim to innervate the orbicular muscle.

The O'Brien block consists of an injection just anterior to the tragus below the zygomatic process and over the condyloid process of the mandible. With a short needle, 2 mL of anesthetic is injected to a depth of about 1 cm (120). This way the facial nerve will be anesthetized while branching at the level of the parotid gland, providing almost complete hemifacial akinesia.

In the Atkinson block the needle is inserted in a location between the Van Lindt and the O'Brien block, below the zygomatic bone toward the zygomatic arch. The exact injection site lies a little posterior to a line descending vertically from the lateral orbital rim. Three milliliters to 10 mL of anesthetic is injected with a 35-mm-long needle along the zygomatic arch (72).

All facial blocks are painful, sometimes requiring intravenous sedation during injection, which may decrease the subsequent collaboration of the patient, who is sedated and disoriented. All of these blocks have been used and provide satisfactory akinesia of the eyelids. The O'Brien block has mostly been abandoned because of the risk of neural injury and the uncomfortable complete semifacial akinesia, although the lid akinesia is more complete with the O'Brien block compared to the other two techniques (121).

TOPICAL ANESTHESIA

Topical anesthesia is now used more frequently since the adoption of phacoemulsification through a corneal incision and folded lens implantation techniques. The drugs used are mostly lidocaine 4% (37) and bupivacaine 0.75% (39). Drops are applied repeatedly shortly prior to surgery, to avoid the epithelial toxicity of all topical anesthetic drugs. This form of anesthesia is the safest method of ocular anesthesia; however, this safety aspect may not pertain to cataract surgery.

Purely topical anesthesia is therefore controversial. It is easy to administer and very safe. There is no danger of injury to orbital structures. Blocking of surface sensibility is excellent. However, there is no akinesia, intraocular sensibility remains intact, and the patient retains vision. The surgeon has to adapt to this particular situation. Verbal communica-

tion with the patient and patient cooperation and selection are extremely important. The cataract surgeon's character and communication skills are as crucial as the surgical capabilities. Because of the patient's retained vision and intraocular sensibility, the surgeon will have to compromise on the surgical techniques. Fine et al (122) reported on the need to initially reduce the light of the operating microscope for the patient to tolerate the procedure since vision is intact. During phacoemulsification when the eye is inflated, the patient feels pain because intraocular sensation remains intact, the authors reported on lowering the infusion bottle. To avoid ciliary spasm pain from miotics, he reduced the amount of epinephrine in the irrigation solution and completely abandoned use of intraocular miotics. Obviously the patient with exclusively topical anesthesia will have "instant vision" and a better visual acuity 24 hours after surgery as well as better cosmesis (122).

However, making all these compromises during surgery is a steep price to pay for the advantages of topical anesthesia. One goal of anesthesia is to prepare the eye for the safest surgery possible. This is obviously not the case with topical anesthesia. It may not even be the most satisfying experience for the patient, who has to see the surgeon operate, fixate on a bright light, and feel repeated intraocular discomfort or even pain (123). Nevertheless, topical anesthesia enjoys wide popularity in the profession.

COMPLICATIONS OF REGIONAL ANESTHESIA

The possible complications of regional anesthesia follow from the anatomic, physiologic, and pharmacologic concepts outlined earlier. They include trauma to the orbital blood vessels leading to a retro-orbital hemorrhage, injury to the optic nerve and spread of anesthetic into the central nervous system, perforation of the globe itself, as well as the rare intra-arterial or intravenous injection of anesthetic. Additionally there may be injury to one or more eye muscles or toxic influence of the anesthetic to an eye muscle, leading to postoperative strabismus or ptosis. Since all these dangers are inherent when using a needle even with the correct technique and the right needle length and shape, there are strong proponents for sub-Tenon's anesthesia (64,124).

The risk of globe perforation is estimated to be 1 per 100 to 1 per 12,000 (73,90) and is up to 1 per 140 in patients with high myopia (99). Therefore, ultrasonographic control may be necessary in myopic patients to exclude an additional staphyloma (125). Perforation has occurred with strictly peribulbar anesthesia (90,94,95,99–103) as well as retrobulbar anesthesia (94,95,99,126). Patients may report pain, and an increase of injection resistance may be felt, followed by hypotony upon withdrawal of the needle. Intraocular complications such as retinal tears, intravitreal bleeding, and retinal detachment will often require immediate intervention from a retinal surgeon. Intravitreally injected steroids and particularly undiluted antibiotics cause more serious damage than intravitreal injection of local anesthetics, which seem to be better tolerated (127–133).

The risk for optic nerve injury and spread of anesthetic to the central nervous system varies from 1 per 350 to 1 per 500 (71,73,78,87,134). Although in most of the patients the symptoms were harmless, serious central nervous depression can occur (135–140). Signs of central nervous system spread of anesthetic include mental confusion, extraocular paresis, amaurosis in the contralateral eye, shivering to convulsion, nausea, dysphagia dyspnea, and sudden swings in the cardiovascular vital signs. If immediate medical support including cardiopulmonary resuscitation is at hand, the outcome is generally favorable.

The risk of retrobulbar hemorrhage has been reported to be 1 per 60 to 1 per 100 (75,141) using retrobulbar and peribulbar anesthesia techniques (142). An arterial hemorrhage will have a quicker onset than a venous hemorrhage and a more intense spread of blood to the conjunctiva and lids (143). Rapidly increasing intraorbital pressure may lead to marked ischemia of the globe (144,145). Management includes osmotic diuresis to lower the intraocular pressure and to maintain a vascular circulation in the globe and a lateral canthotomy to release orbital pressure (143).

Ischemia to the globe may also arise from direct nerve sheath injury resulting in perineural and retrobulbar hemorrhage and optic nerve compression needing optic nerve sheath decompression (79,86,146,147).

Diplopia and strabismus are normal for up to 48 hours after regional anesthesia. Persistent strabismus or ptosis may be due to direct muscle trauma (73,148–155). Apparently the inferior rectus muscle is mostly involved (250, 259–263), providing the rationale to use a curved or bent needle. Additionally, myotoxicity of local anesthetics has been described (156–159). Therefore, direct injection of a toxic agent into the muscle may be responsible for postoperative strabismus and should be avoided (153,157,158, 160).

Postoperative ptosis is also common, the incidence varying from 0% to 20% (161,162). However, 55.5% of patients undergoing cataract surgery have been reported to have a preexisting ptosis (161), which may reflect an already existing degenerated levator aponeurosis that may be exacerbated by surgery. Patients undergoing general anesthesia have a lower risk for postoperative ptosis than do patients receiving local anesthesia (162,163), without there being a difference between the regional anesthesia techniques used (164). The cause of postoperative ptosis may be the myotoxic effects of anesthetic spread to the levator, pressure to the lid exerted by the speculum, traction on the superior and levator muscles, as well as prolonged postoperative patching, though the latter is being abandoned following contemporary cataract surgery (158,161).

REFERENCES

1. Dutton J. *Atlas of clinical and surgical orbital anatomy*. Philadelphia: WB Saunders, 1994.
2. Sacks J. Peripheral innervation of extraocular muscles. *Am J Ophthalmol* 1983;95:520.
3. Stevens J, Giubilei M, Lanigan L, et al. Sub-Tenon, retrobulbar and peribulbar local anesthesia: the effect upon intraocular pressure. *Eur J Implant Ref Surg* 1993;5:25.
4. Koorneef L. The architecture of the musculofibrous apparatus in the human orbit. *Acta Morphol Neerl Scand* 1977;15:35.
5. Gills J, Hustead R, Sanders D. *Ophthalmic anesthesia*. Thorofare, NJ: Slack, 1993.
6. Atkinson W. Local anesthesia in ophthalmology. *Am J Ophthalmol* 1948;31:1607.
7. Liu C, Youl B, Moseley I. Magnetic resonance imaging of the optic nerve in extremes of gaze. Implications for the positioning of the globe for retrobulbar anesthesia. *Br J Ophthalmol* 1992;76:728.
8. Katsev D, Drews R, Rose B. An anatomic study of retrobulbar needle path length. *Ophthalmology* 1989;96:1221.
9. Hayreh S, Dass R. The ophthalmic artery: I. Origin and intracanalicular course. *Br J Ophthalmol* 1962;46:65.
10. De Santis M, Anderson K, King D, Nielsen J. Variability in relationships of arteries and nerves in the human orbit. *Anat Anz* 1984;157:227.
11. Koorneef L. Details of the orbital connective tissue system in the adult. *Acta Morphol Neerl Scand* 1977;15:1.
12. Hogan M, Alvarado J, JE W. *Histology of the human eye: an atlas and textbook*. Philadelphia: WB Saunders, 1971.
13. Stevens JD. A new local anesthesia technique for cataract extraction by one quadrant sub-Tenon's infiltration [see comments]. *Br J Ophthalmol* 1992;76:670.
14. Jay W, Carter H, Williams B, et al. Effect of applying the Honan intraocular pressure in periocular anesthesia. *Am J Ophthalmol* 1985;100:523.
15. Ropo A, Russuvaara P, Paloheimo M, et al. Effect of ocular compression on intraocular pressure. *Acta Ophthalmol (Copenh)* 1990;68:227.
16. Meyer D, Hamilton RC, Loken RG, Gimbel HV. Effect of combined peribulbar and retrobulbar injection of large volumes of anesthetic agents on the intraocular pressure. *Can J Ophthalmol* 1992;27:230.
17. Koorneef L. New insights in the human orbital connective tissue: result of a new anatomical approach. *Arch Ophthalmol* 1977;95:1269.
18. Hill D. *Physics applied to anesthesia*. New York: Appleton-Century-Crofts, 1968.
19. Hessemer V, Wieth K, Heinrich A, Jacobi K. Changes in uveal and retinal hemodynamics produced by retrobulbar anesthesia with different injection volumes. *Fortschr Ophthalmol* 1989;86:760.
20. Hayreh S, Kolder H. Central retinal artery occlusion and retinal tolerance time. *Ophthalmology* 1980;87:75.
21. Hessemer V, Heinrich A, Jacobi K. Ocular circulatory changes induced by retrobulbar anesthesia with and without adrenaline. *Klin Monatsbl Augenheilkd* 1990;197:470.
22. Bucci M, Ducoli P, Manni G, et al. Recovery time after photostress in induced ocular hypertension. *Glaucoma* 1992;14:17.
23. Zabel R, Clarke W, Shirley S, Rock W. Intraocular pressure reduction prior to retrobulbar injection of anesthetic. *Ophthalmic Surg* 1988;19:868.
24. Kothe A, Lovasic J. A parametric evaluation of retinal vascular perfusion pressure and visual neural function in man. *Electroencephalogr Clin Neurophysiol* 1990;75:185.
25. Brunette J, Oliver P, Galeano C, et al. Hyper-response and delay in the electroretinogram in acute ischemia. *Can J Ophthalmol* 1983;18:188.
26. Loken RG, Coupland SG, Deschenes MC. The electroretinogram during orbital compression following intraorbital regional block for cataract surgery. *Can J Anaesth* 1994;41:802.
27. Livingston M, Mackool R, Schneider H. Anesthetic agents used in cataract surgery. *J Cataract Refract Surg* 1990;16:272.
28. Thorburn W, Thorn-Alquist A, Edström H. Etidocaine in retrobulbar anesthesia: a comparison with mepivacaine. *Acta Ophthalmol* 1976;54:591.
29. Smith P, Smith E. A comparison of etidocaine and lidocaine for retrobulbar anesthesia. *Ophthalmic Surg* 1983;14:569.
30. Cohen S. The rational use of local anesthetic mixture. *Reg Anesth* 1979;4:11.
31. Johansen J, Kjeldgard M, Corydon L. Retrobulbar anaesthesia. A clinical evaluation of four different anaesthetic mixtures. *Acta Ophthalmol* 1993;71:787.
32. Bell RW, Butt ZA. Warming lignocaine reduces the pain of injection during peribulbar local anaesthesia for cataract surgery. *Br J Ophthalmol* 1995;79:1015.

33. Ursell PG, Spalton DJ. The effect of solution temperature on the pain of peribulbar anesthesia. *Ophthalmology* 1996;103:839.

34. Brent M, Slomovic A, Easterbrook M. Keratitis associated with the use of proparacaine hydrochloride. *Can Med Assoc J* 1987;136:380.

35. Wilson R. Complications associated with local and general ophthalmic anesthesia. *Int Ophthalmol Clin* 1992;32:1.

36. Rosenwasser G. Complications of topical ocular anesthetics. *Int Ophthalmol Clin* 1989;29:153.

37. Steen W. No-stitch clear-corneal incisions under topical anesthesia. *Ocular Surg* 1993;11:46.

38. Marr W, Wood R, Senterfit L, Sigelman S. Effect of topical anesthesia on regeneration of corneal epithelium. *Am J Ophthalmol* 1957;43:606.

39. Gills JP, Williams DL. Advantage of marcaine for topical anesthesia. *J Cataract Refract Surg* 1993;19:819. Letter.

40. Scott D, Jebson P, Braid D, et al. Factors affecting plasma levels of lignocaine and prilocaine. *Br J Anaesth* 1972;44:1040.

41. Chin G, Almquist H. Bupivacaine and lidocaine retrobulbar anesthesia. A double-blind clinical study. *Ophthalmology* 1983;90:369.

42. Bromage P. *Epidural analgesia.* Philadelphia: WB Saunders, 1978.

43. Hartrick C, Raj P, Dirkes W, Denson D. Compounding of bupivacaine and mepivacaine for regional anesthesia: a safe practice? *Reg Anesth* 1984;9:94.

44. Feitl M, Krupin T. Neural blockade for ophthalmic surgery. In: Cousins M, Bridenbaugh P, eds. *Neural blockade in clinical anesthesia and management of pain.* Philadelphia: JB Lippincott, 1988.

45. Loots JH, Koorts AS, Venter JA. Peribulbar anesthesia. A prospective statistical analysis of the efficacy and predictability of bupivacaine and a lignocaine/bupivacaine mixture [see comments]. *J Cataract Refract Surg* 1993;19:72.

46. Krohn J, Seland JH, Hovding G, et al. Retrobulbar anesthesia with and without hyaluronidase in extracapsular cataract surgery. A prospective, randomized, double-blind study. *Acta Ophthalmol* 1993;71:791.

47. Nathan N, Benrhaiem M, Lotfi H, et al. The role of hyaluronidase on lidocaine and bupivacaine pharmacokinetics after peribulbar blockade. *Anesth Analg* 1996;82:1060.

48. Apel A, Woodward R. Cataract surgery—anesthesia without hyaluronidase. *Aust N Z J Ophthalmol* 1991;19:249. Letter.

49. Atkinson W. Local anesthesia in ophthalmology. *Trans Am Ophthalmol Soc* 1934;32:399.

50. Drews R, Malbran E. Anesthesia, speculum free surgery, intraoperative fundus observation with the surgical microscope. In: Boyd B, ed. *Highlights of ophthalmology.* Vol. I. Cali, Colombia: Carvajal, 1993.

51. Nicoll J, Teuren B, Acharya P, et al. Retrobulbar anesthesia: the role of hyaluronidase. *Anesth Analg* 1986;65:1324.

52. Thomson I. Addition of hyaluronidase to lignocaine with adrenaline for retrobulbar anesthesia in the surgery of senile cataract. *Br J Ophthalmol* 1988;72:700.

53. Morsman CD, Holden R. The effects of adrenaline, hyaluronidase and age on peribulbar anaesthesia. *Eye* 1992;6(pt 3):290.

54. Heyworth P, Seward H. Local anesthesia—the ophthalmologist's view. *Eur Implant Ref Surg* 1993;5:12.

55. O'Brien H. Anesthesia for cataract surgery. *Am J Ophthalmol* 1964;57:751.

56. Pearce J. General and local anesthesia in eye surgery. *Trans Ophthalmol Soc UK* 1982;102:31.

57. Rubin A. Anesthesia for cataract surgery—time for a change. *Anesthesia* 1990;45:717.

58. Hodgkins PR, Luff AJ, Morrell AJ, et al. Current practice of cataract extraction and anaesthesia. *Br J Ophthalmol* 1992;76:323.

59. Backer C, Tinker J, Robertson D. Myocardial reinfarction following local anesthesia for ophthalmic surgery. *Anesth Analg* 1980;59:257.

60. Campbell DN, Lim M, Muir MK, et al. A prospective randomised study of local versus general anaesthesia for cataract surgery. *Anaesthesia* 1993;48:422.

61. Lang D. Morbidity and mortality in ophthalmology. In: Bruce R, McGoldrick K, Oppenheimer P, eds. *Anesthesia for ophthalmology.* Birmingham, AL: Aesculapius, 1982:195.

62. Karteti R, Callahan H, Draper G. Factors leading to hospital admission of elderly patients following outpatient eye surgery: a medical dilemma. *Anesth Analg* 1989;68:S144.

63. Tiret L, Desmond J, Hatton F, et al. Complications associated with anesthesia—a prospective study in France. *Can J Anaesth* 1986;33:336.

64. Greenbaum S. Anesthesia for cataract surgery. In: Greenbaum S, ed. *Ocular anesthesia.* Philadelphia: WB Saunders, 1997:3.

65. Koay P, Laing A, Adams K, et al. Ophthalmic pain following cataract surgery: a comparison between local and general anaesthesia. *Br J Ophthalmol* 1992;76:225.

66. Watts M, Pearce J. Day case cataract surgery. *Br J Ophthalmol* 1988;72:897.

67. Egbert L, Battit G, Turndorf H. The value of the preoperative visit by the anesthetist. *JAMA* 1963;185:553.

68. Scott D. Sedation for local analgesia. Distraction and diazepam. *Anaesthesia* 1975;30:471.

69. Adams A, Jones R. Anesthesia for eye surgery: general considerations. *Br J Anaesth* 1980;52:663.

70. Smith D, Crul J. Oxygen desaturation following sedation for regional anesthesia. *Br J Anaesth* 1989;62:206.

71. Rubin A. Local anesthesia for ophthalmic surgery: an anesthetist's view. *Eur J Implant Ref Surg* 1993;5:8.

72. Atkinson W. *Anesthesia in ophthalmology.* Springfield, IL: Charles C Thomas, 1955.

73. Hamilton R, Gimbel H, Strunin L. Regional anesthesia for 12,000 cataract extraction and intraocular lens implantation procedures. *Can J Anaesth* 1988;35:615.

74. Gills J, Loyd T. A technique of retrobulbar block with paralysis of the orbicularis oculi. *Am Intraocular Implant Surg* 1983;9:339.

75. Morgan C, Schatz H, Vine A, et al. Ocular complications associated with retrobulbar injections. *Ophthalmology* 1988;95:660.

76. Javitt J, Adiego R, Friedberg H, et al. Brain stem anesthesia after retrobulbar block. *Ophthalmology* 1987;94:718.

77. Unsöld R, Stanley J, DeGroot J. The CT-topography of retrobulbar anesthesia. *Arch Klin Ophthalmol* 1981;217:125.

78. Nicoll J, Acharya P, Kjell A, et al. Central nervous system complications after 6000 retrobulbar blocks. *Anesth Analg* 1987;66:1298.

79. Pautler S, Grizzard W, Thompson L, Wing G. Blindness from retrobulbar injection into the optic nerve. *Ophthalmic Surg* 1986;17:334.

80. Abelson M, Paradis A, Mandel E, George M. The effect of hyaluronidase on akinesia during cataract surgery. *Ophthalmic Surg* 1989;20:325.

81. Atkinson W. Use of hyaluronidase with local anesthesia in ophthalmology: preliminary report. *Arch Ophthalmol* 1949;42:628.

82. Khalil S. Local anesthesia for eye surgery. *Anaesthesia* 1991;46:232. Letter.

83. Strauss A. A new retrobulbar needle and injection technique. *Ophthalmic Surg* 1988;19:134.

84. Hustead R, Hamilton R. Techniques. In: Gills J, Hustead R, Sanders D, eds. *Ophthalmic anesthesia.* Thorofare, NJ: Slack, 1993.

85. Martin S, Baker S, Muenzler W. Retrobulbar anesthesia and orbicularis akinesia. *Ophthalmic Surg* 1986;17:232.

86. Grizzard W. Ophthalmic anesthesia. In: Reinecke R, ed. *Ophthalmology annual.* New York: Raven, 1989.

87. Ahn J, Stanley J. Subarachnoid injection as a complication of retrobulbar anesthesia. *Am J Ophthalmol* 1987;103:225.

88. Callahan A. Ultrasharp disposable needles. *Am J Ophthalmol* 1966;62:173. Letter.

89. Davis D, Mandel M. Posterior peribulbar anesthesia: an alternative to retrobulbar anesthesia. *Geriatr Ophthalmol* 1987;86:61.

90. Kimble J, Morris R, Witherspoon C, Feist R. Globe perforation from peribulbar injection. *Arch Ophthalmol* 1987;105:749.

91. Vivian A, Canning C. Scleral perforation with retrobulbar needles. *Eur Implant Ref Surg* 1993;5:39.

92. Galindo A, Keilson L, Mondshine R, Sawelson H. Retro-peribulbar anesthesia. Special technique and needle design. *Ophthalmol Clin North Am* 1990;3:71.

93. Waller S, Taboada J, O'Connor P. Retrobulbar anesthesia risk. Do sharp needles really perforate the eye more easily than blunt needles? *Ophthalmology* 1993;100:506.

94. Hay A, Flynn HJ, Hoffman J, Rivera A. Needle penetration of the globe during retrobulbar and peribulbar injections. *Ophthalmology* 1991;98:1017.

95. Grizzard W, Kirk N, Pavan P, et al. Perforating ocular injuries caused by anesthesia personnel. *Ophthalmology* 1991;98:1011.

96. Wong D. Review article: regional anesthesia for intraocular surgery. *Can J Anaesth* 1993;40:635.

97. Meyers E. Anesthesia. In: Krupin T, Waltman S, eds. *Complications in ophthalmic surgery.* Philadelphia: JB Lippincott, 1984.

98. Leaming DV. Practice styles and preferences of ASCRS members—1993 survey. *J Cataract Refract Surg* 1994;20:459.

99. Duker J, Belmont J, WB B, et al. Inadvertent globe perforation during retrobulbar and peribulbar anesthesia. *Ophthalmology* 1991;98:519.

100. Davis D, Mandel M. Peribulbar: reducing complications. *Ocular Surg News* 1989;7:21.

101. Gentili M, Brassier J. Is peribulbar block safer than retrobulbar? *Reg Anesth* 1992;17:309. Letter.

102. Joseph J, McHugh J, Franks W, Chignell A. Perforation of the globe—a complication of peribulbar anaesthesia. *Br J Ophthalmol* 1991;75:504.

103. Zaturansky B, Hyams S. Perforation of the globe during the injection of local anesthesia. *Ophthalmic Surg* 1987;18:585.

104. Bloomberg L. Anterior periocular anesthesia: five years experience. *J Cataract Refract Surg* 1991;17:508.

105. Bjornstrom L, Hansen A, Otland N, et al. Peribulbar anaesthesia. A clinical evaluation of two different anaesthetic mixtures. *Acta Ophthalmol* 1994;72:712.

106. Sarvela J, Nikki P. Hyaluronidase improves regional ophthalmic anaesthesia with etidocaine. *Can J Anaesth* 1992;39:920.

107. Arora R, Verma L, Kumar A, et al. Peribulbar anesthesia in retinal reattachment surgery. *Ophthalmic Surg* 1992;23:499.

108. Wang H. Peribulbar anesthesia for ophthalmic procedures. *J Cataract Refract Surg* 1988;14:441.

109. Weiss J, Deichmann C. A comparison of retrobulbar and periocular anesthesia for cataract surgery. *Arch Ophthalmol* 1989;107:96.

110. Davis D, Mandel M. Efficacy and complication rate of 16,224 consecutive peribulbar blocks. *J Cataract Refract Surg* 1994;20:327.

111. Tsuneoka H, Ohki K, Taniuchi O, Kitahara K. Tennon's capsule anesthesia for cataract surgery with IOL implantation. *Eur Implant Ref Surg* 1993;5:29.

112. Swan K. New drugs and techniques for ocular anesthesia. *Trans Am Acad Ophthalmol Otolaryngol* 1956;60:368.

113. Snyder C. An operation designated "the extirpation of the eye". *Arch Ophthalmol* 1965;74:429.

114. Mein C, Woodcock M. Local anesthesia for vitreoretinal surgery. *Retina* 1990;10:47.

115. Greenbaum S. Parabulbar anesthesia. *Am J Ophthalmol* 1992;114:776.

116. Stevens J, Restory M. Ultrasound imaging of no-needle 1-quadrant sub-Tenon local anesthesia for cataract surgery. *Eur Implant Ref Surg* 1993;5:35.

117. Stevens JD. Curved, sub-Tenon cannula for local anesthesia. *Ophthalmic Surg* 1993;24:121.

118. Simcock P, Raymond G, Lavin M. Peribulbar injection and direct infiltration for vitreoretinal surgery. *Arch Ophthalmol* 1992;110:1357.

119. Van Lindt A. Paralysie palpebrae temporaire provoquee dans l'operation de la cataracte. *Ann Ocul (Paris)* 1914;151:420.

120. O'Brien C. Akinesis during cataract extraction. *Arch Ophthalmol* 1929;1:447.

121. Schimek F, Fahle M. Techniques of facial nerve block. *Br J Ophthalmol* 1995;79:166.

122. Fine I, Fichman R, Grabow H. *Clear cornea cataract surgery and topical anesthesia.* Thorofare, NJ: Slack, 1993.

123. Duguid IG, Claoue CM, Thamby-Rajah Y, et al. Topical anaesthesia for phacoemulsification surgery. *Eye* 1995;9(pt 4):456.

124. Stewart M, Lambrou F. The management of preoperative, intraoperative and postoperative complications of cataract surgery from the perspective of vitreoretinal surgeons. *Adv Clin Ophthalmol* 1994;1:63.

125. Alberth B, Damjanovich J. Komplikationen retrobulbärer Injektionen. Möglichkeiten der Beseitigung. *Klin Monatsbl Augenheilkd* 1990;196:92.

126. Schneider M, Milsetin D, Oykawa R. Ocular perforation from a retrobulbar injection. *Am J Ophthalmol* 1988;106:35.

127. Brown G, Eagle R, Shakin E, et al. Retinal toxicity of intravitreal gentamicin. *Arch Ophthalmol* 1990;108:1740.

128. Campochiaro P, Conway B. Aminoglycoside toxicity—a survey of retinal specialists: implications for ocular use. *Arch Ophthalmol* 1991;109:946.

129. Jain V, Manes R, McGorray S, Giles C. Inadvertent penetrating injury to the globe with periocular corticosteroid injection. *Ophthalmic Surg* 1991;22:508.

130. Schechter R. Management of inadvertent intraocular injections. *Ann Ophthalmol* 1985;17:771.

131. Schlaegal T, Wilson F. Accidental intraocular injection of depot corticosteroids. *Trans Am Acad Ophthalmol Otolaryngol* 1974;78:847.

132. Berg P, Kroll P, Kuchie H. Iatrogenic eye perforations in para- and retrobulbar injections. *Klin Monatsbl Augenheilkd* 1986;189:170.

133. Lincoff H, Zweifach P, Brodie S, et al. Intraocular injection of lidocaine. *Ophthalmology* 1985;92:1587.

134. Stanley J. Subarachnoid injection of retrobulbar anesthetic as a complication of retrobulbar block. *Saudi Bull Ophthalmol* 1987;2:13.

135. Beltranena H, Vega M, Kirk N, Blankenship G. Inadvertent intravascular bupivacaine injection following retrobulbar block. *Reg Anesth* 1981;6:149.

136. Chang J-L, Gonzalez-Abola E, Larson C, Lobes L. Brain stem anesthesia following retrobulbar block. *Anesthesiology* 1984;1984(61).

137. Hamilton R. Brain stem anesthesia following retrobulbar blockade. *Anesthesiology* 1985;63:688.

138. Mercereau D. Brain stem anesthesia complicating retrobulbar block. *Can J Ophthalmol* 1989;24:159.

139. Rosenblatt R, May D, Barsoumian K. Cardiopulmonary arrest after retrobulbar block. *Am J Ophthalmol* 1980;90:425.

140. Smith J. Retrobulbar marcaine can cause respiratory arrest. *J Clin Neuroophthalmol* 1981;1:171.

141. Peterson W, Yanoff M. Complications of local ocular anesthesia. *Int Ophthalmol Clin* 1992;32:23.

142. Puustjarvi T, Purhonen S. Permanent blindness following retrobulbar hemorrhage after peribulbar anesthesia for cataract surgery. *Ophthalmic Surgery* 1992;23:450.

143. Feibel R. Current concepts in retrobulbar anesthesia. *Surv Ophthalmol* 1985;30:102.

144. Goldsmith M. Occlusion of the central retinal artery following retrobulbar anesthesia. *Ophthalmologica* 1967;153:191.

145. Kraushar M, Seelenfreund M, Freilich D. Central retinal artery closure during orbital hemorrhage from retrobulbar injection. *Trans Am Acad Ophthalmol Otolaryngol* 1974;78:65.

146. Hersch M, Baer G, Dioeckert J, et al. Optic nerve enlargement and central retinal artery occlusion secondary to retrobulbar anesthesia. *Ann Ophthalmol* 1989;21:195.

147. Sullivan K, Brown G, Forman A, et al. Retrobulbar anesthesia and retinal vascular obstruction. *Ophthalmology* 1983;90:373.

148. Carlson B, Emerick S, Komorowski T, et al. Extraocular muscle regeneration in primates. *Ophthalmology* 1992;99:582.

149. Rao V, Kawatra V. Ocular myotoxic effects of local anesthetics. *Can J Ophthalmol* 1988;23:171.

150. de Faber J-T, van Noorden G. Inferior rectus muscle palsy after retrobulbar anesthesia for cataract surgery. *Am J Ophthalmol* 1992;112:209.

151. Grimmett M, Lambert S. Superior rectus muscle overaction after cataract extraction. *Am J Ophthalmol* 1992;116:424.

152. Esswein MB, von Noorden GK. Paresis of a vertical rectus muscle after cataract extraction. *Am J Ophthalmol* 1993;116:424.

153. Ong-Tone L, Pearce W. Inferior rectus muscle restriction after retrobulbar anesthesia for cataract surgery. *Can J Ophthalmol* 1989;24:162.

154. Hamed L, Mancuso A. Inferior rectus muscle contracture syndrome after retrobulbar anesthesia. *Ophthalmology* 1991;98:1506.

155. Hamilton SM, Elsas FJ, Dawson TL. A cluster of patients with inferior rectus restriction following local anesthesia for cataract surgery. *J Pediatr Ophthalmol Strabismus* 1993;30:288.

156. Carlson B, Rainin E. Rat extraocular muscle regeneration. *Arch Ophthalmol* 1985;103:1973.

157. Foster A, Carlson B. Myotoxicity of local anesthetics and regeneration of the damaged muscle fibres. *Anesth Analg* 1980;59:727.

158. Rainin E, Carlson B. Postoperative diplopia and ptosis: a clinical hypothesis on the myotoxicity of local anesthetics. *Arch Ophthalmol* 1985;103:1337.

159. Yadiela J, Benoit P, Buoncristiani R, et al. Comparison of myotoxic effects of lidocaine with epinephrine in rats and humans. *Anesth Analg* 1981;60:471.

160. O'Brien C. Local anesthesia. *Arch Ophthalmol* 1934;12:240.

161. Kaplan L, Jaffee N, Clayman H. Ptosis and cataract surgery. *Ophthalmology* 1985;92:237.

162. Deady J, Price N, Sutton G. Ptosis following cataract and trabeculectomy surgery. *Br J Ophthalmol* 1989;72:238.

163. Alpar J. Acquired ptosis following cataract and glaucoma surgery. *Glaucoma* 1982;4:66.

164. Feibel RM, Custer PL, Gordon MO. Postcataract ptosis. A randomized, double-masked comparison of peribulbar and retrobulbar anesthesia. *Ophthalmology* 1993;100:660.

Intracapsular Cataract Surgery

Henry M. Clayman

Intracapsular cataract extraction (ICCE) is infrequently used nowadays for routine cataract extraction in the United States and is rarely taught in residency programs. However, it is still part of the ophthalmologist's armamentarium and therefore merits discussion. The fundamental difference from extracapsular cataract extraction (ECCE) is that the cataract is completely removed in one maneuver, as compared to the several steps in ECCE or phacoemulsification, and ICCE consequently requires only one piece of sophisticated equipment, namely, a cryoprobe.

Anesthesia is discussed elsewhere (see Chap. 22) but suffice it to say that adequate akinesia is essential. For ICCE, a "soft" eye is desirable and to this end various regimens have been proposed (1). These included pharmaceutical agents such as preoperative hyperosmotic agents administered by either an oral or intravenous route or carbonic anhydrase inhibitors (2). Various devices to administer external pressure on the anesthetized eye preoperatively have been employed and these included a mercury bag acting by weight and inflatable balloons secured uninflated to the eye and then inflated to compress the globe (3). Complications have been associated with pharmaceutical agents and pressure techniques are not completely innocuous (4,5). My personal preference was digital pressure applied by the surgeon in the operating room, after the anesthetic block was administered and when the patient was prepped and draped, as described later.

Cataract surgery is performed in the surgical limbus, except in special cases that require a clear corneal incision. The limbus is the area where clear cornea merges into opaque sclera. Its posterior border is the insertion of Tenon's capsule and the anterior limit is an imaginary line joining the peripheral termination of Bowman's and Descemet's membranes. The limbus is widest superiorly,

narrowing temporally and nasally, then widening inferiorly, though the inferior limbal width is less than the superior width. Anteriorly the limbus has a bluish color that transcends to gray posteriorly. The superior limbus is a logical site for cataract surgery because it provides good surgical exposure and is generally less vascular than more posterior sites.

TECHNIQUE

The actual technique of ICCE varied widely among surgeons and I describe the technique that I used for many years, in the era before the predominance of ECCE. Preoperatively, patients to be operated on in the morning receive nothing orally after midnight. An hour and a half before the scheduled surgery, the eye to be operated on is dilated with cyclopentolate 1% and Neo-Synephrine 10% drops, which are then readministered every 5 minutes for two more doses. There is no consensus on perioperative antibiotics (6) and surgeons generally conform to their community standards. With the anesthetized patient on the operating table and after a standard preparation and draping, intermittent digital pressure is applied to the eye with the lids closed and through a folded 4 × 4-inch gauze. Though portable electronic tonometers are currently available, in the ICCE era the pressure was monitored by a sterile Schiøtz tonometer with a 5.5-g weight until a scale reading of 10 was obtained, which corresponded to an intraocular pressure of approximately 8 mm Hg using the ready-reckon method of 80 divided by the scale reading equals the approximate intraocular pressure. At this point the operation may begin and a suitable lid speculum is inserted.

The first step is placement of the superior rectus traction suture, which enhances surgical exposure by permitting the globe to be rotated inferiorly. This maneuver may be performed by inserting a blunt instrument such as a muscle hook, held in the right hand, in the inferior conjunctival cul-de-sac and rotating the globe down as the rectus superior muscle is grasped by toothed forceps held in the left hand. At this point the instrument held in the right hand is exchanged for a needle holder carrying a 4-0 silk suture, which is passed through the rectus superior muscle, which is slightly elevated as the suture is passed. The suture is then secured under the lid retractor or clamped to the drape so that the eye is rotated inferiorly without causing excessive pressure on the globe. The suture may be placed in a transconjunctival or subconjunctival manner, after the conjunctival flap has been dissected, according to the surgeon's preference. Placement of the rectus superior suture is a straightforward maneuver yet it has been associated with ocular perforation secondary to entrance of the globe by the needle (7).

The conjunctival flap can be dissected according to two techniques, fornix based or limbus based. In the former, the conjunctiva is grasped at the 12-o'clock limbus with 0.12-mm forceps held in the left hand, and incised to the sclera with Westcott scissors held in the right hand. The closed scissors are then inserted through the conjunctival opening to the right and left laterally, to lyse the conjunctival-scleral attachments. The scissors are then withdrawn and reinserted, with one blade under the conjunctiva and the other superior following the arc of the conjunctival-limbal insertion, which is incised to the right and left laterally. Incisions may be made at the lateral extremities of the flap to increase exposure and bleeding is contained with cautery as required.

A limbus-based flap is made by an incision a few millimeters posterior to the limbus through the conjunctiva and Tenon's capsule to bare sclera. In a maneuver as described above, closed scissors are inserted to the right and left to break attachments and then are reinserted with one blade under and the other over the conjunctiva, which is incised laterally to the right and left. There are invariably residual attachments centrad to the line of conjunctival incision and these are dissected to the surgical limbus.

Following satisfactory exposure of the limbus and hemostasis, the initial incision into the anterior chamber is performed with a razor knife or other suitable instrument. If the incision is too anterior, there is the danger of detaching Descemet's membrane as the incision is enlarged (see below) and inducing excessive astigmatism when the incision is sutured. On the other hand, an incision that is too posterior can cause intraoperative bleeding and postoperative hyphema. For this reason, an incision in the gray area of the limbus is desirable and is accomplished by grasping the limbus with 0.12-mm forceps adjacent to the site of the contemplated incision and then entering the anterior chamber with the razor knife at approximately the 11-o'clock position (Fig. 23-1). This initial incision should be of adequate size to accommodate the blade of the corneoscleral scissors, which will be introduced as the next

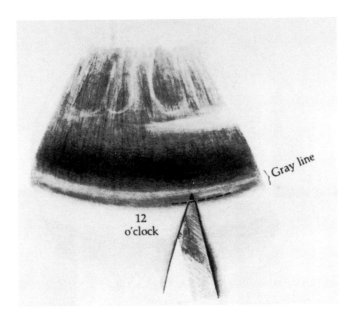

FIGURE 23-1. *Limbal site of initial incision. (Reprinted with permission from HM Clayman, ed.* Atlas of contemporary ophthalmic surgery. *St. Louis: Mosby, 1990.)*

maneuver. The incision described is uniplanar, but there have been advocates of multiplanar incisions who claim more stable wound construction, easier suturing, and more favorable postoperative astigmatism. The surgeon should be cognizant that razor knives and keratome tips are generally triangular and a funnel-shaped incision could result. The inner dimensions of the incision should correspond to the outer dimensions, to minimize the risk of detaching Descemet's membrane as instruments are introduced through the incision.

I next enlarge the incision to the left with one blade of the corneoscleral scissors in the anterior chamber and the other over the surgical limbus. The blade within the eye should always be within the surgeon's view, to avoid the chance that it may inadvertently pass through the iris and precipitate an iridodialysis as attempts are made to enlarge the incision. With the blades correctly placed, the incision is enlarged within the surgical limbus to the left, angulating slightly corneal at the lateral extremity. This conforms to the anatomy of the limbus and avoids hemorrhage from the tributaries of the long choroidal artery. A suture of 8-0 Vicryl or other suitable material is placed through the section at the 12-o'clock position and looped to the surgeon's left. This suture is for later elevation of the cornea or sudden closure of the incision, should an emergency arise. The incision is now enlarged to the right using the same technique as described for enlarging to the left (Fig. 23-2). An incision size of 170 degrees is optimum but the surgeon will not err with a larger incision if in doubt. There was a fad many years ago for performing an ICCE through a "mini-incision." This is an invitation for a broken capsule and vitreous loss and should be avoided.

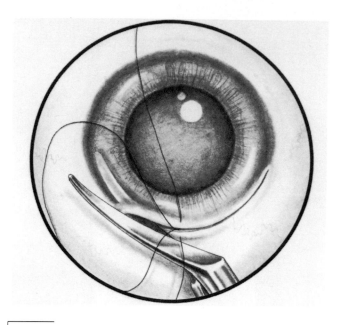

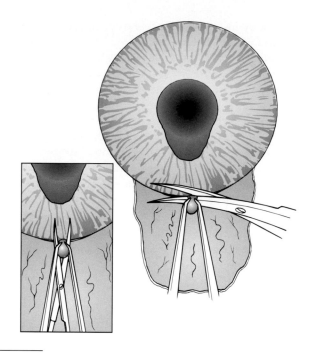

FIGURE 23-3. *Technique of peripheral iridectomy. Inset shows an alternative approach for scissors.*

Peripheral iridectomy or iridotomy is the next step and with ICCE it is prudent to perform this before the cataract is extracted (Fig. 23-3). It was my custom to perform two small iridotomies at the 11- and 1-o'clock positions using small Wescott scissors held in the right hand, while I elevated the cornea by the 12-o'clock suture with tying forceps held in the left hand, after the incision was enlarged. However, a peripheral iridectomy can be performed prior to the cataract section as illustrated in Figure 23-3. In this case the surgeon should take care, as the blade of the corneoscleral scissors can pass inadvertently posterior through the aperture at the peripheral iridectomy site during enlargement of the incision, with a resultant iridodialysis, as noted already. Beware of a peripheral iridectomy that is too posterior as the ciliary processes may be cut with resultant hemorrhage, which could be a consequence of a posterior cataract section as previously discussed. The other caveat concerning the peripheral iridectomy or iridotomy involves the subsequent placement of an anterior-chamber intraocular lens (IOL) if that is the surgeon's intent. The iris openings should be remote from the footplate of the IOL to prevent it from subluxing through the iridectomy with resultant IOL malposition. For this reason, some surgeons prefer a midstromal iridotomy when anterior-chamber IOL placement is planned.

Prior to extraction of the cataract, a bolus of α-chymotrypsin is instilled into the anterior chamber to weaken the zonular attachments (8). This step is not always necessary in older patients but its use is prudent. The usual concentration is 1:5000 to 1:10,000. It is left in the anterior chamber for 1 to 3 minutes, longer in younger

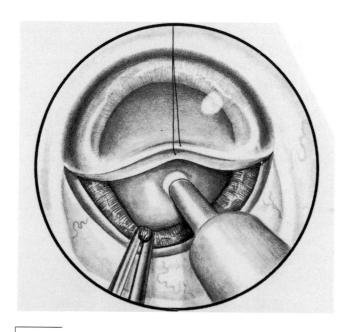

patients and shorter in older patients. It is injected through a fine cannula, which gives the surgeon the opportunity to verify the patency of the iridectomy or iridotomy by injecting a small amount through these sites. The cornea is then elevated by the 12-o'clock suture and the anterior chamber

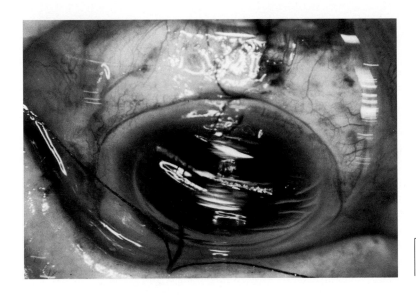

FIGURE 23-5. *Soft eye following cataract extraction. Note the air bubble in the anterior chamber.*

is dried with a cellulose sponge held against the anterior lens capsule. The cornea is then retracted by an assistant as the surgeon retracts the iris with forceps held in the left hand. The cryoprobe is placed on the anterior lens capsule and activated (Fig. 23-4). An ice ball is seen to form and the cataract is gently extracted from the eye with a lateral to-and-fro motion. When ocular hypotension has been achieved prior to incision, an air bubble frequently is sucked into the eye and the cornea may appear concave after the cataract is extracted (Fig. 23-5). Any prolapsed iris is swept back into the anterior chamber, which is re-formed with balanced saline solution, and the 12-o'clock suture is tied and trimmed.

Several points concerning the extraction of the cataract need to the stressed. First, the cryoprobe is placed in the center of the cataract at the junction of its lower two-thirds with the upper one-third (Fig. 23-6). Second, the resultant ice ball should not be too big for it can adhere to the adjacent iris as the cataract is being extracted. If this occurs, one should either irrigate the probe free with a stream of balanced saline solution or deactivate the cryoprobe and reapply, though an adjustment to the freezing temperature may be required. It is only possible to deactivate the freezing mode with the pedal-operated, cylinder-fed, standard operating-room cryoequipment. There are disposable cryounits that have no means for deactivation. If the iris is enveloped by the ice ball while one of these units is used, it may be possible to thaw if free by irrigation with balanced saline solution. The alternative is to wait until the refrigerant is exhausted and then try again. Last, though there are various iris retractors to achieve exposure during cataract extraction, I prefer forceps in the left hand for this purpose, as illustrated in Figure 23-4. This way I have a suitable instrument to strip zonules should that be necessary or a means to lift the cornea if it should be inadvertently dropped. For the same reason, I eschew retracting the iris with a cellulose sponge.

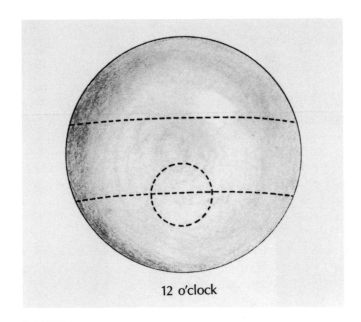

12 o'clock

FIGURE 23-6. *Correct position for cryoprobe placement on the anterior capsule. (Reprinted with permission from HM Clayman, ed. Atlas of contemporary ophthalmic surgery. St. Louis: Mosby, 1990.)*

Various types of sutures and suturing have found favor over the years for the closure of the intracapsular cataract section. Probably the most consistently reliable is the use of interrupted 10-0 nylon sutures. Eight sutures would usually suffice to close a 170-degree incision though some surgeons use more and others less. Certainly if there is an obvious wound leak when the sutured incision is tested in the operating room, then further sutures are indicated. The knots of interrupted sutures can be buried in the needle track and this is easier to do when the knot is slid anteriorly. The 12-o'clock 8-0 Vicryl suture can be left or replaced with a 10-0 nylon suture at the surgeon's discretion. If an anterior-chamber IOL is to be inserted, an appropriate space is left superiorly through which the IOL is passed and after IOL placement this space is sutured. After the wound has been tested for leaks, the superior rectus traction suture is removed and in the case of a fornix-based flap, the flap is pulled down over the wound and tacked in situ with the coaptation forceps of the wetfield cautery or two interrupted absorbable sutures. A limbus-based flap is pulled up over the wound and generally closed with a running absorbable suture, though some surgeons leave the flap unsutured.

The situation in which the pupil does not dilate well or is chronically miotic represents a special contingency for which several techniques are available. One of the most common is to extend the peripheral iridectomy to the pupil (Fig. 23-7) with a resultant *keyhole* pupil (Fig. 23-8). Other alternatives include a sector iridectomy and multiple sphincterotomies. If it is the surgeon's intention to resuture the margins of the iridectomy site, then the suture should be preplaced prior to cataract extraction; otherwise the suture would be passed over an exposed anterior hyaloid face, with the consequent risk of vitreous loss.

POSTOPERATIVE CARE

In the days before IOLs, the usual postoperative care was daily dosage of mydriatic and steroid-antibiotic drops, but because of the danger of dislocation of iris-fixated IOLs, mydriatics were later abandoned. Intraocular pressure is controlled as required with either topical or oral agents, mindful that use of α-chymotrypsin is associated with an increase in intraocular pressure (9). I generally performed an initial refraction at 4 weeks postoperatively and repeated it 4 weeks

later, at which time glasses were prescribed. In the absence of an IOL, an aphakic patient who was previously emmetropic will have an aphakic refraction in the range of +10.00 to +12.00.

COMPLICATIONS

There are three complications that have special relevance to ICCE: retinal detachment (RD), cystoid macular edema (CME), and aphakic bullous keratopathy (ABK). All these complications have a higher incidence after ICCE as compared to ECCE and phakic eyes.

Retinal Detachment

Whereas the incidence of RD in the general public has been estimated to be between 0.005% and 0.010%, after ICCE this increases to about 2% to 3% (10) as compared to 0.5% to 0.9% after ECCE (11), though estimates of the exact incidences following both modalities vary. After ICCE complicated by intraoperative vitreous loss, the incidence of RD approximately doubles (12). The patient's preoperative history also influences the development of a postoperative RD, as axial myopia and the history of RD in the contralateral eye seem to be associated factors.

The definitive reason for the increased incidence of RD after ICCE is not known. It has been proposed that the forward movement of the vitreous after ICCE may produce traction at the vitreous base. Similarly, eye movements in the absence of the crystalline lens may cause vitreous movement, which in turn pulls on the vitreous base. Another theory involves the putative culpability of physical and

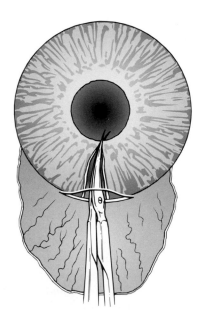

FIGURE 23-7.   *Peripheral iridectomy is extended to the pupil in a patient with miosis.*

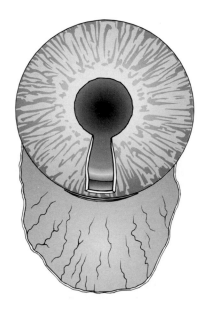

FIGURE 23-8.   *Resultant keyhole pupil.*

biochemical changes within the vitreous following ICCE. Whatever the reasons may be, it is beyond doubt that the chances of postoperative RD are much less after ECCE and this is one of the several reasons for the demise of ICCE as the preferred technique of cataract extraction in the United States.

Cystoid Macular Edema

CME can occur in phakic patients with diabetes mellitus, some retinal degenerations, or uveitis, for example, but until the advent of modern ECCE techniques the most common presentation was in the aphakic eye, following ICCE (13,14), usually uncomplicated. Characteristically the postoperative eye has good vision that decreases in the few months after surgery and then spontaneously improves in about 6 months. Sometimes affected eyes are slightly painful with limbal injection and the anterior hyaloid membrane may or may not be intact. Likewise the presence of vitreous strands adherent to the cataract section is also variable.

Though most cases spontaneously improve, some persist and the treatment is problematic. Corticosteroids or nonsteroidal anti-inflammatory agents are sometimes efficacious in some patients but there is no universally accepted or successful treatment. When vitreous is adherent or incarcerated in the surgical wound, surgery may be beneficial in many patients, even in those with long-standing CME (15). In my experience lysis of vitreous adhesions with the Nd:YAG laser has been difficult and not conspicuously successful.

Aphakic Bullous Keratopathy

Though ABK is not confined to aphakic eyes that have undergone ICCE, it was nevertheless as significant problem in the intracapsular era when it was persistent. Dohlman and Boruchoff (16) stated that a defect in corneal hydration secondary to damage of the corneal endothelium is the etiology of persistent ABK and cite the following as causative factors, either alone or in combination:

1. Preexistent endothelial dystrophy (e.g., Fuchs' dystrophy)
2. Surgical trauma
3. Vitreous contact to the cornea, either central or peripheral
4. Iris adhesion, retrocorneal membrane, Descemet's detachment, epithelial downgrowth
5. Uveitis
6. Glaucoma

Obviously the only factor in this list that is especially peculiar to ICCE is vitreous contact. Even in the absence of intraoperative vitreous loss, it was not unusual in the postoperative period to see free vitreous in the anterior chamber in an eye that heretofore had an intact anterior hyaloid face, and there was no practical means to prevent vitreous adherence to the cornea. If the patient had a preexistent endothelial dystrophy and vitreocorneal adherence, then the chances of ABK were much higher. Beyond intraocular pressure control and topical dehydrating agents, there is no medical therapy for ABK and the only surgical procedure that can restore vision is a penetrating keratoplasty, which is described elsewhere in this text.

INDICATIONS

If ICCE is currently infrequently performed, what might be the indications? The only absolution reason for an ICCE nowadays would be in an eye where the capsular support is compromised or questionable. Examples would include a crystalline lens dislocated into the anterior chamber or obvious phacodonesis. The risk of starting an ECCE procedure and then finding a dislocated lens is undesirable, because by that time the surgeon has committed to a strategy by performing an anterior capsulotomy and therefore in the best of circumstances would have to extract the cataract piecemeal. Whereas if the strategy were to perform ICCE, as the preferred procedure, then there is a good chance of extracting the cataract in entirety without the admixture of vitreous and lenticular components. Where the cataract is frankly subluxed or there is vitreous in the anterior chamber, a pars plana lensectomy is preferable, though there are situations that might be amenable to ICCE followed by an anterior vitrectomy. In these contingencies the surgeon should be mindful that cryoextraction does not work well when there is vitreous adherent to the cryoprobe and anterior lens capsule. A relative indication for ICCE would be in an eye with lens-induced uveitis or the fellow eye when sensitivity to lenticular components is possible.

REFERENCES

1. Kirsch RE, Steinman W. Digital pressure. An important safeguard in cataract surgery. *Arch Ophthalmol* 1955;54:697–703.
2. Kornblueth W, Gombos G. The use of intravenous hypertonic urea in cataract extraction. *Am J Ophthalmol* 1962;54:753–756.
3. Honan PR. New single-use Honan balloon. *Am Intraocular Implant Soc J* 1985;11:496–497.
4. Morgan JE, Chanda A. Intraocular pressure after peribulbar anaesthesia: is the Honan balloon necessary? *Br J Ophthalmol* 1995;79:46–49.
5. Feldman ST, Deutsch TA. Hyphema following Honan balloon use in Fuchs' heterochromic iridocyclitis. *Arch Ophthalmol* 1986;104:967. Letter.
6. Jaanus SD. Prevention of postoperative infection: limits and possibilities. *Br J Ophthalmol* 1996;80:681–682. Editorial.
7. Wong D, Briggs M, Holden R, Needham A. Occult perforation of the globe by superior rectus suture. *J Cataract Refract Surg* 1995;21:238. Letter.
8. Galin MA, Barasch KR, Harris LS. Enzymatic zonulolysis and intraocular pressure. *Am J Ophthalmol* 1996;61:690–696.
9. Anderson DR. Experimental alpha chymotrypsin glaucoma studied by scanning electron microscopy. *Am J Ophthalmol* 1971;71:470–476.
10. Shafer DM. Retinal detachment after cataract surgery. *Int Ophthalmol Clin* 1964;4:1091–1100.
11. Norregaard JC, Thoning H, Andersen TF, et al. Risk of retinal detachment following cataract extraction: results from the International Cataract Surgery Outcomes Study. *Br J Ophthalmol* 1996;80:689–693.
12. Jaffe NS, Jaffe MS, Jaffe GR. *Cataract surgery and its complications.* St Louis: CV Mosby, 1990:657.

13. Wetzig PC, Thatcher DB, Christiansen JM. The intracapsular versus the extracapsular technique in relationship to retinal problems. *Trans Am Ophthalmol Soc* 1979;77:339–345.

14. Jaffe NS, Clayman HM, Jaffe MS. Cystoid macular edema after intracapsular and extracapsular cataract extraction with and without an intraocular lens. *Ophthalmology* 1982;89:25–29.

15. Harbour JW, Smiddy WE, Rubsamen PE, et al. Pars plana vitrectomy for chronic pseudophakic cystoid macular edema. *Am J Ophthalmol* 1995;120:302–307.

16. Dohlman CH, Boruchoff SA. Corneal edema after cataract surgery. *Int Ophthalmol Clin* 1964;4:979–998.

Extracapsular Cataract Extraction

Eduardo C. Alfonso

GENERAL CONSIDERATIONS

Extracapsular cataract extraction (ECCE) was modified in the 1970s when the use of posterior chamber intraocular lenses was shown to be a safe and effective way of correcting aphakia. This method of cataract removal had been previously used in adults and more commonly in children (1). In 1980, it was shown that patients who had undergone ECCE had a lower incidence of retinal detachments compared with those that had undergone intracapsular surgery (2). It was also shown that the incidence of angiographic cystoid macular edema was less in ECCE (3). These and other studies transformed cataract surgery in the mid-1970s, with a subsequent transition to a smaller wound size, enlarged if necessary to extract the dismantled cataract and introduce the intraocular lens (IOL).

The standard ECCE refers to an operation to remove a senile cataract by removing first the nucleus of the lens then the cortex, leaving behind the posterior portion of the capsular bag for implantation of a posterior chamber IOL. With time, many modifications of this procedure have taken place. The Kelman phacoemulsification technique was developed to remove the nucleus by emulsifying it with ultrasound energy (4). Several other techniques have been developed to remove the nucleus in smaller components, in order to achieve a smaller wound size. The nucleus can be stripped of the epinucleus and expressed through a wound of 5mm (5). It can be mechanically divided into pieces to be removed through an incision as small as possible (6,7). By learning the basic ECCE technique, the surgeon can then employ modifications that incorporate intraoperative safety, postoperative improved astigmatic results, and faster rehabilitation of small incision surgery. The removal of the cortex can then be achieved with either a manual aspiration cannula with irrigation or a mechanical aspiration unit (8).

As surgical ideas have evolved and benefits of surgical techniques scientifically documented, instrument development has provided surgeons with the ability to reach the desired outcomes with increasing ease and safety. ECCE instrumentation has evolved with these main ideas in mind. The array of instruments can be few, with the cost based on the use of automated versus manual techniques for cortical removal. I will discuss different available instruments as I outline the different alternatives for each part of the procedure, but because of the number of instruments designed over the years by numerous surgeons, this discussion will not be exhaustive.

ANESTHESIA

Anesthetic modalities for ECCE have evolved from general to local. The choice is based on the medical needs and the surgeon's and patient's preferences. My current technique is to use a peribulbar injection containing 4% lidocaine, using a volume of 5mL or a retrobulbar injection with a volume of 3mL. This method is preferred, especially if the incision size is greater than 6mm and one is concerned with the intraoperative distortion caused by the action of the extraocular muscles. If the incision size is less than 6mm, one could consider using topical anesthesia. If the patient complains of discomfort during the surgical procedure, up to 1mL of nonpreserved 1% lidocaine can be injected into the anterior chamber. A mercury bag to lower the intraocular pressure and decrease the orbital volume is placed over the eye for 15 minutes prior to starting the procedure.

Alternate routes of administering anesthesia can be used, including subtenon's infusions, if discomfort is felt during the procedure.

INCISION

The location and size of the incision can be modified based on the size of the nucleus to be removed and the size of the wound needed for IOL implantation. For standard ECCE in a patient with a senile cataract, the wound can be made following the surgical limbus (Fig. 24-1A). If a self-sealing wound is desired, the scleral incision can be moved to a more posterior location, creating a trifaceted incision by a perpendicular half-scleral thickness, followed by a parallel tunnel scleral incision toward the cornea. Once the incision reaches the cornea, a posterior incision is made into the anterior chamber (Fig. 24-1B). These self-sealing incisions can be left without sutures when they are up to 6mm in length and 3mm in width. The location preferred is superotemporal. A clear cornea incision can be made, usually requiring sutures when the length is greater than 4mm. When the location is temporal, the astigmatic results can be neutral (Fig. 24-1C) (9).

MANAGEMENT OF THE IRIS

Achieving the best possible dilation of the pupil facilitates the surgery. Preoperative pharmacologic dilation is achieved by using drops of 10% neosynephrine, 1% cyclopentolate, and 1% profanol. These can be changed to parent compounds based on medical requirements. If dilation cannot be achieved to 6mm, the pupil can be opened mechanically.

My preferred method is to fill the anterior chamber with a viscoelastic, then using two Kueglen hooks, to stretch the pupil in opposite directions at the same time. Alternatively, one can place iris hooks (De Juan, Griesehaber) or a Graether pupil ring (10). A last resort is to surgically open the pupil by performing a sector iridectomy, which probably would require suturing the iris back at the end of the procedure. I prefer using 10-0 Prolene. It is important to warn the patient that after the procedure he or she may have an irregular pupil.

MANAGEMENT OF THE ANTERIOR CAPSULE

The anterior capsule must be opened in order to allow for the removal of the nucleus and the cortex. The circular opening must be at least 6mm in order to allow for removal of the nucleus. I prefer performing the opening of the anterior capsule after I have filled the anterior chamber with viscoelastic. If possible, I do a continuou tear capsulorrhexis. If the size is smaller than what is necessary to remove the nucleus (see next section), two radial tears toward the equator at 11 and 2 o'clock are made. Because the opening of the anterior capsule is larger, I use forceps to guide the tear. If the tear cannot be visualized, conversion to a can-opener capsulotomy should be considered. Peripheral extensions of the tear can be controlled by reforming the anterior chamber with viscoelastic. Coaxial illumination and retroillumination are helpful for visualizing the tear in the cases of very dense cataracts.

A can-opener capsulotomy can also be used, but a greater risk of extension of a tear radially exists. This procedure can be done by making small punctures circumferentially with the bent tip of a 25-gauge needle. The opening of the ante-

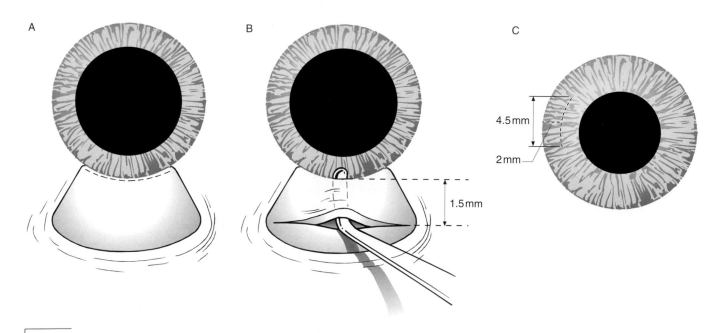

FIGURE 24-1. (A) Incision following surgical limbus. (B) Tunneled incision. (C) Corneal incision.

rior capsule can also be achieved with other cutting and thermal instruments (11).

MANAGEMENT OF THE NUCLEUS

Many surgeons have described various ways of removing the nucleus (12). The general principle is to separate the nucleus from the epinucleus and the cortex. This can be achieved by using hydrodissection and hydrodelineation. I prefer using a syringe with balanced salt solution and a 27-gauge needle. The solution is slowly injected under the anterior capsule until a fluid wave is seen to pass posteriorly. The next step is to inject a fluid wave between the nucleus and epinucleus until separation is achieved, sometimes marked by the presence of the "golden ring sign." The alternative is to engage the nucleus with a needle and rock it from 12 to 6 o'clock and from 9 to 3 o'clock to release its attachments. Once the nucleus is released, it can be removed by different methods. The goals at this stage are to be able to move the nucleus out of the capsule, past the superior edge of the iris, and out of the wound. I will describe the different methods that can be used to remove the nucleus.

The simplest is to prolapse the nucleus out. A wound of adequate size and pupil dilation is necessary. Slight pressure is applied to the wound at 12 o'clock by grasping the sclera 2 mm posterior to the wound with 0.12 forceps and directing the pressure toward the center of the globe. Once the nucleus is seen to prolapse out of the anterior capsule and past the superior iris, as pressure is continued superiorly, counterpressure is applied at the 6 o'clock limbus to help move the nucleus toward the wound. Once the nucleus starts coming out of the wound, it can be engaged with a sharp instrument and helped out of the eye (Fig. 24-2).

Another method is to prolapse the nucleus into the anterior chamber by using an irrigating cannula, passing it under the anterior capsule at 2 o'clock and dissecting the space between the nucleus and cortex posteriorly with the aid of irrigation (13). In this way, the nucleus is brought into the anterior chamber and irrigated toward the wound. The cannulas that can be used are several: I prefer the McIntyre 26-gauge model. Once in the anterior chamber, the nucleus can be brought out of the eye using a Knolle Pearce irrigating lens loop.

A more difficult way is to use the Knolle Pearce irrigating lens loop and to pass it under the nucleus while it is still in the capsular bag (14). First, one must be able to retract the anterior capsule toward 12 o'clock with a Kueglen hook, using the right hand. With the right hand, the irrigating lens loop is introduced into the space between the superior nucleus and posterior cortex and advanced in until it is at least two-thirds of the way under the nucleus. At this point, the irrigation is started and gentle movements of the lens loop toward the cornea apex and the wound helps the nucleus exit.

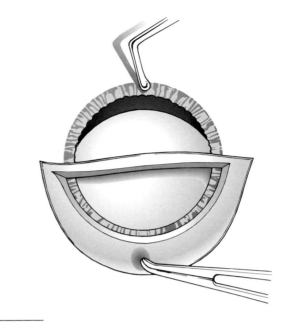

FIGURE 24-2. *Nucleus prolapse.*

Other methods of nucleus removal include dismantling the lens into smaller components, either by removing the epinucleus and breaking up pieces of the nucleus as it is pushed out of the wound (the Blumenthal mininucleus technique) or by using techniques that fracture the nucleus, allowing individual pieces to be removed with forceps (Kansas technique of phacosection) or with an irrigating spoon (McIntyre technique). I have developed a surgical technique that borrows from these methods and allows me to complete the procedure on senile cataracts through an incision of 4 mm through which I can implant a foldable IOL. This technique is described in the section Special Technique.

MANAGEMENT OF THE CORTEX

Before the cortex is removed, the epinucleus, if still present, can be removed either by irrigation into the anterior chamber, forcing the epinucleus out through the wound, or by aspirating it with a cannula with an opening of at least 4 mm. The cortex can then be removed with the use of a manual aspirating cannula or an automated vacuum system. The opening on these aspiration systems is usually 3 mm.

Several manual types are available and have the names of their designers. The Simcoe cannula has a dual-barrel system: one is an irrigating port attached to gravity flow balanced salt solution, and the other is a port attached to a 10- or 20-cc syringe for aspiration (15). Similar systems are available designed by McIntyre, Gills, and others.

The automated systems have vacuum established by a Venturi or peristaltic pump. A pedal control is used to open the irrigation into the anterior chamber and to control the

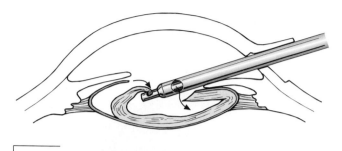

FIGURE 24-3.   *Aspiration of cortex.*

aspiration. The handpiece has an outer irrigating sleeve and an inner aspirating system with a 3-mm opening.

The technique I use is to remove the cortex by engaging it with the aspirating tip at the equator, pulling it toward the center, and then aspirating the piece. I usually aspirate the 12-o'clock cortex first and continue around until all pieces are removed. If there are pieces that cannot be aspirated with ease, I wait until the cortex hydrates and then come back to aspirate it (Fig. 24-3).

Once the entire cortex has been removed, the posterior, equatorial, and anterior capsules can be polished with the same tip or with one developed for posterior capsule polishing (Kratz).

IOL INSERTION

The IOL insertion technique will vary depending on the type of IOL material used. If a PMMA lens is used, the lens is grasped with insertion forceps, and the leading haptic is introduced into the capsular bag by placing it under the anterior leaf of the 6-o'clock area. Once the IOL is in the anterior chamber, the superior or trailing haptic can be introduced with forceps.

The foldable lenses are folded and introduced with special forceps.

I prefer to form the anterior chamber with viscoelastic prior to IOL insertion; others have described the use of continous irrigation or an air bubble.

CLOSURE

If the wound has been constructed with a self-sealing technique, it can be left without sutures if found to be watertight at the end of the procedure. Wounds larger than 5 mm and close to the limbus may slip over time, causing flattening of the area and steepening of the axis of the astigmatism 90 degrees away. If water tightness is not achieved, one can try intrastromal hydration of the edges of the wound using an irrigating cannula. For larger wounds or if concern exists regarding wound slippage, 10-0 nylon sutures can be used for closure. Recently, I have used a 10-0 Vicryl suture where there is concern over the integrity of a small self-sealing wound.

SPECIAL TECHNIQUE (PHACOFRACTURE OR PHACOSECTION)

The following technique allows me to perform an ECCE, with the advantages of low cost, small incision, and excellent postoperative results.

The approach is usually from the superotemporal limbus. The conjunctiva is opened with scissors, creating a fornix-based flap. A groove is made 1.5 to 2.0 mm posterior to the surgical limbus; its length is based on the diameter of the IOL to be used (minimum ~4 mm). A tunnel is made, reaching the anterior edge of the vascular arcade of clear cornea. Temporal and nasal clear corneal valve incisions are made for irrigation and aspiration. Viscoelastic is used to reform the anterior chamber. The anterior chamber is entered through the tunneled incision with a keratome blade and extended to the full width of the desired IOL width. Viscoelastic is again injected into the anterior chamber every time one does not find an adequate separation between corneal endothelium and lens. The capsulorrhexis is made using a cystotome needle and a forceps. Its size should be large enough to be able to prolapse the nucleus into the anterior chamber (remember that the size will be magnified by the viscoelastic), usually 6 mm or greater. Hydrodissection is performed by using a 27-g cannula on a syringe containing balanced salt solution with epinephrine. The anterior cortex and epinucleus are aspirated using irrigation (Lewicky 20-g anterior chamber maintainer) and aspiration handpiece with a 0.5-mm aspirating port.

Once the nucleus is freely loose, its upper pole is gently prolapsed anterior to the superior anterior capsule. I use a Kueglen hook in my right hand to retract the capsule and engage the nucleus, thus prolapsing its superior pole into the anterior chamber. With my left hand, I gently inject viscoelastic under the nucleus to help its superior pole move into the anterior chamber and create a viscoelastic space between the nucleus and posterior epinucleus and cortex (Fig. 24-4). A cushion of viscoelastic is placed anterior and posterior to the nucleus. The flat spatula platform is introduced behind the nucleus (Fig. 24-5). The cutting blade is then brought over the nucleus. Pushing the flat spatula up and the cutting blade down with small seesaw movements, the nucleus is trisected. Both instruments are withdrawn from the anterior chamber gently, using the spatula to slightly depress the scleral lip of the wound, and the middle third of the nucleus usually comes out at this point (Fig. 24-6). If the nucleus is not completely trisected, viscoelastic is placed in the anterior chamber and a nucleus splitter is used to complete the division of the nucleus. Kansas forceps with serrated teeth are used to remove the pieces of nucleus (Fig. 24-7). Alternatively, the McIntyre nucleus spoon (either 3 or 4.5 mm width) is connected to a bottle of 500 mL of balanced salt solution with 0.3 mL of 1:100 intracardiac epinephrine. With irrigation off, the spoon is introduced behind the nucleus. Once it is approximately

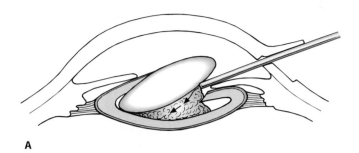

A

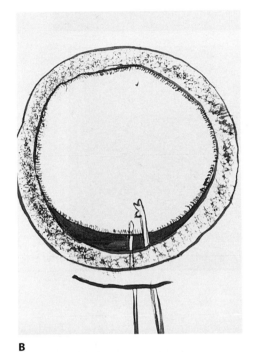

B

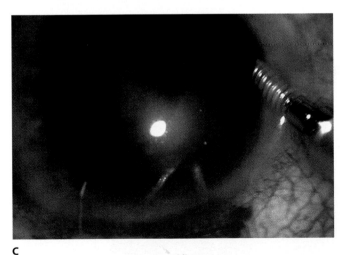

C

FIGURE 24-4. *(A) Space between posterior nucleus and epinucleus/cortex/capsule created with viscoelastic. (B) Nucleus being pushed with hook toward 6 o'clock and up in order to create separation to inject viscoelastic. (C) Intraoperative photograph showing same maneuver.*

one-third of the way under the nucleus, irrigation is started. This keeps the spoon from pushing the nucleus toward 6 o'clock and moves it into the well of the spoon. A second instrument such as a nucleus rotator is useful when introduced through the second site and used to help orient the nucleus to the well of the spoon. Again, slight depression of the posterior lip of the wound with the spoon as it is withdrawn will allow easy exit of the nucleus and spoon. After removal of each nuclear fragment, additional intracameral viscoelastic should be used to recoat the corneal endothelium as well as to help orient each piece of nucleus. If necessary, the wound is closed with 10-0 nylon sutures with temporary loop knots (most of the time it is self-sealing and sutures are not necessary). Removal of the cortex and epinucleus is done using a manual system of aspiration/irrigation. The chamber and capsular bag are reformed with viscoelastic. The loop knots, if present, are released. The IOL is introduced into the capsular bag. The viscoelastic is aspirated. The conjunctiva is then draped over the wound.

COMPLICATIONS

The complications associated with ECCE are similar to those associated with other types of cataract extraction, including conditions that could also happen with the other most common cataract surgical procedure used today, phacoemulsification. These complications include faulty wound construction, which can lead to leaks and induced astigmatism, iris damage, intraoperative hyphema, corneal endothelial damage, capsular dehiscence or rupture, loss of lens material into the vitreous, vitreous prolapse, and IOL dislocations. When complication rates between ECCE and phacoemulsification are compared, it is difficult to isolate all the confounding variables to reach a statistically significant rate comparable between the two procedures. Anecdotal reports confirm the surgeon's preference for a particular surgical procedure. The advantages of phacoemulsification in reducing complications are thus difficult to prove scientifically. A reduction in wound size does lead to reduced surgical astigmatism and faster postoperative rehabilitation of the patient. The postoperative endophthalmitis rate is similar to other cataract extraction procedures. If a large wound is used, the chances of traumatic extrusion of intraocular contents are greater than if a small incision procedure is done.

CONCLUSIONS

ECCE is a procedure that every ophthalmologist should know how to perform. Even when phacoemulsification is the preferred method of removing a cataract, if difficulties arise either with the instrumentation or with an intraoperative complication, conversion to an extracapsular procedure allows the surgeon to provide the patient with an excellent surgical result. The current generation of ophthalmologists is very well trained in extracapsular cataract surgery, and it

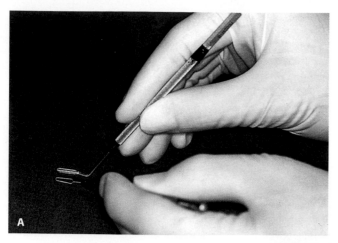

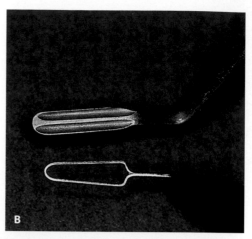

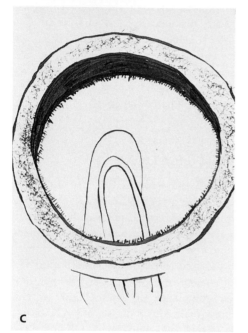

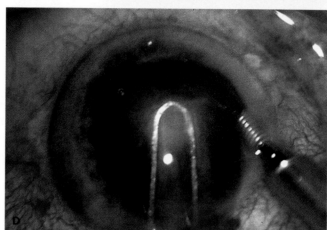

FIGURE 24-5. *Trisection of nucleus with trisector and spatula. (A) Position of spatula and trisector. (B) Close-up of spatula and trisector. (C) Schematic drawing of trisection. (D) Intraoperative photograph of trisection.*

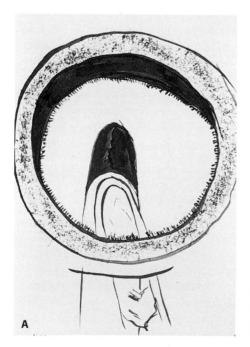

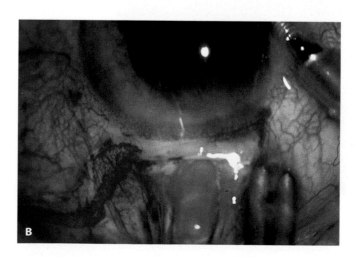

FIGURE 24-6. *Removal of central nuclear piece with the Kansas toothed forceps. (A) Schematic drawing of central third of the nucleus being removed with the trisector. (B) Intraoperative photo of central third of trisected nuclear fragment.*

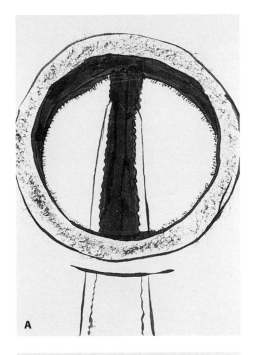

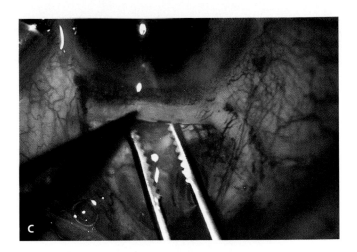

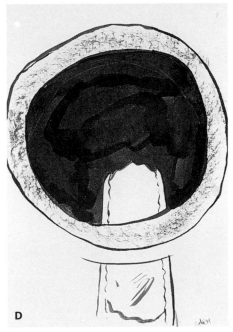

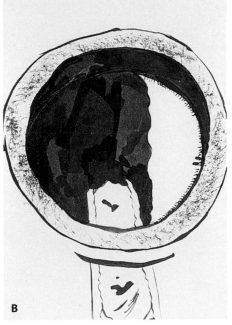

FIGURE 24-7. *Removal of other nuclear pieces with the toothed forceps. (A) Toothed forceps splitting remaining two-thirds of nucleus. (B) Toothed forceps removing piece of nucleus. (C) Intraoperative photograph of piece of nucleus removed with toothed forceps. (D) Toothed forceps removing last piece of nucleus.*

is important for current residents in training to learn this technique of cataract removal.

REFERENCES

1. Emery JM, McIntyre DJ. Extracapsular cataract extraction. In: Emery JM, ed. *Extracapsular cataract extraction.* St. Louis: C.V. Mosby, 1983.

2. Jaffe NS, Clayman HM, Jaffe MS. Retinal detachments in myopic eyes after intracapsular and extracapsular cataract extraction. *Am J Ophthalmol* 1984;97:48–52.

3. Jaffe NS, Clayman HM, Jaffe MS. Cystoid macular edema after intracapsular and extracapsular cataract extraction. *Ophthalmology* 1982;89:25–29.

4. Kelman CD. The history and development of phacoemulsification. *Int Ophthalmol Clin* 1994;34:1–12.

5. Blumentha M. Manual ECCE, the present state of the art. *KLIN Monatsbl Augenheilkd* 1994;205:266–270.

6. Kansas PG, Sax R. Small incision cataract extraction and implantation surgery using a manual phacofragmentation technique. *J Cataract Refract Surg* 1988;14:328–330.

7. McIntyre DJ. Phacosection cataract surgery. In: Steinert RF, ed. *Cataract surgery: technique, complications, and management*. Philadelphia: W.B. Saunders, 1995:119–122.

8. Jaffe NS, Jaffe MS, Jaffe GF, eds. *Cataract surgery and its complications*. St. Louis: C.V. Mosby, 1990:69–86.

9. Steinert RF, Brint SF, White SM, et al. Astigmatism after small incision cataract surgery. A prospective, randomized, multicenter comparison of 4- and 6.5-mm incisions. *Ophthalmology* 1991;98:417.

10. Graether JM. Graether pupil expander for managing the small pupil during surgery. *J Cataract Refract Surg* 1996;22:530–535.

11. Clayman HM, Parel JM. The capsule copeur for automated anterior capsulectomy. *Am Intraocular Implant Soc J* 1984;10:480–482.

12. Emery J. Extracapsular cataract surgery: indications and technique. In: Steinert R, eds. *Cataract surgery: technique, complications, and management*. Philadelphia: W.B. Saunders, 1995:107–108.

13. Knolle G. The Knolle Pierce irrigating loop. *Am Intraocular Implant Soc J* 1982;5:353–355.

14. Simcoe CW. Double barreled irrigation-aspiration unit. *Am Intraocular Implant Soc J* 1981;7:380.

Principles and Techniques of Cataract Surgery Phacoemulsification: Methodology and Complications

David T. Jones   Carol L. Karp   Thomas J. Heigle

Cataract extraction that employs high-frequency ultrasound energy to fragment and emulsify the lens nucleus was developed and first introduced by Charles Kelman in the late 1960s (1). This novel approach revolutionized cataract surgery by permitting cataract extraction through smaller incisions, thereby minimizing surgical trauma to the eye. Small-incision cataract surgery provides optimal wound integrity, allowing for rapid visual recovery while minimizing iatrogenically induced astigmatism (2). Transition to phacoemulsification can be an extremely stressful process for the ophthalmic surgeon. Whether an experienced extracapsular surgeon with years of success or a resident first learning cataract surgery, phacoemulsification presents the challenge of a host of new techniques and potential problems. The beginning phacoemulsification surgeon should endeavor to master two principal areas: 1) acquiring comfort with the new instrumentation and machinery and 2) understanding the surgical techniques unique to the procedure. A thorough understanding of the mechanics of the phacoemulsification machine is critical to the performance of a safe procedure. The successful surgeon soon develops an acute awareness of how the machinery functions and responds, akin to a race car driver knowing the idiosyncrasies of his or her car. From the technical perspective, phacoemulsification comprises a series of steps, each of which is critically dependent on the former, like building a house from the foundation up.

TERMINOLOGY AND INSTRUMENTATION

The goal of phacoemulsification is to emulsify and aspirate the lens while maintaining the structural integrity of the eye. To this end, the phacoemulsification machine provides high-frequency ultrasound energy, vacuum, and fluid inflow

and outflow. Before proceeding, it is important to first clearly define several terms relevant to phacoemulsification (3). The *aspiration flow rate* (measured in mL/min) refers to the rate of fluid flow through the phacoemulsification or irrigation/aspiration (I/A) probe tip and is an indicator of how quickly material will be drawn toward the tip. This represents the attractability of the instrument. Aspiration flow rates on most units vary from 0 to 40 mL/min. More than any other parameter, the aspiration flow rate determines how "fast" objects are going to move within the eye. *Fluid inflow*, delivered from an external bottle, is gravity driven and in a closed system (i.e., tightly conforming surgical wounds) is determined by the fluid outflow rate. *Vacuum* is measured in millimeters of mercury (mmHg). It is the vacuum that gives the surgeon the purchasing or holding power. On most machines, the vacuum ranges from 0 to 150 mmHg for the phacoemulsification component of the surgery although newer models provide greater vacuum levels up to 450 mmHg. The irrigation/aspiration component generally ranges from 0 to 580 mmHg. The *rise time*, or rate at which vacuum will build to a given preset limit, varies for different phacoemulsification systems. In general, the purchase of a piece of lens nucleus allows vacuum to build within the system. Once this piece is emulsified and aspirated, a postocclusion shallowing may occur within the anterior chamber, the degree of which depends upon the inflow rate and the *compliance* of the system. *Compliance* is a measure of the flexibility and compressibility of the system tubing and the fluid within the system. Once the occlusion is cleared, the tubing rebounds to its relaxed state, pulling additional fluid volume from the eye causing the anterior chamber to collapse. Flexible or easily compressible tubing increases the compliance of the system, which can result in large fluctuations in the anterior chamber volume. Similarly, while liquid within the tubing is noncompressible, a gas bubble within the system is highly compressible and increases the compliance of the system, also leading to large fluctuations in anterior chamber dynamics. These problems have been addressed by the equipment manufacturers and are minimized with the newer handpieces and system components currently on the market.

Three principal phacoemulsification systems are currently manufactured. These include peristaltic pump, Venturi pump, and diaphragmatic pump systems. Peristaltic pump units operate via a roller-bearing mechanism that pulls fluid through a flexible line. At low flow rates, this system provides direct and independent control of aspiration flow rates and vacuum levels. At high flow rates, aspiration and vacuum are coupled by the resistance of the tubing and inflow port, which inherently build partial vacuum within the system. Because of the peristaltic mechanism, the aspiration flow rate is not completely smooth. With each turn of the peristaltic pump wheel, the rate increases slightly followed by a slight decrease. Vacuum can be independently manipulated to a predetermined limit, but without tip occlusion in this system, the vacuum will not build. The advantage of this system is the slower vacuum response, which may be safer for the beginning surgeon. In addition, independent control of vacuum and aspiration flow rate allows the surgeon to modulate the speed at which intraocular events occur to a rate that he or she desires. The slow vacuum response time and absence of vacuum without port occlusion are disadvantages that result in slowing the rate of intraocular events and can increase the overall surgical time.

The Venturi pump system is a true vacuum-driven system, in which vacuum is delivered to the tip regardless of port occlusion. The open-ended vacuum system drives aspiration. At a given preset vacuum level, the aspiration rate is dependent on the inflow bottle height (gravity-driven) and the resistance of the phacoemulsification or irrigation/aspiration port and system tubing. Unlike the peristaltic pump system, there is no direct control of the aspiration flow rate. The advantages of this system include rapid vacuum rise times, affording predictable and precise aspiration and thus improving the machine responsiveness to the surgeon. Moreover, the rate of vacuum formation can be adjusted in a linear fashion by the surgeon over a predetermined range. The disadvantage of this system is that it requires a large external gas supply to drive the Venturi mechanism and the enhanced speed of intraocular events can be problematic for beginning surgeons.

The diaphragm pump is the least utilized system. In this system, a valved pump mechanism generates vacuum, which in turn drives aspiration. Like the Venturi system, vacuum drives aspiration, is controlled independently, and increases when the tip is occluded. Similarly, the aspiration rate depends upon the resistance of the phacoemulsification or irrigation/aspiration port and the inflow bottle height. Advantages of the diaphragm pump system include linear control of aspiration and rapid vacuum rise times and

responsiveness at low flow rates. The disadvantages include anterior chamber shallowing due to the constant vacuum and the bulkiness of the system which makes it difficult to store.

One important consideration in the initial transition to phacoemulsification is to optimize all the factors that are within the surgeon's control. An understanding of the instrumentation as described above is essential. Patient selection is another important parameter over which the surgeon has control. The orbital anatomy and general physical health of the patient should be carefully considered. Treatment of patients with deep-set orbits, prominent brows, or enophthalmos should be avoided during the initial learning phase. Patients with severe kyphosis or arthritis, or those who may be uncomfortable or difficult to position lying supine, should also be avoided. Ideally, the body habitus and orbital anatomy should provide easy access to the iris plane with the patient lying supine. Treatment of patients with pulmonary disease, obesity, or an anxious demeanor should also be avoided in the initial transition process. Desirable characteristics with regard to the eye include excellent pupillary dilatation, a low to moderately dense cataract with a clear red reflex, and lack of mitigating factors such as zonular weakness or dehiscence, pseudoexfoliation, or a previous history of trauma.

ANESTHESIA

The surgeon has essentially three anesthetic options to select from for the patient who is undergoing phacoemulsification cataract extraction: topical, local, or general anesthesia. Topical anesthesia consisting of topical tetracaine, lidocaine, proparacaine, or bupivacaine is effective for appropriately selected cooperative patients (4). Topical anesthesia is often used in combination with intravenous sedative agents such as fentanyl and midazolam. In addition, supplemental anesthesia can be achieved with intracameral nonpreserved lidocaine (1% non-preserved intrathecal lidocaine) to provide anesthesia to the iris and ciliary body after the anterior chamber has been entered (5,6). The effects of intraocular lidocaine on the posterior segment are not known and intracameral lidocaine should probably be avoided in cases with posterior capsular rupture or vitreous prolapse. Topical anesthesia has the advantage of avoiding potential complications from retrobulbar/peribulbar and general anesthesia. Moreover, it eliminates the risk of retrobulbar hemorrhage in patients with bleeding diatheses. In order to avoid the danger of sudden movements during the phacoemulsification procedure, topical anesthesia is not recommended for uncooperative patients and those who are unable to fixate on the microscope light.

Local anesthesia in the form of peribulbar or retrobulbar injection has been very popular. Typically, the injection involves a mixture of short-acting lidocaine (2–4%) and longer-acting bupivacaine (0.75%) often combined with hyaluronidase to enhance local diffusion. In high myopes or patients who have undergone scleral buckle procedure, peribulbar anesthesia may be preferred to retrobulbar injection to minimize the likelihood of inadvertent globe penetration. Peribulbar anesthesia usually requires a larger volume of anesthetic and has a slightly slower onset. Another approach is intraoperative sub-Tenon's injection with a blunt-tipped cannula to deliver anesthetic more safely to the muscle cone. Retrobulbar injection administers the anesthetic directly into the muscle cone and is highly effective in producing rapid anesthesia and akinesia. To facilitate diffusion and spread of the anesthetic within the orbit and to decompress the globe, digital compression or compression with an ocular weight such as the Honan balloon or a mercury bag is commonly employed. Many surgeons also employ a lid block to prevent orbicularis contraction during the surgery. Several modifications of this technique have been described, including those by Nadbath, Van Lint, O'Brien, Atkinson, and Spaeth (7). Finally, general anesthesia is certainly effective but carries greater risk and is generally reserved for pediatric patients or adults who may be unable to cooperate.

PATIENT PREPARATION IN THE OPERATING ROOM

By the time the patient reaches the operating room, he or she should be fully anesthetized (unless utilizing general anesthesia) and have maximal pupillary dilatation. The patient should be positioned appropriately for optimal patient and surgeon comfort. The wrist rest should be positioned at a comfortable level for the surgeon operating at either the superior or temporal position. Careful attention to sterile technique throughout the procedure is essential to minimize the risk of postoperative infection (8–11). The surgical field is prepared by cleansing with a sterilizing solution such as povidone-iodine with careful attention to the lashes and lid margins. It is important to remember that time of exposure to the sterilizing solution is more important overall than the amount of solution used. To this end, some authors advocate instillation of povidone-iodine 5% into the cul-de-sac as a part of the routine preoperative preparation (10,11). Draping should be performed with attention to sterile technique and eversion of the lashes out of the surgical field. The placement of 4-0 silk bridle sutures through the superior or inferior rectus muscle insertion sites, or both, is elective and depends on the surgeon's accessibility to the surgical site. A bridle suture is generally not needed when a temporal clear-cornea approach is employed.

INCISION AND WOUND CONSTRUCTION

There are essentially three incision options for the phacoemulsification surgeon. These include limbal, scleral pocket, and clear-corneal incisions. The limbal incision is utilized primarily by the surgeon in transition to pha-

coemulsification from extracapsular techniques. Surgeons who are performing planned extracapsular surgery but are incorporating a few early steps of the phacoemulsification procedure can use the limbal incision to place the phacoemulsification probe into the anterior chamber to acquire familiarity and tactile dexterity with the phacoemulsification instruments.

The scleral pocket incision was developed to provide a self-sealing and astigmatically neutral incision (12,13). The incision size and configuration are determined by the surgeon's preference and the chosen style of intraocular lens. The options for incision configuration include linear (tangential to the limbus), smile (concentric to limbus), or frown (opposite of limbal curvature) (Fig. 25-1). The frown configuration minimizes against-the-rule shift and is reportedly the most astigmatically neutral incision (14,15). A potential disadvantage of the frown incision is the difficulty in enlarging it if conversion to extracapsular cataract surgery is necessary. In order to fashion the scleral pocket, an initial vertical groove of desired length and configuration 50% to 75% in depth is made with a microsurgical steel or diamond blade held perpendicular to the surface of the sclera (Fig. 25-2).

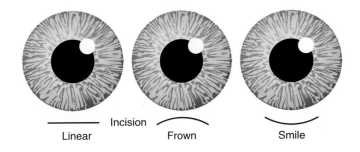

|——— Incision |
Linear   Frown   Smile

FIGURE 25-1. *Optional configurations for scleral tunnel incision.*

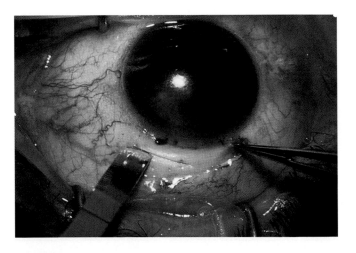

FIGURE 25-2. *Formation of partial-thickness scleral incision of desired length and configuration.*

A rounded crescent blade is then used to dissect a lamellar flap anteriorly through the sclera and 1 to 2 mm into clear cornea (Fig. 25-3). It is important to recall that the curvature of the cornea is steeper than that of the sclera and the tip of the crescent blade must be angled upward away from the iris in order to avoid premature entry into the anterior chamber. Before the eye is entered, while the eye is still firm, a paracentesis incision is fashioned in peripheral clear cornea approximately two to four clock hours away from the scleral tunnel incision (Fig. 25-4). The paracentesis provides the port for the second instrument and its position relative to the scleral tunnel should be based on the comfort of the surgeon. After the paracentesis is created, viscoelastic can be injected into the anterior chamber, depending on the surgeon's preference. The scleral tunnel incision is advanced into the anterior chamber with a diamond or steel keratome

blade by first gently placing the tip within the pocket up to the vascular arcade. The tip of the keratome is then aimed toward the center of the lens, dimpling the cornea, and after entering the chamber is advanced parallel to the iris, thus creating a triplanar self-sealing incision (Figs. 25-5 and 25-6).

The newest option in small-incision phacoemulsification surgery is the clear-cornea incision. This is generally performed temporally where the corneal diameter is greatest and accessibility to the eye is optimal. It can also be performed according to the patient's natural astigmatism, generally reducing the spectacle correction by 0.50 diopters in that meridian (16,17). The incision is created in a uniplanar or triplanar fashion similar to the scleral tunnel incision. The corneal incision is more easily accomplished after the anterior chamber has been filled and stabilized with viscoelastic through the paracentesis site. To create a triplanar incision, an initial groove is incised perpendicular to the corneal surface at or slightly central to the limbal vessels using either a steel or diamond crescent blade (Fig. 25-7). This wound is then advanced approximately 1.75 to 2.0 mm toward the visual axis, dissecting the cornea in a lamellar fashion. To

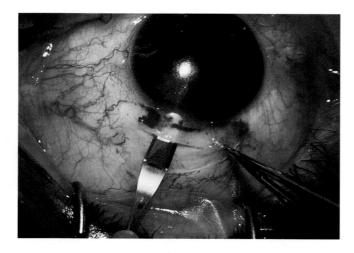

FIGURE 25-3. *A crescent blade is used to dissect a lamellar flap through the sclera and peripheral cornea to the extent of the limbal arcades.*

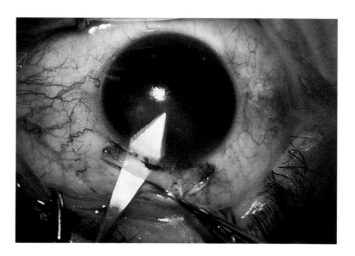

FIGURE 25-5. *Advancement of the scleral tunnel into the anterior chamber with a sharp keratome blade creating a triplanar self-sealing wound.*

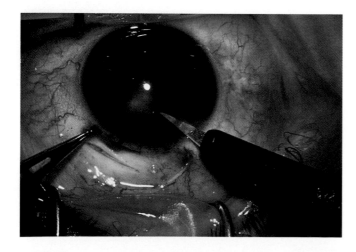

FIGURE 25-4. *A paracentesis tract is fashioned in peripheral clear cornea.*

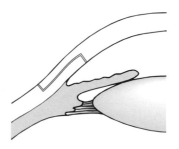

FIGURE 25-6. *Cross section demonstrating the configuration of the self-sealing triplanar wound.*

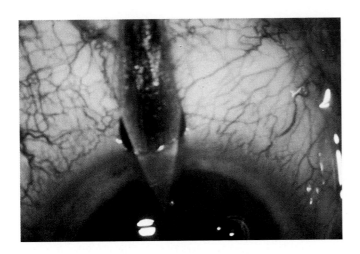

FIGURE 25-7. *A three-plane incision is fashioned in temporal clear cornea with a steel keratome blade. The globe is stabilized with a toothed scleral fixation ring.*

complete the incision, a diamond or steel keratome blade is used to enter the anterior chamber. Stabilization of the globe with a scleral fixation ring greatly facilitates construction of this wound. Generally, the clear-corneal incision is limited to 4 or 5 mm in length in order to be self-sealing.

The clear-cornea approach has several advantages. It facilitates accessibility in patients with deep brows or sunken globes. It avoids any manipulation of the sclera or conjunctiva for patients with bleeding diatheses, scleral thinning, or ocular surface disease (i.e., ocular cicatricial pemphigoid or Stevens-Johnson syndrome). It is also ideal for patients with glaucoma who either have existing blebs or need the conjunctiva to be preserved for future glaucoma surgery. One disadvantage is less flexibility in terms of incision size in order to maintain self-sealing capacity. In addition, if a foldable lens cannot be used, sutures utilized to close a larger corneal incision are closer to the visual axis and may induce significant astigmatism compared with a similar sized scleral wound. In the scenario of a complicated surgery necessitating a large incision, the small corneal incision may be closed and the surgeon can make a scleral incision elsewhere. Finally, compared to scleral incisions, there is potentially a higher risk of wound dehiscence and, perhaps, endophthalmitis.

VISCOELASTICS

The introduction of viscoelastic agents in the late 1970s dramatically improved the quality of anterior segment surgery (18). Viscoelastic materials are nontoxic, elastic, high-viscosity agents that can be utilized to immobilize and protect internal structures during intraocular surgery. Biochemically, the viscoelastic agents in use today consist of

sodium hyaluronate, chondroitin sulfate, hydroxypropyl-methylcellulose, and polyacrylamide either in pure form or in combination. The most commonly used viscoelastic agents include Healon and Healon GV (1% and 1.4% sodium hyaluronate, respectively; Pharmacia & Upjohn, Kalamazoo, MI), Amvisc and Amvisc Plus (1% and 1.6% sodium hyaluronate, respectively; Chiron Vision Corp., Claremont, CA), Viscoat (a combination of 3% sodium hyaluronate and 4% sodium chondroitin sulfate; Alcon Laboratories, Fort Worth, TX), and Ocucoat (2% hydroxypropyl methylcellulose; Storz Ophthalmics, St. Louis, MO). Orcolon (Optical Radiation Corp., Azusa, CA), a 0.5% polyacrylamide polymer, was removed from the market due to a propensity to cause secondary glaucoma (19).

The ideal viscoelastic agent provides excellent anterior chamber stability and endothelial protection while permitting free manipulation of instruments within the anterior segment. In addition, the material should be easily removable from the eye at the close of the procedure to avoid postoperative intraocular pressure elevation. Healon and Amvisc are excellent viscoelastics for routine cataract surgery. The advantage of the higher-viscosity agents, Healon GV and Amvisc Plus, is their capacity to maintain a deep anterior chamber despite positive vitreous pressure. This may be beneficial during pediatric cataract extraction, in the setting of small pupils, or when performing capsulorhexis in the presence of positive vitreous pressure. Viscoat combines the high viscosity and chamber-maintaining properties of sodium hyaluronate with the superior endothelial coating and protection properties of chondroitin sulfate. Viscoat, however, is less cohesive and therefore more difficult to remove entirely at the close of the procedure.

Viscoelastic agents are beneficial to the phacoemulsification surgeon in a variety of ways, including 1) maintenance of the anterior chamber facilitating capsulorrhexis formation and other delicate intraocular maneuvers, 2) protection of the fragile corneal endothelium from the phacoemulsification probe and high velocity nuclear fragments during phacoemulsification, 3) protection of the posterior capsule from sharp edges of broken nuclear fragments during phacoemulsification, 4) tamponade of intraocular structures such as the iris during capsulorrhexis formation and the vitreous body in the event of a posterior capsular rupture, and 5) reformation of the capsular bag before intraocular lens insertion. The main complication of viscoelastic use is the risk of postoperative intraocular pressure elevation. This potential complication is elaborated in the section on short-term postoperative complications.

TECHNIQUES FOR MANIPULATING THE IRIS

Poor pupillary dilatation due to fibrosis, hyalinization, a history of miotic use, or posterior synechiae is associated with an increased risk of intraoperative complications.

Enlargement of the pupillary aperture can be achieved by several different approaches (20). The simplest method is to "nudge" the pupil open by injecting viscoelastic throughout the circumference of the pupillary margin. Alternatively, the pupillary sphincter can be stretched open using two diametrically opposed instruments (i.e., a Sinskey and Kuglen hook) with opposing vector forces at multiple locations around the pupillary border (Fig. 25-8A). Some surgeons prefer to manage the pupil margin proximal to the wound with the sleeve of the phacoemulsification instrument and the distal border with a second instrument in order to gain visualization under the pupil margin. This requires great dexterity and can result in iris chafing and depigmentation. If these approaches are unsuccessful, Vannas or Rappazzo scissors can be utilized to create multiple (4–10) small sphincterotomy incisions in the pupillary margin followed by stretching as described above (Fig. 25-8B). A small pupil can also be enlarged by advancement of a surgical peripheral iridectomy to the pupillary margin. After placement of the IOL, the pupil can be reformed by closure of the pupillary margin with a polypropylene suture. Prosthetic devices have also been developed to assist in enlarging the pupil, including iris hooks made of either titanium or nylon and the iris protector ring. The iris protector ring not only enlarges the pupil but also protects the iris from the phacoemulsification port. Iris hooks passed through peripheral clear cornea at four or five equally spaced sites facilitate centrifugal retraction of the iris at the pupillary margin (Fig. 25-8C). Both disposable and non-disposable iris hooks are available. When using the iris hooks, it is important to place them as peripheral as possible to minimize tenting of the iris, which can interfere with intraocular instrument manipulation. Regardless of the method used, the improved visualization afforded by a larger pupil reduces surgeon anxiety,

facilitates the phacoemulsification process, and reduces the rate of complications. At the completion of the case, the pupil can usually be cosmetically or functionally reformed by the instillation of acetylcholine (Miochol; CIBAVision Ophthalmics, Atlanta, GA) or carbachol (Miostat; Alcon Laboratories) into the anterior chamber.

CAPSULORRHEXIS

Originally, phacoemulsification was performed after the anterior capsule was opened with a can-opener style capsulorrhexis borrowed from the traditional extracapsular technique. The ragged edge was prone to peripheral radial tears during lens manipulation that often extended to the posterior capsule resulting in vitreous loss. This complication was minimized by prolapsing the nucleus into the iris plane for subsequent phacoemulsification. However, the use of the high-energy phacoemulsification tip in the iris plane carried a greater risk of corneal endothelial damage and iris trauma. The evolution of iris plane phacoemulsification to "in-the-bag" phacoemulsification was made possible by the introduction of the continuous-tear curvilinear capsulorrhexis by Gimbel and Neuhann (21–23). A good red reflex and adequate pupillary dilatation greatly enhance the success of this technique. The capsulorrhexis is initiated by creating a small flap tear in the anterior capsule with a cystotome needle (Fig. 25-9A). This tear is advanced in a circular fashion with either the cystotome or capsular (Utrata) forceps (Figs. 25-9B and 25-10). The ideal diameter is about 4.5 to 5.0 mm. The structural and mechanical superiority of this continuous capsulotomy compared with the can-opener style opening allows manipulation of the lens within the bag with minimal risk of creating tears that may extend radially to the posterior capsule. Moreover, should the posterior

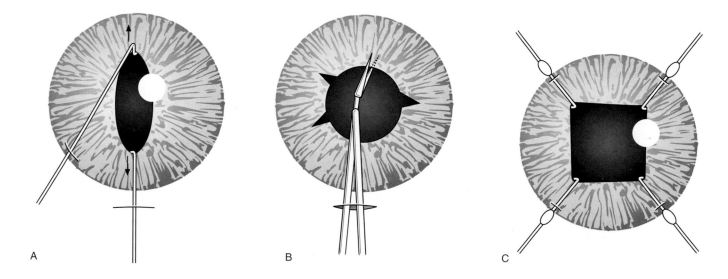

A   B   C

FIGURE 25-8.   *Techniques for iris manipulation. A. Stretching the iris sphincter with opposing iris hooks. B. Creating sphincterotomies with intraocular scissors. C. Pupillary enlargement with iris hooks.*

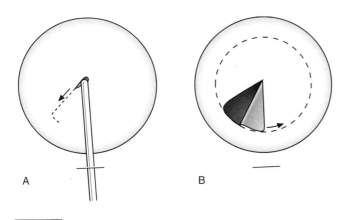

FIGURE 25-9. *Formation of continuous curvilinear capsulorrhexis. A. Initiation of capsular tear with a cystotome. B. Folding over edge of capsular flap.*

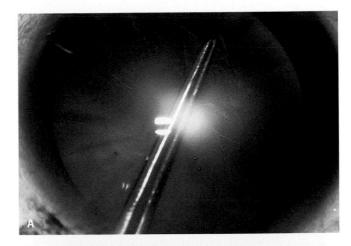

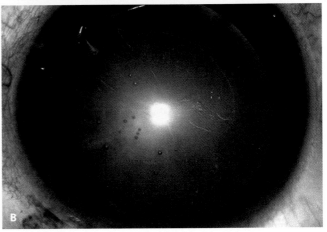

FIGURE 25-10. *Completion of continuous curvilinear capsulorrhexis. A. Advancement of capsular tear with forceps. B. Completed continuous curvilinear capsulorrhexis.*

capsule inadvertently rupture during the procedure, an anterior capsulorrhexis provides sufficient support for placement of a sulcus-fixated posterior chamber intraocular lens provided adequate zonular support is present.

Formation of a continuous-tear capsulorrhexis is a critical step in maintaining capsular integrity through the remainder of the procedure. It is most important that adequate viscoelastic material be used to keep the anterior lens capsule as flat as possible. This will minimize the risk of the tear radiating peripherally. Occasionally, despite one's best efforts, the tear radiates outward under the iris. If the tear is not too peripheral, a second instrument (i.e., a Sinskey or Kuglen hook) can be used to displace the iris so that the tear can be redirected under direct visualization. If this is not possible, attention can be directed to the initial incision, and a second incision with the cystotome can be made, initiating a capsular flap in the opposite direction. Forceps or a cystotome can then be used to bring the capsulotomy around from the opposite direction for completion. If this is not possible, the surgeon has the option of completing the capsulotomy with either a can-opener style capsulorrhexis or cutting the remaining capsule with intraocular scissors. One of these latter techniques will also be necessary if the capsulotomy inadvertently hits a zonular fiber. In this case, the tear will proceed directly along the zonular fiber and the surgeon should immediately release all tension on the flap. Care should be taken to avoid this situation by utilizing enough magnification to identify zonules and by avoiding excessively large capsulotomies. An evaluation of postmortem eyes revealed an average zonular free zone in the central anterior capsule of 6.83 mm diameter (24). In this study, the size of the zonular free zone was independent of patient age or lens diameter. If there is a discontinuity in the capsulorrhexis, such as occurs when the capsule is completed in a spiral pattern from inside to outside, the capsular tag can be folded over, as performed in the initial capsular tear, and simply torn centripetally to blend the capsular

irregularity into a smooth capsular edge. In young patients, the capsule is often extremely elastic and has a tendency to enlarge and extend peripherally. Attempts should be made to initiate these capsulorrhexes as small as possible since they invariably enlarge during the procedure. Further discussion of this topic is available in Chapter 28, "Cataract Surgery in Children."

Capsulorrhexis is often difficult to perform in the setting of a poor red reflex, a mature intumescent lens, or a small pupil. In the case of a poor red reflex, the surgeon should attempt to position the eye and increase the magnification of the microscope to optimize visualization. Indirect illumination from an external light pipe placed near the limbus is sometimes useful in enhancing the reflex. In these difficult scenarios, the capsulotomy should be initiated with a smaller than normal size. With an intumescent or hypermature lens, the increased intralenticular volume creates a convex anterior capsule. It is most important that adequate visoelastic material be used to tamponade the anterior lens capsule to a position that is as flat as possible. In addition, the cystotome-only technique is difficult to perform, as there is no countertraction from the milky lens. The forceps technique, therefore, is optimal in this setting. For hypermature cataracts, an alternative technique creating a triangular anterior capsulotomy with the cystotome and Vannas scissors has also been described (25).

HYDRODISSECTION AND HYDRODELINEATION

In order to perform successful "in-the-bag" phacoemulsification, the lens nucleus must be mobile to allow free rotation within the capsular bag. The purpose of hydrodissection is to break adhesions between the lens nucleus/epinucleus and the peripheral cortical attachments to the capsular bag. Hydrodissection is achieved by injecting balanced salt solution (BSS) peripherally under the anterior capsular rim (Fig. 25-11). In general, a 27- or 30-gauge blunt-tipped cannula is placed under the capsular rim and advanced to the peripheral fornix of the capsular bag in order to direct injected fluid posteriorly. If this is successful, the surgeon may observe a "fluid wave," indicating separation of cortical lens fiber lamellae. A slight diminution in the red reflex may also be observed after successful hydrodissection. Gentle injection of 1 to 2 ml of BSS is usually adequate. To ensure complete hydrodissection, fluid can be injected at multiple sites around the capsulotomy. Too forceful an injection of excessive fluid should be avoided as this can prolapse the lens nucleus into the anterior chamber. If the nuclear diameter exceeds that of the anterior capsulotomy, this may create tears that can extend posteriorly. Hydrodissection effectively separates the lens nucleus and epinucleus from the outer cortex, allowing the nucleus to be freely rotated while still preserving a protective barrier of cortex between the nucleus and posterior capsule.

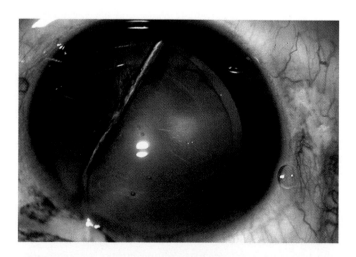

FIGURE 25-11. *Nuclear hydrodissection with a blunt-tipped cannula. Hydrodissection is repeated at different locations around the capsulorrhexis until the lens nucleus is freely mobile.*

Separation of the dense nuclear core that can only be removed by phacoemulsification from softer surrounding epinucleus can be achieved by hydrodelineation (26). After completing the hydrodissection, the cannula tip is placed directly into the body of the nucleus until resistance is encountered and a small amount of fluid is injected. Appearance of the "golden ring" sign indicates successful hydrodelineation. In soft lenses, this step may be superfluous and may simply cause hydrated nuclear lamella to "fluff" into the anterior chamber. Nevertheless, hydrodissection is an important maneuver that may be performed for all types of cataracts.

Some surgeons advocate a further step called "cortical cleavage dissection" (26). The blunt-tipped cannula with balanced salt solution is utilized to tent the anterior capsule superiorly, allowing injected fluid to dissect cortical material from the capsular bag. In practice, this maneuver is not always successful. However, once it is perfected, the surgeon will find that it greatly facilitates cortical cleanup.

MANAGEMENT OF THE NUCLEUS

A wide variety of approaches for removing the lens nucleus have been developed. Regardless of the approach, the ultimate goal is to remove the nucleus with a minimum of phacoemulsification power and intraocular manipulation in order to preserve the corneal endothelium and maintain the integrity of the capsular bag. Although all the techniques are effective, each approaches the task at hand in a different manner. In each approach, the lens nucleus is successively divided into smaller fragments that can be safely manipulated into the phacoemulsification port for emulsification and removal. We next discuss several popular methods for "in the bag" nuclear phacoemulsification.

Divide and Conquer

In the popular "divide and conquer" technique introduced by Gimbel (27,28), a single groove of approximately 85% to 90% depth is created with the phacoemulsification probe along the incisional axis. The nucleus is then rotated 90 degrees and a similar groove is fashioned orthogonal to the first groove (Fig. 25-12). The nucleus is split into four fragments along these grooves and each fragment is purchased and successively moved to the center of the eye, where it is emulsified safely away from the iris, posterior capsule, and corneal endothelium (Fig. 25-13). The cracking process can be achieved with the phacoemulsification probe and a second instrument, such as a cyclodialysis spatula, a Bechert rotator, or a Drysdale spatula. Cracking is performed by placing both instruments deep in the groove and lifting while spreading to avoid straining the posterior capsule. The crack should be easily visualized and must extend past the center of the nucleus so that each fragment will be freely

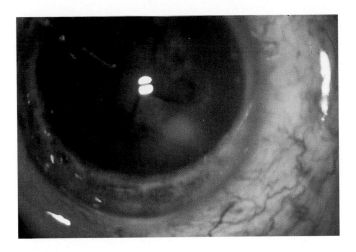

FIGURE 25-12. *Divide and conquer phacoemulsification techniques. The nucleus has been grooved along two orthogonal axes creating a cruciform pattern.*

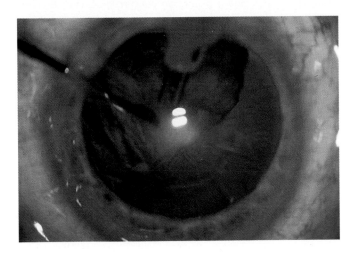

FIGURE 25-13. *Removal of final nuclear fragments with phacoemulsification probe.*

mobile for subsequent removal. If the groove is too narrow to accommodate the phacoemulsification probe and a second instrument, it can be widened, or two instruments alone (i.e., a cyclodialysis and Drysdale spatula) can be placed within the groove to complete the cracking. Nucleus cracking forceps (i.e., Dodick or Salz nuclear cracking forceps) are designed specifically for this purpose and are highly effective but require removal of the phacoemulsification probe and introduction of this instrument. If the nucleus fails to crack, it is usually secondary to inadequate groove depth, and additional sculpting should be performed. Most surgeons complete the initial cross grooves with continuous phacoemulsification ultrasound power and very low vacuum and convert to the high-vacuum pulsed or continuous mode for controlled removal of the individual cracked fragments. The divide and conquer technique is

ideal for firm nuclear sclerotic cataracts, which provide ample resistance for rotation. The disadvantage of this approach is the difficulty encountered in rotating a soft nucleus as is commonly found in young patients and those with posterior subcapsular cataracts and minimal nuclear sclerosis.

Phaco-Chop

The "phaco-chop" technique developed by Nagahara (29) takes advantage of the natural cleavage planes of the lens nucleus. After hydrodissection and removal of the superficial cortex, the lens nucleus is impaled centrally with the phacoemulsification tip to anchor it. A chopping instrument is placed under the capsulorhexis at the border of the nucleus opposite the incision and pulled toward the phacoemulsification probe splitting the nucleus in half. Care should be taken to ensure that the lens chopper does not inadvertently nick the anterior capsule. It is important that the nucleus be completely cleaved along the longitudinal meridian and from anterior to posterior. The nucleus is then rotated approximately three clock hours and a small wedge-shaped fragment is broken free with the chopping instrument and emulsified. The nucleus is successively removed by a combination of nuclear rotation and further fragmentation with the chopping instrument with intervening emulsification of each small wedge-shaped fragment. This technique is highly effective for a wide variety of cataract consistencies. One advantage is that it minimizes phacoemulsification time and the need to perform multiple nuclear rotations. Furthermore, the "cracking" forces are centripetal, minimizing strain on the capsule. This is opposed to divide and conquer, which uses centrifugal cracking forces and can place excess strain on a fragile capsule. The phaco-chop technique can therefore be used for patients with pseudoexfoliation, partial zonular dehiscence, or an imperfect capsulorhexis. Because of the reduced lens manipulation, this technique can also be performed rapidly, thus reducing surgical time.

Stop and Chop

The "stop and chop" technique developed by Koch (30) is a modification of the phaco-chop method in which a single central groove (85% to 90% depth) is first created by phacoemulsification along the incisional meridian of the lens nucleus. The nucleus is then cracked along this groove. The surgeon completes nuclear removal by fragmenting each nuclear half into smaller fragments with a chopping instrument similar to the phaco-chop technique.

Bowling

Soft cataracts are often difficult to crack and therefore do not lend themselves well to the above techniques. Soft cataracts are often best removed by "bowling" in which the central nuclear core is sculpted out in a bowl configuration with the phacoemulsification probe. The remaining epinuclear rim and cortex are then removed by cautiously purchasing an edge with high vacuum and stripping from the posterior capsule toward the center of the bag for safe removal. This final step is delicate and requires using the phacoemulsification probe near the posterior capsule with high vacuum and very little intervening protective lens fiber lamellae. For the inexperienced surgeon, this step is often complicated by posterior capsular rupture with vitreous loss.

Chip and Flip

In the "chip and flip" technique introduced by Fine (31) the central nucleus is first sculpted in a bowl configuration by removal of the central nuclear core. A second instrument is used to pull the remaining nucleus toward the incision and the rim of the nuclear bowl directly opposite the incision is removed with the phacoemulsification probe. This process is continued around the circumference of the nucleus by successively rotating and removing the nuclear rim. After complete removal of the peripheral nuclear rim, a second instrument is swept under the remaining nucleus, elevating the nucleus into the center of the bag where it is emulsified and removed. The remaining soft outer bowl of epinecleus that served as a protective barrier to the previous maneuvers is displaced from the position opposite the incision by purchasing with the phacoemulsification probe and pulling toward the incision with moderate to high vacuum. Once dislodged, it is flipped away from the capsule with a second instrument and removed with low phacoemulsification power or irrigation/aspiration. This technique is effective in removing cataracts with soft nuclei, which are often difficult to rotate.

Modifications

Innovations and modifications of nuclear phacoemulsification techniques are constantly being introduced in an effort to expedite cataract removal while minimizing risk to the capsule and the corneal endothelium. Lindstrom (personal communication, 1997) recently advocated the "tilt and tumble" technique in which the nucleus is partially prolapsed anteriorly out of the capsular bag and tilted toward the phacoemulsification port. Supplemental viscoelastic is injected into the capsular bag and anterior chamber to ensure capsular and endothelial cell protection. The presenting half of the nucleus is then emulsified in the iris plane and the remainder is prolapsed anteriorly, rotated, and similarly removed. While this technique minimizes risk to the posterior capsule, the return to iris plane phacoemulsification may increase the risk of endothelial damage. Another technique, called supracapsular phacoemulsification, involves prolapsing the nucleus anteriorly outside of the capsular bag and returning the upside-down nucleus into

the posterior chamber behind the iris and above the anterior capsule (32). The nucleus is then emulsified in the posterior chamber by one of the above methods. This technique ostensibly minimizes risk to the posterior capsule and endothelium but can lead to capsular tears if the capsulorhexis is not sufficiently large.

Second Instruments

When performing the divide and conquer technique, the second instrument ideally should have a smooth surface, facilitate rotation of the lens nucleus, and permit placement within the groove for cracking. Commonly used instruments include a cyclodialysis spatula, Drysdale spatula, Bechert spatula, or Canoli spatula. When "phaco-chopping" techniques are performed, an instrument that will impale and cut the lens nucleus is required. These include phaco-choppers and other right-angled instruments such as the mushroom or olive. Care should be taken when using the choppers as their sharp point can rupture both the anterior and posterior capsules. The mushroom and olive combine sharp chopping surfaces with smooth, rounded ends compromising the brisk impaling feature of the choppers while optimizing capsule preservation.

MANAGEMENT OF THE CORTEX

The satisfaction and sense of accomplishment afforded by successful removal of the lens nucleus provides a brief respite before one proceeds to cortical cleanup. Vigilance must be maintained, however, as many experienced phacoemulsification surgeons break the capsule or encounter other complications more frequently during cortical cleanup than during phacoemulsification of the lens nucleus.

The effective removal of the lens cortex is dependent on the successful application of prior portions of the procedure, especially capsulorrhexis construction and hydrodissection. A capsulorrhexis that is too small makes the purchase of the subincisional cortex challenging. In addition, adequate hydrodissection earlier in the procedure effectively hydrates the cortex facilitating its removal.

There are several ways to efficiently and effectively remove the cortex that remains after phacoemulsification of the lens nucleus. Choosing the appropriate method depends on the needs, experience, and comfort level of the surgeon. Regardless of which specific technique is chosen, basic principles of cortex removal apply. Following phacoemulsification, the cortex usually lines the inner aspect of the capsular bag. It is most easily removed by engaging the free end of the cortical sheet under the anterior capsule with moderate levels of vacuum and peeling the cortex from anteriorly to posteriorly as the I/A tip is moved toward the center of the pupil. It may be necessary to slowly move the tip back to the periphery periodically to obtain a better purchase on the cortex and therefore better occlusion of the

I/A tip during the cortical stripping. Once one sector of cortex is removed, an adjacent portion usually becomes available for easy purchase and removal. This procedure is repeated until all of the cortex is removed.

Irrigation/aspiration tips are available in many different port diameters, from 0.2 to 0.7 mm; however, 0.3 mm is most commonly used. Tips with larger port diameters are more difficult to occlude, more easily capture the iris and capsule, and can lead to greater variations in chamber depth because of rapid and increased flow through the tip. As a general rule for 0.3-mm I/A tips, 100 to 150 mm Hg vacuum is sufficient to hold the cortex for stripping while levels of 350 to 400 mm Hg will aspirate the cortex through the port (33).

Manual I/A

Many surgeons prefer to use a manual system such as the Simcoe cannula to aspirate the cortex. This method is useful because it provides the surgeon added security through manual control of the aspiration dynamics. Often physicians employ this technique as they transition to phacoemulsification and gain more comfort with the functions of an automated unit. This technique is also ideal in the setting of posterior capsular rupture, as low-flow cortical removal can be performed.

Automated I/A

Straight Tip

The standard automated I/A handpiece is equipped with a straight, blunt-end tip with a 0.3-mm aperture for aspiration on its anterior surface. This tip works well for cortical removal from the 180 degrees of the capsular bag most distal to the incision site. However, as the surgeon progresses closer to the subincisional cortex, obtaining an adequate purchase of the cortex becomes increasingly more difficult. Visualization decreases as the cornea becomes more distorted as a result of striae caused by increased pressure applied to the wound edge by the shaft of the I/A tip. Furthermore, the possibility of tearing the posterior capsule increases as the port is turned more posteriorly in an attempt to engage the subincisional cortex.

Curved Tip

Several manufacturers are now offering I/A handpieces with interchangeable curved aspiration tips. The most commonly available tips include angles of 30, 45, 90, and 180 degrees (Fig. 25-14). These angled tips allow easier access into the capsular bag and facilitate the purchase of subincisional cortex. Because of the angle of the tip, stripping of the cortex may involve a twisting movement of the handpiece instead of the forward-backward motion used with the straight tip. Use of the 180-degree tip can be helpful for subincisional cortex, but requires an extra measure of caution, as the aspiration aperture is usually on the end of

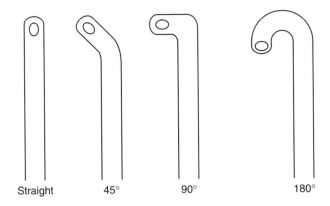

FIGURE 25-14. *Automated irrigation/aspiration handpiece tips.*

the tip and not on its anterior surface, which can easily lead to capsular or zonular rupture. In addition, when retrieving peripheral-subincisional cortex, the surgeon must ensure that the irrigation port remains inside the eye, otherwise, a rapid and significant fluctuation in anterior chamber depth can occur.

Bimanual Automated I/A

One of the newer techniques for cortical removal involves the use of separated ports for irrigation and aspiration (Fig. 25-15). These tips and handpieces are now commercially available in the United States. Some surgeons use the main wound for irrigation with the standard I/A handpiece and attach the aspiration line to a separate aspiration handpiece placed through the paracentesis. Others prefer to make a second paracentesis tract and use the separate irrigation and aspiration handpieces through the paracenteses. The main wound, if constructed properly, is self-sealing when the pressure is increased in the anterior chamber. This system allows easy access to all areas of the capsular bag for safe removal of the cortical remnants but requires bimanual dexterity and forces the surgeon to be cognizant of the location of two instruments simultaneously in the eye.

Subincisional Cortex

The removal of the subincisional cortex is often the most difficult and stressful aspect of cortical cleanup for the cataract surgeon. There are multiple methods that can be used successfully. Some of the more commonly employed techniques include:

Using the straight I/A tip with the port turned more posteriorly to engage the cortex
Using an angled I/A tip
Using the manual I/A tip (Simcoe) through an enlarged paracentesis
Using a bimanual automated I/A technique

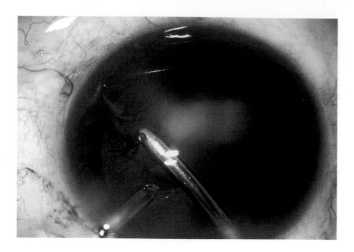

FIGURE 25-15.   *Bimanual technique for automated irrigation/aspiration with separate irrigation and aspiration cannulas.*

Removing the subincisional cortex last to allow time for increased hydration and easier dislodging of the cortex

Implanting the IOL and using the haptic to mechanically dislodge the cortex before aspiration

The most appropriate technique depends on the circumstances of the particular case, the available equipment, and the experience and comfort level of the surgeon.

Capsular Polishing and Vacuuming

Occasionally, following successful cortical cleanup, a plaque or strands of cortex may remain on the posterior capsule. If these remnants are in the visual axis, they can affect postoperative visual acuity. These remnants, especially those that contain epithelial cells, can also contribute to postoperative posterior capsular opacification. By performing capsular polishing or vacuuming one can make a good surgical result even better.

Capsular polishing involves the use of a manual "scratcher" instrument to loosen cortical remnants from the posterior capsule. These remnants can later be removed with an I/A tip. Vacuuming employs the I/A tip itself to remove these remaining bits of cortex. The technique involves combining relatively low flow rates (<5 mL/min) with low vacuum rates (approximately 5 mm Hg) to dislodge and suck the cortical bits into the I/A tip. Flow rates and vacuum levels should be set to draw the posterior capsule to the tip without sucking it into the aperture. Many of the newer phacoemulsification machines have preset values already programmed into the machine's software to make this function faster and less personnel dependent. At appropriate settings, the formation of a 3- to 4-mm "spider" pattern on the posterior capsule should be seen. If the "spider legs" get too long, traction on the capsule is excessive and the incar-

cerated capsule should be released immediately (34). When appropriately engaged, the capsule should be polished with a slow, circular movement of the I/A tip. Special care must be taken to ensure that the I/A tip itself is adequately polished because even small defects can snag and tear the posterior capsule. Some surgeons also prefer to vacuum the undersurface of the anterior capsule with the premise that these remaining epithelial cells contribute to posterior capsular opacification.

Removal of all of the cortex is optimal; however, it is important to remember that a small amount of cortex left behind will usually not lead to significant postoperative inflammation. It is preferable to leave behind a little cortex rather than risk breaking the capsule or causing a zonular dialysis.

INTRAOCULAR LENS

The cataract surgeon today has many options when considering his/her choice of IOL for implantation following successful phacoemulsification. Although the individual choices may be many, those lenses approved for use in the United States can be placed into three basic categories: polymethylmethacrylate (PMMA), silicone, and acrylic. In this section we discuss the advantages and disadvantages of each lens type and the procedures for their implantation. Future lens materials/designs currently in development include hydrogel, multifocal, and other types of injectable lenses.

Regardless of the optic material, several general characteristics are important in the selection of any IOL. First, the optic size should be larger than the undilated pupil to decrease the chance of optical aberrations from the edge of the lens. Thus, optic size should be greater than or equal to 5.0 mm in the elderly and 6.0 to 6.5 mm in younger individuals. Also, the smaller the optic, the greater the effect of even minimal displacement of the IOL postoperatively. Intended lens location is also an important factor in lens selection. The ciliary sulcus has a diameter of 11.5 to 12.0 mm and the capsular bag stretches from 9.5 to 11 mm after cataract surgery. Therefore, lenses with a haptic diameter from 10.5 to 12.5 are best suited for endocapsular placement while the ciliary sulcus better accommodates larger lenses, the total diameter of which ranges from 12.5 to 13.5 mm (35).

Polymethylmethacrylate

Today's PMMA lenses are similar in composition to Harold Ridley's first lenses of the 1940s and 1950s (36). PMMA is a strong, inert, hydrophobic polymer that is rigid at temperatures below 100 degrees. Its refractive index of 1.49 makes it possible to fashion lightweight IOLs that weigh only 3 to 5 mg (37). Using an all PMMA lens gives the surgeon the advantage of implanting a lens made of a sturdy material that is known to be well tolerated by the eye and has produced excellent visual results for many years. PMMA lenses can also accept ultraviolet (UV) coatings to protect the retina from damage associated with UV light exposure. The significant disadvantage of the rigid PMMA lens is the need for a large incision. Even the smallest PMMA lenses require the standard 3.0 to 3.2 mm phacoemulsification wound to be enlarged to at least 5.0 to 5.5 mm before implantation. Enlarging the wound can prolong the recovery of vision and contribute to postoperative astigmatism.

To implant a PMMA lens, the capsular bag is first reformed with viscoelastic. The wound is then enlarged to accommodate the optic. Making the internal incision slightly larger than the external incision usually facilitates insertion. The optic is then held firmly with forceps (Kelman-McPherson or Blaydes type) and placed through the wound into the anterior chamber. Placing BSS or viscoelastic on the lens helps it to pass through the wound. It is important to place the lens within the eye in the proper anterior-posterior orientation. By convention, the proper orientation of the lens is that in which the haptics can be freely rotated clockwise. The leading haptic and optic are directed posteriorly into the capsular bag and released. The trailing haptic can then be directly deposited into the bag with a forceps or lens manipulator or dialed into the capsular bag by placing an instrument (i.e., Sinskey hook) in the haptic-optic junction and rotating the IOL clockwise. Once both haptics are in the capsular bag, the lens should center itself. Failure of the IOL to center within the bag should prompt the surgeon to investigate further. The lens can similarly be placed in the ciliary sulcus by directly placing the haptics between the iris and anterior capsule. Sulcus fixated lenses may require centration with a second instrument. It is best to place both haptics either in the bag or the sulcus. Bag-sulcus haptic placement can lead to decentration.

Silicone

Medical-grade silicone products have many uses in ophthalmology, including contact lenses, scleral buckles, glaucoma shunts, and keratoprostheses, and as a vitreous substitute for retinal tamponade. The elastomers used to make IOLs from silicone give them a refractive index of 1.41 to 1.46 and a flexibility that allows the lens to be folded (38). This characteristic allows a lens with an optic size of 6.0 mm to be placed into the eye through an unenlarged phacoemulsification wound as small as 2.8 mm. The ability to place these lenses through a small incision has been the driving factor in their increasing popularity over the past few years. The patient benefits from faster recovery with minimal iatrogenically induced astigmatism. On the other hand, silicone IOLs are more susceptible to mechanical damage during insertion and to YAG laser damage during capsulotomy than are most PMMA lenses (39). Moreover, the presence of silicone IOLs in patients with vitreoretinal

disease complicates subsequent posterior segment surgery because water droplets condense on the posterior lens surface obstructing the view of the vitreoretinal surgeon. It may be prudent, therefore, to avoid silicone lenses in patients, such as diabetics or high myopes, who may need future vitreoretinal surgery.

Silicone IOLs are produced in two designs: single-plate haptic (Fig. 25-16A) and three-piece lenses. Single-plate haptic IOLs (produced by Staar Surgical Co., Monrovia, CA and Chiron Vision Corp.) and inserted into the capsular bag through an injection system. The lens is placed into a lubricated cartridge and folded. The cartridge is then placed into a metal injector. A V-shaped rod within the injector is advanced until it engages the lens haptic. When the surgeon rotates the threaded injector shaft, the IOL is slowly advanced. With the IOL at the tip of the injector cartridge, the surgeon inserts the cartridge through the wound into a capsular bag inflated with viscoelastic. The IOL is then slowly injected into the bag by clockwise rotation of the threaded injector shaft. The shaft should be advanced until the lens is completely released and lies in the capsular bag.

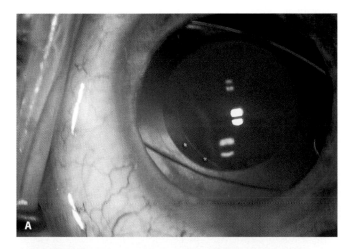

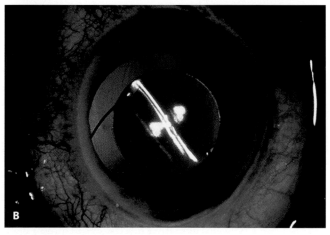

FIGURE 25-16. *A. Silicone IOL centered in the capsular bag. B. Foldable three-piece acrylic IOL unfolding in the capsular bag.*

If one of the haptics remains superior to the anterior capsule, it can be deposited into the bag by pushing it posteriorly with the lens insertion plunger, a smooth hook placed at the haptic-optic junction or the I/A tip. A newer and simpler method for plate haptic IOL insertion is the Passport system (Chiron Vision Corp.). In this system, the IOL is placed flat into a loading chamber. This chamber is then closed and attached to a modified syringe. A V-shaped plastic plunger is then pushed to engage the haptic. The lens is folded as it is advanced through the injector and unfolds as it is released into the bag.

Because of their short overall length, plate haptic lenses must be placed within the capsular bag and require an intact capsulorhexis to assure adequate stabilization. A criticism of plate haptic lenses is their potential for decentration. As the capsular bag fibroses, the lens can migrate. This was thought to be due to poor capsular-haptic adhesion. Newer lenses have larger holes within the haptics to allow better fixation within the bag.

Three-piece silicone lenses can be injected or folded before insertion. To fold a silicone lens, the optic is grasped with a Kelman-McPherson type forceps perpendicular to the axis of the haptics. A lens-folding forceps is then used to fold the IOL in half much like a taco. For convenience, the haptics can be tucked into the folded lens to facilitate insertion. Next, the folded lens is turned horizontally and pushed through the wound. Once inside the eye, the forceps is turned upright and the lens is released. Some surgeons prefer a more controlled release of the IOL and fold the lens parallel to its long axis such that the folded lens resembles a mustache. The three-piece silicone lenses can also be inserted using an injector. In this case, the leading haptic and optic are placed into a cartridge and the trailing haptic is left out at the distal end of the cartridge. The V-plunger is advanced, pushing the leading haptic and optic of the lens into the eye. For all three methods, if the trailing haptic is not in the capsular bag, it can be directly placed or dialed into the bag. Most three-piece silicone lenses have an overall diameter that allows either bag or sulcus fixation.

Flexible Acrylic Lenses

The flexible acrylic lens combines the excellent qualities of PMMA with the benefits of small-incision surgery. The only acrylic lens currently available in the United States is the Acrysof IOL (Alcon Laboratories). These lenses can be folded and inserted through a small incision, and have a temperature-dependent viscoelasticity that regulates their folding and unfolding (Fig. 25-16B). Since, the lens is more pliable at body temperature than at room temperature, it should be warmed before insertion to facilitate folding. This unique property also regulates unfolding within the bag. Acrylic IOLs typically unfold within the eye in a more controlled manner over 3 to 5 seconds compared with less than 1 second for silicone IOLs. The technique for folding and implanting these lenses is similar to that described for three-piece silicone IOLs. To date, there is no injector system for the Acrysof lens. The main disadvantage of the present acrylic lens is its increased cost. Also, these lenses require a slightly larger incision than is required for the foldable silicone lenses.

WOUND CLOSURE

Small incision wounds are usually self-sealing. If after reformation of the anterior chamber the wound is found to be watertight, a suture may not be necessary. If the wound is not watertight, it can be closed with 10-0 nylon in a variety of different styles including simple interrupted, cross, horizontal, or infinity sutures. Care must be taken to avoid placing overly tight sutures in a soft globe to minimize inducing postoperative astigmatism. Once the wound is reapproximated, the anterior chamber can be reformed with BSS through the paracentesis and the wound examined for leaks. The knots are then buried with nontoothed forceps. For scleral tunnel incisions, the conjunctiva is reapproximated over the closed scleral wound at the limbus with mechanical compression of the conjunctiva, wet-field cautery, or dissolvable sutures (i.e., polyglactin or plain gut). Clear-corneal incisions in general do not require suturing. If a leak is present, infiltration of BSS into the corneal stroma at the ends of the wound with a blunt-tipped cannula hydrates and expands the lamella, usually creating a self-sealing wound.

Many surgeons complete the procedure with the administration of subconjunctival antibiotic or steroid, or both. Although the value of this final step has not been clearly demonstrated, it may provide prophylaxis for postoperative endophthalmitis and speed recovery by minimizing the normal postoperative inflammatory response.

INTRAOPERATIVE COMPLICATIONS

The technique of phacoemulsification relies on the skillful execution of each successive step in the procedure. A flawless phacoemulsification surgery can bring gratification to the surgeon and almost instantaneously improve vision for the patient. On the other hand, inadvertent errors can lead to a cascade of complications that often frustrate the surgeon and can lead to vision loss or further surgery for the patient. Every surgeon experiences complications. Good surgeons are able to anticipate and prevent potential complications and quickly recognize and manage existing problems while maintaining composure. The purpose of this section is to discuss some of the more common intraoperative complications that can occur during phacoemulsification surgery with a focus on prevention and management.

The first step to averting complications is to create a professional but relaxed atmosphere in the operating room. A comfortable patient is less likely to move suddenly and a confident, relaxed surgeon can devote his/her energy to performing surgery.

Retrobulbar Hemorrhage

A retrobulbar hemorrhage is caused by the anesthetic needle perforating one of the many vessels that traverse the posterior orbit (Fig. 25-17) (40,41). Although fortunately rare, this complication can cause serious problems for the patient. Surgeons should carefully observe their patients immediately after the administration of the retrobulbar block for subconjunctival and subcutaneous hemorrhage as well as proptosis and tightening of the lids. Should a retrobulbar hemorrhage occur, the first treatment is direct pressure on the globe and orbit for several minutes to expedite clotting and to limit the amount of blood that accumulates in the orbit. This can be done with either digital pressure or with postanesthetic aids such as a mercury bag or Honan balloon. If the intraocular pressure remains normal, the eyelids are freely mobile, and there is no proptosis, the hemorrhage is limited, and the surgeon may wish to proceed with surgery, knowing that some positive posterior pressure may be encountered once the eye is entered (41).

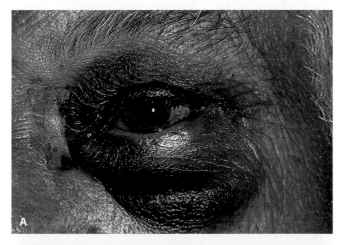

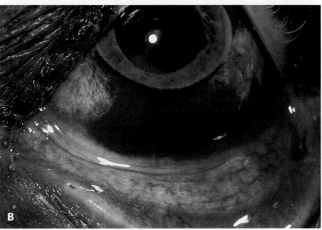

FIGURE 25-17. *A and B. Intraoperative complications: acute retrobulbar hemorrhage after retrobulbar delivery of local anesthetic.*

If, on the other hand, the hemorrhage is extensive, the surgeon should take immediate action to prevent injury to the visual system. Retrobulbar blood can significantly elevate intraocular pressure, tamponade the central retinal artery, and cause acute vision loss. In addition to assessing the intraocular pressure, the surgeon must examine the fundus for evidence of arterial pulsations or occlusion. If the eye is compromised, the first treatment is lateral canthotomy/cantholysis of the lower eyelid. In severe cases both eyelids may need to be disinserted to adequately lower intraocular pressure. Some surgeons also use carbonic anhydrase inhibitors or osmotic agents to further decrease the pressure in the eye. Surgery should be canceled and the patient closely observed until any threat to the visual system is resolved.

Prevention or limitation of retrobulbar hemorrhage can be aided by the cessation of anticoagulants prior to surgery. Aspirin therapy should be stopped 10 to 14 days before the operation. Discontinuation of warfarin (coumadin) 3 or 4 days before surgery often allows coagulation studies to return to normal by the time of the operation. However, before modifying the patient's medical regimen, it is important to consult with the patient's general physician in order to optimize medical management in the perioperative period.

Alternative forms of anesthesia for cataract surgery may also decrease or eliminate the risk of retrobulbar hemorrhage. Peribulbar anesthesia may take longer to produce the desired effect but is quite adequate. Sub-Tenon infusion of anesthetic with a blunt-tipped cannula also decreases the risk of damage to an orbital vessel. Finally, in appropriate patients, topical and/or intraocular anesthesia eliminates the potential for retrobulbar hemorrhage altogether.

Expulsive Hemorrhage

Suprachoroidal or expulsive hemorrhage is due to the rupture of a choroidal vessel with subsequent bleeding into the suprachoroidal space (Fig. 25-18). This event is fortunately rare in phacoemulsification surgery due to the small incisions used and the constant maintenance of intraocular pressure during the procedure. Furthermore, the formation of a self-sealing, tunnel incision also helps to limit choroidal hemorrhage should it occur. Loss of the red reflex, pain, sudden anterior chamber shallowing, or a firming of a previously soft globe may herald the development of a choroidal hemorrhage (42).

If a choroidal hemorrhage develops, the eye must be closed immediately to tamponade the hemorrhage and prevent the expulsion of intraocular contents. If the wound cannot be closed with sutures in a timely fashion, digital pressure should be placed over the wound. It is advisable to wait 30 to 45 minutes before reassessing the status of the eye. During this time, indirect ophthalmoscopy can be performed and intravenous osmotics can be administered to lower the intraocular pressure. If the wound is adequately

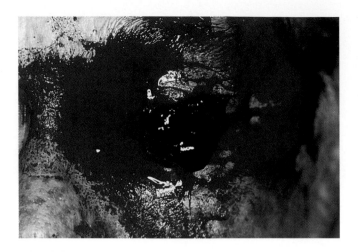

FIGURE 25-18. *Intraoperative complications: expulsive choroidal hemorrhage. (Courtesy of Thomas Johnson, MD, Bascom Palmer Eye Institute, University of Miami, Miami, FL.)*

closed, prolapsed uvea may be reposited with a goal to reforming the anterior chamber. Drainage of the hemorrhage through a scleral incision over the pars plana may be necessary to allow for deepening of the anterior chamber. Once a choroidal hemorrhage develops, other aspects of the planned procedure such as cortical removal and IOL insertion become secondary and can and often should be done at a later date.

Risk factors for expulsive choroidal hemorrhage include elevated intraoperative heart rate, systemic hypertension, atherosclerosis, elevated intraocular pressure, uveitis, aphakia, and increased axial length (43). Those receiving systemic anticoagulants are also at increased risk. The surgeon should be aware of patients in high-risk categories preoperatively and try to plan appropriately. Early recognition of a choroidal hemorrhage and rapid wound closure can limit the hemorrhage and prevent a catastrophe.

Tear in Descemet's Membrane

Descemet's membrane is susceptible to tearing at the wound's internal entry site and at the site of stab incisions (Fig. 25-19A). It is most commonly stripped as an instrument is placed through the wound into the anterior chamber. Tears commonly present as clear, anteriorly scrolled segments of Descemet's membrane and may be mistaken for small pieces of cortex near the wound. The surgeon may note excessive corneal stromal edema in the area of the separation.

These tears can be prevented by placing instruments slowly and cautiously into the eye. The surgeon should train his or her eye to carefully follow the instrument through the wound with each insertion. Directing the tip of the instrument posteriorly as it enters the anterior chamber keeps it away from the cut edge of Descemet's membrane and lessens the chance of inducing a tear.

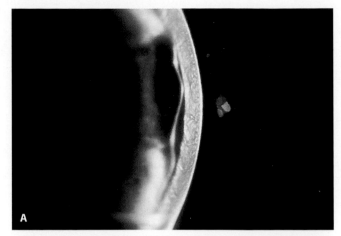

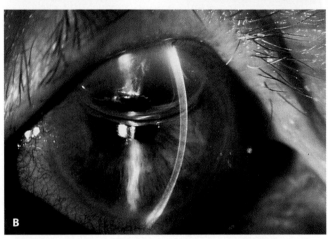

FIGURE 25-19. A. *Intraoperative complications: tear in Descemet's membrane.* B. *Repair of Descemet's membrane detachment by anterior chamber air bubble tamponade.*

Small tears in Descemet's membrane only require unfolding and tamponade with air (Fig. 25-19B) or viscoelastic. Larger tears may require suture fixation. A 10-0 nylon suture is passed full-thickness through the cornea anterior to the tear, through the stripped Descemet's membrane, then back through the cornea to secure it in position.

Peripheral Extension of Capsulorrhexis

One of the most common problems encountered during the capsulorrhexis is peripheral extension. Positive vitreous pressure with anterior bowing of the lens frequently promotes peripheral extensions; therefore, use of sufficient viscoelastic to deepen the anterior chamber and flatten the anterior capsule is helpful.

The technique of capsulorrhexis has been described earlier in this chapter. Both the needle cystotome and forceps techniques have advantages in preventing peripheral extensions. Placing the bent-needle cystotome on the viscoelastic syringe allows for precise tearing of the anterior capsule. Periodic addition of viscoelastic helps to keep the cut edge of the capsule reflected on itself for improved visualization of the tear's leading edge. Capsulorrhexis forceps also allow the tear to be directed with precision by pulling the torn edge "uphill" to counter the tendency for peripheral extension (44).

Should a tear begin to extend peripherally, it can possibly be rescued. Viscoelastic can be used to reinflate the eye, pushing the lens posteriorly to counter the vitreous pressure that may be contributing to the extension. If the tear edge extends under the iris, an iris hook can be employed to lift the iris and improve visualization of the peripheral anterior capsule to better redirect the tear.

Once a tear has extended too far peripherally to be redirected, the surgeon should stop and weigh the two options to complete the capsular opening. First, the surgeon can return to the initial tear site and perform a second capsulorhexis in the other direction, meeting at the area of extension. This option is preferable because it maintains the strength of an intact anterior capsular rim. The other option is to convert to a "can-opener" capsulotomy for the remainder of the capsular opening. Depending on the amount of capsulotomy performed, the density of the nucleus, and surgeon comfort, conversion to an extracapsular technique may be indicated. At the very least, it is best to avoid stressful endocapsular techniques such as cracking if a can-opener capsulotomy is performed.

With time and experience, the surgeon learns to quickly recognize and hopefully prevent significant peripheral extensions, facilitating capsulorrhexis formation.

Posterior Capsular Rupture

The posterior capsule of the lens is an extremely thin basement membrane that measures only 4 μm (45). Yet, preservation of this thin barrier may be the difference between a successful and a complicated cataract surgery. Posterior capsular rupture during surgery (Fig. 25-20) lengthens the procedure and puts the patient at increased risk for vision loss from cystoid macular edema and retinal detachment (46).

There are many potential origins of posterior capsular rents, including:

Posterior extension of an anterior capsular tear
Direct phacoemulsification of the posterior capsule
Piercing of the posterior capsule by the jagged edge of a nuclear fragment
Inadvertent perforation of the posterior capsule with a surgical instrument (nucleus—manipulator, viscoelastic cannula, phacoemulsification probe)
Aspiration of the posterior capsule during cortex removal or polishing
Rupture from excessive manipulation during IOL placement

Early recognition and appropriate management of posterior capsular tears can decrease the potential for serious

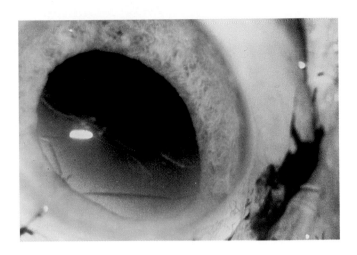

FIGURE 25-20. *Intraoperative complications: posterior capsular tear.*

complications from cataract surgery and sometimes prevent further surgical intervention. The surgeon should always have a heightened awareness of and avoid the situations that increase the risk of posterior capsular rupture. Sudden deepening of the anterior chamber should always raise suspicion of an occult tear. In the presence of a posterior tear, the surgeon should proceed slowly, frequently reassessing the situation and making decisions with the surgeon's comfort level and potential surgical outcome in mind (47).

If the posterior capsule tears during nucleus removal, the first goal is successful removal of all nuclear lens fragments. The surgeon should first assess the extent of the posterior capsular tear and place viscoelastic over the rent to tamponade the vitreous and keep the lens fragments in the anterior segment. The surgeon then must decide whether to convert to an extracapsular technique or to continue with phacoemulsification. If continued phacoemulsification is chosen and the nucleus is not fragmented, the surgeon can lift the nucleus into the anterior chamber and emulsify it with low hydrodynamic flow and a carousel technique. Once the nucleus has been fragmented, the situation becomes more difficult. Placing viscoelastic over the area of torn capsule may push the vitreous back and prevent "nuclear fallout." Placing a lens glide or a second instrument over the torn capsule while emulsifying a fragment elsewhere can also prevent the fragment from falling posteriorly. Another alternative is to spear a fragment with a 25-gauge needle placed through the pars plana to hold it for emulsification. If extracapsular extraction is chosen, the wound should be opened and the fragments removed with a lens loop. Relaxing incisions in the anterior capsule can aid fragment removal if the anterior capsulorrhexis is small. Nuclear expression, which can lead to extension of the posterior tear and vitreous loss, should be avoided.

The following general rules may be helpful in managing posterior capsular rents during cataract surgery:

Try to keep the anterior chamber formed at all times. Chamber collapse can encourage the forward movement of the vitreous.

Decrease the flow rate. Higher flow rates can extend capsular rents and hydrate the vitreous moving it forward.

If vitreous is present in the anterior chamber, remove it. Vitreous caught in the phacoemulsification or I/A tip may pull on the retina and increase the risk of retinal tear.

Anterior vitrectomy is best performed by placing the tip of the vitreous cutter through the rent allowing the vitreous strands to be cut posterior to the capsular tear. A bimanual or low-flow vitrectomy with high cutting rate is preferable.

Remove the cortex most remote from the tear first. Always strip the cortex toward the tear to decrease the stress forces on the rent. Because of improved control, some surgeons prefer to use a manual I/A system to remove the cortex in this situation.

If the rent is small, conversion of the tear into a posterior capsulorhexis can increase the strength of the posterior capsule and allow for placement of the IOL in the capsular bag.

Prevention of posterior capsular rupture can be facilitated by several maneuvers, some of which include:

Adequate hydrodissection to allow easy manipulation of the nucleus for endocapsular phacoemulsification.

Choice of the second instrument may decrease the chance of penetration of the posterior capsule. The Koch spatula is shaped like an oar while the Drysdale manipulator resembles a golf club. Both instruments have large, rounded surfaces which can safely manipulate the posterior capsule. Other manipulators may have sharp or pointed edges and are more prone to damage the capsule. Protective positioning of the second instrument behind the nuclear fragment being emulsified helps to prevent the posterior capsule from being aspirated into the phacoemulsification tip.

Angled I/A tips or bimanual I/A allow easier access to the cortex for safer removal.

Always push viscoelastic or saline ahead of a cannula when inserting it into the eye to prevent inadvertent piercing of the capsule.

It is important to remember that posterior capsular tears happen to both novice and skilled phacoemulsification surgeons. The ability to prevent ruptures and to efficiently and effectively manage this complication when it occurs can significantly decrease the number of poor surgical outcomes.

Zonular Dialysis

The zonules are numerous fine-tissue strands that stretch from the ciliary processes to the lens to hold it in place. These fibers attach to both the anterior and posterior surface of the lens capsule near the equator. The anterior zonules extend slightly more central than the posterior zonules and provide the majority of the capsular support. As mentioned previously, the anterior zonules delimit a circle with an average diameter of 6.83 mm (24), the so-called zonular free zone.

Several conditions including prior ocular trauma, pseudoexfoliation syndrome, Marfan's syndrome, homocystinuria, and Weill-Marchesani syndrome, are associated with weakened or torn zonules (48). Patients with these conditions should be examined closely before surgery for overt phacodonesis or iridodonesis. Patients with focal cortical cataracts should be questioned directly about antecedent ocular trauma. The surgeon may wish to consider an alternative technique (intracapsular or extracapsular) when the zonular support system is known to be disrupted.

Patients with pseudoexfoliation syndrome may have weak zonules. However, the presence of pseudoexfoliation alone does not preclude successful phacoemulsification. The surgeon must consider the density of the nucleus and the potential for excessive intraoperative force on the zonules from nuclear rotation and cracking before proceeding with surgery. Alternative techniques such as anterior chamber or iris plane phacoemulsification may be preferable in these patients.

Zonular dialysis can occur during routine phacoemulsification surgery from excessive nuclear manipulation, aspiration and traction on the capsular bag during I/A, or stress on the bag during IOL insertion. The key to successful management of a zonular dialysis is prompt recognition and implementation of techniques to limit further loss of zonular support. If vitreous has prolapsed into the anterior chamber, it should be removed by either low-flow or dry anterior vitrectomy techniques, placing the tip of the vitrector through the dialysis into the vitreous cavity. If no vitreous is present in the anterior chamber, viscoelastic can be placed over the area of dialysis to tamponade the vitreous body. Once the vitreous has been appropriately managed, the remaining nucleus and cortex can be removed. Cortex most distal to the dialysis should be removed first. All cortical stripping movements should be directed toward the area of dialysis to prevent further stress on the zonules at the edge of the dialysis. Cortex within and adjacent to the dialysis may be difficult to remove due to lack of countertraction on the capsular bag. It is better to leave small amounts of cortex than to risk extending the area of zonular dialysis.

Intraocular lens placement depends on the size of the zonular dialysis. A small dialysis (less than 4 clock hours) allows for lens placement in the capsular bag. Some surgeons prefer to orient the haptics into the dialysis. This orientation expands the capsular bag to its normal size and acts as a barrier to vitreous prolapse. Others choose to orient the haptics away from the dialysis, which places the haptics in areas of greater support. This haptic arrangement may allow for greater postoperative lens decentration from uneven capsular contraction. When the dialysis is moderate (4–6 clock hours), the lens is usually most stable when placed in the ciliary sulcus. If capsular support is inadequate, one of the haptics can be fixated in the ciliary sulcus with a transcleral suture. When the zonular dialysis is extensive (more than 6 clock hours) or complete, both haptics may need to be sutured in the ciliary sulcus, or an anterior chamber IOL can be chosen (49). Alternatively, given sufficient zonular support, an intracapsular support ring may be inserted to support the capsule for in-the-bag IOL placement (discussed further at the end of this chapter).

As with posterior capsular tears, if cases complicated by zonular dialysis are well managed, they often have good visual outcomes.

The "Dropped" Nucleus

The loss of nuclear lens fragments into the posterior segment through a tear in the posterior capsule is a complication feared by all cataract surgeons. The entire support system for the nucleus during phacoemulsification is the posterior capsule, a membrane whose thickness is measured in microns. While the anterior capsule may double in thickness with age, the posterior capsule remains thin with the thinnest portion located posteriorly (50). Although removal of the cataractous lens and cortex without disruption of the posterior capsule is commonplace, given the size and strength of the posterior capsule, it seems remarkable that more "nuclear fallout" does not occur.

A sudden deepening of the anterior chamber or bouncing of the pupil should alert the surgeon to the presence of a posterior capsular tear. Should the nucleus or a portion of it begin to fall, viscoelastic or a lens glide, or both, can be placed behind it. If the nucleus remains in sight, the wound should be enlarged and the nucleus removed with a lens loop. Another technique is to spear the nucleus with a 25-gauge needle placed through the pars plana. The fragment can then be emulsified or delivered through the wound.

Once a portion of the nucleus has fallen posteriorly, heroic attempts at retrieval should not be attempted by the anterior segment surgeon (51). Nuclear fragments in the posterior segment are best handled by a vitreoretinal surgeon through a posterior approach (52–54). Attempts to remove posteriorly dislocated fragments through the anterior wound are associated with posterior segment complications including retinal breaks and detachments and giant retinal tears (52–54). Only an anterior vitrectomy sufficient to remove the prolapsed vitreous from the anterior segment is necessary at the time of cataract surgery. Cortical removal can then be performed with a low-flow system. If anterior

capsular support permits, a posterior chamber IOL can be placed in the ciliary sulcus. If insufficient capsular support is present, the surgeon can choose to suture an IOL in the ciliary sulcus, place an anterior chamber lens, or leave the patient aphakic. If the nucleus was exceptionally hard, it may need to be delivered through the cataract wound by the posterior segment surgeon. Therefore, the cataract surgeon may opt for primary aphakia in these cases.

Thermal Burn

The lens nucleus is disrupted during phacoemulsification by the acoustic shock waves produced from the vibration of the titanium phacoemulsification tip. A portion of the energy produced by the tip is converted to heat. This heat is normally dissipated and the anterior segment spared injury by the constant flow of balanced salt solution. However, only several seconds of interrupted flow into the eye is sufficient to produce a corneoscleral burn.

The most common cause of corneoscleral burns is kinking of the outer sleeve of the phacoemulsification tip in a tight wound or compression of the outer sleeve through an excessively long scleral tunnel. Other causes include machine pump failure and a viscoelastic plug in the aspiration port. Thermal burns can be prevented by adequate wound construction, by checking the irrigation/aspiration system in a test chamber before the surgery, and by chilling the irrigating solution prior to the operation. Should a thermal burn occur, the primary goal becomes adequate wound closure. Thermal burns cause tissue shrinkage and may require multiple sutures to close the wound. If there is significant heat shrinkage of the tissue, a scleral patch graft may be necessary. Eye bank sclera may be utilized if available. If it is not available, a partial-thickness scleral autograft can be harvested. Failure to adequately close the wound may increase the risk of postoperative infection or lead to an inadvertent filtering bleb.

POSTOPERATIVE COMPLICATIONS

Occasionally, despite a flawless and technically uneventful surgery, the patient may experience complications in the postoperative recovery period. These can generally be considered in two categories, those that occur in the short term (first 6 weeks) and those that occur in the long term (greater than 6 weeks).

Short-Term Complications

Postoperative Inflammation

A small degree of postoperative intraocular inflammation is to be expected even after uncomplicated phacoemulsification cataract surgery. The inflammation is limited to the anterior chamber and responds to topical corticosteroids with resolution over several days to weeks. Postoperative inflammation may be more pronounced if the surgical time was prolonged or there was excessive manipulation of the iris, posterior capsular rupture, or vitrectomy performed. Patients with diabetes or preoperative uveitis may also display more pronounced inflammation after surgery.

Severe or prolonged postoperative inflammation, on the other hand, may be a harbinger of significant intraocular pathology. Recognized causes of pathologic postoperative inflammation include retained lens fragments, uveitis (reactivated or new), endophthalmitis, epithelial downgrowth, iris or vitreous incarceration in the wound, IOL malposition, and uveitis-glaucoma-hyphema (UGH) syndrome.

Fragments of the lens nucleus retained in the anterior chamber frequently incite an inflammatory response as phagocytes are recruited to digest and remove this "foreign material" (Fig. 25-21). It is important, therefore, to ensure that no nuclear fragments remain in the anterior chamber, sulcus, or capsular bag at the close of the procedure. Nuclear fragments retained in the anterior segment must often be removed in a second procedure if the inflammation is unresponsive to medical therapy (i.e., topical or sub-Tenon's corticosteroids). Retained cortical fragments are better tolerated and usually do not incite a significant inflammatory response. Cortical lens fiber cells that remain in the peripheral lens capsule often undergo limited cell division, forming a benign Elschnig's pearl that may be evident on slit lamp biomicroscopy. Lens fragments retained in the vitreous cavity can cause substantial inflammation and can be confused with postoperative endophthalmitis (55). This complication is best managed by a referral to a vitreoretinal surgeon (52,54,56–62). With proper treatment these patients often have favorable outcomes.

Iris incarceration in the wound is often associated with wound dehiscence. In general, management of this complication requires a second procedure in which the wound is reapproximated with excision of necrotic uveal tissue and replacement of viable uveal tissue into the anterior

chamber. Complications of wound dehiscence are elaborated below.

Subluxation of the IOL can lead to iris capture or chronic iris irritation with secondary anterior segment inflammation and cystoid macular edema. The haptics of anterior chamber IOLs are supported by the angle or the iris and are more frequently associated with postoperative inflammation than posterior chamber IOLs. Uveitis-glaucoma-hyphema syndrome is believed to be a complication of the IOL rubbing against the iris due to imperfections in the lens implant, improper lens size, or improper lens position (63). It is more common with iris-fixated and anterior chamber IOLs but can also occur with posterior chamber IOLs (64–73). If the inflammation associated with malpositioned IOLs or UGH syndrome cannot be managed medically the IOL may need to be surgically repositioned or replaced. Fortunately, the glaucoma in UGH syndrome may resolve if the trabecular meshwork has not been irreversibly damaged (67,71). Other causes and complications of postoperative inflammation, including epithelial downgrowth, cystoid macular edema, and endophthalmitis, are discussed further in the following sections.

Wound Dehiscence

The estimated incidence of wound dehiscence of between 1% and 5% (74,75) has likely declined in recent years because of the shift toward small-incision surgery. Wound dehiscence can occur spontaneously as a result of poor wound closure or secondary to trauma such as the patient rubbing the eye. The critical elements that affect wound dehiscence are wound construction and wound closure. Creation of a true, triplanar self-sealing scleral tunnel incision minimizes the risk of wound dehiscence (76). Active wound healing begins within 48 hours of surgery. At 1 week postoperatively, wound strength is approximately 10% of that present in normal tissue. By 8 weeks, wound strength has improved to 40% and at 2 years the wound has regained approximately 75% to 80% of its preoperative strength (77–81). Patients at risk for development of wound dehiscence include those who are malnourished (especially vitamin C and protein deficient), those with Werner's syndrome [an autosomal recessive condition of premature aging associated with premature cataract formation (82)], those with peripheral ulcerative keratitis or scleritis associated with systemic collagen vascular disease, and those treated with high-dose systemic steroids (83,84).

Wound dehiscence may manifest as a wound leak, an inadvertent filtering bleb (Fig. 25-22) or complete wound rupture. The clinical signs associated with wound leak include poor vision, hypotony, a shallow anterior chamber, hyphema, choroidal folds or effusions, and optic nerve edema. A wound leak may be identified by painting the suspicious area with a fluorescein strip and viewing with light passed through a cobalt blue filter (Seidel test). A mild wound leak or inadvertent filtering bleb can be managed conservatively if the chamber remains formed and the

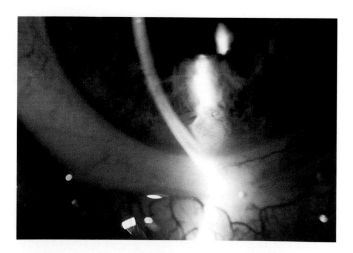

FIGURE 25-21.   *Retained lens fragments in anterior chamber causing inflammation.*

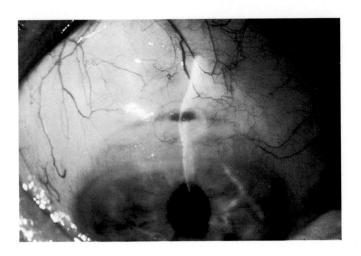

FIGURE 25-22. *Postoperative wound dehiscence causing inadvertent filtering bleb. (Courtesy of William W. Culbertson, MD, Bascom Palmer Eye Institute, University of Miami, Miami, FL.)*

intraocular pressure is adequate. Management options include the administration of prophylactic topical antibiotics in combination with a decrease in or discontinuation of steroid therapy, pressure patching with cycloplegia, application of a large-diameter bandage contact lens or collagen shield, and topical/systemic administration of aqueous fluid suppressants. If these palliative methods are unsuccessful or in the setting of frank wound rupture, definitive closure with sutures may be necessary. Frank wound rupture usually occurs after trauma and is frequently associated with extrusion of intraocular contents, usually the iris. This presentation requires urgent surgical repair with the removal of devitalized tissue in order to minimize the risk of further complications.

Attendance to wound dehiscence is important not only in restoring the integrity of the eye and preserving vision but also in minimizing the risk of further complications including endophthalmitis or epithelial downgrowth, which are ongoing risks in an eye with an active wound leak through an open scleral channel.

Corneal Edema

Postoperative corneal edema is a consequence of inadequate endothelial pump function that results in hydration and opacification of the corneal stroma (85). The overall incidence is less than 1% (86). Damage to the endothelium can occur from a number of different insults (87–89). Surgical trauma secondary to direct injury with an instrument, nuclear fragments, or the IOL, or from excessive ultrasound energy, usually causes a localized patch of edema over the affected area. Endothelial cells have minimal mitotic activity but with time will migrate and enlarge to fill in a devitalized area if it is not too extensive (85,89). Therefore, in healthy eyes, most cases of corneal edema secondary to surgical trauma resolve within a few weeks. Preexisting disease

such as Fuchs' dystrophy or unrecognized low endothelial cell count without guttae can predispose a patient to development of corneal edema if insufficient endothelium is extant to withstand the normal losses associated with surgery. Detachment of Descemet's membrane is another cause of localized edema, the management of which was discussed previously in this chapter. Inadvertent administration of toxic substances such as improperly formulated antibiotics (especially aminoglycosides or vancomycin), detergents from inadequate instrument rinsing, or use of preserved instead of nonpreserved intraocular medications/infusion additives can damage the endothelium causing corneal edema (89). This is generally not reversible but may subside if sufficient endothelium remains to support the cornea. Other rare causes of postoperative corneal edema include prolonged contact with other ocular tissues (flat chamber, iris bombé, suprachoroidal effusion/hemorrhage), trauma from retained foreign material (nuclear fragments or foreign particulate matter), vitreous touch, and epithelial or fibrous downgrowth. Postoperative ocular hypertension is frequently associated with acute corneal edema and is discussed below.

The treatment of postoperative corneal edema is largely palliative unless therapy can be specifically directed to the underlying pathoetiology. Hypertonic solutions, such as 5% sodium chloride preparations, are often effective in improving vision in patients with mild to moderate microcystic epithelial edema. The effect may be most notable in the morning, when edema is maximal due to lack of tear evaporation through closed lids during sleep. Some surgeons advocate the use of topical anti-inflammatory medications such as corticosteroids or nonsteroidal anti-inflammatory drugs (NSAIDs) to reduce postoperative inflammation, which may be compromising the endothelium. There is no proof, however, that this intervention is beneficial in preserving endothelial function. Significant bullous keratopathy can be treated with topical lubricants, hypertonic solutions, and a bandage contact lens, if needed, for pain management. Finally, for those patients with persistent corneal edema (>2–3 months), penetrating keratoplasty is indicated to restore visual function.

Postoperative Ocular Hypertension

An acute rise in intraocular pressure (IOP) is not infrequent following phacoemulsification surgery combined with the use of viscoelastics (90–94). Viscoelastic that remains within the anterior chamber hydrates and swells, occluding the trabecular meshwork and impeding the normal outflow of aqueous (95). This is more common with the higher-viscosity agents, which are difficult to remove completely and swell more extensively when fully hydrated. The IOP rises and peaks between 4 and 7 hours after cataract surgery and generally returns to normal within 24 to 72 hours (92,96). Periocular pain is the typical complaint postoperatively. Corneal microcystic epithelial edema is evident clinically and the angle is open. Eyes with compromised aqueous outflow before surgery may be at higher risk of IOP spike postoperatively (97). Patients with pseudoexfoliation are also at risk for postoperative intraocular pressure spikes. Removal of the viscoelastic at the end of the procedure likely reduces the risk of postoperative IOP spikes (92) and most surgeons attempt to evacuate as much of the viscoelastic agent as possible.

Prophylactic topical beta-adrenergic blockade or treatment with systemic carbonic anhydrase inhibitors is usually effective in controlling moderate postoperative intraocular pressure spikes (98). Significantly elevated IOP can be promptly relieved by "burping" the paracentesis. This usually releases a significant amount of retained viscoelastic material from the anterior chamber. Since this procedure involves opening the paracentesis site it likely carries a low risk of endophthalmitis and must be used judiciously. It may be prudent to treat the eye with prophylactic topical antibiotics or povidone-iodine prior to the procedure.

Topical corticosteroids are routinely used to control normal postoperative inflammation. A certain percentage of patients are "steroid responsive" and will manifest elevated IOP in response to topical steroids (99,100). Generally, the effect is reversible and withdrawal of the medication results in normalization of the IOP in days to weeks. The most common inciting corticosteroids are dexamethasone and prednisolone. Agents that minimize this response, such as fluorometholone or rimexolone, may be most appropriate in this patient population. For those patients who require topical steroids to treat postoperative inflammation, aqueous suppressants can be used in combination with topical steroids to control the IOP until the steroid can be withdrawn.

Infrequent causes of postoperative ocular hypertension or glaucoma include: hyphema, uveitis, lens particle glaucoma, aqueous misdirection (malignant glaucoma), cyclodialysis cleft closure, neovascular glaucoma, and epithelial or fibrous downgrowth. Management of these topics is beyond the scope of this discussion and the reader is referred to in-depth references of cataract surgery (see Bibliography).

Vitreous Prolapse

Vitreous prolapse into the anterior chamber is infrequent following uneventful phacoemulsification surgery with placement of a posterior chamber IOL. However, in the setting of zonular dialysis or posterior capsular rupture, the vitreous body can prolapse forward, extending to the wound (Fig. 25-23) or causing pupillary block. Vitreous incarceration in the wound is associated with cystoid macular edema (101,102) and is evident clinically as a peaked, corectopic pupil with veils of vitreous, with or without pigment, in the anterior chamber extending to the wound. Prolonged contact between the vitreous and anterior segment structures, including the iris, ciliary body and cornea may lead to permanent fibrous adhesions. Surgical lysis of vitreous incarceration or adhesions allows the vitreous to "fall back" into the vitreous cavity and is often associated with

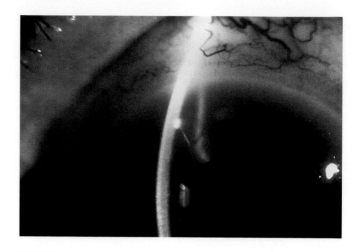

FIGURE 25-23.   *Vitreous incarceration in the wound. (Courtesy of William W. Culbertson, MD, Bascom Palmer Eye Institute, University of Miami, Miami, FL.)*

improved visual acuity and resolution of cystoid macular edema (103). Intervention via neodymium:YAG (Nd:YAG) laser vitreolysis is an alternative treatment method that is often effective and frequently associated with an improvement in visual acuity (104).

Pupillary block glaucoma due to vitreous prolapse is uncommon with an intact posterior capsule and "in-the-bag" placement of a posterior chamber IOL because these structures serve to tamponade and contain the vitreous in the posterior segment. This form of glaucoma can occur after a complicated phacoemulsification procedure with posterior capsular rupture and anterior vitrectomy in which an anterior chamber IOL was implanted because of insufficient capsular support, especially if a surgical peripheral iridectomy is not performed. Occasionally, pupillary block can develop even after placement of a peripheral iridectomy if the intact anterior hyaloid face or formed vitreous prolapses forward occluding the iridectomy. In this instance, Nd:YAG vitreolysis may be effective in relieving the obstruction and restoring aqueous flow from the posterior chamber to the anterior chamber (105).

Long-Term Complications

Epithelial Downgrowth

Epithelial invasion of the anterior chamber is an ominous complication that can follow any violation of the eye wall, including cataract surgery, other anterior segment surgery, or trauma. Although this condition has been recognized since the 1830s (106), management techniques continue to be largely ineffective and the diagnosis carries a grim prognosis. Intractable glaucoma usually develops in the affected eye and eventually progresses to blindness. Pathogenetically, ocular surface epithelium, or in some cases surface fibrous tissue, undergoes atypical growth inward along the wound forming a fistulous tract thereby gaining access to the internal structures of the eye. Three morphologic growth patterns have been described (107): 1) "pearl" tumors of the iris, 2) epithelial inclusion cysts, and 3) sheet-like epithelial ingrowth. Historically, the incidence of cystic and sheet-like epithelial invasion following either trauma or anterior segment surgery has been estimated at 0.06% to 0.11% with cysts considered to be more common (108,109). The current incidence is most likely considerably lower with modern small incision surgical techniques. Risk factors include poor wound closure, incarcerated uvea or vitreous in the wound, and possible exposure to plasmoid aqueous containing proliferative growth factors (110–112). Intraocular lesions that are discontinuous with the wound have been described and can result from direct intraocular implantation by surgical instruments (113).

Pearl tumors usually follow trauma but can occur after intraocular surgery and are the result of implantation of epithelial cells of skin or hair follicles into the anterior chamber (114). These lesions are generally small and circumscribed, and are not connected with the entry site. Pearl tumors are usually benign and enlarge slowly if at all. In rare cases, cyst enlargement affects the visual axis or causes iridocyclitis necessitating removal, which usually results in a favorable outcome.

Epithelial inclusion cysts are thin-walled structures lined with squamous or cuboidal epithelium that may include goblet cells (115). They are typically translucent or gray in appearance and filled with a straw-colored, turbid or mucinous fluid (110,116). Clinically, cysts can remain quiescent for years before enlarging and causing symptoms. The patient typically presents with decreased vision, intraocular inflammation, corneal decompensation, and/or secondary glaucoma. Clinically, epithelial inclusion cysts cover a spectrum that ranges from spontaneous regression (117) to rapid growth. Therefore, it may be prudent to avoid early surgical intervention either with laser treatment or conventional surgery given the documented risk of conversion to the more hazardous sheet-like epithelial downgrowth (115). Conservative management consists of three- to four- month visits with photodocumentation to assess progression. If treatment is necessary, several different modalities have been reported, including direct needling, injection with radioactive or sclerosing agents, diathermy, cryotherapy, surgical removal, and photocoagulation. The ideal treatment modality has not been determined and all carry a risk of conversion to the more serious sheet-like morphology.

Epithelial sheet ingrowth usually presents as a retrocorneal or iris membrane with a gray leading edge. The involved cornea is often clear and may be associated with corneal neovascularization (118). Gonioscopy may reveal peripheral anterior synechiae, epithelialization of the angle, lens remnants, or incarcerated iris or vitreous. The intraocular pressure is usually elevated but one-third of eyes are hypotonous due to a fistulous tract through the wound. The epithelial membrane can extend over many intraocular structures, including the pupil, anterior hyaloid face, and ciliary body, and, in rare cases, can extend to the retina causing retinal detachment. Diagnosis may be facilitated by a positive Seidel test demonstrating a fistulous tract to the anterior chamber and by specular microscopy of the cornea. Argon laser photocoagulation can be used to define the extent of migration over the iris. Treatment of the iris with a 500-µm diameter spot size for 0.2 seconds at 100 to 300 mW produces pathognomonic whitening of the epithelial membrane and can be used to clearly define the membrane borders for future intervention. Surgical therapy, which is beyond the scope of this chapter, endeavors to completely eradicate all intraocular epithelial tissue and often requires extensive tissue removal (119,120).

Posterior Capsule Opacification

Opacification of the posterior capsule is a relatively common event following successful cataract surgery. Retained epithelial cells in the peripheral lens equator proliferate and migrate posteriorly, wrinkling and/or forming a thin plaque along the posterior capsule, thereby degrading the retinal image. The incidence is approximately 30% to 40% by 2 years after surgery (121). In young age groups, the incidence is higher and approaches 100%. The use of a posterior chamber intraocular lens with a convex posterior surface has been reported to reduce the incidence of posterior capsular opacification after cataract surgery (122–124).

The symptomatic patient who experiences glare or reduced visual function as a result of posterior capsular opacification can be treated with the Nd:YAG laser to create a posterior capsulotomy clearing the visual axis (125–128). Before treatment, other possible causes of visual compromise, such as corneal opacification, an epiretinal membrane, or cystoid macular edema, must be ruled out. Neodymium:YAG capsulotomy, which carries a small but finite risk of complications, is effective in alleviating the visual symptoms in the majority of patients. The most common short-term complication is acute intraocular pressure elevation, which is usually transient but can persist (129–133). Intraocular pressure typically begins to rise immediately after the procedure, peaks at 3 to 4 hours and returns to baseline over the ensuing 3 to 7 days. Pilocarpine is effective in reducing this intraocular pressure spike but may be proinflammatory (134). It is therefore recommended that the patient be pretreated with topical beta-adrenergic blocking agents or iopodine and that the pressure be monitored 1 hour after treatment. This is effective in controlling the acute pressure elevation in the majority of patients. Other less frequent complications include retinal detachment (2–4%) (135–142), cystoid macular edema (0.55–2.5%) (125,127,140–142), intraocular lens damage or pitting (15–33%) (126,143,144), macular hole formation (141,145) and endothelial cell loss (2.3–7%) (146,147). Risk factors for retinal detachment following Nd:YAG posterior capsulotomy include axial myopia, a history of retinal detachment in the fellow eye, and younger age (135,148,149). Endophthalmitis due to latent *Propionibacterium acnes* has been reported following Nd:YAG capsulotomy in which quiescent organisms sequestered in the capsule were liberated into the vitreous cavity (150–152).

The ultimate goal is to clear the visual axis using a minimum of laser energy and without damaging the intraocular lens. Two popular strategies for opening the central axis in the opacified membrane include a cruciform pattern and a circular pattern. Ideally, the capsulotomy should be a little larger than the undilated pupil in ambient light. Neodymium:YAG laser posterior capsulotomy results in improved visual acuity in 83% to 96% of treated eyes (125–127,140,153–155).

Cystoid Macular Edema

The evolution from extracapsular to "in-the-bag" phacoemulsification cataract extraction and from anterior chamber and iris-fixated IOLs to posterior chamber IOLs has been associated with a concomitant reduction in the incidence of postoperative cystoid macular edema (CME). Cystoid macular edema is detectable in 16% to 30% of patients after uncomplicated extracapsular cataract extraction by fluorescein angiography. However, fewer than 2.5% of patients suffer permanent visual loss as a consequence of CME (156,157). Complicated cataract surgery involving posterior capsular rupture, iris or vitreous incarceration in the wound, or iris irritation by the IOL is associated with an increased incidence of postoperative CME (158). Examination of the pupil before dilatation may provide clues to the pathoetiology of the CME. A peaked pupil may be an indicator of vitreous prolapse into the anterior chamber with vitreous incarceration in the wound. An elliptic pupil can result from sphincter trauma but can also be associated with iris capture of the IOL or iris tuck by a haptic. Cystoid macular edema can usually be diagnosed clinically with biomicroscopy and a fundus contact lens. Fluorescein angiography may be obtained to confirm the diagnosis in difficult cases (156), however, the extent of staining on the angiogram does not correlate well with the patient's visual function (159). Many patients with CME improve spontaneously without therapy within 6 months (160). However, if CME persists, permanent cellular damage to the retina will ultimately occur with irreversible visual loss (161).

The goal of therapy is to resolve the macular edema before permanent retinal damage occurs. A number of different therapeutic agents have been employed based on the notion that uveal irritation or vitreous incarceration, or both, leads to elevated prostaglandin levels and CME (162–164). Corticosteroids and NSAIDs, both of which inhibit prostaglandin production, have been used to treat postoperative CME. Corticosteroids are clinically effective and commonly used; however, they have never been demonstrated in clinical studies to alter the course of the disease.

In contrast, topical NSAIDs, which inhibit prostaglandin cyclo-oxygenase, have been shown in clinical trials to be effective in restoring visual acuity in patients with CME (165,166). Oral NSAIDs, on the other hand, are not beneficial in treating CME, probably due to poor ocular penetration compared with topical application (164). Carbonic anhydrase inhibitors have been used successfully in the treatment of CME; however, the CME usually recurs when the drug is withdrawn (167).

Currently, there is disagreement over the optimal method of treating postoperative CME (168). If the condition is mild, it may be prudent to observe for 2 to 3 months without treatment awaiting spontaneous resolution. In more severe cases with extensive macular thickening and visual loss below 20/50 treatment can be instituted (169). Some authors recommend starting with combination therapy comprising a topical corticosteroid and a topical NSAID. If no response occurs after 6 to 8 weeks, an oral carbonic anhydrase inhibitor can be added to the regimen. If there is still no response, a sub-Tenon's corticosteroid injection can be administered or oral corticosteroid therapy can be initiated (169). Unfortunately, some cases of CME are refractory to treatment and never respond to medical therapy. Surgical approaches for the treatment of CME are directed to alleviating the presumed inciting cause. Surgical approaches include: 1) Nd:YAG vitreolysis of vitreous strands extending to the wound, 2) repositioning or replacement of the IOL, and 3) vitrectomy. A randomized controlled study of aphakic eyes with CME and vitreous incarceration in the wound demonstrated a significant benefit after vitrectomy (170,171). Nevertheless, vitrectomy is usually reserved as a last resort for cases with clear vitreous adhesions.

Retinal Detachment

Retinal detachment is a well-recognized complication of cataract surgery, with an incidence of 1% to 2% following extracapsular surgery (172–175) and 0.75% to 3.6% following phacoemulsification surgery (135,173,175,176). The increased incidence (3.6%) with phacoemulsification surgery was reported in the late 1970s during the introduction of this methodology (176). With current phacoemulsification techniques, the incidence is approximately 0.75–0.9% (135,175). Nevertheless, a higher incidence has been reported in complicated cases associated with vitreous loss (176) and in patients with high myopia, lattice degeneration, a predisposing systemic disease such as Marfan's and Stickler's syndromes, a family history of retinal detachment, and after blunt trauma (177). The majority of postoperative retinal detachments occur within the first year but rarely are seen during the acute postoperative period (174). Most are the result of a posterior vitreous detachment (PVD) that causes a retinal tear with subsequent progression to a rhegmatogenous retinal detachment. Cataract surgery has been noted to induce structural changes in the vitreous body with loss of hyaluronic acid, increased mobility, and premature synersis that are believed to predispose to earlier

PVD (178). The integrity of the posterior capsule is important to this process with PVD rates being higher in eyes with a disrupted posterior capsule (179). Fortunately, most cases of postoperative retinal detachment are reparable with good outcomes if diagnosed and repaired early before macular detachment has occurred (174).

Endophthalmitis

The development of postoperative endophthalmitis can be devastating for both the patient and the surgeon (Fig. 25-24). Fortunately, postoperative endophthalmitis following cataract surgery is a rare occurrence with an incidence, in retrospective studies, of approximately 0.08% to 0.4% (173,180–185). Although 88% of cases present within the first 6 weeks after surgery, most manifest within the first 1 to 3 postoperative days (186). Risk factors for endophthalmitis include diabetes mellitus, immunocompromised status, chronic alcoholism, complicated or prolonged surgery, wound complications, posterior capsule rupture, vitreous loss, excessive instrumentation, a history of prior ocular surgery, a contaminated IOL, or an IOL with polypropylene haptics (180,181,187). The most commonly isolated organisms are normal ocular adnexal flora such as *Staphylococcus epidermidis* and *Staphylococcus aureus* (188–190). Other less common etiologic agents include other gram-positive organisms such as *Streptococcus* and group D *Enterococcus* species, gram-negative species (*Serratia*, *Proteus*, *Enterobacter*, and *Pseudomonas*), the anaerobic gram-positive bacillus *P. acnes* and fungal species (Table 25-1). Endophthalmitis due to more virulent species, such as *Bacillus*, *Streptococcus*, and the gram-negative species, can progress rapidly, within hours, and the final visual outcome is often poor regardless of therapeutic intervention.

The endophthalmitis vitrectomy study (EVS), a randomized, prospective, multicenter study, evaluated various parameters associated with acute-onset postcataract extraction endophthalmitis (191). In this study, patients in whom endophthalmitis developed within 6 weeks of cataract extraction surgery were randomized to vitrectomy combined with intraocular antibiotics or simple "tap and inject," in which a small sample of vitreous was collected for microbiologic analysis and antibiotics were delivered into the vitreous. Patients were also randomized to systemic intravenous antibiotic therapy with ceftazidime and amikacin or no systemic antibiotic therapy. This study showed that patients who presented with visual acuity better than light perception (LP) in the affected eye responded equally well to either vitrectomy or tap and inject whereas patients with LP or worse vision responded better to vitrectomy. With regard to systemic therapy, outcomes were comparable regardless of the use of intravenous antibiotics. The EVS study concluded that patients who presented with acute postoperative endophthalmitis with LP vision should undergo vitrectomy with administration of intraocular antibiotics and those with better than LP vision can be treated with tap and inject alone. The study also concluded that systemic antibiotic therapy with ceftazidime and amikacin is not necessary in

Table 25-1. Endophthalmitis Vitrectomy Study: Incidence of Pathogens Isolated from Patients Presenting with Acute Postoperative Endophthalmitis After Cataract Surgery (190)

Pathogen	Incidence	
Coagulase-negative micrococci	70.0%	
Staphylococcus aureus	9.9%	
Streptococcus species	9.0%	
S. viridans		3.7%
S. pneumoniae		2.2%
S. agalactiae		0.6%
S. acidominimus		0.3%
Other streptococcal sp.		2.2%
Enterococcus species	2.2%	
E. faecalis		1.2%
E. avium		0.3%
Other enterococcus sp.		0.6%
Miscellaneous gram-positive organisms	3.1%	
Propionibacterium acnes		0.3%
Propionibacterium granulosum		0.3%
Corynebacterium sp.		1.2%
Bacillus sp.		0.6%
Diphtheroid sp.		0.6%
Gram-negative organisms	5.9%	
Proteus mirabilis		1.9%
Pseudomonas aeruginosa		0.9%
Other *Pseudomonas* sp.		0.6%
Morganella morganii		0.6%
Citrobacter diversus		0.6%
Serratia marcescens		0.3%
Enterobacter sp.		0.6%
Flavobacterium sp.		0.3%

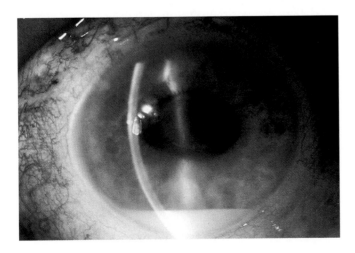

FIGURE 25-24. *Acute fulminant postoperative endophthalmitis. (Courtesy of Harry W. Flynn Jr, MD, Bascom Palmer Eye Institute, University of Miami, Miami, FL.)*

the management of acute postoperative endophthalmitis after cataract extraction surgery. Finally, although visual prognosis was strongly associated with the type of infecting organism, the presenting visual acuity was more important than microbiologic factors in predicting final visual outcome and response to vitrectomy (192).

Endophthalmitis secondary to less virulent species, such as coagulase-negative *Staphylococcus*, *P. acnes*, *Alcaligenes xylosoxidans* (193) and *Acremonium kiliense* (194) often presents with a delayed, low-grade iritis/vitritis and a chronic relapsing time-course. *Propionibacterium acnes* causes characteristic, fluffy intracapsular opacities and/or anterior chamber beading and stranding that are virtually pathognomonic for this infection (195,196). Because the intraocular inflammation associated with these infections often responds to steroid therapy and frequently recurs after the steroid is discontinued, they can easily be mistaken for noninfectious uveitis.

Although the overall incidence of endophthalmitis is small, all measures possible should be taken to prevent the development of this potentially devastating complication. The use of preoperative topical antibiotics and/or iodine preparations to reduce normal flora populations, especially in patients with blepharitis or meibomian gland dysfunction, although of unproven efficacy, seems prudent in selected cases (8–11). The inclusion of antibiotic to the intraoperative irrigation fluid is controversial and also of unproven benefit (197). Improper antibiotic dilution or use of antibiotics that contain preservatives can lead to endothelial toxicity and corneal decompensation. When one also considers the possible selection for antibiotic-resistant strains (198), this practice should perhaps be limited to selected cases or eliminated altogether. Irrigation of the lens before implantation has been shown to reduce bacterial contamination (199) and many surgeons employ this practice prior to IOL implantation in the recipient eye. Finally, although of unproven benefit, many surgeons administer subconjunctival antibiotics at the conclusion of the procedure (8). When endophthalmitis does unfortunately develop, the EVS provides guidelines in selecting the most appropriate course of action to achieve the optimal visual outcome.

SPECIAL SITUATIONS

Capsular Tension Ring

The capsular tension ring (Morcher GmbH) is an open loop PMMA ring that can be introduced into the capsular bag during or after cortical cleanup to support a region of zonular dialysis. These rings are manufactured in several sizes and may be especially useful in a patient with weak zonular support due to pseudoexfoliation or a traumatic cataract with or without preoperative phacodonesis. A properly placed ring supports and stabilizes the capsule preventing vitreous prolapse and allowing for endocapsular placement of an intraocular lens.

Aniridia Intraocular Lens

Patients with enlarged pupils due to aniridia or trauma have traditionally been fitted with aniridic contact lenses which form a substitute pupillary aperture and optimize cosmesis and visual function. However, the necessary pigmentation renders these lenses impermeable to gas exchange. As a consequence, these lenses can generally only be tolerated for short periods of time making them unsatisfactory as a long-term solution. A recently developed alternative for these patients is the aniridic IOL (Morcher GmbH). The aniridic IOL has a permanent aperture formulated into the lens by the incorporation of opaque black pigment into a diaphragm surrounding the lens optic. The pigment is polymerized into the PMMA and is reportedly nontoxic to the eye. These lenses are more fragile than conventional PMMA lenses due to incorporation of pigment into the lens matrix. It is important that this be remembered during intraoperative implantation and manipulation.

Alternatively, a two-piece aniridic diaphragm can be placed within the capsular bag followed by the surgeon's choice of IOL. The two-piece diaphragm is a modification of the capsular tension ring that consists of two interlocking, opaque, black PMMA open-loop rings with teeth. These toothed rings are placed successively into the capsular bag and rotated into a locking position creating an optical aperture. This prosthetic device may be most beneficial in the setting of traumatic cataract with zonular dehiscence and iris/pupillary damage leading to corectopia. Placement of a two-piece aniridic diaphragm serves not only to reform the optical aperture but also to support the capsular bag for subsequent placement of an endocapsular or sulcus-fixated IOL.

CONCLUSION

Cataract surgery, like many fields today, is undergoing constant change and innovation with improvements in surgical machinery and instrumentation, intraocular lenses, patient comfort, postoperative recovery time, and final visual outcomes. This chapter is meant to serve as an introductory guide to phacoemulsification. It is not intended to act as a "cookbook" for cataract surgery. Each surgical case is unique. Prudent surgeons will approach each case with foresight and flexibility so that they can adapt to whatever challenges may arise. To this end it is important for phacoemulsification surgeons to keep abreast of advancements in the field and to incorporate those changes they believe will enhance their surgical finesse and optimize the experience for their patients both during and after the procedure.

BIBLIOGRAPHY

Devine TM, Banko W. Phacoemulsification surgery. New York, NY: Pergamon, 1991.

Jaffe NS, Jaffe MS, Jaffe GF. Cataract surgery and its complications. 6th ed. St. Louis, MO: Mosby, 1997.

Koch PS. Mastering phacoemulsification: a simplified manual of strategies for the spring, crack and stop & chop technique. 4th ed. Thorofare, NJ: Slack, 1994.

Koch PS. Simplifying phacoemulsification. Safe and efficient methods for cataract surgery. Thorofare, NJ: Slack, 1997.

Koch P, Davison J, eds. Phacoemulsification techniques. Thorofare, NJ: Slack, 1991.

Koch PS, Davison JA. Textbook of advanced phacoemulsification techniques. Thorofare, NJ: Slack, 1990.

Maloney WF, Grindle L. Textbook of phacoemulsification. Fallbrook, CA: Lasenda, 1988.

Steinert RF, ed. Cataract surgery: technique, complications and management. Philadelphia, PA: Saunders, 1995.

REFERENCES

1. Kelman CD. Phaco-emulsification and aspiration: a new technique of cataract removal, a preliminary note. *Am J Ophthalmol* 1967;64:23–35.

2. Naus NC, Luyten GPM, Stijnen T, et al. Astigmatism and visual recovery after phacoemulsification and conventional extracapsular cataract extraction. *Doc Ophthalmol* 1995;90:53–59.

3. Seibel BS. Phacodynamics: mastering the tools and techniques of phacoemulsification surgery, 2nd ed. Thorofare, NJ: Slack, 1995.

4. Novak KD, Koch DD. Topical anesthesia for phacoemulsification: initial 20-case series with one month follow-up. *J Cataract Refract Surg* 1995;21:672–675.

5. Gills JP, Cherchio M, Raanan MG. Unpreserved lidocaine to control discomfort during cataract surgery using topical anesthesia. *J Cataract Refract Surg* 1997;23:545–550.

6. Koch PS. Anterior chamber irrigation with unpreserved lidocaine 1% for anesthesia during cataract surgery. *J Cataract Refract Surg* 1997;23:551–554.

7. Wright KW ed. Textbook of ophthalmology. Baltimore, MD: Williams & Wilkins, 1997:784.

8. Starr MB, Lally JM. Antimicrobial prophylaxis for ophthalmic surgery. *Surv Ophthalmol* 1995;39:485–501.

9. Schneider, DM. The role of antibacterial prophylaxis for cataract surgery, *J Cataract Refract Surg* 1993;19:108–111.

10. Apt L, Isenberg SJ, Yoshimori R, et al. Outpatient topical use of povidone-iodine in preparing the eye for surgery. *Ophthalmology* 1989;96:289–292.

11. Speaker MG, Menikoff JA. Prophylaxis of endophthalmitis with topical povidone-iodine. *Ophthalmology* 1991;98:1769–1775.

12. Fine HI. Architecture and construction of a self-sealing incision for cataract surgery. *J Cataract Refract Surg* 1991;17(supp):672–676.

13. Steinert RF, Brint SF, White SM, et al. Astigmatism after small incision cataract surgery: a prospective, randomized, multicenter comparison of 4- and 6.5-mm incisions. *Ophthalmology* 1991;98:417–424.

14. Singer JA. Frown incision for minimizing induced astigmatism after small incision cataract surgery with rigid optic intraocular lens implantation. *J Cataract Refract Surg* 1991;17(Supp):677–688.

15. Koch PS. Mastering phacoemulsification: a simplified manual of strategies for the spring, crack and stop & chop technique. 4th ed. Thorofare, NJ: Slack, 1994:19.

16. Long DA, Monica ML. A prospective evaluation of corneal curvature changes with 3.0- to 3.5-mm corneal tunnel phacoemulsification. *Ophthalmology* 1996;103:226–232.

17. Leyland MD. Corneal curvature changes associated with corneal tunnel phacoemulsification. *Ophthalmology* 1996;103:867–868. Letter.

18. Liesegang TJ. Viscoelastic substances in ophthalmology. *Surv Ophthalmol* 1990;34:268–293.

19. Seigel MJ, Spiro HJ, Miller JA, Siegel LI. Secondary glaucoma and uveitis associated with Orcolon. *Arch Ophthalmol* 1991;109:1496–1497.

20. Koch PS. Simplifying phacoemulsification. Safe and efficient methods for cataract surgery. Thorofare, NJ: Slack, 1997:159–176.

21. Gimbel HV, Neuhann T. Development, advantages and methods of the continuous circular capsulorhexis technique. *J Cataract Refract Surg* 1990;16:31–37.

22. Neuhann T. Theorie und Operationstechnik der Kapsulorhexis. *Klin Monatsbl Augenheilkd* 1987;190:542–545.

23. Gimbel HV, Neuhann T. Continuous curvilinear capsulorhexis. *J Cataract Refract Surg* 1991;17:110. Letter.

24. Sakabe I, Lim SJ, Apple DJ. Anatomical evaluation of the anterior capsular zonular free zone in the human crystalline lens (age range, 50 to approximately 100 years). *Nippon Ganka Gakkai Zasshi* 1995;99:1119–1122.

25. Vajpayee RB, Angra SK, Honavar SG, et al. Capsulotomy for phacoemulsification in hypermature cataracts. *J Cataract Refract Surg* 1995;21:612–615.

26. Koch PS. Mastering phacoemulsification: a simplified manual of strategies for the spring, crack and stop & chop technique. 4th ed. Thorofare, NJ: Slack, 1994:67–77.

27. Gimbel HV. Divide and Conquer. Presented at the European Intraocular Implantlens Council meeting, 1987. Video.

28. Gimbel HV. Divide and conquer nucleofractis phacoemulsification: development and variations. *J Cataract Refract Surg* 1991;17:281–291.

29. Steinert RF, et al. Cataract surgery: technique, complications and management. Philadelphia, PA: Saunders, 1995:166.

30. Koch PS. Mastering phacoemulsification: a simplified manual of strategies for the spring, crack and stop & chop technique. 4th ed. Thorofare, NJ: Slack, 1994:99–103.

31. Fine IH. The chip and flip phacoemulsification technique. *J Cataract Refract Surg* 1991;17:366–371.

32. Maloney WF, Dillman DM, Nichamin LD. Supracapsular phacoemulsification: a capsule-free posterior chamber approach. *J Cataract Refract Surg* 1997;23:323–328.

33. Devine TM, Banko W, eds. Phacoemulsification surgery. New York, NY: Pergamon, 1991:72.

34. Devine TM, Banko W, eds. Phacoemulsification surgery. New York, NY: Pergamon, 1991:77–78.

35. Assia EI, Legler UFC, Libby C, et al. Size and configuration of the capsular bag after short and long term fixation of PC-IOL's in-the-bag. Presented at the American Society of Cataract and Refractive Surgery Annual Meeting, Boston, 1992.

36. Ridley H. Intraocular acrylic lenses: 10 years' development. *Br J Ophthalmol* 1960;44:705–712.

37. Steinert RF, ed. Cataract surgery: technique, complications and management. Philadelphia, PA: Saunders, 1995:273.

38. Mazzocco TR. Progress report: silicone IOL's. *Cataract* 1984;1:18–19.

39. Bath PE, Romberger AB, Brown P. A comparison of Nd-YAG laser damage thresholds for PMMA and silicone intraocular lenses. *Invest Ophthalmol Vis Sci* 1986;27:795–798.

40. Feibel RM. Current concepts in retrobulbar anesthesia. *Surv Ophthalmol* 1985;30:102–110.

41. Cionni R, Osher R. Retrobulbar hemorrhage. *Ophthalmology* 1991;98:1153–1155.

42. Arnold P. Study of acute intraoperative suprachoroidal hemorrhage. *J Cataract Refract Surg* 1992;18:489.

43. Speaker M, Gueirleio P, Reil J, et al. A case control study of risk factors for intraoperative suprachoroidal expulsive hemorrhage. *Ophthalmology* 1991;98:202–210.

44. Steinert RF, ed. Cataract surgery: technique, complications and management. Philadelphia, PA: Saunders, 1995:331.

45. Jaffe N, Horowitz J. Lens and cataract. In: Podos SM, Yanoff M, eds. Textbook of ophthalmology. vol. 3. New York, NY: Raven, 1992:1.4.

46. Jaffe N. Cataract surgery and its complications 3rd ed. St. Louis, MO: Mosby, 1981:368, 576–579.

47. Osher R, Cionni R. The torn posterior capsule: its intraoperative behavior, surgical management and long term consequences. *J Cataract Refract Surg* 1990;16:490–494.

48. Jaffe N, Horowitz J. Lens and cataract. In: Podos SM, Yanoff M, eds. Textbook of ophthalmology. vol. 3. New York, NY: Raven, 1992:17.1–17.8.

49. Steinert RF, ed. Cataract surgery: technique, complications and management. Philadelphia, PA: Saunders, 1995:328.

50. Tripathi RC, Tripathi BJ. Lens morphology, aging, and cataract. *J Gerontol* 1983;38:258.

51. Lambrou FH Jr, Stewart MW. Management of dislocated lens fragments during phacoemulsification. *Ophthalmology* 1992;99:1260–1262.

52. Fastenberg DM, Schwartz PL, Shakin JL, et al. Management of dislocated nuclear fragments after phacoemulsification. *Am J Ophthalmol* 1991;112:535–539.

53. Aaberg TM Jr, Rubsamen PE, Flynn HW Jr, et al. Giant retinal tears as a complication of attempted removal of intravitreal lens fragments during cataract surgery. *Am J Ophthalmol* 1997;124:222–226.

54. Vilar NF, Flynn HW Jr, Smiddy WE, et al. Removal of retained lens fragments after phacoemulsification reverses secondary glaucoma and restores visual acuity. *Ophthalmology* 1997;104:787–792.

55. Irvine WD, Flynn HW Jr, Murray TG, et al. Retained lens fragments after phacoemulsification manifesting as marked intraocular inflammation and hypopyon. *Am J Ophthalmol* 1992;114:610–614.

56. Smiddy WE, Flynn HW Jr. Management of retained lens fragments and dislocated posterior chamber intraocular lenses after cataract surgery. *Semin Ophthalmology* 1993;8:96–103.

57. Blodi BA, Flynn HW Jr, Blodi CF, et al. Retained nuclei after cataract surgery. *Ophthalmology* 1992;99:41–44.

58. Hutton WL, Snyder WB, Vaiser A. Management of surgically dislocated intravitreal lens fragments by pars plana vitrectomy. *Ophthalmology* 1978;85:176–189.

59. Gilliland GD, Hutton WL, Fuller DG. Retained intravitreal lens fragments after cataract surgery. *Ophthalmology* 1992;99:1263–1269.

60. Michels RG, Shacklett DE. Vitrectomy technique for removal of retained lens material. *Arch Ophthalmol* 1977;95:1767–1773.

61. Smiddy WE, Flynn HW Jr. Managing retained lens fragments and dislocated PC-IOLs after cataract surgery. Focal Points (modules), American Academy of Ophthalmology 1996;14, 0.7.

62. Kim JE, Flynn HW, Smiddy WE, et al. Retained lens fragments after phacoemulsification. *Ophthalmology* 1994;101:1827–1832.

63. Steinert RF, ed. Cataract surgery: technique, complications and management. Philadelphia, PA: Saunders, 1995:368.

64. Percival SPB, Das SK. UGH syndrome after posterior chamber lens implantation. *Am Intraocular Implant Soc J* 1983;9:200–201.

65. Berger RO. Fox shield treatment of the UGH syndrome. *J Cataract Refract Surg* 1986;12:419–421.

66. Masket S. Pseudophakic posterior iris chafing syndrome. *J Cataract Refract Surg* 1986;12:252–256.

67. Alpar JJ. Glaucoma after intraocular lens implantation: survey and recommendations. *Glaucoma* 1985;7:241–245.

68. Choyce DP. Complications of the anterior chamber implants of the early 1950's and the UGH syndrome or Ellingson syndrome of the late 1970's. *Am Intraocular Implant Soc J* 1978;4:22–29.

69. Ellingson FT. The uveitis-glaucoma-hyphema syndrome associated with the Mark VIII anterior chamber lends implant. *Am Intraocular Implant Soc J* 1978;4:50–53.

70. Moses L. Complications of rigid anterior chamber implants. *Ophthalmology* 1984;91:819–825.

71. Nicholson DH. Occult iris erosion: A treatable cause of recurrent hyphema in iris-supported intraocular lenses. *Ophthalmology* 1982;89:113–120.

72. Apple DJ, Mamalis N, Loftfield K, et al. Complications of intraocular lenses. A historical and histopathological review. *Surv Ophthalmol* 1984;29:1–54.

73. Pazandak B, Johnson S, Kratz R. Recurrent intraocular hemorrhage associated with posterior chamber lens implantation. *Am Intraocular Implant Soc J* 1983;9:327–329.

74. Swan KC, Campbell L. Unintentional Filtration following cataract surgery. *Arch Ophthalmol* 1964;71:43–49.

75. Lambrou FH, Kozarsky A. Wound dehiscence following cataract surgery. *Ophthalmic Surg* 1987;18:738–740.

76. Koch PS. Structural analysis of cataract incision construction. *J Cataract Refract Surg* 1991;17(supp):661–667.

77. Flaxel JT, Swan KC. Limbal wound healing after cataract extraction. *Arch Ophthalmol* 1969;81:653–659.

78. Flaxel JT. Histology of cataract extractions. *Arch Ophthalmol* 1970;83:436–444.

79. Gliedman ML, Karlson KE. Wound healing and wound strength of sutured limbal wounds. *Am J Ophthalmol* 1955;39:859–865.

80. Masuda K. Tensile strength of corneoscleral wounds repaired with absorbable sutures. *Ophthalmic Surg* 1981;12:110–114.

81. Koch DD, Smith SH, Whiteside SB. Limbal and scleral wound healing. In: Healing processes in the cornea. The Woodlands: Portfolio, 1989:165–181.

82. Jonas JB, Ruprecht KW, et al. Ophthalmic surgical complications in Werner's syndrome: report on 18 eyes of nine patients. *Ophthalmic Surg* 1987;18:760–764.

83. Fechner PU, Wichmann W. Retarded corneoscleral wound healing associated with high preoperative doses of systemic steroids in glaucoma surgery. *Refract Corneal Surg* 1991;7:174–176.

84. Steinert RF, ed. Cataract surgery: technique, complications and management. Philadelphia, PA: Saunders, 1995:353–354.

85. Waring GO, Bourne WM, Edelhauser HF, et al. The corneal endothelium: Normal and pathologic structure and function. *Ophthalmology* 1982;89:531–590.

86. Steinert RF, ed. Cataract surgery: technique, complications and management. Philadelphia, PA: Saunders, 1995:358.

87. Brown SI, McLean JM. Peripheral corneal edema after cataract extraction: A new clinical entity. *Trans Am Acad Ophthalmol Otolaryngol* 1969;73:465–470.

88. Steinert RF, ed. Cataract surgery: technique, complications and management. Philadelphia, PA: Saunders, 1995:358–363.

89. Nuyts RMMA, Edelhauser HF, Pells EII, Breebaart AC. Toxic effects of detergents on the corneal endothelium. *Arch Ophthalmol* 1990;108:1158–1162.

90. Binkhorst CD. Inflammation and intraocular pressure after the use of Healon in intraocular lens surgery. *Am Intraocular Implant Soc J* 1980;6:340–341.

91. Genstler DE, Keates RH. Amvisc in extracapsular cataract extraction. *Am Intraocular Implant Soc J* 1983;9:317–320.

92. Glasser DB, Matsuda M, Edelhauser HF. A comparison of the efficacy and toxicity of and intraocular pressure response to viscous solutions in the anterior chamber. *Arch Ophthalmol* 1986;104:1819–1824.

93. Olivius E, Thorburn W. Intraocular pressure after surgery with Healon. *Am Intraocular Implant Soc J* 1985;11:480–482.

94. Lane SS, Naylor DW, Kullerstrand LJ, et al. Prospective comparison of the effects of Occucoat, Viscoat, and Healon on intraocular pressure and endothelial cell loss. *J Cataract Refract Surg* 1991;17:21–26.

95. Berson FG, Patterson MM, Epstein DL. Obstruction of aqueous outflow by sodium hyaluronate in enucleated human eyes. *Am J Ophthalmol* 1983;95:668–672.

96. Cherfan GM, Rich WJ, Wright G. Raised intraocular pressure and other problems with sodium hyaluronate and cataract surgery. *Trans Ophthal Soc UK* 1983;103:277–279.

97. Handa J, Henry JC, Krupin T, et al. Extracapsular cataract extraction with posterior chamber lens implantation in patients with glaucoma. *Arch Ophthalmol* 1987;105:765–769.

98. Anmarkrud N, Bergaust B, Bulie T. The effect of Healon and timolol on early postoperative intraocular pressure after extracapsular cataract extraction with implantation of a posterior chamber lens. *Acta Ophthalmol* 1992;70:96–100.

99. Armaly MF. Effects of corticosteroids on intraocular pressure and fluid dynamics: 1. The effect of dexamethasone in the normal eye. *Arch Ophthalmol* 1963;70:482–491.

100. Spaeth GL, Rodrigues MM, Weinreb S. Steroid-induced glaucoma: A. Persistent elevation of intraocular pressure. B. Histopathologic aspects. *Trans Am Ophthalmol Soc* 1977;75:353–381.

101. Irvine SR. A newly defined vitreous syndrome following cataract surgery. *Am J Ophthalmol* 1953;36:599–619.

102. Gass JDM, Norton EWD. Cystoid macular edema and papilledema following cataract extraction. *Arch Ophthalmol* 1966;76:646–661.

103. Iliff CE. Treatment of vitreous-tug syndrome. *Am J Ophthalmol* 1966;62:856–859.

104. Steinert RF, Wasson PJ. Neodymium: YAG laser anterior vitreolysis for Irvine-Gass cystoid macular edema. *J Cataract Refract Surg* 1989;15:304–307.

105. Epstein DL, Steinert RF, Puliafito CA. Neodymium-YAG laser therapy to the anterior hyaloid in aphakic malignant (ciliovitreal block) glaucoma. *Am J Ophthalmol* 1984;98:137–143.

106. Mackenzie W. A practical treatise on the disease of the eye. London: Longman, Rees, Orme, Brown and Green, 1830.

107. Perera CA. Epithelium in the anterior chamber of the eye after operation and injury. *Trans Am Acad Ophthalmol Otolaryngol* 1937;42:142–164.

108. Terry TL, Chisholm JF, Schonberg AL. Studies on the surface-epithelium invasion of the anterior segment of the eye. *Am J Ophthalmol* 1939;22:1083–1110.

109. Theobald GD, Haas JS. Epithelial invasion of the anterior chamber following cataract extraction. *Trans Am Acad Ophthalmol Otolaryngol* 1948;52:470–485.

110. Farmer SG, Kalina RE. Epithelial implantation cyst of the iris. *Ophthalmology* 1981;88:1286–1289.

111. Cogan DG. Experimental implants of conjunctiva into the anterior chamber. *Am J Ophthalmol* 1955;39:165–172.

112. Regan EF. Epithelial invasion of the anterior chamber. *Arch Ophthalmol* 1958;60:907–927.

113. Ferry AP. The possible role of epithelial-bearing surgical instruments in pathogenesis of epithelialization of the anterior chamber. *Ann Ophthalmol* 1971;3:1089–1093.

114. Sitchevska O, Payne BF. Pearl cyst of the iris. *Am J Ophthalmol* 1951;34:833–840.

115. Orlin SE, Raber IM, Laibson PR, et al. Epithelial downgrowth following the removal of iris inclusion cysts. *Ophthalmic Surg* 1991;22:330–335.

116. Steinert RF, ed. Cataract surgery: technique, complications and management. Philadelphia, PA: Saunders, 1995:398.

117. Winthrop SR, Smith RE. Spontaneous regression of an anterior chamber cyst: A case report. *Ann Ophthalmol* 1981;13:431–432.

118. Calhoun FP, Jr. The clinical recognition and treatment of epithelialization of the anterior chamber following cataract extraction. *Trans Am Ophthalmol Soc* 1949;47:498–553.

119. Steinert RF, ed. Cataract surgery: technique, complications and management. Philadelphia, PA: Saunders, 1995:401–410.

120. Brown SI. Results of excision of advanced epithelial downgrowth. *Ophthalmology* 1979;86:321–328.

121. Wilhelmus KR, Emery JM. Posterior capsule opacification following phacoemulsification. *Ophthalmic Surg* 1980;11:264–267.

122. Sterling S, Wood TO. Effect of intraocular lens convexity on posterior capsule opacification. *J Cataract Refract Surg* 1986;12:655–657.

123. Downing JE. Long-term discission rate after placing posterior chamber lenses with the convex surface posterior. *J Cataract Refract Surg* 1986;12:651–654.

124. Born CP, Ryan DK. Effect of intraocular lens optic design on posterior capsular opacification. *J Cataract Refract Surg* 1990;16:188–192.

125. Johnson SH, Kratz RP, Olson PF. Clinical experience with the Nd:YAG laser. *Am Intraocular Implant Soc J* 1984;10:452–460.

126. Stark WJ, Worthen D, Holladay JT, et al. Neodymium:YAG lasers. An FDA report. *Ophthalmology* 1985;92:209–212.

127. Bath PE, Frankhouser F. Long-term results of Nd:YAG laser posterior capsulotomy with the Swiss laser. *J Cataract Refract Surg* 1986;12:150–153.

128. Aron-Rosa DS. Pulsed picosecond and nanosecond YAG-lasers-principles and uses. *Cataract* 1984;1:9–18.

129. Slomovic AR, Parrish RK II. Acute elevations of intraocular pressure following Nd:YAG laser capsulotomy. *Ophthalmology* 1985;92:973–976.

130. Richter CU, Arzeno G, Pappas H, et al. Intraocular pressure elevation following Nd:YAG laser posterior capsulotomy. *Ophthalmology* 1985;92:636–640.

131. Flohr MJ, Robin AL, Kelley JS. Early complications following Q-switched neodymium:YAG laser posterior capsulotomy. *Ophthalmology* 1985;92:360–363.

132. Channell MM, Beckman H. Intraocular pressure changes after neodymium:YAG laser posterior capsulotomy. *Arch Ophthalmol* 1984;102:1024–1026.

133. Aron-Rosa DS. Posterior capsulotomy and picosecond pulsed YAG laser influence on eye pressure. *Cataract* 1983;1:13–17.

134. Brown SVL, Thomas JV, Belcher CD, et al. Effect of pilocarpine in treatment of intraocular pressure elevation following neodymium:YAG laser posterior capsulotomy. *Ophthalmology* 1985;92:354–359.

135. Powell SK, Olson RJ. Incidence of retinal detachment after cataract surgery and neodymium:YAG laser capsulotomy. *J Cataract Refract Surg* 1995;21:132–135.

136. Van Westenbrugge JA, Gimbel HV, Souchek J, et al. Incidence of retinal detachment following Nd:YAG capsulotomy after cataract surgery. *J Cataract Refract Surg* 1992;18:352–355.

137. Salvesen S, Eide N, Syrdalen P. Retinal detachment after YAG-laser capsulotomy. *Acta Ophthalmol* 1991;69:61–64.

138. Rickman-Barger L, Florine CW, Larson RS, et al. Retinal detachment after neodymium:YAG laser posterior capsulotomy. *Am J Ophthalmol* 1989;107:531–536.

139. Leff SR, Welch JC, Tasman W. Rhegmatogenous retinal detachment after YAG laser posterior capsulotomy. *Ophthalmology* 1987;94:1222–1225.

140. Keates RH, Steinert RF, Puliafito CA, et al. Long-term follow-up of Nd:YAG laser posterior capsulotomy. *Am Intraocular Implant Soc J* 1984;10:164–168.

141. Winslow RL, Taylor BC. Retinal complications following YAG capsulotomy. *Ophthalmology* 1985;92:785–789.

142. Steinert RF, Puliafito CA, Kumar SR, et al. Cystoid macular edema, retinal detachment, and Glaucoma after Nd:YAG laser posterior capsulotomy. *Am J Ophthalmol* 1991;112:373–380.

143. Shah GR, Gills JP, Durham DG, et al. Three thousand YAG lasers in posterior capsulotomies: an analysis of complications and comparison to polishing and surgical discission. *Ophthalmic Surg* 1986;17:473.

144. Fallor MK, Hoft RK. Intraocular lens damage associated with posterior capsulotomy: a comparison of intraocular lens design and four different Nd:YAG laser instruments. *Am Intraocular Implant Soc J* 1985;11:564–567.

145. Blacharski PA, Newsome DA. Bilateral macular holes after Nd:YAG laser posterior capsulotomy. *Am J Ophthalmol* 1988;105:417–418.

146. Slomovic AR, Parrish RK II, Forster RK, et al. Neodymium:YAG laser posterior capsulotomy. Central corneal endothelial cell density. *Arch Ophthalmol* 1986;104:536–538.

147. Schrems W, Belcher CD III, Tomlinson CP. Changes in the human central corneal endothelium after neodymium:YAG laser surgery. *Ophthalmic Laser Ther* 1986;1:143–152.

148. Koch DD, Liu JF, Gill EP, et al. Axial myopia increases the risk of retinal complications after neodymium:YAG laser posterior capsulotomy. *Arch Ophthalmol* 1989;107:986–990.

149. Dardenne MY, Gerten GJ, Kokkas K, et al. Retrospective study of retinal detachment following neodymium:YAG laser posterior capsulotomy. *J Cataract Refract Surg* 1989;15:676–680.

150. Piest KL, Kincaid MC, Tetz MR, et al. Localized endophthalmitis: a newly described cause of the so-called toxic lens syndrome. *J Cataract Refract Surg* 1987;13:498–510.

151. Carlson AN, Koch DD. Endophthalmitis following Nd:YAG laser posterior capsulotomy. *Ophthalmic Surg* 1988;19:168–170.

152. Tetz MR, Apple DJ, Price FW, et al. A newly described complication of neodymium:YAG laser posterior capsulotomy: exacerbation of an intraocular infection. *Arch Ophthalmol* 1987;105:1324–1325.

153. Chambless WS. Neodymium:YAG laser posterior capsulotomy results and complications. *Am J Intraocular Implant Soc* 1985;11:31–32.

154. Terry AC, Stark WJ, Maumenee AE, et al. Neodymium-YAG laser for posterior capsulotomy. *Am J Ophthalmol* 1983;96:716–720.

155. Wasserman EL, Axt JC, Sheets JH. Neodymium-YAG laser posterior capsulotomy. *Am Intraocular Implant Soc J* 1985;11:245–248.

156. Wright PL, Wilkinson CP, Balyeat HD, et al. Angiographic cystoid macular edema after posterior chamber lens implantation. *Arch Ophthalmol* 1988;106:740–744.

157. Gass JDM, Norton EWD. Follow-up study of cystoid macular edema following cataract extraction. *Trans Am Acad Ophthalmol Otolaryngol* 1969;73:665–682.

158. Steinert RF, ed. Cataract surgery: technique, complications and management. Philadelphia, PA: Saunders, 1995:416.

159. Nussenblatt RB, Kaufman SC, Palestine AG, et al. Macular thickening and visual acuity. Measurement in patients with cystoid macular edema. *Ophthalmology* 1987;94:1134–1139.

160. Jampol LM. Cystoid macular edema following cataract surgery. *Arch Ophthalmol* 1988;106:894–895. Letter.

161. Tso MOM. Pathology of cystoid macular edema. *Ophthalmology* 1982;89:902–915.

162. Jampol LM. Pharmacologic therapy of aphakic cystoid macular edema: a review. *Ophthalmology* 1982;89:891–897.

163. Jampol LM. Pharmacologic therapy of aphakic and pseudophakic cystoid macular edema: 1985 update. *Ophthalmology* 1985;92:807–810.

164. Flach AJ. Cyclo-oxygenase inhibitors in ophthalmology. *Surv Ophthalmol* 1992;36:259–284.

165. Burnett J, Tessler H, Isenberg S, et al. Double-masked trial of fenoprofen sodium: treatment of chronic aphakic cystoid macular edema. *Ophthalmic Surg* 1983;14:150–152.

166. Flach AJ, Jampol LM, Weinberg D, et al. Improvement in visual acuity in chronic aphakic and pseudophakic cystoid macular edema after treatment with topical 0.5% ketorolac tromethamine. *Am J Ophthalmol* 1991;112:514–519.

167. Cox SN, Hay E, Bird AC. Treatment of chronic macular edema with acetazolamide. *Arch Ophthalmol* 1988;106:1190–1195.

168. Flach AJ. Cystoid macular edema following cataract surgery. *Arch Ophthalmol* 1989;107:166. Letter.

169. Steinert RF, ed. Cataract surgery: technique, complications and management. Philadelphia, PA: Saunders, 1995:417–419.

170. Fung WE. Vitrectomy for chronic aphakic cystoid macular edema. Results of a national, collaborative, prospective, randomized investigation. *Ophthalmology* 1985;92:1102.

171. Harbour JW, Smiddy WE, Rubsamen PE, et al. Pars plana vitrectomy for chronic pseudophakic cystoid macular edema. *Am J Ophthalmol* 1995;120:302–307.

172. Davison JA. Retinal tears and detachments after extracapsular cataract surgery. *J Cataract Refract Surg* 1988;14:624–632.

173. Javitt JC, Street DA, Tielsch JM, et al. National outcomes of cataract extraction: Retinal detachment and endophthalmitis after outpatient cataract surgery. *Ophthalmology* 1994;101:100–106.

174. Smith PW, Stark WJ, Maumeneee AE, et al. Retinal detachment after extracapsular cataract extraction with posterior chamber intraocular lens. *Ophthalmology* 1987;94:495–504.

175. Javitt JC, Vitale S, Canner JK, et al. National outcomes of cataract extraction I. Retinal detachment after inpatient surgery. *Ophthalmology* 1991;98:895–902.

176. Wilkinson CP, Anderson LS, Little JH. Retinal detachment following phacoemulsification. *Ophthalmology* 1978;85:151–156.

177. Steinert RF, ed. Cataract surgery: technique, complications and management. Philadelphia, PA: Saunders, 1995:435.

178. Steinert RF, ed. Cataract surgery: technique, complications and management. Philadelphia, PA: Saunders, 1995:434.

179. McDonnell PJ, Patel A, Green WR. Comparison of intracapsular and extracapsular cataract surgery: histopathologic study of eyes obtained postmortem. *Ophthalmology* 1985;92:1208–1225.

180. Javitt JC, Vitale S, Canner JK, et al. National outcomes of cataract surgery: Endophthalmitis following inpatient surgery. *Arch Ophthalmol* 1991;109:1085–1089.

181. Kattan HM, Flynn HW, Pflugfelder SC, et al. Nosocomial endophthalmitis survey. Current incidence of infection following intraocular surgery. *Ophthalmology* 1991;98:227–238.

182. Aaberg TM Jr, Flynn HW, Newton J. Nosocomial endophthalmitis survey: a 10-year review of incidence and outcomes. *Ophthalmology* 1998. Submitted.

183. Weber DJ, Hoffman KL, Thoft RA, et al. Endophthalmitis following intraocular lens implantation: report of 30 cases and review of the literature. *Rev Infect Dis* 1986;8:12–20.

184. Cameron ME, Forster TDC. Endophthalmitis occurring during hospitalization following cataract surgery. *Ophthalmic Surg* 1978;9:52–57.

185. Allen HF, Mangiaracine AB. Bacterial endophthalmitis after cataract extraction. II. Incidence in 36,000 consecutive operations with special reference to preoperative topical antibiotics. *Arch Ophthalmol* 1974;91:3–7.

186. Steinert RF, ed. Cataract surgery: technique, complications and management. Philadelphia, PA: Saunders, 1995:427.

187. Menikoff JA, Speaker MG, Marmor M, Raskin EM. A case-control study of risk factors for postoperative endophthalmitis. *Ophthalmology* 1991;98:1761–1768.

188. Puliafito CA, Baker AS, Haaf J, Foster CS. Infectious endophthalmitis. *Ophthalmology* 1982;89:921–929.

189. Speaker MG, Milch FA, Shah MK, et al. Role of external bacterial flora in the pathogenesis of acute postoperative endophthalmitis. *Ophthalmology* 1991;98:639–650.

190. Han DP, Wisniewski SR, Wilson LA, et al. Spectrum and susceptibilities of microbiologic isolates in the endophthalmitis vitrectomy study. *Am J Ophthalmol* 1996;122:1–17.

191. The Endophthalmitis Vitrectomy Study Group. Results of the endophthalmitis vitrectomy study. A randomized trial of immediate vitrectomy and of intravenous antibiotics for the treatment of postoperative bacterial endophthalmitis. *Arch Ophthalmol* 1995;113: 1479–1496.

192. The Endophthalmitis Vitrectomy Study Group. Microbiologic factors and visual outcome in the endophthalmitis vitrectomy study. *Am J Ophthalmol* 1996;122:830–846.

193. Aaberg TM Jr, Rubsamen PE, Joondeph BC, Flynn HW Jr. Chronic postoperative gram-negative endophthalmitis. *Retina* 1997;17:260–262.

194. Weissgold DJ, Maguire AM, Brucker AJ. Management of postoperative *Acremonium* endophthalmitis. *Ophthalmology* 1996;103:749–756.

195. Roussel TJ, Culbertson WW, Jaffe NS. Chronic postoperative endophthalmitis associated with *Propionibacterium acnes*. *Arch Ophthalmol* 1987;105:1199–1201.

196. Winward KE, Pflugfelder SC, Flynn HW Jr, et al. Postoperative *Propionibacterium acnes* endophthalmitis. *Ophthalmology* 1993;100:447–451.

197. Gimbel HV, Sun R, De Broff BM, et al. Anterior chamber fluid cultures following phacoemulsification. *Ophthalmic Surg Lasers* 1996;27:121–126.

198. Jones DB. Emerging antibiotic resistance: real and relative. *Arch Ophthalmol* 1996;114:91–92.

199. Valfidis GC, March RJ, Stacey AR. Bacterial contamination of intraocular lens surgery. *Br J Ophthalmol* 1984;68:520–523.

Cataract Surgery in Children

Hilda Capó   Michelle Muñoz

Management of pediatric cataracts may involve ophthalmologists with various backgrounds, including pediatric ophthalmic surgeons and anterior segment surgeons with experience in adult cataract surgery. A variety of surgical procedures have been used to treat children with cataracts, and the surgeon's choice of technique may depend on his or her own background and experience as well as the unique characteristics of the case at hand. The following chapter is written considering the experienced adult cataract surgeon who may be involved in treating the child with cataract. A complementary chapter, "Pediatric Cataract Surgery" (Chapter 63), is located in the "Pediatric Ophthalmic and Strabismus Surgery" section.

As a result of the ongoing visual development, the management of cataracts in children has great impact. Difficult issues need to be considered: When is cataract surgery indicated? What kind of optical rehabilitation should be used? In children with monocular cataracts, how does one deal with the ever-present amblyopia?

HISTORY AND LABORATORY EVALUATION[*]

Determining the etiology of infantile cataracts is often an elusive task, even though it is foremost in both the parents' and the physician's minds. A cause can be found in only approximately 50% of bilateral infantile cataracts. In monocular cataracts it is rare to find a cause (1). The most frequently identified cause in patients with bilateral infantile cataracts is genetic, with the most common mode of transmission being autosomal dominant with a high degree of penetrance and variable expression (1). Family members may

have asymptomatic cataracts, thus requiring slit-lamp biomicroscopy before excluding this cause.

Intrauterine Infections

During review of the prenatal history ophthalmologists should explore the possibility of an intrauterine infection, such as rubella, cytomegalovirus (CMV) infection, toxoplasmosis, and herpes simplex, as a cause for the infantile cataracts.

Rubella

Since 1981, following the institution of national vaccination programs, there has been a significant reduction in the incidence of congenital rubella in the United States (2). However, it remains an important cause of infantile cataracts in countries with no immunization programs. The risk of fetal infection is high when maternal rubella is present during the first trimester of pregnancy. The classic signs of clinical rubella—rash, arthralgia, lymphadenopathy, and fever—are often absent in a maternal infection (3). The congenital rubella syndrome consists of the triad of cataract, congenital heart disease, and deafness. Cataracts are found in 39% to 50% of children with congenital rubella syndrome (2). Other ocular findings include corneal haze, which may be transient; glaucoma; microphthalmia; and a salt and pepper retinopathy. If rubella is suspected, the titers of IgM and IgG antibodies against rubella are measured. Approximately 20% of congenital rubella children have declining rubella antibody titers and the diagnosis needs to be confirmed with viral cultures from the throat or urine (3).

Toxoplasmosis

The prevalence of toxoplasmosis shows great variability. The incidence of congenital infection is highest in the countries

---

[*] See also "Embryology, Associated Ocular and Systemic Problems, Inheritance, and Classifications" section in Chapter 63.

with a high prevalence. This protozoan parasite can be transmitted by the consumption of the cyst forms in partially or uncooked infected meat, or the ingestion of oocysts following contact with feces of felines. The fetus is at risk during a primary infection. Signs of disease at birth include toxoplasmic retinitis, cataracts, cerebral calcifications, convulsions, jaundice, and splenomegaly. The principal lesion in toxoplasmic retinitis is white with retinal destruction and becomes surrounded by heavy pigmentation. Most congenitally infected infants show no signs of disease at birth and serologic diagnosis is helpful. When toxoplasmosis is diagnosed, the recommended protocol is treatment for a year with sulfadiazine and pyrimethamine to decrease neurologic and ophthalmic sequelae (4).

Cytomegalovirus Infection

The majority of infections due to CMV are either subclinical or associated with a mild short-lived febrile illness. The best method to establish the diagnosis in an infant is isolation of the virus. Serologic tests are not satisfactory. Isolation of the virus in the first 10 to 14 days of life suggests prenatal infection. Differentiation of prenatal and perinatal infection 4 to 6 weeks after birth or later is difficult (5). Ocular disease in children with congenital CMV infection is far less common than in children with congenital rubella. Eye pathology, cataracts and multiple areas of chorioretinitis, is confined to those with generalized disease in the neonatal period. These infants often demonstrate cerebral calcifications.

Herpes Simplex

Intrapartum herpes simplex infections are usually caused by the genital strain of the virus (type 2), even though clinical disease in the mother may be absent at the time of delivery (5). Vesicular skin lesions are the most common manifestation and the diagnosis is best established by isolation of the virus. The diagnosis of an intrauterine infection is particularly important as a result of its potential for multiple system involvement, specially the central nervous system. The history should be supplemented with serologic testing (TORCH levels). If an intrauterine infection is strongly suspected we should also try to isolate the organism by culture because IgM is not always elevated in the neonatal period (5).

Metabolic Disorders

Metabolic disorders can present with bilateral cataracts at birth or in the first few months of life. The birth weight and general health of the child should be ascertained. As a general rule metabolic disorders associated with cataracts are not seen in healthy children. Hyoglycemia or hypocalcemia can be associated with infantile cataracts. They can occur in the neonatal period in infants with low birth weight and will often result in seizures. In infants suspected of having a metabolic basis for their cataracts serum calcium and glu-

cose levels should be measured. Classical galactosemia or galactose-1-phosphate uridyl transferase deficiency is associated with failure to thrive, hepatomegaly, and cataracts. The only metabolic disorder associated with cataracts in an otherwise asymptomatic child is galactokinase deficiency. These last two conditions can be diagnosed by checking the urine for reducing substances 1 to 2 hours after a galactose containing meal. If galactose is not ingested before the test, a false negative result may be obtained. If reducing substances are present in the urine, the specific enzymatic deficiency can be determined with a red blood cells' assay. Children who fail to thrive and have cataracts should also have their urine screened for amino acids. Lowe syndrome is an X-linked recessive condition associated with aminoaciduria.

The general health of the infant should be assessed by a pediatrician. If in addition to the cataracts there is involvement of two or more organ systems or dysmorphic features, chromosomal studies should be performed. The most common genetic abnormality in association with cataracts in children is trisomy 21 (6).

In summary, a minimum laboratory work-up of a patient with infantile cataracts includes measurements of TORCH titers, serum calcium and phosphorus levels, and blood glucose concentration and tests of urine for reducing substances (and amino acids if appropriate). This work-up can be omitted in the presence of a positive family history. A pediatric evaluation should determine if there are associated abnormalities.

GENETIC COUNSELING

There are some important considerations when one is counseling a family with a history of bilateral infantile cataracts. As mentioned, the most common mode of transmission is autosomal dominant, with high penetrance and variable expression. The risk to an individual with bilateral infantile cataracts of having an affected child is high, even for an isolated case, probably close to 50% with each pregnancy. The risk to the parents of an isolated affected child of having further affected children depends on the findings on slit-lamp biomicroscopy. If the lenses are normal, then the risk of having another affected child is around 10%, because most cases are likely to represent new mutations. A minority may be due to nonpenetrance in the parent, recessive inheritance, or gonadal mosaicism, with higher recurrence risks. If any of the parents has a lenticular opacity, then the risk of having another affected child rises to 50% (7).

CLINICAL EXAMINATION*

Children with congenital cataracts are often referred to the ophthalmologist soon after birth, when an abnormal red reflex is noticed. Often they will not be able to fix and

---

* See also "Descriptive Terminology and Classifications" section in Chapter 63.

follow, yet the ophthalmologist needs to assess the effect of the lenticular opacity on normal visual development. The morphology of the cataract is very helpful in ascertaining the visual prognosis (8). A hungry infant can be examined easily with a portable slit lamp while he or she is being fed. The regular slit lamp can be used as well, by putting the infant in a supine position and bringing the head forward toward the lamp so that the neck is hyperextended and the forehead touches the support band. The morphology, location, density, and size of the cataract can then be adequately assessed and the cataract classified.

Clinical Classification

The clinical classification is as follows (Fig. 26-1) (9).

Lamellar Cataracts

Either present at birth or acquired in the postnatal period, lamellar cataracts include the cortical lamellae surrounding the fetal nucleus. They are usually bilateral, though they can be asymmetric. Their diameter is 5 to 6 mm, but they are often encircled by "riders," spokelike opacified lens fibers

extending toward the periphery. In these cataracts the density of the opacity is critical. In spite of their considerable extension, normal visual development can still occur if they are not dense (Fig. 26-2). They may progress to the point where they require surgery but visual prognosis is good for patients who undergo surgery at a later age (8).

Nuclear Cataracts

Nuclear cataracts are usually bilateral. If dense, they are often associated with microphthalmia. They may consist of a pulverulent translucent opacity in the embryonic nucleus, with minimal impairment of vision (Fig. 26-3). At other times a dense opacity within the Y sutures can result in severe deprivation amblyopia (Fig. 26-4). In these instances, the fetal nuclear cataract is usually combined with an opacity of

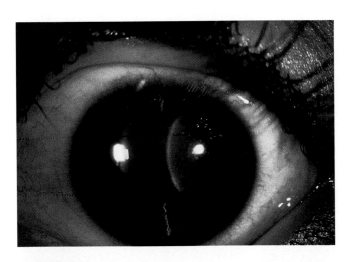

FIGURE 26-2. *Lamellar cataract. Slit-lamp view demonstrates low density. Visual acuity is 20/40.*

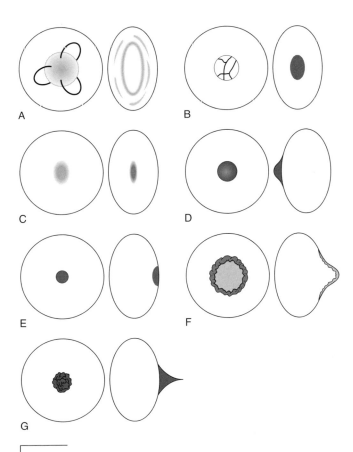

FIGURE 26-1. *Infantile cataracts. A. Lamellar with cortical "riders". B. Nuclear, involving fetal and embryonic nucleus. C. Nuclear, involving embryonic nucleus only. D. Anterior polar. E. Posterior subcapsular. F. Posterior lenticonus. G. Persistent hyperplastic primary vitreous.*

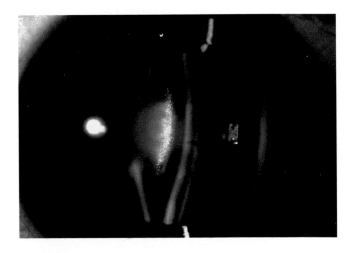

FIGURE 26-3. *Opacity of the embryonic nucleus. The tissue is translucent with visual acuity of 20/30.*

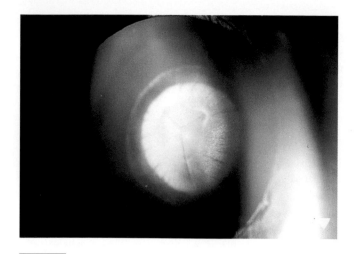

FIGURE 26-4.   *Dense fetal nuclear cataract between the Y sutures. This cataract is very amblyopiogenic.*

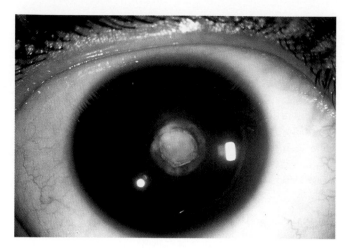

FIGURE 26-6.   *Anterior polar cataract with reduplication of the anterior capsule underneath. Visual acuity has deteriorated.*

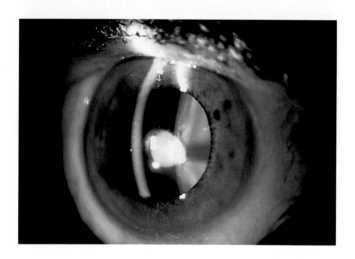

FIGURE 26-5.   *Anterior polar cataract.*

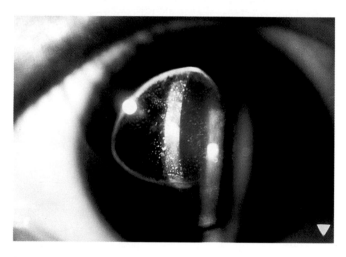

FIGURE 26-7.   *Posterior lenticonus. The bulge in the lens represents a posterior capsular defect.*

the embryonic nucleus, occupying 3.5 mm of axial lens tissue.

Anterior Polar Cataracts

Localized in the anterior capsule, these cataracts rarely affect normal visual development (Fig. 26-5). However, when unilateral or asymmetric they are often associated with anisometropia, which can then result in amblyopia. If 3 mm or larger, they can result in deprivation amblyopia and require surgery. Though usually these cataracts are not progressive, rarely there is reduplication of the capsule underneath the cataract with deteriorating visual acuity (Fig. 26-6).

Posterior Subcapsular Cataracts

These types of cataracts usually involve the posterior cortex. They have a worse prognosis than anterior polar

cataracts as a result of their proximity to the nodal point of the eye. Surgery needs to be considered if they are 3 mm or larger.

Posterior Lenticonus

Posterior lenticonus is usually unilateral and identified around the age of 4 years. A posterior subcapsular ring surrounds a herniation of the posterior capsule toward the vitreous (Fig. 26-7). The etiology is not clear but it may represent a congenitally weak posterior capsule (10). There is progressive opacification of the posterior cortex as the defective capsular area gradually stretches. The opacification of the lens can progress to the point where the typical features of the posterior lenticonus cannot be identified. If suspected, posterior lenticonus can be demonstrated by careful echography. Bilateral posterior lenticonus is usually familial and presents earlier (11,12).

Persistent Hyperplastic Primary Vitreous

Persistent hyperplastic primary vitreous (PHPV) is unilateral, sporadic, and associated with microphthalmia. The clinical picture is typical: There is persistence of the hyaloid system with involvement of the posterior or anterior pole, or both. Remnants of the hyaloid system exit the optic nerve into the vitreous toward the retrolental area. With posterior pole involvement there may be peripapillary glial tissue often accompanied by macular hypoplasia. The characteristic anterior component is a vascularized retrolental plaque. There may be traction on the ciliary body, with elongated ciliary processes. Intralenticular blood vessels and hemorrhages may be observed. The lens may become intumescent and cause narrow-angle glaucoma, which, if untreated, can lead to phthisis bulbi. Patients with severe posterior-pole abnormalities that preclude visual rehabilitation may still undergo surgery to preserve the globe and provide comfort (13). On the other hand, if the PHPV is mild, good vision can be maintained without surgery, with adequate amblyopia therapy.

Total Cataracts

Total cataracts are rare, usually associated with prenatal rubella infection or infants with trisomy 21.

Assessment of Visual Function*

The need for cataract surgery should not be determined on the basis of the distortion of the retinoscopic reflexes or the visual degradation noticed during direct ophthalmoscopy. While retinoscopy provides an estimate of the cataract diameter, it does not assess the density of the opacity adequately enough to determine if surgery is indicated (9). In addition to evaluating the morphology of the cataract with slit-lamp biomicroscopy, careful assessment of visual function is one of the most important facets of the ocular examination in these patients. As mentioned, many of these patients are referred soon after birth before they are able to fix and follow, and the morphology and density of the cataract may be the most important criteria in making a decision regarding surgery at the time. Once the infant is 2 to 3 months old, the fixation pattern needs to be evaluated. This is assessed by comparing fixation saccades induced in each eye separately by a sudden change in the location of the fixation target (9). In the presence of bilateral cataracts, nystagmus is an indication that visual deprivation is interfering with the development of the fixation reflex. With monocular cataracts, nystagmus in the involved eye is a sign of poor vision. Forced-choice preferential looking techniques such as the test with Teller acuity cards can be used to estimate vision in these patients, though these tests will often overestimate the degree of vision, which is also a problem with visual evoked potentials (14,15). In patients with monocular cataracts and gross strabismus, binocular fixation pattern

testing is easily performed; with small or no deviations the 10-diopter (D) base-down test will provide the same information (16,17). In verbal children a visual acuity of less than 20/70 is an indication for surgery (9).

Assessment for Ocular Pathology*

The clinical examination should assess the presence of associated ocular pathology. Evaluation of pupillary responses will disclose the presence of an afferent pupillary defect suggestive of retinal or optic nerve pathology. The measurement of corneal diameters will help in assessing the presence of microphthalmia. Patients with microphthalmia have a higher risk of developing aphakic glaucoma (18). Baseline corneal diameter measurements can also assist in the diagnosis of aphakic glaucoma, often accompanied by corneal enlargement. The presence of synechiae or corneal opacification will often accompany anterior-segment dysgenesis. A cycloplegic refraction will disclose anisometropia in children with asymmetric bilateral partial cataracts or monocular cataracts. Fundus examination, when possible, should assess the anatomic integrity of the posterior pole. An echographic examination is essential when the posterior pole cannot be visualized. In PHPV it will confirm the diagnosis, demonstrating microphthalmia and remnants of the hyaloid system extending from the optic nerve to the retrolental area.

TIMING OF SURGERY†

Time is of essence in the management of these patients. Various animal experiments demonstrated that there is a critical period when visual deprivation will result in permanent loss of vision or irreversible deprivation amblyopia (19). This correlates with loss of binocularly innervated cells in the occipital cortex, as well as loss of monocularly driven cells from the affected eye both in the cortex and in the lateral geniculate body. This critical period in humans probably consists of the first 2 to 3 months of life, as suggested by the development of nystagmus around this age in patients with dense bilateral cataracts. Patients with monocular cataracts have two predisposing factors for the development of amblyopia: binocular rivalry and visual deprivation (19). To prevent otherwise irreversible amblyopia, patients with dense cataracts should have surgery and optical rehabilitation before the age of 17 weeks (16,20). Excellent visual acuity correlates with earlier surgery, earlier contact lens fit, and excellent amblyopia therapy compliance (16). Some authors believe that surgery should be done by the age of 8 weeks for a favorable outcome (21–23). In patients with PHPV the most important indicator for future visual potential is the patient's age at the time of presentation and subsequent surgery, assuming no significant posterior-pole abnormalities (13).

---

* See also "Evaluation" section in Chapter 63.

* See also "Indications for Surgery" section in Chapter 63.
† See also "Timing the Operation" section in Chapter 63.

ACQUIRED CATARACTS

The most common type of acquired cataract in childhood, in addition to traumatic, is posterior lenticonus. Children with mild cases may require only occlusion therapy to prevent or treat an already existing amblyopia. Surgery is required when lenticular involvement is significant; usually the cutoff point is a visual acuity of 20/70 with the Snellen chart. In mild posterior lenticonus the posterior capsule tends to be weak and may easily break at the time of cortical aspiration. Visual prognosis tends to be good in these patients, probably because the opacity usually occurs later in the course of visual development (8,10). The age of the patient when the cataract becomes visually significant is the most important determinant for the development of amblyopia (24). The probability of developing amblyopia is greater the younger the patient is at the onset of the cataract. Patients 6 years or older have a low probability of developing amblyopia from an acquired cataract.

With a cataract of unknown duration, testing tools such as the potential acuity meter or laser interferometer can be helpful, but the results are often confusing. Children with acquired cataracts or progressive congenital cataracts with later development of amblyopia may demonstrate relatively good visual acuity after late cataract surgery, optical rehabilitation, and occlusion therapy (10,13,25–27). Unless there is strong suspicion that a monocular cataract in an older child is congenital, an attempt at visual rehabilitation of the eye is indicated. The absence of strabismus is a good prognostic sign (25). The presence of nystagmus does not appear to be a reliable prognostic indicator of poor results in children with bilateral cataracts (25,28). Microcornea and monocular nystagmus are poor prognostic signs for monocular cataracts when surgery is performed later in life (26). The duration of strabismus, as well as a review of old photographs for the presence of a normal red reflex, can help determine the onset of the cataract. With a history of child abuse the possibility of a traumatic cataract needs to be considered.

SURGICAL TECHNIQUE[*]

Examination Under Anesthesia[†]

An examination under anesthesia just prior to the surgical procedure is recommended for uncooperative children. Of particular interest in cataract patients are measurement of the corneal horizontal diameter, identification of anterior-segment abnormalities, determination of intraocular pressure, and dilated fundus examination. Orbital echography with axial-length measurement should be performed when the fundus is not visualized and when intraocular lens (IOL) implantation is planned.

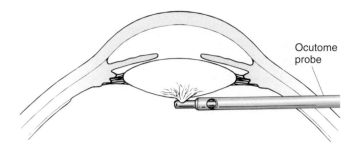

FIGURE 26-8.   *Pars plicata lensectomy—vitreous-cutting instrument is 2.5 mm from the limbus.*

Limbal Versus Pars Plana/Plicata Approach[‡]

Vitreous-cutting instruments are ideal for removing cataracts in children. Most pediatric cataracts can be aspirated without the need of phacoemulsification. Lensectomies may be done either by a limbal or by a pars plana/plicata route. For the pars plana/plicata approach in young children, the sclerotomies are placed 2.0 to 2.5 mm posterior to the limbus to avoid entering the retina, as opposed to 3.5 mm in adult eyes (Fig. 26-8). The pars plana/plicata approach facilitates access for removal of all lens material, but carries the risk of damage to the peripheral aspect of the retina and the risk of vitreous traction and incarceration in the surgical wound. The major drawback is the inability to preserve the posterior capsule for "in-the-bag" placement of an IOL. Implantation of an IOL after pars plana lensectomy can be accomplished by conserving the anterior capsule and positioning the IOL in the sulcus through a limbal incision in front of the intact anterior capsule, followed by a central anterior capsulectomy (29). Other less popular options are IOL implantation in the sulcus prior to the pars plana lensectomy (30) and placement of transscleral anchoring sutures.

The limbal approach is the technique favored by most anterior-segment surgeons.[§] With the limbal approach either a one-port or two-port system can be used. In the one-port system there is a single opening through which the vitrector tip with an infusion sleeve can be introduced (Fig. 26-9), while in the two-port system there is one entry site for the infusion cannula and a second for the vitreous-cutting instrument (Fig. 26-10). The main advantage of the limbal approach is the preservation of the posterior capsule, which facilitates implantation of a posterior-chamber IOL. Disadvantages of this approach include difficulty reaching peripheral lens material behind the iris, compounded by poorly dilating pupils in many of these patients, and the potential damaging effect on the corneal

---

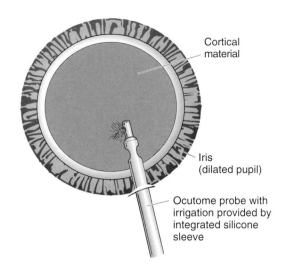

FIGURE 26-9. *Lensectomy through the limbal incision using a vitreous-cutting instrument, with irrigation provided by an integrated silicone infusion sleeve.*

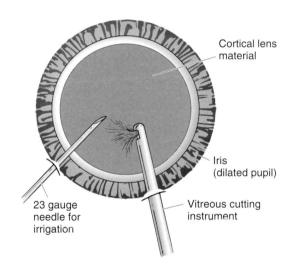

FIGURE 26-10. *Two-handed lensectomy approach with a separate irrigating port through another limbal incision.*

endothelium and the iris tissue. Secondary membranes tend to develop with this technique, especially when a posterior capsulectomy is not performed.

If insertion of an IOL is planned, a limbal approach is preferable. The pars plana/plicata approach can be considered for dislocated lenses, microphthalmic eyes, cataracts due to intrauterine infection or to severe intraocular inflammation, and extensive PHPV (31).★

★ See also "Pars Plana or Pars Plicata Incision" section in Chapter 63.

Anterior Capsulectomy[†]

When IOL implantation is considered, the integrity of the anterior capsulectomy is critical for capsular fixation and centration of the posterior-chamber IOL. Radial tears extending outward from the anterior capsulectomy margin can promote decentration of the IOL by allowing one of the haptics to exit the capsular bag. Because can-opener capsulectomies frequently result in radial tears (32), they are not recommended if IOL implantation is planned. Manual continuous curvilinear capsulorrhexis is less likely to be associated with anterior capsular tears and may be used in children. The capsulorrhexis, however, is generally more difficult to perform in young eyes because the anterior capsule is more elastic and resistant to tearing. If capsulorrhexis is performed, a more central starting position and frequent regrasping of the leading edge may facilitate the procedure (33). Another option is to perform a 5- to 6-mm mechanized circular anterior capsulectomy with the vitrector; this approach is safe, easy to perform, and resistant to radial tearing (Fig. 26-11).[‡] Right-angle edges that predispose to tearing can be avoided if the vitrector is placed just anterior to the capsule with the port directed posteriorly, and the capsule is aspirated into the cutting port (34). Any remaining scalloped capsular tags tend to roll toward the periphery when viscoelastic material is injected into the anterior chamber, resulting in a smooth-edged opening (34).

Posterior Capsulectomy[§]

Posterior-capsule opacification is a frequent complication after cataract surgery in children. A posterior capsulectomy or capsulorrhexis without an accompanying anterior vitrectomy does not prevent the formation of retrolental opacities in young children. Removal of the anterior vitreous face seems to be necessary to eliminate the potential scaffold for remaining lens fiber growth, which leads to secondary-membrane formation (Fig. 26-12). The use of a 3- to 4-mm primary posterior capsulectomy and anterior vitrectomy has been advocated to prevent posterior-capsule opacification in children 5 years old or younger (31,35–38). The posterior capsulectomy (Fig. 26-13) and anterior vitrectomy (Fig. 26-14) can be done either before (31,35,36) or after placement of the IOL. Insertion of the IOL prior to the posterior capsulectomy facilitates the positioning of the lens and decreases the risk of radial tearing of the posterior-capsule opening during IOL insertion. Once the IOL is in place, the posterior capsulectomy and anterior vitrectomy can be done either through the limbal incision by placing the vitrector underneath the IOL (38) or through the pars plana after the limbal wound is closed

---

† See also "Anterior Lens Capsulotomy–Capsulectomy" section in Chapter 63.
‡ See also "Cataract Surgery with Placement of an IOL" section in Chapter 63.
§ See also "Posterior Capsulectomy" section in Chapter 63.

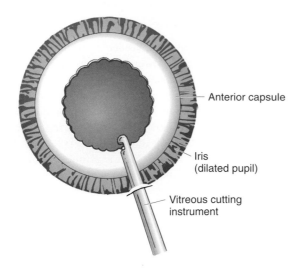

FIGURE 26-11.   *Anterior capsulectomy with vitrector. The cutting port of the vitrector is oriented posteriorly and the center of the anterior capsule is engaged to create an initial opening, which is then enlarged in a circular fashion.*

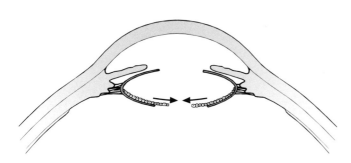

FIGURE 26-12.   *Secondary membranes. When the face of the vitreous remains intact, it acts as a scaffold over which lens fibers may grow, creating a secondary membrane.*

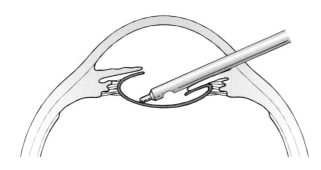

FIGURE 26-13.   *Posterior capsulectomy through a limbal incision. With the cutting port of the vitrector oriented posteriorly, the center of the posterior capsule is engaged and a small opening made. The tip of the vitrector is inserted through the opening and rotated so the cutting port faces anteriorly as the opening is enlarged.*

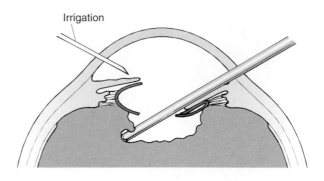

FIGURE 26-14.   *Anterior vitrectomy through a limbal incision. After the posterior capsulectomy is completed, the cutting port of the vitrector is oriented anteriorly and a shallow anterior vitrectomy is performed using low suction and a high cutting rate.*

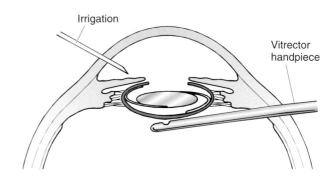

FIGURE 26-15.   *Posterior capsulectomy through the pars plana following placement of an intraocular lens. After the corneoscleral incision is sutured, an irrigation cannula is inserted through the limbal wound. A scleral stab wound is made 2.0 to 2.5 mm posterior to the limbus. The vitrector is inserted behind the posterior capsule to perform the posterior capsulectomy and anterior vitrectomy.*

(Fig. 26-15) (31,39).★ In cases of extensive posterior-capsule opacification (plaques > 4.0 mm) or PHPV remnants attached to the posterior capsule, a pars plana capsulectomy may be preferable (31).

The posterior continuous circular capsulorrhexis (PCCC) is another alternative in the management of the posterior capsule (40,41). After the posterior capsule is punctured with a cystotome posterior to the IOL in the bag, viscoelastic substance is injected through the opening to push the vitreous posteriorly. With capsule forceps the PCCC is extended to a diameter 1 mm smaller than the optic used. The disadvantage of this technique is that secondary membranes covering the initial posterior capsulorrhexis may develop (41,42). Posterior capture of the IOL optic through the PCCC may prevent secondary-membrane formation without the need for an anterior vitrectomy (41). To capture the IOL the optic is slipped inferiorly and then superiorly through the PCCC using a spatula or cannula.

★ See also "Posterior Capsulectomy" section in Chapter 63.

Proponents of this technique suggested two mechanisms by which secondary opacification of the visual axis may be reduced (41). The apposition of anterior- and posterior-capsule leaflets anterior to the optic may limit the migration of Elschnig's pearls. In addition, proliferating lens epithelial cells are released anterior to the IOL into the aqueous humor, which does not provide a scaffold like the vitreous face, reducing the incidence of secondary membranes.

Some authors prefer an intact posterior capsule following the lensectomy (33,40,43,44), with the disadvantage that in children it will most likely opacify. A secondary neodymium (Nd):yttrium-aluminum-garnet (YAG) laser capsulotomy can be performed in adults and most children over the age of 6 years, but cooperation in younger children may be inadequate. For the young or uncooperative child, portable YAG lasers can be mounted vertically and used in the operating room, with the child under general anesthesia in the supine position. A disadvantage of Nd:YAG laser capsulotomies is that an intact anterior vitreous face remains over which residual lens fibers may grow and create a dense secondary membrane, some of which may require surgical treatment. In a series of 45 pseudophakic eyes in patients ranging in age from 1 to 18 years, Nd:YAG laser posterior capsulotomy was performed in 27 (60%) eyes, with 11 (41%) of these requiring a second treatment (33). Atkinson and Hiles (43) reported a 28% rate of recurrence of secondary membranes after laser capsulotomy. The density of the membrane seems to correlate with the time interval between cataract extraction and laser capsulotomy. Some authors advocated YAG laser posterior capsulotomy at the first sign of capsule opacification, usually at 3 postoperative weeks in younger patients, to reduce the energy required for the procedure and allow amblyopia therapy (33,43). To perform YAG capsulotomy the energy level may be initiated at 0.9 mJ and increased up to 2.0 (44) or 2.5 mJ (43).

Peripheral iridectomies are not routinely performed in children. Because the risk of angle closure is significantly decreased when a posterior capsulectomy and anterior vitrectomy accompany the lensectomy, a peripheral iridectomy may not be necessary unless severe inflammation is anticipated. When an intact posterior capsule is preferred, a peripheral iridectomy should be considered unless the child is able to cooperate for a laser peripheral iridectomy, if necessary.★

Postoperative Care†

Subconjunctival steroids and antibiotics are frequently used at the end of the surgery. Either acetylcholine for pupillary miosis or atropine for pupillary dilation may be instilled, according to the surgeon's preference. Because children

develop strong postoperative inflammatory reactions with a fibrinous response, intensive topical corticosteroid therapy is critical. Prednisolone acetate 1% every 2 to 4 hours is commonly used, occasionally in conjunction with oral steroids. Mydriatic drops are important in the prevention of posterior synechiae, to reduce the chance of pupillary block.

OPTICAL CORRECTION★

The main goals of optical rehabilitation after lensectomy in a child are preservation of vision, prevention of amblyopia, and preservation or development of fusion. The different options for optical correction are aphakic spectacles, contact lenses, IOLs, and epikeratophakia. There are features unique to a child's eye that must be considered when deciding on the method of postoperative optical correction. These include changing axial length and corneal curvature, increased tissue reactivity, lower scleral rigidity, smaller globe size, potential for amblyopia, and long life span after cataract removal (45).

Aphakic Spectacles

Aphakic spectacles may be useful for bilateral aphakia, but are unacceptable for unilateral aphakia because of aniseikonia (unequal image size). They provide the highest degree of safety and can be worn immediately after the surgery, but their effectiveness is limited by optical distortion and reduced visual field. They are cosmetically unappealing, but high-refractive-index lenses and aspheric lenses may improve patient tolerance. Good visual acuity may be obtained with aphakic glasses.

Aphakic Contact Lenses

Aphakic contact lenses are the initial choice in most children during the first 2 years of life. Contact lenses are a safe alternative and can be fitted a few days after surgery. The major advantage of the contact lens is the possibility of adjustment as the size of the eye and the refractive error changes. The disadvantages include the expense, high loss rate, risk of irritation, infection, and corneal abrasion or ulcer. The tolerance and compliance tend to decrease with time.

The aphakic contact lens of choice for infants and young children is the silicone lens because of the ease of fitting and the ease of care. These lenses have high oxygen permeability and can be used on an extended-wear basis. They are small and fairly rigid, which makes them easy to insert and more difficult to blink out. The major problem associated with these lenses is their high cost. If the cornea is too steep for a silicone lens, or the silicone lens is too expensive, a daily-wear soft contact lens may be used, with the

---

★ See also "Iridotomy–Iridectomy" section in Chapter 63.
† See also "Postoperative Management" section in Chapter 63.

★ See also "Optical Rehabilitation" section in Chapter 63.

main disadvantage of more difficult handling. Rigid gas-permeable lenses are another option, but they are usually more uncomfortable and associated with increased tearing and rubbing of the eyes.* As a rule, contact lenses should be over-plused by +1.50 to +3.00 D in children under the age of 4 to correct for near vision. Otherwise, bifocal spectacles should be worn over the aphakic contact lens.

Epikeratophakia

Epikeratophakia is a type of refractive surgery in which a partial-thickness corneal lamellar graft is sutured onto the surface of the recipient cornea to produce a change in the anterior corneal curvature. It can be performed as a primary procedure in combination with the lensectomy, or as a secondary procedure. Being an extraocular procedure it is safer than IOL implantation. Bowman's membrane is preserved; thus, it is possible to change the lenticule or to remove it and use another form of optical correction. Disadvantages of this method include delay in corneal healing with a subsequent delay in providing a clear image, and irregular astigmatism. It is not recommended in children under 1 year old because sufficient optical power is usually not attained, and there is rapid growth of the eye resulting in a change in refraction. Presently the lenticules are not commercially available.

Intraocular Lenses[†]

A major problem with pediatric aphakic patients is the poor compliance with contact lenses, and the consequent risks of amblyopia and strabismus. This has contributed to the increasing popularity of posterior-chamber IOL implantation in children. A prospective evaluation of pediatric cataracts in children between 2 and 8 years old examined three methods of management: 1) lensectomy and anterior vitrectomy; 2) extracapsular cataract extraction (ECCE) with IOL implantation; and 3) ECCE with primary posterior capsulotomy, anterior vitrectomy, and IOL implantation. The results showed that the third approach provides optimum refractive correction and a clear visual axis, without increased risk of short-term complications (36).

The minimum age for IOL implantation has been lowered, but implantation of IOLs in children less than 2 years old is still controversial. IOLs should be considered when the parents refuse contact lenses, the child is contact lens intolerant, and social or economic factors preclude adequate contact lens compliance and follow-up. IOLs may also be advantageous for children with traumatic cataracts with corneal scars that preclude successful contact lens wear and those with monocular radiation-induced cataracts. Contraindications include microphthalmia, chronic intraocular inflammation (juvenile rheumatoid arthritis, pars planitis), and dislocated lenses without sufficient capsular support.

In-the-bag placement of the IOL is preferred because it diminishes the risk of lens dislocation or decentration, iris capture, and uveal inflammation. Sulcus placement of the IOL is acceptable. Anterior-chamber IOLs are not recommended in children due to the high complication rate.

Intraocular Lens Size

Reports indicating that 90% of the crystalline lens growth occurs during the first 2 years of life, in conjunction with analysis of IOLs in postmortem eyes, have led to recommendations of downsizing IOLs to approximately 10.0 mm in diameter for children younger than 2 years, and implanting standard, flexible, 12.0- to 12.5-mm-diameter capsular IOLs in children older than 2 years, unless axial-length measurements indicate an unusually small eye (46).

Intraocular Lens Power[‡]

When determining the power of the IOL to be used, one should take into account the changing axial length and refractive power of the eye. The axial length of normal phakic eyes increases from a mean of 16.8 mm at birth, to 20.2 mm by the first year of life, to 21.4 mm by age 2 (47), but eyes with lens extraction during early infancy may grow less (48). Aphakic or pseudophakic eyes in neonatal monkeys grow an average of 2.0 mm less than their fellow phakic eyes (48). However, in spite of the apparent retardation of axial elongation, pseudophakic infant eyes still experience a myopic shift. The degree of postoperative myopic shift seems to be influenced by age at the time of surgery. Patients who have surgery at an average age of 26 months show a myopic shift of 2.90 D after 24 months (27). Children operated on after the age of 7 years show no significant difference between the postoperative increase in axial length in the operated and unoperated eyes (49).

The risk of implanting IOLs with a power appropriate for an adult eye is that severe undercorrection may result during the most important years of visual development. This has prompted recommendations for implantation of IOLs with a power closer to that predicted for immediate emmetropia (40). Some surgeons prefer to target the postoperative refraction to be 1.0 to 2.0 D hyperopic in children under 6 years old, and emmetropic for those over the age of 6 years, avoiding anisometropia greater than 2.5 D (44). Others advocate a postoperative refraction of +4.00 D for children under 2 years, +3.00 D for those 2 to 4 years old, +2.00 D for children 4 to 6 years old, +1.00 D for those 6 to 8 years old, and emmetropia in children over 8 years old, adjusting for the fellow eye to avoid anisometropia greater than 3.00 D and providing bifocal spectacle overcorrection (27,39). BenEzra (50) found that correction of

---

* See Chapter 63, for discussion of rigid gas-permeable contact use.
† See also "The Intraocular Lens" section in Chapter 63.

‡ See also "Lens Style and Power Selection" section in Chapter 63.

aphakia with a +21.0- or +22.0-D IOL yields in most normal-sized eyes of patients over 1 year old a postoperative spherical equivalent of +2.0 ± 1.0 D.

Intraocular Lens Material and Design

Most surgeons prefer the one-piece, all-polymethylmethacrylate (PMMA) IOLs with modified wide C loops (35,46). The one-piece, all-PMMA IOL loops exhibit better memory and hence tend to resist contraction and tend toward outward re-expansion toward the ciliary body. This should help retain the diameter of the capsular bag and lessen the tendency toward zonular stretching (46). The modified C loops are highly flexible, facilitating the insertion of the lens.

Foldable IOLs implanted through a clear 3.5- to 4.0-mm corneal incision may be the way of the future, but the experience in children is limited at the present time.

POSTOPERATIVE COMPLICATIONS*

The surgical complication rate after cataract surgery in children has markedly decreased with the advent of automated lensectomy and vitrectomy. Younger patients are still at an increased risk, with 28% of patients under 2 months old experiencing complications, compared to 10% of those older than 2 months at the time of the surgery (37).

Posterior-Capsule Opacification and Secondary Membranes†

The primary late complication after lensectomy in children is opacification of the posterior capsule. Potential problems generated by a secondary membrane include amblyopia, difficult retinoscopy and fundus examination, as well as possible need of additional surgery. The management of the posterior capsule is discussed earlier in the chapter.

Pigment Deposits on the Intraocular Lens

Pigment deposits are a common abnormality after IOL implantation in children, particularly in those with traumatic cataracts. They have been observed in approximately 43% of patients (27,39).

Intraocular Lens Decentration/Iris Capture

IOL decentration occurs in 3% to 20% of pediatric patients (Fig. 26-16), but lenses are usually easily repositioned (39). In eyes where anterior or posterior capsular tears prevent both haptics from being placed in the capsular bag (Fig. 26-17), it is preferable to place both haptics in the sulcus to minimize IOL decentration.

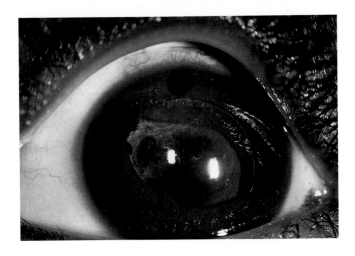

FIGURE 26-16.   *Iris capture of posterior intraocular lens.*

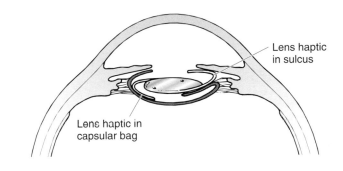

FIGURE 26-17.   *Intraocular lens with one haptic in the capsular bag and the other in the sulcus, predisposing to iris capture.*

Glaucoma‡

Aphakic glaucoma may occur in either an acute or a chronic form and may develop at any time after the surgery. The acute glaucoma is typically of the angle-closure type and usually presents in the early postoperative period. Lens remnants, vitreous, or posterior synechiae block aqueous flow through the pupil, inducing iris bombé. Aphakic and pseudophakic pupillary block glaucoma is a potential complication that can be prevented with a prophylactic peripheral iridectomy.

Chronic open-angle aphakic glaucoma is more common than acute glaucoma. Parks et al (8) reported aphakic glaucoma in 14.9% of aphakic eyes, detected at a mean of 5.3 years after the surgery. Simon et al (51) found aphakic glaucoma in 24% of aphakic eyes detected at a mean of 6.8 years postoperatively. Egbert et al (52) found ocular hypertension in 45% of patients with bilateral cataracts, and 32.5% of patients with unilateral cataracts at least 5 years after pediatric cataract surgery. Owing to the high incidence of ocular hypertension, it is advisable to follow these patients for

---

* See also "Complications" section in Chapter 63.
† See also "Secondary Membranes" section in Chapter 63.

‡ See also "Glaucoma" section in Chapter 63.

glaucoma for the rest of their lives. A sign that may herald the presence of aphakic glaucoma is an excessive loss of hyperopia in pediatric aphakic patients (53).

Several mechanisms have been proposed to explain the development of aphakic glaucoma. It has been speculated that longstanding postoperative inflammation or degenerative lens protein from retained lens material may damage the trabecular meshwork. Parks et al (8) found that 88.5% (23/26) of eyes with aphakic glaucoma had corneal diameters less than 10 mm; aphakic glaucoma developed in only 2.9% of eyes with normal corneal diameters, while 31.9% of eyes with small corneal diameters were affected. Development of aphakic glaucoma was related to nuclear cataracts and PHPV cataracts, both associated with small corneal size. The association between small corneal size and the development of glaucoma suggests the possibility of a developmental abnormality of the anterior segment of the eye that produces the cataracts and also affects outflow, predisposing to an open-angle glaucoma. Another risk factor for the development of glaucoma appears to be surgery at an early age (8).

Hemorrhagic Retinopathy

Retinal hemorrhages may be found postoperatively in up to 40% of children (54). The hemorrhages are predominantly flame shaped and localized to the posterior pole, and may be associated with a vitreous hemorrhage. Retinal hemorrhages occur within 24 hours of surgery, are not progressive, and are clear within 3 weeks postoperatively, with no permanent visual or structural sequelae. Possible etiologies include venous stasis retinopathy, traction on the vessels during anterior vitrectomy, and Valsalva retinopathy. No risk factors such as age, sex, race, duration of surgery, or coagulopathy have been identified.

Cystoid Macular Edema

Clinical cystoid macular edema rarely occurs after cataract surgery in children. The exact incidence is unknown owing to difficulty performing fluorescein angiography in young children.

Retinal Detachment

With the use of automated lensectomy/vitrectomy techniques the incidence of retinal detachments after cataract surgery in children has decreased from 3% to 10% in the past to 1.5% to 3.0% (8). Retinal detachments occurring after congenital cataract surgery usually appear in the second to fourth decades, at an interval of 21 to 33 years between the cataract operation and retinal detachment (55). Aphakic retinal detachments are associated with undetected retinal breaks and vitreous and preretinal traction. Myopia and secondary-membrane procedures increase the risk of retinal detachment (55,56).

Endophthalmitis

The incidence of endophthalmitis following pediatric anterior-segment surgery is estimated at 0.071% (57). It is usually caused by gram-positive organisms, frequently *Staphylococcus epidermidis* and *Streptococcus pneumoniae*. Risk factors for postoperative endophthalmitis include nasolacrimal duct obstruction and upper respiratory tract infection. Visual outcome is generally poor.

Amblyopia

Occlusion therapy is crucial in the prevention and management of amblyopia in most patients following monocular cataract extraction and in a few after bilateral surgery. Regimens for patching are diverse. A popular method is to patch the preferred eye for all but 2 waking hours daily, except in infants younger than 2 months, who are not patched more than half of the waking hours (8). Once fixation preference can be assessed or visual acuity determined by preferential looking tests, the routine is modified. If a strong fixation preference remains, the preferred eye continues to be patched for all but 2 waking hours. Otherwise, the patching is reduced to half the waking hours, and then to 2 to 4 hours daily. Maintenance patching is continued until visual development is complete, usually by the age of 8 to 10 years. Some authors (39) advocate full-time occlusion of the phakic eye for 6 days and of the aphakic eye for 1 day, with no binocular periods, until maximum visual acuity is attained. Regardless of the patching regimen, compliance with occlusion therapy continues to be the major determinant of good visual outcome in unilaterally aphakic children. Although it was initially thought that IOLs would decrease the need for patching, studies done in primates suggest that occlusion therapy is as important in preventing amblyopia in pseudophakic eyes as it is in aphakic eyes corrected with contact lenses (58).[*]

STRABISMUS

Most patients with partial cataracts and relatively good visual acuity will have straight eyes. Patients with bilateral but asymmetric partial cataracts, and patients with significant monocular partial cataracts tend to develop strabismus, usually associated with amblyopia. Patients with monocular aphakia often develop strabismus, in spite of good visual function (21). Patients with dense congenital cataracts in both eyes have a tendency to develop strabismus, irrespective of visual outcome (20,59). In patients with strabismus and amblyopia, visual acuity should be maximally improved before they undergo strabismus surgery. A history of deep amblyopia, even if resolved, will adversely affect the development of binocularity after successful strabismus surgery (19). In patients with intractable amblyopia one should wait

---

[*] See also "Results" section and Tables 63-11 to 63-21 in Chapter 63.

until the angle of deviation is stable before performing strabismus surgery. Some authors (59,60) suggested that even with amblyopia, optical rehabilitation with a contact lens or IOL will help maintain ocular alignment in some of these patients.

It is preferable not to combine cataract and strabismus surgery. Not rarely the ocular alignment will improve when an acquired cataract is removed and the eye is optically rehabilitated with either a contact lens or an IOL. When strabismus is associated with monocular or binocular cataracts, we prefer to wait until visual acuity is maximized after cataract surgery. If needed, strabismus surgery is deferred until the angle of deviation is stable.

REFERENCES

1. Lambert SR, Amaya L, Taylor D. Detection and treatment of infantile cataracts. *Int Ophthalmol Clin* 1989;29:51–56.
2. Cotlier E. Congenital rubella cataracts. In: Cotlier E, Lambert SR, Taylor D, eds. *Congenital cataracts*. Florida: R.G. Landes CRC, 1994:65–76.
3. Wolff SM. The ocular manifestations of congenital rubella. *Trans Am Ophthalmol Soc* 1972;70:577–614.
4. Mets MB, Holfels E, Boyer KM, et al. Eye manifestations of congenital toxoplasmosis. *Am J Ophthalmol* 1996;122:309–324.
5. Marshall WC. Congenital and perinatal infections. In: Wibar K, Taylor D, eds. *Pediatric ophthalmology: current aspects*. New York: Marcel Dekker, 1983:431–446.
6. Merin S, Crawford JS. The etiology of congenital cataracts. *Can J Ophthalmol* 1971;6:178–182.
7. Gibbs ML, Jacobs M, Wilkie AOM, Taylor D. Posterior lenticonus: clinical patterns and genetics. *J Pediatr Ophthalmol Strabismus* 1993;30:171–175.
8. Parks MM, Johnson DA, Reed GW. Long-term visual results and complications in children with aphakia: a function of cataract type. *Ophthalmology* 1993;6:826–840.
9. Parks MM. Visual results in aphakic children. *Am J Ophthalmol* 1982;94:441–449.
10. Crouch ER Jr, Parks MM. Management of posterior lenticonus complicated by unilateral cataract. *Am J Ophthalmol* 1978;85:503–508.
11. Howitt D, Hornblass A. Posterior lenticonus. *Am J Ophthalmol* 1968;66: 1133–1136.
12. Pollard ZF. Familial bilateral posterior lenticonus. *Arch Ophthalmol* 1983;101:1238–1240.
13. Karr DS, Scott WE. Visual acuity results following treatment of persistent hyperplastic primary vitreous. *Arch Ophthalmol* 1986;104:662–667.
14. Sokol S, Hansen VC, Moskowitz A, et al. Evoked potential and preferential looking estimates of visual acuity in pediatric patients. *Ophthalmology* 1983;90:552–562.
15. Mayer DL, Fulton AB, Rodier D. Grating and recognition acuities of pediatric patients. *Ophthalmology* 1984;91:947–953.
16. Drummond GT, Scott WE, Keech RV. Management of monocular congenital cataracts. *Arch Ophthalmol* 1989;107:45–51.
17. Wright KW, Walonker F, Edelman P. 10-Diopter fixation test for amblyopia. *Arch Ophthalmol* 1981;99:1242–1246.
18. Wallace DK, Plager DA. Corneal diameter in childhood aphakic glaucoma. *J Pediatr Ophthalmol Strabismus* 1996;33:230–234.
19. von Noorden GK. Amblyopia: a multidisciplinary approach. *Invest Ophthalmol Vis Sci* 1985;26:1706–1716.
20. Cheng KP, Hiles DA, Biglan AW, Pettapiece MC. Visual results after early surgical treatment of unilateral congenital cataracts. *Ophthalmology* 1991;98:903–910.
21. Beller R, Hoyt CS, Marg E, Odom JV. Good visual function after neonatal surgery for congenital monocular cataracts. *Am J Ophthalmol* 1981;91: 559–565.
22. Gelbart SS, Hoyt CS, Jastrebski G, Marg E. Long-term visual results in bilateral congenital cataracts. *Am J Ophthalmol* 1982;93:615–621.
23. Rogers GL, Tischler CL, Tsou BH, et al. Visual acuities in infants with congenital cataracts operated on prior to 6 months of age. *Arch Ophthalmol* 1981;99:999–1003.
24. Keech RV, Kutschke PJ. Upper age limit for the development of amblyopia. *J Pediatr Ophthalmol Strabismus* 1995;32:89–93.
25. Wright KW, Christensen LE, Naguchi BA. Results of late surgery for presumed congenital cataracts. *Am J Ophthalmol* 1992;114:409–415.
26. Kushner BJ. Visual results after surgery for monocular juvenile cataracts of undetermined onset. *Am J Ophthalmol* 1986;102:468–472.
27. Awner S, Buckley EG, De Varo J, Seaver JH. Unilateral pseudophakia in children under 4 years. *J Pediatr Ophthalmol Strabismus* 1996;33:230–236.
28. Bradford GM, Keech RV, Scott WE. Factors affecting visual outcome after surgery for bilateral congenital cataracts. *Am J Ophthalmol* 1994;117:58–64.
29. Blankenship GW, Flynn HW, Kokame GT. Posterior chamber intraocular lens insertion during pars plana lensectomy and vitrectomy for complications of proliferative diabetic retinopathy. *Am J Ophthalmol* 1989;108:1–5.
30. Tablante RT, Cruz EDG, Lapus JV, Santos AM. A new technique of congenital cataract with primary posterior chamber intraocular lens implantation. *J Cataract Refract Surg* 1988;14:149–157.
31. BenEzra D. The surgical approaches to paediatric cataract. *Eur J Implant Ref Surg* 1990;2:241–244.
32. Assia EI, Apple DJ, Barden A, et al. An experimental study comparing various anterior capsulectomy techniques. *Arch Ophthalmol* 1991;109:642–647.
33. Brady KM, Atkinson CS, Kilty LA, Hiles DA. Cataract surgery and intraocular lens implantation in children. *Am J Ophthalmol* 1995;120:1–9.
34. Wilson ME, Saunders RA, Roberts EL, Apple DJ. Mechanized anterior capsulectomy as an alternative to manual capsulorrhexis in children undergoing intraocular lens implantation. *J Pediatr Ophthalmol Strabismus* 1996;33:237–240.
35. Dahan E, Salmenson BD. Pseudophakia in children: precautions, technique, and feasibility. *J Cataract Refract Surg* 1990;16:75–82.
36. Basti S, Ravishankar U, Gupta S. Results of a prospective evaluation of three methods of management of pediatric cataracts. *Ophthalmology* 1996;103:713–720.
37. Keech RV, Tongue AC, Scott WE. Complications after surgery for congenital and infantile cataracts. *Am J Ophthalmol* 1989;108:136–141.
38. Mackool RJ, Chatiawala H. Pediatric cataract surgery and intraocular lens implantation: a new technique for preventing or excising postoperative secondary membranes. *J Cataract Refract Surg* 1991;17:62–66.
39. Buckley EG, Klomberg LA, Seaber JH, et al. Management of the posterior capsule during pediatric intraocular lens implantation. *Am J Ophthalmol* 1993;115:722–728.
40. Gimbel HV, Ferensowicz M, Raanan M, DeLuca M. Implantation in children. *J Pediatr Ophthalmol Strabismus* 1993;30:69–79.
41. Gimbel HV. Posterior capsulorrhexis with optic capture in pediatric cataract and intraocular lens surgery. *Ophthalmology* 1996;103:1871–1875.
42. Vasavada A, Chauhan MS. Intraocular lens implantation in infants with congenital cataracts. *J Cataract Refract Surg* 1994;20:592–598.
43. Atkinson CS, Hiles DA. Treatment of secondary posterior capsular membranes with the Nd:YAG laser in a pediatric population. *Am J Ophthalmol* 1994;118:496–501.
44. Crouch ER, Pressman SH, Crouch ER. Posterior chamber intraocular lenses: long-term results in pediatric cataract patients. *J Pediatr Ophthalmol Strabismus* 1995;32:210–218.
45. Wilson ME, Bluestein EC, Wang X-H. Current trends in the use of intraocular lenses in children. *J Cataract Refract Surg* 1994;20:579–583.
46. Wilson ME, Apple DJ, Bluestein EC, Wang X-H. Intraocular lenses for pediatric implantation: biomaterials, designs, and sizing. *J Cataract Refract Surg* 1994;20:584–591.
47. Gordon RA, Donzis PB. Refractive development of the human eye. *Arch Ophthalmol* 1985;103:785–789.
48. Lambert SR, Fernandes A, Drews-Botsch C, Tigges M. Pseudophakia retards axial elongation in neonatal monkey eyes. *Invest Ophthalmol Vis Sci* 1996;37:451–458.
49. Kora Y, Shimizu K, Inatomi M, et al. Eye growth after cataract extraction and intraocular lens implantation in children. *Ophthalmic Surg* 1993;24: 467–475.
50. BenEzra D. Cataract surgery and intraocular lens implantation in children. *Am J Ophthalmol* 1996;121:224–225. Letter.
51. Simon JW, Mehta N, Simmons ST, et al. Glaucoma after pediatric lensectomy/vitrectomy. *Ophthalmology* 1991;98:670–674.
52. Egbert JE, Wright MM, Dahlhauser KF, et al. A prospective study of ocular hypertension and glaucoma after pediatric cataract surgery. *Ophthalmology* 1995;102:1098–1101.
53. Egbert JE, Kushner BJ. Excessive loss of hyperopia. A presenting sign of juvenile aphakic glaucoma. *Arch Ophthalmol* 1990;106:1257–1260.
54. Christiansen SP, Muñoz M, Capó H. Retinal hemorrhage following lensectomy and anterior vitrectomy in children. *J Pediatr Ophthalmol Strabismus* 1993;30: 24–27.

55. Toyofuku H, Hirose T, Schepens CL. Retinal detachment following congenital cataract surgery. *Arch Ophthalmol* 1980;98:669–675.

56. Chrousos GA, Parks MM, O'Neill JF. Incidence of chronic glaucoma, retinal detachment and secondary membrane surgery in pediatric aphakic patients. *Ophthalmology* 1984;91:1238–1241.

57. Wheeler DT, Stager DR, Weakley DR. Endophthalmitis following pediatric intraocular surgery for congenital cataracts and congenital glaucoma. *J Pediatr Ophthalmol Strabismus* 1992;29:139–141.

58. Boothe RG, Louden TM, Lambert SR. Acuity and contrast sensitivity in monkeys after neonatal intraocular lens implantation with and without parttime occlusion of the fellow eye. *Invest Ophthalmol Vis Sci* 1996;37:1520–1531.

59. Hing S, Speedwell L, Taylor D. Lens surgery in infancy and childhood. *Br J Ophthalmol* 1990;74:73–77.

60. Kodsi SR, Summers CG, Lavoie JD. The effect of contact lens correction on strabismus in pediatric monocular aphakia. *Binocular Vis Eye Muscle Surg* 1995;10:175–182.

Intraocular Lenses

Henry M. Clayman

HISTORY

The recorded history of an intraocular lens (IOL) begins over 200 years ago. Casanova, the Venetian courtier, is alleged to have discussed this concept with Tadini, an Italian oculist to whom Casanova attributes the idea (1). Casanova is then said to have shared this information with Casaamata, a physician to the Royal Court in Dresden, Germany. Casaamata (2) tried to insert a glass IOL around 1795 but the lens subluxed posteriorly and thereafter no references to IOLs are noted until this century. Foster of Britain wrote a humorous article in 1939 titled "An Oculist in America," which was published in the 1940 Leeds Medical Society magazine and compared the influence of British versus American culture on medical progress. Foster stated, ". . . and thought it was a good idea to see if an intra-ocular glass lens could replace a cataract . . ." (3). Thereafter, in 1940 Marchi attempted animal experiments inserting quartz glass IOLs with platinum fixation haptics (4). These experiments were unsuccessful and during the next 5 years the world was consumed by World War II, which paradoxically provided the catalyst for the modern era of IOL development. Bangerter, in 1947, inserted acrylic anterior-chamber IOLs in the eyes of rabbits but it was Harold Ridley who ushered in lens implantation in humans after an almost 200-year hiatus.

Ridley, while on military duty, noted that intraocular fragments of the plastic canopies of Royal Air Force fighter planes were inert within the eye following penetrating injuries sustained during World War II combat. This plastic was a formulation of polymethylmethacrylate (PMMA) called Perspex and manufactured by Imperial Chemical Industries (ICI). On his return to civilian life, Ridley resumed medical practice and stated that his interest in IOLs was prompted by the question of a medical student who was observing cataract surgery (5). The student inquired why a replacement lens was not inserted into the eye following removal of the crystalline lens. This chance remark led to Ridley's development of a posterior-chamber IOL fabricated from a type of PMMA designated Transpex 1. According to Caudell (6), ICI used various names for their PMMA products such as Perspex, Transpex, and Plexiglas. Ultimately the benchmark IOL material was Perspex CQ, the CQ designating "clinical quality." This material had a refractive index of 1.49 and a specific gravity of 1.19, the actual IOL being manufactured by Rayners of London.

Ridley operated on his first patient on November 29, 1949, performing a planned extracapsular extraction with posterior-chamber IOL insertion. There were some modifications in the design of the lens and in researching another publication I was unable to locate the original blueprints; however, Ridley stated the dimensions as 8.3 mm in diameter, 24 mm in thickness, anterior radius of curvature of 17.8 mm, and posterior radius of curvature of 10.7 mm. The power of the lens was designed to be 74 diopters (D) in air and 24 D in aqueous, but there probably was a miscalculation since Ridley's first patient had a postoperative refraction in excess of -18.00 D and his second patient was likewise highly myopic (7). Ridley persisted and his first eight cases were published in 1951 (3). Thereafter, other reports appeared on patients with Ridley IOLs in situ and several complications became apparent (8). These included iris atrophy and secondary cataract, a particularly bothersome complication because the Ridley IOL design made access to the posterior capsule difficult for a discission. Idiosyncratic shallowing of the anterior chamber also occurred, which in turn sometimes led to secondary glaucoma, and dislocations were also noted, both anterior and posterior.

Another problem was iritis, which was of several possible etiologies including residual lens material, residual sterilizing agent, or IOL induced. Given the obstacles that Ridley faced, it is a miracle that this surgical modality was ever adopted, because in this era there was no operating microscope, no modern pharmaceuticals including corticosteroids, no atraumatic sutures, no automated cataract extraction equipment, and no reliable sterilization technique. Usage of the Ridley lens decreased and over time ophthalmologists searched for other fixation sites. Before I discuss the origins of anterior-chamber and iris-fixated IOLs, a discussion of early sterilization techniques is merited.

STERILIZATION OF IOLs: PAST AND PRESENT

In the early days of IOL surgery, the lenses were soaked in various solutions to effect sterilization. These were usually quaternary ammonium compounds which included Quartamon, Tetraseptan, Zephirol, and Plexiklar, the latter to minimize electrostatic charge on the IOL. Epstein (9) reported his sterilization technique as immersion for 1 hour in Hibitane 1/1000 in a 70% alcohol solution, after which the IOL was transferred to normal saline solution. Many of these cited solutions either are not available or have undergone a name change but were invariably toxic to the eye. Wollensak (10) demonstrated the absorption by PMMA of quaternary ammonium compounds and their propensity to cause inflammation when injected into animal eyes. He also described attempts at ultraviolet sterilization and noted the structural changes induced in PMMA by this radiant energy. Sterilization was a significant problem in the early days of IOL surgery and the profession is indebted to another Ridley, Frederick Ridley, for introducing a reliable method of sterilization colloquially known as the *wet-pack* technique (11). The IOL was immersed in a sodium hydroxide (NaOH) solution that was neutralized with sodium bicarbonate (NaHCO$_3$) solution prior to use, after which the IOL was washed with balanced saline solution prior to insertion. In the 1970s I had personal experience with IOLs sterilized by this technique and recall them shipped for use in two ways. In the first the IOL was sterilized in NaOH by the manufacturer and shipped to the surgeon in a vial or ampule containing the NaHCO$_3$. With the second method the IOL was shipped in a sealed ampule containing the IOL in a NaOH solution and a second sealed ampule contained the neutralizing solution. The neck was filed off of each ampule and the IOL was removed from the NaOH solution and deposited in the NaHCO$_3$ solution prior to use. The Ridley wet pack was generally satisfactory; however, there was an outbreak of fungal endophthalmitis in patients receiving wet-pack sterilized IOLs from a now-defunct manufacturer (12) and the persistence of *Pseudomonas* spores in NaOH solution was also demonstrated (13). Nowadays the only permissible means of sterilizing IOLs is by ethylene oxide, which is a gas at ambient temperatures (the exception is Chiron's practice of using steam sterilization on silicone IOLs with polyimide loops). This cyclic ether does leave residues, which mandates lens quarantine by the manufacturer prior to use. On the other hand, ethylene oxide has no effect on the physical or chemical properties of acrylic materials.

THE ANTERIOR-CHAMBER AND IRIS-FIXATED IOL ERA

Returning to the evolution of IOLs, perhaps because of misgivings on the fixation site of the Ridley posterior-chamber IOLs or because of intellectual curiosity, surgeons began seeking alternative means of IOL fixation and next selected the anterior chamber. The Ridley posterior-chamber IOL was not abruptly abandoned; in fact, a subsequent model, known as the *Saturn*, was being shipped as late as 1966. By that time the evolution of anterior-chamber IOLs was well under way. Baron of France implanted the first angle-supported, anterior-chamber IOL in 1952 and reported his work the following year (14). In 1953, Strampelli implanted an angle-supported, anterior-chamber, one-piece IOL whose design was the basis from which the Choyce anterior-chamber IOLs were developed (15). Though the Choyce IOLs were controversial and not devoid of significant complications, they nevertheless attracted a cadre of devotees and kept this means of fixation viable. Choyce modified his design several times, progressing from the Mark I through the Mark IX (16). These various progressions in design were attempts to obviate corneal decompensation, presumably on the basis of IOL contact with the corneal endothelium at the angle. The Choyce lens had to be sized to the anterior chamber of a given patient. Customarily the patient's horizontal corneal diameter was measured "white-to-white" and 1 mm was added to this, to obtain the corresponding IOL, which was sized in 0.5-mm increments (Fig. 27-1).

While the Choyce IOL was evolving, other surgeons were investigating other potential designs for anterior-chamber fixation. In an attempt to overcome some of the sterilization difficulties alluded to above, autoclavable IOLs with silicate glass optics were proposed and manufactured (17,18). Parenthetically, the concept of glass IOLs was reintroduced by Barasch and Poler in 1979 (19). This proved to be asynchronous with the direction that ophthalmology was taking because glass IOLs were reported to shatter under the impact of neodymium:yttrium-argon-garnet (Nd:YAG) radiation (20) and the concept was abandoned. With concern on the long-term effects of a rigid material in the angle, Supramid (nylon) looped lenses were produced both for angle and external fixation techniques (21). In the short term, gratifying results were obtained in many patients, but with longer follow-up numerous complications became apparent, not the least of which was degradation of the Supramid loops. Again the profession sought a better means of fixation.

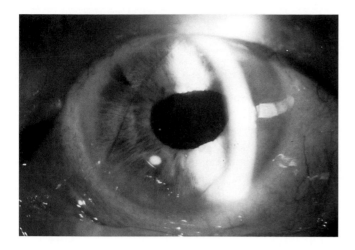

FIGURE 27-1.   *Choyce anterior-chamber IOL.*

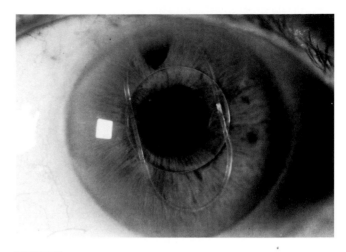

FIGURE 27-2.   *Binkhorst iris-clip IOL.*

Binkhorst and Epstein each considered the iris as a means of IOL fixation. Epstein designed an iris-fixated IOL in the shape of a collar stud and first inserted it in a patient in 1953 (22). Binkhorst, in the meantime, was developing his iris-clip lens, which can be conceptualized as a paper clip with the optic in the center (23). This lens was clipped to the iris diaphragm, with the iris in a position analogous to paper grasped by a paper clip (Fig. 27-2). In some ways, the Epstein IOL was similar to the Copeland iris-fixated IOL, which was used in the United States during the early 1970s until it was supplanted by other iris-fixation lenses, especially the Binkhorst iris-clip IOL, which went through several evolutionary steps. Other surgeons associated with widely used iris-fixated IOLs are Worst, the first to suture an IOL to the iris (Fig. 27-3), and Fyodorov. As noted in a previous chapter, a pivotal event in the evolution of IOLs was Binkhorst's introduction of the iridocapsular IOL (24) in 1972 (Fig. 27-4), and the profession's appreciation of the panocular benefits associated with this type of fixation coincided well with the development of automated techniques of extracapsular cataract extraction (ECCE) including phacoemulsification. It should be understood that the profession did not stop one type of fixation en masse and then abandon that for another type of fixation; on the contrary, various fixation modalities were being used simultaneously according to each surgeon's preference. From the surgeon's point of view, a major problem with the iris-fixated IOLs involved insertion in association with automated ECCE and phacoemulsification, which were closed-chamber techniques. The iris-fixated IOLs were of two planes, with the posterior loops offset from the back surface of the optic, and this caused the incision to gape during insertion, sometimes with anterior-chamber collapse in an era antedating the availability of viscoelastic substances. In the search for a single-plane IOL compatible with ECCE techniques, Kelman introduced a series of anterior-chamber IOLs as the concept of posterior-chamber fixation was being

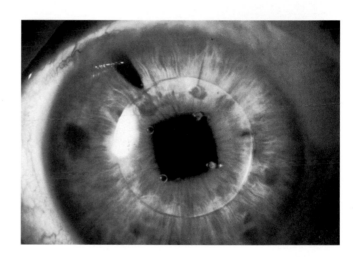

FIGURE 27-3.   *Worst Medallion IOL.*

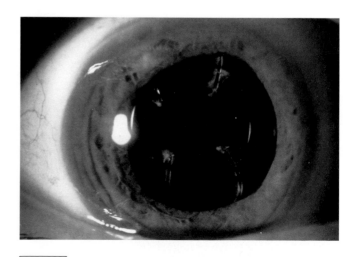

FIGURE 27-4.   *Binkhorst iridocapsular IOL (Duane).*

resurrected. The first of the Kelman anterior-chamber IOLs was shaped in the form of the figure "7" (Fig. 27-5) and could be inserted through a slightly enlarged phaco-emulsification incision (25). These lenses were rigid and still needed to be sized to the diameter of the patient's anterior chamber. The subsequent Kelman anterior-chamber IOLs were semiflexible and a given-length lens was suitable for a range of anterior-chamber diameters. There were two principal models, one with three-point fixation in the angle and the other four-point fixation. The Kelman semiflexible anterior-chamber IOLs are still used today in special situations (Fig. 27-6).

Before leaving the topic of anterior-chamber IOLs, the reader should be familiar with the problems that the profession experienced several years ago with closed-loop anterior-chamber IOLs and the subsequent development of

the uveitis-glaucoma-hyphema (UGH) syndrome in implant recipients (26–29).

POSTERIOR-CHAMBER IOLs

Pearce (30) introduced a posterior-chamber IOL, which he described in 1977. The lens was reminiscent of an anterior-chamber IOL that Ridley had introduced some 20 years previously. The Pearce IOL required an iris-fixation suture for stabilization until capsular fixation occurred. The placement of this suture was an invitation to wound gape with loss of intracameral contents in a time frame antedating viscoelastic agents, and therefore the advantage of its single-plane design was negated. For this reason, the Pearce IOL was not widely embraced by ophthalmic surgeons and it was the Shearing posterior-chamber IOL, described in 1978, that provided the stimulus for the wider adoption of posterior-chamber IOL fixation (Fig. 27-7) with the eventual eclipse of iris and anterior-chamber fixation (31). The results with the Shearing IOL and small-incision cataract surgery were extremely favorable and surgeons began seeking other ways to capitalize on the small incision. The essence of what they were seeking was instant visual recuperation, or close to it, with minimal postoperative convalescence. To further these goals, ways were sought to avoid enlarging the 3-mm phacoemulsification incision to insert a conventional posterior-chamber IOL and the logical solution was a foldable IOL. Mazzocco, having previously filed a patent (32) covering "deformable intraocular lenses" on February 5, 1982, reported on a lens fabricated of silicone (33) in 1985. Though "soft" materials for IOLs had been proposed previously on the premise that they were more suitable to the intraocular environment (34), Mazzocco's concept of folding the IOL was novel and his U.S. patent was issued on March 4, 1986. Before discussing foldable products in detail, I would like to digress at this point to discuss the current status and evolution of IOL materials.

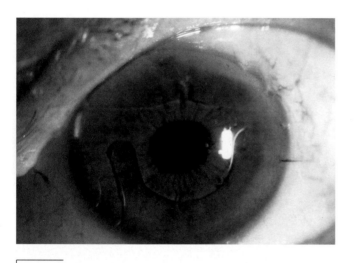

FIGURE 27-5. *Kelman "7" anterior-chamber IOL (2-degree insertion, temporal incision).*

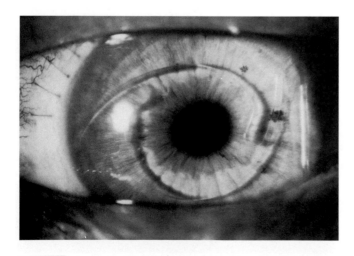

FIGURE 27-6. *Kelman semiflexible anterior-chamber IOL (2-degree insertion, temporal incision).*

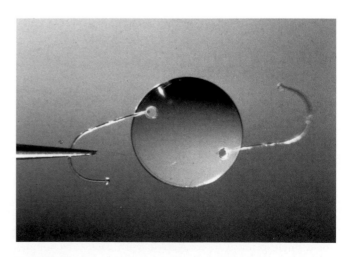

FIGURE 27-7. *Shearing posterior-chamber IOL.*

As mentioned earlier in this chapter the first Ridley IOL was manufactured of a high-molecular-weight PMMA and this thermoplastic material has been used continuously for IOL fabrication for over 45 years. The product initially used by Ridley was manufactured by ICI and ultimately designated Perspex CQ. It is a high-molecular-weight PMMA formulation with a relative high viscosity and therefore is not suitable for injection molding techniques. Therefore, it is supplied as a cast sheet and the IOLs are manufactured by a combination of lathe cutting, machine cutting, compression molding, and tumbling, according to a given manufacturer's preference. Where IOLs are injection molded, a pelletized PMMA of a lower molecular weight is used. This material is introduced into a mold, which under pressure and heat imparts the desired shape and dioptric power to the IOL. Whether cast sheet or pelletized PMMA, the material is prepolymerized, in contradistinction to the cast molding technique wherein methylmethacrylate

(MMA) and a chemical initiator are introduced into a mold. During the mold cycle the MMA is polymerized to PMMA while producing the desired IOL.

Returning to the topic of foldable IOL materials, currently Food and Drug Administration (FDA)–approved silicone and acrylic IOLs are available and a hydrogel IOL has recently been approved. In 1984 Staar Surgical Company introduced the first foldable IOL for clinical investigation in the United States, which was ultimately approved by the FDA in 1991. Two years earlier on October 31, 1989, Allergan Medical Optics (AMO), had two of their three-piece silicone products approved, the SI-18B and SI-18NB. Currently AMO is producing second-generation silicone IOLs with an ultraviolet blocker and a refractive index of 1.46. These models, designated SI-30NB and SI-40NB, are available with either polypropylene or PMMA monofilament loops, respectively (Fig. 27-8). Lens inserters are available for many of the AMO foldable products (Fig. 27-9). In December 1994, Alcon's acrylic foldable IOL was approved by the FDA. The optic is ultraviolet absorbant and has a refractive index of 1.55. Currently the MA30BA with a 5.5-mm optic and the MA60BM with a 6-mm optic are available, both with PMMA loops. Other companies also have acrylics under investigation (Figs. 27-10 and 27-11).

Generally, the results with the foldable IOLs have been very good, though from time to time, reports of complications attributable to the materials have appeared. Since silicone IOLs were the first foldable IOLs to be FDA approved, it is logical that they have had the longest clinical use in the United States and have been the subject of extensive clinical observation. For example, Milauskas (35) and Koch and Heit (36) reported in situ discoloration of silicone IOLs in human patients, but this did not seem to be a significant clinical problem. A few years earlier Newman et al (37) described manufacturing defects in an explanted silicone IOL. However, both the discoloration and IOL quality-control issues seem to have vanished, presumably as a result of better manufacturing practices on the part of both the material and the IOL manufacturers. Perhaps the two most

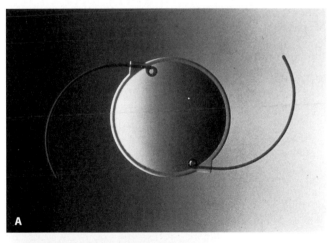

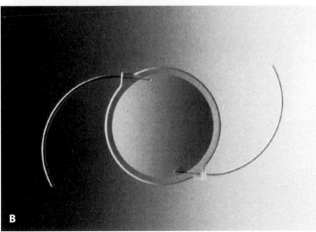

FIGURE 27-8. A. *Second-generation Allergan Medical Optics (AMO) model SI-30NB silicone posterior-chamber IOL with polypropylene haptics. (Courtesy of Allergan Medical Optics.)* B. *Second-generation AMO model SI-40NB silicone IOL with extruded PMMA haptics. (Note the proximal haptic insertion differs from that in A.) (Courtesy of Allergan Medical Optics.)*

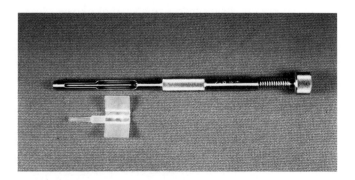

FIGURE 27-9. *AMO PhacoFlex II inserter with disposable chamber cartridge. (Courtesy of Allergan Medical Optics.)*

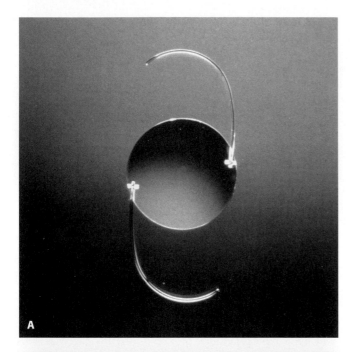

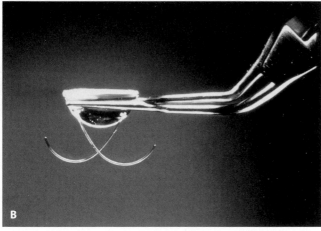

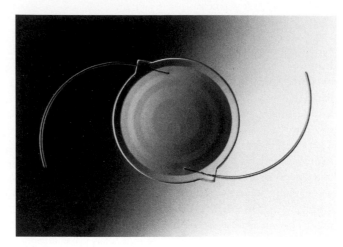

FIGURE 27-11.   *AMO Array multifocal IOL model SA-40N manufactured from AMO's second-generation silicone. (Courtesy of Allergan Medical Optics.)*

FIGURE 27-10.   A. *Alcon's MA30BA acrylic (ACRYSOF) posterior-chamber IOL. (Courtesy of Alcon.)* B. *Alcon MA30BA folded as a prelude to insertion. (Courtesy of Alcon.)*

important clinical disadvantages attributed to silicone are the relative difficulty of performing a Nd:YAG posterior capsulotomy when a silicone IOL is in situ (38,39) and the loss of posterior-segment visualization subsequent to vitreoretinal operative procedures when silicone oil is used in patients with a silicone IOL in situ (40,41).

With acrylic and hydrogel IOLs there is less clinical experience. There have been two reports of cracking of acrylic IOLs during folding or subsequent intracameral maneuvers (42,43) and this has also been seen with silicone IOLs (49). Oshika et al (44) reported excellent results in a series of acrylic IOL recipients and a paucity of problems during postoperative Nd:YAG posterior capsulotomies, but they did comment on the "tackiness" of the material during

intraoperative use. Dhaliwal et al (45) described intralenticular "glistenings" in Alcon acrylic IOLs which seem to be peculiar to IOLs supplied with a specific packaging. Currently this phenomenon does not appear to be of any clinical significance. Hydrogel IOLs have been reported as dislocating into the vitreous following Nd:YAG capsulotomy (46) and in a series of 20 hydrogel IOL–implanted patients with good visual results, Percival and Jaffree (47) noted asymptomatic decentration in 2 patients.

These negative reports on foldable materials should be balanced by the fact that from time to time complications attributed to conventional IOL materials have been reported. For example, in a series of explanted one-piece and three-piece silicone IOLs, the major reasons for explantation were inflammation and decentration, which were no different from the reasons for explantation of PMMA IOLs (48). Flynn and Carlson (49) described the use of laser synechialysis for the management of membranes forming on the surface of silicone IOLs, but this is a phenomenon also seen with PMMA IOLs. The vast majority of both PMMA and foldable IOL recipients have gratifying results.

THE FUTURE

The prospects for breakthroughs in IOL technology and design are muted by the prevailing medical economic climate in the United States. However, it would be reasonable to expect continued refinements in current materials, the search for better materials, and perhaps the introduction of IOLs fabricated from composite materials. Foldable IOL injectors will probably improve (50) and it is conceivable that foldable IOLs will be provided pre-folded, in cartridges. The surgeon will then load the cartridge into an injector as a prelude to intracameral insertion and this would preclude handling of the IOL in the operating room. This presupposes that the IOL will not deform while stored in the cartridge and will have the required memory to return to its desired shape and dioptric power, with good clarity and devoid of persistent striae.

Obviously the future holds the promise of wider adoption of previously proposed indications for IOLs such as myopia and presbyopia. Concerning myopia there would be little debate over the use of IOLs in myopic cataract patients (51) but the use of IOLs as a refractive device in *phakic*, myopic patients is quite controversial (52–54).

Attempts to correct the surgically induced presbyopia of pseudophakia are being addressed by the evaluation of multifocal IOLs. In 1986 the first multifocal IOL was implanted in England (55) and the following year a similar procedure was performed in the United States. The multifocal IOLs being investigated are posterior-chamber models of two general types, diffrative IOLs that focus light by the constructive interference of light waves (56) and refractive IOLs that bend light, according to Snell's law of refraction, as it passes between media of different refractive indices. Problems with loss of contrast sensitivity have been found in some patients (57,58) and Ellingson (59) reported on the explantation of diffractive IOLs in a group of patients. It remains to be seen if multifocal IOLs will be embraced by the profession.

REFERENCES

1. Ascher KW. Prosthetophakia two hundred years ago. *Am J Ophthalmol* 1965;59:445–446.
2. Münchow W. Zur Geschichte der introkularen Korrectur der Aphakie. *Klin Monatsbl Augenheilkd* 1964;145:771–777.
3. Ridley H. Intraocular acrylic lenses. *Trans Ophthalmol Soc UK* 1951;71: 617–621.
4. Strampelli B. L'evolution des lentilles plastique de chambre anterieure. *An Inst Barraquer* 1962;3:519–530.
5. Ridley H. The origin and objectives of intraocular lenticular implants. *Trans Am Acad Ophthalmol Otolaryngol* 1976;81:OP65–OP66.
6. Caudell PM. The first twelve years of intra-ocular lens construction. *An Inst Barraquer* 1962;3:531–542.
7. Ridley H. Intra-ocular acrylic lenses, a recent development in the surgery of cataract. *Br J Ophthalmol* 1952;36:113–122.
8. Jaffe NS, Galin MA, Hirschman H, Clayman HM. *Pseudophakos.* St Louis: CV Mosby, 1978:35.
9. Epstein E. Experiences with modified Ridley lenses and others. *An Inst Barraquer* 1962;3:555–561.
10. Wollensak J. Matières plastiques et lentilles artificielles. *An Inst Barraquer* 1962;3:543–547.
11. Ridley F. Safety requirements for acrylic implants. *Br J Ophthalmol* 1957;41:359–367.
12. O'Day DM. Fungal endophthalmitis caused by *Paecilomyces lilacinus* after intraocular lens implantation. *Am J Ophthalmol* 1977;83:130–131.
13. Galin MA, Turkish L. Sodium hydroxide sterilization of intraocular lenses. *Am J Ophthalmol* 1979;88:560–564.
14. Baron A. Tolerance de l'oeil a la matière plastique: prostheses optiques cristalliennes. *Bull Soc Ophthalmol Fr* 1953;982–988.
15. Strampelli B. Sopportabilità di lenti acriliche in camera anteriore nella afachia e nei vizi di refrazione. *Ann Ottal* 1954;80:75–82.
16. Choyce DP. *Intraocular lenses and implants.* London: HK Lewis, 1964.
17. Emmrich K. Vorderkammerlinsen aus silikatglas. *Klin Monatsbl Augenheilkd* 1958;132:254–256.
18. Strampelli B. Anterior chamber lenses. *Arch Ophthalmol* 1961;66:12–17.
19. Barasch K, Poler S. A glass intraocular lens. *Am J Ophthalmol* 1979;88:556–559.
20. Fritch CD. Neodymium:YAG laser damage to glass intraocular lens. *J Am Intraocular Implant Soc J* 1984;10:225.
21. Dannheim H. Types of anterior chamber lenses with elastic loops. *An Inst Barraquer* 1962;3:570–572.
22. Epstein E. Modified Ridley lenses. *Br J Ophthalmol* 1959;43:29–33.
23. Binkhorst CD, Leonard P. Results in 208 iris-clip pseudophakos implantations. *Am J Ophthalmol* 1967;64:947–956.
24. Binkhorst CD, Katz A, Leonard P. Extracapsular pseudophakos: results in 100 two-loop iridocapsular lens implantations. *Am J Ophthalmol* 1972;73: 625–636.
25. Keates RH, Lichenstein RB. The Kelman and other anterior chamber lenses. *Ophthalmic Surg* 1980;11:708–711.
26. Ellingson FT. The uveitis-glaucoma-hyphema syndrome associated with the Mark VIII anterior chamber lens implant. *Am Intraocular Implant Soc J* 1978;4:50–53.
27. Keates RH, Ehrlich DR. "Lenses of Chance" complications of anterior chamber implants. *Ophthalmology* 1978;85:408–414.
28. Hagan JC III. Complications while removing the Iolab 91Z lens for the UGH-UGH+ syndrome. *Am Intraocular Implant Soc J* 1984;9:209–213.
29. Maynor RC Jr. Five cases of severe anterior chamber lens complications. *Am Intraocular Implant Soc J* 1984;10:223–224.
30. Pearce JL. Experience with 194 posterior chamber lenses in 20 months. *Trans Ophthalmol Soc UK* 1977;97:258–264.
31. Shearing SP. A practical posterior chamber lens. *Contact Intraocular Lens Med J* 1978;4:114–119.
32. Mazzocco TR. US patent no. 4,573,998.
33. Mazzocco TR. Early clinical experience with elastic lens implants. *Trans Ophthalmol Soc UK* 1985;104:578–579.
34. Mehta KR, Sathe SN, Karyekar SD. The new soft intraocular lens implant. *Am Intraocular Implant Soc J* 1978;4:200–205.
35. Milauskas AT. Silicone intraocular lens implant discoloration in humans. *Arch Ophthalmol* 1991;109:913. Letter.
36. Koch DD, Heit LE. Discoloration of silicone intraocular lenses. *Ophthalmology* 1992;110:319–320.
37. Newman DA, McIntyre DJ, Apple DJ, et al. Pathologic findings of an explanted silicone intraocular lens. *J Cataract Refract Surg* 1986;12:292–297.
38. Auffarth CU, Newland TJ, Wesendahl TA, Apple DJ. Nd:YAG laser damage to silicone intraocular lenses confused with pigment deposits on clinical examination. *Am J Ophthalmol* 1994;118:526–528. Letter.
39. Milauskas AT. Posterior capsule opacification after silicone lens implantation and its management. *J Cataract Refract Surg* 1987;13:644–648.
40. Eaton AM, Jaffe GJ, McCuen BW II, Mincey GJ. Condensation on the posterior surface of silicone intraocular lenses during fluid-air exchange. *Ophthalmology* 1995;102:733–736.
41. Kusaka S, Kodama T, Ohashi Y. Condensation of silicone oil on the posterior surface of a silicone intraocular lens during vitrectomy. *Am J Ophthalmol* 1996;121:572–574.
42. Carlson KH, Johnson DW. Cracking of acrylic intraocular lenses during capsular bag insertion. *Ophthalmic Surg Lasers* 1995;26:572–573.
43. Pfister DR. Stress fractures after folding an acrylic intraocular lens. *Am J Ophthalmol* 1996;121:572–574.
44. Oshika T, Suzuki Y, Kizaki H, Yaguschi S. Two year study of a soft acrylic intraocular lens. *J Cataract Refract Surg* 1996;22:104–109.
45. Dhaliwal DK, Mamalis N, Olson RJ, et al. Visual significance of glistenings seen in the AcrySof intraocular lens. *J Cataract Refract Surg* 1996;22:452–457.
46. Levy JH, Pisacano AM, Anello RD. Displacement of bag-placed hydrogel lenses into the vitreous following neodymium:YAG laser capsulotomy. *J Cataract Refract Surg* 1990;16:563–566.
47. Percival SPB, Jaffree AJ. Preliminary results with a new hydrogel intraocular lens. *Eye* 1994;8:672–675.
48. Auffarth GU, Wilcox M, Sims JCR, et al. Analysis of 100 explanted one-piece and three-piece silicone intraocular lenses. *Ophthalmology* 1995;102:1144–1150.
49. Flynn WJ, Carlson DW. Laser synechialysis to prevent membrane recurrence on silicone intraocular lenses. *Am J Ophthalmol* 1996;122:426–428.
50. Habib NE, Singh J, Adams AD, Bartholomew RS. Cracked cartridges during foldable intraocular lens implantation. *J Catarat Refract Surg* 1996;22:630–632.
51. Lyle WA, Jin GJC. Phacoemulsification with intraocular lens implantation in high myopia. *J Cataract Refract Surg* 1996;22:238–242.
52. Fechner PU, Haigis W, Wichmann W. Posterior chamber myopia lenses in phakic eyes. *J Cataract Refract Surg* 1996;22:178–182.
53. Perez-Santonja JJ, Iradier MT, Sanz-Iglesias L, et al. Endothelial changes in phakic eyes with anterior chamber intraocular lenses to correct high myopia. *J Cataract Refract Surg* 1996;22:1017–1022.

54. Perez-Santonja JJ, Iradier MT, Benítez del Castillo JM, et al. Chronic subclinical inflammation in phakic eyes with intraocular lenses to correct myopia. *J Cataract Refract Surg* 1996;22:183–187.

55. Keates RH, Pearce JL, Schneider RT. Clinical results of the multifocal lens. *J Cataract Refract Surg* 1987;13:557–560.

56. Simpson JM. The diffractive multifocal intraocular lens. *Eur J Implant Refract Surg* 1989;1:115–121.

57. Holladay JT, Van Dijk H, Lang A, et al. Optical performance of multifocal intraocular lenses. *J Cataract Refract Surg* 1990;16:413–422.

58. Olsen T, Corydon L. Contrast sensitivity as a function of focus in patients with the diffractive multifocal intraocular lens. *J Cataract Refract Surg* 1990;16:703–706.

59. Ellingson FT. Explantation of 3M diffractive intraocular lenses. *J Cataract Refract Surg* 1990;16:697–702.

Glaucoma Surgery

TODD W. PERKINS AND PAUL L. KAUFMAN
Section Editors

28

Philosophy of Treatment

Douglas E. Gaasterland

The philosophical basis for treating glaucoma can be expressed succinctly: *preserve useful vision*. This statement applies to all forms of the disease, and each word is important. Vision loss from glaucoma goes hand in hand with the optic nerve damage caused by the disease. Glaucomatous optic neuropathy has characteristic clinical and pathological features. There is attenuation within the parapapillary retinal nerve fiber layer and localized loss of thickness of the neural rim tissue on the disk; visual field defects reflect these changes. Without treatment, the damage tends to progress. Glaucomatous optic neuropathy is related to the level of intraocular pressure (IOP); the higher the IOP, the more likely optic nerve damage will be found (1–3). This type of optic neuropathy, characteristic of glaucoma, occurs rarely in other disease processes (4). Glaucoma interventions are designed to reduce IOP. The goal of treatment is to interrupt the progression of glaucomatous optic neuropathy.

GLAUCOMATOUS OPTIC NEUROPATHY

At birth, each normal human eye is endowed with approximately one million or more optic nerve axons (5–7). Each axon arises at a ganglion cell in the retina, courses through the optic nerve to the axonal decussation in the optic chiasm, and ends at a synapse in the lateral geniculate body.

In glaucomatous optic neuropathy, the earliest damage is found at the optic nervehead, both within and slightly anterior to the lamina cribrosa. Individual axons and groups of axons in the bundles in the nervehead show impaired axonal transport (8). Initially, glaucoma tends to damage axons in bundles located in the superior and inferior portions of the nervehead (9–12). When an axon is sufficiently damaged by glaucoma, it and the ganglion cell of its origin degenerate,

probably by apoptosis, and are lost permanently (13). If the damaging stimulus stops, many already weakened axons are lost, while some recover. Unaffected axons are preserved, and progressive vision loss stops. However, when an early glaucomatous defect is first detectable in the threshold visual field test of an eye there has already been a 20% to 40% loss of optic nerve axons (14).

While interrupting the damaging process is likely to save the vision still present in the eye, it will not restore ganglion cells or vision already lost. Based on this, we state three basic principles of glaucoma surgical intervention:

1. Early intervention is better than late.
2. Late intervention is justified if useful vision remains.
3. There is little chance of vision benefit from intervention in an eye that has no perception of light as a result of glaucoma.

Consider an eye (it originally had one million axons) in which glaucoma has killed 650,000 optic nerve axons and weakened 100,000 more. The glaucoma intervention is aimed at saving the 250,000 axons still intact and possibly some of the 100,000 weakened axons. Unfortunately, the intervention itself may damage vision (15,16), and an optic nerve with established moderate to severe damage may show gradual progressive damage despite surgical reduction of IOP to low levels (17).

PATHOPHYSIOLOGY

In order to treat a disease effectively, it helps to understand its pathophysiology. Unfortunately, while we know what happens in the optic nerve and retina, the causes for these events are elusive in some forms of glaucoma. Elevated IOP is one cause. There are others, because not all eyes that develop glaucomatous optic neuropathy have elevated IOP. These other causes appear to be related to the risk factors for a patient developing glaucomatous axonal damage.

Elevated IOP as a Cause of Glaucomatous Optic Neuropathy

In population studies, the most predictive risk factor for glaucomatous optic neuropathy is elevated IOP (1–3). Prevalence increases sharply with increase of IOP (2,3). It is clearly known from clinical experience and from laboratory studies that elevated IOP (i.e., in the mid 20s mmHg and higher) is associated with glaucomatous optic nerve damage. Provided it is sustained, abrupt elevation of IOP high above the normal range causes glaucomatous optic neuropathy. For example, such a rise of IOP is found in untreated acute angle-closure glaucoma.

Sustained elevations of IOP above 35 mmHg eventually cause glaucomatous damage in most, though not all, otherwise normal eyes. While we know less time is required to cause optic nerve damage when the IOP is higher, we have almost no quantitative information about how quickly, at various levels of IOP, sufficient axonal damage accumulates for clinically recognizable glaucomatous optic neuropathy to develop. Laboratory studies show that serious damage to a previously normal primate optic nerve occurs in 2 to 3 weeks when IOP ranges from 36 to 39 mmHg (18). High IOP elevation, sometimes well above 40 mmHg, occurs with abrupt onset in acute angle-closure glaucoma and in some forms of secondary glaucoma. If the elevation persists, glaucomatous optic neuropathy develops and can be expected to progress.

Clinical observations indicate that eyes with previous optic nerve damage from glaucoma are more vulnerable to elevated IOP than are eyes with normal optic nerves (19,20). Clinical observations also suggest that previously damaged eyes deteriorate more quickly than "healthy" eyes when IOP is elevated. Therapeutic reduction of IOP to "subnormal" levels (below the teens) appears to safeguard many, but not all, damaged eyes against progressive optic neuropathy (21).

Other Causes of Glaucomatous Optic Neuropathy

Besides elevated IOP, there are other causes of glaucomatous optic neuropathy. Our knowledge in this area is inadequate, and the evidence is either indirect or anecdotal. The existence of other causes is implied from the well-recognized phenomenon of progression of glaucomatous damage in open-angle glaucoma patients with normal IOP (17,19,20). This can be confusing. For example, one patient with IOP reduced to the high teens from a previous elevation will be stable, while another patient with IOP never observed above the high teens, and usually in the low teens,

will experience progressive loss of visual field due to the glaucomatous process (17).

Epidemiologic studies have shown that about half of untreated patients with glaucoma damage do not have elevation of IOP above the normal range during an initial screening measurement (2). The Normal Tension Glaucoma Study is evaluating the benefit of treatment to reduce IOP 30% from the level associated with progressive damage in patients with normal tension glaucoma (22). Until results are available, there is little documentation of the benefit of reducing IOP below normal with medical or surgical interventions in normal tension glaucoma patients.

In the absence of elevated IOP there are other possible causes of glaucomatous optic neuropathy (23), including but not limited to the following:

- defective blood supply or perfusion to the optic nerve (24)
- abnormal extracellular support tissue in the nervehead (25,26)
- autoimmune phenomena affecting ganglion cells or axons (27)
- intrinsic genetic defects of ganglion cells or their axons, rendering them unusually vulnerable to IOP or other factors (28)

Evidence for each of these has been found in a portion of patients with normal tension glaucoma. Further, other disease processes, including vascular insults, syphilitic optic neuritis, trauma, and compressive injury of the optic nerve within the cranial cavity, may cause an optic neuropathy clinically indistinguishable from that in normal tension glaucoma (4,29–31), although the development of this neuropathy is often faster than in normal tension glaucoma (32). Also, the ophthalmic surgeon must remember that these other disease processes can occur in conjunction with glaucoma or ocular hypertension.

Patients with Inactive Disease

There is another important group of patients with normal IOP and glaucomatous optic neuropathy. We must distinguish these patients who, without using glaucoma medications, currently have both normal IOP and glaucomatous neuropathy acquired previously, during an active process that insulated the optic nerve. An example is a steroid-responder patient who developed glaucomatous optic neuropathy during topical steroid treatment and whose IOP rose with prolonged use of those medications. These patients have inactive disease and do not require medical or surgical glaucoma treatment, though they must be monitored.

TREATING IOP IN GLAUCOMA

Though the pathophysiology is sometimes difficult to determine, one thing is clear: the sole *treatable* factor that causes glaucomatous optic neuropathy is elevated IOP. In primary and secondary glaucoma with high IOP, intervention to reduce pressure to normal levels usually interrupts the progression of damage.

Indications for Surgery

Within the sequence of management maneuvers, an important decision is when to introduce glaucoma surgery to lower IOP. This is not fully defined in the literature. Obviously, immediate surgery is justified in severe situations (e.g., acute angle-closure). Surgery is also justified for medically uncontrollable IOP elevations above the damage threshold–based target level (33), or whenever there is progressive glaucomatous optic neuropathy despite sensible medical management, no matter what the IOP (34).

The appropriate timing for introducing laser and invasive surgery for newly diagnosed primary open-angle glaucoma has been under investigation (Table 28-1). Results from trials in Great Britain suggest that initial intervention with filtering surgery better preserves visual field than does starting with medications or trabeculoplasty (35,36). The Moorfields Trial, Glaucoma Laser Trial, and Glaucoma Laser Trial Follow-up Study show that laser trabeculoplasty is slightly better, in the long term, for preserving visual field (36,37) than is initial medical treatment (37), and less medication is needed. The Fluorouracil Filtering Surgery Trial has shown that adjunctive antifibrotic agents nearly double long-term success rates when added to filtering surgery for eyes with medically uncontrollable glaucoma after previous surgery (38). Ongoing clinical trials are providing more information to answer questions about the role, timing, method, and value of surgical IOP reduction in glaucoma (see Table 28-1) (39).

Surgery for Eyes Without Glaucomatous Optic Neuropathy

Many eyes have elevated IOP and do not develop glaucomatous optic neuropathy, even after years of IOP elevation. Overall, about 90% of otherwise healthy eyes with ocular hypertension do not develop neuropathy during 10 years of follow-up (40). Whether treating such eyes to lower IOP helps to prevent development of glaucomatous optic neuropathy is unclear. The goal of the ongoing Ocular Hypertension Treatment Study (OHTS) is to clarify the value of medical treatment for such eyes. Usually, we do not perform glaucoma surgery for ocular hypertension in the absence of optic neuropathy. It may be justified for rare cases, without neuropathy, where IOP is continually in the upper 30s, or higher, despite medical treatment.

Mechanisms: Effects of Treatment Methods

Whether treatment is medical or surgical, the mechanisms are the same. The goal is to reduce IOP, the level of which reflects the steady-state balance between flow of aqueous humor through the eye and resistance to outflow. Normally, the bulk outflow of aqueous humor responsible for determining IOP level is primarily through the trabecular meshwork to the canal of Schlemm. The physician alters IOP by either enhancing outflow or reducing inflow. The cause of elevated IOP and the patient's previous treatment history guide the choice of procedure.

Table 28-1. Controlled Glaucoma Clinical Trials, Types of Glaucoma Being Studied, Recruitment Goals, Projected Durations of Follow-up, and Current Status

Name	Type of Glaucoma and Types of Intervention	Recruitment Goal	Follow-up Duration	Status
Scottish Glaucoma Trial	Newly diagnosed POAG; trabeculectomy vs. medications	99 patients	3–5 years	C
Moorfields Primary Treatment Trial	Newly diagnosed POAG; trabeculectomy vs. trabeculoplasty vs. medications	168 patients	≥5 years	C
Glaucoma Laser Trial (GLT)*	Newly diagnosed POAG; trabeculoplasty vs. medications	271 patients	2.5–5.5 years	C
Glaucoma Laser Trial Follow-up Study (GLTFS)*	Participants in the GLT	203 patients	6–9 years	C
Fluorouracil Filtering Surgery Study (FFSS)*	Uncontrolled OAG, previous cataract or filtration surgery; another filter w/ or w/o 5-fluorouracil	213 patients	5 years	C
Ocular Hypertension Treatment Study (OHTS)*	Ocular hypertension (glaucoma suspected); observation vs. medications	≥1500 patients	≥5 years	F/U
Normal Tension Glaucoma Study (NTGS)	POAG in eyes with normal IOP; observation then medications vs. trabeculoplasty	200 patients	≥5 years	F/U
Advanced Glaucoma Intervention Study (AGIS)*	OAG after medical treatment failure, no previous surgery; sequences starting with trabeculectomy vs. trabeculoplasty	591 patients (789 eyes)	4–9 years	F/U
Early Manifest Glaucoma Trial (EMGT)*	Newly diagnosed POAG (Sweden); observation vs. medications	300 patients	≥4 years	F/U
Collaborative Initial Glaucoma Treatment Study (CIGTS)*	Newly diagnosed POAG; medications vs. trabeculectomy	600 patients	≥5 years	F/U

* Sponsored by the National Eye Institute.
POAG = primary open-angle glaucoma; C = completed; F/U = follow-up.
SOURCE: Modified from Wilson MR, Gaasterland DE. Translating research into practice: controlled clinical trials and their influence on glaucoma management. *J Glaucoma* 1996;5:139–146.

Elevated IOP caused by a blockage of the aqueous humor's access to the trabecular meshwork, as in angle closure or anterior chamber hemorrhage, responds better to procedures that alleviate the blockade rather than reduce inflow. Filtering procedures, goniotomy, trabeculotomy, and seton drainage procedures, sometimes supplemented with adjunctive antifibrotic agents, address high intrinsic resistance to flow through trabecular tissue in various glaucoma situations. Cyclodialysis, seldom practiced today, provides enhanced drainage via alternative (suprachoroidal) pathways, with associated reduction of IOP.

Cyclodestructive procedures reduce IOP by slowing aqueous inflow. The surgeon coagulates ciliary body tissue by applying energy either directly (from inside the eye) or through the sclera (from the outside). Energy in the form of cryotherapy, diathermy, and light all work, though some have fewer side effects than others. For example, laser transscleral cyclophotocoagulation causes less inflammation than cyclocryotherapy. Cyclodestructive procedures are usually performed only for glaucomatous eyes with an inadequate response to outflow-enhancing surgery that has been supplemented with medicines to reduce inflow. These recalcitrant eyes are management problems.

HISTORY OF SURGICAL GLAUCOMA TREATMENT

Our present day philosophy of treatment rests on the historical recognition of IOP elevation as a cause of blindness and the surgical attempts that followed to reduce the elevation permanently and beneficially. Sir Stewart Duke-Elder details this history masterfully in the glaucoma section of his *System of Ophthalmology*, published in 1969 (41). The following paragraphs provide a brief overview of the early history of glaucoma surgery as told by Duke-Elder, and are supplemented with information about developments during the past three decades.

The teachings of Pierre Demours and his son, Antoine-Pierre Demours led to general acceptance of elevated IOP, identified as a firm globe to palpation, as a cause of glaucomatous loss of vision. They based their teachings on clinical experience with acute, congestive (angle-closure) glaucoma and the later, noncongestive stage of the disease, as published by Antoine-Pierre Demours in 1818.

In the early 1830s, William Mackenzie emphasized that elevated IOP is, first, different from cataract and, second, (like cataract) is another condition arising *within* the eye causing loss of vision. He introduced glaucoma surgical treatment, performing both sclerotomy and paracentesis of the vitreous cavity for elevated IOP.

Using the ophthalmoscope invented by von Helmholtz (1851), both Adolph Weber and Albrecht von Graefe correctly described glaucomatous cupping of the optic nerve in 1855. Müller confirmed the finding histopathologically in 1856. In 1857, von Graefe classified the optic nerve damage associated with inflammatory acute glaucoma (and

its later, noninflamed, residual state) as different from the similar optic nervehead cupping associated with elevated IOP in eyes without inflammation. Frans Cornelis Donders (1862) recognized this latter condition as a form of glaucoma and designated it simple chronic glaucoma. Also, in 1857, von Graefe reported improvement of a staphyloma after basal iridectomy in an eye with acute congestive glaucoma. This introduced iridectomy as surgical treatment for congestive glaucoma. It was soon recognized that iridectomy had little benefit in the chronic forms of the disease.

Louis de Wecker, a student of von Graefe, in the late 1860s conceived anterior sclerectomy with the aim to create, in eyes with chronic glaucoma, a filtering cicatrix to drain the aqueous humor. Many modifications followed, gradually improving the filtering function of the procedures. These include de Wecker's combination of sclerectomy with iridectomy; the Elliot variation of corneoscleral trephining; Scheie's improved wound-cauterizing procedure and the more recent techniques for laser sclerostomy; iridencleisis as introduced by Holth; the various sclerectomy procedures culminating in guarded trabeculectomy as described by both Cairnes in 1967 (42) and Linnér in 1968 (43); numerous seton drainage procedures, starting with implantation of horse hairs and silk threads in the early 1900s; and introduction in recent decades of adjunctive agents to modify wound healing after filtering surgery (38,44,45).

In 1905, Leopold Heine introduced cyclodialysis to reduce IOP by enhancing the function of internal drainage channels (i.e., uveoscleral outflow). In 1893, de Vincentiis conceived transcameral goniotomy in an attempt to enhance drainage to the canal of Schlemm. He was constrained by a lack of ability to visualize the anterior chamber angle recess. In the late 1930s, Otto Barkan perfected the technique by revealing the approach of the surgical knife to the anterior chamber angle with his gonioscopic contact lens and intense illumination, resulting in the goniotomy procedure widely used today for congenital glaucoma (though this has little success in adult glaucoma). Surgeons use a variant of this, the trabeculotomy ab externo introduced in 1960 by Smith (46) and refined by Allen and Burian in 1962 (47), when corneal haze inhibits visualization for goniotomy.

During the early part of the twentieth century, ophthalmologists developed improved understanding of aqueous humor dynamics compared with the knowledge of nineteenth century surgeons. This led to the realization that slowing inflow of aqueous humor by ciliary ablation reduces IOP. Starting in the 1930s, various clinicians described coagulative ciliary ablation, using nearly every imaginable method of energy delivery to the eye to reduce ciliary function. In a 1950 publication, Bietti summarized previous work and described cryotherapy as an alternative to cyclodiathermy for ciliary ablation (48). Beckman reported the first successful transscleral laser ciliary ablation method in 1972, only 12 years after lasers were first described (49). Today, most surgeons only perform ciliary ablation for eyes with recalcitrant glaucoma and severe optic nerve damage after previous surgery and medical treatment have failed. Since the goal of this type of procedure is to bring inflow into balance with the hampered outflow of aqueous humor from the eye there is a risk, in eyes with high outflow resistance, of creating stagnation before IOP is reduced adequately, as emphasized by Spaeth (50). Modern laser ciliary ablation techniques yield control of IOP and preservation of vision for 2 years in 50% to 60% of patients (51).

SUMMARY

1. The goal of glaucoma surgery is to reduce IOP to a level sufficient to preserve useful visual function of the eye; visual function lost to glaucoma cannot be recovered.

2. In some eyes with progressive glaucomatous optic neuropathy, elevation of IOP is clearly the cause. The treatment goal is to reduce IOP well below the level causing damage.

3. Sometimes, glaucomatous optic neuropathy progresses while the IOP is normal. Until a better management technique is identified, we approach these eyes with the aim of reducing IOP substantially below the level found at the time of active damage.

4. Usually, surgery is not justified for eyes with elevated IOP and no glaucomatous optic neuropathy.

5. Usually, surgery is not justified for eyes with normal IOP and stable glaucomatous optic neuropathy.

6. Surgery reduces IOP by enhancing aqueous humor outflow or reducing aqueous humor inflow (or both).

7. Review of the history of glaucoma surgical interventions shows that surgical concepts are comparatively recent and have developed hand in hand with the realization that IOP is elevated in many eyes with glaucomatous optic neuropathy. The IOP elevation in glaucoma reflects increased resistance to outflow; surgical concepts have been directed toward modifying the balance of aqueous dynamics to reduce IOP.

REFERENCES

1. Sommer A. Intraocular pressure and glaucoma. *Am J Ophthalmol* 1989;107:186–188.
2. Sommer A, Teilsch JM, Katz J, et al. Relationship between intraocular pressure and primary open angle glaucoma among white and black Americans. The Baltimore Eye Survey. *Arch Ophthalmol* 1991;109:1090–1095.
3. Leske MC, Connell AMS, Wu S-Y, et al. Risk factors for open-angle glaucoma. *Arch Ophthalmol* 1995;113:918–924.
4. Bianchi-Marzoli S, Rizzo JF III, Brancato R, Lessell S. Quantitative analysis of optic disc cupping in compressive optic neuropathy. *Ophthalmology* 1995;102:439–440.
5. Balazsi AG, Rootman J, Drance SM, et al. The effect of age on the nerve fiber population of the human optic nerve. *Am J Ophthalmol* 1984;97:760–766.
6. Repka MS, Quigley HA. The effect of age on normal human optic nerve fiber number and diameter. *Ophthalmology* 1989;96:26–32.
7. Mikelberg FS, Drance SM, Schulzer M, et al. The normal human optic nerve. Axon count and axon diameter distribution. *Ophthalmology* 1989;96:1325–1328.
8. Minkler DS, Spaeth GL. Optic nerve damage in glaucoma. *Surv Ophthalmol* 1981;26:128–148.
9. Quigley HA, Addicks EM. Regional difference in the structure of the lamina cribrosa and their relation to glaucomatous optic nerve damage. *Arch Ophthalmol* 1981;99:137–144.
10. Quigley HA, Addicks EM, Green WR, Maumenee AE. Optic nerve damage in human glaucoma, II: the site of injury and susceptibility to damage. *Arch Ophthalmol* 1981;99:635–649.
11. Quigley HA, Sanchez RM, Dunkelberger GR, et al. Chronic glaucoma selectively damages large optic nerve fibers. *Invest Ophthalmol Vis Sci* 1987;28:913–920.
12. Jonas JB, Müller-Bergh JA, Schlötzer-Schrehardt UM, Naumann GOH. Histomorphometry of the human optic nerve. *Invest Ophthalmol Vis Sci* 1990;31:736–744.
13. Quigley HA, Nickells RW, Kerrigan LA, et al. Retinal ganglion cell death in experimental glaucoma and after axotomy occurs by apoptosis. *Invest Ophthalmol Vis Sci* 1995;36:774–786.
14. Quigley HA, Dunkelberger GR, Green WR. Retinal ganglion cell atrophy correlated with automated perimetry in human eyes with glaucoma. *Am J Ophthalmol* 1989;107:453–464.
15. Lichter PR, Ravin JG. Risks of sudden visual loss after glaucoma surgery. *Am J Ophthalmol* 1974;78:1009–1013.
16. Kolker AE. Visual prognosis in advanced glaucomas: a comparison of medical and surgical therapy for retention of vision in 101 eyes with advanced glaucoma. *Trans Am Ophthalmol Soc* 1977;75:539–555.
17. Brubaker RF. Delayed functional loss in glaucoma. LII Edward Jackson Memorial Lecture. *Am J Ophthalmol* 1996;121:473–483.
18. Gaasterland D, Tanishima T, Kuwabara T. Axoplasmic flow during chronic experimental glaucoma. I. Light and electron microscopic studies of the monkey optic nervehead during development of glaucomatous cupping. *Invest Ophthalmol Vis Sci* 1978;17:838–846.
19. Abedin S, Simmons RJ, Grant WM. Progressive low-tension glaucoma. Treatment to stop glaucomatous cupping and field loss when these progress despite normal intraocular pressure. *Ophthalmology* 1982;89:1–6.
20. Grant WM, Burke JF. Why do some people go blind from glaucoma? *Ophthalmology* 1982;89:991–998.
21. Lynn JR. Glaucomatous visual field loss and subnormal IOP. In: Mills RP, ed. Perimetry update 1992/93. Proceedings of the Xth International Perimetric Society Meeting, Kyoto, Japan, October 1992. Amsterdam: Kugler, 1993:129–135.
22. Schulzer M. The Normal Tension Glaucoma Study Group. Intraocular pressure reduction in normal-tension glaucoma patients. *Ophthalmology* 1992;99:1468–1470.
23. Van Buskirk EM, Cioffi GA. Perspectives: glaucomatous optic neuropathy. *Am J Ophthalmol* 1992;113:447–452.
24. Ong K, Farinelli A, Billson F, et al. Comparative study of brain magnetic resonance imaging findings in patients with low-tension glaucoma and control subjects. *Ophthalmology* 1995;102:1632–1638.
25. Quigley HA, Addicks EM. Regional differences in the structure of the lamina cribrosa and their relation to glaucomatous optic nerve damage. *Arch Ophthalmol* 1981;99:137–143.
26. Hernandez MR. Ultrastructural immunocytochemical analysis of elastin in the human lamina cribrosa: changes in elastic fibers in primary open-angle glaucoma. *Invest Ophthalmol Vis Sci* 1992;33:2891–2903.
27. Wax MB, Barrett DA, Pestronk A. Increased incidence of paraproteinemia and autoantibodies in patients with normal-tension glaucoma. *Am J Ophthalmol* 1994;117:561–568.
28. Lichter PR. Genetic clues to glaucoma's secrets. The L Edward Jackson Memorial Lecture. Part 2. *Am J Ophthalmol* 1994;117:706–727.
29. Trobe JD, Glaser JS, Cassady J, et al. Nonglaucomatous excavation of the optic disc. *Arch Ophthalmol* 1980;98:1046–1050.
30. Sebag J, Thomas JV, Epstein DL, Grant WM. Optic disc cupping in arteritic anterior ischemic optic neuropathy resembles glaucomatous cupping. *Ophthalmology* 1986;93:357–361.
31. Sonty S, Schwartz B. Development of cupping and pallor in posterior ischemic optic neuropathy. *Int Ophthalmol* 1983;6:213–220.

32. Manor RS. Documented optic disc cupping in compressive optic neuropathy (Letter to the editor). *Ophthalmology* 1995;102:1577.

33. Anderson DR. Glaucoma. The damage caused by pressure. XLVI Edward Jackson Memorial Lecture. *Am J Ophthalmol* 1989;108:485–495.

34. The American Academy of Ophthalmology Preferred Practice Patterns Committee Glaucoma Panel. Preferred practice pattern: Primary open-angle glaucoma. San Francisco: American Academy of Ophthalmology, 1996.

35. Jay JL, Allan D. The benefit of early trabeculectomy versus conventional management in primary open-angle glaucoma relative to severity of the disease. *Eye* 1989;3:528–535.

36. Migdahl C, Hitchings R. Long-term functional outcome of early surgery compared with laser and medicine in open angle glaucoma. *Ophthalmology* 1994;101:1651–1657.

37. Glaucoma Laser Trial Research Group. The Glaucoma Laser Trial and Glaucoma Laser Trial Follow-up Study: 7. Results. *Am J Ophthalmology* 1995;120:718–731.

38. The Fluorouracil Filtering Surgery Study Group. Five-year follow-up of the Fluorouracil Filtering Surgery Study. *Am J Ophthalmol* 1996;121:349–366.

39. Wilson MR, Gaasterland DE. Translating research into practice: controlled clinical trials and their influence on glaucoma management. *J Glaucoma* 1996;5:139–146.

40. Perkins ES. The Bedford glaucoma survey. I. Long-term follow-up of borderline cases. *Br J Ophthalmol* 1973;57:179–185.

41. Duke-Elder S, ed. System of ophthalmology; Volume XI. Diseases of the lens and vitreous; glaucoma and hypotony. St. Louis: Mosby, 1969:379–385.

42. Cairnes JE. Trabeculectomy, preliminary report of a new method. *Am J Ophthalmol* 1968;66:673–679.

43. Linnér E. Microsurgical trabeculectomy "ab externo" in glaucoma. *Trans Ophthalmol Soc* 1969;89:475–479.

44. Skuta GL, Beeson CC, Higginbotham EJ, et al. Intraoperative mitomycin versus postoperative 5-fluorouracil in high-risk glaucoma filtering surgery. *Ophthalmology* 1992;99:438–444.

45. Kitazawa Y, Kawase K, Matsushita H, Minobe M. Trabeculectomy with mitomycin. A comparative study with fluorouracil. *Arch Ophthalmol* 1991;109: 1693–1698.

46. Smith PA. A new technique for opening the canal of Schlemm. *Br J Ophthalmol* 1960;44:370–372.

47. Allen L, Burian HM. Trabeculotomy ab externo. *Am J Ophthalmol* 1962;54: 19–32.

48. Bietti G. Surgical interventions on the ciliary body. New trends for the relief of glaucoma. *J Am Med Assoc* 1950;142:889–896.

49. Beckman H, Kinoshita A, Rota AN, et al. Transscleral ruby laser irradiation of the ciliary body in the treatment of intractable glaucoma. *Trans Am Acad Ophthalmol Otolaryngol* 1972;76:423–435.

50. Spaeth GL. Discussion: Gaasterland DE, Pollack IP. Initial experience with a new method of laser transscleral cyclophotocoagulation for ciliary ablation in severe glaucoma. *Trans Am Ophthalmol Soc* 1992;90:243–246.

51. Kosoko O, Gaasterland DE, Pollack IP, et al. Long term outcome of initial ciliary ablation with contact diode laser transscleral cyclophotocoagulation. *Ophthalmology* 1996;103:1294–1302.

Laser Trabeculoplasty

Jacob T. Wilensky

Shortly after lasers were developed for use in ophthalmology, attempts were made to see if they could be used to help treat glaucoma. The first application involved attempts to create holes from the anterior chamber through the trabecular meshwork into Schlemm's canal, in a manner somewhat analogous to trabeculotomy. Krasnov in Russia (1), using a Q-switched ruby laser, and Worthen and Wickham (2) in the United States, using an argon laser, reported beneficial intraocular pressure (IOP) responses to the treatment. Within a year of Worthen and Wickham's report, however, Gaasterland and Kupfer (3) reported that an experimental glaucoma could be created in monkey eyes by applying laser energy to the trabecular meshwork. This report somewhat dampened the enthusiasm for laser treatment of glaucoma and delayed further clinical work.

In 1979, Wise and Witter (4) reported the results of a somewhat different laser treatment for glaucoma. In their treatment, a series of approximately 100 argon laser burns were scattered over the whole 360 degrees of the trabecular meshwork. These burns were not of sufficient intensity to create penetrating holes through the trabecular meshwork, but rather caused a local area of coagulation and resulted in a decrease in IOP. Other investigators (5,6) quickly confirmed this work and argon laser trabeculoplasty (ALT), as the technique came to be called, rapidly gained widespread acceptance within the ophthalmic community as a treatment for open-angle glaucoma.

The mechanism by which laser trabeculoplasty lowers IOP is still the subject of debate (7). Wise and Witter (4) proposed that the coagulation caused by the laser burns results in contracture of the adjacent tissues, thereby tightening the trabecular ring and perhaps widening the adjacent trabecular pores. A second theory is that the laser induces physiologic changes in the activity of the trabecu-

lar cells. Differences in cellular glycosaminoglycan measured by radiolabeled sulfate incorporation were detected in treated autopsy eyes. Others (8) reported increased phagocytic activity of the trabecular meshwork cells in laser-treated eyes. A third theory is that ALT induces division of trabecular meshwork cells as has been demonstrated in human organ transplant culture systems (9). Whatever the mechanism by which it is accomplished, multiple observers have documented that ALT increases the tonographic facility of aqueous outflow from the anterior chamber (5,6) and this is how IOP is lowered.

TECHNIQUES

The initial Wise and Witter treatment protocol consisted of placing approximately 100 laser burns in the middle of the pigmented trabecular meshwork. The burns were 50 μm in size and one-tenth of a second in duration at an initial power level of 1000 mW, increasing to 1500 mW depending on the tissue response. Since then, there have been multiple articles reporting the results of various alterations in this technique. Even today there is not a complete consensus about all of the treatment parameters (9).

One early study reported that a significant IOP response could be achieved with treatment of as little as 90 degrees of the trabecular meshwork with 25 laser burns. Increasing the amount of meshwork treated to 180 degrees seems to achieve greater lowering of IOP. Studies comparing treatment of 180 versus 360 degrees of the trabecular meshwork failed to show any significant difference in the response. Wise (10) believes that after 2 years or longer, eyes receiving full treatment maintain the pressure-lowering effect better than do those having half the angle treated, but at least one study comparing 50 versus 100 burns failed to show any major difference after 5 years of follow-up (11).

Different investigators (12) have placed their burns over almost all aspects of the trabecular meshwork, ranging anteriorly from the nonpigmented trabecular meshwork just below Schwalbe's line all the way to the ciliary body band posteriorly. In general, there does not seem to be any major difference in pressure-lowering effect, but with more posteriorly placed burns there was more patient discomfort, inflammatory response, and late synechial formation. For these reasons I recommend placing the burns anteriorly at the junction between pigmented and nonpigmented meshwork.

Most studies of laser trabeculoplasty utilized argon lasers emitting energy of several wavelengths in the blue-green spectrum. There have been reports of treatments with green-only argon lasers, diode lasers, and Nd:YAG lasers in the infrared range. All of these were found to be effective but do not have any advantages over the blue-green argon lasers (12).

Energy density is determined by a combination of the duration, power, and diameter of the burns placed. There have been reports of 0.2-second burns, but they do not offer an advantage over the 0.1-second standard. Although Wise (4) initially treated with 1000 mW or more, other investigators determined that a pressure-lowering response could be achieved with energy levels as low as 500 mW. Rouhianen et al (13) found no difference in pressure lowering when the laser power was varied from 500 to 800 mW. Although the majority of investigators treated to a tissue reaction of either blanching or small bubble formation and varied the energy level to achieve such a reaction, others found that good pressure lowering can be achieved even in the absence of a visible tissue response and advocate a standard 800-mW power setting for all eyes (12).

When the diameter of the laser beam is doubled at a constant power setting, the energy density is reduced by a factor of four. Therefore, it is important to make sure that the aiming beam is sharply focused on the trabecular meshwork during treatment. If the gonioscopy lens is tilted or if the slit lamp itself is not parfocal with the aiming beam, the density of the energy delivered at the level of the trabecular meshwork will be reduced significantly.

RESULTS

Many observers found that the greatest absolute percentage of IOP reduction occurred in eyes with exfoliation syndrome glaucoma (14). It is not unusual to achieve IOP decreases of 20 mm Hg. However, there seems to be a much greater "rebound" of IOP in eyes with exfoliation syndrome (15). In 2 or 3 years in a significant percentage of patients, the IOP may be back near the pretreatment level or even higher.

In patients with primary open-angle glaucoma (POAG), most studies indicated that one can expect a reduction in IOP of 20% to 30% (12). Although the absolute magnitude of the pressure drop will be greater the higher the initial IOP, the percentage drop seems to be fairly constant over a wide pressure range. A number of studies suggested that ALT is much less effective for aphakic open-angle glaucoma, although others refuted this. There have been relatively few reports of the results of ALT in pseudophakic eyes, but there is a suggestion that the results are better in pseudophakia than in aphakia. The beneficial effects of ALT are not diminished by subsequent cataract extraction (16).

Good results have also been found in patients with pigmentary glaucoma, but laser trabeculoplasty may be less effective in the older somewhat atypical pigmentary glaucoma patient (17).

There is a tendency for the IOP to creep upward over time. Whether this is a loss of treatment effect or a slow worsening of the glaucoma is uncertain. Shingleton et al (18) reported that IOP control was lost after 4 years in about half of their patients. Schwartz et al (19) presented data suggesting that this loss of control may occur even faster in black patients.

ALT is somewhat less beneficial and more risky for a number of the secondary glaucomas. In uveitic glaucoma, even when there is sufficient open angle to allow treatment, there is a risk that the trabeculoplasty may cause a flare-up of the uveitis, and some experience suggests that there is a greater risk of peripheral anterior synechial formation. Similarly, very mixed results have been reported for angle recession glaucoma. Severe acute rises in pressure have been seen after such treatment, although a beneficial response occurs in a small number of eyes. There is also a lower response rate and significant complications in juvenile glaucoma patients (20). In general, ALT is more effective in older individuals than younger ones (21). In addition, a higher complication rate has been reported in younger patients. Whether this is related to age or the type of glaucoma is not completely clear.

Many studies tried to correlate the degree of trabecular pigmentation with the effectiveness of ALT (22). Several, but not all, reports indicated a higher success rate in eyes with greater pigmentation (12). It has been suggested that the pigmentation of the trabecular meshwork allows a sharper or more precise focusing of the laser beam and that the pigment better absorbs the laser energy so less energy is required to obtain a tissue response. However, two entities showing a particular good response to ALT, exfoliation syndrome glaucoma and pigmentary glaucoma, have densely pigmented trabecular meshworks, and one could argue that the disease entity rather than the presence of the pigment promotes the good result.

As with all therapeutic modalities, the greatest reduction in IOP occurs in eyes with the highest initial pressures. However, if one defines success as the absence of progression of visual field loss or cupping, then eyes with lower initial pressures would probably achieve this criterion more often.

POAG and many of the secondary glaucomas are usually bilateral diseases, although they may be somewhat asymmetric in presentation. Accordingly, a reasonable number of patients will require ALT bilaterally. Most investigators believe that there is a strong correlation between the response in the two eyes (23) so that a favorable response in the first eye predicts a good result in the second. Similarly, a lack of response in the first eye tends to predict a poor response in the second.

COMPLICATIONS

The single most common complication of ALT is an acute rise in IOP immediately after the treatment. Depending on the treatment technique and other variables, 10% to 30% of patients may experience a rise in IOP equal to or greater than 10 mm Hg 1 to 7 hours after the treatment (24). In most studies the rise occurred within the first 3 hours, but there have been a few reports of delayed IOP elevation. A number of studies suggested that both the incidence and magnitude of pressure rise can be reduced by treating only 180 degrees of the trabecular meshwork with approximately 50 burns in a treatment session instead of treating the entire circumference of the eye with 100 burns (25).

The pathophysiology of this acute pressure rise is unclear. No strong experimental evidence exists to support any of the theories. Steroidal and nonsteroidal anti-inflammatory drugs have not prevented the pressure rise. One study suggested that the use of additional pilocarpine at the time of the laser treatment blunts the pressure elevation (26), as do α_2-adrenergic agents such as apraclonidine and brimonidine (27).

There have also been several reports of more long-term pressure elevations after ALT. They have occurred days to weeks after the treatment and have persisted for weeks to months. In an early series 3% of patients were found to have IOP greater than their pretreatment value at 1 month (14). In at least some of these eyes, the elevated pressure had been associated with the development of posttreatment uveitis.

There have been several reports of central vision loss immediately after ALT (14,25). Most of these losses occurred early in the history of ALT and appeared to be associated with acute pressure elevations that were not aggressively treated. There have not been similar reports during the last few years, indicating that close monitoring of IOP and aggressive intervention with α_2-agonists, carbonic anhydrase inhibitors, and osmotics, when needed, protect even vulnerable small central islands of vision.

Peripheral anterior synechiae (PAS) have been observed in 12% to 47% of eyes that have undergone ALT. In the Glaucoma Laser Trial, PAS to the level of pigmented trabecular meshwork were seen in 33% of the eyes (24). In that study the only factor that correlated with a higher incidence of PAS formation was denser pigmentation of the trabecular meshwork. There was no correlation with laser power. Other studies suggested a higher incidence of PAS formation when the laser burns were placed more posteriorly in the angle (27). To date there have been no data to support any deterimental effects from these small PAS, and the effectiveness of the treatment is comparable in patients both with and without PAS formation.

Mild iritis is an almost universal sequela of ALT. Rarely, severe iritis after laser treatment persists for months (5). Eyes in which "significant" iritis develops are more prone to PAS formation (28). Most clinicians use topical cortical steroids during the immediate period after laser treatment in an attempt to minimize this problem.

An unusual and unexpected complication of ALT has been syncope, with the patient "passing out" at the laser or within minutes of the treatment (29). Most of the patients who experience syncopal episodes have been younger men with no apparent cardiac disease or other predisposing illnesses.

REPEAT TRABECULOPLASTY

As was previously mentioned, the effects of ALT appear to diminish with time. In one study, the IOP in 77% of the eyes was considered to be successfully controlled 2 years after treatment, but this percentage decreased to only 46% at the end of 5 years (19). The results were worse in black patients (32% success rate) than in white patients. In another larger series (18), the mean decrease in IOP after 5 years was about the same as after 1 year (9.3 mm Hg versus 10.3 mm Hg), but only 44% of the eyes treated initially were considered to have successful IOP control. These investigators stated that although failure was most common in the first year after treatment (23%), control of IOP in additional eyes failed at a rate of 7% to 10% per year (18).

A natural question is whether repeat trabeculoplasty might be beneficial in these patients. In less selective early series, only approximately a third of individuals showed a significant beneficial response to the treatment and the glaucoma in several patients appeared to have been made worse (30,31). When retreatment was restricted to individuals who had shown a very good initial response to ALT that persisted for at least a year or two, the success rate for retreatment was, at least initially, higher (32). Even in these patients, however, there seems to be a fairly rapid loss of adequate IOP control. Therefore, retreatment does not appear to be a major long-term option for most patients.

INDICATIONS FOR TREATMENT

Laser trabeculoplasty offers certain advantages over both medical and conventional surgical therapy. It is safer than medications. There is no risk of inducing asthma, slowing the heart rate, or causing severe depression as can occur with some of the glaucoma medications. Similarly, because it is a noninvasive procedure, there is no risk of endophthalmitis or progression of cataracts as can occur with conventional filtration surgery. This safety profile enhances the indications for its use.

Laser trabeculoplasty should be considered in most patients with primary open-angle glaucoma, exfoliation syndrome glaucoma, pigmentary glaucoma, and angle-closure glaucoma successfully treated with laser iridectomy but having a residual elevated IOP and open angles. It also may be indicated in many patients with normotensive (low-tension) glaucoma and aphakic/pseudophakic glaucoma. It is much less commonly indicated in uveitic glaucoma, angle recession glaucoma, and juvenile glaucoma, and then only with the patient being aware that there is a substantial risk that treatment will worsen the glaucoma.

In addition to the glaucoma diagnosis, other factors must be taken into consideration in deciding whether to use ALT. In general, the older the patient, the lower the IOP, and the less advanced the glaucoma damage, the greater likelihood that ALT will be successful in controlling the glaucoma. Conversely, the younger the patient, the higher the IOP, and the more advanced the damage, the less likely that ALT will be adequate treatment.

Initially, ALT was used only when IOP was not controlled with maximal medical therapy. With experience, there is a trend toward using it earlier in the therapeutic regimen. It is now often used before carbonic anhydrase inhibitors, as a substitute for miotics in symptomatic patients, or before cataract extraction in otherwise controlled eyes. With the growing number of reports on the successful use of ALT as an initial treatment for glaucoma, and especially the results (31) of the Glaucoma Laser Trial showing that it was at least as effective as, and possibly superior to, initial medical treatment, laser trabeculoplasty should be considered as a first-line treatment in many glaucoma patients. This is particularly true in older patients and those with obstructive lung disease and cardiovascular disease. There are still many glaucoma specialists, however, who believe that medical therapy should always be tried first.

RECOMMENDED TREATMENT TECHNIQUE

Because many patients achieve a significant (sometimes maximal) IOP reduction with treatment of only half of the angle with a reduced risk of posttreatment IOP elevation, many ophthalmologists now perform ALT in divided sessions. The second treatment is usually performed about a month after the initial one, but occasionally the IOP reduction exceeds the treatment objective and the second treatment can be deferred. If the pressure rises above the target level at some point in the future, then the second half of the angle can be treated at that time.

The laser burns should be placed anteriorly straddling the border of the pigmented and nonpigmented trabecular meshwork. This seems to result in less pain during treatment, fewer PAS, and less postoperative inflammation than do more posteriorly placed burns. A 50-μm laser spot

and a duration of 0.1 second should be used. I use standard power setting (e.g., 800 mW) for all treatments, but even if one chooses to treat to tissue reaction (blanch or small bubble formation) the laser power should not exceed 1000 mW.

After laser treatment, patients continue their usual glaucoma medications. In eyes with very advanced visual field loss or cupping of the optic nerve head, a drop of apraclonidine is instilled before or after, or before and after, the laser treatment. In all patients the IOP is measured hourly for 2 to 4 hours after the treatment. If a significant elevation of IOP is detected (generally defined as a rise equal to or greater than 10 mm Hg), apraclonidine, a carbonic anhydrase inhibitor, or a hyperosmotic agent, or a combination of these drugs, is administered. In all patients topical cortical steroids are administered for several times daily for several days and the patient is seen for follow-up in 1 to 2 weeks. At that time, depending on the amount of reduction in IOP, the patient's previous glaucoma medication can be reduced as indicated.

REFERENCES

1. Krasnov MM. Laseropuncture of the anterior chamber angle in glaucoma. *Am J Ophthalmol* 1973;75:674–678.
2. Worthen DM, Wickham MG. Laser trabeculoplasty in monkeys. *Invest Ophthalmol Vis Sci* 1973;12:707–711.
3. Gaasterland De, Kupfer C. Experimental glaucoma in the rhesus monkey. *Invest Ophthalmol Vis Sci* 1974;13:455–457.
4. Wise JB, Witter SL. Argon laser therapy for open-angle glaucoma; a pilot study. *Arch Ophthalmol* 1979;97:319–322.
5. Wilensky JT, Jampol LM. Laser therapy for open-angle glaucoma. *Ophthalmology* 1981;88:213–217.
6. Schwartz AL, Whitten ME, Bleiman B, Martin D. Argon laser trabeculoplasty in uncontrolled phakic open-angle glaucoma. *Ophthalmology* 1981;88:203–212.
7. Van Buskirk EM. Pathophysiology of laser trabeculoplasty. *Surv Ophthalmol* 1989;33:264–272.
8. Byslma SB, Samples JR, Acott TS, Van Buskirk EM. Trabecular cell division after argon laser trabeculoplasty. *Am J Ophthalmol* 1988;106:544–547.
9. Wilensky JT, Weinreb RN. Low dose trabeculoplasty. *Am J Ophthalmol* 1983;95:423–426.
10. Wise JB. Ten year results of laser trabeculoplasty. *Eye* 1985;1:45–50.
11. Grayson DK, Ritch R, Camras C, et al. Influence of treatment protocol on long-term efficacy of argon laser trabeculoplasty. *J Glaucoma* 1993;2:7–12.
12. Reiss GR, Wilensky JT, Higginbotham EJ. Laser trabeculoplasty. *Surv Ophthalmol* 1991;36:407–428.
13. Rouhiainen HJ, Terasvirta ME, Tuovinen EJ. The effect of some treatment variables on the results of trabeculoplasty. *Arch Ophthalmol* 1988;106:611–614.
14. Thomas JV, Simmons BJ, Belcher CD. Argon laser trabeculoplasty in the presurgical glaucoma patient. *Ophthalmology* 1982;89:187–197.
15. Higginbotham EJ, Richardson TM. Response of exfoliation glaucoma to laser trabeculoplasty. *Br J Ophthalmol* 1986;709:837–839.
16. Brown SLV, Thomas JV, Budenz DV, et al. Effect of cataract surgery on intraocular pressure reduction obtained with laser trabeculoplasty. *Am J Ophthalmol* 1985;100:373–376.
17. Lieberman MF, Hoskins HD, Hetherington J. Laser trabeculoplasty and the glaucomas. *Ophthalmology* 1983;90:790–795.
18. Shingleton BJ, Richter CU, Bellows AR, et al. Long-term efficacy of argon laser trabeculoplasty. *Ophthalmology* 1987;94:1513–1518.
19. Schwartz AL, Love DC, Schwartz MH. Long-term follow-up of argon laser trabeculoplasty for uncontrolled glaucoma. *Arch Ophthalmol* 1985;103:1482–1484.
20. Wilensky JT, Weinreb RN. Early and late failures of argon laser trabeculoplasty. *Arch Ophthalmol* 1983;101:895–897.
21. Safran MJ, Robin AL, Pollack IP. Argon laser trabeculoplasty in younger patients with primary open-angle glaucoma. *Am J Ophthalmol* 1984;97:292–295.

22. Traverso CE, Spaeth GL, Starita RJ, et al. Factors affecting the results of argon laser trabeculoplasty in open-angle glaucoma. *Ophthalmic Surg* 1986;17:554–559.

23. Bishop KI, Krupin T, Feitl ME, et al. Bilateral argon laser trabeculoplasty in primary open-angle glaucoma. *Am J Ophthalmol* 1989;107:591–595.

24. Glaucoma Laser Trial Research Group. The Glaucoma Laser Trial. 1. Acute effects of argon laser trabeculoplasty on intraocular pressure. *Arch Ophthalmol* 1989;107:1135–1142.

25. Weinreb RN, Ruderman J, Justin R, Zweig K. Immediate intraocular pressure response to argon laser trabeculoplasty. *Am J Ophthalmol* 1983;95:279–281.

26. Ofner S, Samples JR, Van Buskirk EM. Pilocarpine and the increase in intraocular pressure after trabeculoplasty. *Am J Ophthalmol* 1984;97:647–649.

27. Traverso CE, Greenedge KC, Spaeth GL. Formation of peripheral anterior synechiae following argon laser trabeculoplasty. *Arch Ophthalmol* 1984;102:861–863.

28. Pappas HR, Berry DP, Partamian L, et al. Topical indomethacin therapy before argon laser trabeculoplasty. *Am J Ophthalmol* 1985;99:571–575.

29. Hoskins HD, Hetherington J, Minckler DS, et al. Complications of laser trabeculoplasty. *Ophthalmology* 1983;90:796–799.

30. Starita RJ, Fellman RL, Spaeth GL, Poryzees E. The effect of repeating full-circumference argon laser trabeculoplasty. *Ophthalmic Surg* 1984;15:41–43.

31. Brown SVL, Thomas JV, Simmons RJ. Laser trabeculoplasty retreatment. *Am J Ophthalmol* 1985;99:8–10.

32. Grayson DK, Camras CB, Podos SM, Lustgaiten JS. Long-term reduction of intraocular pressure after repeat argon laser trabeculoplasty. *Am J Ophthalmol* 1988;106:312–321.

33. Glaucoma Laser Trial Study Group. The Glaucoma Laser Trial and Glaucoma Laser Trial Follow-up Study (GLT and GLTFS): 7 final results. *Am J Ophthalmol* 1995;120:718–731.

Laser Iridotomy and Peripheral Iridoplasty

Robert Ritch   Jeffrey M. Liebmann

HISTORICAL OVERVIEW

In 1916, Verhoeff and Bell (1) first focused sunlight on the iris and retina. In 1956, Meyer-Schwickerath (2) first reported the creation of a patent iridotomy using the xenon arc photocoagulator. Patent iridotomies were created in 1958 using high-intensity radiant energy from a copper-coated carbon arc (3). These and other (4,5) early attempts at thermal iridotomy were characterized by a high rate of complications, such as lens opacity and inflammation.

The advent of laser technology enabled the use of monochromatic focused light. Iridotomy using the pulsed ruby laser required less energy than previous methods (6–11). In 1973, Beckman and Sugar (12) attempted unsuccessfully to use the neodymium laser in human irides.

The development of the continuous-wave argon laser initiated the era of laser treatment of glaucoma. Khuri (13) achieved successful argon laser iridotomy in rabbits and Beckman and Sugar (12), in humans. Others soon reported successful iridotomy in eyes with angle-closure glaucoma (14,15). Elimination of the difficulties associated with penetration of dark-brown and blue irides led to virtually 100% success in penetration with this procedure and revolutionized the treatment of angle-closure glaucoma (16–21). By the early 1980s, argon laser iridotomy had replaced incisional surgical iridectomy as the procedure of choice for angle-closure glaucoma (17,21–37).

Many clinicians now use the neodymium:yttrium-aluminum-garnet (Nd:YAG) laser because of the relative simplicity of the procedure, compared to the more subtle techniques necessary to produce an iridotomy with the argon laser (38–43). However, complications, particularly hyphema and inflammation, are more common and severe.

DIFFERENTIAL DIAGNOSIS OF ANGLE-CLOSURE GLAUCOMA

Determination of the specific pathophysiologic mechanism responsible for the angle closure is crucial in arriving at an accurate diagnosis and in planning appropriate therapy. It is not just differentiation of angle-closure from open-angle glaucoma that is important, but accuracy of diagnosis within the group of glaucomas characterized by angle closure.

Angle-closure glaucoma is an anatomic disorder comprising a final common pathway of iris apposition to the trabecular meshwork resulting from various abnormal relationships of anterior-segment structures. These in turn result from one or more abnormalities in the relative or absolute sizes or positions of anterior-segment structures or posterior-segment forces that alter anterior-segment anatomy (44).

Angle closure results from blockage of the meshwork by the iris, but the forces causing this blockage may be viewed as originating at four successive anatomic levels: the iris (pupillary block), the ciliary body (plateau iris), the lens (phacomorphic glaucoma), and posterior to the lens (malignant glaucoma) (44). The more posterior the level at which the angle closure occurs, the more complex are the diagnosis and treatment, since each level may have a component of the mechanism peculiar to each of the levels preceding it. Understanding these mechanisms makes appropriate treatment in any particular case an exercise in deductive logic.

Indentation gonioscopy provides the advantage of a dynamic view of the anterior-chamber angle and is mandatory when evaluating an angle for the presence of peripheral anterior synechiae (PAS) (Figs. 30-1 and 30-2) (45).

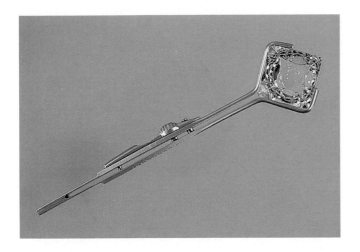

FIGURE 30-1. *Zeiss indentation gonioprism.*

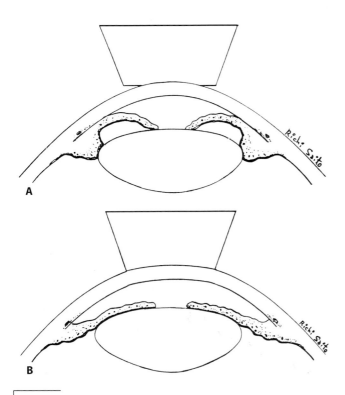

FIGURE 30-2. A. *During gonioscopy with the Zeiss gonioprism, the cornea retains its normal configuration. B. During indentation, gentle pressure on the central part of the cornea causes it to bow posteriorly, shallowing the central part of the anterior chamber. The displaced aqueous is forced into the angle recess, open areas of appositional angle closure. Regions of synechial angle closure will remain closed.*

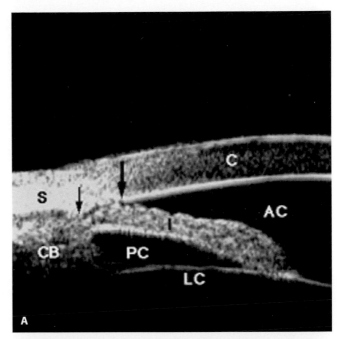

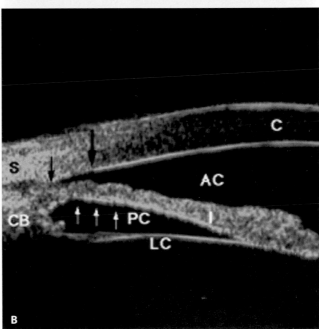

FIGURE 30-3. A. *Ultrasound biomicrograph of the anterior-chamber angle in bright illumination. The cornea (C), iris (I), anterior chamber (AC), posterior chamber (PC), ciliary body (CB), lens capsule (LC), scleral spur (thin black arrow), and Schwalbe's line (thick black arrow) are visible. The iris is slightly convex (white arrows), consistent with relative pupillary block. Aqueous has access to the trabecular meshwork, which is between Schwalbe's line and sclera spur. B. In dim illumination, the peripheral iris has now moved against the trabecular meshwork, closing the angle.*

When one is attempting to determine whether or not a narrow angle is occludable, gonioscopy should always be performed in a completely darkened room using the smallest square of slit-lamp illumination possible, which will enable a view of the angle. The difference in the angle in light and dark conditions may be much greater than

expected and can be demonstrated by ultrasound biomicroscopy (UBM) (Fig. 30-3). UBM is extremely useful for explaining the nature of angle closure and the rationale of treatment to patients who may be confused between open-angle and angle-closure glaucomas and different types of laser surgery.

Pupillary Block (Aqueous Pressure)

In pupillary block, aqueous humor flow from the posterior chamber to the anterior chamber is limited by resistance to aqueous flow through the pupil by iridolenticular contact. This creates a relative pressure gradient between the two chambers, and forces the iris anteriorly, causing bowing of the anterior part of the iris, narrowing of the angle, and acute or chronic angle-closure glaucoma. During indentation gonioscopy, pressure on the cornea forces aqueous into the angle, widening it to permit viewing over the iris convexity. Since only aqueous in the posterior chamber offers resistance, the angle opens easily (Fig. 30-4). The anterior-segment structures and their anatomic relationships appear otherwise normal.

Pupillary block may be either relative or absolute. Relative pupillary block typically occurs in hyperopic eyes, which have a shorter than average axial length, shallower anterior chamber, thicker lens, more anterior lens position, and smaller radius of corneal curvature (46–50). In absolute pupillary block, posterior synechiae between the iris and lens are responsible. When pupillary block develops, the iris assumes a bombé configuration, creating an angle that is narrow throughout its approach (Fig. 30-5). Relative pupillary block underlies approximately 90% angle closure. The rest have one or more mechanisms other than or in addition to pupillary block. Some can be worsened by miotic therapy, particularly in patients with intumescent or anteriorly subluxated lenses or malignant glaucoma.

Laser iridotomy eliminates the pressure differential between the anterior and posterior chambers and relieves

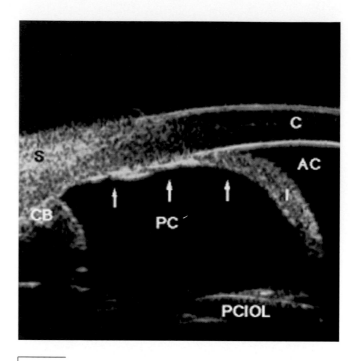

FIGURE 30-5.   *In more severely affected eyes, the iris (I) convexity achieves a bombé configuration, as is present in this pseudophakic eye. The* arrow *indicates the force of aqueous pressure.*

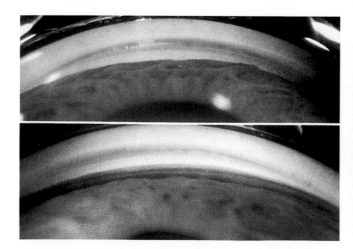

FIGURE 30-4.   *Goniophotograph of an appositionally closed angle in an eye with relative pupillary block* (top). *With gentle pressure during indentation gonioscopy, the angle opens uniformly, revealing the angle structures* (bottom).

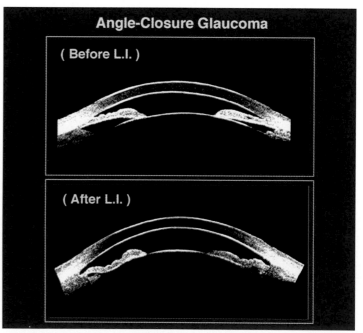

FIGURE 30-6.   A. *Relative pupillary block angle closure prior to laser iridotomy.* B. *Following laser iridotomy, the iris assumes a flat configuration* (white arrow) *and the angle opens* (black arrows *at scleral spur and Schwalbe's line*).

the iris convexity. This results in several changes in anterior-segment anatomy. The iris assumes a flat or planar configuration and the iridocorneal angle widens. The region of iridolenticular contact actually increases, as aqueous flows through the iridectomy rather than the pupillary space (Fig. 30-6) (51).

Plateau Iris (Ciliary Body Pressure)

A large or anteriorly positioned ciliary body can maintain the iris root in proximity to the trabecular meshwork, creating a configuration known as *plateau iris* (52–55). The anterior chamber is usually of medium depth and the iris surface slightly convex. On gonioscopy, the iris root angulates forward and then centrally. With indentation

gonioscopy, the ciliary processes prevent posterior movement of the peripheral iris, resulting in a configuration in which the slit beam follows the curvature of the iris to its deepest point at the periphery of the lens where the ciliary processes begin, then rises agian over the ciliary processes before dropping peripherally (Σ sign) (Figs. 30-7 and 30-8).

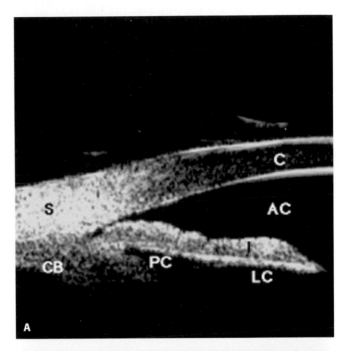

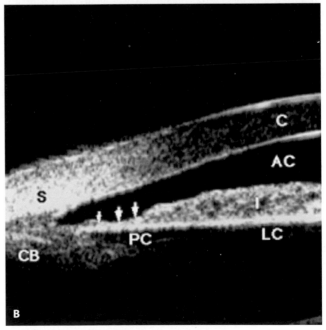

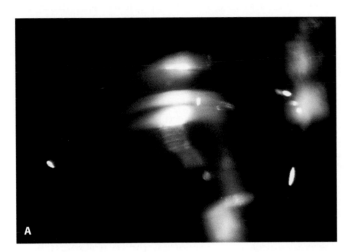

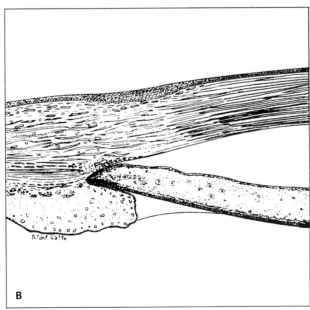

FIGURE 30-7.   A. *In plateau iris with indentation, the deepest displacement of the iris occurs at the lens equator.* B. *Diagram of an eye with plateau iris showing anterior extension of the ciliary processes, supporting the iris root against the trabecular meshwork.*

FIGURE 30-8.   *Ultrasound biomicrograph of an eye with plateau iris which has already undergone laser iridotomy. The iris surface is flat and the chamber appears normally deep. The iris root is thick and the entire periphery of the iris is supported by large and anteriorly positioned ciliary processes.*

Greater force is needed to open the angle than in pupillary block because the ciliary processes must be displaced, and the angle does not open as widely.

Plateau iris *syndrome* refers to the development of angle closure, either spontaneously or after pupillary dilation, in an eye with plateau iris configuration despite the presence of a patent iridectomy or iridotomy. Acute angle-closure glaucoma may develop (56–59). The extent, or the "height" to which the plateau rises, determines whether or not the angle will close completely with a rise in intraocular pressure (IOP) (complete plateau iris syndrome) or only partially without a rise in IOP (incomplete plateau iris syndrome) (60). The angle can narrow further with age due to enlargement of the lens, so that an angle with plateau configuration that does not close after iridotomy may do so some years later. Periodic gonioscopy is required.

Treatment must be targeted at the cause of angle closure, in this case the ciliary body and iris root. If pupillary block either is not a component mechanism of the angle closure or has been eliminated by iridotomy, it is necessary to find a way to eliminate the physical blockage of the angle. This is accomplished by argon laser peripheral iridoplasty (ALPI), which compresses the iris root and creates a space where none was before (61).

Phacomorphic Glaucoma (Lens Pressure)

Lens swelling may convert a medium-depth anterior chamber into a very shallow one and precipitate acute angle-closure glaucoma (phacomorphic glaucoma) from the lens forcing the iris and ciliary body anteriorly. Paradoxical reactions to pilocarpine treatment, which increases axial lens thickness and causes anterior lens movement, further shallowing the anterior chamber, are common (62–66). ALPI is effective in breaking attacks of phacomorphic angle closure (67).

The eye may be severely inflamed, as these patients are often referred after being treated unsuccessfully for a few days. Treatment must be oriented at the level of the lens. Lens removal is indicated for intumescent cataracts, but is prone to complications if performed during an acute angle-closure attack. Breaking the attack with ALPI allows 2 to 3 weeks for the inflammation and cornea to clear, permitting cataract extraction under conditions much closer to ideal (67). Any element of pupillary block is treated as soon as possible (usually within 2–3 days) after breaking the attack.

In anterior lens subluxation due to trauma or such hereditary disorders as Weill-Marchesani syndrome, ALPI is less successful because the pressure of the lens against the iris continues, with or without an iridotomy, as long as the underlying cause is present. Cycloplegics are useful if the zonules are intact, but this may not always be so (68). A more complete discussion of this subject can be found elsewhere (69,70). If not treated in time, forward lens movement can lead to malignant glaucoma.

Malignant Glaucoma (Posterior-Segment Pressure)

Also termed *ciliary block* or *posterior aqueous misdirection*, angle closure caused by forces posterior to the lens that push the lens-iris diaphragm forward presents the greatest diagnostic and treatment challenge of the angle-closure glaucomas. Analogous to pupillary block, in which the angle is occluded by iris because of a pressure differential between the posterior and anterior chambers, in ciliary block a pressure differential is created between the vitreous and aqueous compartments by aqueous misdirection into the vitreous (Fig. 30-9).

Swelling or anterior rotation of the ciliary body with forward rotation of the lens-iris diaphragm and relaxation of the zonular apparatus causes anterior lens displacement. UBM often reveals a shallow supraciliary detachment not evident on routine B-scan examination (Figs. 30-10 and 30-11). This effusion appears to be the cause of the anterior rotation of the ciliary body and the forward movement of the lens-iris diaphragm. This, combined with aqueous misdirection into the vitreous, increases vitreous pressure, pushing the lens-iris diaphragm forward and causing angle closure by physically pushing the iris against the trabecular meshwok in a manner similar to that in phacomorphic glaucoma (71).

The effusions in many of these conditions, such as angle closure after PRP or scleral buckling, is self-limited, but treatment is indicated to prevent PAS formation and to lower IOP. A component of pupillary block is often present and the opposite angle often narrow, and if the cornea is clear, laser iridotomy can be performed. If appositional closure remains after iridotomy or if the cornea is not clear, ALPI again is almost always successful at opening the angle.

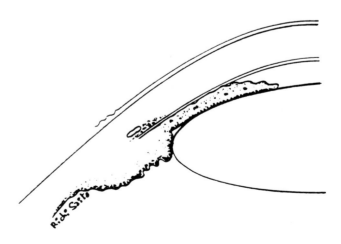

FIGURE 30-9.   *In aqueous misdirection, an abnormality of the vitreociliary relationship causes a posterior diversion of aqueous into the vitreous. The resultant increased posterior-segment pressure is the cause of angle closure.*

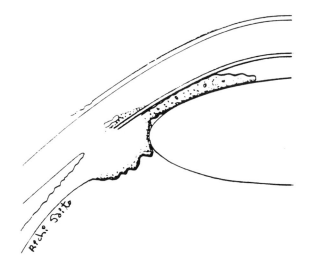

FIGURE 30-10.   *In some patients with a clinical diagnosis of malignant glaucoma, annular detachment of the ciliary body is the cause of the angle closure.*

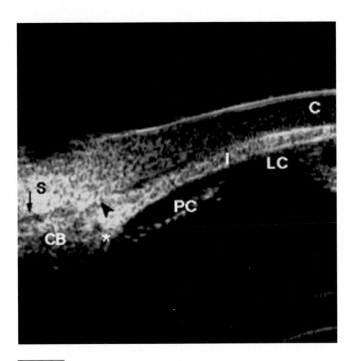

FIGURE 30-11.   *Ultrasound biomicrograph of an eye with malignant glaucoma. Anterior rotation of the ciliary processes (star) has forced the peripheral iris against the trabecular meshwork (arrowheads). A shallow supraciliary effusion is present (arrow).*

LASER IRIDOTOMY

Indications

Acute Angle-Closure Glaucoma

Laser iridotomy is the procedure of choice for all angle-closure glaucomas with a component of pupillary block. All eyes with acute angle-closure glaucoma require laser iridot-

omy. Therapy can be assumed successful only when the angle can be determined to be open gonioscopically, as transient lowering of IOP may occur with medial therapy. Ideally, iridotomy should be performed after the acute attack has been terminated and the eye is no longer inflamed. If this is not possible but the iris can be adequately visualized, iridotomy can be attempted, preferably with the argon laser because of the greater chance of iris bleeding with the Nd:YAG laster (72). Alternatively, pretreatment with the argon laser may allow safe application of the Nd:YAG laser with minimal bleeding. If an argon laser is not available and the Nd:YAG laser is to be used, an attempt should be made to perforate the iris with a single application, as bleeding at the iridotomy may preclude a second laser application at that site. Acute angle-closure glaucoma that is unresponsive to medical treatment, or in which iridotomy is not possible due to hazy media, may be successfully aborted with ALPI (see below) (32,67,73).

Eyes with phacomorphic glaucoma usually have some element of pupillary block, but the response to treatment with miotics is often paradoxical, resulting in worsening of the attack (25). Ciliary muscle contraction further loosens the zonules and causes lens thickening and anterior lens movement, further narrowing the angle. ALPI will almost always break the attack (61,67,74).

Chronic Angle-Closure Glaucoma

Eyes with chronic appositional closure with or without PAS are at risk for progressive synechial closure, trabecular damage, elevated IOP, and acute angle closure. Iridotomy can eliminate the progression of PAS in eyes with chronic angle closure caused by pupillary block. Even if the angle structures cannot be visualized by indentation gonioscopy prior to treatment (which may occur when IOP is over 40 mm Hg), areas of functional meshwork may become apparent after iridotomy, particularly when there is "hamstringing" of the iris between PAS. In essence, all eyes with angle closure should be given the benefit of iridotomy before filtration surgery is considered.

The effect of iridotomy on IOP control depends on the degree of trabecular dysfunction. In eyes with minimal damage, iridotomy alone may reduce or control IOP. Failure of medications to control IOP prior to iridotomy does not necessarily mean that this will be so afterward. Quigley (75) found reduced IOP following iridotomy in 44% of eyes with chronic angle closure. After elimination of pupillary block by iridotomy, repeat gonioscopy may permit a more complete evaluation and assessment of the extent of trabecular injury and synechial closure (17,28,76,77).

Aphakic or Pseudophakic Pupillary Block

Aphakic and pseudophakic pupillary block can be relieved by laser iridotomy (78–83). Loculation of pockets of both aqueous and vitreous may be present posterior to the iris, owing to iridovitreal, iridocapsular, or iridolenticular adhesions. An iridotomy made over an area of vitreous-iris adhesion or apposition will not relieve the pupillary block (78). Multiple iridotomies may be required before a pocket of aqueous humor is located and the block relieved (17,78,84,85). In situations in which more than one loculated area is present, at least one iridotomy will be required for each area of loculation. Iridotomy helps to rule out pupillary block in cases of suspected malignant glaucoma, which requires disruption of the anterior hyaloid face or vitrectomy (84,86).

Prophylactic Iridotomy

With rare exceptions, prophylactic iridotomy should be performed in the fellow eye of a patient with either acute or chronic angle-closure glaucoma. Given similar refractive errors and globe size, the fellow eye of a high proportion of such individuals will eventually develop angle closure. Angle closure associated with an intumescent or anteriorly subluxated lens may present with an open, nonoccludable angle in the fellow eye. This may also occur in patients with anisometropia, with angle closure developing in the more hyperopic eye. Eyes with normal IOP and spontaneous appositional closure of at least one full quadrant on darkroom gonioscopy should also have prophylactic iridotomy.

In a retrospective study of 50 eyes treated with laser iridotomy or surgical iridectomy and 64 eyes treated medically to assess the long-term outcome of surgical and medical treatment of narrow angles, eyes treated by iridotomy or iridectomy showed a greater number of improved anterior-chamber configurations (74% versus 28%), had a lower incidence of PAS (2% versus 10%) and required fewer antiglaucoma medications (87). The overall percentages of eyes with increased IOP, decreased visual acuity, and abnormal visual fields were similar in the two groups.

Malignant Glaucoma

When acute angle closure occurs because of malignant glaucoma, medical treatment or iridotomy or both are usually insufficient to relieve the glaucoma. ALPI can open the angle, at least temporarily, and lower IOP. Prophylactic iridotomy usually protects the fellow eye against both acute angle-closure glaucoma and possibly subsequent malignant glaucoma which could be triggered by opening and decompressing the globe. Pilocarpine, which increases lens thickness and shallows the anterior chamber, may trigger an episode of malignant glaucoma (88,89).

To Facilitate Argon Laser Trabeculoplasty

Argon laser trabeculoplasty (ALT) may be difficult to perform in open but anatomically narrow angles. In these cases, irdotomy will facilitate the trabeculoplasty. If the angle is narrow because of plateau iris, ALPI is a better alternative for improving visualization of the angle structures.

Nanophthalmos

Nanophthalmos, characterized by high hyperopia, short axial length, small corneal diameter, thick sclera, and narrow angles (90), represents one end of a spectrum of disease, and many hyperopic eyes have crowded anterior segments. Patients with nanophthalmos are anatomically predisposed to angle-closure glaucoma due to anterior-chamber crowding. Angle-closure glaucoma usually appears between the ages of 20 and 50 years. Laser iridotomy is usually unsuccessful or only temporarily successful. Bilateral nonrhegmatogenous retinal detachments have occurred following laser iridotomy (91) and may be attributable to worsening of preexisting retinal or choroidal disease (92).

Pigment Dispersion Syndrome

Laser iridotomy eliminates the iris concavity often found in pigment dispersion syndrome (93–95). The concave iris configuration is due to reverse pupillary block, in which aqueous passing from the posterior to the anterior chamber cannot equilibrate because of extensive iridolenticular contact. The sudden increase of aqueous volume into the anterior chamber pushes the iris back against the zonular bundles. Iridotomy provides an additional pathway for aqueous equilibration between the chambers (Fig. 30-12).

Contraindications

Iridotomy is contraindicated when angle closure is caused by contraction of the iris against the trabecular meshwork, such as in uveitis, neovascular glaucoma, or iridocorneal endothelial syndrome. It should not be performed in eyes with corneal edema or opacification precluding a view of the iris, or a grade 2 or 3 flat anterior chamber.

Techniques of Laser Iridotomy

Preoperative Preparation

Contact lenses reduce saccades and extraneous eye movements that can interfere with accurate superimposition of burns, keep the lids separated, focus the beam, and minimize reflective loss of laser power, while the gonioscopy solution absorbs excess heat, decreasing the chance of corneal burns (16,28,96,97). The Abraham lens consists of a fundus contact lens with a +66-diopter (D) planoconvex lens button on its anterior surface. This provides magnification without loss of depth of focus and reduces the effective size of a 50-μm spot on the iris surface to approximately 30 μm, providing higher energy per unit area and permitting the procedure to be performed with a lower total energy. The beam is rapidly defocused posterior to the site of focus, decreasing potential injury to the posterior segment (98,99). The Wise lens is similar but has a +103-D button, allowing even greater concentration of laser energy (100).

Topical anesthesia virtually always suffices. If the pupil is not already maximally miotic, 2% or 4% pilocarpine should be administered to minimize iris stromal thickness. Perioperative apraclonidine decreases the magnitude and frequency of postlaser IOP spikes (101–104), for which

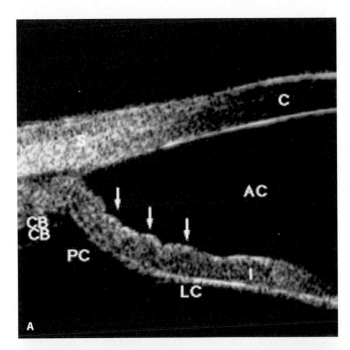

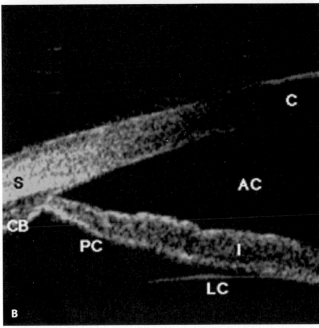

FIGURE 30-12.   A. *In the untreated eye with pigment dispersion syndrome, the iris assumes a concave configuration* (white arrows) *due to pressure differential between the anterior and posterior chambers. B. Following laser iridotomy, elimination of the pressure gradient across the iris allows it to assume a planar, or flat, configuration.*

the density of the arcus causes a drop in laser power across the cornea, and the arcus itself interferes with clear focusing of the beam. This is less of a problem with the Nd:YAG laser than with the argon laser. The beam should be perpendicular to the contact lens surface to maximize energy delivery. Since focus is critical to efficient laser energy delivery, all lenses should be clean. Medium-brown irides are generally the easiest to penetrate with the argon laser, the energy of which is readily absorbed by the iris pigment. Light-blue and dark-brown irides are more difficult (30,77). Lighter irides are more easily penetrated with the Nd:YAG laser than are darker, thicker irides.

The iridotomy should be made peripherally between the 11- and 1-o'clock positions, where it will be covered by the upper lid, to minimize glare and diplopia. If the iridotomy is bisected by either the lid or the tear meniscus, the patient may be bothered by glare or a "white line" in the superior visual field (105). The beam should be aimed to avoid accidental foveal injury; performing the iridotomy nasally eliminates this possibility.

Types of Argon Laser Burns

Various types of burns, including contraction, penetrating, punch, and cleanup burns, and their uses in particular circumstances have been fully described elsewhere (100). Low-power, large-spot-size, and long-duration *contraction burns* (500-μm spot size, 0.5-second duration, and 200–400-mW power) compact the stroma at the site of the burn and are used to 1) increase the density of iris stroma to facilitate laser energy absorption in blue or light-brown irides, 2) create a "hump" on which penetrating burns are placed, and 3) perform ALPI or pupilloplasty. One should begin with 200 mW in brown irides and 300 mW in light ones and adjust the power as necessary. If bubbles or pigment release occur, the power should be reduced. In very light irides, a 200-μm spot size may be more effective.

Penetrating burns are higher-power, small-spot-size (50-μm) burns designed to vaporize iris tissue and create an opening. In the late 1970s and early 1980s, burns of 0.1- to 0.2-second duration and 1000 to 2000-mW power were common. These produce charring and penetration failure in darkly pigmented irides, while lower-power, shorter-duration burns are more successful at penetrating the surface layer of the iris and densely pigmented stroma (18). Burns of 0.01- or 0.02-second duration were formerly termed *punch burns*. The optimal power is 600 to 1200 mW and varies depending on the duration of the burn and the consistency and pigmentation of the iris. In many eyes, the iris surface layer has denser pigment than the stroma. Charring is minimal or absent when punch burns are used.

In most blue, hazel, and light-brown irides, burns of 0.05-second duration, 50-μm spot size, and 600- to 800-mW power can be used after the initial contraction burns. Failure of tissue to vaporize with each laser application implies that laser energy is being applied without effect. A second site may need to be chosen or a Nd:YAG laser employed.

patients with more extensive synechial closure or trabecular dysfunction are at higher risk. The greater the energy used, the greater the risk of postoperative IOP spike.

Iris variations in thickness, color, and number and size of crypts should be taken into account. It is usually easier to perform iridotomy in the base of an iris crypt, where the stroma is thinner. An arcus senilis should be avoided because

Shorter-duration (0.01- or 0.02-second) burns are optimal for use in dark irides, particularly in black and Asian patients, to avoid charring at the base of the iridotomy site (18,26,106–110). Once the surface layer of fibroblasts and melanocytes has been penetrated and the stroma is being chipped away, the duration can be increased to 0.05 second. Posterior synechiae may occur less frequently after short-duration burns (26).

After the stroma has been eliminated, cleanup burns (about 200-mW power, 100-200-μm spot size, and 0.2-second duration) are used to remove residual iris pigment epithelium without dislodging more pigment into the opening. If shock waves due to high-energy absorption are created, pigment from surrounding areas will often move into the opening (landsliding).

Linear Evaporation

This technique, originally described by Wise (111,112), uses the radial orientation of the dilator muscle to enlarge the iridotomy. Punch burns are used to make a straight-line incision in the iris, perpendicular to the dilator muscle. The incision should be about 500 μm long, full thickness throughout its length, and only as wide as a single row of laser burns. When the stroma is fully incised, the dialator muscle assists in separating the pigment epithelium, reducing the amount of pigment epithelium that must be lasered and creating a larger opening.

Drumhead Technique

In this approach, developed in the 1970s (28), six to eight burns of 0.2 second, 200 mW, and 200 μm are placed in a circle around the site selected for penetration to thin the iris stroma in the center of the ring and make it more taut. Penetrating burns are then applied in the center of the ring.

Helpful Hints

Improvisation and flexibility in technique and choice of laser settings for different types of irides are the keys to success. The entire procedure may require anywhere from 1 to 300 burns. It should be remembered that 200 applications of 0.02-second duration and 600-mW power equal 10 applications of 0.2-second duration and 1200-mW power, the latter settings often requiring 100 to 200 burns to penetrate a dark iris.

For any iridotomy, the first burn often serves as an indicator for the ease of the procedure. The desired result from the first burn is the appearance of a small hole with a darker base and dispersion of a small amount of debris into the anterior chamber. Bubble formation indicates stromal vaporization. One then continues to deliver burns until the stroma has been penetrated.

In the absence of stromal pigmentation, bubble formation and pigment release may be minimal. One clue to the gradual deepening of the iridotomy is a gradual darkening of the base. An orange reflex at the time of beam impact, most commonly seen in irides with little stromal pigmentation, signifies that one is nearing the pigment epithelium.

When the pigment epithelium is reached, denser bursts of fine pigment appear in the anterior chamber. A cloud of pigment mixed with aqueous often slowly balloons into the anterior chamber, indicating passage of aqueous from the posterior chamber. Simultaneously, the iris stroma floats backward and the peripheral anterior chamber deepens. This can be quite marked in eyes with greater degress of relative pupillary block. After penetration, the iridotomy may be enlarged and pigment removed with cleanup burns. At completion, the lens capsule should be visible through the opening. Gonioscopy should be performed to ensure that the angle is open.

Transillumination through the pupil or the iridotomy is not a reliable indicator of success in light irides, as it is possible to destroy pigment epithelium without penetrating the stroma. Once this happens, the overlying stroma cannot be penetrated except with a Nd:YAG laser, and the surgeon may mistakenly assume that the procedure has been successful.

Nd:YAG Laser Iridotomy

The Nd:YAG laser creates a plasma of free ions and electrons at the site of optical breakdown. This photodisruption releases shock waves that mechanically cause tissue rupture, as opposed to the thermal effect of the argon laser (113,114). Iris color and density are much less important than with argon laser iridotomy. By the mid 1980s, several series had described the easily obtained, successful results of Nd:YAG laser iridotomy (40,115–119).

One should begin with a single pulse at approximately 1.5 to 3.0 mJ to assess the response of both the patient and the iris to the laser application. An increase in energy to 4 to 6 mJ is often sufficient to create a patent iridotomy with one to three additional applications. We prefer a linear incision technique using lower-power burns, on the order of 1 mJ (112,120), and never to use the multiple-pulse mode. The importance of precise focus on the anterior iris stroma cannot be overemphasized; maximal photodisruption is obtained and the possibility of lens injury minimized (121). Since the anterior lens surface is further from the iris in the periphery, the chance of accidental lens injury is reduced by choosing a peripheral location.

Other Wavelengths

Combining argon laser to thin the iris stroma and coagulate blood vessels followed by Nd:YAG completion has been advocated as an approach that takes advantage of the photothermal effects of the first and easier penetration achieved via photodisruption of the latter (92,122–124). The risk of hemorrhage is also reduced (125). Iridotomies may also be successfully created with combined dye and argon (126), diode (127,128), krypton (129), and picosecond (130,131) lasers.

Postoperative Management

The eye should be irrigated to remove excess methylcellulose and a drop of prednisolone applied. An additional drop of apraclonidine can be administered. The patient should be reassured that the visual blur will dissipate. We often suggest that the patient relax for a short period of time and then return in 60 to 90 minutes for a postlaser pressure check. If the IOP is lower, which is often the case due to the previously administered pilocarpine and apraclonidine, the patient is discharged and instructed to return for follow-up from 1 day to 1 week, depending on the severity of preexisting damage and the complexity of the angle-closure mechanisms. The pupil can be dilated at that time if desired. Although the follow-up schedule needs to be individualized, all patients should be evaluated 4 to 6 weeks postoperatively to determine continued patency of the iridotomy. If a postoperative IOP rise occurs, oral hyperosmotics usually suffice to control it. Rarely, is paracentesis required.

Histopathology

Initial changes in the iris near the iridotomy site include edema, necrosis, loss of melanocytes, the presence of pigment-laden macrophages, and irregular clumps of granules on the pigment epithelial surface (15,28,132). Histopathologic examination of Nd:YAG laser iridotomies reveals circumscribed holes with limited tissue alteration at the margin, compared with more extensive early edema and tissue destruction after argon laser iridotomy (133). Pigment debris accumulates in the trabecular meshwork and decreases with time (134). The pigment granules initially are located in the extracellular and intracellular spaces and are phagocytosed by the trabecular cells. The pigment becomes more concentrated in the juxtacanalicular meshwork and is progressively absorbed. Histopathology of Nd:YAG laser iridotomy, obtained at the time of cataract surgery 3 to 5 years later, reveals the edges to contain loosely arranged melanocytes, fibrocytes, and vessels without evidence of pigment proliferation or scarring (135). Inflammatory changes in the meshwork have been noted histologically after persistent elevation of pressure following laser iridotomy (136). Any increase in tonographic outflow facility after iridotomy is probably related to relief of pupillary block and reversal of appositional angle closure (28).

Postlaser Iris Configuration and Anterior-Chamber Depth

Increased peripheral chamber depth has been shown ultrasonographically (137). Central anterior-chamber depth is unaffected (138). This has been confirmed with Scheimpflug photography (139), which also shows a decrease in iris convexity (140). Iridolenticular contact increases following laser iridotomy (51). Any apparent deepening of the central anterior chamber may be the result of the postlaser use of cycloplegia and discontinuation of miotics and their respective effects on lens position.

Complications

Corneal Damage

Corneal edema may prevent achievement of a patent iridotomy with either the argon or the Nd:YAG laser. Scattering to the beam diffuses the laser power and precise focusing on the iris may be imposssible. Greater energy is usually necessary and may cause corneal damage. If the angle is closed, ALPI can usually open it and lower the IOP, buying time until the cornea can clear. If ALPI has been performed, but corneal edema is persistent, pupilloplasty to peak the pupil may eliminate pupillary block.

The argon laser can cause epithelial and endothelial thermal burns. Both were far more common when settings of 0.1 and 0.2 second were used. These rarely occur with the use of lower-energy burns. Epithelial coagulation and whitening are transient, but may interfere with the delivery of laser energy and make the creation of a patent iridotomy difficult. If this occurs, an attempt can be made to angle the beam around the burn to complete the iridotomy (141). It may be necessary to choose another location for the iridotomy or use a Nd:YAG laser. Stromal edema and striate keratopathy may also occur. If the anterior chamber is extremely shallow, corneal endothelial injury may develop rapidly. This may be circumvented by using contraction burns to deepen the chamber before the placement of punch burns or penetrating burns. When the anterior chamber is extremely shallow, the power should be reduced and applications not performed too rapidly.

Endothelial burns are generally dense white with sharp margins. They require more time for resolution and may result in focal endothelial cell loss. Although endothelial cell loss following argon laser iridotomy has not been statistically significant during follow-up periods of up to 1 year (142–146), an increase in mean cell size and cell loss associated with the use of greater laser powers has been documented (147). Although the endothelial cell number after Nd:YAG iridotomy reportedly is unchanged (148,149), focal loss occurs when photodisruption takes place less than 1 mm from the endothelium and at the site of treatment (149,150). The area of focal loss is reduced with the use of an Abraham lens (151). Damage to Descemet's membrane occurs when this distance is reduced to 0.1 mm. Progressive corneal edema requiring penetrating keratoplasty has occurred following Nd:YAG (152) or argon (153–156) therapy. Risk factors appear to include preexisting guttata and excessive laser energy (153,154).

Intraocular Pressure Elevations

Prior to apraclonidine, transient postlaser pressure spikes were common. A rise greater than 6 mm Hg occurred in up to 40% of patients and to over 30 mm Hg in as many as 30%

(41,157–159). Approximately two-thirds of patients had a maximal elevation in the first hour and one-third in the second (40,158). Rapid elevation to high levels occurred immediately after both argon and Nd:YAG iridotomies (40,106,157,160–163). Perioperative apraclonidine decreases the duration and magnitude of the rise and most IOP elevations are mild and easily controlled (103,104,164–166).

No significant difference in postoperative pressure rises has been found between the two types of lasers (159). The elevation may be related to the amount of energy used, the degree of pigment dispersion, and the preoperative outflow facility. Eyes in which iridotomies are performed prophylactically may have a lower incidence of postoperative IOP spikes (37). Before or after laser treatment, administration of miotics, β-blocking agents, carbonic anhydrase inhibitors, or oral hyperosmotic agents can also reduce the severity of the rise (162,167–169).

Closure of the Iridotomy Site

Closure of a previously patent iridotomy may be immediate or delayed. Early closure is caused by occlusion of the opening by circulating debris or landsliding of the pigment epithelium surrounding the iridotomy site (17,170) and is typically visible immediately following the procedure or at the time of the first postoperative visit.

Delayed closure is usually caused by localized pigment proliferation occluding the opening. Pigment proliferation is more prominent after argon laser iridotomy (17,171) and usually occurs within the first 6 to 12 weeks. As many as one-third of patients have required retreatment. The iris opening after Nd:YAG laser iridotomy is more irregular, with less pigment dispersion, but retreatment may be necessary in about 9% of patients (41). Closure after either type of laser treatment is extremely common in patients with uveitis. Other causes of late failure include the development of a transparent, thin fibrous membrane occluding the opening and regeneration of iris pigment epithelium from the margins of the iridotomy. This characteristically grows in evenly from the margins of the iridotomy toward the center and does not come forward to occlude the portion of the opening through the stroma. Functional closure may occur with the formation of posterior synechiae between the iridotomy site and the lens. Retreatment to open the iridotomy is simple. Argon laser iridotomies that repeatedly close may remain open after Nd:YAG treatment (172).

Other Complications

Blurred Vision Patients routinely experience transient postlaser blurring of vision. Patients should be informed preoperatively that when the argon laser is used, retinal pigment bleaching limits vision for 20 to 30 minutes and makes everything appear red. Other factors that contribute to blurring include the use of methylcellulose, pigment dispersion, anterior-segment inflammation, residual pilo-carpine effect, and hyphema when the Nd:YAG laser has been used.

Pupillary Abnormalities Slight contraction of the iris toward the site of iridotomy is common, generally minor, and transient and does not produce visual complaints. It is more prominent with the argon laser than with the Nd:YAG laser. The extent of the peaking is greater the closer the iridotomy is to the pupil, the lighter the iris is, and the greater the total energy used.

Diplopia and Glare These are uncommon given the small size of most iridotomies, but may develop or worsen if the iridotomy enlarges over time (173). Diplopia is more common if the iridotomy is placed nasally or temporally, but may occur anywhere if it is not covered by the upper lid. The sensation of a horizontal line in the upper visual field, occasionally accompanied by glare, is common. It occurs when the iridotomy is partially covered by the lid margin and is relieved when it is completely covered or completely exposed (105). There is also a "shutter effect" created by the lid crossing the iridotomy site during blinking. Patients often no longer notice it after a few months. Tinted soft contact lenses to ameliorate diplopia have been described (174). Opaque contact lenses to cover the iridotomy site may be used to reduce the amount of stray light entering through it (175).

Inflammation Postlaser anterior-segment inflammation is typical, is usually mild, and ceases within several days. Breakdown of the blood-aqueous barrier has been demonstrated with both the argon and Nd:YAG lasers (176,177). Topical corticosteroids are outinely prescribed for a few days.

Posterior synechiae may form between the pupil and the lens or the iridotomy site and the lens (178). Their formation may be less common after Nd:YAG laser iridotomy (40), can be minimized by postoperatively administering topical steroids, by minimizing the total energy applied, and by dilating the pupil at the time of the first postoperative visit if the iridotomy is patent and the angle is adequately open.

Hemorrhage Bleeding is rare with the argon laser because the iris tissue undergoes thermal coagulation. However, hyphema may occur (179) and may even occur days after the iridotomy, accompanied by increased IOP (180). Nd:YAG photodisruption does not coagulate iris vessels, and a small hemorrhage at the iridotomy site may occur in up to 50% of patients (158,181,182). Bleeding can occasionally be more substantial (172). Gentle pressure on the eye with the contact lens may help control the bleeding. The argon laser may be used to coagulate bleeding vessels or may be used before the Nd:YAG laser to coagulate the iris vessels in the location of the anticipated Nd:YAG iridotomy. Iridotomy in eyes with rubeosis or uveitis should be performed with the argon laser.

Lens Opacities Focal, nonprogressive, anterior subcapsular opacities may occur after both argon and Nd:YAG iridotomy in up to 45% of eyes (41,159). However, no increased incidence of visual impairment from cataracts in patients having had laser iridotomy compared to the general population has been presented. The possibility that the permanently altered aqueous flow pattern may adversely affect lens physiology has not been proved or disproved.

Although rare cases of capsular rupture with Nd:YAG iridotomy have been described (183), the earlier widespread fear of acute onset of cataract after Nd:YAG iridotomy has not been substantiated. Limiting the use of the Nd:YAG laser to the single-burst mode, performing the iridotomy peripherally, and focusing on the anterior iris stroma minimize the chance of lens damage. These localized lens changes do not affect visual acuity. Small ruptures of the anterior lens capsule after Nd:YAG iridotomy have been documented histopathologically in patients undergoing subsequent intracapsular cataract extraction (184). Animal studies suggest that fibrous proliferation covers the small anterior capsular breaks (185). Pitting of the anterior lens capsule by the Nd:YAG laser also occurs (184).

Retinal Damage   The possibility of photocoagulation of the periphery of the retina between the equator and the ora serrata, which usually occurs when an opening is being enlarged (75,186) is greatly reduced by the use of a contact lens (98,100). Inadvertent foveal photocoagulation has been reported (187), and proper positioning of the laser beam is essential. Choroidal and retinal detachment (188) and non-rhegmatogenous retinal detachment in nanophthalmic eyes (91) have also been reported. Microperforations of the retina may occur with use of the Nd:YAG laser if the beam is inadvertently focused to within 2 to 3 mm of the retina (189).

Miscellaneous Complications   Sterile hypopyon (141,190, 191), cystoid macular edema (192), unexplained loss of central visual acuity (193), lens capsule rupture (121), pupillary pseudomembranes (194), phacoanaphylactic endophthalmitis (195), and malignant (aqueous misdirection) glaucoma (89,196–202) have been reported.

ARGON LASER PERIPHERAL IRIDOPLASTY

This is a simple and effective means of opening an appositionally closed angle in situations in which laser iridotomy either cannot be performed or does not physically eliminate appositional angle closure because mechanisms other than pupillary block are present. Contraction burns (long duration, low power, and large spot size) placed in the extreme periphery of the iris withdraw the iris stroma from the angle and compress it, mechanically opening the angle (16,32,61,67,203). ALPI is highly successful in reversing acute angle-closure glaucoma when medical treatment fails (67,204). A technique for direct treatment of 360 degrees of the peripheral iris through a gonioscopy lens, termed *gonioplasty*, served as the conceptual basis for the modern procedure (205). Although ALPI is simple to perform, important aspects of technique must be followed for a successful result.

Approach to Acute Angle-Closure Glaucoma

Copious miotic treatment was, and still is, common in the treatment of acute angle-closure glaucoma. This, however, is undesirable for several reasons. When the IOP is over 60 mm Hg, the pupil becomes unresponsive to miotics because of ischemia and paralysis of the iris sphincter. Pilocarpine may paradoxically worsen the block (65–67,206). Miotics cause forward motion of the lens-iris diaphragm, and overtreatment can exacerbate acute angle closure when it is due to block at the level of or behind the lens. The following is our approach to acute angle-closure glaucoma (25):

1. Examine the affected eye and fellow eye, particularly noting central and peripheral anterior-chamber depth, the shape of the peripheral iris, and the appearance on indentation gonioscopy.
2. Administer an oral hyperosmotic agent and, if desired, aqueous suppressants.
3. Place the patient supine. This permits the lens to fall backward to whatever extent possible when the hyperosmotic shrinks the vitreous. Remember that the vitreous volume is reduced only about 3%, but this 0.12 cm^3 equals twice the volume of the posterior chamber and half the volume of the anterior chamber.
4. Reassess ocular findings after 1 hour. The IOP is usually decreased, but the angle remains appositionally closed. One drop of 4% pilocarpine is given and the patient re-examined 30 minutes later.
   a. If the IOP is reduced and the angle is open, pupillary block or plateau iris or both are responsible for the angle closure, and the patient may be treated medically with topical low-dose pilocarpine, β-blockers, and steroids until the eye quiets and laser iridotomy can be performed.
   b. If the IOP is unchanged or elevated and the angle remains closed, level 3 or 4 block should be suspected, further pilocarpine withheld, and the attack broken by ALPI (67,73,207).

We have performed ALPI for nearly 100 attacks of angle-closure glaucoma unresponsive to medical therapy, even after several days. All but one eye, which had total synechial closure, responded with at least transient normalization of IOP and opening of the angle. ALPI does not eliminate pupillary block and is not a substitute for laser iridotomy, which must be performed as soon as the eye is quiet. However, even in eyes with extensive synechial closure, the IOP is lowered sufficiently for a few days for the inflammation to resolve. The alternative of prolonging a paradoxical reaction to medical therapy for several days seriously increases the possibility of irreversible damage to the iris, lens, cornea, trabecular meshwork, and optic nerve.

Up to one-third of angles without PAS remain narrow after iridotomy, and approximately half of these are capable of closure with mydriasis (208). Continued appositional angle closure in the presence of a patent iridotomy is an indication for ALPI (32,61). If extensive PAS are present after ALPI, goniosynechialysis may be performed. This procedure is successful if the PAS have been present for less than 1 year (209). Promising results have been reported in both phakic and pseudophakic eyes (210–212). It is effective both alone and in conjunction with other surgical procedures (213). ALPI can be used postoperatively to further flatten the peripheral iris and prevent synechial reattachment (214).

Indications

Medically Unbreakable Attacks of Angle-Closure Glaucoma

An attack of angle-closure glaucoma that is unresponsive to medical therapy outlined above and in which corneal edema, a shallow anterior chamber, or marked inflammation precludes laser iridotomy, or that is unresponsive to successful iridotomy, may be broken with ALPI (67,204, 215,216).

Circumferential treatment of the iris opens the angle in those areas in which there are no PAS. All published series have reported virtually 100% success. In a prospective study of 10 eyes with medically unbreakable attacks of 2 to 5 days' duration, the mean prelaser IOP was 54.9 mm Hg and 2 to 4 hours after laser treatment the mean IOP was 18.9 mm Hg (216). Even when extensive PAS are present, the IOP is usually normalized within an hour or two, perhaps because of associated secretory hypotony. The effect lasts sufficiently long for the cornea and anterior chamber to clear, so that iridotomy can be performed. In cases in which an intumescent lens is responsible for the angle-closure attack, cataract extraction can be postponed until the intraocular inflammation has sufficiently resolved.

Plateau Iris Syndrome

In this condition, discussed already, the angle remains appositionally closed or occludable following laser iridotomy because of abnormally anteriorly positioned ciliary processes (53,54).

Angle Closure Related to Size or Position of the Lens

Angle closure caused by an enlarged lens or pressure posterior to the lens (malignant glaucoma) is not often responsive to iridotomy, although iridotomy should be performed to eliminate any component of pupillary block. Appositional closure remaining after iridotomy can be partially or entirely eliminated by ALPI (32,203,217,218). After the angle has been opened and the IOP reduced, cycloplegics may be given cautiously to ascertain the mechanism of the angle closure.

Adjunct to Laser Trabeculoplasty

If a narrow but open angle results from plateau iris or angle crowding, ALPI can retract the iris away from the trabecular meshwork (16).

Retinopathy of Prematurity

Angle closure in young children with retinopathy of prematurity occurs owing to forward shifting of the lens-iris diaphragm (219–224). These children do not respond to iridotomy. In young adults with this condition, there appears to be a superimposed element of pupillary block, and iridotomy may be successful (225,228).

Nanophthalmos

Flattening of the peripheral iris by argon laser was first reported in 1979 by Kimbrough et al (205). Combined iridotomy and ALPI often brings the angle closure under control (227). Uveal effusions have occurred after both laser iridotomy (91) and ALT (228). The risks of surgical intervention include malignant glaucoma, expulsive suprachoroidal hemorrhage, and retinal detachment (229). Posterior sclerotomy may or may not be successful at preventing uveal effusion (227,230).

Contraindications

Corneal edema is not a contraindication to ALPI when it is performed in order to break a medically unresponsive attack of angle-closure glaucoma. Extensive corneal opacification may present difficulties, because higher powers necessary to cause contraction of the iris may injure the cornea as well. Glycerin may help clear the cornea temporarily.

If the anterior chamber is flat with iris-corneal apposition, any attempt at photocoagulation will result in damage to the corneal endothelium. If the anterior chamber is very shallow, laser applications should be timed enough apart so that the heat generated can dissipate.

Although ALPI has been reported to break PAS (231), we have been unable to accomplish this. ALPI should not be used to relieve synechial angle closure, especially in eyes with uveitis, neovascular glaucoma, or iridocorneal-endothelial syndrome.

Technique

ALPI is performed on an outpatient basis using topical anesthesia and an Abraham lens. Apraclonidine is administered perioperatively. Shortly before treatment, 4% pilocarpine is applied topically to put maximal stretch on the iris. In eyes predisposed to a paradoxical reaction to pilocarpine, the risk is minimized by the timing of the pilocarpine application close to the laser procedure. Miotics should not, however, be continued following the procedure.

Contraction burns (500-μm spot size, 0.5-second duration, and 200–400-mW power) are used to pull the surrounding iris tissue toward, and compact the stroma at the site of the burn (Figs. 30-13 and 30-14). The short-term effect appears to be related to the heat shrinkage of collagen and the long-term effect secondary to contraction of a fibroblastic membrane in the region of the laser burn (232).

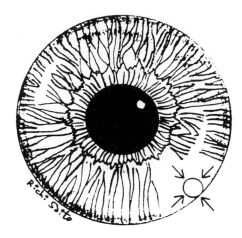

FIGURE 30-13.   *Correct placement of the ALPI burn in the extreme periphery allows for contraction of the iris toward the burn and away from the angle.*

The aiming beam should be directed to the most peripheral portion of the iris possible. Spot placement short of the iris root is ineffective. The patient should look in the same direction as the quadrant of iris being treated. It is useful to allow a thin crescent of the aiming beam to overlap the sclera at the limbus. The surgeon should begin with 200 mW for dark irides and 300 mW for light ones and adjust the power as necessary to obtain visible stromal contraction. Contraction is accompanied by deepening of the peripheral region of the anterior chamber at the site of the burn. If bubbles form or if pigment is released, the power should be reduced. Occasionally, in light-gray irides, a 200-μm spot size may be more effective.

Twenty to 24 spots are placed over 360 degrees, leaving approximately two spot-diameters between each spot and avoiding large visible radial vessels if possible. Although rare, iris necrosis may occur if too many spots are placed too closely together. If this is insufficient, more spots may be given at a later time. The presence of an arcus senilis should be ignored. An extremely shallow anterior chamber and corneal edema, relative contraindications to laser iridotomy, do not preclude ALPI.

Other laser settings that have been advocated in the past, most commonly 20 μm, 0.1- or 0.2-second duration, and 200-mW power, and burns placed through the angled mirror of a gonioscopy lens, often provide insufficient contraction and result in tissue vaporization. In those uncommon angles with a very sharp peripheral drop-off that do not respond well to the above treatment, one of the angled mirrors of a Goldmann or Ritch lens and a 200-μm spot size directly onto the peripheral iris can be used.

Gonioscopy should be performed to assess the effect of the procedure. Patients are treated with topical steroids four to six times daily for 3 to 5 days. IOP is monitored postoperatively as after any other anterior-segment laser proce-

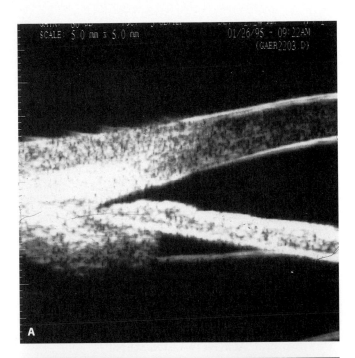

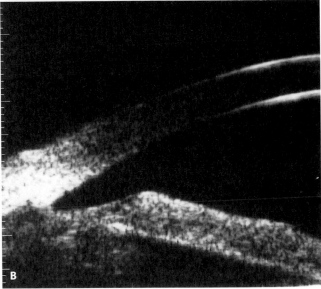

FIGURE 30-14.   *A. Ultrasound biomicroscopic image of an eye with plateau iris prior to ALPI. B. A similar eye after ALPI. Note the compression of the iris root, creating a space between it and the trabecular meshwork.*

dure and patients treated as necessary if an increase occurs after laser treatment.

Complications

Mild postoperative iritis is common and responds to topical steroid treatment. The patient may experience transient ocular irritation. Hemorrhage does not occur. A transient rise in IOP can occur as with other anterior-segment laser procedures. Because ALPI is often performed on patients with extremely shallow peripheral anterior chambers, ill-defined, diffuse corneal endothelial burns may occur. We have seen only one case of corneal decompensation following ALPI in a patient with preexisting Fuchs' dystrophy. Lenticular opacification has not occurred and theoretically would be highly unlikely.

The duration of success depends on the mechanism of the cause of angle closure. Eyes with plateau iris rarely if ever require retreatment. However, angle closure may recur on the basis of lens enlargement with time. Pressure from the lens against the posterior iris may lead to gradual narrowing of the angle, possibly because of further anterior lens movement or stretching of the iris stroma. Necessity for retreatment is most common in eyes in which angle closure is due to forward lens movement, particularly those with malignant glaucoma. Patients in whom angle closure results from intumescent lenses usually undergo cataract extraction. Patients should be observed gonioscopically at regular intervals and further treatment given if necessary.

ACKNOWLEDGMENT

Supported in part by the New York Glaucoma Research Foundation.

REFERENCES

1. Verhoeff FH, Bell L. The pathological effects of radiant energy on the eye. *Proc Am Acad Arts Sci* 1916;51:630.
2. Meyer-Schwickerath G. Erfahrungen mit der Lichtkoagulation der Metzhaut und der Iris. *Doc Ophthalmol* 1966;10:91.
3. McDonald JE, Light A. Photocoagulation of the iris and retina. *Arch Ophthalmol* 1958;60:384.
4. Hogan MF, Schwartz A. Experimental photocoagulation of the iris in guinea pigs. *Am J Ophthalmol* 1960;49:629.
5. Burns RP. Improvement in technique of photocoagulation of the iris. *Arch Ophthalmol* 1965;74:306.
6. Beckman H, et al. Laser iridectomies. *Am J Ophthalmol* 1971;72:393.
7. Flocks M, Zweng HC. Laser coagulation of ocular tissues. *Arch Ophthalmol* 1964;72:604.
8. Perkins ES, Brown NA. Iridotomy with a ruby laser. *Br J Ophthalmol* 1973;57:487.
9. Perkins ES. Laser iridotomy. *BMJ* 1970;2:580.
10. Zweng HC, et al. Laser photocoagulation of the iris. *Arch Ophthalmol* 1970;84:193.
11. Zweng HC, et al. Experimental laser photocoagulation. *Am J Ophthalmol* 1964;58:353.
12. Beckman H, Sugar HS. Laser iridectomy therapy of glaucoma. *Arch Ophthalmol* 1973;90:453.
13. Khuri CH. Argon laser iridectomies. *Am J Ophthalmol* 1973;76:490.
14. Abraham RK, Miller GL. Outpatient argon laser iridectomy for angle-closure glaucoma: a two-year study. *Trans Am Acad Ophthalmol Otol* 1975;79:OP529.
15. Pollack IP, Patz A. Argon laser iridotomy: an experimental and clinical study. *Ophthalmic Surg* 1976;7:22.
16. Ritch R. *Techniques of argon laser iridectomy and iridoplasty.* Palo Alto: Coherent Medical, 1983.
17. Ritch R, Podos SM. Argon laser treatment of angle-closure glaucoma. *Perspect Ophthalmol* 1980;4:129.
18. Ritch R, Palmberg P. Argon laser iridectomy in densely pigmented irides. *Am J Ophthalmol* 1982;94:800.
19. Stetz D, Smith HJ, Ritch R. A simplified technique for laser iridectomy in blue irides. *Am J Ophthalmol* 1983;96:249.
20. Hoskins HD Jr, Migliazzo CV. Laser iridectomy—a technique for blue irises. *Ophthalmic Surg* 1984;15:488.
21. Pollack IP. Laser iridotomy: current concepts in techniques and safety. *Int Ophthalmol Clin* 1984;21:137.
22. Abraham RK, Miller GL. Outpatient argon iridectomy for angle-closure glaucoma: a 3$^1/_2$ year study. *Adv Ophthalmol* 1977;34:186.
23. Go FJ, Akiba F, Yamamoto T, Kitazawa Y. Argon laser iridectomy and surgical iridectomy in the treatment of primary angle-closure glaucoma. *Jpn J Ophthalmol* 1984;28:36.
24. Harrad RA, Stannard KP, Shilling JS. Argon laser iridotomy. *Br J Ophthalmol* 1985;69:368.
25. Kramer P, Ritch R. The treatment of angle-closure glaucoma revisited. *Ann Ophthalmol* 1984;16:1101–1103. Editorial.
26. Mishima S, Kitazawa Y, Shirato S. Laser therapy for glaucoma. *Aust N Z J Ophthalmol* 1985;13:225.
27. Podos SM, et al. Continuous wave argon laser iridectomy in angle-closure glaucoma. *Am J Ophthalmol* 1979;88:836.
28. Pollack IP. Use of argon laser energy to produce iridotomies. *Ophthalmic Surg* 1980;11:506.
29. Quigley HA, Maumenee AE. Long-term follow-up of treated open-angle glaucoma. *Am J Ophthalmol* 1979;87:519.
30. Ritch R. The treatment of angle-closure glaucoma. *Ann Ophthalmol* 1979;11:1373–1375. Editorial.
31. Ritch R. The treatment of chronic angle-closure glaucoma. *Ann Ophthalmol* 1981;13:21–23. Editorial.
32. Ritch R, Solomon IS. Glaucoma surgery. In: L'Esperance FA, ed. *Ophthalmic lasers.* 3rd ed. St. Louis: CV Mosby 1989.
33. Robin AL, Pollack IP. Argon laser peripheral iridotomies in the treatment of primary angle closure glaucoma: long-term follow-up. *Arch Ophthalmol* 1982;100:919.
34. Schwartz LW, et al. Argon laser iridotomy in the treatment of patients with primary angle-closure or pupillary block glaucoma: a clinicopathologic study. *Ophthalmology* 1978;85:294.
35. Schwartz L, Spaeth G. Argon laser iridotomy in primary angle closure or pupillary block glaucoma. *Trans Ophthalmol Soc U K* 1979;99:257.
36. Yamamoto T, Shirato S, Kitazawa Y. Treatment of primary angle-closure glaucoma by argon laser iridotomy: a long-term follow-up. *Jpn J Ophthalmol* 1985;29:1.
37. Yassur Y, Melamed S, Cohen S, Ben-Sira I. Laser iridotomy in closed-angle glaucoma. *Arch Ophthalmol* 1979;97:1920.
38. Klapper RM. Q-switched neodymium:YAG laser iridotomy. *Ophthalmology* 1984;91:1017.
39. Latina MA, Puliafito CA, Steinert RR, Epstein DL. Experimental iridotomy with the Q-switched neodymium:YAG laser. *Ophthalmology* 1984;102:1211.
40. Moster MR, et al. Laser iridectomy: a controlled study comparing argon and neodymium:YAG. *Ophthalmology* 1986;93:20.
41. Schwartz LW, et al. Neodymium-YAG laser iridectomies in glaucoma associated with closed or occludable angles. *Am J Ophthalmol* 1986;102:41.
42. Tomey KF, Traverso CE, Shammas IV. Neodymium-YAG laser iridotomy in the treatment and prevention of angle closure glaucoma: a review of 373 eyes. *Arch Ophthalmol* 1987;105:476.
43. Wishart PK, Hitchings RA. Neodymium YAG and dye laser iridotomy—a comparative study. *Trans Ophthalmol Soc U K* 1986;105:521.
44. Ritch R, Liebmann J, Tello C. A construct for understanding angle-closure glaucoma: the role of ultrasound biomicroscopy. *Ophthalmol Clin North Am* 1995;8:281–293.
45. Forbes M. Gonioscopy with corneal indentation: a method for distinguishing between appositional closure and synechial closure. *Arch Ophthalmol* 1966;76:488–497.
46. Lowe RF. Primary angle-closure glaucoma: a review of ocular biometry. *Austral J Ophthalmol* 1977;5:9–17.
47. Delmarcelle Y, et al. Biometrie oculaire clinique (oculometrie). *Bull Soc Ophthalmol Belge* 1976;fascicule 1:172.
48. Tomlinson A, Leighton DA. Ocular dimensions in the heredity of angle-closure glaucoma. *Br J Ophthalmol* 1973;57:475–486.
49. Lowe RF, Clark BAJ. Posterior corneal curvature: correlations in normal eyes and in eyes involved with primary angle-closure glaucoma. *Br J Ophthalmol* 1973;57:475.
50. Lee DA, Brubaker RF, Illstrup DM. Anterior chamber dimensions in patients with narrow angles and angle-closure glaucoma. *Arch Ophthalmol* 1984;102:46–50.
51. Caronia RM, Liebmann JM, Stegman Z, et al. Iris-lens contact increases following laser iridotomy for pupillary block angle-closure glaucoma. *Am J Ophthalmol* 1996;122:53–57.
52. Tornquist R. Angle-closure glaucoma in an eye with a plateau type of iris. *Acta Ophthalmol* 1958;36:413.
53. Pavlin CJ, Ritch R, Foster FS. Ultrasound biomicroscopy in plateau iris syndrome. *Am J Ophthalmol* 1992;113:390–395.

54. Ritch R. Plateau iris is caused by abnormally positioned ciliary processes. *J Glaucoma* 1992;1:23–26.

55. Wand M, Pavlin CJ, Foster FS. Plateau iris syndrome: ultrasound biomicroscopic and histological study. *Ophthalmic Surg* 1993;24:129.

56. Godel V, Stein R, Feiler-Ofry V. Angle-closure glaucoma following peripheral iridectomy and mydriasis. *Am J Ophthalmol* 1968;65:555–560.

57. Lowe RF. Primary angle-closure glaucoma: postoperative acute glaucoma after phenylephrine eye-drops. *Am J Ophthalmol* 1968;65:552.

58. Lowe RF. Plateau iris. *Aust J Ophthalmol* 1981;9:71.

59. Wand M, Grant WM, Simmons RJ, Hutchinson BT. Plateau iris syndrome. *Trans Am Acad Ophthalmol Otol* 1977;83:122.

60. Lowe RF, Ritch R. Angle-closure glaucoma. Clinical types. In: Ritch R, Shields MB, Krupin T, eds. *The glaucomas*. Vol. 2. St Louis: CV Mosby, 1989:839–853.

61. Ritch R. Argon laser peripheral iridoplasty: an overview. *J Glaucoma* 1992;1:206–213.

62. Bleiman B, Schwartz AL. Paradoxical response to pilocarpine. *Arch Ophthalmol* 1979;97:1305.

63. Abramson DH, Franzen LA, Coleman DJ. Pilocarpine in the presbyope: demonstration of an effect on the anterior chamber and lens thickness. *Arch Ophthalmol* 1973;89:100–102.

64. Abramson DH, Chang S, Coleman DJ, et al. Pilocarpine-induced lens changes: an ultrasonic biometric evaluation of dose response. *Arch Ophthalmol* 1974;92:464.

65. Gorin G. Angle-closure glaucoma induced by miotics. *Am J Ophthalmol* 1966;62:1063.

66. Rieser JC, Schwartz B. Miotic induced malignant glaucoma. *Arch Ophthalmol* 1972;87:706.

67. Ritch R. Argon laser treatment for medically unresponsive attacks of angle-closure glaucoma. *Am J Ophthalmol* 1982;94:197.

68. Ritch R, Solomon LD. Argon laser peripheral iridoplasty for angle-closure glaucoma in siblings with Weill-Marchesani syndrome. *J Glaucoma* 1992;1:243–247.

69. Liebmann JM, Ritch R. Lens-associated angle-closure glaucoma. In: Ritch R, Shields MB, Krupin T, eds. *The glaucomas*. 2nd ed. St Louis: CV Mosby, 1996.

70. Ritch R. Angle-closure glaucoma. Treatment overview. In: Ritch R, Shields MB, Krupin T, eds. The glaucomas. 2nd ed. St Louis: CV Mosby, 1996:••.

71. Phelps CD. Angle-closure glaucoma secondary to ciliary body swelling. *Arch Ophthalmol* 1974;92:287.

72. Fleck BW, et al. A randomized, prospective comparison of Nd:YAG laser iridotomy and operative peripheral iridectomy in fellow eyes. *Eye* 1991;5:315–321.

73. Shin DH. Argon laser treatment for relief of medically unresponsive angle-closure glaucoma attacks. *Am J Ophthalmol* 1982;94:821.

74. Tomey KF, Al-Rajhi AA. Neodymium:YAG laser iridotomy in the initial management of phacomorphic glaucoma. *Ophthalmology* 1992;99:660–665.

75. Quigley HA. Long-term follow-up of laser iridotomy. *Ophthalmology* 1981;88:218.

76. Gieser D, Wilensky J. Laser iridectomy in the management of chronic angle-closure glaucoma. *Am J Ophthalmol* 1984;98:446.

77. Rivera AH, Brown RH, Anderson DR. Laser iridotomy vs surgical iridectomy: have the indications changed? *Arch Ophthalmol* 1985;103:1350–1354.

78. Anderson DR, Forster RK, Lewis ML. Laser iridotomy for aphakic pupillary block. *Arch Ophthalmol* 1975;93:343–346.

79. Cinotti DJ, Reiter DJ, Maltzman BA, Cinotti AA. Neodymium:YAG laser therapy for pseudophakic pupillary block. *J Cataract Refract Surg* 1986;12:174.

80. Forman JS, Ritch R, Dunn MW, Szmyd L. Pupillary block following posterior chamber lens implantation. *Ophthalmic Laser Ther* 1987;2:85.

81. Patti JC, Cinnoti AA. Iris photocoagulation therapy of aphakic pupillary block. *Arch Ophthalmol* 1975;93:347.

82. Samples J, et al. Pupillary block with posterior chamber intraocular lenses. *Am J Ophthalmol* 1987;105:335.

83. Werner D, Kaback M. Pseudophakic pupillary-block glaucoma. *Br J Ophthalmol* 1977;61:329.

84. Shrader CE, et al. Pupillary and iridovitreal block in pseudophakic eyes. *Ophthalmology* 1984;91:831.

85. Melamed S, Wagoner MD. Recurrent closure of neodymium:YAG laser iridotomies requiring multiple treatments in pseudophakic pupillary block. *Ann Ophthalmol* 1988;20:105–108.

86. Epstein DL, Steinert RF, Puliafito CA. Neodymium-YAG laser therapy to the anterior hyaloid in aphakic malignant glaucoma. *Am J Ophthalmol* 1984;98:137.

87. Schwartz GF, Steinmann WC, Spaeth GL, Wilson RP. Surgical and medical management of patients with narrow anterior chamber angles: comparative results. *Ophthalmic Surg* 1992;23:108–112.

88. Cashwell LF, Martin TJ. Malignant glaucoma after laser iridotomy. *Ophthalmology* 1992;99:651–658.

89. Merritt JC. Malignant glaucoma induced by miotics postoperatively in open-angle glaucoma. *Arch Ophthalmol* 1977;95:1988.

90. O'Grady RB. Nanophthalmos. *Am J Ophthalmol* 1971;71:1251.

91. Karjalainen K, Laatikainen L, Raitta C. Bilateral nonrhegmatogenous retinal detachment following neodymium-YAG laser iridotomies. *Arch Ophthalmol* 1986;104:1134.

92. Singh OS, Belcher CD, Simmons RJ. Nanophthalmic eyes and neodymium-YAG laser iridectomies. *Arch Ophthalmol* 1987;105:455.

93. Potash SD, Tello C, Liebmann J, Ritch R. Ultrasound biomicroscopy in pigment dispersion syndrome. *Ophthalmology* 1994;101:332–339.

94. Pavlin CJ, Macken P, Trope G, et al. Ultrasound biomicroscopic features of pigmentary glaucoma. *Can J Ophthalmol* 1994;29:187–192.

95. Lagreze WD, Funk J. Iridotomy in the treatment of pigmentary glaucoma: documentation with high resolution ultrasound. *Ger J Ophthalmol* 1995;4:162–166.

96. Abraham RK. Protocol for single-session argon laser iridectomy for angle-closure glaucoma. *Int Ophthalmol Clin* 1981;21:145.

97. L'Esperance FA, James WA. Argon laser photocoagulation of iris abnormalities. *Trans Am Acad Ophthalmol Otolaryngol* 1975;79:OP321.

98. Bongard B, Pederson JE. Retinal burns from experimental laser iridotomy. *Ophthalmic Surg* 1985;16:42.

99. Schirmer KE. Argon laser surgery of the iris, optimized by contact lenses. *Arch Ophthalmol* 1983;101:1130.

100. Wise JB, Munnerlyn CR, Erickson PJ. A high-efficiency laser iridotomy-sphincterotomy lens. *Am J Ophthalmol* 1986;101:546.

101. Hill RA, Minckler DS, Lee M, et al. Apraclonidine prophylaxis for postcycloplegic IOP spikes. *Ophthalmology* 1991;98:1083–1086.

102. Krupin T, Stank T, Feitl ME. Apraclonidine pretreatment decreases the acute intraocular pressure rise after laser trabeculoplasty or iridotomy. *J. Glaucoma* 1992;1:79–86.

103. Robin AL. The role of apraclonidine hydrochloride in laser therapy for glaucoma. *Trans Am Ophthalmol Soc* 1989;87:729.

104. Robin AL, Pollack IP, DeFaller JM. Effects of topical ALO 2145 (p-aminoclonidine hydrochloride) on intraocular pressure rise following argon laser iridotomy. *Arch Ophthalmol* 1987;105:1208–1211.

105. Murphy PH, Trope GE. Monocular blurring: a complication of YAG laser iridotomy. *Ophthalmology* 1991;98:1539–1542.

106. Yamamoto T, Shirato S, Kitazawa Y. Argon laser iridotomy in angle-closure glaucoma: a comparison of two methods. *Jpn J Ophthalmol* 1982;29:387.

107. Mandelkorn RM, Mendelsohn AD, Olander KW, Zimmerman TJ. Short exposure times in argon laser iridotomy. *Ophthalmic Surg* 1981;12:805.

108. Ritch R. Overview of laser iridectomy with particular reference to the dark brown iris. *Trans Asia Pacific Acad Ophthalmol* 1984;10:160–163.

109. Ritch R, Podos SM. Laser treatment of glaucoma. *Proc Asia Pacific Acad Ophthalmol* 1982;8:658–672.

110. Yamamoto T, Shirato S, Kitazawa Y. Argon laser iridotomy: short-burn technique. *Jpn Rev Clin Ophthalmol* 1983;77:8–11.

111. Wise JB. Iris sphincterotomy, iridotomy, synechiotomy by linear incision with the argon laser. *Ophthalmology* 1985;92:641.

112. Wise JB. Large iridotomies by the linear incision technique using the neodymium:YAG laser at low energy levels. A study using cynomolgus monkeys. *Ophthalmology* 1987;94:82–86.

113. Prum BEJ, Shields SR, Shields MB, et al. In vitro videographic comparison of argon and Nd:YAG laser iridotomy. *Am J Ophthalmol* 1991;111:589–594.

114. Goldberg MF, Tso MO, Mirolovich M. Histopathological characteristics of neodymium-YAG laser iridotomy in the human eye. *Br J Ophthalmol* 1987;71:623–638.

115. Haut J, et al. Study of the first hundred phakic eyes treated by peripheral iridotomy using the Nd:YAG laser. *Int Ophthalmol* 1986;9:227–235.

116. Albuquerque M, Belcher CDI, Tomlinson CP. Success of neodymium:YAG laser iridectomy. *Ophthalmic Laser Ther* 1987;2:239–244.

117. Rockwood EJ, Meyers SM, et al. Treatment of selected cases of pupillary block with YAG laser iridotomies. *Ophthalmic Surg* 1984;15:968.

118. Schrems W, Belcher CDI, Tomlinson CP. Neodymium:YAG laser iridectomy: a report of 200 cases. *Ophthalmic Laser Ther* 1987;2:33–42.

119. Wand M, Clark JA, Hill DA. Nd:YAG laser iridectomies: 100 consecutive cases. *Ophthalmic Surg* 1988;19:399–402.

120. Wise JB. Low-energy linear-incision neodymium:YAG laser iridotomy versus linear-incision argon laser iridotomy: a prospective clinical investigation. *Ophthalmology* 1987;94:1531.

121. Fernandez-Bahamonde JL. Iatrogenic lens rupture after a neodymium: yttrium aluminum garnet laser iridotomy attempt. *Ann Ophthalmol* 1991;23:346–348.

122. Ho T, Fan R. Sequential argon-YAG laser iridotomies in dark irides. *Br J Ophthalmol* 1992;76:329–331.

123. Damerow A, Utermann D. Combined thermal-photodisruptive iridotomy using the argon and Nd:YAG laser. *Klin Monatsbl Augenheilkd* 1989;195: 61–67.

124. Zborowski-Gutman L, Rosner M, Blumenthal M, Naveh N. Sequential use of argon and Nd:YAG lasers to produce an iridotomy—a pilot study. *Metab Pediatr Syst Ophthalmol* 1988;11:58–60.

125. Goins K, Schmeisser E, Smith T. Argon laser pretreatment in Nd:YAG iridotomy. *Ophthalmic Surg* 1990;21:497–500.

126. Hitchings RA. Combined dye and argon laser treatment for narrow angle glaucoma. *Trans Ophthalmol Soc U K* 1985;104:52.

127. Emoto I, Okisaka S, Nakajima A. Diode laser iridotomy in rabbit and human eyes. *Am J Ophthalmol* 1992;113:321–327.

128. Schuman JS, Puliafito CA, Jacobson JJ. Semiconductor diode laser peripheral iridotomy. *Arch Ophthalmol* 1990;108:1207–1208. Letter.

129. Yassur Y, David R, Rosenblatt I, Marmour U. Iridotomy with red krypton laser. *Br J Ophthalmol* 1986;70:295–297.

130. Frangie JP, Park SB, Aquavella JV. Peripheral iridotomy using ND:YLF laser. *Ophthalmic Surg* 1992;23:220–221.

131. Oram O, Gross RL, Severin TD, et al. Picosecond neodymium:yttrium lithium fluoride (Nd:YLF) laser peripheral iridotomy. *Am J Ophthalmol* 1995;119:408–414.

132. Rodrigues MM, Streeten B, Spaeth GL, Schwartz LW. Argon laser iridotomy in primary angle closure or pupillary block glaucoma. *Arch Ophthalmol* 1978;96:2222.

133. Rodrigues MM. Histopathology of neodymium:YAG laser iridectomy in humans. *Ophthalmology* 1985;92:1696.

134. Robin AL, et al. Histologic studies of angle structures after laser iridotomy in primates. *Arch Ophthalmol* 1982;100:1665.

135. Tetsumoto K, Küchle M, Naumann GOH. Late histopathological findings of neodymium:YAG laser iridotomies in humans. *Arch Ophthalmol* 1992;110:1119–1123.

136. Greenidge KC, et al. Acute intraocular pressure elevation after argon laser trabeculoplasty and iridectomy: a clinicopathologic study. *Ophthalmic Surg* 1984;15:105.

137. Schrems W, Hofmann G, Krieglstein GK. Biometry of the anterior chamber of the eye in Nd:YAG laser iridectomy. *Klin Monatsbl Augenheilkd* 1990;196:128–131.

138. Jacobs IH. Anterior chamber depth measurement using the slit-lamp microscope. *Am J Ophthalmol* 1979;88:236.

139. Morsman CD, Lusky M, Bosem ME, Weinreb RN. Anterior chamber angle configuration before and after iridotomy measured by Scheimpflug video imaging. *J Glaucoma* 1994;3:114–116.

140. Jin JC, Anderson DR. The effect of iridotomy on iris contour. *Am J Ophthalmol* 1990;110:260–263.

141. Cooper RL, Constable IJ. Prevention of corneal burns during high-energy laser iridotomy. *Am J Ophthalmol* 1981;91:534.

142. Wishart PK, et al. Corneal endothelial changes following short pulsed laser iridotomy and surgical iridectomy. *Trans Ophthalmol Soc U K* 1986;105:541.

143. Panek WC, Lee DA, Christensen RE. Effects of argon laser iridotomy on the corneal endothelium. *Am J Ophthalmol* 1988;105:395–397.

144. Hirst LW, et al. Corneal endothelial changes after argon-laser iridotomy and panretinal photocoagulation. *Am J Ophthalmol* 1982;93:473.

145. Smith J, Whitted P. Corneal endothelial changes after argon laser iridotomy. *Am J Ophthalmol* 1984;98:153.

146. Thoming C, van Buskirk EM, Samples JR. The corneal endothelium after laser therapy for glaucoma. *Am J Ophthalmol* 1987;103:518.

147. Hong C, Kitazawa Y, Tanishima H. Influence of argon laser treatment of glaucoma on corneal endothelium. *Jpn J Ophthalmol* 1983;27:567.

148. Schrems W, Belcher CD, Tomlinson CP. Changes in the human central corneal endothelium after neodymium:YAG laser surgery. *Ophthalmic Laser Ther* 1986;1:143.

149. Panek WC, Lee DA, Christensen RE. The effects of Nd:YAG laser iridotomy on the corneal endothelium. *Am J Ophthalmol* 1991;111:505–507.

150. Meyer KT, Pettit TH, Straatsma BR. Corneal endothelial damage with neodymium:YAG laser. *Ophthalmology* 1984;91:1022.

151. Power WJ, Collum LMT. Electron microscopic appearances of human corneal endothelium following Nd:YAG laser iridotomy. *Ophthalmic Surg* 1992;23:347–350.

152. Wilhelmus KR. Corneal edema following argon laser iridotomy. *Ophthalmic Surg* 1992;23:533–537.

153. Jeng S, Lee JS, Huang SCM. Corneal decompensation after argon laser iridotomy—a delayed complication. *Ophthalmic Surg* 1991;22:565–569.

154. Zabel RW, MacDonald IM, Mintsioulis G. Corneal endothelial decompensation after argon laser iridotomy. *Can J Ophthalmol* 1991;26:367–373.

155. Kalnins LY, Mandelkorn RM. Corneal decompensation after argon laser iridectomy. *Arch Ophthalmol* 1989;107:792. Letter.

156. Schwartz AL, Martin NF, Weber PA. Corneal decompensation after argon laser iridectomy. *Arch Ophthalmol* 1988;106:1572–1574.

157. Krupin T, et al. Acute intraocular pressure response to argon laser iridotomy. *Ophthalmology* 1985;92:922.

158. Pollack IP, et al. Use of the neodymium:YAG laser to create iridotomies in monkeys and humans. *Trans Am Ophthalmol Soc* 1984;82:307.

159. Robin AL, Pollack IP. A comparison of neodymium:YAG and argon laser iridotomies. *Ophthalmology* 1984;91:1011.

160. Henry JC, Krupin T, Schultz J, Wax M. Increased intraocular pressure following neodymium-YAG laser iridotomy. *Arch Ophthalmol* 1986;104:178. Letter.

161. Robin AL. Intraocular pressure rise after iridotomy. *Arch Ophthalmol* 1986;104:1117. Letter.

162. Schrems W, Eichelbronner O, Krieglstein GK. The immediate IOP response of Nd-YAG-laser iridotomy and its prophylactic treatability. *Acta Ophthalmol* 1984;92:673.

163. Taniguchi T, Rho SH, Gotoh Y, Kitazawa Y. Intraocular pressure rise following Q-switched neodymium:YAG laser iridotomy. *Ophthalmic Laser Ther* 1987;2:99.

164. Kitazawa Y, Taniguchi T, Sugiyama K. Use of apraclonidine to reduce acute intraocular pressure rise following Q-switched Nd:YAG laser iridotomy. *Ophthalmic Surg* 1989;20:49–52.

165. Hong C, Song KY, Park WH, Sohn YH. Effect of apraclonidine hydrochloride on acute intraocular pressure rise after argon laser iridotomy. *Korean J Ophthalmol* 1991;5:37–41.

166. Brown RH, et al. ALO 2145 reduces the IOP elevation after anterior segment laser surgery. *Ophthalmology* 1988;95:378.

167. Brown SVL, Thomas JV, Belcher CDI, Simmons RJ. Effect of pilocarpine in treatment of intraocular pressure elevation following neodymium:YAG laser posterior capsulotomy. *Ophthalmology* 1985;92:354–359.

168. Liu PF, Hung PT. Effect of timolol on intraocular pressure elevation following argon laser iridotomy. *J Ocul Pharmacol* 1987;3:249.

169. Hsieh JW. Effects of timolol and acetazolamide on intraocular pressure elevation following argon laser iridotomy. *J Formosa Med Assoc* 1992;91:29–33.

170. Brainard JO, Landers JH, Shock JP. Recurrent angle closure glaucoma following a patent 75 micron laser iridotomy: a case report. *Ophthalmic Surg* 1982;13:1030.

171. Del Priore LV, Robin AL, Pollack IP. Neodymium:YAG and argon laser iridotomy. Long-term follow-up in a prospective, randomized clinical trial. *Ophthalmology* 1988;95:1207–1211.

172. Gilbert CM, Robin AL, Pollack IP. Hyphema complicating neodymium:YAG iridotomy. *Ophthalmology* 1984;91:1123. Letter.

173. Sachs SW, Schwartz B. Enlargement of laser iridotomies over time. *Br J Ophthalmol* 1984;68:570.

174. Kublin J, Simmons RJ. Use of tinted soft contact lenses to eliminate monocular diplopia secondary to laser iridectomies. *Ophthalmic Laser Ther* 1987;2:111.

175. Fresco BB, Trope GR. Opaque contact lenses for YAG laser iridotomy occlusion. *Optom Vis Sci* 1992;69:656–657.

176. Sanders DR, et al. Studies on the blood-aqueous barrier after argon laser photocoagulation of the iris. *Ophthalmology* 1983;90:169.

177. Schrems W, van Dorp HP, Wendel M, Krieglstein GK. The effect of YAG laser iridotomy on the blood aqueous barrier in the rabbit. *Graefes Arch Clin Exp Ophthalmol* 1984;221:179.

178. Lederer CMJ, Price PK. Posterior synechiae after laser iridectomy. *Ann Ophthalmol* 1989;21:61–64.

179. Hodes BL, Bentivegna JF, Weyer NJ. Hyphema complicating laser iridotomy. *Arch Ophthalmol* 1982;100:924.

180. Rubin L, Arnett J, Ritch R. Delayed hyphema after argon laser iridectomy. *Ophthalmic Surg* 1984;15:852.

181. Dragon DM, Robin AL, Pollack IP, et al. Neodymium : YAG laser iridotomy in the cynomolgus monkey. *Invest Ophthalmol Vis Sci* 1985;29:789.

182. McAllister JA, Schwartz LW, Moster M, Spaeth GL. Laser peripheral iridectomy comparing Q-switched neodymium : YAG with argon. *Trans Ophthalmol Soc U K* 1984;104:67.

183. Berger CM, Lee DA, Christensen RE. Anterior lens capsule perforation and zonular rupture after Nd : YAG laser iridotomy. *Am J Ophthalmol* 1989;107:674–675.

184. Welch DB, et al. Lens injury following iridotomy with a Q-switched neodymium-YAG laser. *Arch Ophthalmol* 1986;194:123.

185. Gaasterland DG, Rodrigues MM, Thomas G. Threshold for lens damage during Q-switched Nd : YAG laser iridectomy: a study of rhesus monkey eyes. *Ophthalmology* 1985;92:1616.

186. Watts GK. Retinal hazards during laser irradiation of the iris. *Br J Ophthalmol* 1971;55:60.

187. Berger BB. Foveal photocoagulation from laser iridotomy. *Ophthalmology* 1984;91:1029.

188. Corrineau LA, Nasr Y, Fanous S. Choroidal and retinal detachment following argon laser iridotomy. *Can J Ophthalmol* 1986;21:107.

189. Jampol LM, Goldberg MF, Jednock N. Retinal damage from a Q-switched YAG laser. *Am J Ophthalmol* 1983;96:326.

190. Shin DH. Another hypopyon following laser iridotomy. *Ophthalmic Surg* 1984;15:968.

191. Cohen JS, Bibler L, Tuckher D. Hypopyon following laser iridotomy. *Ophthalmic Surg* 1984;15:604.

192. Choplin NT, Bene C. Cystoid macular edema following laser iridotomy. *Ann Ophthalmol* 1983;15:172.

193. Balkan RJ, Zimmerman TJ, Hesse RJ, Steigner JB. Loss of central visual acuity after laser peripheral iridectomy. *Ann Ophthalmol* 1982;14:721.

194. Geyer O, Mayron Y, Rothkoff L, Lazar M. Pigmented pupillary pseudomembranes as a complication of argon laser iridotomy. *Ophthalmic Surg* 1991;22:162–164.

195. Margo CE, Lessner A, Goldey SH, Sherwood M. Lens induced endophthalmitis after Nd : YAG laser iridotomy. *Am J Ophthalmol* 1992;113:97–98. Letter.

196. Go FJ, Kitazawa Y. Complications of peripheral iridectomy in primary angle closure glaucoma. *Jpn J Ophthalmol* 1981;25:222.

197. Aminlari A, Sassani J. Simultaneous bilateral malignant glaucoma following laser iridotomy. *Graefes Arch Clin Exp Ophthalmol* 1993;231:12–14.

198. Brooks AMV, Harper CA, Gillies W. Occurrence of malignant glaucoma after laser iridotomy. *Br J Ophthalmol* 1989;73:617–620.

199. Fourman S. "Malignant" glaucoma post laser iridotomy. *Ophthalmology* 1992;99:1751–1752. Letter.

200. Robinson A, et al. The onset of malignant glaucoma after prophylactic laser iridotomy. *Am J Ophthalmol* 1990;110:95–96.

201. Geyer O, Rothkoff L, Lazar M. Malignant glaucoma after laser iridectomy. *Br J Ophthalmol* 1990;74:576. Letter.

202. Hodes BL. Malignant glaucoma after laser iridotomy. *Ophthalmology* 1992;99:1641–1642. Letter.

203. York K, Ritch R, Szmyd LJ. Argon laser peripheral iridoplasty: indications, techniques and results. *Invest Ophthalmol Vis Sci* 1984;25(suppl):94.

204. Lim AS, Tan A, Chew P, et al. Laser iridoplasty in the treatment of severe acute angle closure glaucoma. *Int Ophthalmol* 1993;17:33–36.

205. Kimbrough RL, Trempe CS, Brockhurst RJ, Simmons RJ. Angle-closure glaucoma in nanophthalmos. *Am J Ophthalmol* 1979;88:572.

206. Mapstone R. Closed-angle glaucoma: theoretical considerations. *Br J Ophthalmol* 1974;58:36–40.

207. Ritch R, Solomon IS. Laser treatment of glaucoma. In: L'Esperance FAJ, ed. *Ophthalmic lasers.* Vol. 2. 3rd ed. St Louis: CV Mosby, 1989:650–748.

208. Lowe RF. Primary angle-closure glaucoma investigations after surgery for pupillary block. *Am J Ophthalmol* 1964;57:931.

209. Campbell DG, Vela A. Modern goniosynechialysis for the treatment of synechial angle-closure glaucoma. *Ophthalmology* 1984;91:1052–1060.

210. Ando H, Kitagawa K, Ogino N. Results of goniosynechialysis for synechial angle-closure glaucoma after pupillary block. *Folia Ophthalmol Jpn* 1990;41:883–886.

211. Nagata M, Nezu N. Goniosynechialysis as a new treatment for chronic angle-closure glaucoma. *Jpn J Clin Ophthalmol* 1985;39:707–710.

212. Tanihara H, Nishiwaki K, Nagata M. Surgical results and complications of goniosynechialysis. *Graefes Arch Clin Exp Ophthalmol* 1992;230:309–313.

213. Shingleton BJ, Chang MA, Bellows AR, Thomas JV. Surgical goniosynechialysis for angle-closure glaucoma. *Ophthalmology* 1990;97:551–556.

214. Tanihara H, Nagata M. Argon-laser gonioplasty following goniosynechialysis. *Graefes Arch Clin Exp Ophthalmol* 1991;229:505–507.

215. Matai A, Consul S. Argon laser iridoplasty. *Indian J Ophthalmol* 1987;35:290–292.

216. Chew P, Chee C, Lim A. Laser treatment of severe acute angle-closure glaucoma in dark Asian irides: the role of iridoplasty. *Lasers Light Ophthalmol* 1991;4:41–42.

217. Burton TC, Folk JC. Laser iris retraction for angle-closure glaucoma after retinal detachment surgery. *Ophthalmology* 1988;95:742–748.

218. Koster HR, Liebmann JM, Ritch R, Hudock S. Acute angle-closure glaucoma in a patient with acquired immunodeficiency syndrome successfully treated with argon laser peripheral iridoplasty. *Ophthalmic Surg* 1990;21:501–502.

219. Cohen J, Alfano JE, Boshes LD, Palmgren C. Clinical evaluation of school age children with retrolental fibroplasia. *Am J Ophthalmol* 1964;57:41–57.

220. Hittner HM, Rhodes LM, McPherson AR. Anterior segment abnormalities in cicatricial retinopathy of prematurity. *Ophthalmology* 1979;86:803–816.

221. Pollard ZF. Secondary angle-closure glaucoma in cicatricial retrolental fibroplasia. *Am J Ophthalmol* 1980;89:651.

222. McCormick AQ, Pratt-Johnson JA. Angle-closure glaucoma in infancy. *Can J Ophthalmol* 1971;6:38–41.

223. Laws DE, et al. Axial length biometry in infants with retinopathy of prematurity. *Eye* 1994;8:427–430.

224. Kushner BJ. Ciliary block glaucoma in retinopathy of prematurity. *Arch Ophthalmol* 1982;100:1078.

225. Ueda N, Ogino N. Angle-closure glaucoma with pupillary block mechanism in cicatricial retinopathy of prematurity. *Ophthalmologica* 1988;196:15–18.

226. Smith J. Angle-closure glaucoma in adults with cicatricial retinopathy of prematurity. *Arch Ophthalmol* 1984;102:371.

227. Jin JC, Anderson DR. Laser and unsutured sclerotomy in nanophthalmos. *Am J Ophthalmol* 1990;109:575–580.

228. Good WV, Stern WH. Recurrent nanophthalmic uveal effusion syndrome following laser trabeculoplasty. *Am J Ophthalmol* 1988;106:234–235.

229. Hyams S. *Angle-closure glaucoma.* Amsterdam: Kugler and Ghedini, 1990.

230. Calhoun FP. The management of glaucoma in nanophthalmos. *Trans Am Ophthalmol Soc* 1975;73:97.

231. Wand M. Argon laser gonioplasty for synechial angle closure. *Arch Ophthalmol* 1992;110:353–367.

232. Sassani JW, Ritch R, McCormick S, et al. Histopathology of argon laser peripheral iridoplasty. *Ophthalmic Surg* 1993;24:740–745.

Cyclophotocoagulation, Cryotherapy, and Ultrasound

M. BRUCE SHIELDS

In the 1930s and 1940s Weve (1), Vogt (2), and others introduced the concept of destroying portions of the ciliary body to reduce aqueous humor production, and thereby control intraocular pressure in unusually difficult cases of glaucoma. These surgeons used various forms of diathermy as the destructive element. In 1950 Bietti (3) suggested freezing the ciliary body to produce the tissue damage, and cyclocryotherapy became the cyclodestructive procedure of choice for the next several decades. Coleman et al (4) introduced another destructive element, therapeutic ultrasound, in 1985. However, all of these modalities are significantly limited by unpredictable pressure results and a high rate of complications, including marked inflammation, pain, and visual loss. With the advent of laser energy as the cyclodestructive element, pioneered by Beckman et al (5,6) in the 1970s and 1980s, these limitations have not been eliminated, but have been reduced to the point that cyclophotocoagulation has now become the cyclodestructive procedure of choice. This chapter focuses primarily on the various methods of cyclophotocoagulation, with brief reference to cryotherapy and therapeutic ultrasound.

CYCLOPHOTOCOAGULATION

Routes of Delivery

Unlike other cyclodestructive operations that are limited to the transscleral mode of energy delivery, laser energy can be delivered to the ciliary body by several routes: transpupillary, intraocular, and transscleral.

Transpupillary Cyclophotocoagulation

This concept, introduced by Lee and Pomerantzeff in 1971 (7), involves the direct application of laser energy to individual ciliary processes with the use of a gonioscopic lens.

This technique is limited to eyes in which a sufficient number of ciliary processes can be visualized gonioscopically. Such visualization is not possible in most glaucomatous eyes, especially those in which long-term miotic therapy prevents wide dilation. However, there are some situations, such as a large iridectomy or retraction of the iris in the presence of advanced neovascular glaucoma, that may provide adequate gonioscopic visualization of the ciliary processes.

The procedure typically involves use of the argon laser with settings of 0.1 to 0.2 second, 100 to 200 μm, and an energy level that is sufficient to produce white discoloration, as well as a brown concave burn, often with pigment dispersion or gas bubbles or both (usually 700–1000 mW). Special contact lenses with scleral depressors have been developed to rotate the processes into better view, although the value of this has yet to be established. All visible portions of the ciliary process should be treated, which usually requires three to five applications per process. It is customary to treat up to a 180-degree arc of processes at one session, with additional treatment at subsequent sessions if required.

Experience with transpupillary cyclophotocoagulation has been disappointing. The success rate is low even in the small percentage of patients in whom gonioscopic visualization allows treatment of a large number of ciliary processes. Nevertheless, transpupillary cyclophotocoagulation may be worth trying in some patients, such as those with refractory neovascular glaucoma, before going to more aggressive therapy.

Intraocular Cyclophotocoagulation

Another method by which laser energy can be applied directly to individual ciliary processes is with an endophotocoagulator through a pars plana incision. This is most commonly performed in conjunction with vitreous surgery for diabetic retinopathy in eyes with intractable neovascular glaucoma (8). After the vitrectomy (and lensectomy if the eye is not already aphakic) is performed, the intraocular pressure is lowered and scleral indentation is used to bring the ciliary processes into transpupillary view. The individual processes are then treated under direct visualization with the endophotocoagulator that is inserted through the same cannula as used for the vitrectomy instrument (Fig. 31-1). The endophotocoagulator is attached to an argon laser, and the tip of the laser probe is positioned 2 to 3 mm from the processes. Standard laser settings include an exposure time of 0.1 to 0.2 second and a power level that is sufficient to produce a white reaction and shallow tissue disruption (usually 1000 mW). Three to five laser exposures are then applied to each process in the two quadrants opposite the entry site.

Although the main value of intraocular cyclophotocoagulation with transpupillary visualization is as an adjunct to pars plana vitrectomy, endoscopic visualization has also been evaluated as a primary surgical procedure for eyes with refractory glaucoma. Early attempts employed a direct-viewing ocular endoscope to which an argon laser fiber-optic was attached (9). Endo Optiks (Little Silver, NJ) developed a newer ophthalmic laser microendoscope system for intraocular cyclophotocoagulation, in which fiberoptics for a television monitor, diode laser delivery, and an illumination source are all housed in an 18-gauge probe (10). The probe can be introduced through either a pars plana or scleral tunnel incision into an aphakic eye with prior anterior vitrectomy (Fig. 31-2). While the ciliary processes are visualized on the television monitor, the diode laser energy is applied to the processes in the same manner as described

previously for argon laser intraocular cyclophotocoagulation. Although this technique has the advantage of allowing direct visualization and precise treatment of individual ciliary processes, it is an incisional procedure with the associated risks, and its role in the treatment of difficult glaucomas has yet to be delineated.

Transscleral Cyclophotocoagulation

The early work of Beckman et al (5,6) was with transscleral ruby laser cyclophotocoagulation. Although their initial experience was encouraging, it was not until the availability of specially designed neodymium:yttrium-aluminum-garnet (Nd:YAG) lasers that widespread interest developed in transscleral cyclophotocoagulation.

Instruments

The lasers that have been evaluated for transscleral cyclophotocoagulation differ according to 1) wavelength (currently Nd:YAG or semiconductor diode), 2) laser mode (pulsed, thermal, or continuous-wave mode), and 3) the delivery system (noncontact, slit-lamp system or contact probe, fiberoptic system). The Microruptor II (H-S Meridian, formerly Lasag) is an example of the noncontact, Nd:YAG system that operates in the free-running, thermal mode of 20-msec pulses. Two additional features of the unit are 1) an adjustable offset between the focal points of the helium-neon aiming beam and the therapeutic beam, and 2) high energy levels of up to 8 to 9 J. This unit is no longer commercially available, but is still used by many surgeons, and the experience gained with it has formed the basis for much of the continued study in this surgical field (11–13).

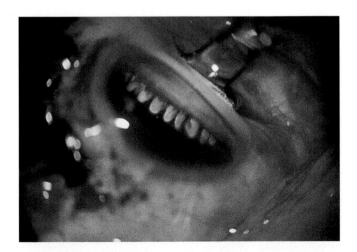

FIGURE 31-1.   *Intraocular cyclophotocoagulation with transpupillary visualization. Ciliary processes are brought into view with a scleral depressor and treated with a laser endophotocoagulator via a pars plana incision. (Reprinted with permission from Shields MB. Cyclodestructive surgery for glaucoma: past, present and future. Trans Am Ophthalmol Soc 1985;83:285.)*

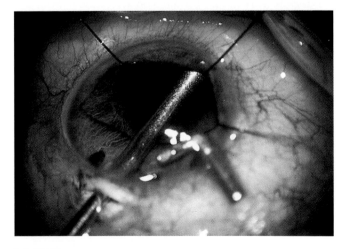

FIGURE 31-2.   *Endoscopic cyclophotocoagulation in an aphakic eye performed with an Endo Optiks diode laser microendoscope through a scleral tunnel incision. Iris retractors are used inferiorly to improve the endoscopic visualization by pulling the iris anteriorly.*

Several laser units are now available for contact transscleral cyclophotocoagulation, although the one that has been most extensively evaluated is the SLT CL60 (Surgical Laser Technologies, Oaks, PA), which is a Nd:YAG laser that operates in the continuous-wave mode with a range of 0.1 to 10.0 seconds (14). A 2.2-mm sapphire-tip, handheld probe, which is focused at 1.5 to 2.0 mm in air, is coupled to a fiberoptic delivery system. The unit can provide powers in excess of 10 W (energy in joules = power in watts × duration in seconds).

More recently, the Microruptor III (H-S Meridian) was introduced; it also provides continuous-wave Nd:YAG laser energy with contact probe delivery. In addition, semiconductor diode lasers are being evaluated for transscleral cyclophotocoagulation. These operate in a continuous-wave mode and can be delivered by either contact probe with the OcuLight SLX (Iris Medical Instruments, Mountain View, CA) (15) or the Multilase (Keeler, Broomall, PA) or by slit lamp with the Microlase (Keeler) (16).

Histologic Observations

Histologic studies in animal and human eyes showed that the laser-induced tissue damage is limited primarily to the ciliary epithelium, with minimal damage to other ocular structures. Studies with the noncontact, pulsed laser in human autopsy eyes revealed a blister-like elevation of the epithelial layers from the adjacent stroma, with marked disruption primarily of the pigmented epithelium, but minimal change in the ciliary muscle and sclera in the path of the laser beam (17). Similar histologic findings, with the addition of fibrin and scant inflammatory cells between the disrupted epithelial layers and stroma, were seen in human eyes that were enucleated a few days after the procedure (18). In the latter study, no significant changes were observed in the ciliary body vasculature or adjacent sclera. In contrast to the lesions created by the noncontact, pulsed laser, the histologic appearance of lesions created by the contact, continuous-wave Nd:YAG laser was a smaller, more coagulative effect on the epithelium with less of the blister-like elevation (19).

The histologic observations in animal and human eyes suggest that the most likely mechanism by which transscleral Nd:YAG cyclophotocoagulation reduces aqueous production is through destruction of the ciliary epithelium. However, since intraocular pressure reduction is also observed when the laser lesions are applied posterior to the pars plicata (20), alternative mechanisms of pressure reduction have also been considered. These include ciliary vascular disruption, with reduced aqueous production, or chronic inflammation, which could either reduce inflow or increase uveoscleral outflow.

Techniques

Unlike most other laser procedures, the intraoperative pain associated with transscleral cyclophotocoagulation is such that retrobulbar anesthesia is usually required. With the Microruptor II noncontact, pulsed technique, the patient is positioned at the slit lamp and the lids are separated manually with a special contact lens (Fig. 31-3). The lens also compresses and blanches the conjunctiva and provides measurements from the limbus (12). Standard laser settings include a pulse of 20 msec and a maximum offset between the aiming and therapeutic beams, which is 3.6 mm in air. Placement of the laser lesions 1.0 to 1.5 mm behind the limbus is optimum for damaging the pars plicata and is preferred by most surgeons. Preferred energy levels vary considerably from 2 to 8 J, and the optimum energy level has yet to be established. In a prospective study comparing 4 and 8 J, the higher energy level was associated with a trend toward better intraocular pressure control, although this did not reach statistical significance, and there was no clinical or statistical difference in the final visual outcome (13). The total number of laser applications also varies among surgeons, with most using 30 to 40 evenly spaced lesions for 360 degrees.

The contact, continuous-wave, Nd:YAG technique with the SLT generally utilizes exposure times of 0.5 to 0.7 second. The laser focus is fixed by the design of the probe tip, which is held perpendicular to the surface of the conjunctiva with the anterior edge of the probe 0.5 to 1.5 mm behind the limbus (Fig. 31-4). As with the noncontact system, preferred power settings vary considerably from 4 to 9 W, with 30 to 40 applications for 360 degrees (14). The Microruptor III Nd:YAG laser and the semiconductor diode laser have been evaluated with similar protocols, although durations of exposure of 1 to 2 seconds have been studied with these units. The Iris diode laser has a specialized probe (G-Probe) that allows measurement of fiberoptic placement from the limbus and between applications, and the benefit of these features may be enhanced by using the magnification at the slit lamp (Fig. 31-5). The duration of laser exposure appears to influence the nature of tissue response even among the continuous-wave

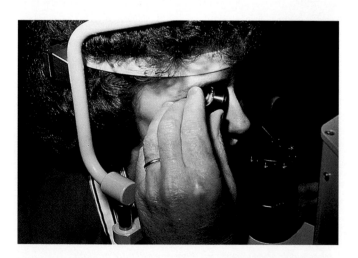

FIGURE 31-3. *Technique of noncontact, transscleral Nd:YAG cyclophotocoagulation performed with the Microruptor II laser and contact lens.*

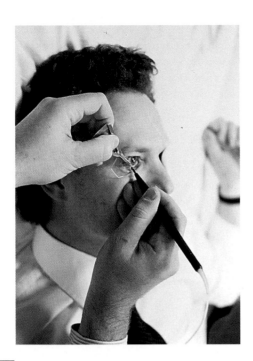

FIGURE 31-4. *Technique of contact, transscleral Nd:YAG cyclophotocoagulation performed with the SLT CL60. (Reprinted with permission from Schuman JS, Puliafito CA. Laser cyclophotocoagulation.* Int Ophthalmol Clin *1990;30:111.)*

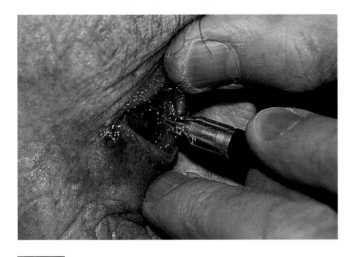

FIGURE 31-5. *Technique of performing contact, transscleral diode cyclophotocoagulation at a slit lamp.*

units, although the optimum clinical protocol has yet to be established (21).

Postoperative management is directed primarily at inflammation, which is always present and can be severe. One approach is to use a subconjunctival injection of dexamethasone and administration of topical atropine and prednisolone for approximately 10 days (11). A transient rise in intraocular pressure is not a common problem, although it is advisable to check the pressure a few hours after the procedure and the following day. Preoperative antiglaucoma

medications, with the exception of miotics, are continued postoperatively and are gradually discontinued as the decline in pressure allows. Postoperative pain is usually mild and transient, requiring only a mild analgesic.

Clinical Experience

Preliminary experience with both the noncontact and contact techniques reveals satisfactory intraocular pressure reduction in approximately two-thirds or more of the patients following the initial treatment session, with the pressure in most of the remainder coming under control with one or more repeat treatments (11,14). Maximum pressure reduction is typically achieved in 1 month, and it is usually desirable to wait at least this long before re-treating. The contact technique requires less total energy and appears to have a slightly better efficacy in lowering intraocular pressure and a lower complication rate with regard to reduction in visual acuity. Both techniques have significant advantages over cyclocryotherapy, which include a less transient rise in intraocular pressure, less inflammation, and less pain. However, reduced visual acuity remains a significant problem, which may be related to macular edema. Efforts to reduce the visual loss associated with macular edema have included the use of nonsteroidal anti-inflammatory agents, such as oral indomethacin or topical ketorolac. However, there have been no controlled studies to evaluate the efficacy of these measures with transscleral cyclophotocoagulation. The patient, therefore, must be informed that visual loss is a significant risk with this operation, and it should only be recommended when alternative treatments are not thought to offer a better outcome.

CRYOTHERAPY

Technique

With the standard 2.5-mm tip, the center of the probe is placed 1.0 to 1.5 mm from the limbus (Fig. 31-6). The temperature is reduced to −80°C and maintained for 60 seconds (22). Some surgeons will refreeze in the same site, although the value of this was never established. Cryoapplications are placed at each clock-hour position for 180° to 270°. Postoperatively, the eye is treated with subconjunctival steroids and topical steroid and atropine. Antiglaucoma medications, with the exception of miotics, are continued and are tapered as intraocular pressure decline permits. If the pressure is not adequate after approximately 1 month, the procedure can be repeated.

Results

Early postoperative complications include a transient but often marked rise in intraocular pressure, profound inflammation and uveitis, severe pain, and occasional hyphema. Late complications include hypotony and phthisis, and visual reduction, the incidence of which exceeds 50% in most studies. It is for these reasons that cryotherapy

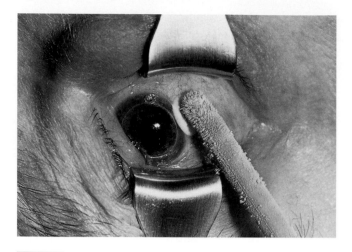

FIGURE 31-6.   *Technique of cryotherapy with the typical appearance of an ice ball. (Reprinted with permission from Shields MB. Textbook of glaucoma. 3rd ed. Baltimore: Williams & Wilkins, 1992:615.)*

has been considered by most surgeons to be a "last resort" effort, usually more for relief of painful pressure elevation than preservation of vision. Nevertheless, in certain difficult situations, such as an eye with a penetrating keratoplasty, especially when the laser is not available, cryotherapy may be useful (23).

THERAPEUTIC ULTRASOUND

Technique

The original therapeutic ultrasound apparatus utilized a water bath, through which the transducer is aimed at the treatment location over the sclera, after a diagnostic transducer has been used to localize the specific area of treatment. The transducer system was designed to provide a focal zone 0.4 mm in diameter and 3.0 mm in length at a distance centered 90 mm from the transducer. An average of six to seven exposures of ultrasound at an intensity level of $10 kW/cm^2$ for 5 seconds is delivered to scleral sites near the limbus (4).

Results

Preliminary reports were encouraging (4,24) but complications are only slightly less than those noted for cryotherapy, and the procedure never achieved wide acceptance.

PRESENT STATUS AND FUTURE ROLE OF CYCLOPHOTOCOAGULATION

At the present time, there is sufficient evidence to claim that transscleral cyclophotocoagulation is the cyclodestructive

procedure of choice. However, whether it will assume a broader role in the treatment of glaucoma, than has been the case with cyclodestructive surgery of the past, awaits further evaluation of new lasers and refined techniques.

REFERENCES

1. Weve H. Die zyklodiatermie das corpus ciliare bei glaukom. *Zentralbl Ophthalmol* 1933;29:256.
2. Vogt A. Cyclodiathermy puncture in cases of glaucoma. *Br J Ophthalmol* 1940;24:288–297.
3. Bietti G. Surgical intervention on the ciliary body: new trends for relief of glaucoma. *JAMA* 1950;142:889–896.
4. Coleman DJ, Lizzi FL, Driller J, et al. Therapeutic ultrasound in the treatment of glaucoma. II. Clinical applications. *Ophthalmology* 1985;92:347–353.
5. Beckman H, Sugar HS. Neodymium laser cyclophotocoagulation. *Arch Ophthalmol* 1973;90:27–28.
6. Beckman H, Waeltermann J. Transscleral ruby laser cyclocoagulation. *Am J Ophthalmol* 1984;98:788–795.
7. Lee P-F, Pomerantzeff O. Transpupillary cyclophotocoagulation of rabbit eyes. An experimental approach to glaucoma surgery. *Am J Ophthalmol* 1971;71:911–920.
8. Zarbin MA, Michels RG, de Bustros S, et al. Endolaser treatment of the ciliary body for severe glaucoma. *Ophthalmology* 1988;95:1639–1648.
9. Shields MB, Chandler DB, Hickingbotham D, Klintworth GK. Intraocular cyclophotocoagulation. Histopathologic evaluation in primates. *Arch Ophthalmol* 1985;103:1731–1735.
10. Uram M. Ophthalmic laser microendoscope ciliary process ablation in the management of neovascular glaucoma. *Ophthalmology* 1992;99:1823–1828.
11. Hampton C, Shields MB, Miller KN, Blasini M. Evaluation of a protocol for transscleral neodymium:YAG cyclophotocoagulation in 100 patients. *Ophthalmology* 1990;94:910–917.
12. Simmons RB, Shields MB, Blasini M, Wilkerson M. Transscleral neodymium:YAG cyclophotocoagulation with a contact lens. *Am J Ophthalmol* 1991;112:671–677.
13. Shields MB, Wilkerson MH, Echelman DA. A comparison of two energy levels for noncontact transscleral neodymium:YAG cyclophotocoagulation. *Arch Ophthalmol* 1993;111:484–487.
14. Schuman JS, Puliafito CA, Allingham RR, et al. Contact transscleral continuous-wave neodymium:YAG laser cyclophotocoagulation. *Ophthalmology* 1990;97:571–580.
15. Gaasterland DE, Abrams DA, Belcher CD, et al. A multicenter study of contact diode laser transscleral cyclophotocoagulation in glaucoma patients. *Invest Ophthalmol Vis Sci* 1992;33 (suppl):1019–1023.
16. Stroman GA, Stewart WC, Hamzari S, et al. Contact versus noncontact diode laser transscleral cyclophotocoagulation in cadaver eyes. *Ophthalmic Surg Lasers* 1996;27:60–65.
17. Hampton C, Shields MB. Transscleral neodymium:YAG cyclophotocoagulation. A histologic study of human autopsy eyes. *Arch Ophthalmol* 1988;106:1121–1123.
18. Blasini M, Simmons R, Shields MB. Early tissue response to transscleral neodymium:YAG cyclophotocoagulation. *Invest Ophthalmol Vis Sci* 1990;31:1114–1118.
19. Prum BE, Shields SR, Simmons RB, et al. The influence of exposure duration on transscleral Nd:YAG cyclophotocoagulation. *Am J Ophthalmol* 1992;114:560–567.
20. Schubert HD. Non-contact and contact pars plana transscleral neodymium:YAG laser cyclophotocoagulation in postmortem eyes. *Ophthalmology* 1989;96:1471–1475.
21. Echelman DA, Nasisse MP, Shields MB, et al. Influence of exposure time on inflammatory response to neodymium:YAG cyclophotocoagulation in rabbits. *Arch Ophthalmol* 1994;112:977–981.
22. Prost M. Cyclocryotherapy for glaucoma. Evaluation of techniques. *Surv Ophthalmol* 1983;28:93–100.
23. Brindley G, Shields MB. Value and limitations of cyclocryotherapy. *Graefes Arch Ophthalmol* 1986;224:545–548.
24. Maskin SL, Mandell AI, Smith JA, et al. Therapeutic ultrasound for refractory glaucoma. A three-center study. *Ophthalmic Surg* 1989;20:186–192.

Laser Sclerectomy and Trephination

JOEL S. SCHUMAN

The use of lasers to perform filtering surgery is of great interest in glaucoma surgery. Laser filtering surgery, or laser sclerectomy (as tissue is actually being *removed* by the laser), offers the opportunity to reduce intraoperative and postoperative complications, reduce surgical time, and prolong the success of the filtration surgery itself. By using a laser, it is possible to create a sclerectomy with a 1-mm conjunctival incision, or even with no incision at all, and manipulation of the conjunctiva is minimized or eliminated.

Unfortunately, laser sclerectomy is actually a step backward rather than a great advance in glaucoma surgery. It is a return to full-thickness filtering surgery but does not provide the benefits of that procedure. It does, however, include all of the risks attendant to full-thickness filtering surgery, including shallow or flat anterior chambers; hypotony, which can lead to maculopathy, choroidal effusion, and cataract; and suprachoroidal hemorrhage, which may have disastrous results (1–4).

CONVENTIONAL FILTRATION SURGERY

Filtration surgery has been performed for nearly 100 years. The objective is to create a fistula between the anterior chamber of the eye and the subconjunctival space, thereby decreasing resistance to aqueous outflow and lowering the intraocular pressure. The ultimate goal has always been the preservation of visual function. In the early 1900s, an operation utilizing a trephine to create a full-thickness sclerectomy was described by Major Robert Elliot (5). This procedure was modified by Scheie (6), who introduced the use of a thermal cautery. This thermal sclerostomy was also a full-thickness procedure. Posterior lip sclerectomy was introduced in an effort to simplify the sclerectomy procedure by making a slit incision into the eye (with subsequent

removal of the posterior scleral lip), thus minimizing the risk of incision into the ciliary body.

Perhaps the greatest advance in conventional filtration surgery was the introduction of the trabeculectomy, which is a guarded filtration procedure. In this operation, a partial-thickness scleral flap is dissected anteriorly, and a block of corneoscleral tissue is removed underneath this flap. The flap is then sutured into place, providing some resistance to outflow and helping to reduce hypotony, with its attendant risks.

Complications

All of these operations have potential complications. Leaks can occur at the conjunctival wound or in the bleb. Shallow or flat anterior chambers can occur, especially with the full-thickness procedures. Hypotony is a serious problem, because it can lead to choroidal effusion and cataract. Choroidal effusion can lead to suprachoroidal hemorrhage. In addition, any of these procedures may fail, primarily because of subconjunctival fibrosis but also because of occlusion or closure of the scleral ostium, or possibly due to episcleral fibrosis, especially with the trabeculectomy procedure.

LASER SCLERECTOMY

Rationale

Laser sclerectomy offers an alternative to conventional filtration surgery. Some laser sclerectomy techniques offer the advantage of fistulizing surgery with no conjunctival incision. Others offer the advantage of minimal conjunctival manipulation. Most types of laser sclerectomy can be performed either ab interno, from the inside out, or ab externo, from the outside in. Ab interno lasers include the continuous-wave Nd:YAG (neodymium:yttrium-aluminum-garnet) laser (7–10); the Nd:YLF picosecond laser (11–13); the dye-enhanced, flash lamp–pumped, microsecond-pulsed–dye laser (2,14–18); the excimer laser (19); the diode laser; the erbium:YAG and erbium:YSGG lasers (20,21); the holmium:YAG laser (20,21); and the argon laser (22,23). Only the continuous-wave Nd:YAG laser is approved by the United States Food and Drug Administration (FDA) for ab interno laser sclerectomy. Ab externo lasers include the holmium:YAG laser (1,3,4,20,24–35), the erbium:YAG and erbium:YSGG lasers (20,21,31,36–39), the excimer laser (40–45), and the diode laser (46,47). Only the holmium:YAG laser is approved by the FDA for ab externo laser sclerectomy.

The laser offers the potential for sclerectomy with little or no conjunctival manipulation through the lack of a conjunctival incision with the ab interno techniques, or a small conjunctival incision with the ab externo techniques. The small or absent conjunctival incision minimizes or eliminates the risk of a conjunctival wound leak, possibly permitting the earlier use of 5-fluorouracil (5-FU) or other antimetabolites (see below under Antimetabolites). In addition, these lasers offer access to areas that are difficult to reach in conventional surgery, and the procedures are often technically simpler than conventional surgery. However, laser sclerectomy techniques (as stated above) represent a return to full-thickness filtration surgery and all of the risks of that operation, including flat anterior chamber, hypotony, suprachoroidal hemorrhage, and cataract formation (1).

Holmium and Nd:YAG Laser Sclerectomy

The holmium and Nd:YAG lasers are the two devices approved by the FDA for laser sclerectomy. While the holmium is used primarily ab externo and the Nd:YAG primarily ab interno, the two lasers perform in a similar fashion and produce similar results.

Both the holmium and Nd:YAG lasers create a thermal sclerectomy; that is, each laser heats water, resulting in thermal removal of tissue and the creation of a sclerectomy. Both lasers have reported success rates in the 60% to 80% range, and both can cause serious complications, including flat anterior chamber, cataract, hypotony, choroidal effusion, maculopathy, and suprachoroidal hemorrhage, due to the full-thickness nature of the sclerectomies created (1,3,4,7,9,21,25,26,28,30,32,35,48).

The Role of Thermal Damage

When lasers came under intense investigation for their utility in filtering surgery, one debate centered on whether collateral thermal damage was beneficial or detrimental. Most investigators thought that collateral thermal damage

(i.e., thermal coagulation necrosis on either side of the ostium) would incite an inflammatory response, making the filtering surgery more likely to fail. Several lasers, most notably the erbium and the excimer, received special attention due to the low (with the erbium) and absent or nearly absent (with the 193-nm excimer) thermal damage (Figs. 32-1 to 32-3) (20,31,36–45,49).

However, the studies show similar success rates with all types of lasers for sclerectomy, suggesting that the minimal thermal damage associated with excimer and erbium lasers does not significantly affect the overall outcome of the surgery. If anything, the clinical results with the erbium and excimer laser are even more discouraging than those with the holmium and Nd:YAG lasers.

The excimer laser is photoablative, breaking chemical bonds and forcing the ejection of ablated tissue. There is

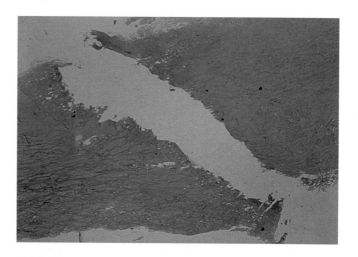

FIGURE 32-1.   *Holmium laser sclerectomy. Note prominent collateral thermal injury along either side of the ostium.*

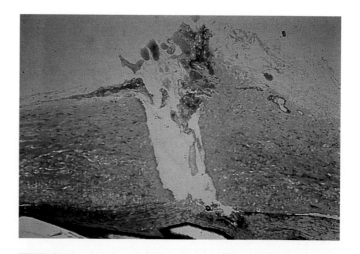

FIGURE 32-2.   *Erbium laser sclerectomy. Markedly less collateral thermal injury surrounds the ostium, as compared to the holmium laser lesion in Figure 32-1.*

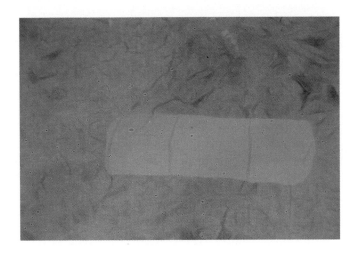

FIGURE 32-3. *Sclerectomy using 193-nm argon fluoride excimer laser. Note absence of thermal damage.*

little or no thermal damage with this laser using argon fluoride gas, with a wavelength of 193 nm. In addition, ablation supposedly does not proceed in an aqueous environment.

This last point was used to develop partial external trabeculectomy (PET), the guiding concept of which is that an unroofing of Schlemm's canal, or a sinusotomy, could be performed, leaving the inner wall of Schlemm's canal and trabecular meshwork intact. In theory, this would eliminate hypotony and flat anterior chambers and would greatly decrease the other complications associated with laser sclerectomy.

While he did not comment on this, Seiler showed that the inner wall and the juxtacanalicular trabecular meshwork are ablated with PET; ablation does not abruptly stop when aqueous fluid is released (40,42). The incidence of hypotony and flat anterior chamber is just as high clinically with PET as with the other laser sclerectomy techniques. Even more discouraging, the success rate (about 50% with the excimer laser) is not even as high as for holmium or Nd:YAG laser sclerectomy, despite the lack of thermal damage (41,43,44).

The erbium laser heats water in the sclera to create a thermal sclerectomy. The laser has a wavelength of 2.9 µm and a pulse width in the microsecond range, but the area of the surrounding sclera suffering thermal damage is in the tens of microns, as opposed to the hundreds of microns damaged with the holmium laser. Despite this minimal thermal damage, success rates with the erbium laser have been approximately 30% (36).

Gonioscopic Ab Interno Laser Sclerectomy

Gonioscopic ab interno laser sclerectomy, in theory, offers an office filtering procedure. The concept is that the patient sits at a slit-lamp mounted laser, the surgeon applies a contact lens and fires the laser, and the patient goes home with a new filter. In reality, it's not that simple.

There are two primary types of gonioscopic ab interno laser sclerectomy. One uses the pulsed-dye laser, and the other uses the picosecond laser. The success rate with the pulsed-dye laser is dismal: 12.5% at 15 months. Only half of the patients who sit for the procedure actually receive patent sclerectomies. Of those who have a patent fistula, only 25% remain successful at 15 months (2,16,18).

While the concept is cleaver—using a dye matched to the peak spectral absorption of the dye laser and iontophoresing that dye into the sclera as a target (14,15)—in practice this technique does not prove to be beneficial to the patient for three reasons. First, the iontophoresis technique is cumbersome and time-consuming. If inadequate dye is introduced, the procedure will fail. Second, the procedure has a poor success rate, as mentioned above. Finally, the pulsed-dye laser technique produces a tremendous cavitation bubble that can wreak havoc in the anterior chamber (17).

In a study performed using high-speed photography, Namazi showed that a cavitation bubble expands and contracts in the anterior chamber extremely rapidly with each exposure from the pulsed-dye laser (Figs. 32-4 and 32-5) (17). This bubble is large and powerful enough to deform the overlying cornea and to locally denude the corneal endothelium. Clinically, the results of this cavitation bubble may be seen as corneal edema in the area of the fistula, angle recession, and hyphema.

The picosecond laser has also been investigated for gonioscopic ab interno laser sclerectomy (11–13). However, the problem with this laser is nearly opposite of that with the pulsed-dye laser. Inadequate power is available with the picosecond laser to reliably produce a full-thickness fistula in an intact, in vivo human eye.

Antimetabolites

An important advance in conventional glaucoma filtering surgery is the use of adjunctive antimetabolites. Aside from topical steroids, there was little to prevent postoperative fibrosis prior to the introduction of 5-FU into filtration surgery in 1984 (50,51). Several agents have been evaluated for this purpose since the beginning the antimetabolite era. However, most were found to be too toxic to use or inferior to 5-FU in efficacy until mitomycin C (MMC) was suggested by Chen in 1983 (52) as a means to prevent postoperative scarring in filtration surgery. Widespread use began in the U.S. following a report by Palmer in 1991 (53). This agent has proven much more potent than 5-FU and requires only a single 3.5-minute application to the sclera at the time of surgery. Conversely, 5-FU must be given as subconjunctival injections for as long as two weeks postoperative or more (54,55).

Since laser sclerectomy may fail in 20% to 88% of cases (1,2,9,10,25,26), it would be beneficial to employ these

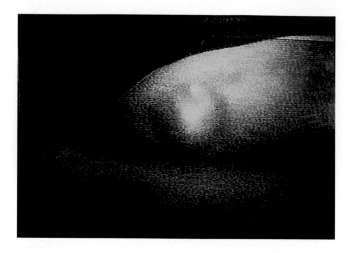

FIGURE 32-4. *Cavitation bubble in the anterior segment produced using pulsed-dye laser and captured with high-speed photography. Note deformity of the cornea overlying the bubble.*

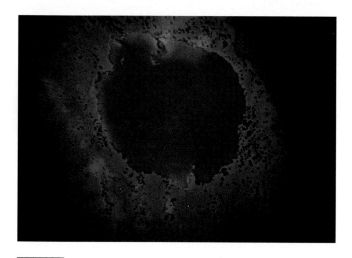

FIGURE 32-5. *Corneal endothelial denudation due to cavitation bubble. This effect is* thermal.

adjunctive agents to reduce the postoperative fibroblastic proliferation that is responsible for failure in the majority of cases. Unfortunately, agents such as 5-FU injected postoperatively and MMC applied to the sclera intraoperatively, which have been used in conjunction with conventional filtering surgery, are technically difficult to administer with laser sclerectomy.

The problem with the use of MMC in conjunction with laser sclerectomy is the route of delivery. In conventional trabeculectomy, the drug is applied to the sclera at the time of surgery. This is not feasible in the laser procedure due to the small conjunctival wound, which is some distance from the sclerectomy site. Recent work on animal models has indicated that it may be feasible to deliver MMC by an alternate route (transconjunctivally) and thereby prolong the success of this procedure (27,34,47). Surgical success

rates may also be enhanced by 5-FU administered intraoperatively or postoperatively (1,3,4,56).

TREPHINATION

The first successful filters, by Elliot (5), utilized a trephine to create the communication between the anterior chamber and the subconjunctival space. Since that time, however, we have progressed to having greater control over aqueous outflow through the use of a guarding scleral flap, while maintaining low postoperative intraocular pressures through the use of antimetabolites.

Since Elliot's time trephination procedures have been introduced and discarded, usually due to an unsatisfactory risk-to-benefit ratio (5,57–74). Nearly every one of these procedures, however, used an ab externo approach. One procedure that differs was introduced by Brown, and it uses a new instrument called a trabecuphine (75,76).

The device consists of an irrigating trephine with a rotating head. It is introduced through a paracentesis or a limbal incision and passed across the anterior chamber. The sclera opposite the insertion site is drilled through, resulting in a full-thickness sclerectomy.

Though a clever idea, the risks are all the same as those discussed above for laser sclerectomy. This is a full-thickness procedure; it does not provide the same degree of success as a guarded filter, yet has a greater risk. It is difficult, therefore, to see an indication for this surgery except in the extremely highly-select case, as for laser sclerectomy (4).

CONCLUSIONS

For the most part all of the lasers, whether operating ab interno or ab externo, and trephination as well, have similar potential benefits and risks. The purpose with each of the devices is to make a hole in the eye which will remain patent indefinitely, in order to stabilize the intraocular pressure and control the glaucoma. The question that one must ask with any new technology, however, is whether or not it is superior in some way to existing techniques in terms of risks and/or benefits. In nearly every instance, the answer for laser sclerectomy and for trephination must be no. There are certain *theoretical* advantages to these procedures, namely the lack of conjunctival manipulation that supposedly would result in less fibrosis, but in reality these procedures actually have greater risk than trabeculectomy, with inferior surgical results to guarded filtration surgery. The only advantage is an often simpler and faster, and perhaps more interesting, surgical technique.

The future may produce laser sclerectomy procedures with a more favorable risk-to-benefit ratio as investigation into these techniques proceeds. A guarded filter that can be made quickly and easily with a laser, with optimal delivery of an appropriate antimetabolite, is a goal for those of us who continue to study this problem. At this point, however, conventional trabeculectomy with MMC, or even glaucoma implant surgery, remains the treatment of choice for nearly all glaucoma patients requiring filtering surgery.

REFERENCES

1. Schuman JS, Stinson WG, Hutchinson BT, et al. Holmium laser sclerectomy. Success and complications. *Ophthalmology* 1993;100:1060–1065.

2. Latina MA, Melamed S, March WF, et al. Gonioscopic ab interno laser sclerostomy: a pilot study in glaucoma patients. *Ophthalmology* 1992;99:1736–1744.

3. Iwach AG, Hoskins HD Jr, Drake MV, Dickens CJ. Update of the subconjunctival THC:YAG (holmium) laser sclerostomy ab externo clinical trial: 30-month report. *Ophthalmic Surg* 1994;25:13–21.

4. Friedman DS, Katz LJ, Augsburger JJ, Lean M. Holmium laser sclerostomy in glaucomatous eyes with prior surgery: 24-month results. *Ophthalmic Surg Lasers* 1998;29:17–22.

5. Elliot RH. Preliminary note on a new operative procedure for the establishment of a filtering cicatrix in the treatment of glaucoma. *Ophthalmoscope* 1909;7:804.

6. Scheie HG. Retraction of scleral wound edges as a fistulizing procedure for glaucoma. *Am J Ophthalmol* 1958;45:220–228.

7. Federman JL, Wilson RP, Anso F. Contact laser thermal sclerostomy ab interna. *Ophthalmic Surg* 1987;18:726–727.

8. Higginbotham EJ, Kao G, Peyman G. Internal sclerostomy with the Nd:YAG contact laser versus thermal sclerostomy in rabbits. *Ophthalmology* 1988;95:385–390.

9. Javitt JC, O'Connor SS, Wilson RP, Federman JL. Laser sclerostomy ab interno using a continuous wave Nd:YAG laser. *Ophthalmic Surg* 1989;20:552–556.

10. Wilson RP, Javitt JC. Ab interno laser sclerostomy in aphakic patients with glaucoma and chronic inflammation. *Am J Ophthalmol* 1990;110:178–184.

11. Zysset B, Fujimoto JG, Puliafito CA, et al. Picosecond optical breakdown: tissue effects and reduction of collateral damage. *Lasers Surg Med* 1989;9:193–204.

12. Cooper HM, Schuman JS, Puliafito CA, et al. Picosecond Nd:YLF sclerectomy. *Am J Ophthalmol* 1993;115:221–224.

13. Woods WJ, Schuman JS, Wang N, et al. Gonioscopic picosecond Nd:YLF laser sclerectomy ab interno in the feline model. *Invest Ophthalmol Vis Sci* 1993 (suppl.);34:173.

14. Latina MA, Goode S, de Kater AW, et al. Experimental ab interno sclerotomies using a pulsed-dye laser. *Lasers Surg Med* 1988;8:233–240.

15. Latina MA, Dobrogowski M, March WF, Birngruber R. Laser sclerostomy by pulsed-dye laser and goniolens. *Arch Ophthalmol* 1990;108:1745–1750.

16. Melamed S, Solomon A, Neumann D, et al. Internal sclerostomy using laser ablation of dyed sclera in glaucoma patients: a pilot study. *Br J Ophthalmol* 1993;77:139–144.

17. Namazi N, Fleckner M, Feld JR, et al. Effects of cavitation bubbles created by pulsed laser ablation in the anterior chamber. *Invest Ophthalmol Vis Sci* 1993 (suppl.);34:1070.

18. Ruben S, Migdal C, De Vivero C. Ab interno pulsed dye laser sclerostomy for the treatment of glaucoma: preliminary results of a new technique. *Eye* 1993;7:436–439.

19. Muller-Stolzenburg M, Muller GJ. Transmission of 308 nm excimer laser radiation for ophthalmic microsurgery—medical, technical and safety aspects. *Biomed-Tech (Berlin)* 1989;34:131–138.

20. Ozler SA, Hill RA, Andrews JJ, et al. Infrared laser sclerostomies. *Invest Ophthalmol Vis Sci* 1991;32:498–503.

21. Gaasterland DE, Hennings DR, Boutacoff TA, et al. Ab interno and ab externo filtering operations by laser contact surgery. *Ophthalmic Surg* 1987;18:254.

22. Jaffe GJ, Williams GA, Mieler WF, et al. Ab interno sclerostomy with a high-powered argon endolaser. *Am J Ophthalmol* 1988;106:391–396.

23. Jaffe GJ, Mieler WF, Radius RL, et al. Ab interno sclerostomy with a high-powered argon endolaser. Clinicopathologic correlation. *Arch Ophthalmol* 1989;107:1183–1185.

24. Hoskins HD, Iwach AG, Drake MV, et al. Subconjunctival THC:YAG laser limbal sclerostomy ab externo in the rabbit. *Ophthalmic Surg* 1990;21:589–592.

25. Hoskins HD Jr, Iwach AG, Vassiliadis A, et al. Subconjunctival THC:YAG laser thermal sclerostomy. *Ophthalmology* 1991;98:1394–1399, discussion 1399–1400.

26. Iwach AG, Hoskins HD Jr, Drake MV, Dickens CJ. Subconjunctival THC:YAG ("holmium") laser thermal sclerostomy ab externo. A one-year report. *Ophthalmology* 1993;100:356–365, discussion 365–366.

27. Schuman JS, Namazi N, Wang N, et al. Transconjunctival mitomycin C with holmium laser sclerectomy in rabbits and humans. *Invest Ophthalmol Vis Sci* 1993 (suppl.);34:1808.

28. Luntz MH, Fliegler RD, Mastrobattista J. Subconjunctival THC:YAG laser sclerostomy under a partial thickness flap. *Eur J Ophthalmol* 1996;6:268–272.

29. Hara T, Adachi M, Shirato S. Thalium-holmium-chromium-doped YAG laser sclerostomy ab externo in uncontrollable glaucoma. *Nippon Ganka Gakkai Zasshi* 1994;98:787–791.

30. Fliegler RJ, Mastrobattista J, Luntz MH. Subconjunctival THC:YAG laser sclerostomy under a partial-thickness corneal flap. *Ophthalmic Surg* 1994;25:28–33.

31. Brinkmann R, Droge G, Schroer F, et al. Ablation dynamics in laser sclerostomy ab externo by means of pulsed lasers in the mid-infrared spectral range. *Ophthalmic Surg Lasers* 1997;28:853–865.

32. Bonomi L, Perfetti S, Marraffa M, et al. Subconjunctival THC:YAG laser sclerostomy for the treatment of glaucoma: preliminary data. *Ophthalmic Surg* 1993;24:300–303.

33. Saheb NE. Short-term results of holmium laser sclerostomy in patients with uncontrolled glaucoma. *Can J Ophthalmology* 1993;28:317–319.

34. Namazi N, Schuman JS, Wang N, et al. Acute and long-term effects of THC:YAG sclerostomy with adjunctive antimetabolite therapy in rabbits. *Invest Ophthalmol Vis Sci* 1992 (suppl.);33:1266.

35. McAllister JA, Watts PO. Holmium laser sclerostomy: a clinical study. *Eye* 1993;7:656–660.

36. Beckman RL, Baerveldt G, Beckman H, et al. Erbium-YAG laser sclerostomy in humans—an update. *Invest Ophthalmol Vis Sci* 1993 (suppl.);34:1071.

37. Kampmeier J, Burgass W, Schutte E, et al. Comparative study of ab-externo sclerostomy with the excimer and Er:YAG laser. *Ophthalmologe* 1993;90:594–598.

38. Kampmeier J, Klafke M, Hibst R, et al. Ab externo sclerostomy with the Er:YAG laser: report of outcome after 2 years. *Klin Monatsbl Augenheilkd* 1996;208:218–223.

39. Wetzel W, Scheu M. Experimental laser sclerostomy ab externo with erbium:YAG laser. *Ophthalmologe* 1993;90:40–44.

40. Schuman JS, Chang W, Wang N, et al. Excimer laser effects on outflow facility and outflow pathway. *Invest Ophthalmol Vis Sci* 1992 (suppl.);33:1017.

41. Traverso CE, Murialdo U, Venzano D, et al. Excimer laser photoablative filtration surgery for primary open angle glaucoma. *Invest Ophthalmol Vis Sci* 1992 (suppl.);33:1017.

42. Seiler T, Kriegerowski M, Bende T, Wollensak J. Partial external trabeculectomy. *Klin Monatsbl Augenheilkd* 1989;195:216–220.

43. Kampmeier J, Schutte E, Schroder D, et al. Excimer laser sclerostomy of secondary glaucoma. *Ophthalmologe* 1993;90:35–39.

44. Brooks AM, Samuel M, Carroll N, et al. Excimer laser filtration surgery. *Am J Ophthalmol* 1995;119:40–47.

45. Aron-Rosa D, Maden A, Ganem S, et al. Preliminary study of argon fluoride (193 nm) excimer laser trabeculectomy. Scanning electron microscopy at five months. *J Cataract Refract Surg* 1990;16:617–620.

46. Karp CL, Higginbotham EJ, Edward DP, Musch DC. Diode laser surgery. Ab interno and ab externo versus conventional surgery in rabbits. *Ophthalmology* 1993;100:1567–1573.

47. Karp CL, Higginbotham EJ, Griffin EO. Adjunctive use of transconjunctival mitomycin-C in ab externo diode laser sclerostomy surgery in rabbits. *Ophthalmic Surg Lasers* 1994;25:22–27.

48. Kendrick R, Kollarits CR, Khan N. The results of ab interno laser thermal sclerostomy combined with cataract surgery versus trabeculectomy combined with cataract surgery 6 to 12 months postoperatively. *Ophthalmic Surg Lasers* 1996;27:583–586.

49. Wetzel W, Duncker G, Schumacher C, Dolle W. Laser sclerostomy: an alternative to current surgical filtering procedures. Experimental studies. *Klin Monatsbl Augenheilkd* 1989;194:170–172.

50. Heuer DK, Parrish RKI, Gressel MG, et al. 5-Fluorouracil and glaucoma filtering surgery. II. A pilot study. *Ophthalmology* 1984;91:383.

51. The FFSS Group. Fluorouracil filtering surgery study one-year follow-up. *Am J Ophthalmol* 1989;108:625–635.

52. Chen CW. Enhanced intraocular pressure controlling effectiveness of trabeculectomy by local application of mitomycin C. *Trans Asia-Pacific Acad Ophthalmol* 1983:9.

53. Palmer SS. Mitomycin as an adjunct chemotherapy with trabeculectomy. *Ophthalmology* 1991;98:317–321.

54. Kitazawa Y, Kawase K, Matsushita H, Minobe M. Trabeculectomy with mitomycin. *Arch Ophthalmol* 1991;109:1693–1698.

space. As described in this chapter, the goal of fistulization surgery is to establish this connection between the anterior chamber and the subconjunctival space.

Creating the fistula is not technically difficult, and in some European ophthalmology training programs, guarded fistulization is used as a resident physician's first intraocular surgery experience (2). But the fistula itself is not the most significant part. The difficult portion of the surgery is keeping the fistula open as long as possible, and maintaining just the right amount of resistance of flow to maintain an acceptable IOP. The history of this procedure first centers around the simple creation of the fistula, and has shifted increasingly to the development of methods to maintain the opening as long as possible.

HISTORY

From MacKenzie's sclerotomy (1830) to Watson's "tra-beculectomy" (1970), the process of surgically lowering the IOP has taken several forms.

MacKenzie (1830) performed sclerectomies and paracen-teses, but successful flow was short-lived (3). This approach persisted because in some patients with secondary glaucoma, the paracenteses permanently relieved the pupillary block and were therefore successful.

During von Graefe's era in the late 1800s, peripheral iri-dectomy was the standard treatment for all forms of glau-coma. von Graefe noted that although not all peripheral iridectomies successfully lowered the IOP, some did indeed control pressure over the long run. Although he described transparent vesicles that appeared at the limbus in these successful eyes, apparently indicating transscleral flow of aqueous, he did not make the association of these vesicles with surgical success (4). In fact, he "regarded the persis-tence of a flat or shallow anterior chamber to indicate the persistence of high pressure, which forced aqueous to trickle out of the wound" (5). These incisions were at the corneal limbus, not beneath the conjunctiva. He correctly made the association of chronic leaks with endophthalmi-tis, and advised that inadvertent vesicles be excised. The relationship between vesicle formation and surgical success was further obscured by the fact that surgical methods of the day may have resulted in cyclodialyses, resulting in permanently lowered IOP without the formation of visible vesicles.

The same year, DeWecker noted that more than iris needed to be excised for long-term success. He described the sclerectomy, and considered successes only those sur-geries that continued to filter fluid in the long term. The name *filter* became associated with this surgery because DeWecker believed that the aqueous filtered through the loose scar tissue that formed in this incision (5). He also contributed to a more refined approach for surgical treat-ment of glaucoma, noting that several diagnoses did not fare well with the simple iridectomy that had been used for all types of glaucoma until this time.

Herbert (1903) (6) and Holth (1906) (7) also realized the importance of maintaining flow through the hole that was created surgically and began intentionally placing iris in the wound to help prevent cicatricial closure. While Holth had developed a punch to entrap iris in the sclera, LaGrange introduced scleral excision as a means of creating an open hole without inclusion of iris.

Between 1909 and the 1940s, Elliot's method of limbal trephination (8,9) was the predominant operation. The depth of tissue trephined and removed was varied based on the type of glaucoma diagnosed. The incidence of late endophthalmitis led to replacement of trephination by scle-rostomies created by cautery, as described by Presiozi (1924) (10) and Scheie (11).

Many of the problems of these procedures were due to their full-thickness nature—too much filtration too early in the postoperative period led to flat anterior chambers, corneal clouding and cataract, and hemorrhagic choroidal detachments.

In 1961, Sugar (12) tried to bypass the meshwork and send fluid directly to Schlemm's canal. In this procedure, a scleral flap was created, the trabecular meshwork removed, and the flap tightly secured to its bed. The goal was to allow aqueous to pass from the anterior chamber directly into Schlemm's canal. This was a true trabeculectomy, and Sugar utilized the term. Unfortunately, most of these procedures failed owing to internal fibrosis.

In the course of searching for an improvement, Cairns (13) in 1968 reported success in 17 eyes, with development of vesicular filtering blebs in 6 of the eyes. As with Sugar's procedure, the flaps were intended to be securely fixed and watertight.

In 1970, Watson (14) found success in 25 of 44 eyes with a similar procedure. For both Cairns's and Watson's surgeries, the filtration that resulted in success was unintended. No attempt was made to connect the anterior chamber with the subconjunctival space, but rather to Schlemm's canal. It gradually became appreciated that this procedure allowed partial filtration, in a "guarded" fashion, from the anterior chamber to outside the sclera, and to this day, work has con-tinued to promote aqueous flow in a titratable fashion. As surgeons sought to avoid iris incarceration and flat anterior chambers resulting from direct flow, the site of the sclerectomy was moved forward toward clear cornea anterior to Schwalbe's line. This site gave better IOP control and more consistent results.

As this principle matured, the term did not change to reflect the modification of the procedure. It is more correct to use the term *peripheral (or posterior) keratectomy*, since the tissue removed is usually anterior to the meshwork. Spaeth (15) suggested the term *guarded filtration procedure*, but noted his affection for the nickname "trab." Teichmann (16) agreed with Spaeth and elaborated further, pointing out that since the biologic filter, the trabecular meshwork, is bypassed, a term more proper than *guarded filter* is *guarded fistula*. The name *trabeculectomy* continues to be common parlance.

conventional trabeculectomy with MMC, or even glaucoma implant surgery, remains the treatment of choice for nearly all glaucoma patients requiring filtering surgery.

REFERENCES

1. Schuman JS, Stinson WG, Hutchinson BT, et al. Holmium laser sclerectomy. Success and complications. *Ophthalmology* 1993;100:1060–1065.
2. Latina MA, Melamed S, March WF, et al. Gonioscopic ab interno laser sclerostomy: a pilot study in glaucoma patients. *Ophthalmology* 1992;99:1736–1744.
3. Iwach AG, Hoskins HD Jr, Drake MV, Dickens CJ. Update of the subconjunctival THC:YAG (holmium) laser sclerostomy ab externo clinical trial: 30-month report. *Ophthalmic Surg* 1994;25:13–21.
4. Friedman DS, Katz LJ, Augsburger JJ, Lean M. Holmium laser sclerostomy in glaucomatous eyes with prior surgery: 24-month results. *Ophthalmic Surg Lasers* 1998;29:17–22.
5. Elliot RH. Preliminary note on a new operative procedure for the establishment of a filtering cicatrix in the treatment of glaucoma. *Ophthalmoscope* 1909;7:804.
6. Scheie HG. Retraction of scleral wound edges as a fistulizing procedure for glaucoma. *Am J Ophthalmol* 1958;45:220–228.
7. Federman JL, Wilson RP, Anso F. Contact laser thermal sclerostomy ab interna. *Ophthalmic Surg* 1987;18:726–727.
8. Higginbotham EJ, Kao G, Peyman G. Internal sclerostomy with the Nd:YAG contact laser versus thermal sclerostomy in rabbits. *Ophthalmology* 1988;95:385–390.
9. Javitt JC, O'Connor SS, Wilson RP, Federman JL. Laser sclerostomy ab interno using a continuous wave Nd:YAG laser. *Ophthalmic Surg* 1989;20:552–556.
10. Wilson RP, Javitt JC. Ab interno laser sclerostomy in aphakic patients with glaucoma and chronic inflammation. *Am J Ophthalmol* 1990;110:178–184.
11. Zysset B, Fujimoto JG, Puliafito CA, et al. Picosecond optical breakdown: tissue effects and reduction of collateral damage. *Lasers Surg Med* 1989;9:193–204.
12. Cooper HM, Schuman JS, Puliafito CA, et al. Picosecond Nd:YLF sclerectomy. *Am J Ophthalmol* 1993;115:221–224.
13. Woods WJ, Schuman JS, Wang N, et al. Gonioscopic picosecond Nd:YLF laser sclerectomy ab interno in the feline model. *Invest Ophthalmol Vis Sci* 1993 (suppl.);34:173.
14. Latina MA, Goode S, de Kater AW, et al. Experimental ab interno sclerotomies using a pulsed-dye laser. *Lasers Surg Med* 1988;8:233–240.
15. Latina MA, Dobrogowski M, March WF, Birngruber R. Laser sclerostomy by pulsed-dye laser and goniolens. *Arch Ophthalmol* 1990;108:1745–1750.
16. Melamed S, Solomon A, Neumann D, et al. Internal sclerostomy using laser ablation of dyed sclera in glaucoma patients: a pilot study. *Br J Ophthalmol* 1993;77:139–144.
17. Namazi N, Fleckner M, Feld JR, et al. Effects of cavitation bubbles created by pulsed laser ablation in the anterior chamber. *Invest Ophthalmol Vis Sci* 1993 (suppl.);34:1070.
18. Ruben S, Migdal C, De Vivero C. Ab interno pulsed dye laser sclerostomy for the treatment of glaucoma: preliminary results of a new technique. *Eye* 1993;7:436–439.
19. Muller-Stolzenburg M, Muller GJ. Transmission of 308 nm excimer laser radiation for ophthalmic microsurgery—medical, technical and safety aspects. *Biomed-Tech (Berlin)* 1989;34:131–138.
20. Ozler SA, Hill RA, Andrews JJ, et al. Infrared laser sclerostomies. *Invest Ophthalmol Vis Sci* 1991;32:498–503.
21. Gaasterland DE, Hennings DR, Boutacoff TA, et al. Ab interno and ab externo filtering operations by laser contact surgery. *Ophthalmic Surg* 1987;18:254.
22. Jaffe GJ, Williams GA, Mieler WF, et al. Ab interno sclerostomy with a high-powered argon endolaser. *Am J Ophthalmol* 1988;106:391–396.
23. Jaffe GJ, Mieler WF, Radius RL, et al. Ab interno sclerostomy with a high-powered argon endolaser. Clinicopathologic correlation. *Arch Ophthalmol* 1989;107:1183–1185.
24. Hoskins HD, Iwach AG, Drake MV, et al. Subconjunctival THC:YAG laser limbal sclerostomy ab externo in the rabbit. *Ophthalmic Surg* 1990;21:589–592.
25. Hoskins HD Jr, Iwach AG, Vassiliadis A, et al. Subconjunctival THC:YAG laser thermal sclerostomy. *Ophthalmology* 1991;98:1394–1399, discussion 1399–1400.
26. Iwach AG, Hoskins HD Jr, Drake MV, Dickens CJ. Subconjunctival THC:YAG ("holmium") laser thermal sclerostomy ab externo. A one-year report. *Ophthalmology* 1993;100:356–365, discussion 365–366.
27. Schuman JS, Namazi N, Wang N, et al. Transconjunctival mitomycin C with holmium laser sclerectomy in rabbits and humans. *Invest Ophthalmol Vis Sci* 1993 (suppl.);34:1808.
28. Luntz MH, Fliegler RD, Mastrobattista J. Subconjunctival THC:YAG laser sclerostomy under a partial thickness flap. *Eur J Ophthalmol* 1996;6:268–272.
29. Hara T, Adachi M, Shirato S. Thalium-holmium-chromium-doped YAG laser sclerostomy ab externo in uncontrollable glaucoma. *Nippon Ganka Gakkai Zasshi* 1994;98:787–791.
30. Fliegler RJ, Mastrobattista J, Luntz MH. Subconjunctival THC:YAG laser sclerostomy under a partial-thickness corneal flap. *Ophthalmic Surg* 1994;25:28–33.
31. Brinkmann R, Droge G, Schroer F, et al. Ablation dynamics in laser sclerostomy ab externo by means of pulsed lasers in the mid-infrared spectral range. *Ophthalmic Surg Lasers* 1997;28:853–865.
32. Bonomi L, Perfetti S, Marraffa M, et al. Subconjunctival THC:YAG laser sclerostomy for the treatment of glaucoma: preliminary data. *Ophthalmic Surg* 1993;24:300–303.
33. Saheb NE. Short-term results of holmium laser sclerostomy in patients with uncontrolled glaucoma. *Can J Ophthalmology* 1993;28:317–319.
34. Namazi N, Schuman JS, Wang N, et al. Acute and long-term effects of THC:YAG sclerostomy with adjunctive antimetabolite therapy in rabbits. *Invest Ophthalmol Vis Sci* 1992 (suppl.);33:1266.
35. McAllister JA, Watts PO. Holmium laser sclerostomy: a clinical study. *Eye* 1993;7:656–660.
36. Beckman RL, Baerveldt G, Beckman H, et al. Erbium-YAG laser sclerostomy in humans—an update. *Invest Ophthalmol Vis Sci* 1993 (suppl.);34:1071.
37. Kampmeier J, Burgass W, Schutte E, et al. Comparative study of ab-externo sclerostomy with the excimer and Er:YAG laser. *Ophthalmologe* 1993;90:594–598.
38. Kampmeier J, Klafke M, Hibst R, et al. Ab externo sclerostomy with the Er:YAG laser: report of outcome after 2 years. *Klin Monatsbl Augenheilkd* 1996;208:218–223.
39. Wetzel W, Scheu M. Experimental laser sclerostomy ab externo with erbium:YAG laser. *Ophthalmologe* 1993;90:40–44.
40. Schuman JS, Chang W, Wang N, et al. Excimer laser effects on outflow facility and outflow pathway. *Invest Ophthalmol Vis Sci* 1992 (suppl.);33:1017.
41. Traverso CE, Murialdo U, Venzano D, et al. Excimer laser photoablative filtration surgery for primary open angle glaucoma. *Invest Ophthalmol Vis Sci* 1992 (suppl.);33:1017.
42. Seiler T, Kriegerowski M, Bende T, Wollensak J. Partial external trabeculectomy. *Klin Monatsbl Augenheilkd* 1989;195:216–220.
43. Kampmeier J, Schutte E, Schroder D, et al. Excimer laser sclerostomy of secondary glaucoma. *Ophthalmologe* 1993;90:35–39.
44. Brooks AM, Samuel M, Carroll N, et al. Excimer laser filtration surgery. *Am J Ophthalmol* 1995;119:40–47.
45. Aron-Rosa D, Maden A, Ganem S, et al. Preliminary study of argon fluoride (193 nm) excimer laser trabeculectomy. Scanning electron microscopy at five months. *J Cataract Refract Surg* 1990;16:617–620.
46. Karp CL, Higginbotham EJ, Edward DP, Musch DC. Diode laser surgery. Ab interno and ab externo versus conventional surgery in rabbits. *Ophthalmology* 1993;100:1567–1573.
47. Karp CL, Higginbotham EJ, Griffin EO. Adjunctive use of transconjunctival mitomycin-C in ab externo diode laser sclerostomy surgery in rabbits. *Ophthalmic Surg Lasers* 1994;25:22–27.
48. Kendrick R, Kollarits CR, Khan N. The results of ab interno laser thermal sclerostomy combined with cataract surgery versus trabeculectomy combined with cataract surgery 6 to 12 months postoperatively. *Ophthalmic Surg Lasers* 1996;27:583–586.
49. Wetzel W, Duncker G, Schumacher C, Dolle W. Laser sclerostomy: an alternative to current surgical filtering procedures. Experimental studies. *Klin Monatsbl Augenheilkd* 1989;194:170–172.
50. Heuer DK, Parrish RKI, Gressel MG, et al. 5-Fluorouracil and glaucoma filtering surgery. II. A pilot study. *Ophthalmology* 1984;91:383.
51. The FFSS Group. Fluorouracil filtering surgery study one-year follow-up. *Am J Ophthalmol* 1989;108:625–635.
52. Chen CW. Enhanced intraocular pressure controlling effectiveness of trabeculectomy by local application of mitomycin C. *Trans Asia-Pacific Acad Ophthalmol* 1983:9.
53. Palmer SS. Mitomycin as an adjunct chemotherapy with trabeculectomy. *Ophthalmology* 1991;98:317–321.
54. Kitazawa Y, Kawase K, Matsushita H, Minobe M. Trabeculectomy with mitomycin. *Arch Ophthalmol* 1991;109:1693–1698.

55. Skuta GL, Beeson CC, Higginbotham EJ, et al. Intraoperative mitomycin versus postoperative 5-fluorouracil in high-risk glaucoma filtering surgery. *Ophthalmology* 1992;99:438–444.

56. Schmidbauer JM, Hoh H, Jahnig T, Daberkow I. Antiproliferative therapy with 5-fluorouracil in erbium:YAG laser sclerostomy ab externo. *Ophthalmologe* 1996;93:569–575.

57. Mawas E, Parizot H. A simple and effective operation for glaucoma: Elliot's trephine combined with an iridencleisis. *Trans Ophthalmol Soc UK* 1964;84:139–154.

58. Kutschera E, Seher K. Iridencleisis of Elliot's trephining? A comparative study. *Klin Monatsbl Augenheilkd* 1968;153:305–313.

59. Hollwich F. Trephining by the Elliot method (indication, successful and unsuccessful results). *Klin Monatsbl Augenheilkd* 1969;155:645–658.

60. Sugar HS. Further experience with limboscleral trephination. *Eye, Ear, Nose & Throat Monthly* 1968;47:165–170.

61. Kroner B. Elliot's trepanation and iridencleisis of the university eye clinic Tuebingen. Attempt at retrospective documentation. *Doc Ophthalmol* 1969;27:90–95.

62. Dellaporta A, Fahrenbruch RC. Trepano-trabeculectomy. *Trans Am Acad Ophthalmol Otolaryngol* 1971;75:283–295.

63. Fronimopoulos J, Lambrou N, Christakis C. Goniotrepanation with scleral cover. Development of the surgical technic and postoperative results. *Klin Monatsbl Augenheilkd* 1971;159:565–574.

64. Sugar HS. Limboscleral trepanation; eleven years' experience. *Arch Ophthalmol* 1971;85:703–708.

65. Dellaporta A. Combined trephine-trabeculectomy and cataract extraction. *Klin Monatsbl Augenheilkd* 1972;160:49–56.

66. Hommer K. Elliot's trepanation with scleral flap and mitred incision in combined glaucoma cataract operation. *Klin Monatsbl Augenheilkd* 1972;160:327–329.

67. Schmidt-Mumm E. Fenestrated microtrephine for Elliot's glaucoma surgery. *Klin Monatsbl Augenheilkd* 1972;161:239.

68. Jackson AH. Lamellar limboscleral trephination in the surgical treatment of glaucoma. *Ann Ophthalmol* 1973;5:1137–1140.

69. Egerer I. A new type of trephine (screw trephine). *Klin Monatsbl Augenheilkd* 1975;167:907–908.

70. Fronimopoulos J, Christakis C. Goniotrepanation (gotrep) and further observations on this operation for chronic glaucoma. *Albrecht Von Graefes Archiv Klin Experimentelle Ophthalmologie* 1975;193:135–143.

71. Gliem H, Pedal W. Experiences with trepano-trabeculectomy (goniotrepanation). *Klin Monatsbl Augenheilkd* 1975;166:598–601.

72. Stangos N, Papathanassiou AP, Psilas K, et al. Trabeculectomy and trephining under the scleral flap: results and comparison of the methods in simple chronic glaucoma, secondary open-angle and closed-angle glaucomas. *Cesk Oftalmol* 1976;32:335–340.

73. Jacob M, Thomas A. Subscleral goniotrepanation in primary glaucoma. *Indian J Ophthalmol* 1984;32:69–72.

74. Prasad VN, Narain M, Bist HK, Khan MM. Trepano-trabeculectomy (a combined operation for glaucoma). *Indian J Ophthalmol* 1984;32:73–75.

75. Brown RH, Denham DB, Bruner WE, et al. Internal sclerectomy for glaucoma filtering surgery with an automated trephine. *Arch Ophthalmol* 1987;105:133–136.

76. Brown RH, Lynch MG, Denham DB, et al. Internal sclerectomy with an automated trephine for advanced glaucoma. *Ophthalmology* 1988;95:728–734.

Trabeculectomy

GREGG A. HEATLEY

Trabeculectomy is the mainstay of surgical treatment for glaucoma. Typically used if medical or laser treatments fail to control glaucoma progression, this surgery is performed by both glaucoma specialists and comprehensive ophthalmologists. Trabeculectomy may be appropriate for nearly all causes of elevated intraocular pressure (IOP). In its role as the primary initial surgery for glaucoma, this procedure has been the subject of intensive development in the past 20 years. The recent availability of adjuvant antimetabolite therapy has created a large amount of confusing data, which makes it difficult for the practitioner to know how to apply this information to an individual patient. This chapter presents the underlying principles of this procedure, describes the historical background, sorts the recent additions to the literature, and discusses the nuances of each step of trabeculectomy. As for few other procedures in ophthalmology, it is these seemingly picayune details that separate a short-lived reward from a long-term success. To set a fastidious tone, consider even the name of the procedure.

DEFINITION

Stedman's Medical Dictionary defines *trabeculectomy* as "a filtering operation for glaucoma by creation of a fistula between the anterior chamber of the eye and the subconjunctival space, through a subscleral excision of a portion of the trabecular meshwork" (1). This definition is incorrect. A fistula is indeed created, a subscleral incision is used, and the goal of the surgery is to create a communication between the anterior chamber and the veins draining the subconjunctival space, but little if any of the trabecular meshwork is excised. As currently performed, the ostomy is created in the posterior and peripheral aspect of the cornea, anterior

to the meshwork. Although some anterior meshwork may be removed in some patients, *peripheral keratectomy* would be a more accurate term.

When beginning to describe and understand a procedure, it is important to specify the intended result. Simply put, successful fistulization surgery lowers the IOP. It is accepted that elevation of IOP is a major risk factor for the development of glaucomatous optic nerve damage. Until research elucidates more about the mechanism of retinal ganglion cell death, lowering the IOP will remain the major treatment.

IOP is determined by the rate of formation of aqueous humor by the ciliary body and the ease with which aqueous humor exits the eye by the trabecular meshwork and the uveoscleral pathways. In ocular hypertension, the resistance to outflow through the meshwork is increased, and the IOP rises to the level needed to drive the fluid across that higher resistance. Medical therapy can reduce the amount of fluid created by the ciliary body, reduce meshwork resistance, and increase uveoscleral outflow. Laser treatments can decrease trabecular outflow resistance and aqueous production by the ciliary body.

When medical or laser treatments are insufficient to reduce IOP, it becomes necessary to create an outflow tract of lower resistance. Patients understand this concept of creating a "new drain." When searching for a destination for the fluid, several spaces are available—extraocular, subconjunctival, venous, and lymphatic. Ideally, the final site of the fluid accumulation should be isolated from the ocular surface, to minimize the risk of infection; it should be fairly vascular, to drain the fluid from the orbit into the venous system; it should be able to provide enough outflow resistance to avoid ocular collapse; and it should remain viable for years. The space that best meets these criteria is the subconjunctival space. As described in this chapter, the goal of fistulization surgery is to establish this connection between the anterior chamber and the subconjunctival space.

Creating the fistula is not technically difficult, and in some European ophthalmology training programs, guarded fistulization is used as a resident physician's first intraocular surgery experience (2). But the fistula itself is not the most significant part. The difficult portion of the surgery is keeping the fistula open as long as possible, and maintaining just the right amount of resistance of flow to maintain an acceptable IOP. The history of this procedure first centers around the simple creation of the fistula, and has shifted increasingly to the development of methods to maintain the opening as long as possible.

HISTORY

From MacKenzie's sclerotomy (1830) to Watson's "trabeculectomy" (1970), the process of surgically lowering the IOP has taken several forms.

MacKenzie (1830) performed sclerectomies and paracenteses, but successful flow was short-lived (3). This approach persisted because in some patients with secondary glaucoma, the paracenteses permanently relieved the pupillary block and were therefore successful.

During von Graefe's era in the late 1800s, peripheral iridectomy was the standard treatment for all forms of glaucoma. von Graefe noted that although not all peripheral iridectomies successfully lowered the IOP, some did indeed control pressure over the long run. Although he described transparent vesicles that appeared at the limbus in these successful eyes, apparently indicating transscleral flow of aqueous, he did not make the association of these vesicles with surgical success (4). In fact, he "regarded the persistence of a flat or shallow anterior chamber to indicate the persistence of high pressure, which forced aqueous to trickle out of the wound" (5). These incisions were at the corneal limbus, not beneath the conjunctiva. He correctly made the association of chronic leaks with endophthalmitis, and advised that inadvertent vesicles be excised. The relationship between vesicle formation and surgical success was further obscured by the fact that surgical methods of the day may have resulted in cyclodialyses, resulting in permanently lowered IOP without the formation of visible vesicles.

The same year, DeWecker noted that more than iris needed to be excised for long-term success. He described the sclerectomy, and considered successes only those surgeries that continued to filter fluid in the long term. The name *filter* became associated with this surgery because DeWecker believed that the aqueous filtered through the loose scar tissue that formed in this incision (5). He also contributed to a more refined approach for surgical treatment of glaucoma, noting that several diagnoses did not fare well with the simple iridectomy that had been used for all types of glaucoma until this time.

Herbert (1903) (6) and Holth (1906) (7) also realized the importance of maintaining flow through the hole that was created surgically and began intentionally placing iris in the wound to help prevent cicatricial closure. While Holth had developed a punch to entrap iris in the sclera, LaGrange introduced scleral excision as a means of creating an open hole without inclusion of iris.

Between 1909 and the 1940s, Elliot's method of limbal trephination (8,9) was the predominant operation. The depth of tissue trephined and removed was varied based on the type of glaucoma diagnosed. The incidence of late endophthalmitis led to replacement of trephination by sclerostomies created by cautery, as described by Presiozi (1924) (10) and Scheie (11).

Many of the problems of these procedures were due to their full-thickness nature—too much filtration too early in the postoperative period led to flat anterior chambers, corneal clouding and cataract, and hemorrhagic choroidal detachments.

In 1961, Sugar (12) tried to bypass the meshwork and send fluid directly to Schlemm's canal. In this procedure, a scleral flap was created, the trabecular meshwork removed, and the flap tightly secured to its bed. The goal was to allow aqueous to pass from the anterior chamber directly into Schlemm's canal. This was a true trabeculectomy, and Sugar utilized the term. Unfortunately, most of these procedures failed owing to internal fibrosis.

In the course of searching for an improvement, Cairns (13) in 1968 reported success in 17 eyes, with development of vesicular filtering blebs in 6 of the eyes. As with Sugar's procedure, the flaps were intended to be securely fixed and watertight.

In 1970, Watson (14) found success in 25 of 44 eyes with a similar procedure. For both Cairns's and Watson's surgeries, the filtration that resulted in success was unintended. No attempt was made to connect the anterior chamber with the subconjunctival space, but rather to Schlemm's canal. It gradually became appreciated that this procedure allowed partial filtration, in a "guarded" fashion, from the anterior chamber to outside the sclera, and to this day, work has continued to promote aqueous flow in a titratable fashion. As surgeons sought to avoid iris incarceration and flat anterior chambers resulting from direct flow, the site of the sclerectomy was moved forward toward clear cornea anterior to Schwalbe's line. This site gave better IOP control and more consistent results.

As this principle matured, the term did not change to reflect the modification of the procedure. It is more correct to use the term *peripheral (or posterior) keratectomy*, since the tissue removed is usually anterior to the meshwork. Spaeth (15) suggested the term *guarded filtration procedure*, but noted his affection for the nickname "trab." Teichmann (16) agreed with Spaeth and elaborated further, pointing out that since the biologic filter, the trabecular meshwork, is bypassed, a term more proper than *guarded filter* is *guarded fistula*. The name *trabeculectomy* continues to be common parlance.

The mechanics of the surgery have changed little since the Watson-Cairns era. The recent developments in glaucoma surgery have been chemical rather than physical. In the immediate postoperative period, without much fibrosis yet in place, the resistance to flow is very low and aqueous will flow easily from the anterior chamber to the conjunctival bleb. But after several days to weeks, as fibrosis mounts, the resistance increases, flow decreases, and the pressure will rise, hopefully to a plateau that is low enough to avoid further ganglion cell loss (Fig. 33-1).

Therefore, the crux of the surgical goal is to avoid the early hypotony and yet not allow the final plateau to be dangerously high. Ideally, this means being able to mechanically avoid early overfiltration, so that the starting point of the curve is above approximately 5 mm Hg, and to minimize fibrosis, making the curve of IOP increase due to scarring relatively flat. Inhibiting fibrosis and managing the progressive healing with staged intervention (e.g., suture release or lysis) is the key to successful fistula surgery, with the ultimate goal of preserving vision.

The recent availability of chemicals that retard wound healing has greatly affected the likelihood that these outcomes will be realized. Over the past decade, use of antimetabolite drugs has become routine, with significant ramifications. Many steps of this surgery that had been inconsequential in the years before antimetabolite use are now of paramount importance. Before one can appreciate the relevance of surgical details, it is necessary to fully understand the mechanism and impact of these drugs on the wound-healing process.

MODULATION OF WOUND HEALING GENERAL PRINCIPLES

The major site of fibrosis after a guarded filtration procedure is the episcleral surface, owing to a high density of fibroblasts. Beginning with the initial incision, the injured

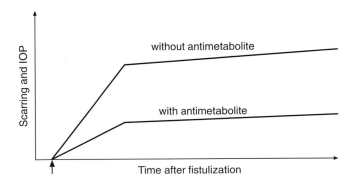

FIGURE 33-1. *Development of scarring at the fistula site creates increased resistance to the flow of aqueous and increased intraocular pressure (IOP). Eventually, the bleb matures, and resistance stabilizes. Use of an adjuvant antimetabolite minimizes scar formation, allowing lower initial and final IOP.*

scleral tissues secrete cytokines and allow leakage of plasma proteins into the tissue bed. This process activates cells in the area, and attracts cells from remote areas (17). The plasma proteins may clot and provide an organized network of tissue to act as a scaffold for later collagen deposition. Most of the wound-healing activity comes from the cells originally present, through cell division and replication, as shown by animal studies (18–21). Therefore, the amount of scar tissue ultimately produced is determine by both the number of activated cells and the activity of each cell to produce structural proteins. Limitation of either or both of these steps will result in less wound healing. For guarded-fistula surgery, less wound healing translates into lower final IOP.

The inciting step of the activation process is the tissue damage from cautery, incision, and crush. Both steroids and nonsteroidal compounds are capable of reducing the cellular response to these injuries, and steroids have the additional advantage of inhibiting cellular migration into the wound area. As described later in this chapter, intraoperative subconjunctival injection of steroid is a routine component of fistulization surgery, and postoperative treatment with steroid drops significantly increases the rate of success (22). Some surgeons prefer to begin steroid treatment preoperatively, so that the anti-inflammatory effect is present from the moment of the initial surgical incision (23,24).

Once the cells are activated and beginning to secrete cytokines and the area fills with plasma proteins, the released proteins may coagulate. This step is very similar to the classic blood clotting cascade. Compounds that interfere with this process, such as tissue plasminogen activator (tPA) and streptokinase, may become clinically significant modulators in fistulization surgery as delivery systems are developed (25).

It is difficult to completely suppress the chemical reaction of the injured cells, but the next step, cell division, can be directly inhibited. This phase begins to become important in the first few days after surgery, as the cells begin the mitotic process. Chemicals can be applied directly to the tissues during surgery, or delivered to the operative area in the early postoperative period. The selection of drug depends on its efficacy and side effects on surrounding tissues. Most of the antineoplastic agents work by inhibiting cell division, by altering either DNA or the proteins involved in mitosis. Two such compounds, used systemically for cancer therapy in the past, have come to widespread use in glaucoma surgery: 5-fluorouracil (5-FU) and mitomycin C. Each works by interfering with DNA replication. These are the major adjuvants used in fistulization surgery.

5-FU, through an intracellular metabolite, inhibits thymidylate synthetase, an enzyme that converts deoxyuridine phosphate to thymidine phosphate. Through this inhibition, DNA synthesis is markedly suppressed. This enzyme is inactive or absent except when the cell is actively dividing. Timing of the dose of 5-FU is therefore critical. The tissue levels must be high postoperatively, when the cells are responding to the injury stimulus by active proliferation.

Mitomycin C is an antibiotic derived from *Streptomyces caespitosus* and works by directly binding DNA. Since this process is not dependent on the cell-division phase, mitomycin can be applied to cells that are in any phase of the cell cycle and still have effect. This makes timing of the dose of mitomycin less critical. Thus, although 5-FU inhibits mitosis best when applied postoperatively, effective limitation of cell division can be achieved with intraoperative doses of mitomycin C.

Histopathologic and cell-culture studies have confirmed that mitomycin C and 5-FU minimize proliferation of fibroblasts of Tenon's capsule and the episclera (26–35). In cell culture, these drugs adversely affect conjunctival cells (36).

These antimetabolites may also directly attenuate the inflammatory response (29), even in the presence of severe inflammatory events (37). 5-FU has also been used as subconjunctival injections to ameliorate anterior uveitis unrelated to glaucoma surgery (38).

Other chemicals have been investigated, with some success in cell-culture, animal, and human models. These include tPA (39,40), taxol, cytochalasin B and colchicine (41), minoxidil (42), interferon gamma (43), cytarabine (44), and daunorubicin (45). The presence of ascorbic acid in the aqueous humor may correlate positively with long-term success of blebs (46–48). Various growth factors and cellular receptors have also been investigated (28,49–51).

Investigations into modulation of the final step of the fibrotic process, collagen cross-linking, are ongoing (50).

Techniques of Drug Delivery to Tissues

Given that antimetabolite agents are identified, consideration of the application of these drugs in a surgical setting then turns to defining the timing and methods of administration.

Preoperative administration can occur by topical, oral, or injectable routes. Both topical and oral routes have been used for one class of antimetabolites: steroids. No reports of preoperative injections of other antimetabolites have been published. Advantages of preoperative administration are ease of use and a nonselective effect on the entire globe.

The advantages of intraoperative application are numerous. The antimetabolite effect is nonselective—any tissue exposed to the chemical will be affected. However, success of fistulization surgery requires healing to be very selective—the conjunctival incision is required to heal completely and quickly after surgery to keep the bleb inflated and avoid hypotony. Less than 6 mm away, the scleral flap and bed are required to heal as little as possible. Intraoperative administration of an antimetabolite allows for selective

exposure of only the scleral flap, avoiding the conjunctival margins. Compared to subconjunctival injections, the time and concentration of drug exposure at the precise surgical site can be fairly well controlled, theoretically allowing a knowledgeable titration appropriate to the clinical situation. For example, reoperations on uveitic eyes clearly need more antifibrosis than a first operation on a quiet eye. Intraoperatively, the drug can be delivered as a single exposure, as on a pledget (52), or as an implanted system (53,54) that is allowed to remain in place postoperatively, continuously releasing drug to the scleral surface. Either method of intraoperative application allows only one try at getting the dose correct, and requires fastidious avoidance of contact of the drug with the conjunctival margins.

Postoperative delivery methods usually consist of subconjunctival injections of the drug, as topical delivery can be extremely toxic to the surface (55). Since delivery of the drug to the intraocular spaces has markedly damaging effects on corneal endothelium and other intraocular tissues (43,56,57), it is necessary to place the injection far enough away from the scleral flap so as to avoid retrograde flow into the anterior chamber. Diffusion of the drug within the subconjunctival space achieves a therapeutic level in the fistula site.

The significant advantage of postoperative administration protocols is that it is possible to titrate the amount of drug given based on the clinical appearance of the eye. Variables such as intrableb hemorrhage, anterior-chamber inflammation, and vascularity of the bleb surface are often not apparent intraoperatively, and the dose given intraoperatively may be inappropriate to the appearance of the eye as the patient recovers. As these ominous factors develop postoperatively, the amount of drug given can be adjusted. Similarly, doses can be adjusted downward if none of the threats develop (Table 33-1).

The original clinical trials of 5-FU were performed with multiple postoperative subconjunctival injections. Since

Table 33-1.   Factors Influencing the Choice of Intraoperative or Postoperative Application of Antimetabolite

	Intraoperative Application	Postoperative Application
Advantages	Contact only with intended tissue	Allows titration of dose based on postoperative appearance
	Control of dose and time of exposure	
	Painless	
Disadvantages	Cannot titrate exposure postoperatively	Diffusion to other tissues (corneal epithelium)
	Does not treat cells arriving at site postoperatively	Painful
	Requires meticulous avoidance of conjunctival margins	May result in fresh postoperative hemorrhage

diffusion occurs in all directions from the injection site, more than the flap tissue achieves therapeutic levels. The corneal limbus and conjunctival incision may also be considered to have been treated by that injection. In clinical trials utilizing similar postoperative injections, conjunctival wound leaks were common, and the dose-limiting side effect of the drug was often corneal epithelial defect due to inhibition of limbal stem-cell division (58–68).

These theoretical factors are important in consideration of whether intraoperative or postoperative administration is selected for a given patient. But equally important is a more pragmatic question: Which one works better? A large, confusing literature revolves around the comparison of fistulization surgery with the antimetabolites mitomycin C and 5-FU.

Clinical Effects of 5-Fluorouracil and Mitomycin C

Mitomycin C greatly improves the success of guarded fistulization in animal (69–72) and human (73–82) procedures. Similar improvements in success rates of fistulization surgeries have been shown for 5-FU (83–113).

Historically, studies with 5-FU predated the mitomycin investigations. The drugs had a similar process of evolution—the initial reports were encouraging, and in each case the complication rates of the early trials prompted work to lower the doses to minimize these complications without losing the beneficial effects. Each drug was first investigated in high-risk eyes, and then expanded into use in uncomplicated glaucoma surgeries. Although each study defined outcomes in different ways, the final "success" rates of each of these studies were based on IOP reduction.

Clinical work on 5-FU began in earnest in the mid 1980s. Heuer et al (114) reported improvement in success (IOP < 21 mm Hg) of fistulization surgery in high-risk eyes in an uncontrolled study. Kitazawa et al (111) found a success rate of 10% after repeat fistulization without 5-FU, which improved to 68% with the inclusion of postoperative high-dose 5-FU. Rockwood et al (115) found 3-year success rates in high-risk eyes of 64% (aphakia), 75% (failed first surgery), and 68% (neovascular glaucoma). Taniguchi et al (112) found a 60% success rate without antimetabolite and a 75% success rate with 5-FU in eyes undergoing either the first or second guarded fistulization surgery. Both of these studies had relatively short follow-up periods. Nakano et al (110) studied a similar group of patients and found IOPs less than 20 mm Hg at 3 years postoperatively in 90% of the eyes treated with 5-FU and only 40% of the eyes treated without 5-FU.

The most widely known examination of the effects of 5-FU was done by the Fluorouracil Filtering Surgery Study Group (FFSS) (84,109,116,117). As one of the initial trials, eyes considered for study were only those at high risk for fistulization failure, and were randomized to receive high-dose 5-FU injections postoperatively or fistulization without

antimetabolite treatment. Two hundred thirteen eyes were studied and the rates of success (IOP < 21 mm Hg) at 1 year were 73% in the 5-FU group and 50% in the control group. By 3 years, the difference was maintained but many eyes had failed in both groups—50% success rate in the treated group and 26% success rate in the controls. At the 5-year follow-up, 49% of the 5-FU–treated eyes had IOPs less than 22 mm Hg, compared with 26% of the untreated eyes (118). The late complications of bleb leak and thin bleb walls prompted the authors to warn against using the antimetabolite in patients with good surgical prognoses, and to recommend that 5-FU only be used in patients with prior cataract surgery or failed fistulization (84,118).

As the FFSS was progressing, Ophir and Ticho (119) published an evaluation of five patients who had failed prior 5-FU fistulization surgery and underwent repeat 5-FU–augmented surgery. With 6 to 19 months of follow-up, the IOP was less than 20 mm Hg with or without medication in all five patients. This indicated that the eyes which had failed antimetabolite-assisted surgery could still respond favorably to a repeat of the same procedure. Wilson and Steinmann (106) showed that very low final IOPs could be obtained with 5-FU use, although there was an associated loss of visual acuity. In 1992, 5-year follow-up data were published, indicating success rates in chronic open-angle glaucoma patients of 95% with 5-FU and 78% without 5-FU, and in refractory glaucoma patients, success rates of 58% with 5-FU and 28% without 5-FU.

Additional studies looked at specific categories of high-risk eyes and found a greater likelihood of success when 5-FU was used. These categories include inflammatory glaucoma (108,120), neovascular glaucoma (121), young patients (98,103), prior encircling band surgeries (86), irido-corneal-endothelial syndrome (104), and even after failed glaucoma drainage implants (122).

This success led some to investigate the use of 5-FU in patients who did not fit the high-risk category. Liebmann et al (105,123) found lower IOP, less medication requirement, and higher success rate (IOP < 21 mm Hg) for uncomplicated glaucoma. Ophir and Ticho (124) found good success (IOP < 21 mm Hg) in uncomplicated glaucomas, but the follow-up time was short. A prospective, randomized, multicenter study (100) with a 1-year follow-up showed that in initial guarded fistulization, the final IOP and number of medications needed were significantly lower with surgery and 5-FU treatment than with surgery without an antimetabolite.

The work with mitomycin C evolved in a pattern similar to that of 5-FU. Initial studies were done in the mid 1980s using the technique of intraoperative pledget application described by Chen in 1983 (52). These studies were done in high-risk eyes, with fairly high doses and prolonged intraoperative mitomycin exposure (71,73–75,101,125–128). The success rates were equivalent to or slightly better than those in the 5-FU studies, but largely without the surface toxicity side effects. For example, Chen et al (81) reported a success rate (IOP $<$ 21 mm Hg) of 78% in a population of high-risk prior-surgery eyes, using a dose of 100 to 400 µg/mL for 5 minutes. The next year, Palmer (129) studied a similar high-risk group and found success (IOP at target, no VF progression) in 84% of patients followed for 6 to 42 months. In African-American patients, Kupin et al (77) found significantly lower IOPs at all follow-up visits after mitomycin procedures than after historical control procedures performed without antimetabolite. It is very difficult to meta-analyze such studies into a coherent group because there was no standard for defining "successful IOP control." Some authors allowed pressure-lowering medications and some did not; some used 21 mm Hg as a goal, while others used arbitrary target pressures for each patient. However, the studies provided evidence that the effect of mitomycin was a lower final IOP in these high-risk eyes.

COMPLICATIONS OF ANTIMETABOLITE USE

Given that these drugs can do an impressive job minimizing fibrosis after fistulization surgery, it is tempting to consider using them routinely. The decision to include antimetabolite therapy for a given patient is not a small one, for the potential complications and side effects are many.

Perhaps the most frustrating complication is that the antimetabolite therapy may work too well, prevent even minimal scarring, and result in profound hypotony (77,82, 126,127,130–147). Histopathologic studies have shown that mitomycin can greatly inhibit the fibrovascular response, in some cases well after the original surgical application (27,28,30,37).

This hypotony was noted even in high-risk eyes. When mitomycin began being used in initial surgeries in low-risk eyes, hypotony was even more frequent. For example, Mirza et al (78) reported in 1994 that patients with uncomplicated glaucoma who had fistulas created with mitomycin had an average postoperative IOP of 4 mm Hg at 17 months after surgery. Mitomycin was applied at a concentration of 500 µg/mL for 3 minutes to the episclera and 2 minutes under the scleral flap. Patients who had identical surgeries performed without mitomycin had an average IOP of 10 mm Hg.

The prevalence of postoperative hypotony led to a search for the lowest mitomycin dose that would still maintain the antifibrotic effect. Unfortunately, differences in patient populations and variability of relevant intraoperative techniques (such as ostomy and flap size) make direct comparisons across studies difficult. Mitomycin doses in these studies have ranged from 20 to 500 µg/mL for times of 2 to 5 minutes. Kitazawa et al (138) showed that 20 µg/mL applied for 5 minutes is substantially less effective than 200 µg/mL applied for a similar time. Several studies indicated that doses between 200 and 500 µg/mL may have equivalent effects (79,140), and that lower doses for shorter

exposure times are associated with fewer immediate postoperative complications (140).

Despite the pattern toward lower doses of mitomycin C, hypotony is still a significant problem. Methods of dealing with prolonged hypotony have shown variable success and are discussed in another chapter in this text.

Hypotony is a major concern with use of mitomycin but corneal problems are rare. When postoperative 5-FU is used, the chief concern is corneal epithelial toxicity, a very common problem (58–68). Suggestions for minimizing corneal complications of 5-FU are dose regulation or dose delay (97,148–152), use of a bandage soft contact lens to protect the corneal epithelium (153), incising the conjunctiva well back from the corneal limbus (97), and waiting until fairly late in the postoperative course so that the true necessity for 5-FU injections can be established (94). Work has been done to deliver 5-FU intraoperatively, to minimize the need for postoperative injections and the surface problems associated with that system (71,85,87,88, 91,96).

While corneal epithelial complications are common with 5-FU, they are usually only a nuisance in the greater picture of the patient's ongoing care. Vision-threatening complications such as endophthalmitis are also more likely in eyes having undergone antimetabolite-aided surgeries (37,79,103,147,154–160). This may be due in part to the higher incidence of thin bleb walls and bleb leaks that occur both early after surgery and in the late postoperative period (29,34,35,68,78,84,126,137,142,161–167).

At this point of the evolution of antimetabolite use, it was accepted that each agent improved the likelihood of success of fistulization surgery to reduce IOP over the long term. Compared to surgery without an antimetabolite, use of each drug carried an increased risk of endophthalmitis. Use of mitomycin caused more hypotony, and postoperative 5-FU injections caused more corneal toxicity. A significant question remained: Which one "worked" better?

Studies directly comparing the two antimetabolites have shown mixed results. Kitazawa et al (89) compared 32 high-risk eyes and found success (IOP $<$ 21 mm Hg without drops) rates of 88% for mitomycin C and 47% for 5-FU in a follow-up period that ranged from 7 to 12 months. In a randomized clinical trial, Skuta et al (74) compared postoperative 5-FU administration with intraoperative mitomycin C in 39 eyes. The mitomycin group showed significantly lower IOPs at 6 months postoperatively, less corneal toxicity, and less need for pressure-reducing medications. Lamping and Belkin (99) studied pseudophakic eyes and found significantly lower IOPs and fewer antiglaucoma medications in the mitomycin group at 1-year of follow-up. Katz et al (128) reported increased success with fewer medications in the mitomycin group, in a long-term (32 months) study in high-risk eyes. However, Prata et al (113) found no difference in final IOP or complication rates between mitomycin-treated and 5-fluorouracil–treated pseudophakic eyes. Most of these studies had comparable rates of short-term complications, with mitomycin causing a slightly increased risk of choroidal detachment or encapsulated filtering blebs compared with 5-FU groups. Specific long-term complications of cataract formation and corneal endothelial cell loss were comparable between the two drugs (80).

Because of these results, most surgeons regard mitomycin as a superior choice over 5-FU in many situations. The ease of application, greater antifibrotic effect, and minimal corneal toxicity outweigh the increased chance of postoperative hypotony. Most surgeons have responded to the risk of hypotony by more secure closure of the scleral flap and reducing the time and concentration of intraoperative mitomycin exposure. With use of either agent, it must be remembered that thin blebs pose a risk for late endophthalmitis (37,79,103,147,154–160). These patients must be monitored closely. At present, many surgeons use a low dose of intraoperative mitomycin and augment with postoperative 5-FU injections if the clinical course dictates.

Once the choices of antimetabolite usage and dose have been completed, the surgeon's attention turns to the fistulization procedure itself. It may be seductive, especially to the inexperienced glaucoma physician, to think that the antimetabolite use will be so effective at inhibiting healing that careful attention to surgical detail is not required. Even antifibrotic agents cannot overcome sloppy surgical technique, and the tissues must be respected. Rather than being "forgiving," use of antimetabolites may actually decrease the margin for error, since hypotony may be longer-lived. The surgical healing process is similar to a metabolic cascade— tissue injury leads to inflammation which results in scarring. In glaucoma surgery, scarring is often synonymous with failure. It is far easier to control the magnitude of the final steps if the cascade has been limited earlier in the process. Since the antimetabolites affect only the latest stages of the healing response (scarring), if the tissues have been abused and inflammation is excessive, even a maximal dose of antimetabolite may not be sufficient to prevent surgical failure. The key to good results is to keep the cascade from beginning, by minimizing tissue injury and inflammation. In filtration surgery, this is achieved through minimal and gentle tissue manipulation, light scleral and ciliary body cautery sufficient to preclude postoperative hemorrhage, and avoidance of excessive iris trauma. Conversely, poor surgical technique can contribute to excessive filtration and conjunctival wound leaks, especially in the presence of antimetabolites.

INDICATIONS FOR GUARDED FISTULIZATION

The decision to perform guarded fistulization surgery can be very difficult. As for any surgery, the decision to proceed is based on an estimate of the risk–benefit ratio. The same analysis must be considered for the other treatment options, including no treatment, continued medical treatment, laser therapy, and placement of implant devices.

The list of potential complications of guarded fistulization with or without antimetabolite is long and includes loss of vision, suprachoroidal hemorrhage, endophthalmitis, retinal detachment, and cataract (139,157,158,168–181). Over the years, a fairly stable consensus has been derived that incisional surgery carries too high a risk to be considered as a first step in chronic open-angle glaucoma treatment, although some authors disagree (182–185). The CIGT Study is under way to address this question. Some authors found early surgery to be less expensive than chronic use of medications (186). There is evidence that long-term use of topical medications may decrease the success rate if surgery is eventually required (187–190). However, the IOP in some patients is well controlled with long-term medications and these eyes may never need surgery. Thus, this potential advantage does not apply to the majority of patients, while the risk of early surgery does apply to all eyes undergoing surgery. Spirited comparisons of opinion are fascinating to read and provide a range of perspectives (50,191). Some authors favored simultaneous bilateral fistulization to minimize hospital costs and patient rehabilitation time (192). A well-accepted paradigm for stepped glaucoma care begins with those medications each individual patient tolerates with a minimum of side effects, and if pressure is uncontrolled on these medications, laser trabeculoplasty is then considered. When both laser and pharmaceutical options have been exhausted, surgery is often appropriate. An important variable to consider in each case is the rate of loss of vision. Patients with rapid visual loss may benefit from surgery far earlier in the course of treatment than elderly patients with a very slow visual decline, for whom the amount of visual loss would never significantly affect their daily activities. The timing of surgery for any given patient must be individualized and is based on the amount of visual field loss, the rate of change, level of IOP control with nonsurgical treatment, and the effect on the patient's lifestyle over his or her lifetime.

Once the decision to proceed to surgery is made, and the consideration of antimetabolite use completed, attention is turned to the procedure itself.

PREOPERATIVE PREPARATIONS

Antiglaucoma Medications

Most patients coming to surgery will be taking antiglaucoma medications preoperatively, and aqueous production will be suppressed. In the immediate postoperative period, aqueous production falls further due to the inflammation from the surgery, and temporary hypotony may result. Discontinuation of carbonic anhydrase suppression and β-blockade for several days preoperatively can help to minimize the ciliary body shutdown. Some surgeons use pilocarpine preoperatively to constrict the pupil and help minimize or prevent any intraoperative lens-corneal touch during the creation of the scleral fistula. This postoperative advantage must be weighed against the increased risk of suprachoroidal hemorrhage in eyes with elevated IOP (117).

Anti-inflammatory Agents

Steroids do not have immediate anti-inflammatory effects, requiring time to modulate expression of inflammatory-control genes. Therefore some surgeons prefer to begin steroid treatment before the day of surgery. Three to 5 days of topical or oral steroids in anticipation of the surgery date is usually enough time to have maximally developed inhibitory effects (23,24).

Antibiotics

Preoperative antibiotics can be given for several days before surgery to minimize colonization of the conjunctiva, as is sometimes done in preparation for cataract surgery. Gentamicin should be avoided owing to its toxic inflammatory effects on the conjunctiva, and neomycin is avoided because of its allergic effects.

Site Selection

It is important to plan the surgery before entry into the operating room. At the clinic slit lamp, the topically anesthetized conjunctiva can be manipulated with a moist cotton-tipped applicator, and a quadrant where the conjunctiva is mobile and free of adhesions to the sclera can be chosen. Nasal trabeculectomies are associated with lower IOP postoperatively (193), and it is wise to decenter the incision to the middle of the quadrant, leaving untouched as much conjunctiva as possible in consideration of needs for future surgeries. Placing the fistula site in the nasal quadrant also allows easier temporal access if subsequent cataract extraction should become necessary. Trabeculectomies in the inferior quadrant have similar (194) or worse (195) success rates than do those in superior-quadrant sites. Blebs at the inferior limbus have a higher rate of endophthalmitis (195), presumably because the constant rubbing of the lower eyelid against the bleb surface allows more access of bacteria into the anterior chamber (196).

ANESTHETIC CONSIDERATIONS AND DRAPING THE EYE

General anesthesia is usually avoided for ocular surgery, because the patient population is often older and in poor health. In addition, the risk of awakening with nausea or coughing is higher with general anesthesia than with local anesthetic techniques. This increases the risk of suprachoroidal hemorrhage in freshly fistulized eyes, especially if the preoperative IOP pressure is high (117).

Local anesthesia is often the best choice for these cases. Most patients need some sort of orbicularis block, be it by the Atkinson, Nadbath, Van Lint, or O'Brien method. Injecting 1 to 3 mL of a 1 : 1 mixture of 2% lidocaine with hyaluronidase and 0.75% bupivacaine into the temporal canthal region is enough to paralyze the orbicularis for these procedures. Using this peripheral approach minimizes the danger of perforating major blood vessels and the parotid gland compared to blocks administered more centrally.

Retrobulbar and peribulbar injections of similar mixtures of local anesthetics have been used for years in guarded fistulization procedures, with great success. Recently, the move to subconjunctival or even topical anesthesia for cataract extraction has been investigated for glaucoma surgery (197–199). In general, these techniques require very particular attention to patient selection, as patient cooperation is critical. These superficial blocks also tend to have a shorter duration of action. If the surgeon is inexperienced, or the patient's condition makes complicated, difficult surgery more likely, the longer-acting peribulbar or retrobulbar methods should be chosen.

Patients with very vascular conjunctiva and Tenon's capsule present a significant anesthetic problem. The local anesthetic agent is carried out of the tissues quickly upon injection, so less of the tissue itself is anesthetized, and the surgery tends to require more time. These factors lead to incomplete and short-lived anesthesia. A common result is patient discomfort during closure of Tenon's layer and the conjunctiva. Irrigation of the orbital or posterior aspect of the subconjunctival space with more local anesthetic agent on a blunt cannula is usually adequate to control this recovery of sensation.

Because filtration surgery involves incising conjunctiva deep in the fornix, exposure and draping are important. The speculum should provide maximum separation of the lids without creating any external pressure on the globe. Since cilia are extremely hard to disinfect, it is important to isolate them from the operative field. This can be accomplished by trimming the lashes prior to the iodine scrub, or by covering the lashes with a fold of the plastic drape. Some specula infraduct the eye by exerting pressure on the lower conjunctival fornix, obviating the need for a traction suture (200). Not all eyes are sufficiently infraducted with this technique, and often more definitive methods of traction are needed.

SURGICAL TECHNIQUES

The Traction Suture

Good exposure of the surgical field facilitates guarded fistulization. Most trabeculectomies are performed in the superior hemifield, requiring downward displacement of the globe. Two structures are strong enough to provide sufficient traction to supply this downward force: the rectus superior muscle and the cornea.

Superior Rectus Bridle Suture Technique

Placement of a superior rectus bridle suture, usually 4-0 silk on a tapered or cutting needle, is a common technique for cataract surgery. These sutures are placed 8 to 9 mm behind the limbus and supply good downward traction. The conjunctival incision for the fistulization is made anterior to the suture (Fig. 33-2).

There are three main drawbacks to this method:

1. **Hemorrhage.** The anterior ciliary arteries follow the course of the superior rectus tendon, and the forceps or needle may lacerate the vessels. Bleeding in this area makes identification of Tenon's capsule and conjunctiva very difficult for both dissection and closure, and any blood near the fistula brings fibroblasts, which can cause ultimate failure of the surgery.

2. **Distortion of landmarks.** Placement of a superior rectus suture may incorporate a wide area of conjunctiva. This "bunching" can be minimized by keeping the forceps closed until contacting the conjunctiva, then maintaining gentle pressure on the conjunctiva as the tips are allowed to open. In this way, the conjunctiva is stretched over the tendon, rather than being gathered by the open tips.

3. **Placement of incision.** The superior rectus muscle inserts 6.5 to 7.0 mm behind the limbus, and a common goal of fistulization surgery is to incise at 10 mm from the limbus. It can be very difficult to incise cleanly behind this type of suture and maintain sufficient downward traction. Therefore, use of a superior rectus bridle suture may force the incision to be anterior to 10 mm. By decreasing the distance from the ostomy to the conjunctival incision, the surgeon increases the risk of postoperative wound leak and hypotony.

Corneal Stroma Suture Technique

An alternative to the superior rectus suture is to place a traction stitch in the superior aspect of the cornea. A 5-0 or 6-0 polyglycolic acid (Dexon) or silk suture, on a spatulated side-cutting needle (e.g., Davis+Geck 7505-13) supplies sufficient traction for a posterior incision, without conjunctival distortion or hemorrhage. Silk sutures have also been used (201). Before beginning, a surgical marking pen is used to place small marks on the conjunctival limbus at the two quadrant edges (i.e., at 9- and 12-o'clock positions for a temporal filter on a right eye) (Fig. 33-3). This keeps landmarks visible for the rest of the procedure. If the anterior ciliary arteries can be visualized through the conjunctiva,

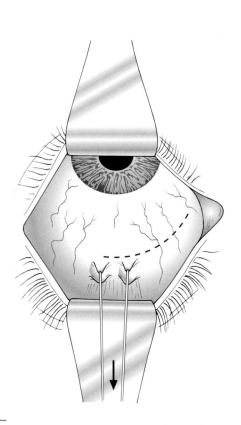

FIGURE 33-2. *Placement of superior rectus bridle suture.*

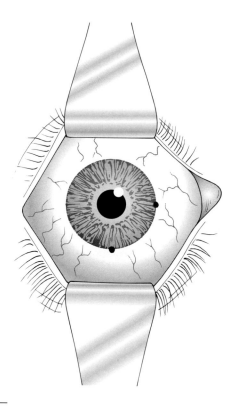

FIGURE 33-3. *Marking the meridians. Without manipulation of the position of the eye in the orbit, the cardinal meridians of the quadrant are marked. To avoid spread of the surgical ink, careful drying with cellulose sponges is required prior to marking.*

they can also be used as markers of the quadrant. Then, with either a toothed forceps to grasp corneal stroma, or a muscle hook placed into the conjunctival fornix directly behind the intended penetration angle, the suture is placed for 3 to 5 mm into half the depth of the cornea (Fig. 33-4). If it becomes evident that the anterior chamber has been entered, it is necessary to remove the suture, re-form the chamber if needed, and replace the stitch in a new corneal track.

The suture is placed 2 mm inside the corneal limbus to avoid the visual axis and yet allow room for dissection of the sclerocorneal flap, and is centered directly anterior to the intended site of the flap where it functions as a landmark to guide dissection.

With either of these traction sutures in place, the suture is then clamped to the inferior drape with a mosquito snap or fixed to the lower blade of the lid speculum, allowing exposure of the bulbar conjunctiva as far into the superior fornix as possible (Fig. 33-5). If a superior rectus bridle suture is used, good infraduction of the eye might be obtained by fixing the suture to the superior drape.

Conjunctival Incision

Creation of the conjunctival incision is an important factor in the success of guarded fistulization, both to avoid short-term complications and to allow long-term success.

Limbus-Based Versus Fornix-Based Conjunctival Incision

The goal of this surgery is to create an anterior-chamber fistula, and access to the subconjunctival limbal tissues is required. The conjunctiva can be incised at the limbus and drawn posteriorly, or incised posteriorly and elevated to expose the underside of the limbal insertion.

Neither incision is dramatically superior in terms of either final IOP control or percentage of cases that are successful (202–206). However, the characters of the blebs are quite different, as are the short-term problems (207,208).

Limbus-based flaps usually result in a high, localized bleb, and if incised far enough behind the limbus, rarely leak. They require far more conjunctival incision and dissection, are more likely to result in conjunctival hemorrhage, and take more time and surgical effort to close adequately.

Fornix-based flaps are quickly dissected, with less need for cautery, and usually result in a more flattened, diffuse bleb. They are more likely to leak in the early postoperative phase, until the corneal margin re-epithelializes (206,209–213).

Technique

Fornix-Based Conjunctival Flaps   With smooth or serrated forceps, limbal peritomy of the conjunctiva and Tenon's capsule is performed with rounded-tip Wescott scissors. With the scissor tips kept flat against the sclera on both sides of the conjunctival insertion, small bites are used to free the conjunctiva, with care not to leave any tags at the insertion. It is easiest to cut both Tenon's capsule and the con-

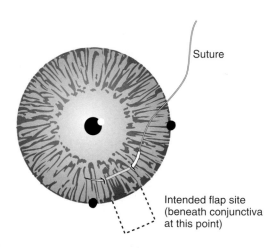

Suture

Intended flap site
(beneath conjunctiva
at this point)

FIGURE 33-4.   *Placement of the corneal traction stitch. With the limits of the quadrant marked at the limbus, a suture is placed into the cornea to provide traction. The track is parallel to the limbus, far enough from the conjunctival insertion to allow creation of the scleral flap. The entry and exit points of the track should correspond to the intended width of the sides of the scleral flap. The track is then used as a guide during creation of the scleral flap.*

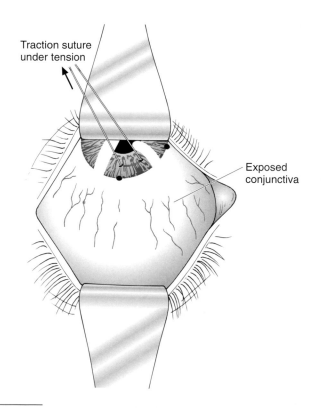

Traction suture
under tension

Exposed
conjunctiva

FIGURE 33-5.   *Infraduction of the eye, corneal traction stitch. With the track completed, the needle is removed and the traction suture tied. Force is applied to the stitch to expose the intended quadrant, and the suture is clipped to the drape or speculum.*

junctiva simultaneously, but this may be done in two layers (Fig. 33-6).

An alternative is to use a rounded-tip Beaver blade (No. 69 or 66). The conjunctiva is grasped several millimeters behind the limbus with smooth forceps and elevated from the sclera. The blade is held parallel to the corneoscleral junction, aiming posteriorly, and the conjunctiva and Tenon's insertions are lysed. Angling the blade away from a parallel position may result in cutting into the sclera (Fig. 33-7).

The incision is widened until enough exposure is created to dissect and secure the planned flap. This is usually 2 to 3 mm on each side of the intended flap edges.

Limbus-Based Conjunctival Flap With the eye maximally rotated away from the intended incision site, an arc of conjunctiva 8 to 10 mm posterior to the limbus is marked with a surgical pen (Fig. 33-8). The ends of this arc should overlie the rectus muscles on either side of the quadrant. The line is made wide enough to be useful to identify the anterior and posterior edges of the conjunctiva during closure.

With the marked line as a guide, smooth forceps and rounded-tip scissors are used to incise conjunctiva only. Conjunctiva is separated from Tenons's layer by undermining in all directions, particulary anteriorly and posteriorly. This step allows easy closure of the conjunctival layer separately from Tenon's layer. Inadvertent dog-ear flaps are excised.

The incision into Tenon's capsule is made parallel to the conjunctival incision, but 2 to 3 mm more posteriorly. Staggering the incisions helps to avoid wound leaks. Tenon's capsule is incised more posteriorly because the anterior edge tends to fray and roll during the manipulations during the rest of the procedure. By incising away from the limbus, one can easily identify Tenon's capsule and close it at its edge, avoiding "dragging" the incision forward and allowing formation of as large a bleb as possible.

Incising Tenon's capsule while avoiding hidden rectus muscles and orbital fat takes attention and care. It is best to work from the center of the quadrant out toward the muscles. Tenon's capsule is grasped with the smooth forceps and elevated from the globe, and round-tipped scissors are

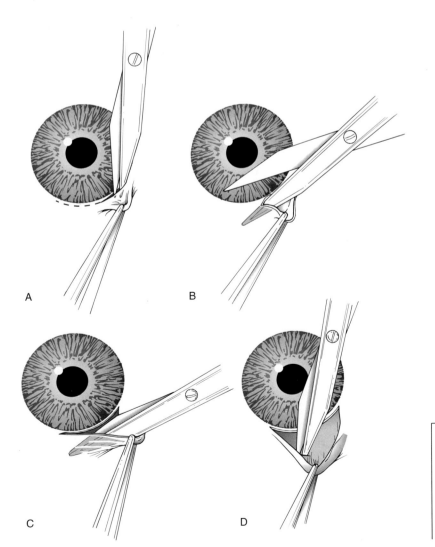

A   B

C   D

FIGURE 33-6. *Limbal peritomy, scissors technique. The conjunctiva and Tenon's capsule tissues are elevated with smooth forceps, and the limbal insertion of each is lysed with rounded-tip scissors. Care is taken to avoid creation of dog-ear flaps and to completely remove Tenon's insertion. The width is appropriate to barely expose the sides of the intended flap and allow for placement of flap sutures.*

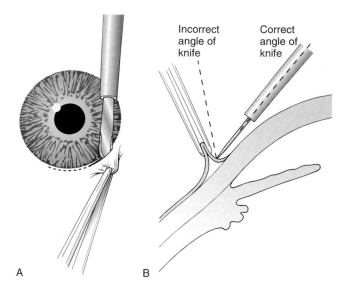

FIGURE 33-7. *Limbal peritomy, blade method. A. While the conjunctiva and Tenon's capsule are elevated with a smooth forceps, a rounded-tip blade is used to lyse insertions of each tissue at the limbus. B. Care is taken to hold the blade parallel to the scleral surface, cutting posteriorly.*

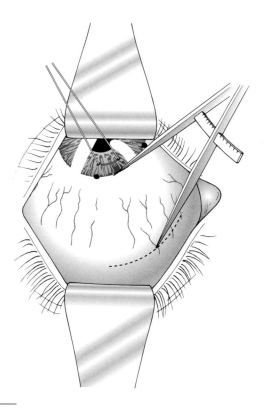

FIGURE 33-8. *Marking intended conjunctival insertion, for limbus-based flap. As the quadrant is exposed with traction inferiorly, the conjunctival surface is dried completely with cellulose sponges. A surgical marking pen and calipers are used to mark a line 10 mm behind the limbus, extending just beyond the muscles on either side of the quadrant. This line is wide enough to be used as a landmark when the conjunctiva is closed later during the procedure.*

used to sharply and bluntly dissect perpendicularly toward the scleral surface until sclera is seen. Often, the assistant may grasp one edge of the Tenon's layer to help evert the incision (Fig. 33-9).

Once sclera is identified, the anterior margin of Tenon's layer is undermined to free up a visible flap. With care to stay superficial to the muscles, Tenon's layer is then bluntly and sharply dissected in both directions toward the limit of the quadrant. Especially in the area of the superior rectus, it is important to pick up the tissue with one jaw of the scissors, and elevate it clearly off the sclera before closing the jaws and cutting. With this technique, it is possible to visualize and avoid the muscle tendon and anterior ciliary arteries.

To allow a large posterior bleb, the adhesions of Tenon's capsule posterior to the incision are then bluntly dissected in the entire quadrant. Maximal bleb size is promoted by dissection posteriorly with Westcott scissors until the hub of the scissors is buried.

With the conjunctival-Tenon's circumferential incision created, attention is then turned to dissecting Tenon's capsule free from the episclera anteriorly. This is done by both blunt and sharp dissection, with care to preserve the conjunctival insertion at the limbus. It is helpful to watch the scissor tips through the conjunctiva to ensure that no conjunctival buttonholes are created. To avoid forcing a tip of the scissors through the delicate conjunctival insertion, the scissors must be pointed directly radially at all times. This evenly distributes the force to each tip and minimizes the possibility of creating a buttonhole at the conjunctival insertion. It will be necessary to pivot the scissors around the limbus as the margins of the quadrant are being dissected (Fig. 33-10).

Dissection of this sub-Tenon's space all the way to the limbus makes creation of the scleral flap much easier. Because the area of dissection stimulates wound-healing responses in the tissues, some attention has been given to techniques that minimize dissection anteriorly, with the thought that these blebs would be less inflamed and therefore function for longer periods (214). With the further development and success of antimetabolite use, this approach has not become popular.

It may become obvious that the intended scleral flap area cannot be fully exposed unless the original conjunctival incision is widened. This should be done in two layers, similar to the original technique.

There is often a remnant of Tenon's insertion at the limbus that is difficult to remove with scissors dissection. A Gill knife can be used to stretch the last few fibers of Tenon's insertion without putting the conjunctival insertion at risk of perforation. The blade is held perpendicular to the scleral surface, and without sawing side to side, the fibers are pushed forward radially until they lyse. This is continued until only the conjunctival insertion is left (Fig. 33-11).

Dry cellulose sponges can also be used to free Tenon's

insertion if the layers are not tightly adherent. If prior surgery has been performed, dissection of the conjunctiva and Tenon's capsule from the episclera can be very difficult. Sodium hyaluronate may be useful to bluntly dissect this plane, particularly after extracapsular cataract surgery (215).

It is possible to perform guarded fistulization without conjunctival incision, accessing the iris and peripheral cornea through a corneal incision. However, these surgeries have mixed results in terms of long-term control of IOP (216–222).

Cautery

In fistulization surgery, hemorrhage is a much bigger problem than in almost any other ocular surgery. The same amount of bleeding that helpfully "stimulates wound healing" in cataract surgery incisions may be enough hemorrhage to cause a guarded fistulization to fail. If only an intraoperative antimetabolite is used, those cells brought to the site by late intraoperative or postoperative bleeding are untreated and freely make scar tissue.

This argues for extensive cautery of the operative site. However, balancing the concern for complete hemostasis is the effect of overcauterization and tissue necrosis. Few things are as chemotactic for healing and scarring as necrosis, and excessive fibroblast migration may overwhelm the fibroblastostatic effect of the antimetabolite. Cautery to the point of tissue char negates the benefit of hemostasis.

The correct balance is enough cautery to provide a white operative field, with the major scleral feeder vessels well cauterized. Char is to be avoided, especially near the limbus. Cauterizing the larger vessels posteriorly first will limit how much anterior cautery is needed. A bipolar eraser tip with enough power to constrict the larger vessels and enough surface area to gently close the capillaries works particularly well at this stage. The final step of cautery is to outline the intended scleral flap area, with the goal of a bloodless flap bed. Cautery tips have been designed especially for guarded fistulization, allowing cautery of both surface sclera and intraocular iris and ciliary body vessels (223).

Antimetabolite Administration and Scleral Flap Construction

Opinions have been divided about which step to perform next—create the scleral flap to allow treatment with an antimetabolite above and below the flap itself, or treat with an antimetabolite first.

Rationale for Applying an Antimetabolite First

Proponents of antimetabolite application before flap creation cite two major reasons for this sequence. First, the layer most responsible for fibrosis, and therefore most needing antimetabolite treatment, is the episclera–inner Tenon's

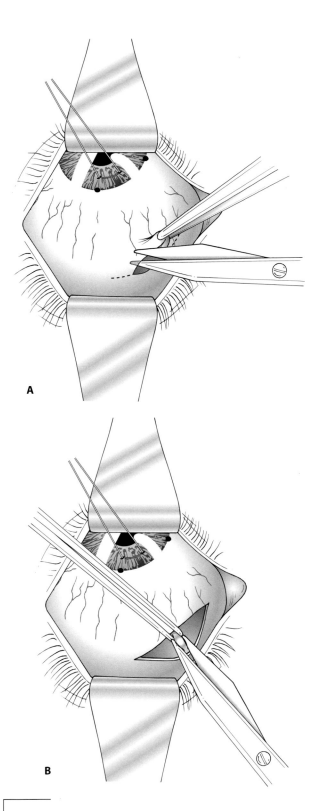

FIGURE 33-9. *Staggering incisions in conjunctiva and tenon's capsule. After opening the conjunctiva along the inked line and undermining in all directions to separate Tenon's capsule from the conjunctiva, an incision is made into Tenon's capsule. The incision should be parallel to and 1 to 2 mm posterior to the conjunctival incision.*

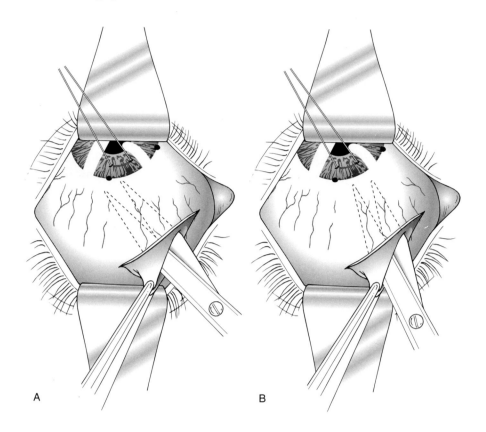

FIGURE 33-10. *Lysing Tenon's insertion at the corneal limbus. As Tenon's layer is separated from episclera toward the limbus, care must be taken when Tenon's insertion is encountered. The scissors must be rotated, keeping the two tips in gentle contact with the limbus before each spreading or cutting action. Spreading the jaws when only one tip is in contact with the insertion may cause sufficient force to create a limbal buttonhole.*

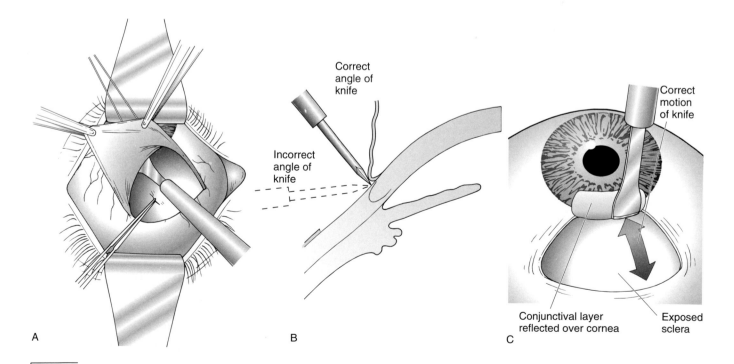

FIGURE 33-11. *Use of a Gill knife for Tenon's disinsertion. Lysing the final remnants of the limbal insertion of Tenon's capsule may require use of blunt force with a rounded knife. The knife is kept perpendicular to the scleral surface, and care is taken to keep a radial motion, not cutting the insertion with circumferential cuts.*

layer. Placing the antimetabolite under the flap may not significantly affect the cells on the flap's episcleral surface.

The second reason is the risk of intraocular penetration of the antimetabolite if applied after the eye has been entered surgically. Kee et al (224) showed that exposure of monkey eyes to mitomycin, without any incisional surgery, significantly reduced aqueous production. Mietz and Addicks (225) found histopathologic evidence of damage to the ciliary nerves after application of mitomycin over full-thickness sclera in rabbit eyes. Seah et al (226) measured intraocular levels of mitomycin C after above-flap and below-flap applications, and found a sevenfold greater intraocular concentration with below-flap application. Mietz and Rump (227) found a wide range of intraocular concentrations of mitomycin in sclera, vitreous, and aqueous humor that did not correlate with the amount of mitomycin given. These findings indicate that some intraocular penetration may occur through even full-thickness sclera, but other studies did not find significant intraocular levels or damage (228,229).

Since mitomycin is also very toxic to the corneal endothelium (43,56,225), its use is relatively contraindicated if the eye has been accidentally entered during creation of the scleral flap (43). If the antimetabolite is applied before flap creation, there is no risk of inadvertent penetration and the drug can safely be applied as planned.

Rationale for Creating the Scleral Flap First

Proponents of the under-the-flap treatment believe that they achieve lower IOP postoperatively. This may be due to decreased production of aqueous from penetration of mitomycin into the ciliary body, to better limitation of fibroblastic activity, or both.

Application of the Antimetabolite

Prior to application of the antimetabolite, the limbus, conjunctival flap edges, and the fornix should be completely dried with cellulose sponges. It is important to clear these fluid menisci, as they can act to wick the antimetabolite to the incision margins.

Any porous material that can transfer fluid to the sclera may be used as a pledget for the antimetabolite. Weck Cel and Merocel sponges work well (76). Two factors are most important: the size of the pledget and the amount of saturation.

Size of the Pledget

The pledget should be just large enough to extend slightly beyond the edges of the planned flap. Its thickness is less important, as long as it is thin enough to allow easy placement beneath the conjunctival margins. Some surgeons trim and discard the distal end of the cellulose spear and then cut several more thin strips from the trimmed end, selecting the best size following hydration. If all of the strips seem to thick, it is possible to cut the spear in half parallel to the longest width with an iris scissors, and then trim the strips (164). This method creates a very thin pledget, most appro-

priate for use with fornix-based flaps with more difficult access to the limbal sclera.

Saturation of the Pledget

In early papers describing the results of fistulization with mitomycin C, a wide variability of antifibrotic effect was seen. With delivery by a pledget, three variables influence the tissue effect: concentration of the drug in the solution, duration of pledget contact with the tissues, and the amount of drug in the pledget. Exposure time and concentration are easily controlled, but saturation of the pledget is difficult to standardize, and the amounts remaining in the pledgets after application vary widely (230). Mietz et al (231) suggested a scleral shield device to limit the penetration of mitomycin through the sclera. Surgery employing this device showed fewer toxic changes in a rabbit model (231). Whether by device or consistent technique, each surgeon needs a system to reproducibly load the pledget, so that the time and concentration variables can be used to titrate the effect desired. Simply tapping the flat side of the pledget against the wall of the container is usually enough to ensure consistent saturation.

Once sized and loaded with antimetabolite, the pledget is transferred to the operative site and applied to the sclera. To avoid wound leaks, contact of the pledget with the conjunctival edges must be carefully avoided. With the pledget in place, timing is begun, and any fluid is meticulously dried.

If exposure of Tenon's capsule to the antimetabolite is desired, the conjunctiva-Tenon's flap is then draped over the pledget, avoiding any contact of the pledget with the conjunctival edges. If the conjunctiva is extremely thin and the patient has no risk factors for copious postoperative scarring, it may be enough to treat only the scleral surface.

On completion of the planned exposure time, the conjunctiva-Tenon's flap is carefully elevated and the pledget removed (232). The area is copiously irrigated with 15 to 45 mL of balanced salt solution.

To avoid contaminating tissue forceps with mitomycin, it is useful to use different forceps exclusively to handle the pledget and then remove those forceps from the operative field.

Creation of the Scleral Flap

Historically, full-thickness procedures provided direct outflow of aqueous, with lower final pressures and less chance of surgical failure (233). The natural history of these holes was of dramatic flow of fluid in the first weeks after the procedures, and a gradual decrease of flow as long-term scarring occurred. The period of high flow resulted in many flat anterior chambers, cataracts, decompensated corneas, and prolonged choroidal effusions. Lens-corneal touch after surgery causes dramatic changes in the corneal endothelium and lens and should be avoided at all costs (234). Flat anterior chambers can be prevented with intraoperative titration of aqueous flow or by placement of chamber-retaining sutures (235).

Although the good long-term pressure control of full-thickness procedures is very desirable, most surgeons believe that the short-term complication and reoperation rates are unacceptably high. The half-thickness procedures, with the ostomy guarded by some other tissue, such as Tenon's capsule or sclera, were developed to minimize the period of overfiltration. The resistance to flow in the early postoperative period can be affected by every variable of this portion of the surgery: the size of the flap, the thickness of the flap, and the size and location of the ostomy. This step is where the art begins.

The flap is first outlined with light cautery, both to minimize bleeding during the flap dissection and to serve as a landmark for the flap-edge cuts.

Flap shape varies from rectangular, with the long axis parallel to the limbus, to triangular, to trapezoidal (i.e., a truncated triangle), to square. The flap should be large enough to completely seal the intended ostomy, with enough room to secure it with several black 10-0 nylon sutures. The exact size and shape of the flap vary among surgeons, and differences of shape have not been correlated with overall success.

A rough guideline for the size of the flap is 2 to 4 mm both limbally and radially. The globe needs to be well fixated for flap creation, and either a firm grasp with 0.12-mm toothed forceps or a scleral twistpick can be used (Fig. 33-12). The pick has the advantage of rarely needing to be adjusted and affords great control over the globe in all directions. The 0.12-mm forceps has the advantage of being familiar to most surgeons, but if many grasp-regrasp motions are necessary, the sclera may become thinned and

irregular, making flap sutures difficult to place later in the procedure. The twistpick is far less likely to fragment the scleral tissues.

Depth perception is important when beginning the flap dissection, and increased microscope magnification is helpful to judge the depth of the cuts. It is also beneficial to keep the flap edges dry throughout this step, to avoid any optical distortion of the cutting plane.

The edges of the flap are then cut with a sharp blade (Beaver blade No. 69, 57, or 66, or a diamond knife) to approximately half the scleral depth (Fig. 33-13). Olsen et al (236) studied 55 eye bank eyes and found the thickness of sclera near the limbus to be approximately 500 μm. Care is taken to ensure that the depth of the flap at the corners is the same as at the center of the sides. It is important to keep the blade perpendicular to the scleral surface while all three sides are cut, to allow good control of aqueous flow and firm tissues for flap closure. The sides of the flap are advanced as far as the conjunctival insertion will allow, with care taken not to cut through the conjunctiva itself. If all of Tenon's capsule has been released, the blue color of the corneal insertion should be seen in the anterior side cuts.

Once the depth is adequate on all sides, the edge of the flap is gently lifted and the half-depth plane followed anteriorly into the corneal blue line. The No. 57 blade makes the initiation of the flap particularly easy, for its hockey-stick shape allows the surgeon to start the cut "under the corner" of the flap without needing to grasp the flap itself (and so minimizing distortion of the flap tissues). Attention then turns to establishing a good and uniform flap thickness.

The standard technique to help ensure uniform depth of the flap along its entire course is to cut only those fibers "on stretch." With 0.12-mm toothed forceps the flap edge is gently raised until the base of the flap looks slightly rounded, like a fluid meniscus. This indicates that the scleral fibers at the anterior margin of the dissection are being stretched (Fig. 33-14).

By very gentle lysing of these fibers with the sharp blade, the lamella of sclera is followed forward to the limbus. If the same point on the arc of stretched scleral fibers is consistently lysed with the knife, the flap will maintain uniform thickness all the way up to the corneal limbus. The end point is visualization of clear-blue cornea anteriorly in the base of the flap. It is useful to periodically set the blade gently in the apex of the flap bed, allow the flap to fall over the blade, and move the conjunctival flap to allow visualization of the blade tip through the corneal surface. In this manner, the end point is visualization of the blade within clear cornea.

An alternative method is to create the flap in a scleral-tunnel fashion. With standard cataract instruments, the standard tunnel technique is used, incising only the posterior margin of the intended flap and creating a tunnel with a crescent or similar blade. The width of the flap, and the posterior starting point are adjusted to create a fistulization-

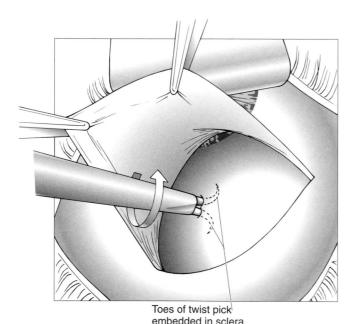

Toes of twist pick
embedded in sclera

FIGURE 33-12. *Scleral twistpick. The curved teeth of this instrument provide a gentle, secure method of fixing the globe during scleral flap creation. The two tips are placed in contact with the sclera, and gentle pressure is exerted while the pick is twisted.*

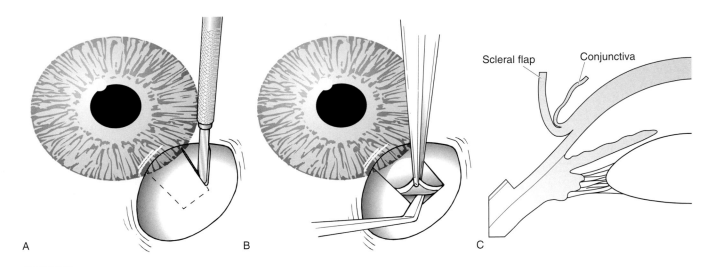

FIGURE 33-13. *Cutting the sides of the scleral flap. A sharp knife is used to create perpendicular, half-depth cuts into sclera to outline a flap. The limbal edge of the flap should be as far into cornea as the conjunctival insertion allows.*

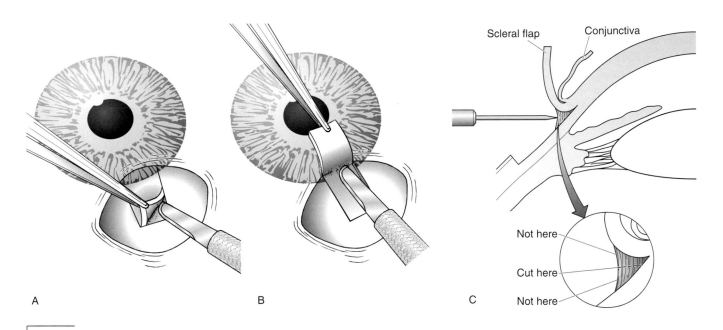

FIGURE 33-14. *Creation of the half-thickness flap. The scleral flap is cut forward into the limbus. Maintaining a uniform depth is key and can be accomplished by cutting those fibers "on stretch." As the flap is gently elevated with a toothed forceps, the tissue at the base of the flap creates a curved "meniscus" of tension. Cutting in the middle of the meniscus allows maintenance of uniform depth throughout the cut.*

sized half-thickness scleral flap. The end point is similar to that of a cataract surgery incision, ending when the crescent blade tip is visualized just into clear cornea. A Vannas scissors is then used to snip the sides of the tunnel, releasing the roof of the tunnel to create the scleral flap (237,238). The advantages of this method are its uniform depth, and that most surgeons may be more familiar with the technique. The disadvantages are the difficulty of cutting anteriorly into the cornea without harming the conjunctival insertion, and the difficulty of cutting the edges perfectly

perpendicular to the scleral bed. Flap sides that are not perpendicular may allow overfiltration in the immediate postoperative period. Perpendicularity can be accomplished by using multiple small cuts of the Vannas scissors, alternating cuts on each side of the flap as the roof is released toward the limbus.

With either method, the farther forward the dissection extends into clear cornea, the less likely the ostomy punch will incorporate ciliary body or iris root, minimizing the chance of hyphema (239,240). Many beginning surgeons stop when the blue limbus is reached, but it is helpful to extend the dissection a half millimeter beyond that landmark, into clear cornea itself. The factor that limits forward dissection is the conjunctival insertion, which must not be cut as the flap is extended. This is the importance of completely lysing Tenon's insertion with the Gill knife when the conjunctival flap is created, earlier.

Although scleral tissue is much more durable than conjunctiva, buttonholes or disinsertions of the scleral flap can still occur. Several methods are used to deal with these intraoperative problems, and include patching the hole with Tenon's layer (241) and placement of horizontal mattress sutures at the anterior flap margin (242,243). If the sclera is extremely thin, it may be impossible to create a half-thickness flap at all, and techniques have been described by which donor sclera can be used to cover a full-thickness hole in the thin host sclera (242).

The Paracentesis Incision

It is necessary to create a paracentesis in the peripheral cornea for two intraoperative reasons: maintenance of the anterior chamber once the flap and ostomy are created, and to provide fluid to assess flow as the scleral flap tension is being adjusted during closure. Any size paracentesis sufficient to permit passage of a 30- or 27-gauge cannula will be adequate. Often a 25- or 26-gauge needle is used, with its site marked with the surgical marker or the needle coated with fluorescein. This is an adequate size for both intraoperative uses.

However, it is wise to think ahead to a third use for the paracentesis: re-formation of the anterior chamber during the first few postoperative days if overfiltration occurs (244,245). The optimum size for these considerations is an opening that will allow easy passage of a viscoelastic cannula (27 gauge) under conditions of hypotony for several days postoperatively. A 25-gauge needle track may close too early postoperatively, and a larger slit is useful. A No. 75 blade can be used to create a larger but still self-sealing track. Making the sides of the track square will allow easy passage of the cannula later. Because these re-formations are often best done at the slit lamp, creating the ostomy in the temporal region of the cornea makes postoperative access much easier. A site near a larger subconjunctival blood vessel or other landmark facilitates finding the site at the slit lamp.

Regardless of the instrument chosen, the track is made parallel to the iris surface, to avoid contact with the iris or lens capsule below. Fixation of the globe is obtained by grasping the exposed scleral surface at the flap bed, or using a small toothed forceps to grasp cornea 180 degrees away from the track.

Releasing tension on the traction stitch before creation of the paracentesis will help avoid sudden loss of the anterior chamber.

Use of Viscoelastic Substance

Michielsens and Hennekes (246) investigated the use of intracameral viscoelastic substance during routine guarded fistulization, in an effort to protect the lens and cornea from shallowing of the anterior chamber intraoperatively and in the immediate postoperative period. Barak et al (247) found less damage of corneal endothelium and fewer shallow chambers, but increased numbers of postoperative pressure elevations. Raitta et al (248,249) found less severe postoperative chamber shallowing, more pressure elevations (statistically insignificant), and more hyphemas (250) when viscoelastic agents were used. Wand (251) proposed placing viscoelastic substance in the anterior chamber as the initial step of fistulization, to avoid hypotony even intraoperatively. No convincing data regarding protection from cataract progression have been published. Use of intraocular viscoelastic makes intraoperative titration of flow through the scleral flap very difficult.

Creation of the Ostomy

Determining the size and location of the sclerocorneal ostomy is the second step that makes the difference between a short- and long-lived fistula.

While gently fixating the flap with toothed forceps, the surgeon uses a No. 75 blade to make a cut at the anterior-most margin of the flap, nearly from one end of the flap to

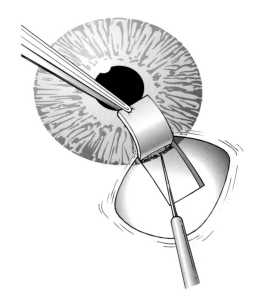

FIGURE 33-15.   *Cutting the ostomy. Once the flap has been dissected into the corneal tissue, a small, sharp blade is used to enter the peripheral region of the cornea. The cut should be slightly beveled but perpendicular enough to the iris to allow engagement of the posterior edge of the corneal incision by the punch. Care is taken not to extend all the way to the end of the flap, but to stop 1 mm from each end of the flap.*

the other. The slit must be long enough to allow passage of the corneal punch or Vannas scissors into the anterior chamber. To avoid a full-thickness hole, the slit should stop well within the bed of the flap (Fig. 33-15).

The knife should be held perpendicular to the scleral surface, and care is taken to cut only deep enough to penetrate the corneal tissue, avoiding iris, ciliary body, and lens zonules. As the anterior chamber is entered, aqueous will well into the flap bed.

Once the slit is completed, the ostomy itself is created, with a punch device or with Vannas scissors and a toothed forceps. The Kelly Descemet punch is a semicircular punch well suited to create a half-round opening. After the first punch of tissue is removed, the wound is directly inspected. Additional punches are made until the ostomy opening is adequate to allow free aqueous flow and avoid blockage by fibrin. For most flaps, a total of two full punch widths is adequate (Fig. 33-16). It is helpful to inspect the wound

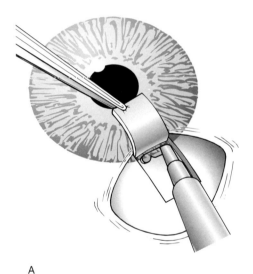

A

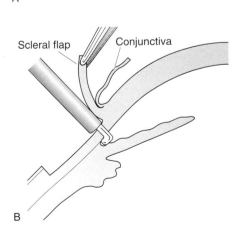

Scleral flap   Conjunctiva

B

FIGURE 33-16. *Completion of the ostomy. The Kelly Descemet punch is used to widen the corneal ostomy. For most flaps, a final ostomy equal to two full punch bites is adequate to allow sufficient flow of aqueous.*

after every punch to avoid incorporation of ciliary body or iris. It is also useful to pull up very slightly on the punch before cutting—if iris is inadvertently engaged in the punch, it will be seen to move slightly when viewed through the cornea, and the punch can be repositioned before the cut is made.

One of the main determinants of aqueous flow postoperatively is the distance the fluid travels between the ostomy edge and the flap edge. If this distance is short, little resistance is encountered and the fluid escapes readily, as in a full-thickness procedure. If the flap is large and the ostomy small and central, the tissue resistance is high, and the IOP will be higher postoperatively. Therefore, immediate IOP can be controlled by the size and location of the ostomy.

Recently, some surgeons (233) discussed offsetting the ostomy to one side of the flap. This maximizes flow once the flap is released by suture lysis or suture release but maintains the immediate pressure control postoperatively. This technique has the advantages of the full-thickness procedures for long-term IOP control, with a means of avoiding the early hypotony that full-thickness ostomies create.

New techniques being tested for ostomy creation include excimer laser ablation of the sclera overlying Schlemm's canal, leaving the meshwork intact to help control postoperative IOP (252).

The Iridectomy

The flow of aqueous through the scleral ostomy will pull along iris fibers into the opening. To keep the iris from plugging the hole, some of the iris tissue must be removed.

The optimum site for the iridectomy is directly under the ostomy, and the optimum size is slightly larger than the ostomy itself. This requires pulling the iris out of the eye to cut it at the level of the ostomy. It is easy to mistakenly incorporate ciliary body or iris root during this maneuver. The iris should be grasped through the anterior border of the ostomy with a toothed forceps, grasping only anterior iris stroma so as to avoid incorporating lens zonules. Withdrawing the forceps and tenting the iris stroma, the surgeon uses an angled scissors to press the sides of the ostomy gently down, and the iris is cut. The tips of the scissors must be closely watched to avoid cutting conjunctiva, the scleral flap, or the distal edge of the ostomy. Grasping sufficient stroma to allow this pull is most easily accomplished if the two arms of the forceps are kept truly radial, incorporating a full radial pillar of iris (Fig. 33-17).

Assessment of the patency of the iridectomy is accomplished by direct visualization of the ciliary body through the ostomy, and by establishment of the presence of transillumination. The ciliary body and iris root are then inspected for hemorrhage.

There are several accepted ways to control ciliary body

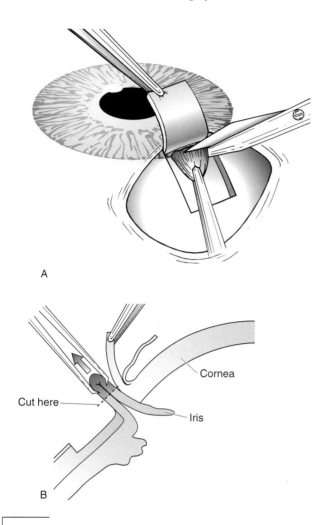

A

Cornea

Cut here

Iris

B

FIGURE 33-17. *Iridectomy technique. The surgical assistant gently elevates the scleral flap. A toothed or serrated iris forceps is used to grasp a pillar of iris. To avoid incorporation of the ciliary body, the jaws should be opened parallel to the limbus, so that a single pillar of iris is grasped. The jaws should be pressed gently against the pupillary margin of the ostomy, intending to grasp iris well away from the ciliary body and zonules. The iris is gently drawn into the ostomy, and scissors used to cut both iris stroma and pigment layers. Upon completion, the scleral flap is released, and the iridectomy inspected for transillumination and direct visualization of ciliary processes.*

hemorrhage—benign neglect, use of vasoconstrictors, and cautery. Benign neglect is often effective if bleeding is mild. For vigorous bleeding, cold balanced salt solution or preservative-free phenylephrine can be dropped directly onto the ciliary body. This works well but may have the unwanted side effect of mydriasis, which may allow capture of the iris into the ostomy overnight. Specialized 23-gauge needle-tip intraocular cautery devices (e.g., Mentor 22-1265) allow pinpoint application of cautery power. It is easy to cause shrinkage of the scleral ostomy tissue with overcautery, and this may result in a larger ostomy closer to the flap edge than originally intended. In rare cases,

the ciliary processes may be incarcerated in the ostomy, requiring resection (253).

Once the bleeding has ceased, the anterior-chamber depth is rechecked and re-formed by instillation of balanced salt solution through the paracentesis if necessary.

If vitrectomy is required in aphakic or pseudophakic eyes, it is best accomplished at this stage, so that any vitreous that might prolapse through the iridectomy can be removed (254).

Closure of the Scleral Flap

Closure of the scleral flap requires planning for the immediate postoperative period. If the patient needs immediate maximal IOP reduction, the flap should be secured loosely, and the sutures placed so as to be easily found with the laser for early lysis. If the patient is aphakic and immediate hypotony is to be avoided at all costs, the flap should be very securely fixed with multiple sutures, allowing many suture lyses and more control over daily IOP.

Some surgeons (255–257) place a loop of suture beneath the flap, passing through sclera outside the bled. The ends of this loop pass under the conjunctival surface and into the corneal surface, as for a releasable flap suture. Pulling this loop postoperatively causes lysis of the adhesions between the flap and the scleral bed.

In planning for early postoperative care, the surgeon has several choices of suture style. There are many excellent techniques for securing the flap, each with advantages. The easiest sutures to place are simple interrupted 10-0 nylon loops. Melting these with any colored laser source postoperatively releases traction on the flap, allowing more fluid flow and lower IOP (258). However, hemorrhage within the bleb may obscure these loops and prevent laser lysis (259). Use of polypropylene (Prolene) sutures may have a theoretical advantage, as they stretch before breaking, which may allow titration of increased aqueous flow without sudden hypotony (260). The same effect can be approximated by tying several sutures to different tensions, and lysing the tightest ones first. Blok et al (261) found a lower incidence of flat anterior chambers and corneal-lens touch postoperatively in patients with seven to nine flap sutures than in those with two to six sutures. Geijssen and Greve (134) found less hypotony with placement of at least seven flap sutures in eyes treated with mitomycin C intraoperatively, whereas Savage et al (262) found good titration of postoperative IOP with five sutures. Many devices have been designed to facilitate visualization and lysis of these sutures postoperatively (137,162,263–266).

Releasable sutures are an excellent idea if intrableb hemorrhage is anticipated. There are many ways to place these sutures (267–271) but all methods result in an end of the suture being fixed in the cornea, anterior to the conjunctival insertion. At the appropriate postoperative indication, this free end is gently pulled, undoing the knot and allowing the flap to separate from the scleral bed. These sutures have drawbacks: They are technically difficult to place without perforating the conjunctival insertion, the corneal ends of the stitch may cause foreign body irritation, and they provide a track through which infection can enter the bleb if they are not removed in the first few weeks after surgery.

Before antimetabolites were commonly used, releasability was a major concern, for healing occurred quickly. If laser lysis could not be performed in the first few postoperative days, by the time the hemorrhage cleared, cutting the stitch made no difference—the flap would have scarred to the scleral bed already.

But with the use of an antimetabolite, the "window" during which cutting the suture still affects the IOP can be weeks rather than days. This is usually enough time for the hemorrhage to clear, and has made the necessity of releasable sutures far less significant. In fact, with early use of high-dose mitomycin C, the window of useful lysis can extend several months postoperatively (272).

Flap sutures should be placed through the flap first, then placed through the scleral bed. A long scleral pass makes for a longer loop, which is easier to find under the slit lamp for lysis. For rectangular or square flaps, it is usually sufficient to secure the flap corners with two interrupted simple stitches. If the ostomy is large or decentered, or the flap is small, it may be necessary to limit flow further by adding sutures on the radial sides of the flap. Placing sutures as close to the limbus as possible will maximize the restriction of flow. After the corners are secure, the anterior chamber is reinflated with balanced salt solution, and the flap is dried with cellulose spears. Fresh sponges are then gently placed next to or directly on the flap-bed junction, and fluid flow into the sponge is monitored visually (Fig. 33-18). Some flow should occur without compressing the flap or bed. Titration of this flow is accomplished by adjust-ing or adding flap sutures. If an antimetabolite is used, less flow at this stage will help to avoid hypotony. There appears to be no advantage to attempting to avoid the requirement of laser suture lysis by sewing the flap sutures loosely—if suture lysis is carried out appropriately postoperatively, no difference in final IOP is seen (273–275).

When the flow is adequate, the sutures are rotated into the sclera to bury the knots, using a tying forceps or Kelman angled forceps. Although "cheese wiring" of the flap may occur during burial, it is important to bury all the knots to avoid erosion of the antimetabolite-treated conjunctiva. If tissues do not allow burial, an alternative is to trim the suture flush on the knot and rotate the knot away from the flap. Because manipulation of the sutures may stretch the flap and thereby loosen them, the flow of fluid around the flap edges should be reassessed following burial and immediately before closure of Tenon's capsule. It will likely be necessary to reinflate the anterior chamber with balanced salt solution to adequately assess flow. Some surgeons have used air to re-form the anterior chamber, with the idea that its higher surface tension would allow manipulation of the flap during sewing without allowing the chamber to fully deflate. Asamoto and Yablonski (276) found an increased incidence of anterior subcapsular cataract with the use of air and recommended use of either balanced salt solution or a viscoelastic substance.

Modifications of the flap have been recommended to allow additional flow through the fistula site by "tenting" the flap with a superficial stitch (277). Two studies investigating the effect of placing viscoelastic beneath the scleral flap have been published. One (278) found no effect on postoperative IOP, bleb size, or ultimate success of the surgery, but noted maintenance of a deeper anterior chamber postoperatively, with development of a thin, loculated bleb. The other study

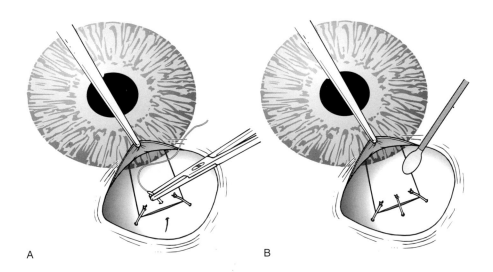

A   B

FIGURE 33-18. *Assessing the flow of aqueous. Following closure of the flap with sutures, flow is assessed by refilling the anterior chamber with saline solution through the paracentesis and monitoring the appearance of aqueous at the flap margins. Use of cellulose sponges, gently touched to the flap, can aid in visualization of the rate of flow.*

(279) found lower IOP, less need for postoperative timolol, and improved bleb appearance. These studies were performed prior to the availability of antimetabolite drugs.

Exactly how much flow is "enough" can be difficult to assess both intraoperatively and postoperatively. Many surgeons have thought that increased flow of aqueous in the immediate postoperative period would cause a larger, more succulent bleb to form and result in better long-term pressure control. Batterbury and Wishart (280) found no correlation with final IOP and this "high-flow" method of guarded fistulization.

With an appropriate amount of flow established, bleeding controlled, and the anterior chamber re-formed and stable, attention can then turn to closure of the conjunctiva and Tenon's capsule (Table 33-2).

Closure of Tenon's Capsule of the Limbus-Based Flap

The marking pen has identified the conjunctival edges, and these should be easily seen. Serrated forceps and cellulose sponges can be used to unroll anterior and posterior edges of both Tenon's capsule and conjunctiva. The anterior margin of Tenon's capsule is likely to be very thin owing to

the multiple manipulations during the surgery, and finding the true margin often is difficult. Having staggered the incision lines earlier will leave a longer margin of Tenon's capsule anteriorly, making it much easier to find and sew. While some surgeons prefer to perform a partial tenonectomy to help form a larger bleb, evidence suggests that this step does not significantly alter the final outcome (281,282).

Intraoperatively, Tenon's capsule is forgivingly watertight, and closure with a cutting needle is straightforward (Fig. 33-19). Absorbable sutures such as polyglactin (Vicryl)

Table 33-2.   Intraoperative Factors Influencing Final Intraocular Pressure (IOP)

Factors Favoring Low Final IOP	Factors Favoring High Final IOP
Large ostomy	Small ostomy
Small scleral flap	Large scleral flap
Short ostomy-to-flap edge distance (e.g., decentered ostomy)	Long ostomy-to-flap edge distance
Thin scleral flap	Thick scleral flap
Loosely secured flap	Tightly secured scleral flap
Few scleral flap sutures	Multiple flap sutures

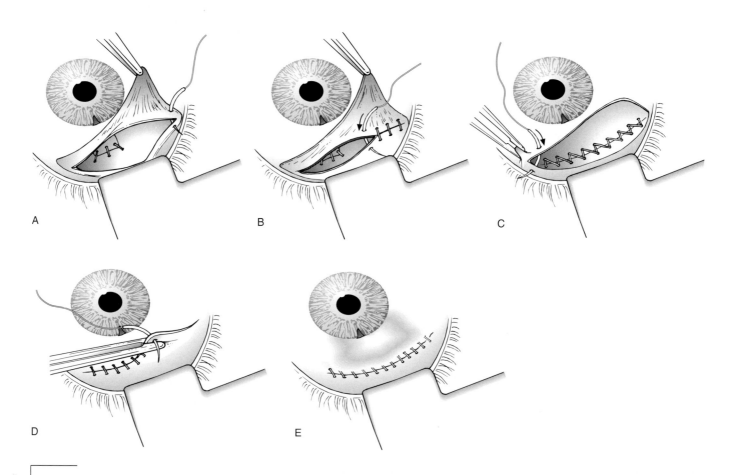

A   B   C

D   E

FIGURE 33-19.   *Closure of Tenon's capsule and conjunctiva, limbus-based flaps. Running simple or mattress sutures are used. Only enough tissue to create adequate closure is used, allowing as much tissue as possible to form a large bleb.*

provide adequate adhesion. The suture can be moderately sized, such as 8-0 or 9-0, and a TG-140 or similar needle allows easy manipulation and closure. Dual-layer closures can utilize a simple running stitch. A mattress closure will result in additional tissue eversion, which is more watertight. With any kind of stitch, watertight closure necessitates that the knot loop be passed just beyond the opening, into uncut tissue, and the first running loop be passed just beneath the knot, also into uncut tissue. Without this precaution, a gap will be created when the suture is put under tension as closure proceeds.

Placement of the bites should incorporate as little tissue from the edges as is practical, because as much surface area as possible is desired for the internal surface of the bleb. Tenon's tissue that becomes folded into the suture line will not be available to filter aqueous flow. Many small bites of Tenon's capsule will ensure a watertight closure. Occasionally locking a suture pass can help maintain constant tension on the tissue margins. The same effect can be achieved by having the assistant gently "follow" the suture by grasping the suture loop after each pass, slightly elevating the tissue off of the globe. An advantage of this maneuver is that it "shows" the tissue edge to the surgeon to facilitate placement of the following passes more easily.

By the time Tenon's capsule is closed, a bled should be seen beginning to form. The final stitch should mirror the initial loop, and be entirely within uncut tissue beyond the incision's end. Before the final step of conjunctival closure, the anterior chamber should be reinflated with balanced salt solution if necessary.

Closure of Conjunctival Layer of a Limbus-Based Flap

Conjunctival closure is very similar to closure of Tenon's capsule, with one significant exception: when antimetabolite has been used, a cutting needle is contraindicated. The preferred needle is a tapered-tip one, widely used in vascular surgery, because the hole left behind the swedge is no larger than the suture itself, minimizing fluid leak.

A common choice for closure after antimetabolite use is a 9-0 monofilament polyglactin suture on a BV-100 needle. This needle can be difficult to handle and a fine-jawed titanium nonmagnetic nonlocking needle holder makes manipulation of the needle much easier.

The same principles of Tenon's closure apply to closing conjunctiva: Use small bites, leaving as much tissue to become bleb as possible; and start and end beyond the incised tissue to ensure a watertight closure. Care is required to ensure that the conjunctival margins have not rolled onto themselves, and a moistened cellulose spear can be used to unroll any edges.

After completion of the conjunctival closure, the anterior-chamber depth is rechecked and the chamber re-formed if necessary.

Closure of Fornix-Based Flaps

It would seem that a fornix-based flap would be easier and faster to close than a longer, two-layer limbus-based flap. However, the cornea and conjunctiva are of very different densities, and making the small, precise bites required for watertight closure can be very time-consuming. These closures are very close to the fistula site, and tend to leak in the early postoperative period.

Denuding the corneal epithelium before closure greatly enhances the likelihood that the conjunctival undersurface will seal to the cornea. The epithelium can be removed before the scleral flap is created, or immediately prior to closure. A rounded sharp blade such as a No. 69 blade is scraped along the surface, avoiding the anterior flap sutures, for the length of the limbal incision (Fig. 33-20). The surface is then rinsed with balanced salt solution.

The conjunctiva can be sewn to the cornea in a running fashion (283) or with several interrupted mattress sutures. A tapered-tip needle can be used to minimize leaks through the conjunctival surface, but these needles are extremely challenging to pass through corneal stroma (165). A small-caliber cutting needle works well, especially in a mattress style. Both styles have been used with success in eyes in which an antimetabolite was applied.

Techniques have been developed to create a groove in the corneoscleral margin, to give a more watertight closure in the immediate postoperative period (284).

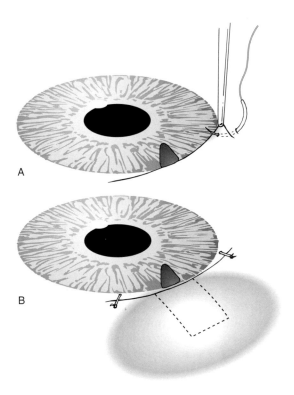

FIGURE 33-20. *Closure of fornix-based flap. The limbal corneal epithelium is scraped away with a rounded blade. The conjunctival flap is secured to cornea on both sides of the scleral flap.*

SUBCONJUNCTIVAL INJECTIONS AND DRESSING MEDICATIONS

As with any intraocular surgery, antibiosis and suppression of excessive inflammation is paramount. Suppression of intraocular inflammation is especially important in guarded fistulization, since scarring at the ostomy or flap edges is the major cause of long-term failure.

Use of an injectable antibiotic into the subconjunctival space is recommended. Cefazolin is less toxic if it gains access to intraocular contents, and so may be preferred over gentamicin or similar drugs.

Injection of steroids beneath Tenon's capsule are common, to help minimize inflammation and potentiate the inhibition of fibroblastic activity of the intraoperative antimetabolite. These injections are usually placed between 90 and 180 degrees away from the filtration site. Loftfield and Ball (285) found that injection of dexamethasone directly over the flap site did not improve pressure control, and may have contributed to an increased rate of development of encapsulated blebs. Steroids with moderate duration of effect such as betamethasone sodium phosphate (Celestone) are preferable.

Dressing medications typically consist of atropine ointment and antibiotic-steroid ointments. Keenan and Hakin (286) compared patients given atropine as a postoperative dressing with those who began atropine on the first postoperative day, and found no difference in the two groups except for larger pupils on the first postoperative day in the treated group.

POSTOPERATIVE FOLLOW-UP AND MEDICATION REGIMEN

The postoperative period may include intense inflammation, hyphema, hypotony, or shallow anterior chamber. Frequent examinations are necessary, often daily until problems are improved. It is insufficient to check the eye only weekly, until the eye has stabilized. Early prognostic factors are seen in the first 2 postoperative days, and may affect management of the specific eye (287).

Medications include steroid drops every 1 to 2 hours while the patient is awake, cycloplegics, and antibiotics.

Use of topical steroids after filtering surgery can improve long-term success, but systemic steroids do not improve the outcome of routine cases (288). Gwin et al (289) found similar results in rabbits that received systemic nonsteroidal compounds or steroids postoperatively.

Cycloplegics help to minimize iridocyclitis, to provide patient comfort during the inflammatory phase, to deepen the anterior chamber to minimize the likelihood of lens-corneal touch, and potentially to avoid development of aqueous misdirection syndrome (286). Surgeons differ in their opinions on the minimum frequency of cycloplegic administration, but a minimum of twice per day seems necessary to have positive effects. Often, these can be discontinued at the same time as the antibiotics, at 2 weeks postoperatively. Careful attention to the deleterious effect on the mental and emotional status of elderly patients is required with high-dose or long-term use of these cycloplegics.

The duration of use of these medications has been controversial. Cycloplegics may be discontinued when inflammation is controlled and the likelihood of shallow chambers has passed. Since steroids function to delay and minimize scar formation, maintaining high postoperative doses (every 2 hours while awake) for 4 to 6 weeks is recommended. While exact doses should be individualized based on bleb vascularity and postoperative course, it is wise to taper steroids very slowly, often spending several weeks to months each at doses given four times a day, three times a day, twice a day, and daily.

Broad-spectrum antibiosis is recommended as it is for cataract or other intraocular surgery. Antibiotics that increase inflammation such as gentamicin are contraindicated because of the increased scarring this inflammation can cause.

REFERENCES

1. *Stedman's medical dictionary*. Baltimore: Williams & Wilkins, 1982.
2. Morrell AJ, Searle AE, O'Neill EC. Trabeculectomy as an introduction to intraocular surgery in an ophthalmic training program. *Ophthalmic Surg* 1989;20:557–560.
3. MacKenzie W. *A practical treatise on diseases of the eye*. London: Longman, Rees, Orm, Brown & Green, 1830.
4. von Graefe A. Uber die Wirkung der Iridectomie bei Glaucom. *Arch Ophthalmol* 1857;1:371–382.
5. Kronfeld P. The rise of the filter operations. *Surv Ophthalmol* 1972;17:168.
6. Herbert H. Subconjunctival fistula operation in the treatment of primary chronic glaucoma. *Trans Ophthalmol Soc UK* 1903;23:324–346.
7. Holth S. Sclerectomie avec la pince emportepiece dans le glaucome, de preference apres incision a la pique. *Ann Ocul* 1909;141:1.
8. Elliot R. A preliminary note on a new operative procedure for the establishment of a filtering cicatrix in the treatment of glaucoma. *Ophthalmoscope* 1909;7:804.
9. Elliot G. *Sclero-corneal trephining in the operative treatment of glaucoma* London: George Pulman and Sons, 1913.
10. Presiozi C. The electrocautery in the treatment of glaucoma. *Br J Ophthalmol* 1924;8:414.
11. Scheie H. Retraction of scleral wound edges: a fistulizing procedure for glaucoma. *Am J Ophthalmol* 1958;45:220.
12. Sugar HS. Experimental trabeculectomy in glaucoma. *Am J Ophthalmol* 1961;51:623.
13. Cairns J. Trabeculectomy. Preliminary report of a new method. *Am J Ophthalmol* 1968;66:673–679.
14. Watson P. Trabeculectomy. A modified ab externo technique. *Ann Ophthalmol* 1970;2:199–205.
15. Spaeth GL. "Guarded filtration procedure"—not "trabeculectomy." [see comments]. *Ophthalmic Surg* 1992;23:583. Editorial.
16. Teichmann KD. "Guarded filtration procedure"—not "trabeculectomy." *Ophthalmic Surg* 1993;24:136. Letter; comment.
17. Clark R, RB C. Wound repair. In: McDoonagh J, ed. *Plasma fibrinogen structure and function*. New York: Marcel Dekker, 1985.
18. Miller M. An animal model of filtration surgery. *Trans Ophthalmol Soc UK* 1985;104:893.
19. Seetner A, Morin J. Healing of trabeculectomies in rabbits. *Can J Ophthalmol* 1979;14:121.
20. Desjardins D. Wound healing after filtering surgery in owl monkeys. *Arch Ophthalmol* 1986;104:1835.
21. Gressel M. 5-Fluorouracil and glaucoma filtering surgery, I. An animal model. *Ophthalmology* 1984;91:1242.

22. Starita RJ, et al. Short- and long-term effects of postoperative corticosteroids on trabeculectomy. *Ophthalmology* 1985;92:938–946.

23. Giangiacomo J, Dueker D, Adelstein E. The effect of preoperative subconjunctival triamcinolone administration on glaucoma filtration. I. Trabeculectomy following subconjunctival triamcinolone. *Arch Ophthalmol* 1986;104:838.

24. Giangiacomo J, Adelstein E, Dueker D. The effect of preoperative subconjunctival triamcinolone on glaucoma filtration. *Invest Ophthalmol Vis Sci* 1984;26:126.

25. Piltz JR, Starita RJ. The use of subconjunctivally administered tissue plasminogen activator after trabeculectomy. *Ophthalmic Surg* 1994;25:51–53.

26. Jampel H. Effect of brief exposure to mitomycin C on viability and proliferation of cultured human Tenon's capsule fibroblasts. *Ophthalmology* 1992;99:1471–1476.

27. Nuyts RM, et al. Histopathologic effects of mitomycin C after trabeculectomy in human glaucomatous eyes with persistent hypotony. *Am J Ophthalmol* 1994;118:225–237.

28. Mullaney P, et al. Fibroblast and endothelial outgrowth from human Tenon's explants: inhibition of fibroblast growth by 5HT receptor antagonism. *Res Commun Chem Pathol Pharmacol* 1991;74:201–213.

29. Hutchinson AK, et al. Clinicopathologic features of excised mitomycin filtering blebs. *Arch Ophthalmol* 1994;112:74–79.

30. Madhavan H, et al. In vitro sensitivity of human Tenon's capsule fibroblasts to mitomycin C and its correlation with outcome of glaucoma filtration surgery. *Ophthalmic Surg* 1995;26:61–67.

31. Rivera A, et al. Trifluorothymidine and 5-fluorouracil: antiproliferative activity in tissue culture. *Can J Ophthalmol* 1987;22:13–16.

32. Senderoff R, et al. Evaluation of antiproliferative agents using a cell-culture model. *Invest Ophthalmol Vis Sci* 1990;31:2572–2578.

33. Wong V, et al. Inhibition of rabbit ocular fibroblast proliferation by 5-fluorouracil and cytosine arabinoside. *J Ocul Pharmacol* 1991;7:27–39.

34. Khaw P, et al. Prolonged localized tissue effects from 5-minute exposures to fluorouracil and mitomycin C. *Arch Ophthalmol* 1993;111:263–267.

35. Khaw P, et al. Intraoperative and post operative treatment with 5-fluorouracil and mitomycin-C: long term effects in vivo on subconjunctival and scleral fibroblasts. *Int Ophthalmol* 1992;16:381–385.

36. Takahashi N, Ikoma N. The cytotoxic effect of 5-fluorouracil on cultured human conjunctival cells. *Lens Eye Toxicity Res* 1989;6:157–166.

37. Yaldo MK, Stamper RL. Long-term effects of mitomycin on filtering blebs. Lack of fibrovascular proliferative response following severe inflammation [published erratum appears in *Arch Ophthalmol* 1993;111:1358]. *Arch Ophthalmol* 1993;111:824–826.

38. Ophir A, Ticho U. Remission of anterior uveitis by subconjunctival fluorouracil. *Arch Ophthalmol* 1991;109:12–13. Letter.

39. Fourman S, Wiley L. Tissue plasminogen activator modifies healing of glaucoma filtering surgery in rabbits. *Ophthalmic Surg* 1991;22:718–723.

40. Ozment R, Laiw Z, Latina M. The use of tissue plasminogen activator in experimental filtration surgery. *Ophthalmic Surg* 1992;23:22–30.

41. Joseph J, Grierson I, Hitchings RA. Taxol, cytochalasin B and colchicine effects on fibroblast migration and contraction: a role in glaucoma filtration surgery? *Curr Eye Res* 1989;8:203–215.

42. Handa JT, Murad S, Jaffe GJ. Minoxidil inhibits ocular cell proliferation and lysyl hydroxylase activity. *Invest Ophthalmol Vis Sci* 1993;34:567–575.

43. Lee Y, Park M, Baek N. Effect of gamma-interferon on fibroblast proliferation and collagen synthesis after glaucoma filtering surgery. *Korean J Ophthalmol* 1991;5:59–67.

44. Lee D, Shapourifar-Tehrani S, Kitada S. The effect of 5-fluorouracil and cytarabine on human fibroblasts from Tenon's capsule. *Invest Ophthalmol Vis Sci* 1990;31:1848–1855.

45. Demailly P, Kretz G. Daunorubicin versus 5-fluorouracil in surgical treatment of primary open angle glaucoma: a prospective study. *Int Ophthalmol* 1992;16:367–370.

46. Jampel H, Ascorbic acid is cytotoxic to dividing human Tenon's capsule fibroblasts—a possible contributing factor in glaucoma filtration surgery success. *Arch Ophthalmol* 1990;108:1323–1325.

47. Jampel H. Ascorbic acid is cytotoxic to dividing human Tenon's capsule fibroblasts—a possible contributing factor in glaucoma filtration surgery success. *Arch Ophthalmol* 1991;109:318–319. Letter.

48. Shin D, et al. Ascorbic acid is cytotoxic to dividing human Tenon's capsule fibroblasts—a possible contributing factor in glaucoma filtration surgery success. *Arch Ophthalmol* 1991;109:318–319. Reply.

49. Cunliffe I, Rees R, Rennie I. The effect of TGF-beta 1 and TGF-beta 2 on the proliferation of human Tenon's capsule fibroblasts in tissue culture. *Acta Ophthalmol Scand* 1996;74:31–35.

50. Sharir M, Zimmerman T. In vitro inhibition of collagen formation by 2,4-pyridine dicarboxylate and minoxidil in rabbit corneal fibroblasts. *Curr Eye Res* 1993;12:553–559.

51. Gillies M, Su T. Cytokines, fibrosis and the failure of glaucoma filtration surgery. *Aust N Z J Ophthalmol* 1991;19:299–304.

52. Chen C. Enhanced intraocular pressure controlling effectiveness of trabeculectomy by local application of mitomycin-C. *Trans Asia Pacific Acad Ophthalmol* 1983;9:172–177.

53. Simmons S, et al. Pharmacokinetics of a 5-fluorouracil liposomal delivery system. *Br J Ophthalmol* 1988;72:688–691.

54. Trope G, et al. Depot drug delivery system for 5-fluorouracil after filtration surgery in the rabbit. *Can J Ophthalmol* 1994;29:263–267.

55. Heuer D, et al. Topical fluorouracil. II. Postoperative administration in an animal model of glaucoma filtering surgery. *Arch Ophthalmol* 1986;104:132–136.

56. Mannis M, Sweet E, Lewis R. The effect of fluorouracil on the corneal endothelium. *Arch Ophthalmol* 1988;106:816–817.

57. McDermott ML, Wang J, Shin DH. Mitomycin and the human corneal endothelium. *Arch Ophthalmol* 1994;112:533–537.

58. Thomas R, et al. Incidence of complications following 5-fluorouracil with trabeculectomies. *Indian J Ophthalmol* 1993;41:185–186.

59. Hurvitz L. Corneal opacification after 5-fluorouracil injections. *Ophthalmic Surg* 1994;25:130. Letter.

60. Hayashi M, Ibaraki N, Tsuru T. Lamellar keratoplasty after trabeculectomy with 5-fluorouracil. *Am J Ophthalmol* 1994;117:268–269. Letter.

61. Oram O, et al. Necrotizing keratitis following trabeculectomy with mitomycin. *Arch Ophthalmol* 1995;113:19–20. Letter.

62. Hickey-Dwyer M, Wishart P. Serious corneal complication of 5-fluorouracil. *Br J Ophthalmol* 1993;77:250–251.

63. Franks WA, Hitchings RA. Complications of 5-fluorouracil after trabeculectomy [see comments]. *Eye* 1991;5(Pt 4):385–389.

64. Phelan MJ, Skuta GL. Reversible corneal keratinization following trabeculectomy and treatment with 5-fluorouracil. *Ophthalmic Surg* 1990;21:296–298.

65. Peterson MR, et al. Striate melanokeratosis following trabeculectomy with 5-fluorouracil [see comments]. *Arch Ophthalmol* 1990;108:1216–1217. Letter.

66. Patitsas C, et al. Infectious crystalline keratopathy occurring in an eye subsequent to glaucoma filtering surgery with postoperative subconjunctival 5-fluorouracil. *Ophthalmic Surg* 1991;22:412–413.

67. Knapp A, et al. Serious corneal complications of glaucoma filtering surgery with postoperative 5-fluorouracil. *Am J Ophthalmol* 1987;103:183–187.

68. Lee D, et al. Complications of subconjunctival 5-fluorouracil following glaucoma filtering surgery. *Ophthalmic Surg* 1987;18:187–190.

69. Pasquale L, et al. Effect of topical mitomycin C on glaucoma filtration surgery in monkeys. *Ophthalmology* 1992;99:14–18.

70. Herschler J. Primate trabeculectomies with 5-fluorouracil collagen implants. *Am J Ophthalmol* 1990;110:579–580. Letter.

71. Khaw P, et al. Effects of intraoperative 5-fluorouracil or mitomycin C on glaucoma filtering surgery in the rabbit. *Ophthalmology* 1993;100:367–372.

72. Wilson M, et al. The effects of topical mitomycin on glaucoma filtration surgery in rabbits. *J Ocul Pharmacol* 1991;7:1–8.

73. Prata J Jr, et al. Trabeculectomy with mitomycin C in glaucoma associated with uveitis. *Ophthalmic Surg* 1994;25:616–620.

74. Skuta G, et al. Intraoperative mitomycin versus postoperative 5-fluorouracil in high-risk glaucoma filtering surgery. *Ophthalmology* 1992;99:438–444.

75. Mermoud A, Salmon JF, Murray AD. Trabeculectomy with mitomycin C for refractory glaucoma in blacks. *Am J Ophthalmol* 1993;116:72–78.

76. Bank A, Allingham R. Application of mitomycin C during filtering surgery. *Am J Ophthalmol* 1993;116:377–379. Letter.

77. Kupin TH, et al. Adjunctive mitomycin C in primary trabeculectomy in phakic eyes. *Am J Ophthalmol* 1995;119:30–39.

78. Mirza GE, et al. Filtering surgery with mitomycin-C in uncomplicated (primary open angle) glaucoma. *Acta Ophthalmol* 1994;72:155–161.

79. Megevand GS, et al. The effect of reducing the exposure time of mitomycin C in glaucoma filtering surgery. *Ophthalmology* 1995;102:84–90.

80. Dreyer E, Chaturvedi N, Zurakowski D. Effect of mitomycin C and fluorouracil-supplemented trabeculectomies on the anterior segment. *Arch Ophthalmol* 1995;113:578–580.

81. Chen CW, et al. Trabeculectomy with simultaneous topical application of mitomycin-C in refractory glaucoma. *J Ocul Pharmacol* 1990;6:175–182.

82. Costa VP, et al. Effects of topical mitomycin C on primary trabeculectomies and combined procedures. *Br J Ophthalmol* 1993;77:693–697.

83. Watanabe J, et al. Trabeculectomy with 5-fluorouracil. *Acta Ophthalmol* 1991;69:455–461.

148. Weinreb R. Adjusting the dose of 5-fluorouracil after filtration surgery to minimize side effects. *Ophthalmology* 1987;94:564–570.

149. Krug J, Melamed S. Adjunctive use of delayed and adjustable low-dose 5-fluorouracil in refractory glaucoma. *Am J Ophthalmol* 1990;109:412–418.

150. Ticho U, Ophir A. Regulating the dose of 5-fluorouracil to prevent filtering bleb scarring. *Ann Ophthalmol* 1991;25:225–229.

151. Rabowsky J, Ruderman J. Low-dose 5-fluorouracil and glaucoma filtration surgery. *Ophthalmic Surg* 1989;20:347–349.

152. Loane M, Weinreb R. Reducing corneal toxicity of 5-fluorouracil in the early postoperative period following glaucoma filtering surgery. *Aust N Z J Ophthalmol* 1991;19:197–202.

153. Beckman R, et al. Bandage contact lens augmentation of 5-fluorouracil treatment in glaucoma surgery. *Ophthalmic Surg* 1991;22:563–564.

154. Wolner B, et al. Later bleb-related endophthalmitis after trabeculectomy with adjunctive 5-fluorouracil. *Ophthalmology* 1991;98:1053–1060.

155. Del Piero E, Pennett M, Leopold I. *Pseudomonas cepacia* endophthalmitis. *Ann Ophthalmol* 1985;17:753–756.

156. Katz LJ, Cantor LB, Spaeth GL. Complications of surgery in glaucoma. Early and late bacterial endophthalmitis following glaucoma filtering surgery. *Ophthalmology* 1985;92:959–963.

157. Lee K, Pien F. Endophthalmitis caused by nutrient variant streptococci after filtering bleb surgery (case report). *Ann Ophthalmol* 1993;25:51–53.

158. Lipman RM, Deutsch TA. Late-onset *Moraxella catarrhalis* endophthalmitis after filtering surgery (case report). *Can J Ophthalmol* 1992;27:249–250.

159. Lobue TD, Deutsch TA, Stein RM. *Moraxella nonliquefaciens* endophthalmitis after trabeculectomy. *Am J Ophthalmol* 1985;99:343–345.

160. Wallace RT, O'Day DM. Restoration of intraocular pressure after streptococcus endophthalmitis with vitrectomy. *Ophthalmic Surg* 1994;25:110–111.

161. Munden PM, Alward WL. Combined phacoemulsification, posterior chamber intraocular lens implantation, and trabeculectomy with mitomycin C. *Am J Ophthalmol* 1995;119:20 29.

162. Schwartz AL, Weiss HS. Bleb leak with hypotony after laser suture lysis and trabeculectomy with mitomycin C [see comments]. *Arch Ophthalmol* 1992;110:1049. Letter.

163. Smith MF, Magauran R, Doyle JW. Treatment of postfiltration bleb leak by bleb injection of autologous blood. *Ophthalmic Surg* 1994;25:636–637.

164. Wand M. Minimizing conjunctival wound leaks in filtration surgery with mitomycin C. *Ophthalmic Surg* 1993;24:708–709. Letter.

165. Liss RP, Scholes GN, Crandall AS. Glaucoma filtration surgery: new horizontal mattress closure of conjunctival incision. *Ophthalmic Surg* 1991;22:298–300.

166. Brown R, et al. Treatment of bleb infection after glaucoma surgery. *Arch Ophthalmol* 1994;112:57–61.

167. Wolner B, et al. Treatment of bleb infection after glaucoma surgery. *Arch Ophthalmol* 1994;112:1277–1278. Letter.

168. Costa VP, et al. Loss of visual acuity after trabeculectomy. *Ophthalmology* 1993;100:599–612.

169. Watson PG, et al. The complications of trabeculectomy (a 20-year follow-up). *Eye* 1990;4:425–438.

170. Drake M. Complications of glaucoma filtration surgery. *Int Ophthalmol Clin* 1992;32:115–130. Review.

171. Ariano ML, Ball SF. Delayed nonexpulsive suprachoroidal hemorrhage after trabeculectomy. *Ophthalmic Surg* 1987;18:661–666.

172. Canning CR, et al. Delayed suprachoroidal haemorrhage after glaucoma operations. *Eye* 1989;3(Pt 3):327–331.

173. Deady JP, Price NJ, Sutton GA. Ptosis following cataract and trabeculectomy surgery. *Br J Ophthalmol* 1989;73:283–285.

174. Clarke MP, Vernon SA, Sheldrick JH. The development of cataract following trabeculectomy. *Eye* 1990;4(Pt 4):577–583.

175. Lavin M, Franks W, Hitchings RA. Serous retinal detachment following glaucoma filtering surgery. *Arch Ophthalmol* 1990;108:1553–1555.

176. Grossniklaus HE, et al. Iris melanoma seeding through a trabeculectomy site. *Arch Ophthalmol* 1990;108:1287–1290.

177. Fechtner RD, et al. Complications of glaucoma surgery. Ocular decompression retinopathy. *Arch Ophthalmol* 1992;110:965–968.

178. Nuyts RM, Van Diemen HA, Greve EL. Occlusion of the retinal vasculature after trabeculectomy with mitomycin C. *Int Ophthalmol* 1994;18:167–170.

179. Detry-Morel M, Kittel B, Lemagne JM. Surface-wrinkling maculopathy as a potential complication of trabeculectomy: a case report. *Ophthalmic Surg* 1991;22:38–40.

180. Vesti E. Development of cataract after trabeculectomy. *Acta Ophthalmol* 1993;71:777–781.

181. Bonomi L, et al. Prospective study of the lens changes after trabeculectomy. *Dev Ophthalmol* 1989;17:97–100.

182. McHam ML, Migdal CS, Netland PA. Early trabeculectomy in the management of primary open-angle glaucoma. *Int Ophthalmol Clin* 1994;34:163–172. Review.

183. Migdal C. What is the appropriate treatment for patients with primary open angle glaucoma: medicine, laser, or primary surgery? *Ophthalmic Surg* 1995;26:108–109. Editorial.

184. Jay JL, Murray SB. Early trabeculectomy versus conventional management in primary open angle glaucoma. *Br J Ophthalmol* 1988;72:881–889.

185. Jay JL, Allan D. The benefit of early trabeculectomy versus conventional management in primary open angle glaucoma relative to severity of disease. *Eye* 1989;3(Pt 5):528–535.

186. Ainsworth JR, Jay JL. Cost analysis of early trabeculectomy versus conventional management in primary open angle glaucoma. *Eye* 1991;5(Pt 3):322–328.

187. Sherwood M, et al. Long-term morphologic effects of antiglaucoma drugs on the conjunctiva and Tenon's capsule in glaucomatous patients. *Ophthalmology* 1989;96:327–335.

188. Broadway DC, et al. Adverse effects of topical antiglaucoma medication. II. The outcome of filtration surgery. *Arch Ophthalmol* 1994;112:1446–1454.

189. Lavin MJ, et al. The influence of prior therapy on the success of trabeculectomy. *Arch Ophthalmol* 1990;108:1543–1548.

190. Gwynn DR, et al. Conjunctival structure and cell counts and the results of filtering surgery. *Am J Ophthalmol* 1993;116:464–468.

191. Sherwood M, Migdal C, Hitchings R. Initial treatment of glaucoma: surgery or medications? Part I: filtration surgery. *Surv Ophthalmol* 1993;37:293–305.

192. Hugkulstone CE, Stevenson L, Vernon SA. Simultaneous bilateral trabeculectomy. *Eye* 1994;8(Pt 4):398–401.

193. Sanders R, MacEwen CJ, Haining WM. Trabeculectomy: effect of varying surgical site. *Eye* 1993;7(Pt 3):440–443.

194. Vesti E, Raitta C. Trabeculectomy at the inferior limbus. *Acta Ophthalmol* 1992;70:220 224.

195. Caronia R, et al. Trabeculectomy at the inferior limbus. *Arch Ophthalmol* 1996;114:387–391.

196. Gollamudi S, et al. Photographically documented access of tear film to the anterior chamber through a leaky filtering bleb (photo essay). *Arch Ophthalmol* 1993;111:394–395.

197. Dinsmore S. Drop, then decide approach to topical anesthesia. *J Cataract Refract Surg* 1995;21:666–671.

198. Ritch R, Liebmann JM. Sub-Tenon's anesthesia for trabeculectomy. *Ophthalmic Surg* 1992;23:502–504.

199. Buys YM, Trope GE. Prospective study of sub-Tenon's versus retrobulbar anesthesia for inpatient and day-surgery trabeculectomy. *Ophthalmology* 1993;100:1585–1589.

200. Yamabayashi S, Tsukahara S. New lid speculum for glaucoma filtering surgery. *Ophthalmic Surg* 1994;25:128–129.

201. Conklin JD, Goins KM, Smith TJ. Corneal traction suture in trabeculectomy [see comments]. *Ophthalmic Surg* 1991;22:494. Letter.

202. Brincker P, Kessing SV. Limbus-based versus fornix-based conjunctival flap in glaucoma filtering surgery. *Acta Ophthalmol* 1992;70:641–644.

203. Reichert R, Stewart W, Shields MB. Limbus-based versus fornix-based conjunctival flaps in trabeculectomy. *Ophthalmic Surg* 1987;18:672–676.

204. Khan AM, Jilani FA. Comparative results of limbal based versus fornix based conjunctival flaps for trabeculectomy. *Indian J Ophthalmol* 1992;40:41–43.

205. Robinson DI, et al. Long-term intraocular pressure control by trabeculectomy: a ten-year life table. *Aust N Z J Ophthalmol* 1993;21:79–85.

206. Shuster JN, et al. Limbus- v fornix-based conjunctival flap in trabeculectomy. A long-term randomized study. *Arch Ophthalmol* 1984;102:361–362.

207. Freedman J. Flap selection in glaucoma filtering surgery. *Ann Ophthalmol* 1987;19:449–452.

208. Agbeja AM, Dutton GN. Conjunctival incisions for trabeculectomy and their relationship to the type of bleb formation—a preliminary study. *Eye* 1987;1(Pt 6):738–743.

209. Luntz MH. Limbal- vs fornix-based conjunctival trabeculectomy flaps. *Am J Ophthalmol* 1988;105:100–101. Letter.

210. Traverso CE, Tomey KF, Antonios S. Limbal- vs fornix-based conjunctival trabeculectomy flaps. *Am J Ophthalmol* 1987;104:28–32.

211. Traverso C, Tomey K, Antonios S. Limbal- vs fornix-based conjunctival trabeculectomy flaps. *Am J Ophthalmol* 1988;105:219–220. Reply to letter.

212. Traverso C. Limbal- vs fornix-based conjunctival trabeculectomy flaps. *Am J Ophthalmol* 1988;105:100–101. Reply to letter.

213. Kaushik NC. Limbal- vs fornix-based conjunctival trabeculectomy flaps. *Am J Ophthalmol* 1988;105:219–220. Letter.

214. Smith AD, Hesse RJ, Terry AP. The partial dissection trabeculectomy. *Ophthalmic Surg* 1991;22:171–174.

215. Eichenbaum JW. Sodium hyaluronate dissection of conjunctival flap for trabeculectomy after extracapsular cataract extraction. *Ophthalmic Surg* 1993;24:632–633. Letter.

216. Cairns JE. Clear-cornea trabeculectomy. *Trans Ophthalmol Soc U K* 1985;104(Pt 2):142–145.

217. Cioffi GA, Van Buskirk EM. Corneal trabeculectomy without conjunctival incision. Extended follow-up and histologic findings [see comments]. *Ophthalmology* 1993;100:1077–1082.

218. Elder MJ, Molteno AC. Five-year follow-up of clear cornea trabeculectomy. *Aust N Z J Ophthalmol* 1992;20:19–22.

219. Elder MJ. Corneal trabeculectomy. *Ophthalmology* 1993;100:1603–1604. Letter; comment.

220. Van Buskirk EM. Trabeculectomy without conjunctival incision. *Am J Ophthalmol* 1992;113:145–153.

221. Phillips CI. Trabeculectomy without conjunctival incision. *Am J Ophthalmol* 1992;114:108–109.

222. Fahmy IA, Ali MA, Spaeth GL. Long-term follow up of clear cornea trabeculectomy. *Ophthalmic Surg* 1990;21:294–295.

223. Shields MB. Evaluation of a tapered, blunt, bipolar cautery tip for trabeculectomy. *Ophthalmic Surg* 1994;25:54–56.

224. Kee C, Pelzek CD, Kaufman PL. Mitomycin C suppresses aqueous human flow in cynomolgus monkeys. *Arch Ophthalmol* 1995;113:239–242.

225. Mietz H, Addicks K. Intraocular toxicity to ciliary nerves after extraocular application of mitomycin C in rabbits. *Int Ophthalmol* 1995;19:89–93.

226. Seah SK, et al. Mitomycin-C concentration in human aqueous humour following trabeculectomy. *Eye* 1993;7(Pt 5):652–655.

227. Mietz H, Rump A. Ocular concentrations of mitomycin C after extraocular application in rabbits. *J Ocul Pharmacol Ther* 1995;11:49–55.

228. Rump A, et al. Mitomycin-C concentration in human ocular aqueous humor after topical administration during trabeculectomy. *Arzneimittelforschung* 1995;45:1329–1330.

229. Hollo G, Suveges I. The effect of brief intrascleral or episcleral application of mitomycin C on the ciliary epithelium and pressure in the rabbit eye. *Acta Ophthalmol* 1994;72:739–742.

230. Yamamoto T, Kitazawa Y. Residual mitomycin C dosage in surgical sponges removed at the time of trabeculectomy. *Am J Ophthalmol* 1994;117:672–673. Letter.

231. Mietz H, Addicks K, Krieglstein GK. A scleral shield for the application of mitomycin C during trabeculectomy: a rabbit model. *Ophthalmic Surg* 1994;25:466–470.

232. Shin DH, et al. Retained cellulose sponge after trabeculectomy with adjunctive subconjunctival mitomycin C. *Am J Ophthalmol* 1994;118:111–112. Letter.

233. Wilson MR. Posterior lip sclerectomy vs trabeculectomy in West Indian blacks. *Arch Ophthalmol* 1989;107:1604–1608.

234. Smith DL, et al. The effect of glaucoma filtering surgery on corneal endothelial cell density. *Ophthalmic Surg* 1991;22:252–255.

235. Wilson R, Moster M. The chamber-retaining suture revisited. *Ophthalmic Surg* 1990;21:625–627.

236. Olsen T, et al. Human sclera: dimensions of the cadaver eye. (Submitted for publication.) 1996.

237. Luntz MH, Schlossman A. Trabeculectomy: a modified surgical technique. *J Cataract Refract Surg* 1994;20:350–352.

238. Schumer R, Odrich S. A scleral tunnel incision for trabeculectomy (brief report). *Am J Ophthalmol* 1995;120:528–530.

239. Konstas AG, Jay JL. Modification of trabeculectomy to avoid postoperative hyphaema. The "guarded anterior fistula" operation. *Br J Ophthalmol* 1992;76:353–357.

240. Saari KM, Heikkila LA. Early post-operative pressure rise with ciliary body incarceration into Watson type trabeculectomy fistula. *Acta Ophthalmol Suppl* 1987;182:30–33.

241. Brown SV. Management of a partial-thickness scleral-flap buttonhole during trabeculectomy. *Ophthalmic Surg* 1994;25:732–733.

242. Riley SF, Smith TJ, Simmons RJ. Repair of a disinserted scleral flap in trabeculectomy. *Ophthalmic Surg* 1994;24:349–350.

243. Palmer RM, Burgoyne CF. Applications for a corneal mattress suture in anterior limbal wound repairs. *Ophthalmic Surg* 1994;25:726–729.

244. Goins K, et al. Axial anterior chamber depth after trabeculectomy. *Ophthalmologica* 1990;200:177–180.

245. Austin MW, Wishart PK. Reformation of the anterior chamber following trabeculectomy. *Ophthalmic Surg* 1993;24:461–466.

246. Michielsens A, Hennekes R. The use of hyaluronic acid of different viscosities in preventing postoperative hypotony after trabeculectomy. *Bull Soc Belge Ophtalmol* 1993;250:17–23.

247. Barak A, et al. The protective effect of early intraoperative injection of viscoelastic material in trabeculectomy. *Ophthalmic Surg* 1992;23:206–209.

248. Raitta C, Setala K. Trabeculectomy with the use of sodium hyaluronate. One year follow-up. *Acta Ophthalmol* 1987;65:709–714.

249. Raitta C, Vesti E. The effect of sodium hyaluronate on the outcome of trabeculectomy. *Ophthalmic Surg* 1991;22:145–149.

250. Raitta C, et al. A randomized, prospective study on the use of sodium hyaluronate (Healon) in trabeculectomy. *Ophthalmic Surg* 1994;25:536–539.

251. Wand M. Viscoelastic agent and the prevention of post-filtration flat anterior chamber. *Ophthalmic Surg* 1988;19:523–524.

252. Brooks A, et al. Excimer laser filtration surgery. *Am J Ophthalmol* 1995;119:40–47.

253. Melamed S, et al. Trabeculectomy with resection of ciliary processes in glaucoma following scleral buckling. *Ophthalmic Surg* 1988;19:506–507.

254. Melamed S, Neumann D, Blumenthal M. Trabeculectomy with anterior vitrectomy in aphakic and pseudophakic glaucoma. *Int Ophthalmol* 1991;15:157–162.

255. Gross P. A temporary dissecting seton for trabeculectomy: delayed re-creation of the glaucoma filtering sclerostomy bleb. *Ophthalmic Surg* 1993;24:775–779.

256. Gross P. Temporary dissecting seton for trabeculectomy. *Ophthalmic Surg* 1994;25:412–413. Reply to letter.

257. Ullman S. Temporary dissecting seton for trabeculectomy. *Ophthalmic Surg* 1994;25:412–413. Letter; comment.

258. Melamed S, et al. Tight scleral flap trabeculectomy with postoperative laser suture lysis [see comments]. *Am J Ophthalmol* 1990;109:303–309.

259. Shin DH, Parrow KA, Presberg-Greene SE. Tight scleral flap trabeculectomy with postoperative laser suture lysis. *Am J Ophthalmol* 1990;110:325–326. Letter; comment.

260. Hugkulstone CE, Spencer AF, Vernon SA. Argon laser suture lysis with different suture materials. An experimental study. *Br J Ophthalmol* 1994;78:390–391.

261. Blok MD, et al. Scleral flap sutures and the development of shallow or flat anterior chamber after trabeculectomy. *Ophthalmic Surg* 1993;24:309–313.

262. Savage JA, et al. Laser suture lysis after trabeculectomy. *Ophthalmology* 1988;95:1631–1638.

263. Hoskins H Jr, Migliazzo C. Management of failing filtering blebs with the argon laser. *Ophthalmic Surg* 1984;15:731–733.

264. Menage MJ. Use of a glass rod in argon laser suture cutting after trabeculectomy. *Eye* 1993;7(Pt 4):599. Letter.

265. Mandelkorn R, Crossman J. A new argon laser suture lysis lens. *Ophthalmic Surg* 1994;25:480–481.

266. Ritch R, Potash SD, Liebmann JM. A new lens for argon laser suture lysis. *Ophthalmic Surg* 1994;25:126–127.

267. Hsu CT, Yarng SS. A modified removable suture in trabeculectomy. *Ophthalmic Surg* 1993;24:579–584.

268. Maberley D, Apel A, Rootman DS. Releasable "U" suture for trabeculectomy surgery. *Ophthalmic Surg* 1994;25:251–255.

269. Kolker AE, Kass MA, Rait JL. Trabeculectomy with releasable sutures. *Arch Ophthalmol* 1994;112:62–66.

270. Johnstone M, Wellington D, Ziel C. A releasable scleral-flap tamponade suture for guarded filtration surgery. *Arch Ophthalmol* 1993;111:398–403.

271. Jacob P, et al. Releasable suture technique for trabeculectomy. *Indian J Ophthalmol* 1993;41:81–82.

272. Pappa KS, et al. Late argon laser suture lysis after mitomycin C trabeculectomy. *Ophthalmology* 1993;100:1268–1271.

273. Asamoto A, Yablonski ME, Matsushita M. A retrospective study of the effects of laser suture lysis on the long-term results of trabeculectomy. *Ophthalmic Surg* 1995;26:223–227.

274. Bluestein EC, Stewart WC. Tight versus loose scleral flap closure in trabeculectomy surgery. *Doc Ophthalmol* 1993;84:379–385.

275. Lieberman MF. Tight scleral flap trabeculectomy with postoperative laser suture lysis. *Am J Ophthalmol* 1990;110:98–99. Letter; comment.

276. Asamoto A, Yablonski ME. Posttrabeculectomy anterior subcapsular cataract formation induced by anterior chamber air. *Ophthalmic Surg* 1993;24:314–319.

277. Berger RR, McGrath EJ. A "tent trabeculectomy" (T.T)—surgical alternative for countries of Third World. *Int Ophthalmol* 1992;16:195–196.

278. Teekhasaenee C, Ritch R. The use of PhEA 34c in trabeculectomy. *Ophthalmology* 1986;93:487–491.

279. Alpar JJ. Sodium hyaluronate (Healon) in glaucoma filtering procedures. *Ophthalmic Surg* 1986;17:724–730.

280. Batterbury M, Wishart PK. Is high initial aqueous outflow of benefit in trabeculectomy? *Eye* 1993;7(Pt 1):109–112.

281. Miller KN, et al. A comparison of total and partial tenonectomy with trabeculectomy. *Am J Ophthalmol* 1991;111:323–326.

282. Kapetansky F. Trabeculectomy or trabeculectomy with tenonectomy. A comparative study. *Glaucoma* 1980;2:451.

283. Wise JB. Mitomycin-compatible suture technique for fornix-based conjunctival flaps in glaucoma filtration surgery. *Arch Ophthalmol* 1993;111:992–997.

284. Pfeiffer N, Grehn F. Improved suture for fornix-based conjunctival flap in filtering surgery. *Int Ophthalmol* 1992;16:391–396.

285. Loftfield K, Ball SF. Filtering bleb encapsulation increased by steroid injection. *Ophthalmic Surg* 1990;21:282–287.

286. Keenan J, Hakin J. Atropine after trabeculectomy. *Ann Ophthalmol* 1992;24:225–229.

287. Stewart WC, et al. Early postoperative prognostic indicators following trabeculectomy. *Ophthalmic Surg* 1991;22:23–26.

288. Roth SM, et al. The effects of postoperative corticosteroids on trabeculectomy and the clinical course of glaucoma: five-year follow-up study. *Ophthalmic Surg* 1991;22:724–729.

289. Gwin T, Stewart W, Gwynn D. Filtration surgery in rabbits treated with diclofenac or prednisolone acetate. *Ophthalmic Surg* 1994;25:245–250.

Glaucoma Implants

Todd W. Perkins

TERMINOLOGY

Glaucoma implants were designed to treat glaucoma in eyes failing trabeculectomy. These devices consist of a tube that shunts aqueous from the anterior chamber across the limbus along the subconjunctival scleral surface to a plate located near the equator of the eye. The term implant is used to describe these lumenated devices rather than the term seton (*L. seta* "bristle") which more correctly describes hairs or other solid material meant to keep a wound open. The plate portion of implants creates and maintains a filtration bleb that surrounds the plate. The amount of drainage through the implant is determined by the size of the plate, and hence the minimum bleb surface area, and the degree of wound healing, which determines the thickness of the bleb wall.

Because an increasing number of implants of differing sizes and properties are available to the glaucoma surgeon, an attempt is made to describe most fully the implants likely to be useful to the reader.

HISTORICAL REVIEW AND DEVELOPMENT

After development of the classic glaucoma drainage operations of sclerectomy (1), iridencleisis (2), and corneoscleral trephination (3), it became clear that many of these procedures would fail due to excessive scarring, particularly in cases of secondary glaucoma. These failures led to the investigation of artificial drainage devices for use in eyes unresponsive to the classic operations. A great number of devices and materials have been tried over the years; most received the attention of only a single report with limited follow-up and then disappeared. Surgeons interested in attempting new approaches would do well to learn from the numerous creative and colorful failures of their predecessors. Devices

may be categorized as paracentesis devices, vitreo-Tenon's drains, cyclodialysis implants, translimbal setons, translimbal tubes, bleb-maintaining devices, shunts to distant sites, and combination tube-plate devices.

Paracentesis devices, first described in 1906 by Rollet and Moreau (4) who used a horsehair across the limbus, drained aqueous from the anterior chamber to the conjunctival sac. Although these devices posed the unacceptable risk of endophthalmitis and sympathetic ophthalmia, they had been described as recently as 1965 for treatment of neovascular glaucoma (5).

For vitreo-Tenon's devices, described by Vail (6), a silk thread was passed from the vitreous cavity into the sub-Tenon's space. This type of device could be expected to be ineffective because aqueous was not adequately drained from the vitreous cavity, and no subsequent success has been described for this approach.

Cyclodialysis implants were designed to maintain the patency of a cyclodialysis cleft. This approach had the theoretical advantage of increasing uveoscleral outflow with an intraocular surgery that did not permanently violate the integrity of the globe. Row (7) described the use of a platinum wire in 1934 for this purpose. A number of other materials have been attempted, including magnesium, tantalum, Supramid, gelatin film, Teflon, silicone, and most recently, polymethylmethacrylate (PMMA) (8–13). Although the biologically less reactive plastics were well tolerated by the eye, the operation had poor results, due to either scarring around the device preventing flow into the suprachoroidal space or perhaps the inherent limitations of uveoscleral outflow.

Translimbal setons consisted of solid stents that bridged the eye wall from the anterior chamber to the subconjunctival space. Theoretically, aqueous flowed along the surface or within the body (as a wick) of the seton out of the eye.

Zorab (14) used a silk thread in 1912 in a procedure he called *aqueoplasty*. A number of other materials were attempted, including gold, glass, tantalum, platinum, protoplast, autologous lacrimal canalicular material, cartilage, and silicone (5,10,15–19). These devices failed because the surrounding tissues fibrosed intimately to the implant and prevented fluid flow.

Anterior-chamber shunts to distant sites were attempted to obviate the difficulties of subconjunctival scarring. Aqueous has been shunted to the lacrimal sac (20), the superficial temporal vein (21), an intrascleral vortex vein (22), and an angular vein (23). Theoretically, since the one-way valve function of the trabecular meshwork is bypassed, reflux of blood or tears could have posed problems, but no long-term reports are available for these rarely performed procedures.

Bleb-maintaining devices were designed to prevent contraction of the filtering bleb after a classic drainage operation. Use of a silver tripod (24) and Gelfoam (25) was attempted, but no long-term success has been reported using this approach.

Translimbal tubes have been used to shunt aqueous across the limbus over the years and have been made of gold (15), tantalum (26,27), polyethylene (28), polyvinyl (29,30), silicone (10,31,32), and PMMA (33). These devices were an important step forward in the development of successful glaucoma implants, as they effectively shunted aqueous across the limbus into the subconjunctival space. Some degree of success was shown with the device designed by Krupin (34), which contained a pressure-sensitive, unidirectional valve, but these devices generally failed due to the formation of a fibrous cap at the distal end of the tube (28).

Molteno was the first investigator to address both problems of transscleral fluid flow and bleb maintenance, by adding to a translimbal tube a bleb-maintaining plate to prevent the end of the tube from fibrosing closed. An 8.5-mm-diameter acrylic limbal plate was attached to a translimbal tube implant to form a device that would both shunt aqueous across the limbus and limit the degree of bleb contraction to the size of the plate (35). Molteno then used the new device as an experimental system to develop a chemotherapy regimen to limit the thickness of the bleb that formed around the implant (see Adjunctive Wound-Healing Modulators) (36,37). The limbal location of the plate caused problems of discomfort and corneal dellen and so was moved posteriorly, which also allowed enlargement. This version became known as the *long-tube implant* and is currently in use (38).

DEVELOPMENT AND RATIONALE FOR TUBE-PLATE IMPLANTS

Development of the Molteno Implant

The long-tube implant, the archetype for current glaucoma implants, was first described by Molteno et al in 1976 (38).

It consisted of a 13-mm polypropylene episcleral plate connected to a translimbal silicone tube (Fig. 34-1). Since the plate was sutured posterior to the equator of the eye and the tube passed under deep scleral flaps, problems of erosion, dellen formation, and exposure found in the short-tube implant were minimized.

To avoid problems associated with postoperative hypotony related to unrestricted flow through the tube, a two-stage implantation procedure was first described (39), followed by a Vicryl-tie technique (40). Subsequently, a dual-chamber device was developed that allows limited early flow, limited to a small surface area by Tenon's capsule and an inner plate wall (Fig. 34-2) (41).

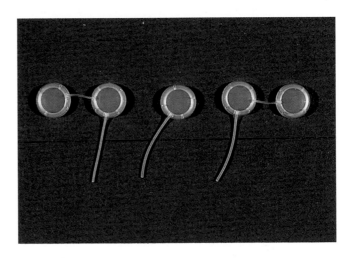

FIGURE 34-1. *Molteno implants: single plate, right and left double plate.*

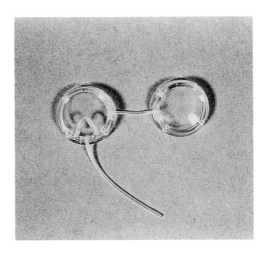

FIGURE 34-2. *Molteno implant with pressure ridge. (Courtesy of IOP, Costa Mesa, CA.)*

Device Design and Physiology

A number of implants were developed following the principles of Molteno's original device. These include the Schocket, Joseph, Krupin, Baerveldt, White, Ahmed, and Optimed implants. They share the essential features of a translimbal tube and a posteriorly sutured plate. Aqueous flows through the tube across the limbus and exits onto the superior surface of the plate and forms a bleb cavity that surrounds the plate (Fig. 34-3). Some devices also include a valve or other flow-resistive feature.

Translimbal Tube

The translimbal tube in each of the devices is made of silicone, a biologically low-reactive material (42), and functions to transport aqueous from the anterior chamber to the posterior plate. The tube has the advantage of preventing blockage of filtration at the limbus by a fibrovascular or cellular membrane as occurs in neovascular and iridocorneal endothelial (ICE) syndromes (43,44).

Episcleral Plate

The episcleral plate prevents wound healing from reducing the size of the bleb to less than that of the plate (35). Plates are composed of biologically low-reactive materials (silicone, polypropylene, Silastic, or PMMA) that are hard enough to resist deformation by subconjunctival contractile elements during wound healing.

Bleb Fluidics and Physiology

Glaucoma implant devices provide pressure control by formation of a permeable bleb consisting of collagen and fibrous tissue that surrounds the episcleral plate (37,45). Aqueous flows through the translimbal tube, passes above the plate, then filters through the wall of the bleb into the orbital tissues where capillaries and lymphatics drain the fluid from the orbit (42,45,46). When the bleb wall is well developed, the episcleral plate actually floats within the bleb and is surrounded by aqueous (Fig. 34-4) (47,48). The rate of aqueous flow across the bleb wall is entirely pressure dependent, without active transport (45), and depends on the thickness of the bleb wall and the surface area of the filtering capsule (45,46,49,50).

Adjunctive Wound-Healing Modulators

Molteno concluded from implant development work that an antifibrosis regimen consisting of oral prednisone 10 mg three times a day, colchicine 300 μg three times a day, and flufenamic acid (a prostaglandin synthetase inhibitor) was essential to the success of the implant (36,37). Since the healing response of the subconjunctival tissues determined the thickness of the bleb, this pharmacologic modulation of the healing response was thought to minimize the resultant cyst wall thickness (36). Subsequent surgeons abandoned use of the regimen, citing poor tolerance by patients and lack of effect (51). Subsequently, several investigators presented retrospective evidence that wound-healing inhibition with the adjunctive intraoperative antimetabolite mitomycin C improved the success of Molteno implants (52,53). However, preliminary prospective studies failed to show the efficacy of mitomycin C at lower doses in improving success in Molteno implant surgery (54,55). Studies in rabbits found only a temporary effect of mitomycin in delaying wound healing after placement of the Molteno implant and indications of toxicity to extraocular muscles were present (56).

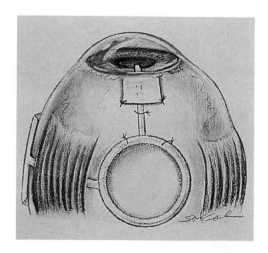

FIGURE 34-3.   *Molteno implant. Schematic diagram of a Molteno implant that shows the transscleral tube connecting to the episcleral plate.*

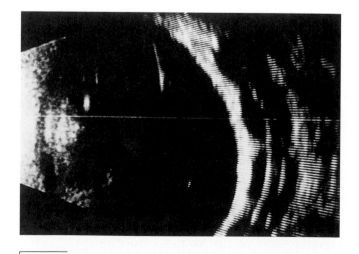

FIGURE 34-4.   *Bleb cavity. Ultrasound view of the cystic bleb cavity with the plate floating inside. (Courtesy of Iolab.)*

Size

Another question addressed by Molteno was the optimal size of an implant. He experimented with implants consisting of one (135 mm^2), two (270 mm^2), and four plates (540 mm^2) and concluded that the two-plate (270-mm^2) configuration allowed good pressure control while avoiding early hypotony (49). A subsequent prospective study confirmed the conclusion that two plates (270 mm^2) provided better control of intraocular pressure (IOP) than did one plate (135 mm^2) (50). Animal studies also suggested that pressure lowering after implants was proportional to implant size (57). Work with both the Baerveldt and the Joseph implant in humans demonstrated that there may be an optimum upper limit to surface area (350–383 mm^2 for a single surface) that represents the best compromise between IOP control and operative difficulty and risk (58–60). Larger plate size (up to 765 mm^2) reduced the dependence on postoperative glaucoma medication, thereby improving the quality of IOP control, but was associated with increased operative complexity and postoperative complications due to device size. This information suggests that the optimal surface area for an implant may be between 270 and 380 mm^2 (Table 34-1).

Flow Resistance

During the first 2 to 6 weeks following placement of a glaucoma implant, the bleb wall is being formed and provides little resistance to flow. Flow through the implant must be resisted by external means during this wound-healing phase, in order to prevent severe overfiltration and hypotony (39). Free-flow tubes are usually temporarily ligated (37). However, uneven pressure control with very high or very low pressure is not uncommon during this period (61). To avoid these extremes of IOP in the immediate postoperative period, valves and flow-decreasing elements have been developed to permanently resist flow through the tube (62–64). It has been a technical challenge to develop devices that limit flow at the extremely low rates (2–3 μL/min) found in the eye yet avoid occlusion from fibrin and debris.

Krupin was the first investigator to develop a valved device for pressure control in the eye (31,34,62,65). The original device consisted of a Supramid tube with horizontal and vertical slits in the end of the tube that functioned as a unidirectional valve with an opening pressure of 11 mm Hg and a closing pressure of 9 mm Hg in air. The most recent version (62) uses a Silastic tube with a similar slit arrangement. Ahmed developed a silicone sheet valve that uses a Venturi chamber to allow the valve to function at very low flows (63).

Laboratory investigation of these valves suggests that when immersed in fluid, they function more as flow-resistance elements than as true valves. Neither have measurable opening or closing pressures (66). When perfused at physiologic flow rates, they provide less than the advertised pressures, except for the Optimed device (Table 34-2). However, when used in the eye, they usually produce the desired moderate IOPs because of the additional resistance of the tissues around the plates (see Table 34-2) (66).

The utility of valves is debated by surgeons. Proponents cite ease of use and fewer perioperative pressure problems (62,63). Other surgeons note that valves do not eliminate early pressure problems and are undesirable after the initial postoperative period. Since they interfere with the tidal motion of aqueous that may keep the tube open, the tube may become occluded by fibrin or blood and may even require amputation for late occlusion (67).

THE DEVICES

Commonly Used Implants

Implants can be divided into those in widespread use related to their ease and efficacy of use (Molteno, Baerveldt, Krupin, Ahmed), and those used less commonly. In addition, implants can be divided into those that allow free flow

Table 34-1.   Implants

Device	Material	Surface Area (mm^2)	Height (mm)	Width/Length (mm)	Chamber Anterior Tube (outer/inner diameter, mm)
Free flow					
Molteno, 2 plate (49,68)	Polypropylene	270	1.5 (74)	13/13	0.63/0.30
Baerveldt (59)	Silicone	350 (250, 425)	1.0	32/14	0.64/0.30
Resisted flow					
Krupin (62)	Silicone	180	1.75	18/14	0.58/0.38
Ahmed (63)	Polypropylene	184	1.9	13/16	0.64/0.32

Table 34-2. Flow Resistance Devices

Device	IOP (mmHg) in Rabbit Eyes Perfused at 2 μL/min	IOP (mmHg) with Bench Perfusion at 2 μL/min
Ahmed	7.5 ± 0.8	2.6 ± 0.3
Krupin	3.8 ± 0.6	0.6 ± 0.2
Optimed	19.6 ± 5.6	3.9 ± 0.8
Baerveldt (no valve)	4.6 ± 1.5	0.3 ± 0.8*

IOP = intraocular pressure.
* Partially ligated.
SOURCE: Prata JA, et al. In vitro and in vivo flow: characteristics of glaucoma drainage implants. *Ophthalmology* 1995;102:894–904.

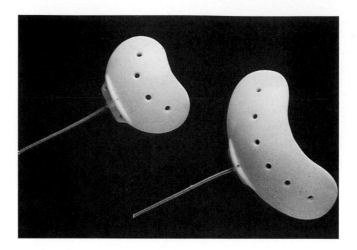

FIGURE 34-5. *Baerveldt implant with fenestrations.*

(Molteno, Baerveldt, Schocket) and those that resist flow (Krupin, Ahmed, Joseph, White, Optimed).

Free-Flow Implants

Molteno Implant

In its present form, the Molteno implant (IOP, Costa Mesa, CA, and Staar Surgical, Monrovia, CA) consists of a 16-mm silicone tube with an outer diameter of 0.63 mm and an inner diameter of 0.30 mm connected to a 13-mm diameter polypropylene (originally PMMA) plate (45,68) (see Fig. 34-1). The plate has a thickened rim 0.7 mm in height that is perforated for suture placement. The more commonly used double plate uses another segment of silicone tube to connect to a second plate, creating a surface area of 270 mm² (49) (see Table 34-1). The plates are designed to straddle the superior rectus muscle and to not encroach on the other muscles or the posterior ciliary arteries (49). The double-plate device is available in right- and left-eyed versions. A pediatric version (8-mm-diameter plate) is available, but is rarely used.

Baerveldt Implant

To simplify placement of a device with a large surface area, the Baerveldt implant (Iovision, Irvine, CA) was designed to be implanted in one quadrant (69) (Fig. 34-5). The device consists of a silicone tube (0.64-mm external diameter, 0.30-mm bore) attached to a barium-impregnated silicone plate with a surface area of 250 mm², 350 mm² (32 × 14 mm), or 425 mm² (59). Owing to early problems of strabismus caused by a very large bleb cavity (70), fenestrations were added to the plate to facilitate the formation of a lower, multiloculated bleb with a larger surface area (69) (Baerveldt G, personal communication, 1996). Other versions have included devices with surface areas of 200, 450, or 500 mm².

Resisted-Flow Implants

Krupin Implant

The Krupin Eye Disc (Hood Laboratories, Pembroke, MA) consists of a 20-mm silicone tube (0.58-mm outer diame-

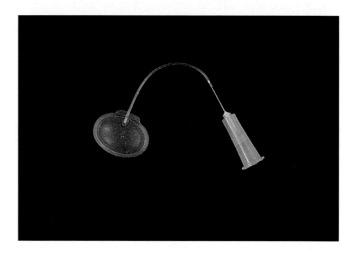

FIGURE 34-6. *Krupin valve with disk.*

ter, 0.38-mm bore) connected to an oval silicone episcleral plate, 13 × 18 mm, with a 1.75-mm-high side wall (Fig. 34-6) (62). The plate is contoured to the curvature of the globe and measures approximately 180 mm². The distal end of the tube has horizontal and vertical slits that are designed to function as a unidirectional valve. However, experimental work suggested that very little resistance is added by the slits and that some degree of reflux also occurs (66).

Ahmed Implant

The Ahmed Glaucoma Valve Implant (New World Medical, Rancho Cucamonga, CA) consists of a silicone tube, outer diameter of 0.64 mm and bore of 0.32 mm, connected to a polypropylene episcleral plate measuring 16 × 13 mm with a surface area of 184 mm² (Fig. 34-7) (63). The distal end of the tube is connected to a silicone sheet valve mounted on a plate to form a chamber shaped to take advantage of the

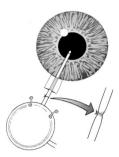

FIGURE 34-17. *Free-flow tube occluded with a Vicryl ligature in association with a venting slit.*

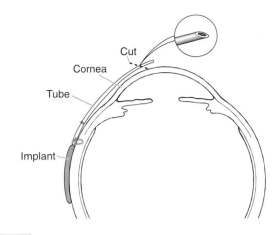

FIGURE 34-18. *Implant tube trimmed to the appropriate length with the bevel facing anteriorly.*

The tube is trimmed to the proper length by estimating a distance 2 to 3 mm past the limbus (Fig. 34-18). The tube is held with tube introducer forceps (92) or tying forceps and is cut with a bevel facing anteriorly to prevent iris incarceration and to facilitate tube entry. Stretching the tube makes a beveled cut easier to obtain, although the location of the cut on the tube must be selected prior to stretching so that the resulting contracted tube is long enough. It is better to have the tube too long than too short. If the tube is cut too short, the plate must be advanced closer to the limbus to allow adequate tube length for the anterior chamber.

Translimbal Incision

The anterior chamber is prepared for placement of the tube. Generally, a paracentesis is performed and the iris and lens positions are noted. If vitreous was noted in the anterior chamber on the preoperative planning examination, an anterior vitrectomy is performed through a lateral limbal incision. If a pars plana vitrectomy with pars plana tube placement is planned, then the vitrectomy is performed at this point.

A 23-gauge needle attached to a syringe containing a viscoelastic agent is passed through the limbus underneath the scleral flap as posteriorly as possible while remaining anterior to the iris in a plane parallel to the iris (Fig. 34-19). A small bolus of viscoelastic substance is injected to prevent anterior movement of the iris and to limit bleeding. Lateral motion during needle removal is avoided to prevent undesired enlargement of the opening.

Tube Insertion

The tube is then passed through the opening with tube introducer forceps (92) or tying forceps (Fig. 34-20). Tubes with internal suture stents for occlusion or those with a temporary suture stent are easier to pass (88,93). The ideal position for the tube is parallel to, and just anterior to, the iris (Fig. 34-21). If the tube is in poor position, it should be repositioned through another entry site and the original

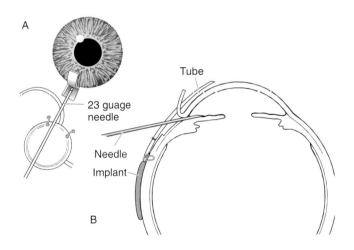

FIGURE 34-19. *Insertion of a 23-gauge needle into the anterior chamber just anterior to and parallel to the iris.*

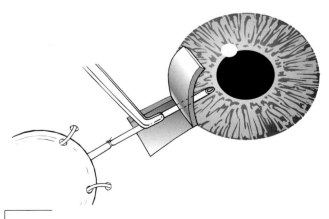

FIGURE 34-20. *Introduction of the tube into the anterior chamber with introducer forceps.*

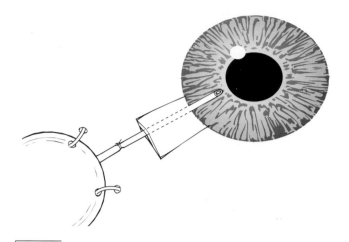

FIGURE 34-21.   *Proper tube placement in the anterior chamber.*

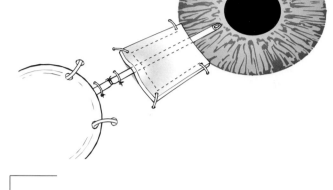

FIGURE 34-22.   *The scleral flap is reapproximated with the edges inset, and donor sclera or banked material is placed over the tube.*

opening sutured if necessary. Proper tube placement obviates many postoperative complications and justifies any extra intraoperative time required.

Eyes with chronic angle closure related to prior penetrating keratoplasty may have very high PAS. The tube may be passed through the iris without significant bleeding in these eyes.

Tube Coverage and Closure

The lamellar scleral flap, if present, is reapproximated with interrupted 10-0 nylon sutures, with the corners inset slightly to reduce tension over the tube and minimize erosion. A glycerin- or alcohol-preserved donor scleral patch graft (37,94) measuring at least 4 × 6 mm is sewn into place with 10-0 nylon interrupted sutures (Fig. 34-22). A vertical mattress suture through peripheral cornea and anterior graft can be helpful to place the graft anteriorly enough to prevent limbal erosion of the tube in cases where no lamellar scleral flap is present. Preserved human dura mater (95), preserved fascia lata, or pericardium (Staar Surgical) folded in two may be used instead of sclera and may have advantages of cost and sterility. Another author (96) suggested autologous fascia lata.

Tenon's capsule is closed with interrupted 9-0 polyglactin sutures at the edges of a limbal peritomy or with a running suture if a limbus-based peritomy was used. Conjunctiva is closed using a running 9-0 polyglactin suture (Fig. 34-23). The anterior chamber is repressurized, if necessary, with balanced salt solution administered through the paracentesis site and the wound inspected. Injections of a steroid and an antibiotic are made subconjunctivally, and topical combination steroid-antibiotic and atropine ointments are applied.

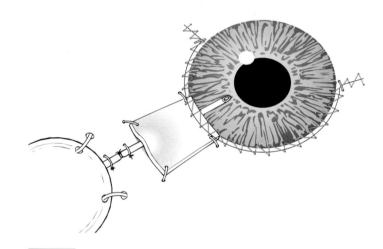

FIGURE 34-23.   *Conjunctival closure.*

Postoperative Management

Postoperative topical medications include steroids every 2 hours while awake and an ointment at bed time, antibiotics four times a day, and atropine four times a day. Patients with prior uveitis are given oral prednisone 40 to 60 mg/day 1 day prior to and for 5 days after sugery. Patients with prior herpes are also given a 3-month course of acyclovir 1200 mg/day. If an oral antifibrosis cocktail is planned, it is started immediately postoperatively.

Patients with ligated free-flow devices usually require reinstitution of preoperative glaucoma medications, depending on the pressure postoperatively. Occasionally, leakage around the tube or an incomplete ligation allows aqueous egress and a low pressure.

Patients are seen for follow-up weekly the first month, then every 2 weeks the second month, then at three months. Ligated tubes may be opened if need be at 1 week, but preferably at 2 to 4 weeks. For double-plate Molteno devices with mitomycin C, one should wait 6 weeks prior to tube opening, to avoid postoperative hypotony (53). Patients with tubes ligated with polyglactin may be told to expect a sudden softening of the eye when the ligature is absorbed, at approximately 4 weeks. Restricted-flow devices require few postoperative adjustments if there are no complications. Steroids are tapered over 3 months, although some surgeons use them once a day indefinitely.

RESULTS

Comparison of results of different implant devices based on existing literature is difficult. There is a paucity of prospective studies and interpretation of the available retrospective studies is unreliable because of differences in patient selection, criteria for reporting success, and use of statistics. Table 34-3 shows a general comparison of the various devices. Although it is generally accepted that adequate protection of the optic nerve from pressure-related damage in advanced disease requires IOPs of 15 mm Hg or lower (97), most literature still reports successful IOP control as 21 mm Hg or below and so that value is used here only for comparative purposes.

Molteno Implant

Molteno's originally reported success rates with the double-plate implant in maintaining pressure 20 mm Hg or below were 91% (50% success without additional medication) in 64 patients at 1.5 to 3.0 years and 75% (42% success without medication) in 24 patients at 2.5 to 3.0 years (38). Subsequent authors reported success rates using similar criteria ranging from 43% to 95% (12%–75% without medication) at follow-up times of 6 to 84 months, depending on the severity of disease and time postoperatively (39,50,53, 61,88,98–103). Loss of two or more lines of acuity occurred

in 8% to 47% of eyes, while reoperations for complications were required in 3% to 47%.

Neovascular glaucoma carries the poorest surgical prognosis and success rates range from 58% to 83% (IOP < 22 mm Hg), with most reported rates closer to 60% (51,68, 78,104). Many eyes lose light perception irrespective of pressure control (78). Success rates with the single- and double-plate Molteno implants in juvenile glaucoma vary from 23% to 95% (IOP < 21 mm Hg) (105–108), while the success rate in one series of patients with epithelial ingrowth was 78% (IOP < 21 mm Hg) (109).

Baerveldt Implant

The Baerveldt implant produced success rates ranging from 72% to 84% in larger studies (IOP < 22 mm Hg with or without glaucoma medications) at a follow-up time of 6 to 24 months (59,110,111). Success rates without glaucoma medications ranged from 15% to 53% in those studies. In a randomized comparison of the Baerveldt 500-mm^2 implant versus the 350-mm^2 implant, patients receiving the 500-mm^2 device required fewer glaucoma medications (0.7 versus 1.3, $p = 0.006$), and a greater proportion maintained an IOP of 21 mm Hg or less without medication (38% versus 15%, $p = 0.05$), although the overall success rates with or without medications were equal (59).

A nonrandomized comparison of case series of the double-plate Molteno implant versus the Baerveldt 350-mm^2 implant showed no significant difference in postoperative IOPs. Pressure lower than 20 mm Hg was found in 89% of Molteno implant patients and 100% of Baerveldt implant patients (103).

One early report of the original version of the Baerveldt implant found an unacceptably high rate of strabismus (77%) (70). Subsequently, the manufacturer designed a fenestrated implant to minimize this complication by encouraging the creation of a smaller, multiloculated bleb (Baerveldt G, personal communication, 1996). Rates of strabismus in more recent series ranged from 3% to 8% (60,103,110,111). Reoperation rates for complications ranged from 17% to 25% in these same series. Loss of two or more lines of

Table 34-3.   Implant Results

Device	IOP < 21 mm Hg	IOP < 21 mm Hg No Medications	Reoperative Rate	Complication Follow-up (mo)
Free flow				
Molteno (50)	75%	12%	20%	7–30
Baerveldt (59)	84%	15%	19%	6–24
Resisted flow				
Krupin (62)	80%	50%	18%	6–36
Ahmed (63)	78%	—	22%	12

IOP = intraocular pressure.

Snellen acuity occurred in 8% to 38% of patients (59,69, 110,111).

As with other implants, the success rate of the Baerveldt in neovascular glaucoma patients is less than that in non-neovascular glaucoma patients. The rate ranged from 44% to 56% in one study (60).

Krupin Implant

A multicenter trial reported placement of the Krupin valve with disk to result in successful pressure control (IOP < 20 mm Hg) in 80% of patients (50% without glaucoma medications) at 1 year postoperatively (62). Another study found 64% of patients with an IOP of 6 to 21 mm Hg (28% off medications) at a follow-up time of 4 to 19 months (67). Pressures the first day postoperatively were below 6 mm Hg in 8% to 24% of patients, indicating that the presence of the valve does not eliminate early postoperative hypotony. In 24% to 30% of patients, complications resulted in loss of two lines of vision, while 18% to 28% had reoperations for complications. Amputation of an obstructed valve was performed in three of the patients in this series (67).

Ahmed Implant

The Ahmed implant results in pressures of 5 to 21 mm Hg (with at least a 20% reduction of IOP) in 78% of patients with one year follow-up (63). Patients were considered failures when their pressure remained above these criteria for greater than two months. Pressures less than 5 mm Hg occurred in 13% of patients on postoperative day one. Complications resulting in loss of two or more lines of vision occurred in 33%, while reoperations for complications were performed in approximately 22%.

Schocket ACTSEB

The original reports of the Schocket implant involved patients with active neovascular glaucoma. In spite of this, success (IOP < 22 mm Hg) was 96% at 14 months or more, although 60% of patients developed flat or shallow anterior chambers, and 23% required revisions for complications (72). Other surgeons have obtained success rates of 63% to 81% (IOP < 22 mm Hg) at 8 to 33 months with a reoperation rate for complications of 38% to 40% (111,112).

Results of a modified Schocket technique for connecting an anterior chamber tube to a previously placed encircling element indicated that 85% of patients were controlled (IOP < 22 mm Hg) (46% off medications) at 6–21 months (113). Reoperations for complications occurred in 38% of patients, most commonly for an occlusion of the distal end of the tube at its insertion against the encircling element.

In randomized studies the Schocket implant with a No. 20 (300-mm^2) encircling element provided equivalent IOP control to the Molteno implant (74). Use of the larger No. 220 element (450 mm^2) also resulted in IOP control similar to that with the Molteno implant (90% versus 95% of patients, ≤21 mm Hg), but only half as many patients (33% versus 68%) required postoperative glaucoma medications (61).

Joseph Implant

The Joseph 360-degree (765-mm^2) implant resulted in successful pressure control (IOP < 22 mm Hg) in 96% to 100% (91% without medications) of patients at a follow-up time of 6 months (58,75). The 180-degree implant (383 mm^2) was slightly less effective, with a rate of 91% (64% without medications) (58). Loss of acuity occurred in 11% to 55% of eyes and reoperations for complications in 27%.

White Pump Shunt

White presented a series of 37 patients with the follow-up time ranging from 6 to 60 months in which 89% had IOPs of 22 mm Hg or lower and none required reoperations for complications (64). Another study using the same device found 31% of eyes to have an IOP of 21 mm Hg or lower, with a reoperation rate for complications of 38% (115). An additional study in neovascular patients found the device to be equivalent to trabeculectomy with 5-fluorouracil (5-FU), but with a higher rate of complication (76).

Optimed Implant

The Optimed implant provided successful pressure control (IOP < 22 mm Hg) in 75% of patients (44% without medications) at 6 to 52 months' follow-up (33). Reoperations were required in 28% of patients for complications. Results of a version that includes an episcleral plate are not yet available.

COMPLICATIONS AND MANAGEMENT

Early Postoperative

Overfiltration and Hypotony

Overfiltration with hypotony, a flat anterior chamber, or choroidal detachments may occur whether or not a resistive element is present. Causes include flow around the tube if an overly large translimbal incision was made, inadequate resistance from a flow-modulating element, and inadequate ligation of a free-flow tube. The incidence and consequences of hypotony are greater when an antimetabolite such as mitomycin C is used (53). Surgical intervention for hypotony is indicated for tube contact with the cornea or lens, serous choroidal effusions that remain in contact with each other ("kissing") for more than 1 to 2 weeks, and most hemorrhagic choroidal detachments. Surgery requires, at a minimum, drainage of choroidal fluid and re-formation of the anterior chamber. In addition, it may be necessary to limit flow through the tube by suture ligation if, in the surgeon's judgment, an inadequate amount of wound healing has occurred around the tube and plate to prevent a recurrence. Presence of a limbal bleb suggests leakage around the tube; this form of overfiltration may be expected to persist 1 to 2 weeks until the limbal sclera heals enough to form a seal. If surgical repair is required, the tube is reinserted through a new needle track and the old opening sutured closed. If inadequate function of a flow-resisting implant is suspected, as is common owing to the incomplete valve effect of these devices (see Flow Resistance), surgical repair may require placement of a temporary external ligature to prevent recurrence of the hypotony, especially if mitomycin C was used. If an incomplete external ligature is suspected, repair involves religating the tube.

Underfiltration and Increased Intraocular Pressure

Elevated IOP may be anticipated when external ligatures have been placed around a free-flow tube. Early release of the ligature may be performed if medical therapy is unsuccessful in maintaining safe pressures. As a normal part of wound healing, a transient elevation in IOP at 1 to 2 months postoperatively can occur and may respond to temporary medical treatment (37,50).

Proximal Tube Occlusion

During the early postoperative period, the tube may be occluded by blood, fibrin, iris, or vitreous. Tissue plasminogen activator can be used to lyse clots that have formed (116,117). The yttrium-aluminum-garnet (118) (YAG) or neodymium:yttrium-lithium-fluoride (YLF) (119) laser can be used to cut iris, membranes, or vitreous strands, although it is often necessary to sweep iris away from the tube with a spatula or to remove vitreous with a vitreous cutter. Small strands of vitreous that enter the tube but create no pressure problems and no retinal traction may be left without consequence (Fig. 34-24).

Distal Occlusion

Occasionally, devices with flow-restricting elements may have blockage of those elements with fibrin or blood. It is possible to irrigate these blockages with a 27- or 30-gauge cannula passed across the anterior chamber (120). The 27-gauge cannula creates a tight seal with the tube and allows the delivery of maximum pressure during irrigation.

Wound Dehiscence

Since eyes that receive implants often have severe conjunctival scarring, contraction of the sparse reamaining conjunctiva may lead to dehiscence of the wound. It is wise to repair these openings as best as possible to prevent epithelial ingrowth and formation of a leaking fistula (121). If fistulization occurs, excision of ingrown conjunctiva and cautery are performed with closure of the freshened edges (121) (Fig. 34-25).

Late Postoperative

Elevated Intraocular Pressure

Elevated IOP in the late postoperative period may be due to blockage of the tube at its proximal or distal end, but more usually is due to bleb fibrosis and thickening. Occlusion of the proximal end is usually obvious and is related to iris, fibrin, or vitreous entering the tube. As in the early postoperative period, revision may be attempted with a YAG laser followed by vitrectomy or mechanical manipulation if unsuccessful.

Distal tube occlusion is indicated by the lack of a visible or palpable bleb over the episcleral plate and lack of a cyst on B-scan ultrasound (47). This type of occlusion may be more common if a flow-resisting element is present, because the element may function as a scaffold for fibrin adhesions or cellular proliferation. Flow may be re-established by manipulation of the valve with a muscle hook (122),

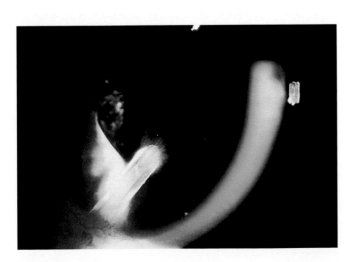

FIGURE 34-24. *Vitreous incarcerated in the tip of the tube.*

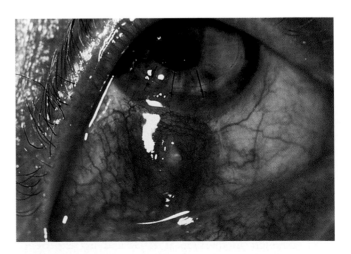

FIGURE 34-25. *Exposure of the tube due to wound dehiscence.*

cannular flush (120), or failing those maneuvers, amputation of the valve element (67).

Bleb fibrosis is the primary mode of late failure of implant devices, as in trabeculectomy. Although Molteno (37) commented that late implant failure due to bleb fibrosis is rare, most other investigators noted an attrition of success over time (50,53). Surgical options include revision of the bleb, implantation of a second device, or a cyclodestructive procedure. Implantation of a second device is usually the best alternative as reports of successful bleb revision are not available, and my experience has been disappointing.

Tube Erosion

Erosion of the tube or plate may occur as with any implanted material, especially in the setting of chronic inflammation and through incision sites (see Fig. 34-25). This complication may be minimized by use of a scleral (or fascial, dural, or pericardial) graft at the time of initial surgery. In addition, placement of conjunctival incisions over areas of future grafting rather than directly over the tube will prevent exposure after a minor wound dehiscence. The major risk of tube exposure is endophthalmitis (123). Erosions should be repaired by use of a scleral (124), dural (94), pericardial, or fascial (125) patch graft. In situations where scleral melt has or is likely to occur, corneal patch grafts may be more resistant to breakdown.

Corneal Decompensation and Graft Failure

Decompensation of an otherwise normal cornea following placement of an implant device is rare, unless tube-cornea touch has occurred. Endothelial cell counts following tube placement decrease by a clinically insignificant amount (126). Several large series described an incidence of 2% to 3% corneal decompensation, but the majority of these eyes had numerous surgical insults (98,127).

The incidence of corneal graft failure following glaucoma implants ranges between 41% and 51% (128–130). Possible causes include intermittent corneal touch, chronic mechanical irritation leading to chronic inflammation, and an alteration of the blood-aqueous barrier. One study showed a trend for better graft survival in eyes that received implants prior to penetrating keratoplasty (129).

Strabismus

Strabismus and diplopia can occur after placement of any of the common implants. Implants with plates designed to minimize the chance of contact with the extraocular muscles, such as the Molteno and the Ahmed implants, seem to have the lowest prevalence of postoperative strabismus (0%–6%) (63,70,103). Placement of the Molteno implant inferiorly increased the prevalence up to 56% in one report (131), although another report (103) and my experience suggest a much lower number. The highest rates of strabismus are associated with larger implants that contact the extraocular muscles such as the Baerveldt and the Krupin

implants. The original version of the Baerveldt implant had a reported rate of strabismus of as high as 77% (70) and so was modified with fenestrations to minimize cyst size. Reported rates with the fenestrated version ranged between 6% and 19% (59,103,111). The Krupin implant has a higher ridge (1.5mm) than some of the other devices (see Table 34-1), and barely contacts the muscles if placed in the temporal quadrants but may underlie them if placed nasally without trimming the implant. The Krupin implant has resulted in rates of diplopia of 2% to 14% (62,67,132). The Krupin implant is now available with a lower ridge to minimize this complication. Rates of strabismus for all implants increase with placement in the nasal quadrants and many surgeons recommend only temporal placement of the larger devices.

The cause of strabismus following implant placement is most commonly a mass effect of the cyst wall that both stretches an overlying muscle and restricts it from relaxing by incorporating it in the cyst scar (70,131–136). This mechanism has most often been observed with the larger implants. Other mechanisms that have been described included a "Faden" effect of the Molteno tube underlying a muscle (137), a Brown's syndrome (138,139), and a progressive fat adherence syndrome (140).

Treatment of strabismus usually requires removal of the implant and replacement with a smaller device or placement of a device in a location less likely to result in strabismus (70), although a lesser degree of recalcitrant strabismus may remain (70,136).

Cataract

If the implant tube touches the lens in the postoperative period, a cataract may form. Usually, a superficial, nonprogressive opacity develops and requires no treatment (141) (Fig. 34-26).

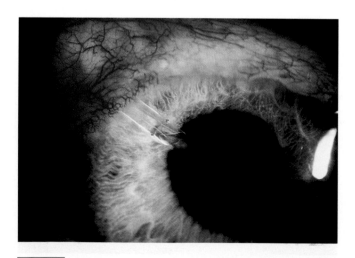

FIGURE 34-26. *Nonprogressive cataract following tube-lens touch.*

Uveitis

A chronic, low-grade uveitis can develop, albeit rarely, following implant surgery, especially if the tube remains in contact with the iris. Occasionally, fibrin deposits may form around the tube and an anterior-chamber tap may be required to exclude endophthalmitis (Fig. 34-27) (142). Most cases of uveitis related to tubes respond to topical steroids, although occasional patients may require chronic use.

Hypotony

Late onset of hypotony following implant surgery suggests a secondary cause, such as uveitis, retinal detachment, cyclitic membrane, or erosion of the plate. After these possibilities are excluded, it is usually concluded that aqueous production has been reduced by the effects of multiple interventions below the drainage capacity of the implant. Treatment requires lowering that capacity by reducing the effective surface area of the device and is indicated only if complications such as choroidal detachment or maculopathy develop. If the hypotony is profound, complete ligation of the translimbal tube with a permanent suture such as polypropylene may be indicated, and allows easy reversal should additional pressure control become required in the future. Alternatively, the device can be removed. For milder hypotony, a double-plate Molteno implant can be ligated at the interplate junction to isolate the distal plate and reduce the filtration area of the plates by one-half. Eyes with prior cyclocryotherapy are particularly prone to hypotony (143).

Tube Migration

During wound healing, the implant is encapsulated in a fibrous cocoon that usually restricts any motion away from its original position. Occasionally however, contraction of the wound may place great stress on the implant device and move it if it is not adequately anchored. The episcleral plate may be pulled posteriorly, causing the tube to slip out of the eye, or the plate may be forced toward the limbus, causing apparent tube elongation and corneal touch inside the anterior chamber. In addition, the tube may move laterally, such that its original straight, radial orientation to the limbus is altered to an S shape that also may cause the tube to slip out of the anterior chamber (141). Surgical repair is best achieved with an incision over the scleral graft (to prevent later dehiscence) and repositioning of the tube with adequate suture fixation.

Retinal Detachment

Retinal detachment occurs after implant surgery in approximately 2% of patients, although it is not usually causally related to the procedure (50,98). In one series of 350 patients, 5% of the patients with Molteno implants developed retinal detachments, the majority of which were believed to relate to prior surgery and underlying disease (144). Repair may be difficult, as only 56% of patients in this series achieved anatomic reattachment.

Endophthalmitis

As in any eye surgery, endophthalmitis may complicate implant placement in the early postoperative period (50,98,145). In the late postoperative period, endophthalmitis may occur related to implant erosion and exposure (123) or subsequent operation (146). In many situations the infection can be controlled with the implant in place (98,146), while in others, it may be best to remove the implant to avoid abscess formation (145). Sterile endophthalmitis may occur in the absence of erosion and may mimic infectious endophthalmitis. Although sterile endophthalmitis responds to steroid treatment, anterior-chamber or vitreous tap may be required to differentiate the two (142).

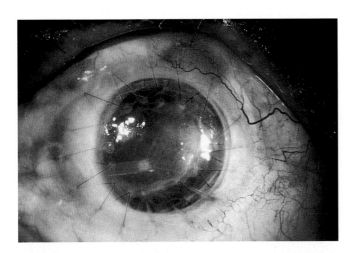

FIGURE 34-27. *Fibrinoid anterior-chamber reaction must be distinguished from endophthalmitis.*

REFERENCES

1. Herbert H. Subconjunctival fistula formation in the treatment of primary chronic glaucoma. *Trans Ophthalmol Soc UK* 1903;23:324–346.
2. Holth S. Iridencleisis antiglaucoma. *Ann d'Ocul* 1907;137:345.
3. Elliot R. A preliminary note on a new operative procedure for the establishment of a filtering cicatrix in the treatment of glaucoma. *Ophthalmoscope* 1909;7:804–806.
4. Rollett M, Moreau M. Traitment de le hypopyon par le drainage capillaire de la chambre anterieure. *Rev Gen Ophthalmol* 1906;25:481–489.
5. MacDonald RK, Pierce MBE. Silicone setons. *Am J Ophthalmol* 1965;59:635–646.
6. Vail DT. Retained silk thread or 'seton' drainage from vitreous chamber to Tenon's lymph channel for the relief of glaucoma. *Ophthalmol Rec Chicago* 1915;24:184–186.
7. Row H. Operation to control glaucoma: preliminary report. *Arch Ophthalmol* 1934;12:325.
8. Troncosco MU. Cyclodialysis with insertion of a metal implant in the treatment of glaucoma: a preliminary report. *Arch Ophthalmol* 1940;23:270–300.
9. Troncosco MU. Use of tantalum implants for inducing a permanent hypotony in rabbits' eyes. *Am J Ophthalmol* 1949;32:499–508.
10. Ellis RA. Reduction of intraocular pressure using plastics in surgery. *Am J Ophthalmol* 1960;50:733–742.
11. Pinnas G, Boniuk M. Cyclodialysis with Teflon tube implants. *Am J Ophthalmol* 1969;68:879–883.

12. Portney GL. Silicone elastomer implantation cyclodialysis. *Arch Ophthalmol* 1973;89:10–12.
13. Lee KY, et al. Magnetic resonance imaging of the aqueous flow in eyes implanted with the trabeculo-suprachoroidal glaucoma seton. *Invest Ophthalmol Vis Sci* 1992;33(suppl):948.
14. Zorab A. The reduction of tension in chronic glaucoma. *Ophthalmoscope* 1912;10:258–261.
15. Stefansson J. An operation for glaucoma. *Am J Ophthalmol* 1925;8:681–693.
16. Blumenthal M, Harris LS, Galin MA. Experimental study of cartilage setons. *Br J Ophthalmol* 1970;54:62–65.
17. Bock RH. Subconjunctival drainage of the anterior chamber by a glass seton. *Am J Ophthalmol* 1950;33:929–939.
18. Gibson GG. Transscleral lacrimal-canaliculus transplants. *Am J Ophthalmol* 1944;27:258–269.
19. Muldoon WE, Ripple PH, Wilder HC. Platinum implant in glaucoma surgery. *Arch Ophthalmol* 1951;45:666–672.
20. Mascati NT. A new surgical approach for the control of a class of glaucomas. *Int Surg* 1967;47:10.
21. Rajah-Sivayoham ISS. Camero-venous shunt for secondary glaucoma following orbital venous obstruction. *Br J Ophthalmol* 1968;52:843–845.
22. Lee PF, Wong WT. Aqueous-venous shunt for glaucoma: report on 15 cases. *Ann Ophthalmol* 1974;6:1083–1088.
23. Welsh NH. Veno-cameral shunt in end-stage glaucoma. Presented at the International Glaucoma Symposium, Jerusalem, 1991.
24. Roig A. Artefacto operatorio in la operacion de Elliott. *Arch Soc Oftal Hispano-AM* 1954;14:797–798.
25. Laval J. The use of absorbable gelatin film (Gelfilm) in glaucoma filtration surgery. *Arch Ophthalmol* 1955;54:677–682.
26. Bick MW. Use of tantalum for ocular drainage. *Arch Ophthalmol* 1949;42:373–388.
27. Stone W. Alloplasty in surgery of the eye. I. *N Engl J Med* 1958;258:486–490.
28. Epstein E. Fibrosing response to aqueous—its relation to glaucoma. *Br J Ophthalmol* 1959;43:641–647.
29. La Rocca V. Gonioplasty in glaucoma: a preliminary report. *Br J Ophthalmol* 1962;46:404–415.
30. Richards RD, Van Bijsterveld OP. Artificial drainage tubes for glaucoma. *Am J Ophthalmol* 1965;60:405–408.
31. Krupin T, Podos SM, Becker B, Newkirk JB. Valve implants in filtering surgery. *Am J Ophthalmol* 1976;81:232–235.
32. Honrubia FM, Grijalbo MP, Gomez ML, Lopez A. Surgical treatment of neovascular glaucoma. *Trans Ophthalmol Soc UK* 1979;99:89–91.
33. Hauber F. Artificial drainage implants in glaucoma. *Ophthalmic Pract* 1994;12:114–118.
34. Krupin T, Kaufman P, Mandell AI, et al. Long-term results of valve implants in filtering surgery for eyes with neovascular glaucoma. *Am J Ophthalmol* 1983;95:775–782.
35. Molteno ACB. New implant for glaucoma, clinical trial. *Br J Ophthalmol* 1969;53:606–615.
36. Molteno ACB, Straughan JL, Ancker E. Control of bleb fibrosis after glaucoma surgery by anti-inflammatory agents. *S Afr Med J* 1976;50:881–885.
37. Molteno ACB. Use of Molteno implants to treat secondary glaucoma. In: Cairns JE, ed. *Glaucoma*. London: Grune & Stratton, 1986:211–238.
38. Molteno ACB, Straughan JL, Ancker E. Long tube implants in the management of glaucoma. *S Afr Med J* 1976;50:1062–1066.
39. Molteno ACB, Van Biljon G, Ancker E. Two-stage insertion of glaucoma drainage implants. *Trans Ophthalmol Soc N Z* 1979;31:17–26.
40. Molteno ACB, Polkinghorne PJ, Bowbyes JA. The Vicryl tie technique for inserting a draining implant in the treatment of secondary glaucoma. *Aust N Z J Ophthalmol* 1986;14:343–354.
41. Molteno ACB. The dual-chamber single-plate implant. *Aust N Z J Ophthalmol* 1990;18:431–436.
42. Schocket SS. Investigations of the reasons for success and failure in the anterior shunt-to-the-encircling-band procedure in the treatment of refractory glaucoma. *Trans Am Ophthalmol Soc* 1986;84:743–798.
43. Krupin T, Mandell A, Ritch R, et al. Filtering valve implant surgery for eyes with neovascular glaucoma. *Am J Ophthalmol* 1980;89:338–343.
44. Loeffler KU, Jay JL. Tissue response to aqueous drainage in a functioning Molteno implant. *Br J Ophthalmol* 1988;72:29–35.
45. Minckler DS, Shammas A, Wilcox M, Ogden TE. Experimental studies of aqueous filtration using the Molteno implant. *Trans Am Ophthalmol Soc* 1987;85:368–392.
46. Wilcox MJ, Minckler DS, Ogden TE. Pathophysiology of artificial aqueous drainage in primate eyes with Molteno implants. *J Glaucoma* 1994;3:140–151.
47. Lloyd MAE, Minckler DS, Heuer DK, et al. Echographic evaluation of glaucoma shunts. *Ophthalmology* 1993;100:919–927.
48. Crighton ACS, Kasper DM, Kirker GEM, et al. Ultrasonography to assess patency of the tube in Molteno seton implantation. *Ophthalmology* 1993;28:273–275.
49. Molteno ACB. The optimal design of drainage implants for glaucoma. *Trans Ophthalmol Soc N Z* 1981;33:39–41.
50. Heuer DK, Lloyd MA, Abrams DA. Which is better? One or two? A randomized clinical trial of single-plate versus double-plate Molteno implantation for glaucomas in aphakia and pseudophakia. *Ophthalmology* 1992;99:1512–1519.
51. Brown RD, Cairns JE. Experience with the Molteno long tube implant. *Trans Ophthalmol Soc UK* 1983;103:297–312.
52. Susanna R, Nicolela MT, Takahashi WY. Mitomycin C as adjunctive therapy with glaucoma implant surgery. *Ophthalmic Surg* 1994;25:458–462.
53. Perkins TW, Cardakli UF, Eisele JR, et al. Adjunctive mitomycin C in Molteno implant surgery. *Ophthalmology* 1995;102:91–97.
54. Cantor LB, Sanders S, Bhavenani V, et al. The effect of mitomycin-C on Molteno implant surgery. *Invest Ophthalmol Vis Sci* 1996;37(suppl):255.
55. Kalenak JW, Ripkin DJ, Mendendorp SV. A randomized controlled trial of the Molteno implant with and without mitomycin-C. *Invest Ophthalmol Vis Sci* 1996;37(suppl):155.
56. Prata JA, Minckler DS, Mermoud A, Baerveldt G. Effects of intraoperative mitomycin-C on the function of Baerveldt glaucoma drainage implants in rabbits. *J Glaucoma* 1996;5:29–38.
57. Prata JA, Santos RCR, LaBree L, Minckler DS. Surface area of glaucoma implants and perfusion flow rates in rabbit eyes. *J Glaucoma* 1995;4:274–280.
58. Hitchings RA, Joseph NH, Sherwood MB, et al. Use of one-piece valved tube and variable surface area explant for glaucoma drainage surgery. *Ophthalmology* 1987;94:1079–1084.
59. Lloyd MAE, Baerveldt G, Fellenbaum PS, et al. Intermediate-term results of a randomized clinical trial of the 350-mm² vs the 500-mm² Baerveldt implant. *Ophthalmology* 1994;101:1456–1464.
60. Sidoti PA, Dunphy TR, Baerveldt G, et al. Experience with the Baerveldt glaucoma implant in treating neovascular glaucoma. *Ophthalmology* 1995;102:1107–1118.
61. Smith M, Sherwood MB, McGorray SP. Comparison of the double-plate Molteno drainage implant with the Schocket procedure. *Arch Ophthalmol* 1992;110:1246–1250.
62. Krupin Eye Valve Filtering Surgery Study Group. Krupin eye valve with disk for filtration surgery. *Ophthalmology* 1994;101:651–658.
63. Coleman AL, Hill R, Wilson MR, et al. Initial clinical experience with the Ahmed glaucoma valve implant. *Am J Ophthalmol* 1995;120:23–31.
64. White TC. Clinical results of glaucoma surgery using the White glaucoma pump shunt. *Ann Ophthalmol* 1992;24:365–373.
65. Krupin T. Setons in glaucoma surgery. In: Waltman SR, et al, eds. *Surgery of the eye*. New York: Churchill Livingstone, 1988:377–385.
66. Prata JA, et al. In vitro and in vivo flow: characteristics of glaucoma drainage implants. *Ophthalmology* 1995;102:894–904.
67. Fellenbaum PS, Almeida AR, Minckler DS, et al. Krupin disk implantation for complicated glaucomas. *Ophthalmology* 1994;101:1178–1182.
68. Molteno ACB, Van Rooyen MMB, Bartholomew RS. Implants for draining neovascular glaucoma. *Br J Ophthalmol* 1977;61:120–125.
69. Lloyd MAE, Baerveldt G, Heuer DK, et al. Initial clinical experience with the Baerveldt implant in complicated glaucomas. *Ophthalmology* 1994;101:640–650.
70. Smith SL, Starita RJ, Fellman RL, Lynn JR. Early clinical experience with the Baerveldt 350-mm² glaucoma implant and associated extraocular muscle imbalance. *Ophthalmology* 1993;100:914–918.
71. Freedman J. Clinical experience with the Molteno dual-chamber single-plate implant. *Ophthalmic Surg* 1992;23:238–241.
72. Schocket SS, Lakhanpal V, Richards RD. Anterior chamber tube shunt to an encircling band in the treatment of neovascular glaucoma. *Ophthalmology* 1982;89:1188–1194.
73. Schocket SS, Nirankari VS, Lakhanpal V, et al. Anterior chamber tube shunt to an encircling band in the treatment of neovascular glaucoma and other refractory glaucomas: a long-term study. *Ophthalmology* 1985;92:553–562.
74. Wilson RP, Cantor L, Katz LJ, et al. Aqueous shunts: Molteno versus Schocket. *Ophthalmology* 1992;99:672–678.
75. Joseph NH, Sherwood MB, Trantas G, et al. A one piece drainage system for glaucoma surgery. *Trans Ophthalmol Soc UK* 1986;105:657–664.
76. Chihara E, Kubota H, Takanashi T, Nao-i N. Outcome of White pump shunt surgery for neovascular glaucoma. *Ophthalmic Surg* 1992;23:666–671.
77. Bluestein EC, Stewart WC. Trabeculectomy with 5-fluorouracil versus single-plate Molteno implantation. *Ophthalmic Surg* 1993;24:669–673.

78. Mermoud A, Salmon JF, Alexander P, et al. Molteno tube implantation for neovascular glaucoma: long-term results and factors influencing outcome. *Ophthalmology* 1993;100:897–902.

79. El Sayyad F, Helal M, Elsherif Z, El-Maghraby A. Molteno implant versus trabeculectomy with adjunctive intraoperative mitomycin-C in high-risk glaucoma patients. *J Glaucoma* 1995;4:80–85.

80. Perkins TW. Surgery in the face of adherent Teno-conjunctival scarring: which augmented approach is best? Presented at the American Academy of Ophthalmology Meeting, Atlanta, GA, Nov. 1, 1995.

81. Caronia RM, Liebmann JM, Friedman R, et al. Trabeculectomy at the inferior limbus. *Arch Ophthalmol* 1996;114:387–391.

82. Higginbotham EJ, Stevens RK, Musch DC. Bleb-related endophthalmitis after trabeculectomy with mitomycin C. *Ophthalmology* 1996;103:650–656.

83. Wolner B, Liebmann JM, Sassani JW, et al. Late bleb-related endophthalmitis after trabeculectomy with adjunctive 5-fluorouracil. *Ophthalmology* 1991;98:1053–1060.

84. Traverso CE, Tomey KF, Al-Kaff A. The long-tube single-plate Molteno implant for the treatment of recalcitrant glaucoma. *Int Ophthalmol* 1989;13:159–162.

85. Price FW, Whitson WE. Polypropylene ligatures as a means of controlling intraocular pressure with Molteno implants. *Ophthalmic Surg* 1989;20:781–783.

86. Liebmann JM, Ritch R. Intraocular suture ligature to reduce hypotony following Molteno seton implantation. *Ophthalmic Surg* 1992;23:51–52.

87. El-Sayad F, El-Maghraby A, Helal M, Amayem A. The use of releasable sutures in Molteno glaucoma implant procedures to reduce postoperative hypotony. *Ophthalmic Surg* 1991;22:82–84.

88. Hoare Nairne JEAH, et al. Single stage insertion of the Molteno tube for glaucoma and modifications to reduce postoperative hypotony. *Br J Ophthalmol* 1988;72:846–851.

89. Susanna R. Modifications of the Molteno implant and implant procedure. *Ophthalmic Surg* 1991;22:611–613.

90. Latina MA. Single stage Molteno implant with combination internal occlusion and external ligature. *Ophthalmic Surg* 1990;21:444–446.

91. Sherwood MB, Smith MF. Prevention of early hypotony associated with Molteno implants by a new occluding stent technique. *Ophthalmology* 1993;100:85–90.

92. Fechtner RD, Acland RD. Tubing introducer forceps for glaucoma drainage-tube implants. *J Glaucoma* 1994;3:79–80.

93. Wright MM, Singh K, Grajewski AL. Polypropylene suture stent for insertion of glaucoma tube shunt implants. *Ophthalmic Surg* 1994;25:743–744. Letter.

94. Freedman J. Scleral patch grafts with Molteno setons. *Ophthalmol Surg* 1987;18:532–534.

95. Brandt JD. Patch grafts of dehydrated cadaveric dura mater for tube-shunt glaucoma surgery. *Arch Ophthalmol* 1993;111:1436–1439.

96. Lieberman MF. Autologous fascial grafts. *Arch Ophthalmol* 1992;110:1685. Letter.

97. Preferred Practice Pattern, AAO Primary Open Angle Glaucoma 1995, San Francisco, CA.

98. Molteno ACB. The use of draining implants in resistant cases of glaucoma—late results of 110 operations. *Trans Ophthalmol Soc N Z* 1983;35:94–97.

99. Ward WJ, Cooper RL. Molteno tube implants: long-term results. *Aust N Z J Ophthalmol* 1987;15:109–112.

100. Goldberg I. Management of uncontrolled glaucoma with the Molteno system. *Aust N Z J Ophthalmol* 1987;15:97–107.

101. Downes RN, Flanagan DW, Jordan K, Burton RL. The Molteno implant in intractable glaucoma. *Eye* 1988;2:250–259.

102. Price FW, Wellemeyer M. Long-term results of Molteno implants. *Ophthalmic Surg* 1995;26:130–135.

103. Smith MF, Doyle JW, Sherwood MB. Comparison of the Baerveldt glaucoma implant with the double-plate Molteno drainage implant. *Arch Ophthalmol* 1995;113:444–447.

104. Ancker E, Molteno ACB. Molteno drainage implant for neovascular glaucoma. *Trans Ophthalmol Soc UK* 1982;102:122–123.

105. Molteno ACB, Ancker E, Van Biljon G. Surgical technique for advanced juvenile glaucoma. *Arch Ophthalmol* 1984;102:51–57.

106. Billson F, Thomas R, Aylward W. The use of two-stage Molteno implants in developmental glaucoma. *J Pediatr Ophthalmol Strabismus* 1989;26:3–8.

107. Hill RA, Heuer DK, Baerveldt G, et al. Molteno implantation for glaucoma in young patients. *Ophthalmology* 1991;98:1042–1046.

108. Netland PA, Walton DS. Glaucoma drainage implants in pediatric patients. *Ophthalmic Surg* 1993;24:723–729.

109. Fish LA, Heuer DK, Baerveldt G, et al. Molteno implantation for secondary glaucomas associated with advanced epithelial ingrowth. *Ophthalmology* 1990;97:557–561.

110. Fellenbaum PS, Sidoti PA, Heuer DK, et al. Experience with the Baerveldt implant in young patients with complicated glaucomas. *J Glaucoma* 1995;4:91–97.

111. Hodkin MJ. Early clinical experience with the Baerveldt implant in complicated glaucoma. *Am J Ophthalmol* 1995;120:32–40.

112. Sherwood MB, Joseph NH, Hitchings RA. Surgery for refractory glaucoma: results and complications with a modified Schocket technique. *Arch Ophthalmol* 1987;105:562–569.

113. Spiegel D, Shrader RR, Wilson RP. Anterior chamber tube shunt to an encircling band (Schocket procedure) in the treatment of refractory glaucoma. *Ophthalmic Surg* 1992;23:804–807.

114. Sidoti PA, Minckler DS, Baerveldt G, et al. Aqueous tube shunt to a preexisting episcleral encircling element in the treatment of complicated glaucomas. *Ophthalmology* 1994;101:1036–1043.

115. Davidovski F, Stewart RH, Kimbrough RL. Long-term results with the White glaucoma pump-shunt. *Ophthalmic Surg* 1990;21:288–293.

116. Pastor SA, Schumann SP, Starita RJ, Fellman RL. Intracameral tissue plasminogen activator: management of a fibrin clot occluding a Molteno tube. *Ophthalmic Surg* 1993;24:853–854.

117. Richards DW. Intracameral tissue plasminogen activator to treat blocked glaucoma implants. *Ophthalmic Surg* 1993;24:854–855.

118. Fiore PM, Melamed S. Use of neodymium:YAG laser to open an occluded Molteno tube. *Ophthalmic Surg* 1989;20:373–374.

119. Oram O, Gross R, Severin TD, et al. Opening an occluded Molteno tube with the picosecond neodymium-yttrium lithium fluoride laser. *Arch Ophthalmol* 1994;112:1023.

120. Krawitz PL. Treatment of distal occlusion of Krupin eye valve with disk using cannular flush. *Ophthalmic Surg* 1994;25:102–104.

121. Sidoti PA, Minckler DS, Baerveldt G, et al. Epithelial ingrowth and glaucoma drainage implants. *Ophthalmology* 1994;101:872–875.

122. Weiss HS. Postoperative manipulation of the Krupin valve. *Ophthalmic Surg Lasers* 1996;27:151–153.

123. Krebs DB, Liebmann JM, Ritch R, Speaker M. Late infectious endophthalmitis from exposed glaucoma setons. *Arch Ophthalmol* 1992;110:174–175.

124. Watzke R. Scleral patch graft for exposed episcleral implants. *Arch Ophthalmol* 1984;102:114–115.

125. Dresner DB, Boyer DS, Feinfeld RE. Autogenous fascial grafts for exposed retinal buckles. *Arch Ophthalmol* 1991;109:288–289.

126. McDermott ML, Swendris RP, Shin DH, et al. Corneal endothelial cell counts after Molteno implantation. *Am J Ophthalmol* 1993;115:93–96.

127. Minckler DS, Heuer DK, Hasty B, et al. Clinical experience with the single-plate Molteno implant in complicated glaucomas. *Ophthalmology* 1988;95:1181–1188.

128. McDonnell PJ, Robin JB, Schanzlin DJ, et al. Molteno implant for control of glaucoma in eyes after penetrating keratoplasty. *Ophthalmology* 1988;95:364–369.

129. Beebe WE, Starita RJ, Fellman RL, et al. The use of Molteno implant and anterior chamber tube shunt to encircling band for the treatment of glaucoma in keratoplasty: the risks and advantages. *Ophthalmology* 1990;97:1414–1422.

130. Sherwood MB, Smith MF, Driebe WT, et al. Drainage tube implants in the treatment of glaucoma following penetrating keratoplasty. *Ophthalmic Surg* 1993;24:185–189.

131. Wilson-Holt N, Franks W, Nourredin B, Hitchings R. Hypertropia following inferiorly sited double-plate Molteno tubes. *Eye* 1992;6:515–520.

132. Frank JW, Perkins TW, Kushner BJ. Ocular motility defects in patients with the Krupin valve implant. *Ophthalmic Surg* 1995;26:228–232.

133. Munoz M, Parrish RK II. Strabismus following implantation of Baerveldt devices. *Arch Ophthalmol* 1993;111:1096–1099.

134. Kooner KS, Cavanagh HD, Zimmerman CF, Itani K. Eye movement restrictions after Molteno implant surgery. *Ophthalmic Surg* 1993;24:498–499.

135. Prata JA, Minckler DS, Green RL. Pseudo-Brown's syndrome as a complication of glaucoma drainage implant surgery. *Ophthalmic Surg* 1993;24:608–611.

136. Cardakli UF, Perkins TW. Recalcitrant diplopia after implantation of a Krupin valve with disc. *Ophthalmic Surg* 1994;25:256–258.

137. Christmann LM, Wilson ME. Motility disturbances after Molteno implants. *J Pediatr Ophthalmol Strabismus* 1992;29:44–48.

138. Ball SF, Herrington RG, Liang K. Brown's superior oblique tendon syndrome after Baerveldt glaucoma implant. *Arch Ophthalmol* 1992;110:1368.

139. Dobler AA, Sondhi N, Cantor LB, Ku S. Acquired Brown's syndrome after a double-plate Molteno implant. *Am J Ophthalmol* 1993;116:641–642.

140. Munoz M, Parrish R. Hypertropia after implantation of a Molteno drainage device. *Am J Ophthalmol* 1992;113:98–100.

141. Rosenberg LF, Krupin T. Implants in glaucoma surgery. In: Ritch R, Shields MB, Krupin T, eds. *The glaucomas.* Vol 3. St. Louis: Mosby, 1996: 1783–1807.

142. Heher KL, Lim JI, Haller JA, Jampel HD. Late-onset sterile endophthalmitis after Molteno tube implantation. *Am J Ophthalmol* 1992;114:771–772.

143. Wellemeyer ML, Price FW. Molteno implants in patients with previous cyclocryotherapy. *Ophthalmic Surg* 1993;24:395–398.

144. Waterhouse WJ, Lloyd MAE, Dugel PU. Rhegmatogenous retinal detachment after Molteno glaucoma implant surgery. *Ophthalmology* 1994;101:665–671.

145. Perkins TW. Endophthalmitis after placement of a Molteno implant. *Ophthalmic Surg* 1990;21:733–734.

146. Ellis BD, Varley GA, Kalenak JW, et al. Bacterial endophthalmitis following cataract surgery in an eye with a preexisting Molteno implant. *Ophthalmic Surg* 1993;24:117–118.

Surgical Iridectomy and Goniosynechialysis

ROBERT M. SCHERTZER   DAVID G. CAMPBELL

HISTORY

In 1857, von Graefe first introduced surgical sector iridectomy for the treatment of acute glaucoma. Until Curran (2) explained the mechanism of relative pupillary block in 1920, peripheral iridectomy did not gain widespread acceptance. Shortly after Barkan (3) introduced an anatomic classification for glaucoma in 1938, surgical peripheral iridectomy became the treatment of choice for primary angle-closure glaucoma. It remained the treatment of choice for pupillary block in eyes with angle-closure glaucoma prior to the alternatives offered by laser therapy. There are still patients in whom laser iridotomy is inadvisable or impossible such as those with flat anterior chambers or cloudy corneas not cleared with topical glycerin.

Surgical reduction of synechial angle closure has evolved since 1957 when Shaffer (4) recommended synechialysis, inverse cyclodialysis, or iridencleisis for synechial angle closure under operating-room gonioscopy. Chandler and Simmons (5) proposed a chamber-deepening procedure in 1965 to improve assessment of the extent of closure to decide whether iridectomy would suffice or if trabeculectomy would be required. They also noted the chamber-deepening procedure itself sometimes broke recently formed synechiae. Campbell and Vela (6) in 1984 described a surgical goniosynechialysis technique that takes advantage of the development of viscoelastic substances to break peripheral synechiae in a well-controlled manner.

INDICATIONS

Surgical peripheral iridectomy is indicated to eliminate pupillary block (7,8) in situations where laser iridotomy has failed or is not feasible (Table 35-1).

Goniosynechialysis is indicated for the treatment of complete or near-complete synechial angle closure (≥270 degrees), present for 6 months or less (6,9). It can be combined with or follow a surgical iridectomy or laser iridotomy.

ANESTHESIA

Difference of opinion exists as to the ideal anesthesia for a surgical iridectomy. A retrobulbar or peribulbar block combined with a lid block provides excellent anesthesia and akinesia. There is also the potential pressure-lowering effect of the inhibition of the sympathetic supply to the eye. Spaeth (7) advocated a facial nerve block combined with topical anesthesia to be ideal, avoiding retrobulbar or peribulbar blocks that risk retrobulbar hemorrhage which could delay surgery, resulting in permanent visual loss.

PREOPERATIVE MANAGEMENT

Maximal medical therapy is attempted, along with laser iridotomies, to break the acute angle-closure attack. The preoperative medications include pilocarpine for pupillary constriction and a topical antibiotic for antimicrobial prophylaxis. Each of these agents can be instilled every 10 to 30 minutes for three doses, with 5 minutes between each drop. Pilocarpine strengths greater than 2% are best avoided because they risk an exuberant accommodative response that could further shallow the anterior chamber in susceptible eyes.

Another important factor in preoperative care is to minimize inflammation. There is a balance in timing the surgery between the degree of inflammation and the level of intraocular pressure. Certainly, the greater the preoperative

Table 35-1.   Indications for Surgical Peripheral Iridectomy (7,8)

Laser iridotomy not feasible
    Corneal edema or opacity precluding adequate iris visualization
    Flat anterior chamber with broad iridocorneal contact
    Patient unable or unwilling to cooperate
    Lack or breakdown of laser equipment
    Dislocated lens
Laser iridotomy failed
    Uveitis closing iridotomies
In association with other surgery
    Cataract extraction
    Keratoplasty
    Glaucoma filtration surgery
    Chamber deepening and goniosynechialysis
Iris pathologic specimen required

inflammation, the poorer the postoperative result. Hourly prednisolone acetate (1%) provides excellent anti-inflammatory action. As the delay until surgery would likely not exceed 2 weeks, the risk of steroid-induced pressure rise is minimal (7).

Intraocular pressures higher than 30 mm Hg increase the risk of malignant glaucoma or expulsive choroidal hemorrhage. Therefore preoperative paracentesis may be required to bring the pressure into the range of 15 to 30 mm Hg (7). Following instillation of several drops of an antibiotic-steroid, with any anesthesia method of choice, a horizontal rectus muscle is firmly grasped with toothed forceps. Under visualization with surgical loupes or an operating microscope, a No. 75 blade enters at the temporal limbus, angled toward the 6-o'clock position to avoid lens trauma. In our experience, this bedside technique provides excellent temporary relief of elevated pressure.

The "fellow eye" should be examined for signs of early angle closure and treated appropriately with low-dose pilocarpine (0.5%–1.0%) until a laser iridotomy can be performed.

SURGICAL TECHNIQUE FOR IRIDECTOMY

The iridectomy consists of five steps: 1) incision, 2) exteriorization of the iris, 3) excision of the iris, 4) repositioning of the iris, and 5) closure of the incision. Scleral and clear corneal incisions are described. A rectus superior bridle suture of 4-0 or 5-0 silk is placed and fastened to the drapes. A paracentesis through clear cornea is performed temporally.

Incision

The incision is made either under a conjunctival flap or through clear cornea. Although it is more difficult to pro-

lapse the iris tissue through a clear corneal incision, conjunctiva will be spared for future trabeculectomy if required (8). Other considerations for a clear corneal incision include extensive peripheral anterior synechiae and a need to minimize bleeding (7).

Initial penetration to one-half to two-thirds thickness (10) allows for the preplacement of a 9-0 white virgin silk suture or a 9-0 nylon suture through the groove (Fig. 35-1). The suture needs to be strong enough for traction (7) but fine enough for precise wound closure.

Scleral Approach

A small fornix-based conjunctival flap is made supratemporally or supranasally and hemostasis is achieved with cautery. A shelved incision 2 to 3 mm long is made (7,8,11) using a No. 75 blade at the posterior edge of the surgical limbus, 1.0 to 1.5 mm behind the corneolimbal junction (Fig. 35-2).

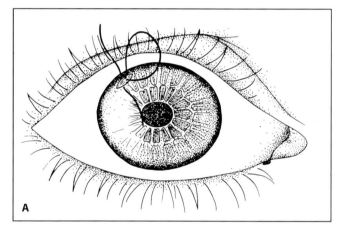

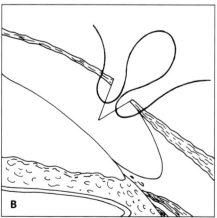

FIGURE 35-1.   *Preplacement of a suture in a two-thirds' thickness corneal wound. A. Anterior view. B. Cross-sectional view. (Redrawn with permission from Wilson MR. Peripheral iridectomy and chamber deepening. In: Albert DM, Jakobiec FA, eds. Principles and practice of ophthalmology. Philadelphia: WB Saunders, 1994: 1618.)*

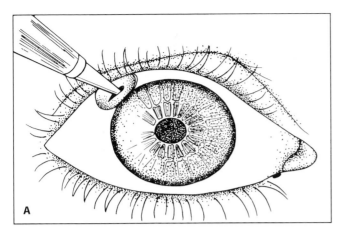

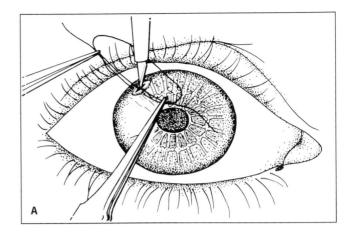

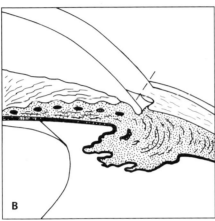

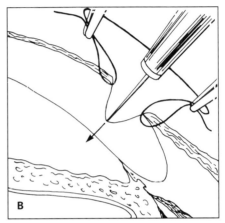

FIGURE 35-2. *A scleral incision 1.0 to 1.5 mm behind the corneolimbal junction. A. Anterior view. B. Cross-sectional view. (Redrawn with permission from Spaeth GL. Glaucoma surgery. In: Spaeth GL, ed. Ophthalmic surgery: principles and practice. Philadelphia: WB Saunders, 1990.)*

Clear Corneal Approach

The corneal incision should be perpendicular to the corneal tangent to facilitate iris prolapse, and should be just anterior to the limbal vessels. With the assistant spreading open the wound with the preplaced suture or tying forceps, Descemet's membrane is penetrated the full length of the wound (8) with the No. 75 blade, to enter the anterior chamber (Fig. 35-3).

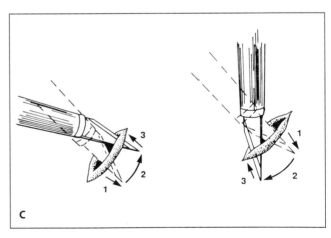

FIGURE 35-3. *A, B. The preplaced sutures facilitate access to the inner depths of the cornea. C. Descemet's membrane is penetrated the full length of the corneal wound by entering centrally (1), rotating the blade through an arc (2), and exiting with the cutting edge perpendicular to the wound (3). (B, C redrawn with permission from Wilson MR. Peripheral iridectomy and chamber deepening. In: Albert DM, Jakobiec FA, eds. Principles and practice of ophthalmology. Philadelphia: WB Saunders, 1994:1618.)*

Exteriorization of the Iris

Gentle pressure on the posterior lip of the scleral wound will usually prolapse the iris into the wound (11). When sutures are preplaced, the assistant can provide traction with these sutures (8) while gentle pressure is applied to the posterior lip of the incision (Fig. 35-4). If the anterior-chamber entry wound is too small, this maneuver will be difficult and the original incision should be enlarged.

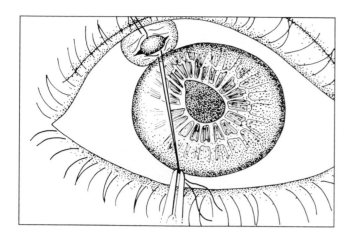

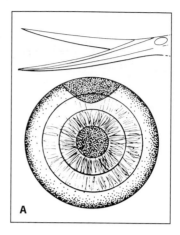

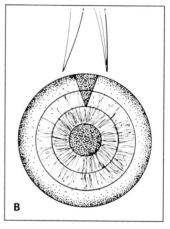

FIGURE 35-4.   *Preplaced sutures in the scleral wound assisting in access to the anterior chamber for iridectomy.*

FIGURE 35-5.   A. *Keeping the scissors parallel to the limbus results in a broad-based iridectomy.* B. *With the scissors perpendicular to the limbus, a narrow, sharply peaked iridectomy results.*

Excision of the Iris

The prolapsed iris is grasped with fine curved iris forceps and cut with Vannas or de Wecker scissors kept parallel to the iris-corneal plane (8,11). Keeping the scissors parallel to the wound ensures a broad-based iridectomy (Fig. 35-5A). Cutting perpendicular to the wound yields a more cosmetically appealing narrow-based sector (Fig. 35-5B). If the tissue is near the tips of the scissors, the iris will tend to slip, resulting in a ragged edge (7). The posterior surface of the specimen is examined to ensure that pigmented epithelium has been excised. If the iris does not prolapse, then the anterior chamber must be entered with fine nontoothed forceps to grasp the iris (8).

Repositioning of the Iris

The iris will usually spontaneously return into the anterior chamber after iridectomy unless it has suffered ischemic damage from the acute attack of glaucoma (10). If the iris remains prolapsed, one should massage in circular motions around the limbal wound (11) (Fig. 35-6A) or in radial motions over the peripheral clear cornea (8) using a blunt instrument (Fig. 35-6B), such as a muscle hook or cannula, to reposit the iris. Intracameral injection of acetylcholine can also be useful (11). Occasionally, an iris spatula is required to push the iris back into the anterior chamber. Care must be taken to avoid inadvertent damage to the lens.

Closure of the Incision

If a preplaced suture was used, it can be tightened and tied to reapproximate the wound edges (8). Otherwise, one or two interrupted 10-0 nylon sutures can be used to close the incision (11). The knot is buried, and if a limbal approach was used, the conjunctiva is closed with a 9-0 absorbable

suture. Subconjunctival corticosteroids and antibiotics are injected (topical application of these medications may supplement or replace this regimen).

SURGICAL TECHNIQUE OF GONIOSYNECHIALYSIS

This technique can be combined with surgical peripheral iridectomy or perioperative laser iridotomy to relieve the relative pupillary block. Iridectomy or iridotomy in a patient with 360-degree synechial closure would be ineffective without goniosynechialysis. If the goniosynechialysis fails, trabeculectomy or placement of a seton would be required.

The steps in goniosynechialysis include 1) chamber deepening with viscoelastic substance, 2) intraoperative gonioscopy, 3) goniosynechialysis with a cyclodialysis spatula, and 4) closing steps. Rectus superior and inferior 4-0 silk bridle sutures are recommended to facilitate stabilization and rotation of the globe (6).

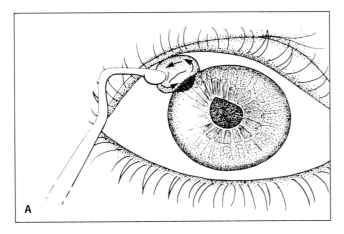

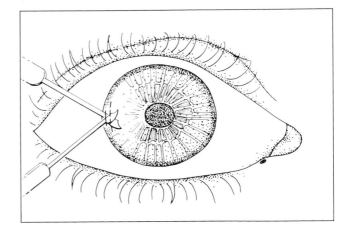

FIGURE 35-7. *The paracentesis incision should be wider at its internal aspect than its external aspect. The wide internal aspect allows unhindered rotation of instruments within the anterior chamber while the narrower external aspect prevents excess loss of viscoelastic substance.*

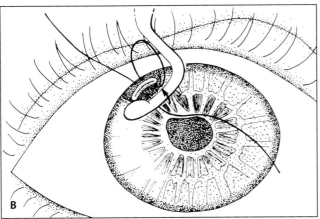

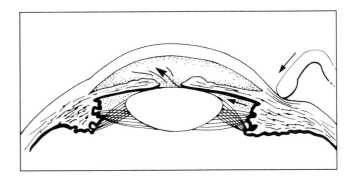

FIGURE 35-8. *Aqueous humor trapped behind the iris is expressed with a muscle hook. (Redrawn with permission from Campbell DG, Vela A. Modern goniosynechialysis for the treatment of synechial angle closure glaucoma.* Ophthalmology *1984;91: 1052–1060.)*

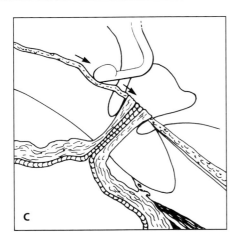

FIGURE 35-6. *Two approaches to repositing the iris. A. Massaging in circular motions. (Redrawn with permission from Baerveldt G. Surgical peripheral iridectomies. In: Minckler DS, Van Buskirk EM, eds.* Color atlas of ophthalmic surgery: glaucoma. *Philadelphia: JB Lippincott, 1992:29.) B, C. Massaging radially. (B, C redrawn with permission from Wilson MR. Peripheral iridectomy and chamber deepening. In: Albert DM, Jakobiec FA, eds.* Principles and practice of ophthalmology. *Philadelphia: WB Saunders, 1994: 1618.)*

Chamber Deepening with Viscoelastic Substance

Anterior-chamber deepening as described by Chandler and Simmons (5) in 1965 converts a previously slit-like or closed angle into an artificially widened angle to vastly improve visualization.

A temporal paracentesis site just below the horizontal meridian is made (5,6) with a sharp blade such as the No. 75 blade or Wheeler or Ziegler knife (Fig. 35-7). The incision should be two to three times longer than its width to prevent iris prolapse and should be angled inferiorly to enter the very shallow anterior chamber and minimize the risk of damage to the iris and lens. Depressing the posterior lip of the wound with the blade handle will allow aqueous to escape. A muscle hook is then used to depress the limbus 360 degrees (6), forcing the trapped aqueous behind the iris to go into the anterior chamber (Fig. 35-8). This fluid is then allowed to exit the paracentesis site. The anterior chamber is now deepened with viscoelastic substance, forcing the iris and lens back to a depth of six to eight corneal thicknesses.

The benefits of sodium hyaluronate to anterior-segment surgery have been well established since its first experimental use in animal models (12) and human eyes (13). Other viscoelastic substances have also gained acceptance since that time; these include mixtures of sodium hyaluronate with chondroitin sulfate (e.g., Viscoat, Alcon). The properties of viscoelastic substances that are of particular benefit to anterior-chamber deepening are indicated in Table 35-2 (6,14).

Intraoperative Gonioscopy

At this point, direct visualization using a Koeppe lens, headlight, and surgical loupes or indirect visualization with a Sussman lens through the operative microscope should be performed. This will confirm synechial angle-closure glaucoma and will be curative for those patients with less adherent synechiae.

During the synechialysis, visualization should be with the Barkan lens replacing the Koeppe lens. The truncated side of the Barkan lens allows access to the paracentesis site for the cyclodialysis spatula, similar to its use in goniotomy. In many cases, the operative microscope can be tilted to near a horizontal position to allow its use as the light source and the magnification system, should the surgeon not feel comfortable with the headlight and loupe technique. The indirect-visualization technique with the Sussman lens can be confusion during synechialysis because of the inverted image.

Goniosynechialysis with a Cyclodialysis Spatula

A curved, smooth-tipped cyclodialysis spatula is used for goniosynechialysis. With the advent of the more viscous viscoelastic substances, an irrigating spatula as originally described (6) is no longer necessary to maintain the chamber depth. The spatula enters the temporal incision, crossing through the anterior chamber, thus avoiding

Table 35-2.   Viscoelastic Properties (6,14)

Remains in the eye during surgery
Easily injected and aspirated
Coats tissues for protection and lubricates instruments
Localizes and limits bleeding to droplets
Optically clear, but visible for removal
Does not significantly elevate intraocular pressure if left in the eye
Rapidly clears from the eye
Noninflammatory, nonpyrogenic, and nonantigenic
Economical

corneal endothelium and lenticular contact to access the angle.

Delicate teasing of the iris away from the angle is performed with the smooth tip of the cyclodialysis spatula in an anterior-to-posterior direction (Fig. 35-9). Care must be taken to avoid inadvertent cyclodialysis, or angle recession. The assistant, while guiding the glob's position with the bridle sutures, must advise when the spatula threatens the corneal endothelium or the lens (6).

Once the nasal 165- to 180-degree angle is opened, the procedure is repeated for the temporal angle. To do this, a paracentesis site is created nasally and the surgeon and assistant must reposition themselves. The creation of a third paracentesis site ensures access to all 360 degrees of the angle.

Closing Steps

The viscoelastic substance is removed by vigorous irrigation with balanced salt solution through each paracentesis site while the posterior lip of the wound is depressed to allow the irrigant to escape (6). The paracentesis sites are closed with interrupted 10-0 nylon sutures, burying the knots.

POSTOPERATIVE MANAGEMENT

Postoperative management begins with a decision as to whether the patient requires admission to the hospital. If the patient is frail, with congestive heart failure, or requires systemic pressure-lowering agents, then he or she may be safer in the hospital for postoperative monitoring (10) with the assistance of an internist.

Most patients can be managed on an outpatient basis. Slit-lamp examination is performed on the first postoperative day. The patency of the iridectomy and the intraocular pressure are determined. Examination should be repeated within 1 week to repeat the intraocular pressure assessment and rule out postoperative endophthalmitis. Most patients can be successfully managed with a topical combination of

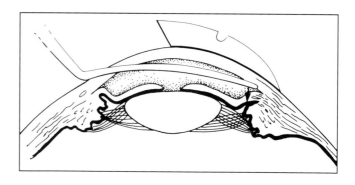

FIGURE 35-9.   *The cyclodialysis spatula tip is used to peel the synechially apposed iris from the trabecular meshwork in an anterior-to-posterior direction under direct visualization with a Barkan lens.*

antibiotic and steroid four times daily. To prevent synechiae, pilocarpine should not be continued in the postoperative period, while tropicamide (1%) may be administered twice daily (8,10).

Gonioscopy should be performed in the early postoperative period to evaluate the success of the procedure (8). If goniosynechialysis has been combined with the iridectomy, then careful assessment of the angle for new synechiae is required with aggressive control of inflammation by using steroids or nonsteroidal anti-inflammatory agents.

COMPLICATIONS

A number of intraoperative and postoperative complications should be kept in mind during the surgery and follow-up period.

Intraoperative

Incomplete Iridectomy

Once it is excised, the iris specimen should be examined for the presence of pigmented epithelium by brushing it lightly against a surgical sponge. With the scleral approach, the iris must be prolapsed through the wound again to remove the pigment epithelium with Pierce-Hoskins forceps or a spear-tipped sponge. If the iris does not prolapse, the scleral wound may need to be extended. With the clear corneal approach, direct visualization by retracting the anterior corneal incision is possible, allowing regrasping of the iris and repeating the iridectomy (11).

Bleeding from the Iris

Bleeding from the iris can occur and is usually self-limited (8). More exuberant bleeding can occur if the iris is rubeotic or inflamed. For rubeosis, the iris vessels can be cauterized with diathermy prior to excision of tissue (8,15). Bleeding can be controlled by injection of chilled viscoelastic substance or air into the anterior chamber, or by topical application of 1:1000 epinephrine. Viscoelastic substance should be removed prior to completion of the surgery, to minimize the chances of an intraocular pressure spike (8). Small amounts of bleeding can be controlled with simple anterior-chamber irrigation with chilled balanced salt solution.

Bleeding from the Ciliary Body

If the approach is too posterior, exuberant bleeding into the anterior chamber is most likely from the ciliary body (11). Hemostasis, as suggested for iris bleeding, can be used (8).

Vitreous Loss

Should vitreous present at the time of surgery, then the surgical incision is likely too posterior (in the otherwise nontraumatized anterior segment). This surgical site should be closed and a new site created with a more anterior approach (8).

Postoperative

Hyphema

Persistent iris or ciliary body bleeding can result in a hyphema. This is usually self-limited, requiring no treatment. In the event of profuse bleeding, an eight-ball hyphema may result. The clot often extends into the posterior chamber as well, blocking aqueous flow and significantly raising the intraocular pressure (10). A hyphemectomy can be performed through a 4- to 5-mm incision just anterior to the limbus, and the clot gently expressed (10). An alternative approach using a Simcoe cannula assisted by viscoelastic dissection of the clotted blood from the corneal endothelium can be utilized.

Cataract

Cataract formation can occur rapidly following direct surgical trauma to the lens (11). Even without obvious direct lens damage at the time of surgery, numerous cases of cataract formation following peripheral iridectomy have been described (8,16–19).

Leaking Incision

Seidel's test should be performed intraoperatively to ensure proper wound closure and should be repeated postoperatively, especially in the presence of a shallow anterior chamber. Any wound leak should be repaired (11). If the anterior chamber is shallow, and Seidel's test result is negative for a wound leak, then aqueous misdirection or choroidal effusion should be suspected (8).

Persistent Elevated Intraocular Pressure

Intraocular pressure may remain elevated in the postoperative period in the presence of aqueous misdirection, imperforate or incarcerated iridectomy, synechial angle closure, or plateau iris syndrome.

A shallow anterior chamber with an intraocular pressure higher than expected and no wound leak is suspicious for aqueous misdirection syndrome. Appropriate measures include the use of topical atropine, aqueous suppression with carbonic anhydrase inhibitors, disruption of the vitreous face, and aqueous tap or vitrectomy. When available, the ultrasound biomicroscope may confirm aqueous misdirection.

The imperforate iridectomy should be avoided by ensuring the presence of the pigmented epithelium in the excised iris specimen at the time of surgery. In unusual circumstances such as severe inflammation or bleeding, or another medical reason to stop surgery, this may not have been possible. The imperforate iridectomy may respond well to adjunctive surgical or laser treatment to remove vitreous incarcerated in the iridectomy.

Intraoperative gonioscopy should indicate the presence of synechial angle closure. As discussed, goniosynechialysis can then be performed in conjunction with the surgical iridectomy. Not only does this allow arresting of the pupillary block by performing the iridectomy, but also it repairs the damage to the outflow track by peeling away the synechiae.

If the intraocular pressure remains elevated following iridectomy in a patient with plateau iris configuration, then pupillary block was not playing a significant role in the patient's mechanism of glaucoma, and their plateau iris syndrome may require laser gonioplasty (8,20).

Other

The complications common to all intraocular surgery should always be kept in mind during the postoperative period. These include retrobulbar hemorrhage, allergy to topical medications or soaps used in surgical preparation, and the toxicity of systemic medications used to lower intraocular pressure.

Postoperative endophthalmitis, although extremely rare, should always be suspected because of its potential for devastating consequences. The presence of persistent or recurrent postoperative inflammation or decreased visual acuity would be highly suspicious. Comanagement with a vitreoretinal surgeon for vitreous aspiration or vitrectomy may be required.

Complaints of uniocular diplopia, glare, and photophobia following peripheral iridectomies have been recorded (8,21,22). Much of this can be prevented by placing the iridectomy superiorly where it will be covered by the upper lid (11).

RESULTS

Recent reports confirmed the long-term success of nonfiltering surgery for angle-closure glaucoma. In a study following 13 primary angle-closure patients for at least 18 months after undergoing goniosynechialysis as a primary procedure, 12 (92%) maintained an intraocular pressure lower than 21 mm Hg; 4 patients required a repeat procedure (23). In 70 eyes for which laser iridotomy or surgical iridectomy failed, 34 (87%) of 39 aphakic eyes maintained an intraocular pressure lower than 20 mm Hg following goniosynechialysis, versus 13 (42%) of 31 phakic eyes (24).

ACKNOWLEDGMENTS

We thank Luanna R. Bartholomew, PhD, for research and editorial assistance and Joan E. Thomson for the illustrations.

REFERENCES

1. Graefe A. Veber die Iridectomie be: Glaucom und uber den glaucomatosen process. *Graefes Arch Clin Exp Ophthalmol* 1857;3:456.
2. Curran EJ. A new operation for glaucoma involving a new principle in the etiology and treatment of chronic primary glaucoma. *Arch Ophthalmol* 1920;49:131.
3. Barkan O. Glaucoma: classification, causes, and surgical control. *Am J Ophthalmol* 1938;21:1099.
4. Shaffer RN. Operating room gonioscopy in angle closure glaucoma surgery. *Trans Am Ophthalmol Soc* 1957;55:59–64.
5. Chandler PA, Simmons RJ. Anterior chamber deepening for gonioscopy at time of surgery. *Arch Ophthalmol* 1965;74:177–190.
6. Campbell DG, Vela A. Modern goniosynechialysis for the treatment of synechial angle closure glaucoma. *Ophthalmology* 1984;91:1052–1060.
7. Spaeth GL. Glaucoma surgery. In: Spaeth GL, ed. *Ophthalmic surgery: principles and practice.* Philadelphia: WB Saunders, 1990.
8. Wilson MR. Peripheral iridectomy and chamber deepening. In: Albert DM, Jakobiec FA, eds. *Principles and practice of ophthalmology.* Philadelphia: WB Saunders, 1994:1618.
9. Shingleton BJ, Chang MA, Bellows AR, et al. Surgical goniosynechialysis for angle-closure glaucoma. *Ophthalmology* 1990;97:551–556.
10. Spaeth GL, Katz LJ, Terebuh AK. Glaucoma surgery. In: Tasman W, Jaeger EA, eds. *Duane's clinical ophthalmology.* Vol. 6. Hagerstown, MD: JB Lippincott, 1995:14.
11. Baerveldt G. Surgical peripheral iridectomies. In: Minckler DS, Van Buskirk EM, eds. *Color atlas of ophthalmic surgery: glaucoma.* Philadelphia: JB Lippincott, 1992:29.
12. Miller D, O'Connor P, Williams J. Use of Na-hyaluronate during intraocular lens implantation in rabbits. *Ophthalmic Surg* 1977:58.
13. Miller D, Stegmann R. Use of Na-hyaluronate in anterior segment eye surgery. *J Am Intraocul Implant Soc* 1980;6:13.
14. Schertzer RM, Pang DX, Bartholomew LR. Multimedia teaching module for phacoemulsification cataract surgery. *Ophthalmology* 1995;102(9A):180.
15. Hersh SB, Kass MA. Iridectomy in rubeosis iridis. *Ophthalmic Surg* 1976;7:19.
16. Sugar HS. Cataract formation and refractive changes after surgery for angle-closure glaucoma. *Am J Ophthalmol* 1970;69:747.
17. Godel V, Regenbogen L. Cataractogenic factors in patients with primary angle-closure glaucoma after peripheral iridectomy. *Am J Ophthalmol* 1977;83:180.
18. Floman N, Berson D, Landau L. Peripheral iridectomy in closed angle glaucomas: late complications. *Br J Ophthalmol* 1977;61:101.
19. Krupin T, Mitchell KB, Johnson MF, et al. The long-term effects of iridectomy for primary acute angle-closure glaucoma. *Am J Ophthalmol* 1978;86:506.
20. Hager H. Besondere mikrochirurgische eingriffe. *Klin Monatsbl Augenheilkd* 1973;162:437.
21. Go FJ, Kitazawa Y. Complications of peripheral iridectomy in primary angle-closure glaucoma. *Jpn J Ophthalmol* 1981;25:222.
22. Luke S. Complications of peripheral iridectomy. *Can J Ophthalmol* 1969;4:346.
23. Tanihara H, Negi A, Akimoto M, Nagata M. Long-term results of non-filtering surgery for the treatment of primary angle-closure glaucoma. *Graefes Arch Clin Exp Ophthalmol* 1995;233:563.
24. Tanihara H, Nishiwaki K, Nagata M. Surgical results and complications of goniosynechialysis. *Graefes Arch Clin Exp Ophthalmol* 1992;230:309.

Combined Phacoemulsification and Trabeculectomy

Joseph Caprioli

The approach to glaucoma patients who require cataract extraction has evolved with the development of small-incision cataract surgery. Trabeculectomy previously was combined with both intracapsular and extracapsular cataract extraction, and enjoyed a renewed interest after the incorporation of extracapsular cataract extraction into common surgical practice in the early 1980s. However, the procedure did not become widely accepted because of disappointment with the long-term reduction in intraocular pressure (IOP) compared with trabeculectomy alone, and prolonged visual recovery compared to cataract surgery alone. Over the past decade, surgical techniques for both trabeculectomy and cataract extraction have evolved with the advent of antimetabolites, laser suture lysis, releasable sutures, small-incision phacoemulsification, and foldable lenses. Combined procedures are once again enjoying a revival in the form of trabeculectomy combined with small-incision phacoemulsification, together with the possible enhancement of this procedure with antimetabolites. On the basis of the potential benefits of trabeculectomy combined with phacoemulsification and encouraging early results, the indications for combined procedures have been somewhat liberalized in recent years.

INDICATIONS FOR COMBINED CATARACT AND GLAUCOMA SURGERY

An algorithm for the choice of surgery in patients with glaucoma who require visual rehabilitation with cataract surgery is shown in Figure 36-1. This algorithm, similar to that offered by Shields (1), will doubtless need revision as we learn more about the long-term risks and benefits of combined phacoemulsification and glaucoma surgery. In this scheme, patients with early glaucomatous damage and stable, acceptable IOPs at or near their target range would undergo

cataract extraction only. Cataract surgery would preferably be performed in such a way as not to disturb the superior conjunctiva and allow for subsequent trabeculectomy if it were required. Combined surgery is recommended for patients with moderate to advanced glaucomatous damage, but with IOPs at or near the target pressure range. The number of glaucoma medications can be reduced and the possibility of a postoperative rise in IOP is minimized to protect an already damaged optic nerve. Patients with early glaucomatous damage in whom IOPs are not adequately controlled are also good candidates for combined surgery. The additional pressure lowering from the combined surgery will often achieve an adequate target IOP with or without supplemental medications. Many surgeons still recommend only trabeculectomy in patients with advanced progressive glaucomatous damage, or with glaucoma that is likely to be progressive because IOPs are not at or near their target level. These patients would have trabeculectomy only, and have cataract surgery several months after a mature filtering bleb has developed. Recommendations for this last group remain somewhat controversial; some surgeons prefer combined surgery for this group as well (indicated by a dashed line in the algorithm of Fig. 36-1). Unfortunately, the data are not yet in with respect to which of these two alternatives is best in this group.

SURGICAL TECHNIQUES

Phacoemulsification and Trabeculectomy Through the Same Incision

There are several variations on phacoemulsification and trabeculectomy at the same incision site. The conjunctival flap may be fornix based or limbus based. Fornix-based flaps are easier to use and generally provide better exposure.

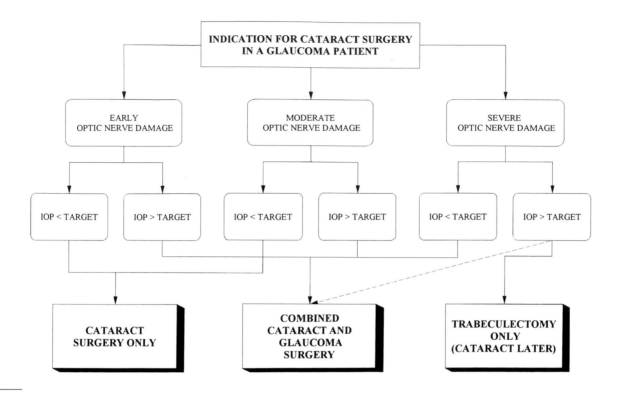

FIGURE 36-1. *Algorithm for the selection of cataract surgery alone, trabeculectomy alone, or combined surgery for patients with cataract and glaucoma. This algorithm depends on the severity of optic nerve damage and whether the intraocular pressure (IOP) has been controlled at or near the target level. Those with early optic nerve damage typically have detectable structural changes to the optic nerve but little or no visual field loss. Those with moderate optic nerve damage have typical visual glaucomatous field defects in one hemifield only. Those with advanced optic nerve damage have extensive visual field loss involving both hemifields. The dotted line indicates an area of changing indications because of the evolution of small-incision phacoemulsification.*

Limbus-based flaps offer better protection against postoperative leaks, especially when antimetabolites are used. There are no data to indicate which is the better approach, and either can be used successfully. Figure 36-2 demonstrates the use of a scleral tunnel through which phacoemulsification is performed and a lens implant inserted. This tunnel is converted into a scleral flap by radial scleral incisions, and a standard trabeculectomy is performed. The corneal incision could be extended somewhat to the left and right if required to accommodate a rigid intraocular lens implant. Alternatively, phacoemulsification can be performed after the scleral flap for trabeculectomy is fashioned, but before trabeculectomy is performed. Viscoelastic substance should be removed by aspiration as thoroughly as possible. After completion of the cataract extraction, standard trabeculectomy is performed. An iridectomy should always be performed as part of the standard trabeculectomy procedure. It is important, when using a fornix-based flap, to suture the conjunctiva tightly with a nasal and temporal suture that includes a small bite of sclera. This produces a right seal at the limbus and reduces the incidence of significant or persistent leaks.

Phacoemulsification and Trabeculectomy Through Separate Incisions

An approach that separates the cataract and trabeculectomy incisions has some theoretical advantage. Reduced tissue manipulation at the trabeculectomy site may increase the success of bleb formation. If extracapsular cataract extraction combined with trabeculectomy reduces long-term filtration because of local tissue manipulation, it seems reasonable to separate the two incisions entirely. The conjunctival and scleral manipulation during the trabeculectomy portion of the separate-incision combined procedure described below is no greater than that during trabeculectomy alone.

Cataract extraction is performed before trabeculectomy, during the same operating session, with phacoemulsification through a temporal clear-corneal approach and a small incision (3.2 mm) with no manipulation of the conjunctiva. Pupils less than 4 mm in diameter after dilatation are enlarged through a small temporal sphincterectomy and a nasal sphincterotomy. A foldable silicone posterior-chamber intraocular lens is inserted into the capsular bag. One-piece

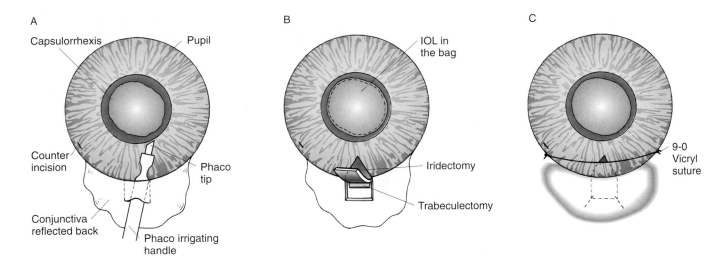

FIGURE 36-2. *Technique for combined phacoemulsification and trabeculectomy through the same incision. The conjunctival flap may be fornix based or limbus based. A fornix-based flap is shown here. A. Phacoemulsification is performed through a scleral tunnel, and a foldable intraocular lens is inserted through the tunnel. A foldable intraocular lens can be inserted through this incision, or the incision can be extended at the limbus slightly to the left and right to accommodate a rigid intraocular lens. B. The scleral tunnel is then converted by radial incisions into a scleral flap. The trabeculectomy and a basal iridectomy is then performed. The scleral flap is sutured at each of its corners with a single 10-0 nylon suture. C. The conjunctiva is pulled down toward the limbus and sutured securely at each corner with a 9-0 absorbable suture. The conjunctiva should be held by these sutures taut against the cornea to reduce possible leakage at the limbus. The bleb is raised by injection of balanced salt solution through the clear-corneal counter incision.*

or three-piece silicone lenses, or three-piece acrylic lenses can be used for capsule fixation. Three-piece acrylic lenses are used for ciliary sulcus fixation when indicated. Carbachol is injected intracamerally. This wound is then closed with a single 10-0 nylon suture, and a standard trabeculectomy is performed superiorly, with or without antimetabolites (Fig. 36-3) (2,3). It is important to make the eye firm (about 20 mm Hg) at the conclusion of the cataract portion of the operation, by instillation of balanced salt solution. This step facilitates the dissection of the scleral flap for trabeculectomy. An eye with a typical postoperative appearance is shown in Figure 36-4.

RESULTS OF COMBINED SURGERY

In the preantimetabolite and prephacoemulsification era, most ophthalmologists would agree that combined extracapsular extraction–trabeculectomy did not provide the same level of long-term IOP control as trabeculectomy alone (1,4,5). Nevertheless, combined surgery did provide some protection against short-term postoperative pressure spikes, and resulted in lower long-term IOP and less requirement for long-term antiglaucoma medication than did extracapsular cataract extraction alone (6). One commonly used approach in the cataract patient with uncontrolled glaucoma in whom long-term filtration was desired was to perform filtration surgery first, followed by cataract extraction 3 to 6 months after a mature bleb had formed. Methods of enhancing the long-term IOP-lowering effect

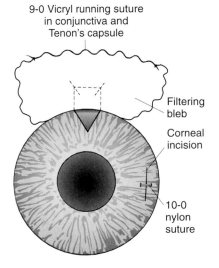

FIGURE 36-3. *Separate-incision phacoemulsification and trabeculectomy. With a separate-incision phacoemulsification and trabeculectomy technique, clear-corneal phacoemulsification is performed and a foldable intraocular lens is implanted in the bag. The clear-corneal wound is sutured with a single 10-0 nylon suture. Next, standard trabeculectomy is performed superiorly. It is helpful to make sure the eye is firm by instillation of balanced salt solution through the clear-corneal counterincision before the scleral flap is dissected. This approach is usually performed with a limbus-based conjunctival flap, which provides for the safer use of antimetabolites.*

of combined surgery, without increasing the short-term complications, have been sought.

The results of studies of combined-procedure outcomes with either extracapsular extraction or phacoemulsification are summarized in Table 36-1. Several conclusions are apparent from inspection of this table. The comparison of one study with another is difficult. Absolute IOP reduction is only partially satisfactory as an outcome parameter because

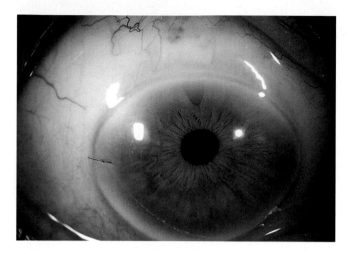

FIGURE 36-4.   *Postoperative appearance of eye after combined phacoemulsification and trabeculectomy. This slit-lamp photograph was taken 3 weeks after combined phacoemulsification and trabeculectomy, and shows a quiet diffuse bleb and clear-corneal incision closed with a single 10-0 nylon suture. The intraocular pressure was 12 mm Hg without glaucoma medications.*

preoperative and target IOPs differ from population to population and from patient to patient. Similarly, follow-up duration varies from one study to another. There is a generally apparent trend toward rising IOP with increasing follow-up time. This is true not only for combined procedures, but also for trabeculectomy alone. The IOP reduction achieved with phacoemulsification coupled with trabeculectomy augmented with low-dose 5-fluorouracil does not appear significantly greater than that obtained with extracapsular cataract extraction combined procedures, though some articles did not specify the number of glaucoma medications used and whether this medical burden was reduced postoperatively.

Most studies of primary trabeculectomy demonstrated a 1-year success rate of approximately 80% without antimetabolites (7,8). The reasons for the reduced long-term success of extracapsular extraction combined with trabeculectomy are not completely understood, but are commonly attributed to the increased incision size and additional conjunctival manipulation with subsequent fibrosis and scarring. The development of mature functional blebs is apparently not as well served under these conditions as with trabeculectomy alone. A separate-incision technique has previously been described with a corneal section extracapsular cataract extraction (9). At least one study suggested that smaller incisions with less tissue manipulation improve filtration: Single-site phacotrabeculectomy with a 6-mm incision was compared to that with a 3-mm incision, and a lower 1-year IOP and less need for medication in the smaller-incision group were reported (10).

Table 36-1.   Comparison of Data from Previous Studies

	Mean IOP Reduction (mm Hg)	No. (%) with Reduction of Medication	Eyes (n)	Follow-up (mo)	Cataract Extraction	Other
Shields (1986) (1)	6.5	—	34	10	ECCE	—
Simmons et al (1987) (4)	3.0	—	58	12	ECCE	—
Murchison and Shields (1989) (5)	1.7	—	22	21	ECCE	—
Percival (1985) (15)	6.0	—	21	6	ECCE	—
McCartney et al (1988) (6)	6.0	—	10.8	16.8	ECCE	—
Williamson et al (1989) (9)	9.0	—	35	12	ECCE	Separated entry
Cohen (1990) (16)	4.1	1.1 (65%)	22	5.4	Phaco and ECCE	5-FU: 17.3 mg
Hennis and Stewart (1991) (17)	3.0	1.6 (70%)	15	3.0	ECCE	5-FU: 43.7 mg
Lyle and Jin (1991) (10)	8.9	—	94	6	Phaco	3-mm incision
Pasquale and Smith (1992) (18)	4.4	1.1 (58%)	35	12	Phaco	—
Wishart and Austin (1993) (19)	5.2	—	34	12.6	Phaco	—
O'Grady et al (1993) (11)	4.7	1.5 (68%)	38	13.2	Phaco	5-FU: 24.8 mg
Hurvitz (1993) (20)	6.2	1.9 (79%)	38	12	Phaco	Low dose (?)
Park et al (1996) (3)						
Combined-surgery group	6.8	1.6 (73%)	40	17.3	Phaco	5-FU: 16 mg
Trabeculectomy control group	10.3	2.0 (87%)	40	17.5	Phaco	5-FU: 16 mg

IOP = intraocular pressure; Phaco = phacoemulsification; ECCE = extracapsular cataract extraction; 5-FU = 5-fluorouracil (total postoperative dose is indicated).

The role of antimetabolites in phacotrabeculectomy remains largely unproved. Several controlled studies failed to find an effect of low-dose 5-fluorouracil injection (11,12) or mitomycin C application (13) on lasting IOP control or reduction of medications. These studies employed single-incision combined surgery and their conclusions may not be applicable to a separate-incision technique.

To compare the IOP-lowering effects of temporal corneal phacoemulsification combined with separate-incision superior trabeculectomy with those of trabeculectomy alone, a retrospective case-control study was performed (2). Forty consecutive patients who underwent combined temporal corneal phacoemulsification and superior trabeculectomy with low-dose 5-fluorouracil served as cases, and 40 eyes matched with respect to age, race, preoperative medications, and preoperative IOP who had trabeculectomy alone with low-dose 5-fluorouracil served as controls. Survival analyses for IOP were performed for the cases and controls.

The mean postoperative IOP was statistically higher in the combined-surgery group than in the trabeculectomy group at each follow-up interval ($p < 0.05$). Kaplan-Meier survival analysis showed that the cumulative success rates at 2 years were 62.1% in the combined-surgery group and 85.8% in the trabeculectomy group. The survival time was significantly shorter ($p = 0.04$) in the combined-surgery group, as determined by the log-rank test (Fig. 36-5). In this study, combined surgery for cataract and glaucoma did not reduce IOP as well as did trabeculectomy alone despite the use of identical trabeculectomy techniques in both groups.

Nevertheless, combined surgery is effective in lowering IOP and reduces the long-term requirement for antiglaucoma medications without significant additional complications. This technique is appropriate in selected patients with coexisting cataract and glaucoma, as suggested in Figure 36-1.

Factors in addition to subconjunctival manipulation must be involved in the reduction of filtration seen with combined surgery. Perhaps intraocular differences, such as additional breakdown in the blood-aqueous barrier after cataract extraction, are involved. Lens-related growth factors released after cataract surgery may diffuse into the bleb and stimulate fibroblast activity. Despite the smaller filtration effect obtained with the combined procedure, the majority of patients had significant pressure reduction 1 year after the surgery. The absence of significant complications related to the trabeculectomy itself is also encouraging. It is my belief that more widespread application of combined surgery is appropriate with these newer techniques. Future work in understanding the mechanisms by which cataract surgery compromises filtration will hopefully produce techniques to improve IOP reduction.

SPECIAL CONSIDERATIONS OF CATARACT SURGERY IN GLAUCOMA PATIENTS

Small pupil and posterior synechiae are the technical problems most frequently encountered by the cataract surgeon in glaucoma patients. Experienced phacoemulsification surgeons can successfully and safely remove even a hard lens through a pupil of 4mm or more. In general, small pupils should be enlarged for safe and effective cataract removal. In patients who have small pupils with extensive posterior synechiae and a small rigid and fibrotic iris sphincter from years of miotic use, stretching the pupil often causes multiple sphincter tears and a postoperative fibrinous exudate, which may form a fibrin clot in the anterior chamber and lead to secondary problems. In such patients, it is my preference to employ a small temporal sphincterectomy followed by a nasal sphincterotomy after installation of viscoelastic substance in the anterior chamber, and after sweeping the iris adhesions with an iris or Barraquer spatula (Fig. 36-6). When the pupil is very small, but where extensive posterior synechiae are not present and the iris sphincter is not fibrotic, iris hooks can be successfully employed to provide adequate exposure. Care must be taken to place the hooks in proper position and to avoid enhancing the possibility of iris prolapse through the phacoemulsification wound.

The tight junctions between the vascular endothelial cells of the iris and of the nonpigmented epithelial cells of the ciliary body form the blood-aqueous barrier of the anterior segment. Miotics, particularly strong miotics, are known to weaken these tight junctions (14). The additional insult of cataract surgery can result in frank breakdown of the blood-aqueous barrier and lead to serious exudation and fibrinous

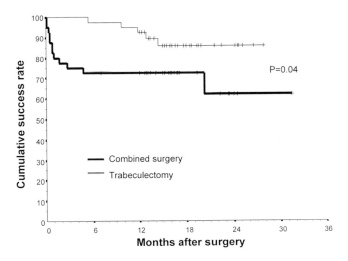

FIGURE 36-5. *Survival curves for separate-incision phacoemulsification and trabeculectomy versus trabeculectomy alone. Based on Kaplan-Meier survival analysis, the cumulative intraocular pressure success rate was statistically lower (p = 0.04) in the combined-surgery group than in the trabeculectomy group (log-rank test). (Reprinted with permission from Caprioli J, Park HF, Weitzman M. Temporal corneal phacoemulsification combined with superior trabeculectomy: a controlled study. Arch Ophthalmol 1997;115:318–323.)*

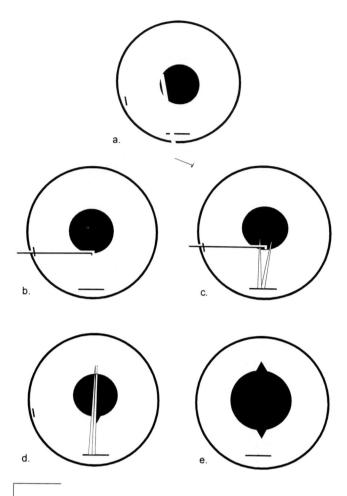

FIGURE 36-6.   *An approach to the patient with a small pupil and extensive posterior synechiae. A 3.0-mm incision is located temporally. The synechiae were swept with an iris or Barraquer spatula (a) after instillation of a viscoelastic substance into the anterior chamber. A clear-corneal counterincision is made, and the temporal iris is tented with a straight intraocular lens hook (b). With the iris tented, long intraocular scissors are used to perform a small temporal sphincterectomy (c). A small sphincterotomy is made on the nasal side with the same scissors (d). Additional viscoelastic substance is instilled and the pupil size becomes quite adequate for continuing phacoemulsification (e).*

clots in the anterior chamber. These can further lead to synechiae between the iris and the lens or the lens capsule, or even to the anterior-chamber angle. Preoperative treatment with topical steroids for 4 to 7 days seems prudent to reduce this effect, as does gentle treatment of the iris and the avoidance of gripping or tearing this tissue.

The atrophic iris can easily prolapse through the cataract wound. The atrophic iris is usually found in patients who have been on long-term miotic treatment and in diabetic patients. The intraoperative complication of iris prolapse can best be avoided by proper structure of a corneal wound that is not too peripheral and therefore not near the base of the iris; creating a shelf on this wound helps, but does not necessarily prevent iris prolapse. The placement of a small amount of viscoelastic substance at the base of the iris just

under the corneal wound will also help prevent this complication.

The presence of a loose lens should be ascertained preoperatively whenever possible. Preoperative knowledge and appropriate surgical care could avert frank zonular dehiscence and subsequent vitreous loss during surgery. Loose lenses should be suspected in an eye that has previously undergone trabeculectomy, particularly in those that may have a flat or shallow anterior chamber postoperatively. The presence of pseudoexfoliation should also alert the examiner to the possibility of a loose lens. Unless there is a frank zonular dehiscence, phacoemulsification can successfully be performed under these conditions without incident. Care should be taken not to overly manipulate the lens or the lens nucleus, and to perform gentle surgery.

Proper preoperative evaluation, which includes an assessment of corneal status, macular status, and the extent of glaucomatous visual field loss, should always be performed. Corneal endothelial cell counts can be reduced by long-term glaucoma treatment. Patients who had a previous trabeculectomy, particularly those with a flat or shallow anterior chamber postoperatively, can have a severely compromised cornea. The macular status should be evaluated as in any preoperative patient undergoing cataract surgery. In glaucoma patients one should make sure that advanced field loss does not involve fixation and that this, rather than the cataract, is the cause of decreased vision.

In the presence of a functional filtering bleb, cataract extraction should be undertaken at a location remote from the filtering bleb to help avoid the risk of reducing the function of the bleb. I prefer a clear-corneal temporal approach in these patients. Cataract extraction could be supplemented by the additional use of postoperative injections of 5-fluorouracil to help avoid reduction of the function of the filtering bleb, but no clear-cut evidence of the efficacy of this approach has been presented. Antimetabolites, particularly mitomycin, are routinely used in conjunction with combined procedures performed in patients in whom a previous trabeculectomy failed. The postoperative rise in IOP can be reduced by thorough removal of viscoelastic substance and the instillation of carbachol intraoperatively. In selected patients with advanced optic nerve damage, β-adrenergic antagonists or apraclonidine may be used at the conclusion of the procedure. If appropriate measures are taken, it is not necessary to routinely measure IOP in the first postoperative hours after cataract surgery in most patients.

POSTOPERATIVE CARE

Cycloplegia is usually not used after combined procedures, particularly because the incidence of flat anterior chamber is very low. Patients who have undergone a combined procedure often show additional intraocular inflammation compared with those who have had cataract surgery alone, especially compared to patients without glaucoma. Patients are maintained on a tapering dose of topical corticosteroids for a period of 8 to 12 weeks. This reduces the accumulation of pigmented inflammatory deposits on the intraocular lens, especially silicone lenses, which are more prone to this occurrence. Laser suture lysis is employed as necessary to increase filtration, as is done after trabeculectomy alone. Sutures can often be cut earlier because of the reduced chance of a flat chamber in the pseudophakic eye.

SURGICAL COMPLICATIONS

The risk of flat anterior chamber is considerably reduced in the pseudophakic eye compared to the phakic eye that has undergone trabeculectomy. Flat anterior chamber is treated as it is after trabeculectomy alone, although corneal endothelial damage by pseudophakic touch is likely to be more severe.

Hypotony and choroidal detachment do not occur more frequently after combined procedures than after trabeculectomy alone. These are treated as for trabeculectomy alone. Postoperative exudation of fibrin into the anterior chamber can occur after combined procedures, particularly if the iris sphincter is ripped or excessively traumatized. Intensive topical corticosteroids usually provide adequate resolution of this problem. High postoperative IOP can be treated by application of pressure near the scleral flap to increase filtration, and occasionally laser suture lysis may be required, particularly if the flap has been sutured tightly. Encapsulated blebs are treated as for trabeculectomy alone. Ciliary block glaucoma can occur after combined procedures, though it probably occurs less frequently than after trabeculectomy alone in eyes at risk for this complication. Eyes at risk usually include hyperopic eyes, those with preexisting primary angle-closure glaucoma, or those with a lax zonule or large, loose lens.

CONCLUSIONS

The advent of small-incision cataract surgery and the increased proficiency in the use of phacoemulsification are changing the indications for combined cataract and glaucoma surgery. While patients with far-advanced, progressing damage may do better with trabeculectomy alone, followed by cataract surgery at a later date, those with stable disease or less severe damage will usually benefit from combined surgery, when sufficient indications exist for removal of cataract. Trabeculectomy combined with nonphaco-

emulsification extracapsular cataract surgery is not recommended in most instances. Phacoemulsification can be combined with trabeculectomy at the same site, or the incisions may be separate. While the separate-incision approach has theoretical advantages, and has a measured 1-year outcome (3), it is not yet clear which of these techniques is preferred, and both seem acceptable in current practice.

REFERENCES

1. Shields MB. Combined cataract extraction and guarded sclerotomy. Reevaluation in extracapsular era. *Ophthalmology* 1986;93:366–370.
2. Weitzman M, Caprioli J. Temporal corneal phacoemulsification combined with separate incision superior trabeculectomy. *Ophthalmic Surg* 1995;26:271–273.
3. Park HJ, Weitzman M, Caprioli J. Temporal corneal phacoemulsification combined with superior trabeculectomy: a controlled study. *Arch Ophthalmol* 1997;115:318–323.
4. Simmons ST, Litoff D, Nichols DA, et al. Extracapsular cataract extraction and posterior chamber intraocular lens implantation combined with trabeculectomy in patients with glaucoma. *Am J Ophthalmol* 1987;104:465–470.
5. Murchison JF Jr, Shields MB. An evaluation of three surgical approaches for coexisting cataract and glaucoma. *Ophthalmic Surg* 1989;20:393–398.
6. McCartney DL, Memmen JE, Stark WJ, et al. The efficacy and safety of combined trabeculectomy cataract extraction intraocular lens implantation. *Ophthalmology* 1988;95:754–763.
7. Lamping KA, Bellows AR, Hutchinson BT, Afran SI. Long-term evaluation of initial filtration surgery. *Ophthalmology* 1986;93:91–101.
8. Nouri-Mahdavi K, Brigatti L, Weitzman M, Caprioli J. Outcomes of initial trabeculectomy for open-angle glaucoma. *Ophthalmology* 1995;102:1760–1769.
9. Williamson TH, Bacon AS, Flanagan DW, et al. Combined extracapsular cataract extraction and trabeculectomy using a separated corneal incision. *Eye* 1989;3:547–552.
10. Lyle WA, Jin JC. Comparison of a 3- 6-mm incision in combined phacoemulsification and trabeculectomy. *Am J Ophthalmol* 1991;111:189–196.
11. O'Grady JM, Juzych MS, Shin DH, et al. Trabeculectomy, phacoemulsification, and posterior chamber lens implantation with and without 5-fluorouracil. *Am J Ophthalmol* 1993;116:594–599.
12. Wong PC, Ruderman JM, Krupin T, et al. 5-Fluorouracil after primary combined filtration surgery. *Am J Ophthalmol* 1994;117:149–154.
13. Shin DH, Simone PA, Song MS, et al. Adjunctive subconjunctival mitomycin C in glaucoma triple procedures. *Ophthalmology* 1995;102:1550–1558.
14. Mori M, Araie M, Sakurai M, Oshika T. Effects of pilocarpine and tropicamide on blood-aqueous barrier permeability in man. *Invest Ophthalmol Vis Sci* 1992;33:416–423.
15. Percival SPB. Glaucoma triple procedure of extracapsular cataract extraction, posterior chamber lens implantation, and trabeculectomy. *Br J Ophthalmol* 1985;69:99–102.
16. Cohen JS. Combined cataract implant and filtering surgery with 5-fluorouracil. *Ophthalmic Surg* 1990;21:181–186.
17. Hennis HL, Stewart WC. The use of 5-fluorouracil in patients following combined trabeculectomy and cataract extraction. *Ophthalmic Surg* 1991;22:451–454.
18. Pasquale LR, Smith SG. Surgical outcome of phacoemulsification combined with the Pearce trabeculectomy in patients with glaucoma. *J Cataract Refract Surg* 1992;18:301–305.
19. Wishart PK, Austin MW. Combined cataract extraction trabeculectomy. *Ophthalmic Surg* 1993;24:814–821.
20. Hurvitz LM. 5-FU supplemented phacoemulsification, posterior chamber intraocular lens implantation, and trabeculectomy. *Ophthalmic Surg* 1993;24:674–680.

Trabeculectomy and Glaucoma Drainage Devices: Special Considerations in Children

Paul A. Sidoti   Dale K. Heuer

The need to perform aqueous outflow surgery for the management of childhood glaucomas is governed by several factors. The etiology of the glaucoma will often determine whether angle surgery (trabeculotomy or goniotomy) or aqueous outflow surgery (trabeculectomy or drainage implant surgery) should be undertaken as the primary surgical procedure. Congenital and primary infantile glaucoma as well as glaucoma associated with anterior-segment dysgeneses of mild degree are generally best managed with primary angle surgery. The success rates with these procedures are relatively high and the intraoperative and postoperative risks are relatively small in comparison with more extensive intraocular procedures. Outflow surgery is generally undertaken in such patients when one or more angle surgeries have failed to control the intraocular pressure. The management of more complicated glaucomas such as those associated with more severe acquired or developmental angle anomalies, retinopathy of prematurity, and aphakia or pseudophakia favors an outflow procedure as the initial surgical option. The degree of intraocular pressure elevation, the severity of disk damage, the age of the patient, and the patient's prior surgical history should also be considered in determining the type of surgery and timing of intervention.

This chapter discusses some of the decision-making and technical considerations involved in the planning, execution, and postoperative management of both trabeculectomy and glaucoma drainage implant surgery in young children.

GENERAL CONSIDERATIONS

Wound Healing in Children

The ability of trabeculectomy and drainage implants to successfully control intraocular pressure is, in large part, determined by the fibroproliferative healing response that occurs

postoperatively. The most common cause of filtration failure following trabeculectomy is the formation of subconjunctival and episcleral scar tissue with closure of the surgical fistula (1–5). The degree of intraocular pressure reduction achieved with a drainage tube device is influenced by the thickness, permeability, and inner surface area of the fibrous capsule surrrounding the scleral explant (6,7).

The occurrence of more rapid and exuberant scar tissue formation following ocular surgery in children as compared with adults has never been unequivocally demonstrated (1). Clinical experience, however, has shown that a more vigorous wound-healing response occurs in young patients following all forms of ocular surgery. Experimental studies of soft tissue wound healing in rats (8–10) and of collagen synthesis by human fibroblasts in culture (11) support the concept of a more rapid and vigorous wound-healing response associated with youth.

Gressel et al (12) demonstrated a significantly lower success rate for trabeculectomy in patients with primary glaucoma who were younger than 30 years compared with patients who were older. The success rate for patients between 30 and 50 years old was similar to that reported for older adults with primary glaucoma (13–17). Therefore, youth itself may be a risk factor for surgical failure after trabeculectomy. In their retrospective study of mitomycin C trabeculectomy, Susanna et al (18) found that younger patients (age ≤ 1 year) showed a significantly lower rate of successful intraocular pressure control at final follow-up than did the older ones. Miller and Rice (19) similarly identified age less than 7 years as a factor associated with an increased risk of failure following trabeculectomy.

Ocular and Orbital Development

The choice of procedure in children younger than 6 months is influenced by the sizes of the globe and the orbit. In very young children with small palpebral fissures and orbits, any surgical procedure performed at the superior limbus is technically difficult. This is particularly true in infants with abnormal and disproportionately enlarged corneas. It may be reasonable to consider primary angle surgery (i.e., goniotomy or trabeculotomy) even in complicated cases in which the success rate of these procedures is low. Performing these procedures at the temporal limbus obviates the need for good exposure superiorly. Even partial or temporary reduction of intraocular pressure is beneficial in this setting, allowing time for the eye and orbit to grow. Trabeculectomy and drainage implant installation are more easily performed on a larger eye in a more developed orbit, as access to the superior limbal and equatorial regions of the globe is improved. Additionally, the risks and potential morbidity of angle surgery are considerably less than those of trabeculectomy or drainage implant insertion, thereby helping to justify primary angle surgery despite the small likelihood of long-term success in some types of glaucoma.

Visual Development

The ultimate goal of any medical or surgical intervention in a child with glaucoma is the preservation of all aspects of visual function. The glaucoma surgeon must therefore be concerned with the prevention of amblyopia as well as the preservation of visual field. The various treatment modalities available must be considered in terms of both their ability to control the intraocular pressure as well as their potential for further compromising vision or visual development.

Control of intraocular pressure is usually the more immediate goal in the management of these patients. However, the issue of visual development must also be considered in the planning of any surgical procedure on a child in the amblyogenic age range, particularly between the ages of 3 and 5 years. Successful intraocular pressure control does not guarantee successful preservation of vision, as a myriad of factors may contribute to the development of amblyopia in children with glaucoma. Compromised vision during the early postoperative period following even uncomplicated glaucoma surgery has the potential to result in amblyopia. Surgical complications resulting in visually significant media opacity or impaired visual function (e.g., cataract, hyphema, corneal decompensation, retinal detachment, choroidal effusion) may prolong the interval during which vision is compromised. The potential for irreversible visual loss secondary to amblyopia is great. In some situations, careful planning and aggressive amblyopia management can avoid unnecessary visual loss. Owing to time constraints imposed by the developing visual system, treatment of amblyopia must be undertaken concurrently with glaucoma management. This is particularly true in children with monocular glaucoma.

Consideration should be given to postponing surgery, when possible, until the child is beyond the age of 9 years, at which point the risk of amblyopia development is substantially reduced. Although medical therapy has a limited role in the management of childhood glaucomas, it may provide temporary reduction of the intraocular pressure to acceptable levels. Postoperative management is also facilitated in older children, owing to improved cooperation with office examination, medication use, and amblyopia therapy. This approach is particularly valuable in children who have already undergone one or more glaucoma surgical procedures with only partial surgical success. Careful follow-up, with possible supplementation of pressure control using topical medications, and postponement of further surgery may provide the best long-term visual outcome in such situations.

Associated Ocular Anomalies

Glaucoma in children is often associated with other ocular anomalies. Some of these, such as cataract and corneal opacification, can significantly interfere with vision and result in the development of amblyopia if not eliminated at an early age. Surgical planning must include consideration of all coexisting anomalies that threaten the visual axis. Cataract extraction or corneal transplantation may be indicated at the same time as or shortly after glaucoma filtering surgery or drainage implant insertion. The need for, sequence of, and timing of multiple surgical procedures should be anticipated and planned at the time of the initial office evaluation or examination under anesthesia.

Risk of General Anesthesia

The administration of general anesthesia by an experienced anesthesiologist is relatively free of complications even in very young children and infants. When the need for surgery is anticipated based on prior office evaluation, inhalation anesthetics via endotracheal intubation are used from the outset. Limited examination under anesthesia to make or confirm a diagnosis or for postoperative assessment may be performed following the administration of intramuscular ketamine. Conversion to general endotracheal anesthesia is possible if the need for surgery is determined at the time of examination.

Variability in intraocular pressure readings will occur, depending on the type of anesthetic used and the timing of the pressure measurement in relation to anesthetic administration and intubation. Intramuscular ketamine can cause some elevation in intraocular pressure, while halothane and other inhalational agents can result in intraocular pressure reduction, depending on the depth of anesthesia. The intraocular pressure can also be artificially elevated by crying prior to anesthetic administration as well as immediately following endotracheal intubation—in both cases due to elevation of the central venous pressure. The optimal time for intraocular pressure measurement is immediately after the patient is sedated by administration of an inhaled anesthetic via a face mask and prior to intubation. The Tonopen (Mentor O & O, Norwell, MA) is particularly useful for intraocular measurement in this situation. The pressure should be rechecked 5 to 10 minutes after intubation before deep anesthesia is achieved. When ketamine is used, the intraocular pressure should be checked 5 minutes after administration.

Although general anesthesia can be safely administered to children of all ages, the risk of a life-threatening complication is substantially greater in very young infants (i.e., <3 months old following full-term delivery) as compared with older children (20,21). The majority of such complications involve respiratory failure and hypoxemia due to the immaturity of the infant respiratory system (22). The risk of adverse cardiac or pulmonary complications associated with general anesthesia is significantly reduced beyond the ages of 3 to 4 months, and it is best to postpone surgery until this time, if possible. Unfortunately, the severe intraocular pressure elevations associated with congenital glaucomas generally necessitate immediate surgical intervention to ensure the best visual outcome. In this situation, the availability of an experienced pediatric anesthesiologist and facilities for neonatal intensive care are imperative.

Unilateral Versus Bilateral Surgery

The decision to perform unilateral versus bilateral glaucoma surgery in a young child is governed by several factors. The severity and refractory nature of the intraocular pressure elevation often warrant simultaneous bilateral surgery. As discussed already, the potential for life-threatening systemic complications related to general anesthesia also supports the case for bilateral surgery. These considerations are balanced by the risk of serious, vision-threatening complications either intraoperatively or during the early postoperative period (such as acute postoperative endophthalmitis). The risk of such untoward occurrences is, in theory, greater when more complicated surgical procedures such as mitomycin-augmented trabeculectomy and drainge tube implantation are undertaken. The nature of the underlying glaucoma may also allow prognostication regarding the likelihood of surgical complications. The probability of serous choroidal detachment, choroidal hemorrhage, and associated flat anterior chamber following trabeculectomy in a child with Sturge-Weber syndrome is greater than in a child with primary congenital glaucoma.

The risk of death or serious systemic morbidity from general anesthesia, particularly in infants, is probably greater than the risk of bilateral, vision-threatening complications related to intraocular surgery. This may, in fact, be true for children of all ages. However, there are no unequivocal data to support or refute this hypothesis (23). Certainly, in healthy infants under 3 months old, and those born prematurely or with significant systemic anomalies, the risks associated with general anesthesia are substantially increased and simultaneous bilateral surgery is indicated more often.

CHOICE OF PROCEDURE

The optimal surgical procedure for children in whom angle surgery (i.e., goniotomy or trabeculotomy) has failed to control the intraocular pressure or is unlikely to succeed is unclear. Treatment options include conventional filtering surgery, installation of a glaucoma drainage implant, or cyclodestructive surgery. No prospective, randomized clinical studies offer comparative data regarding the relative outcomes and efficacy of these modalities.

Transscleral cyclodestructive procedures (cyclocryotherapy or cyclophotocoagulation) are generally reserved for eyes with extremely poor visual potential or eyes that have failed to achieve adequate intraocular pressure reduction following trabeculectomy or drainage tube surgery or both (24). The risk of significant visual loss, the difficulty titrating the amount of treatment to the desired intraocular pressure level, and the concern regarding the effects of severe aqueous humor suppression on the long-term health of the eye have resulted in the limited use of cyclodestructive procedures until other options have been exhausted. Recent reports of sympathetic ophthalmia following transscleral cyclophotocoagulation with the neodymium: yttrium-aluminum-garnet (Nd:YAG) laser also warrant consideration when contemplating this treatment modality (25–27).

Trabeculectomy is the conventional filtering procedure of choice in young children, especially with the availability of adjunctive intraoperative antimetabolic agents. The potential benefit of full-thickness filtering procedures in terms of sustained intraocular pressure reduction is outweighed by the significantly higher incidence of early postoperative complications due to overfiltration and ocular hypotony associated with these procedures. Difficulty with the nonsurgical management of complications such as shallow or flat anterior chambers, and the need for general anesthesia for any postoperative manipulations, further mitigate against the use of unguarded filtering procedures in young children.

Trabeculectomy with adjunctive mitomycin C is currently preferred by most surgeons as the initial outflow procedure in the management of pediatric glaucomas refractory to goniotomy or trabeculotomy, or in situations in which angle surgery is unlikely to succeed. However, the choice between mitomycin C–augmented trabeculectomy and drainage implantation is not necessarily so straightforward and is guided by a very limited body of published clinical data. Although the intraoperative episcleral application of mitomycin C appears to enhance the rate of successful intraocular pressure control following pediatric trabeculectomy, it may adversely affect the complication profile of this procedure. The risks of bleb leak, hypotony, and delayed-onset blebitis and endophthalmitis appear to be substantially increased following the use of mitomycin C (28–31).

Therefore, the use of drainage implants in children prior to trabeculectomy may be reasonable, especially considering the significant rate of filtering bleb failure following the application of mitomycin C during trabeculectomy in several small series (18,32,33). However, the occurrence of bleb leaks and ocular hypotony is replaced by the long-term risk of tube-related and plate-related complications such as extrusion, conjunctival erosion, anterior tube migration with corneal decompensation, and tube obstruction. The frequency of such complications, especially those related to thinning and erosion of the overlying limbal tissues, is higher in young children as compared with adults, owing to the greater scleral elasticity and (in buphthalmic eyes) thinness.

The risks associated with trabeculectomy are, in general terms, the same as those associated with adult filtering surgery. As the use of adjunctive mitomycin C has become a routine part of trabeculectomy in young children, the frequency and severity of certain of these complications are expected to increase. Because of the paucity of published clinical data regarding mitomycin C trabeculectomy in the pediatric age group, incidence data for specific complications are not yet available. The most common postoperative complication, despite the use of a potent antimetabolite, is filtration failure due to subconjunctival and episcleral fibrosis overlying the scleral fistula. Late bleb leaks, ocular hypotony, and hypotony-related complications (i.e., maculopathy, serous and hemorrhagic choroidal detachment) in the early and late postoperative periods are likely to occur with greater frequency and be more difficult to treat following the use of mitomycin C as compared with no antimetabolite. Attenuation and irregularity of the overlying conjunctival epithelium and the resultant thin, avascular filtering blebs associated with the use of mitomycin (30,34,35) are also likely to increase the incidence of delayed-onset blebitis and bleb-related endophthalmitis (29).

Several general considerations should affect the choice between trabeculectomy and drainage implantation in the management of childhood glaucomas. These include the anticipated severity of the postoperative wound-healing response, the technical ability to perform the procedures, the potential for postoperative complications, and the predetermined target intraocular pressure.

Specific circumstances that favor the use of a drainage implant over trabeculectomy include a history of prior unsuccessful trabeculectomy with adjunctive mitomycin C in the operative or the fellow eye, the presence of extensive conjunctival scarring, a history of other prior intraocular or conjunctival incising surgical procedures, and the need for other procedures at the time of glaucoma surgery. Prior surgery on the conjunctiva, sclera, and anterior segment predisposes the eye to a more pronounced inflammatory response and a more severe fibroproliferative healing response following subsequent surgical procedures. Previously failed filtering surgery, even if performed without technical difficulties (i.e., intraoperative or postoperative complications such as serous choroidal detachment, flat anterior chamber, conjunctival wound leak, etc.), increases the likelihood of a similar outcome should the same surgical procedure be repeated. An indication of the inherent wound-healing properties of the eye is provided by this history, in addition to the fact that the eye has already undergone at least one intraocular procedure. To the extent that surgical complications may adversely affect the long-term outcome of trabeculectomy, documentation of such an event may make repeat filtering surgery more reasonable. If surgical complications can be avoided, a more favorable outcome may result. Failure of a technically flawless and complication-free trabeculectomy on one eye of a patient with bilaterally symmetric disease bodes poorly for the outcome of the identical procedure on the fellow eye. Primary drainage tube implantation on the fellow eye should be considered in such situations. Given the paucity of comparative data regarding the outcome of trabeculectomy with mitomycin C versus drainage tube implantation, consideration should be given to performing a trabeculectomy in one eye and inserting a drainage device in the fellow eye of a child with bilateral, symmetric disease in whom angle surgery failed or is unlikely to be of benefit.

Other factors influencing the choice between trabeculectomy and drainage tube implantation include the type of glaucoma, the presence of associated ocular abnormalities, the desired target intraocular pressure, and certain socioeconomic factors. In managing glaucoma associated with severe disorganization of the anterior segment, as in Peter's anomaly, the primary use of a drainage device may be indicated. The technical difficulties in performing trabeculectomy, the need for concurrent procedures such as penetrating keratoplasty, vitrectomy, and lens extraction, and the propensity toward severe postoperative inflammation make drainage tube insertion reasonable as an initial surgical option. Similarly, when subsequent surgical procedures are anticipated, there is less risk of compromising intraocular pressure control in the presence of a glaucoma drainage implant as compared with a trabeculectomy. Gressel et al (12) demonstrated a significantly higher failure rate of trabeculectomy in young patients with secondary glaucomas than in those with primary glaucomas. Among patients with secondary glaucomas, those who had undergone previous intraocular surgery were significantly less likely to achieve successful intraocular pressure control following trabeculectomy. Poor results were also noted for patients with developmental glaucomas (possibly due to the frequency of prior intraocular surgery and the younger average age) and neovascular glaucoma.

The potential for obtaining an intraocular pressure in the low-normal range for patients with advanced optic nerve head damage is greater following trabeculectomy with mitomycin C than drainage device implantation. An intraocular pressure in the range of 8 to 12 mm Hg is an uncommon long-term result of drainage tube surgery, even with the adjunctive use of antiglaucoma medications. Furthermore, even in patients in whom adequate intraocular pressure control is ultimately achieved with a drainage device, the occurrence of a prolonged hypertensive phase may result in difficulty maintaining an acceptable intraocular pressure or necessitate the use of multiple antiglaucoma medications for weeks to months following the initiation of flow through the tube. Therefore, a trabeculectomy is preferred in patients with extensive optic nerve head cupping in whom an extremely low intraocular pressure is desired to reduce the risk of further damage.

Conditions predisposing to an increased likelihood of serious bleb-related intraocular infection (such as poor hygiene, the need for long-term soft contact lens wear, or severe ocular surface disease) militate against a decision to perform a trabeculectomy, especially with an adjunctive antimetabolite. The risk of delayed-onset bleb-related intraocular infection is significantly reduced following drainage implant surgery as compared with trabeculectomy. The presence of subconjunctival aqueous filtration and an anterior scleral fistula after trabeculectomy results in significant compromise of the normal barrier to the intraocular spread of bacteria. Excessively thin conjunctiva, as occurs following full-thickness surgery or with antimetabolite use, increases the risk of intraocular infection. Glaucoma drainage implants are not associated with this complication, except in cases where tube erosion or scleral plate extrusion results in breakdown of the overlying conjunctiva with direct continuity between the external ocular surface and the anterior or posterior chamber.

The silicone tube of a glaucoma drainage device serves as a permanent conduit for aqueous humor between the anterior or posterior chamber and the equatorial fibrous capsule surrounding the scleral plate. A vigorous fibroproliferative healing response with rapid encapsulation of the scleral explant is desirable, especially with the use of a nonvalved tube. This provides resistance to aqueous outflow and ensures a physiologic intraocular pressure following tube ligature release. Unlike trabeculectomy, fibrous tissue encapsulation of the drainage site is necessary and is not detrimental to the surgical outcome, although excessive fibrosis may result in transient or permanent elevation of the intraocular pressure. A successful outcome is, therefore, more likely with the use of a drainage implant than with trabeculectomy in situations in which excessive inflammation and postoperative scarring are expected.

TECHNICAL CONSIDERATIONS

Trabeculectomy

The incidence of successful, long-term intraocular pressure control following trabeculectomy in young children is rela-

tively poor compared with the outcome of this procedure in adults (12,36–40). Outcome assessment and monitoring for disease progression require serial intraocular pressure measurements, optic nerve head examinations, and measurement of refractive error and axial length (often under general anesthesia). Visual field assessment is generally precluded by the young age and poor cooperation of the patients, until at least the age of 5 years.

The poor success rate of pediatric trabeculectomy may be attributed to several factors, including the complexity of the associated pathology, multiple previous surgeries, a propensity toward vigorous wound healing, and difficult preoperative and postoperative management. Anatomic factors such as buphthalmos with scleral thinning and decreased scleral rigidity, the presence of a deep anterior chamber with lens subluxation or other associated ocular anomalies, and limbal ectasias and staphylomas make surgery technically more difficult and also contribute to its poor success rate (36,41). The increased thickness of infantile Tenon's capsule may also play a role in the failure of the surgical procedure, owing to an enhanced proclivity to fibrovascular proliferation and scarring postoperatively (1). Prior ocular surgeries often result in conjunctival adherence to the sclera in addition to enhancement of the postoperative inflammatory response. Preoperative preparation may be difficult. Administration of intravenous ocular hypotensive or hyperosmotic agents prior to surgery may be dangerous and even contraindicated in some children. Postoperative management is also complicated because of the problems associated with proper eyedrop administration, clinical evaluation, and manipulations such as digital ocular massage, laser suture lysis, and transconjunctival needle revision.

Beauchamp and Parks (36) reported final intraocular pressures lower than 25 mm Hg following 13 (50%) of 26 trabeculectomies performed on 25 eyes of 16 patients, at a mean follow-up interval of 15.5 months. Primary congenital glaucoma was present in the majority of their patients, although a variety of secondary glaucomas were also represented. Significant complications including intraoperative vitreous loss, postoperative scleral ectasia, retinal detachment, choroidal effusion, and endophthalmitis were noted in this small series. In contrast, Burke and Bowell (37) reported an 87% incidence of average intraocular pressures of 18 mm Hg or lower after trabeculectomy was performed as the primary intraocular procedure in 21 eyes of 15 patients with primary or secondary infantile glaucoma. The mean follow-up time in this series was 3.9 years. Most patients were younger than 1.5 years at the time of surgery and all had a preoperative intraocular pressure less than or equal to 30 mm Hg. No significant intraoperative or postoperative complications were encountered. Fulcher et al (38) presented more extended follow-up data on a subgroup of patients from the study of Burke and Bowell (37). After a mean follow-up period of 7.9 years, 18 (90%) of 20 eyes maintained the intraocular pressure at 18 mm Hg or lower following a single trabeculectomy without use of an antimetabolite.

Debnath et al (39) reported a more modest 54% incidence of intraocular pressure of 16 mm Hg or lower after primary trabeculectomy in 30 eyes of 16 patients at a mean follow-up time of 11.2 months. The mean preoperative intraocular pressure was 35 mm Hg in this series. Serious complications including vitreous loss, endophthalmitis, and shallow anterior chamber were noted. Cadera et al (40) reported a similarly poor rate of intraocular pressure control (<22 mm Hg) after thermal sclerostomy (46 cases) and trabeculectomy (8 cases) in 38 eyes of 24 children with a variety of primary and secondary glaucomas. Six (35%) of 17 eyes in which the filtering procedure was the primary surgical procedure achieved an intraocular pressure lower than 22 mm Hg. The preoperative intraocular pressure was 35 mm Hg or higher in 35 eyes.

Gressel et al (12) reported a series of 117 trabeculectomies performed on 98 patients under the age of 50 years. The overall rate for achieving an intraocular pressure below 25 mm Hg without medications or 21 mm Hg or lower with medications was 51% at a mean follow-up interval of 36 months. The rate was significantly better for patients with primary glaucoma (74%) as compared with the rates for secondary (48%), developmental (35%), and neovascular (9%) glaucomas. Prior ocular surgery and younger age were associated with a poorer outcome in this series. A successful outcome was noted in 25 (83%) of 30 patients with primary glaucomas between the ages of 30 and 49 years, but only in 4 (44%) of 9 patients under the age of 30 years. Among the patients in the younger age group, those with no prior ocular surgery demonstrated a higher success rate (4/5 patients). However, the number of patients in this category was too small to draw any meaningful conclusions. Six trabeculectomies were performed on patients younger than 9 years. All of these were failures, requiring further glaucoma surgery or resulting in loss of light perception. Nineteen patients between 10 and 19 years old were included. Only 7 (37%) of these achieved successful intraocular pressure control.

Sturmer et al (41) identified a lower overall success rate of trabeculectomy in young patients compared with reported success rates in older adults. They attributed the poorer outcome in young patients to the common occurrence or exaggerated effect of several risk factors including aphakia, previous argon laser trabeculoplasty, previous glaucoma surgery, and preoperative intraocular pressure higher than 40 mm Hg, rather than age alone. This series included only 12 patients younger than 20 years and none younger than 11 years. In contrast, other studies evaluated the outcome of initial trabeculectomy in young patients and concluded that the success rate is comparable to that demonstrated for older adults with primary glaucoma (12,42). However, these studies included patients with a wide range of ages and only small numbers of young children. In fact, the series of Costa et al (42) specifically excluded patients under 15 years old.

It is generally accepted (as has been our experience) that children (i.e., <18 years) exhibit a more vigorous wound-healing response and a greater propensity toward filtration failure than do young adults (i.e., 18–50 years). This appears to be due to an inherent, age-related proclivity toward exuberant scar tissue formation, although a contribution from coexisting ocular risk factors as identified in the study of Sturmer et al (41) may play a role in some patients. Moreover, accepted risk factors for surgical failure may have a more pronounced adverse effect on surgical outcome in younger patients (43).

Adjunctive therapy with the antiproliferative agents 5-fluorouracil and mitomycin C can enhance the success rate and effectiveness of trabeculectomy in adult patients (44–53). This is primarily due to a pronounced inhibitory effect on fibroblast proliferation (54–58). The use of such adjunctive agents in pediatric trabeculectomy would be expected to be of particular benefit, given the exaggerated wound-healing response in this age group. An increased incidence of postoperative complications in comparison with non-antimetabolite-augmented trabeculectomy (i.e., late bleb leak, bleb-related endophthalmitis, and hypotony) is expected, in proportion with the incidence of avascular, thin-walled filtering blebs (30,31,34,35,59,60). Whiteside-Michel et al (61) reported a 95% incidence of intraocular pressure of 20 mm Hg or lower without antiglaucoma medications, following initial trabeculectomy with postoperative 5-fluorouracil in a series of 20 patients between 13 and 40 years old. The mean intraocular pressure at final follow-up was 10.5 mm Hg. Significant postoperative complications included bleb-related endophthalmitis in 2 patients and hypotony maculopathy in 1 patient.

There are limited published data on the clinical efficacy of either 5-fluorouracil or mitomycin C in conjunction with pediatric trabeculectomy (18,32,33,62,63). The use of 5-fluorouracil following trabeculectomy in children has been reported (62). In general, however, the use of this adjunctive agent is limited by the difficulty of repeated subconjunctival injections in young, uncooperative patients. Good results have been obtained with the intraoperative application of 5-fluorouracil to the episcleral surface during trabeculectomy in adults (64–67). However, the need for supplemental subconjunctival injections postoperatively is not predictably eliminated.

A distinct advantage of mitomycin C over 5-fluorouracil, particularly in pediatric patients, is its administration in a single intraoperative dose, obviating the need for repeated postoperative subconjunctival injections. In vitro studies demonstrated a more pronounced effect of mitomycin C relative to 5-fluorouracil on the inhibition of fibroblast proliferation (54,56). Additionally, mitomycin C can offer a better success rate, when compared to 5-fluorouracil, in eyes at high risk for failure of the trabeculectomy (68–73). In several small series, successful control of intraocular pressure was established in 60% to 70% of pediatric patients following trabeculectomy with mitomycin C (18,32,33). Susanna et al (18) retrospectively studied 56 patients (79 eyes) who were followed for at least 6 months after trabeculectomy with mitomycin C. Fifty-three of these patients were 18 years or younger and a variety of congenital and developmental glaucoma diagnoses were represented. After a mean follow-up time of 17 months, 53 (67%) of the eyes demonstrated an intraocular pressure of 21 mm Hg or lower.

Preoperative Assessment

Nasolacrimal System Congenital obstruction of the lacrimal drainage system may become clinically evident in as many as 2% to 4% of newborn infants (74). The incidence of lacrimal insufficiency and both acute and chronic dacryocystitis in the pediatric age group may be even higher. Careful evaluation of the functional status of the lacrimal drainage system is imperative prior to undertaking surgical procedures that carry a high long-term risk of intraocular infection. The use of adjunctive mitomycin C at the time of trabeculectomy may significantly compromise the normal barriers to the intraocular spread of bacteria, thereby enhancing the risk of bleb-related infections (28,29). Prior to undertaking filtering surgery in children, the surgeon should routinely elicit from each patient (or the parents) a careful history of excessive tearing without rhinorrhea, punctal discharge, or matting of the lashes. The preoperative examination should include inspection of the medial canthal area for evidence of inflammation, the application of digital pressure over the lacrimal sac, and the appropriate culture of any resultant discharge. If there is any question regarding the functional integrity of the lacrimal drainage apparatus based on history or clinical findings, formal diagnostic testing should be performed, and surgical correction of confirmed nasolacrimal duct obstruction should be undertaken prior to any intraocular procedure.

Conjunctival Assessment In patients who have undergone previous ocular surgery, careful preoperative assessment of the degree and location of conjunctival scarring is essential to the planning of trabeculectomy. In older children, inspection of the conjunctiva at the slit lamp and gentle manipulation with a cotton-tipped applicator may be possible. Younger or uncooperative children may require examination under anesthesia immediately prior to the intended surgery. A thorough ophthalmic history is crucial, as the potential need for alternative surgical procedures (i.e., drainage implantation) must be anticipated.

Trabeculotomy should be performed at the nasal or temporal position, thereby leaving the superior conjunctiva and sclera undisturbed should future trabeculectomy be necessary. Although a superior location allows for conversion to a trabeculectomy if technical difficulties (i.e., inability to identify Schlemm's canal, inadvertent anterior-chamber entry) are encountered, a trabeculectomy performed under such circumstances is generally suboptimal. Intraoperative antimetabolite use is contraindicated if deep limbal dissection or frank entry into the anterior chamber has already occurred, unless the wound can be adequately closed or the anterior chamber "pressurized" with viscoelastic substance or air.

Surgical Technique

Selection of Surgical Site As in adults, the superior quadrants are preferred to the inferior quadrants for trabeculectomy. The superior quadrant with the least conjunctival scarring will allow the procedure to be performed with the greatest technical ease and will ensure the best chance of a successful outcome. The inferior quadrants should be avoided owing to the greater risk of postoperative bleb-related infection as compared with superiorly positioned filtering blebs (29,75–77). This is especially true following the adjunctive use of mitomycin C, owing to the increased likelihood of developing an avascular, thin-walled filtering bleb. The cumulative lifetime risk of developing such a devastating complication in a young child is probably high. Moreover, difficulties with the postoperative care and monitoring of the filtering bleb make the early detection of a severe intraocular infection unlikely. Therefore, many surgeons consider an inferior location for pediatric trabeculectomy to be contraindicated. Noninfectious anterior and posterior scleritis has also been reported following inferior trabeculectomy with mitomycin C in adults (78).

The superonasal quadrant is generally the preferred location for a primary trabeculectomy in a phakic eye. This places the resultant filtering bleb as far as possible from the temporal limbus, where cataract extraction can be performed at a later date. Moreover, this location preserves the superotemporal sclera and conjunctiva, facilitating repeat trabeculectomy or drainage tube implantation should the initial procedure fail. Some surgeons prefer to position the trabeculectomy flap such that it overlaps or straddles the 12-o'clock meridian. This ensures maximal protection of the resultant filtering bleb by the upper lid.

Conjunctival Incision Although there is no proven benefit in terms of successful intraocular pressure control of limbus-based over fornix-based conjunctival flaps in adult trabeculectomy (79,80), several considerations make the limbus-based approach more desirable in the pediatric age group. The incision for a limbus-based flap and the resultant conjunctival wound lies in the superior conjunctival fornix where it is protected from inadvertent eye rubbing and exposure.

In the early postoperative period, there is a significant incidence of transient aqueous leak from beneath the anterior edge of a fornix-based conjunctiva-Tenon's flap (79). In adult patients, such leaks are of variable duration and generally resolve spontaneously, but they occur more frequently and are more prolonged following the use of mitomycin C. The occurrence of an aqueous leak at the limbus in the early postoperative period may significantly compromise the formation of a filtering bleb, as the aqueous will exit the subconjunctival space anteriorly without elevating the conjunctiva. Failure to separate the conjunctiva from the episcleral surface with aqueous increases the likelihood of subconjunctival and episcleral scar tissue formation at the filtering site. This is of particular importance during the early postoperative period when the wound-healing response is most vigorous. The mechanical as well as the antifibroblastic effect (81) of the aqueous humor is of crucial importance to the ultimate development of a successful filtering bleb.

In adults, there are various interventions that enable the surgeon to minimize the duration and severity of such early postoperative aqueous leaks. These include soft bandage contact lens wear (82), use of collagen shields (83), application of tissue adhesive (84,85), and use of a symblepharon ring (86) or a Simmons' tamponade shell (87,88). In young children, however, such interventions may not be possible, depending on the patient's age and level of cooperation. Moreover, careful follow-up examinations in the office may be difficult.

Another potential difficulty with the fornix-based conjunctival flap results from its closure at the limbus, if nonabsorbable sutures, such as 10-0 nylon, are used. The knots of the wing sutures used to anchor the anterior corners of the conjunctival flap to the peripheral cornea are often left unburied and the cut ends of the sutures are left long. Removal of these sutures is usually necessary at some point postoperatively, after the anterior conjunctival edge has healed sufficiently. In young children, this necessitates a return to the operating room. Failure to remove these sutures may result in persistent ocular irritation. More significant, however, is the tendency of the exposed sutures to trap mucus and surface debris, in an area of persistent surface breakdown that they create. The increased risk of local bacterial keratitis and secondary blebitis or endophthalmitis dictates careful follow-up, continued prophylactic use of a topical antibiotic, and suture removal as soon as adequate healing has occurred. Closure of the limbal incision with an absorbable suture, such as 9-0 polyglactin, or careful burial of the knots of the nylon wing sutures eliminates the need for suture removal.

As in adult trabeculectomy, the conjunctiva-Tenon's incision for a limbus-based flap should be made as far posterior as possible without disturbing orbital fat. This is to minimize the effect of inflammation evoked by the incision itself and the suture material (particularly polyglactin) used to close the wound on the healing response in the area of the trabeculectomy. Moreover, this posterior location positions the conjunctival incision as far as possible from the area of mitomycin exposure. As the conjunctival wound often delimits the posterior aspect of the resultant filtering bleb, the more posterior location permits the development of a larger, more diffuse area of filtration.

In certain situations, a fornix-based conjunctival flap may be advantageous. Easier conjunctival dissection and better limbal exposure are possible with this approach. This may be particularly useful in children with extremely large corneas or small palpebral fissures. If the decision is made to proceed with trabeculectomy in the presence of extensive anterior conjunctival scarring, a limbal incision will facilitate the conjunctival dissection.

Scleral Flap Dissection Scleral thinning in young children, especially in the setting of buphthalmos, dictates caution during scleral flap preparation, dissection, and closure. Anterior-chamber entry during outlining of the scleral flap with a sharp blade may occur, especially at the corneoscleral junction. This can lead to difficulty in maintaining the anterior chamber during subsequent flap dissection. Also, application of mitomycin C to the ocular surface may be contraindicated in this situation. The use of mitomycin prior to any scleral incision is recommended for this reason, as well as those discussed below.

Particular attention to the dissection of a thick scleral flap is important, owing to the baseline scleral thinning as well as the possibility of further scleral attenuation secondary to the effect of mitomycin C. Damage to a thin scleral flap can occur in several ways during dissection and manipulation. Tearing or full-thickness hole formation at the posterior or middle aspect of the flap can result from the application of and excessive tension with a toothed forceps. This can preclude adequate coverage of the internal ostium, resulting in excessive aqueous outflow and secondary postoperative hypotony.

If disruption of the flap occurs prior to excision of the internal block, several options are available. The initial site can be abandoned and a new flap created adjacent to it. This may require extension of the original conjunctiva-Tenon's incision. If there is no suitable alternative site or if the discontinuity in the flap is relatively posterior or localized, the position of the internal ostium can be adjusted such that it lies as far from the flap defect as possible. The advantage of a large scleral flap in allowing for adjustment in the position of the internal section is obvious. It may also be necessary to make the internal section smaller than usual. As long as the flap defect does not lie directly over the internal section, a suture may be placed through the flap between the tear and a point that overlies the posterior edge of the internal ostium. The flap can then be sutured to the underlying scleral bed in a manner that minimizes flow through the flap defect (Fig. 37-1). If excessive aqueous flow persists through a scleral flap tear, a patch of Tenon's fascia may be harvested from a distant site and sutured over the flap defect to provide some additional resistance to aqueous flow (89). Most important, however, is taking measures to prevent the occurrence of such complications. Use of nontoothed forceps (such as Pierce-Hoskins style) and avoidance of excessive tension in the manipulation of thin scleral flaps will minimize the incidence of flap damage.

Complete avulsion of the scleral flap occurs infrequently, but is more commonly encountered during flap dissection through an area of thin sclera. Several options may be exercised in the management of this complication. Resuturing of the torn scleral edges is possible if the dehiscence is at least 1 to 2 mm from the conjunctival insertion. The use of 9-0 polyglactin, 10-0 nylon, or 10-0 polypropylene (Prolene) suture on a vascular needle is most effective in this situation. This may, however, result in foreshortening of the

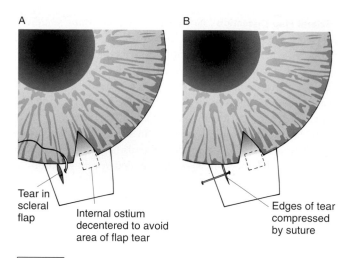

FIGURE 37-1. *Closure of a scleral flap tear. A. A 10-0 nylon suture is passed through the flap between the central edge of the tear and a point overlying the closest edge of the internal ostium. Note that the internal ostium (dashed line) has been decentered so that it does not lie directly beneath the flap tear. B. The suture is tied tightly, compressing the adjacent edges of the tear together and securing the flap to the underlying scleral bed in the area of the tear.*

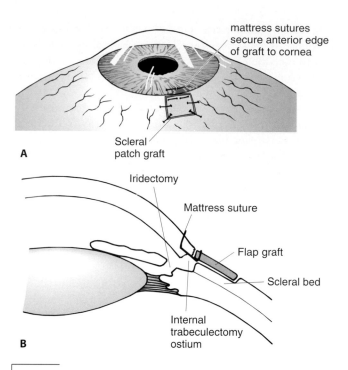

FIGURE 37-2. *Repair of an avulsed scleral flap. The donor material is cut to an appropriate size and sutured to the limbus with two 10-0 nylon mattress sutures at its anterior edge. The three remaining sides of the graft are secured as a normal trabeculectomy flap, to allow controlled flow from the limbal fistula. A. Surface view of the scleral flap graft in place. B. Cross section through the flap graft in the meridian of the internal trabeculectomy ostium. The path of the mattress suture through the graft and the torn anterior edge of the host flap is diagrammed.*

flap and compromised tamponade over the internal fistula. If the flap is avulsed at its base, it can sometimes be resutured directly to the limbus using one or two horizontal mattress sutures of 10-0 nylon or polypropylene (Fig. 37-2) (90). If the torn scleral edge is excessively attenuated (as is usually the case), a new flap may be fashioned from one of several sources and sutured to the limbus with one or more horizontal mattress sutures. An autologous piece of lamellar sclera from a distant site or a piece of donor sclera, fascia lata, dura mater, or pericardium can be used depending on availability. Occasionally, the avulsed flap can be rotated 180 degrees so that its thicker, posterior edge lies over the trabeculectomy fistula. It can then be secured with one or two vertical mattress sutures as with a free graft. This latter option is most likely to be technically feasible when working with a large, rectangular scleral flap.

Distortion of the normal limbal anatomy due to stretching of the ocular coats or other primary structural anomalies can lead to difficulty in identifying external landmarks. This can result in improper incision placement and premature or posterior entry into the anterior chamber. Posterior placement of the internal fistula is associated with an increased incidence of vitreous loss, intraocular hemorrhage, and obstruction of the ostium by ciliary processes. The management of vitreous loss is discussed later. Obstruction of the internal fistula by ciliary processes should be recognized and corrected prior to conjunctival closure, as this can be a difficult problem to manage postoperatively, especially in a child. Generally the ciliary processes will present themselves at the fistula following iridectomy. They can be mistaken for

residual iris and excised, a situation that frequently leads to excessive intraocular hemorrhage. Direct application of cautery using a micropoint bipolar probe (Mentor O & O, Norwell, MA) or diathermy using an intraocular probe (MIRA, Waltham, MA) can coagulate and shrink the ciliary processes, clearing the ostium. If the ostium does not appear to be completely obstructed by the ciliary processes, the anterior chamber should be irrigated both before and after scleral flap closure to demonstrate aqueous flow through the trabeculectomy site. Further anterior dissection of the trabeculectomy flap and internal ostium, although technically difficult, can also be performed to clear the ciliary processes and establish unimpeded aqueous flow.

Antimetabolite Application In young children, a 3- to 5-minute episcleral application of mitomycin C at a concentration of 0.5 mg/mL provides maximal effectiveness without an unacceptably high incidence of complications. A pledget is fashioned from a thin piece of a cellulose surgical sponge (i.e., a surgical spear or instrument wipe). A large pledget size (i.e., 4–5 mm × 8–10 mm) is desirable to promote the development of a diffuse filtering bleb. The sponge is soaked in the mitomycin solution and placed on the episcleral surface over the intended trabeculectomy site. The flap of conjunctiva and Tenon's capsule is draped posteriorly over the sponge. Care should be taken to avoid exposure of the cut edge of conjunctiva to the mitomycin. This can be accomplished by elevating the flap off of the ocular surface with two nontoothed forceps or by everting the posterior edge of the flap.

Mitomycin C can be applied either before or after dissection of the lamellar scleral flap, but always prior to incision into the anterior chamber, owing to its potent corneal endothelial toxicity (91). Detectable concentrations of mitomycin C in the aqueous humor have been demonstrated following episcleral application both before and after scleral dissection (92,93). Aqueous levels were significantly higher when the mitomycin was applied after scleral flap dissection. In buphthalmic eyes with thin sclera, mitomycin should be applied prior to incising the sclera, because of the risk of early anterior-chamber entry during flap dissection, as well as the potential for enhanced intraocular penetration through the intact sclera. This can lead to corneal endothelial damage as well as ciliary body toxicity (94,95).

The use of mitomycin C in young adults with enlarged eyes should also be undertaken with caution. The scleral thinning and decreased healing response in young adults seem to predispose these eyes to prolonged hypotony and hypotony-related complications (30,96). As patients in this age group tend to be more cooperative, the use of intraoperative 5-fluorouracil with supplemental postoperative subconjunctival injections may be a safer approach. If mitomycin C is used, consideration should be given to decreasing the concentration (i.e., 0.2–0.4 mg/mL) or the duration of application (i.e., 2–4 minutes) or both.

Scleral Flap Closure   The particular suturing technique used for scleral flap closure is determined, in large part, by the age and cooperativeness of the patient. By the age of 5 to 6 years, most children can cooperate for slit-lamp examination. The manipulations involved in laser suture lysis are somewhat more involved and may not be possible for several more years. As a general rule, if it is possible to perform gonioscopy in the office, laser suture lysis via a conventional slit-lamp delivery system should be possible. In such children, trabeculectomy can be performed and managed postoperatively as in adults, with relatively tight initial flap closure and serial laser suture lysis. Vertically mounted lasers and special laser lens holders in conjunction with fiberoptic laser probes (97) make laser suture lysis an option even in very young children. This specialized equipment is not widely available and a monitored setting for administration of inhalational anesthetics via face mask or intramuscular ketamine by an anesthesiologist is necessary.

In very young or otherwise uncooperative children, several alternatives to postoperative laser suture lysis should be considered, to allow tight initial flap closure and decrease the risk of early postoperative hypotony. Absorbable suture material, such as polyglactin, may be used for some or all of the scleral flap sutures. The absorbable sutures will eventually dissolve, allowing for loosening of the scleral flap in the

meridian of the suture. Enhanced aqueous egress from the eye will result if permanent subconjunctival and episcleral fibrosis has not already occurred.

There are several disadvantages to this technique. First, the time interval between surgery and suture dissolution is variable and unpredictable. The longer the suture remains in position, the greater the likelihood that episcleral scarring will occur prior to suture release. In this regard, the finer 10-0 polyglactin suture may be preferable to the 9-0 suture. This dissolves in approximately 3 to 4 weeks, but probably loosens significantly prior to this time. Dissolution time for this suture material in the subconjunctival space may be shorter than that for the same suture on the ocular surface. Second, it is not possible to prevent suture dissolution in patients who have adequate aqueous flow with all of the sutures in place. The risk of ocular hypotony following suture dissolution in such situations is enhanced, especially following the application of mitomycin C. Third, the potential for the polyglactin suture material to incite inflammation, thereby promoting scar tissue formation in the vicinity of the scleral flap, is greater than that for the more inert nylon sutures. In our experience, however, the additional amount of inflammation induced by the polyglactin suture material is not clinically significant. A combination of nylon and polyglactin sutures may offer the best compromise between uncontrolled suture release and a total inability to augment flow postoperatively. For example, polyglactin may be used for the two anterior sutures of a rectangular or trapezoidal flap and nylon for the two posterior sutures. The anterior sutures can be tied tightly to avoid early overfiltration.

Releasable scleral flap sutures are another alternative to conventional interrupted nylon sutures and postoperative laser lysis (Fig. 37-3) (98–100). The flap sutures can be released at one or more examinations under anesthesia within the first 4 postoperative weeks. Minimal anesthesia is required; insufflation with a face mask or intramuscular ketamine is usually sufficient. In young children, rapid subconjunctival/episcleral fibrosis sometimes results in difficulty with suture removal after only 2 to 3 weeks. The initial postoperative examination under anesthesia should, therefore, be scheduled no later than 2 weeks after the initial procedure.

Thin scleral flaps are also prone to the development of large suture tracks following closure with a spatulated or side-cutting needle as found with most 10-0 nylon and polyglactin sutures. These may be accompanied by excessive aqueous leakage and difficulty maintaining a deep anterior chamber. This is particularly problematic with sutures placed anteriorly at the sides of the flap. A suture track leak can often be managed by removal of the involved suture, which exerts tension on the flap defect and acts to pull the hole more widely open. A new suture of 10-0 nylon or 9-0 polyglactin can then be placed with a vascular needle, taking care to incorporate the original needle track in the second pass.

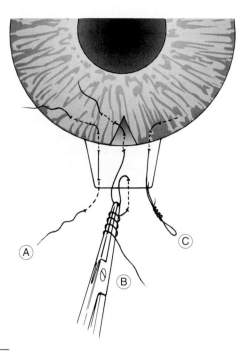

FIGURE 37-3.   *Releasable scleral flap sutures (99). A. The needle is passed through the posterior sclera and scleral flap. It is then passed through the base of the flap, beneath the conjunctival insertion, and up through peripheral clear cornea. A second, partial-thickness corneal pass is made at an angle to the first, as diagrammed. B. A slipknot is then tied, pulling the loop of suture overlying the flap through four throws of the free posterior end. C. After final adjustments have been made, the anterior end of the suture is cut flush with the corneal surface. The suture is released by grasping the exposed portion between the two corneal bites with fine forceps, and pulling tangential to the ocular surface and in a direction opposite to the site of scleral fixation. The dashed lines indicate buried segments of suture.*

If suture track leaks are large, multiple, or difficult to close in the manner just described, consideration may be given to the use of a Tenon's patch over the trabeculectomy site (90). Filling the anterior chamber with viscoelastic substance or air or both may be helpful if excessive filtration persists. Suture track leaks are best avoided by using a vascular needle when closing thin scleral flaps. Also, care should be taken to create a small square knot without incorporation of tissue fragments, to facilitate its burial and avoid enlargement of the suture track. Rotation and knot burial away from the scleral flap should generally be attempted first. The knots can also be left unburied as long as the free suture ends are cut long, to prevent trauma and perforation of the overlying conjunctiva.

Conjunctival Closure   A limbus-based conjunctiva-Tenon's flap may be closed in one or two layers with polyglactin or nylon suture. Use of an absorbable suture eliminates the need for suture removal at a later date as well as the prolonged presence of foreign material adjacent to the filtering bleb. The 8-0 or 9-0 polyglactin sutures with a vascular needle may be used.

A fornix-based flap of conjunctiva and Tenon's capsule is also best closed with an absorbable suture such as 9-0 polyglactin. The flap is advanced anteriorly over the trabeculectomy site and secured to the far periphery of the cornea with interrupted wing sutures. Relaxing incisions at one or both ends of the peritomy can be closed with running extensions of the wing suture using the same suture material. One or more horizontal mattress sutures (depending on the circumferential extent of the conjunctival opening) should be used to secure the anterior edge of the flap to the cornea. Aqueous leaks from beneath the anterior edge of the flap are common, especially following the use of mitomycin C, and are particularly difficult to manage in young children. A running suture of 9-0 or 10-0 nylon or polyglactin may be used to ensure tight anterior conjunctival closure and minimize the incidence of aqueous leak (101).

Tenonectomy is generally not recommended in pediatric trabeculectomy. Excessive thinning and avascularity of the conjunctival bleb may be more likely after the intraoperative removal of Tenon's fascia. In young children there is some concern, as discussed already, about the increased lifetime risk of serious bleb-related infection. Moreover, there is no proven beneficial effect of tenonectomy on the outcome of filtering surgery (102). Improved visualization of scleral flap sutures is not a consideration in young children unless special equipment is available to perform postoperative laser suture lysis.

Following conjunctival closure, attention to several details will assist in postoperative assessment and help to minimize postoperative complications. In many young children, especially those with enlarged, thin corneas, aqueous leak through the corneal paracentesis track, either spontaneously or with minimal pressure on the globe, is common. Routine placement of an interrupted 10-0 nylon or polyglactin suture to close the paracentesis at the conclusion of the procedure is advisable. In children for whom slit-lamp examination is difficult or impossible, placement of a small air bubble into the anterior chamber at the conclusion of the procedure permits easier assessment of anterior-chamber depth on the first 1 to 2 postoperative days. Posterior sub-Tenon's injection of a depot steroid such as triamcinolone acetonide (Kenalog) should be considered when reliable administration of topical steroids may not be possible.

Complications

The eyes of patients with childhood glaucomas are prone to certain intraoperative complications due to characteristic structural abnormalities. The thin sclera of buphthalmic eyes predisposes them to collapse and infolding following decompression. Placement of scleral flap sutures can be difficult under such circumstances. Rapid flap closure and re-formation of the anterior chamber can be facilitated by preplacing two of the flap sutures prior to entering the anterior chamber and excising the internal trabeculectomy block. If a trapezoidal or rectangular flap is used, placement of a suture at the anterior aspect of each side of the flap is most beneficial. These may be tied tightly in a temporary locking fashion immediately after the iridectomy is performed, allowing compression across the internal fistula. Re-formation of the anterior chamber with air or balanced salt solution may then be accomplished followed by placement of additional flap sutures. Tension on the initial side sutures can then be adjusted to optimize aqueous flow from beneath the scleral flap, and these can then be tied permanently.

Aphakic eyes and eyes that have previously undergone vitrectomy are particularly prone to collapse following decompression during trabeculectomy. Placement of a self-retaining anterior-chamber infusion cannula prior to performance of the internal section may assist in stabilizing the globe. Generally, however, fluid egress through the trabeculectomy fistula occurs at a rate equal to the inflow through the cannula and scleral infolding may still occur. Placement of a Flieringa's ring is of much greater benefit in establishing scleral support at the trabeculectomy site (Fig. 37-4). The ring is positioned on the surface of the globe after dissecton of the conjunctiva-Tenon's flap and lamellar scleral flap. It should be placed eccentrically, centered over the trabeculectomy site. Three 6-0 silk interrupted sutures are used to secure the ring to the episcleral surface—two within the area of conjunctival dissection posterior to the trabeculectomy site, and a third at the corneoscleral limbus directly opposite the surgical site. The ring is removed after closure of the scleral flap.

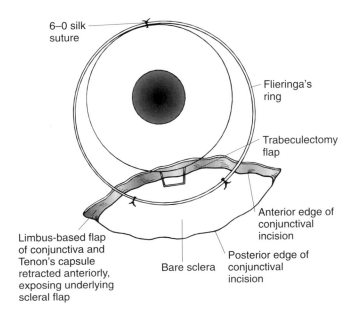

6–0 silk suture

Flieringa's ring

Trabeculectomy flap

Anterior edge of conjunctival incision

Posterior edge of conjunctival incision

Bare sclera

Limbus-based flap of conjunctiva and Tenon's capsule retracted anteriorly, exposing underlying scleral flap

FIGURE 37-4. *Positioning of Flieringa's ring during trabeculectomy. The ring is decentered superiorly to surround the area of scleral dissection. Adequate room is left for placement of the scleral flap sutures.*

Vitreous loss is more frequent in pediatric than in adult trabeculectomy. This may be related to the tendency toward scleral collapse as well as the attenuation of the zonule and anterior hyaloid face in buphthalmic eyes. In very large eyes, stabilization of the globe with a Flieringa's ring may help to minimize the occurrence of this complication. Maintenance of the anterior chamber with continuous infusion of balanced salt solution or a viscoelastic substance (especially in pseudophakic or aphakic eyes) will also help to minimize anterior-segment collapse and anterior-vitreous prolapse.

Prolapse of vitreous through the trabeculectomy fistula, if not grossly evident, may be identified by application of a cellulose sponge to the ocular surface overlying the fistula. This maneuver should be performed routinely prior to closure of the trabeculectomy flap. A limited anterior vitrectomy is necessary if vitreous loss is identified. Disruption of the anterior hyaloid face with herniation of vitreous through the trabeculectomy ostium must be distinguished from presentation of an intact anterior hyaloid face at the inner aspect of the ostium, as may occur in association with scleral collapse or posterior placement of the fistula. If the anterior hyaloid face is intact and the trabeculectomy fistula properly positioned, vitrectomy should be avoided. The vitreous face will move posteriorly when the eye is repressurized and the globe re-formed.

Following vitreous loss, a limited anterior vitrectomy with a cellulose sponge and sharp scissors is generally the safest approach. This may be quite effective at clearing the fistula and allowing the remainder of the vitreous gel to fall posteriorly after the scleral flap is closed and the globe is repressurized. Passing instruments into the eye under these circumstances risks damage to the crystalline lens, zonule, and ciliary processes and should generally be avoided. In pseudophakic eyes, mechanical vitrectomy can be performed through the trabeculectomy site. Continuous infusion of balanced salt solution through a separate corneal paracentesis is recommended. Simultaneous infusion and vitrectomy through the same site is inefficient, as continuous hydration of the vitreous at the site of prolapse results in further prolapse, necessitating a longer and more extensive vitrectomy. Although several of the modern anterior vitrectomy hand pieces combine an infusion sleeve with the vitreous cutting and aspiration apparatus, removal of the infusion sleeve and use of a separate infusion port is advised. Vitrectomy with intermittent manual infusion should be avoided, given the predisposition of these eyes to scleral collapse and further anterior vitreous prolapse.

In aphakic eyes, planned anterior vitrectomy at the time of trabeculectomy is generally best performed through two small corneal incisions, one for the vitreous cutter and the other for the infusion cannula, prior to performing the internal scleral section. This prevents deformation of the globe and the continued anterior movement of vitreous associated with scleral collapse.

Glaucoma Drainage Devices

Selection of Implant

Size/Surface Area   The use of glaucoma drainage devices in young patients with various types of complicated, nonneovascular glaucoma has resulted in intraocular pressure control in 26% to 86% of patients (103–111). Comparison of the results from different studies is difficult because of the small patient numbers, variable follow-up periods, varied glaucoma diagnoses, and use of different devices. Several studies prospectively evaluated the effect of scleral explant size on surgical outcome. Their results suggest better intraocular pressure control with larger-surface-area devices (6,107,108). The facility of aqueous filtration and the resultant steady-state intraocular pressure appear to be proportional to the bleb surface area and its permeability to passive flow. Children, in particular, with their tendency toward exuberant fibrovascular proliferation and thick bleb capsule formation, are likely to attain lower postoperative intraocular pressures with larger-surface-area devices. The "surface area" of a glaucoma drainage device in this context refers to the two-dimensional scleral contact area of the drainage plate. The plate acts as a scaffold for fibrovascular proliferation, thereby determining the size or internal surface area of the resultant bleb capsule.

Earlier studies using the single-plate Molteno implant in the treatment of childhood glaucomas demonstrated a frequent requirement for additional plates to achieve adequate intraocular pressure control. Hill et al (105) reported final intraocular pressures between 6 and 21 mm Hg in 40 (62%) of 65 patients younger than 25 years, at a mean follow-up time of 22.7 months after single-plate Molteno implantation. However, in only 22 (34%) patients the pressure was controlled with the initial single-plate implant. In the other 18 patients, the pressure was controlled after installation of one additional Molteno plate or more, thereby increasing the effective surface area for aqueous drainage. Sixteen patients failed to achieve intraocular pressure control despite the use of additional plates. Minckler et al (110) described a 54% rate of intraocular pressure control in 13 patients younger than 13 years with a variety of complicated glaucomas, at a mean follow-up time of 22.8 months. Lloyd et al (111) analyzed a series of 16 patients under 13 years old with childhood glaucomas, updating the results of the previous study. Life-table analysis revealed intraocular pressures between 5 and 21 mm Hg in 56% of the patients at 4 years after placement of a single-plate Molteno implant. Inclusion of data from patients who underwent installation of a second single-plate Molteno implant after failure of the first plate to adequately control the intraocular pressure resulted in an increase in the 4-year life-table success rate to 69%. Nesher et al (106) evaluated the results of single- and double-plate Molteno implantation in 27 eyes of 20 children, ranging from 2 months to 13 years old. Final intraocular pressures at 21 mm Hg or lower were attained in 16 (59%) of the eyes at an average follow-up time of 20 months. The mean post-operative intraocular pressure for all patients at 1 year was 19 mm Hg.

A significant number of patients in the above-cited studies required antiglaucoma medications to maintain adequate control of intraocular pressure following glaucoma drainage implant insertion. Adjunctive medical therapy, usually with a topical β-blocker, a systemic carbonic anhydrase inhibitor, or both, was required in 58% to 73% of successfully controlled patients following Molteno implantation (105,106,110,111).

The use of devices with a larger surface area for aqueous drainage, such as the double-plate Molteno (Optomat Supplies, Dunedin, New Zealand; 270mm^2) and the Baerveldt Glaucoma Implant (Pharmacia/Iovision, Irvine, CA; currently available in 250-, 350-, and 425-mm^2 sizes), may result in an improved surgical outcome. Several small series using such devices demonstrated a higher incidence of intraocular pressure control or a decreased requirement for postoperative antiglaucoma medications when compared with earlier studies using single-plate Molteno implants (135 mm^2). Netland and Walton (103) reported on 20 eyes of 13 patients younger than 10 years with a variety of complicated glaucomas treated with either the single-plate Molteno implant or the 350-mm^2 Baerveldt Glaucoma Implant. After an average of 32 months of follow-up, a final intraocular pressure of 21 mm Hg or lower (mean = 19 mm Hg) was maintained in 10 (77%) of 13 eyes with the single-plate Molteno implant. Six (86%) of the 7 eyes that had a Baerveldt implant placed demonstrated a mean intraocular pressure of 15 mm Hg, although the mean follow-up period for this group was substantially shorter (11 months). Postoperative antiglaucoma medications were required in 12 (92%) patients in the Molteno group versus 3 (43%) patients in the Baerveldt group. Fellenbaum et al (104) described a series of 30 patients (30 eyes) under 21 years old with complicated glaucomas who underwent installation of the Baerveldt Glaucoma Implant (200, 350, or 500 mm^2). Life-table success rates at 6 and 12 months were 93% and 86%, respectively. Nine (36%) of the 25 patients with intraocular pressure control required one or more antiglaucoma medications at final follow-up. The mean intraocular pressure at final follow-up for patients with the pressure controlled was 13.5 mm Hg.

Use of drainage devices with large-surface-area scleral explants (i.e., double-plate Molteno, or Baerveldt implants) appears to afford the greatest likelihood of achieving long-term intraocular pressure control with a minimum requirement for postoperative medications. These devices are preferred in children in whom normal ciliary body function is anticipated postoperatively and in whom insertion of a large scleral explant is technically feasible.

Valved Versus Nonvalved Devices   Currently, two drainage devices are designed to provide restriction to aqueous flow in the early postoperative period prior to fibrous encapsulation of the scleral plate—the Ahmed Glaucoma Valve (New World Medical, Rancho Cucamonga, CA) and the

Krupin Eye Disk (HOOD Laboratories, Pembroke, MA). Both clinical and in vitro studies showed that the "valves" in these devices perform more like flow restrictors than true valves (112–115). Their ability to maintain the intraocular pressure within strictly defined limits is inconsistent. Both excessively high intraocular pressures (as might occur with a nonvalved, ligatured tube) and hypotony (as might result from an incompletely ligatured, nonvalved tube) occur in a significant proportion of eyes containing either of these devices (113–115).

Hypotony can be difficult to manage, and may lead to significant complications such as serous or hemorrhagic choroidal detachment, flat anterior chamber, and cataract formation, particularly in eyes with recalcitrant glaucoma that have undergone multiple prior intraocular surgeries and may have had very high preoperative intraocular pressures. Management of hypotony is problematic especially in young children in whom activity restriction and avoidance of the Valsalva maneuver are difficult to control. Frequent office examinations can be difficult without undue manipulation of a soft globe, and multiple examinations under general anesthesia may be necessary. Interventions such as anterior-chamber re-formation with air or a viscoelastic substance are generally not possible in an office setting.

High pressures secondary to valve obstruction or malfunction can be equally problematic. Manipulations such as the application of digital pressure to the globe and the anterior-chamber injection of balanced salt solution (116), and use of tissue plasminogen activator (117,118) usually require general anesthesia in young children. Unidirectional valve mechanisms are also limited by their inability to prevent episodic hypotony associated with mechanical compression of the globe or a sudden Valsalva maneuver (i.e., during extubation, emesis, or vigorous crying). This is a significant theoretical disadvantage of valved drainage devices, especially in eyes at high risk for suprachoroidal hemorrhage and other postoperative complications.

The above-mentioned concerns regarding the use of drainage devices with flow-restriction modifications must be assessed in the context of their potential functional advantage. Their primary benefit is the ability to provide immediate reduction in intraocular pressure. Moreover, there is no need for temporary tube ligatures or stents. This reduces the operating time and eliminates the need for a second operation to release a ligature or remove a stent should this become necessary prior to spontaneous release. However, fibrous encapsulation of the scleral plate occurs as early as 1 week postoperatively. Once this has occurred, it is the capsule that provides resistance to aqueous outflow and determines the steady-state intraocular pressure. The valve mechanism no longer serves any useful purpose, but it does remain a potential source of complications. Obstruction from particulate debris, fibrin, blood, or fibrous tissue is more likely to occur at the valve site and lead to malfunction. Additionally, the currently available valved devices contain relatively small-surface-area scleral plates. To the extent that a large surface area for aqueous drainage is beneficial in maintaining intraocular pressure control, this is a further disadvantage of these devices. In a patient with very high preoperative intraocular pressure in whom immediate pressure reduction is desired, consideration should be given to using a ligatured, nonvalved drainage device and performing a concurrent "bridge" trabeculectomy (without antimetabolite). The trabeculectomy will provide intraocular pressure control during the period between surgery and tube ligature release.

There are several situations in which a valved tube may, at least in theory, provide some long-term benefit. These include conditions in which aqueous hyposecretion is anticipated for an abnormally long postoperative interval, as with chronic and recurrent uveitis and ocular ischemia. The intraocular pressure in such conditions may be limited by poor aqueous production rather than excessive bleb capsule size or permeability. A second situation in which valved devices may provide some prolonged advantage involves the adjunctive use of antimetabolic agents, such as mitomycin C, with drainage implantation. This can result in a significant and unpredictable delay in scleral plate encapsulation. Spontaneous or planned release of the tube ligature might, therefore, occur prior to adequate fibrous capsule formation and result in hypotony and related complications with a nonvalved tube. The use of a valved tube to restrict aqueous flow independent of the bleb capsule is recommended in this setting.

Surgical Technique

Selection of Surgical Site

The quadrant of the globe where the drainage device is to be implanted is determined by several factors. Conjunctival scarring, scleral thinning, the presence of other scleral explants (i.e., scleral buckle, prior glaucoma drainage implant), the specific device being used, and the presence of silicone oil may affect the choice of a quadrant for scleral explant fixation. In general, it is best to avoid the superonasal quadrant because of the presence of the obliquus superior muscle and the relatively high incidence of strabismus following drainage implant insertion in this location (119–121). Consideration must also be given to the proximity of the optic nerve to the nasal side of the globe (especially in children with small eyes) when working with devices that extend well past the equator of the globe. The anteroposterior dimension of the Baerveldt 250-, 350-, and 425-mm² implants, the Molteno implants, and the Krupin disk is 13 mm, while that of the Ahmed Glaucoma Valve is 16 mm. The anterior aspect of the Ahmed implant should be placed no more than 8 mm posterior to the limbus when operating on the nasal side of the globe.

Orbital access is generally optimal in the superotemporal quadrant, especially in young children with underdeveloped orbits. This is the preferred quadrant for drainage device implantation. If excessive conjunctival scarring the presence of a prior drainage implant, or intravitreal silicone oil precludes the use of the superotemporal quadrant, the inferonasal or inferotemporal quadrant should be utilized. The inferonasal quadrant is preferable when using implants that are large in both the circumferential and the anteroposterior dimension such as the Baerveldt Glaucoma Implant. The scleral plate may be placed further posteriorly in this quadrant, as compared with the inferotemporal quadrant, without limitation by the obliquus inferior muscle as it approaches its point of scleral insertion.

Scleral Explant Insertion Care should be taken to avoid incorporation of the obliquus superior tendon during insertion of the Baerveldt Glaucoma Implant in the superotemporal quadrant. This can lead to postoperative motility dysfunction of the pseudo-Brown's variety. After plate placement and prior to suture fixation, the scleral plate should be grasped with forceps and advanced anteriorly under direct visualization. Difficulty advancing the plate to a position immediately behind the rectus superior insertion generally indicates placement of the nasal wing of the implant over the obliquus superior tendon. The plate should be removed and reinserted beneath both the rectus superior and obliquus superior muscles after isolation of the rectus superior with two muscle hooks.

If an implant must be placed over a preexisting scleral buckle, the Baerveldt implant provides a distinct advantage over the other available devices because of its low profile (0.9-mm thickness) and flexibility. The scleral plate may be placed over the encircling element and beneath the adjacent rectus muscles, and sutured directly to the silicone tire. Extensive scar tissue sometimes prevents adequate isolation of the rectus muscles overlying a wide scleral buckling element. In this situation, the wings of the Baerveldt implant can be trimmed so that the scleral plate fits entirely between the two adjacent rectus muscles. The plate is then sutured to the encircling band. Before the plate is secured, the fibrous capsule surrounding the encircling band is excised. This permits encapsulation of the encircling band and drainage plate as a unit, possibly augmenting the effective surface area for aqueous outflow.

If a large solid silicone encircling element is present, consideration should also be given to implanting a silicone tube alone to shunt aqueous from the anterior or posterior chamber to the fibrous capsule surrounding the previously placed band (122). This obviates the need to install another piece of hardware as well as the need for a temporary tube ligature, since a mature fibrous capsule already surrounds the scleral band.

Scleral Explant Fixation The scleral explant of any drainage device should be secured to the surface of the globe with nonabsorbable suture material. This is to counter any tendency for the plate to migrate anteriorly or posteriorly as a result of fibrous tissue contraction during the later stages of wound healing. Eye rubbing in young children may increase the likelihood of scleral plate displacement. We prefer to use an 8-0 nylon suture for this purpose.

The sclera is relatively thin in the vicinity of scleral explant fixation just posterior to the rectus muscle insertions. In young children, particularly those with abnormally high axial lengths, the sclera is even more thin and elastic compared with that in adults, and is therefore more prone to perforation during suture placement. Perforation of the sclera and choroid at this anteroposterior location may result in a retinal hole with or without some degree of vitreous hemorrhage. Transscleral cryoretinopexy should be performed over the perforation site immediately, after any prolapsed vitreous is excised with sharp scissors. The perforation site should be visualized by indirect ophthalmoscopy at the time of cryopexy if media clarity permits. Following suture fixation, the anterior edge of the plate should be grasped with forceps and moved side to side to ensure adequate fixation.

Several precautions during explant fixation will help to minimize the incidence of this complication, especially when exposure of the surgical site is poor. Scleral sutures can be preplaced, prior to explant insertion. When one is suturing after explant insertion, it is generally safest to pass the sutures in two steps. A scleral bite is taken first. The needle is then retrieved and the needle holder rearmed. A second pass is then made through the fixation hole of the scleral plate. Alternatively, the scleral pass can be made parallel, rather than perpendicular, to the limbus. If excessively thin sclera is encountered in any location, the scleral plate can be anchored to the adjacent rectus muscle tendons. Finally, use of a relatively small-caliber needle, such as that provided with an 8-0 nylon suture, is preferable. The larger needle of sutures such as 5-0 Mersilene can be difficult to control and offer no advantage in terms of explant fixation.

Tube Ligature Techniques Single-stage implantation of nonvalved drainage devices should always be accompanied by complete occlusion of the tube lumen using one of a variety of suture ligature techniques (123–130). These techniques are the same as those employed during drainage implant surgery in adults. In older children who are particularly cooperative, a releasable stent can be used (127–130). This can be removed in the office at the slit lamp as early as 1 to 2 weeks postoperatively if the intraocular pressure is unacceptably high. In younger children, a releasable stent might also be considered, as ligature removal will then necessitate only ketamine or face-mask anesthesia, and a small conjunctiva-Tenon's incision well away from the tube and drainage plate. A single, absorbable suture (8-0 or 7-0 polyglactin) positioned between the patch graft and the scleral plate is sufficient in younger children, although planned release will entail a somewhat more involved procedure. A subconjunctival releasable stent should generally be removed at some point (even if early, planned ligature release is not required for intraocular pressure control), as erosion of the relatively large-caliber suture through the overlying conjunctiva occasionally occurs. Externalized releasable stents also require removal.

Normal aqueous humor production is desirable following ligature release, and ciliary body function can be significantly reduced for a prolonged period after the discontinuation of medications such as topical β-blockers. However, medical therapy is usually instituted to moderate postoperative intraocular pressure elevations until the tube opens. More rapidly reversible agents such as topical α₂-agonists or systemic or topical carbonic anhydrase inhibitors may be preferable if medical control of intraocular pressure is necessary during the interval between surgery and ligature release. After the first postoperative week, ligature release rather than medical therapy should be considered if the intraocular pressure is unacceptably high.

Scleral Fistulization and Tube Insertion Insertion of a tube into the anterior chamber through a limbal sclera fistula can result in several long-term complications. Anterior migration or rotation of an initially well-positioned tube can ultimately lead to corneal endothelial contact and corneal decompensation. Progressive thinning of the overlying limbal sclera can lead to erosion of the tube through the conjunctiva and tube exposure. These complications are more common in young children because of the relative elasticity and thinness of the sclera compared with adults. These general properties of young sclera are compounded in the buphthalmic eye in which further stretching and thinning of the sclera with loss of rigidity have taken place. Silicone tubing, although flexible, has an inherent tendency to straighten over time. The abrupt, artificial bend created in the tube at its point of entry into the eye produces an anterior vector force due to the "memory" within the silicone material and the tendency of the tube to assume its original straight configuration. This results in forward rotation of the anterior portion of the tube around its point of angulation at the scleral fistula. Normal adult sclera is generally able to resist this tendency toward anterior tube migration.

Several technical considerations should help to minimize the incidence of complications related to limbal tube insertion. The scleral fistula should be made as posterior as possible without contacting the anterior surface of the iris. Generally, a point approximately 0.5 to 1.0 mm posterior to the blue line in either superior quadrant results in good tube positioning. A 23-gauge needle should be used to create a tight fit and minimize aqueous leak around the tube. Additionally, the orientation of the needle (and, therefore, the resulting fistula) should be parallel to the iris plane or angled slightly posteriorly (Fig. 37-5). Although the external scleral entry point may be adequately posterior, if the fistula is angled anteriorly, the proximal tube tip may lie too close to the posterior corneal surface. This is especially true in young children in whom the tube should be left slightly long to allow for subsequent growth of the eye.

In pseudophakic eyes, the tube may be positioned further posteriorly, given the increased anterior-chamber depth and the lack of concern about contact with the intraocular lens. Insertion directly over an existing iridectomy just anterior

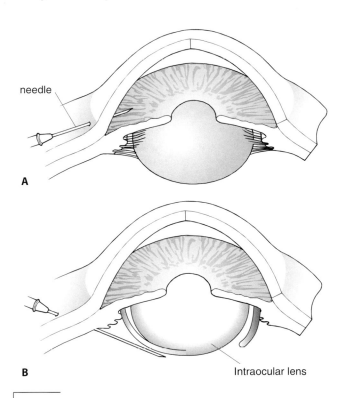

needle

A

B   Intraocular lens

FIGURE 37-5. *Needle orientation during scleral fistulization. A. Limbal fistula. B. Pars plana fistula. Note that the needle is directed slightly posterior to the iris plane for pars plana fistulization.*

to the front surface of the intraocular lens allows for even more posterior placement of the tube, while eliminating the possibility of iris-tube block. If the iris has been drawn anteriorly by corneal adhesions, resulting in diffuse or focal obliteration of the anterior-chamber angle, the tube is best positioned between the iris and the lens implant. In a phakic eye, the meridian of a preexisting iridectomy should be avoided, as scleral fistulization and tube insertion in this location risk damage to the crystalline lens. Nonradial insertion, which places the tube in the "gutter" of the anterior chamber, may be preferable. In this position, tube-cornea touch will cause peripheral corneal damage rather than central, vision-threatening decompensation. However, tube-cornea touch may be more likely because of the closer proximity between the tube and cornea in the peripheral anterior chamber. Contact between the tube and the lens is also more predictably avoided as the tube overlies the periphery of the iris, even with the pupil in the dilated position.

Pars plana tube insertion is advantageous because it minimizes complications related to the anterior portion of the tube (131–133). There are, however, two prerequisites for pars plana insertion. First, a complete pars plana vitrectomy with attention to the vitreous base must be performed either concurrent with or prior to the drainage implant procedure. Second, the eye must be aphakic or pseudophakic. There is a significant risk of cataract formation and lens damage or intumescence following pars plana tube insertion in a phakic eye (122).

The desire to place the tube through a pars plana scleral fistula is generally not a sufficient indication for performing a vitrectomy, which adds considerable time, expense, and potential morbidity from intraoperative and postoperative complications to the surgical procedure. If another indication exists, such as aphakia with anterior vitreous prolapse, pars plana vitrectomy and tube insertion should be considered. Owing to the complicated nature of these cases and the need for careful dissection of the vitreous base, the vitrectomy should be performed by an experienced vitreoretinal surgeon. The posterior infusion cannula should be left in place until scleral fistulization and tube placement are completed, to protect against collapse of the globe and development of choroidal separation during tube insertion.

Scleral fistulization for pars plana tube insertion should be performed approximately 3.0 to 3.5 mm posterior to the corneoscleral limbus in a normal-sized globe. This distance should be decreased to 2.0 to 2.5 mm in microphthalmic eyes. As with limbal insertion, a 23-gauge sharp disposable needle should be used to minimize the chance of aqueous leak around the tube. The needle should be radially oriented relative to the visual axis and angled slightly posteriorly with respect to the iris plane (see Fig. 37-5). Insertion perpendicular to the scleral surface, as recommended by some authors (133), should be avoided, as this can result in kinking of the tube with luminal obstruction due to the sharp angle at the scleral entry site. Prior to insertion, the tube should be trimmed with a bevel facing posteriorly. This will prevent obstruction of the proximal opening should the tube tip migrate anteriorly and contact the posterior surface of the iris, lens capsule, or intraocular lens.

In contrast to limbal tube insertion, pupillary dilatation is helpful when working through the pars plana. The tube should be left long enough so that it can be visualized through the dilated pupil. Visualization of the tube through the pupil in the operating room is critical. The pliability of the silicone tube can result in misdirection into the suprachoroidal space or beneath the vitreous base as it is passed through the scleral fistula. Depending on the length of the tube within the eye, the pupillary diameter, the media clarity, and the direction of insertion, scleral indentation over the fistula may be necessary to bring the proximal tip into view. If the tube is not visualized, it should be removed and reinserted through the same track after repeat fistulization with the 23-gauge needle. Failure to visualize the tube after two or more such attempts may necessitate abandoning the initial site and attempting fistulization and tube insertion at a new location. Closure of the original fistula with an 8-0 polyglactin (Vicryl) suture may be necessary if there is excessive fluid leak. Insertion of the tube through the sclerotomy used for the pars plana vitrectomy should be avoided because of the large size of this opening relative to the external diameter of the tube and the likelihood of substantial fluid leak around the tube postoperatively.

Pars plana tube insertion is contraindicated in phakic eyes, owing to the risk of damage to the crystalline lens. In eyes in which intravitreal silicone oil has been used to repair a complicated retinal detachment, and those in which the use of silicone oil is anticipated, the drainage tube should be inserted through a limbal scleral fistula in either inferior quadrant of the globe. Tube placement in this location minimizes the chance of silicone oil drainage through the tube.

Several factors must be considered in determining the optimal intraocular tube length. In general, extension of the tube 2 mm past the site of conjunctival insertion when laid over the ocular surface in the meridian in which it will be inserted will result in optimal positioning within the anterior chamber. The tube should be placed as far posteriorly as possible without contacting the iris or crystalline lens. In young children, in whom further growth of the eye is expected, an additional 1 to 2 mm of intraocular tube length should be provided. Retraction of the tube into the anterior-chamber angle or out of the eye may result if the tube is trimmed too short at the time of initial implantation.

Aphakic and vitrectomized eyes, as in adults, are particularly problematic owing to the immediate and often profound softening and scleral collapse that occur following scleral fistulization. The tube will always extend farther into the globe in its hypotonus state than it does when the globe is fully expanded at a physiologic pressure. Thus, the appearance of the tube in the anterior chamber immediately after insertion can be misleading as a guide to its appropriate length. Retraction of the tube can occur postoperatively when the eye is repressurized. The surgeon should estimate the tube length prior to scleral fistulization, and verify the tube position and length only after re-forming the globe and normalizing the intraocular pressure with balanced salt solution.

A viscoelastic substance can be used to stabilize the anterior chamber during tube insertion. However, complete removal at the conclusion of the case is difficult. Also, care must be taken not to artificially overdeepen the anterior chamber, as this can result in placement of the tube too far posteriorly with iridial contact postoperatively when the anterior chamber returns to its normal depth. Continuous infusion of balanced salt solution via a self-retaining anterior-chamber maintainer inserted through a corneal paracentesis is another option for stabilizing the globe during scleral fistulization and tube placement. This is particularly useful in aphakic, vitrectomized eyes.

If the most appropriate tube length or scleral fistula location is unclear, it is advisable to leave additional tubing on the scleral surface. This can be done by routing the tube between the scleral plate and the scleral fistula over a sinuous course (Fig. 37-6). Multiple vertical mattress sutures of 8-0 polyglactin should be used to anchor the tubing to the epi-

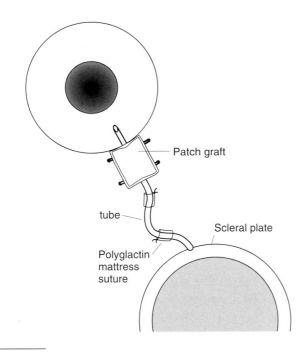

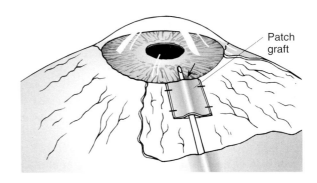

FIGURE 37-7. *Proper positioning of the patch graft with its anterior edge (arrow) at the level of the original conjunctival insertion. The edge of the conjunctival flap will be positioned anterior to the graft during final wound closure.*

FIGURE 37-6. *Excess tubing secured to the episcleral surface following scleral fistulization and tube insertion. The excess can be utilized if repositioning of the tube becomes necessary.*

scleral surface when its course deviates from the straight radial path. If retraction of the tube from the anterior or posterior chamber occurs postoperatively (or if revision is required for any other reason), the episcleral portion of the tube can be straightened, providing increased length and permitting appropriate repositioning and insertion through a new scleral fistula.

Patch Graft Use of a patch graft to cover the anterior portion of the tube and scleral fistula is preferable to placing the tube beneath a lamellar host scleral flap. A free graft provides greater reinforcement of the already thin, pliable limbal tissue, where the majority of tube-related complications occur. As in adults, a variety of materials can be used. Glycerin- or ethyl alcohol–preserved donor sclera (134) can be obtained from a local eye bank on a per case basis. Recently, dehydrated cadaveric dura mater (135), fascia lata (136), and pericardium (Tutoplast Processed Pericardium, Biodynamics International, U.S., Tampa, FL) were used with excellent results. The thinness and uniformity of these latter materials make them easier to work with than sclera, and their long shelf-life permits the convenience of storage in the operating room. Moreover, the risk of microbial contamination with these materials is less than that with sclera as they are sterilized by solvent dehydration and γ-irradiation—processes that kill or inactivate all microorganisms, including the human immunodeficiency virus. Additionally, the unit cost of fascia lata, dura mater, and

pericardium may be significantly less than that of sclera (136). Limited clinical data show good host compatibility in humans, without any graft-induced inflammation, rejection, melting, tube erosion, or infection (135,136).

Proper positioning of the graft is important in preventing long-term complications related to tube erosion through the overlying sclera and conjunctiva. The graft should be placed with its anterior edge at the site of conjunctival insertion, overlying the far periphery of the cornea and covering the angled portion of the tube and the scleral fistula (Fig. 37-7). Conjunctiva and Tenon's capsule are then secured to the peripheral clear cornea anterior to the front edge of the graft during final wound closure. The anterior edge of the graft should be as thin as possible with a posterior bevel to reduce the risk of dellen formation postoperatively. The thinnest area of the piece of donor sclera (usually in the vicinity of the rectus muscle insertions) should be used. Thicker portions of donor sclera may need to be manually thinned prior to placement on the eye. All grafting materials may be secured to the episclera with 7-0 or 8-0 polyglactin or 10-0 nylon sutures, one at each of its four corners. An additional modified mattress suture securing the anterior edge of the graft to the underlying limbus may be useful in cases in which conjunctival scarring might cause conjunctival retraction postoperatively. Absorbable sutures are preferred, as the graft tissue becomes fixed in place with fibrovascular scar tissue rather quickly and sutures are not needed for an extended period.

Conjunctival Closure Meticulous technique and attention to several procedural details during closure of the conjunctiva-Tenon's flap will help to limit the occurrence of certain postoperative complications and facilitate reoperation, should this become necessary. During the first stage of a two-stage installation, preservation of both the conjunctiva and Tenon's capsule and good reapproximation of both tissue layers at the limbus allows for easier tissue dissection and better wound closure during the second-stage surgery. The nonsurgical management of wound-related complications is particularly difficult in young children. Therefore, it is better to spend some additional time to ensure a tight and secure wound at the time of the initial surgery.

Retraction of the anterior edge of a fornix-based conjunctival flap in the early postoperative period occurs more commonly in children than adults, particularly after surgery in the inferior quadrants. This is generally limited in extent and results in baring of the anterior portion of the scleral graft (Fig. 37-8). Greater exposure of the inferior limbus as compared to the superior limbus, owing to the normal position of the corresponding eyelid, combined with the increased tendency of children to rub the recently operated eye probably account for the frequency of this complication. Therefore, care should be taken to position the scleral

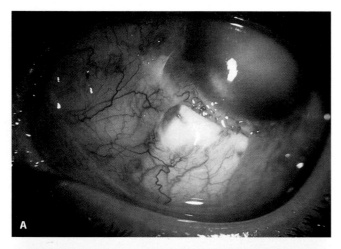

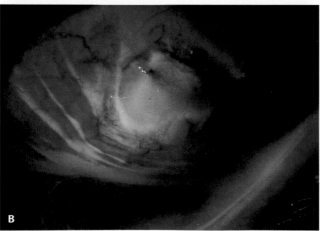

FIGURE 37-8.   *Retraction of a fornix-based conjunctival flap 2 weeks postoperatively in a 7-year-old child. The drainage device and scleral patch graft were placed in the inferonasal quadrant. A. The anterior edge of the scleral patch graft is exposed. B. The same patient after the application of fluorescein dye to highlight the conjunctival defect. Conservative treatment with antibiotic ointment resulted in stabilization with complete epithelialization over a 2-week period.*

graft anterior to the tube insertion site and the anterior edge of the conjunctiva well anterior to the scleral graft. The conjunctiva should be stretched tightly against the cornea anterior to the graft; indentation of the conjunctiva and cornea at this location is a desirable visual end point. For inferiorly placed implants, or when tight conjunctival-corneal apposition is not achieved with anchoring sutures at the anterior corners of the conjunctival flap, one or more horizontal mattress sutures of 8-0 polyglactin or 10-0 nylon should be placed to anchor the conjunctiva to the cornea anterior to the scleral graft. The use of eyeglasses or a protective shield for several weeks postoperatively may also help to prevent inadvertent manipulation of the eye, thereby minimizing the occurrence of conjunctival retraction.

Management of conjunctival retraction depends on its extent, stability, and the structures exposed. Frequently administered topical lubricants (drops, ointments), reduction in the use of topical steroids, and avoidance of repeated trauma to the ocular surface are generally effective in stabilizing the retraction and allowing epithelialization of the exposed graft and episcleral surfaces. Excessive retraction, particularly with exposure of the silicone tube, may require resuturing.

The prior or concurrent placement of a large silicone tire for repair of a retinal detachment may also increase the difficulty of conjunctival closure following drainage implantation. Undue tension on the anterior wound edge in such situations increases the likelihood of wound dehiscence and retraction. When possible, the use of deep 7-0 or 8-0 polyglactin sutures to advance and secure Tenon's capsule to the perilimbal sclera or surface of the patch graft will prevent excessive tension on the overlying conjunctiva. This helps to prevent wound dehiscence, limbal retraction, and epithelial ingrowth (137).

In general, a limbus-based conjunctival flap should be closed in two separate layers to ensure a stable, watertight closure. This is essential for valved devices and desirable for nonvalved, ligatured tubes in case early ligature release becomes necessary or inadvertent leak around or through the tube occurs in the early postoperative period. A careful, two-layer closure is particularly important when working with conjunctiva that is thin, scarred, or under excessive tension. If insufficient anterior Tenon's capsule is present, the posterior flap of Tenon's capsule can be sutured directly to the episcleral surface and patch graft using a running or multiple interrupted suture of 7-0 or 8-0 polyglactin.

A fornix-based flap is best secured with deep episcleral mattress sutures through conjunctiva and Tenon's capsule at the two anterior corners of the flap. The edge of conjunctiva should be carefully positioned anterior to the scleral graft. Running extensions of the anchoring sutures are then used to close the radial relaxing incisions. When a valved drainage device is used, care should be taken to ensure that the conjunctival closure is watertight. A two-layer closure of the radial relaxing incisions using 8-0 or 9-0 polyglactin suture, preferably with a vascular needle, generally provides excellent wound integrity. A single-layer closure, incorporating both conjunctiva and Tenon's capsule, can also be used. In areas of excessively thin conjunctiva, deep suture passes through episclera can anchor and stabilize the conjunctiva and promote more rapid wound healing.

Corneal Paracentesis Closure Postoperative aqueous leak through a corneal paracentesis incision is common in young children. This is probably due to the low rigidity of the external ocular tissues in children under 3 to 4 years old. This tendency is probably further exacerbated by stretching and thinning of the cornea and sclera in the buphthalmic eye. Routine placement of a single interrupted 10-0 nylon or 10-0 polyglactin corneal suture will ensure stability of the paracentesis incision in the early postoperative period and eliminate a potential source of aqueous leak and hypotony. An absorbable suture material such as polyglactin is preferred as this will eliminate the long-term occurrence of exposed or broken corneal sutures. An exposed nylon suture represents a nidus for infection and may cause significant ocular discomfort and inflammation. It should be removed promptly, using sedation or general anesthesia as necessary.

Adjunctive Antimetabolite Use The degree of intraocular pressure reduction achieved with a glaucoma drainage device is determined, in large part, by the thickness and permeability of the fibrous capsule surrounding the scleral plate. Antifibrotic agents can be used to modify the wound-healing response and potentially alter the thickness and hydraulic conductivity of the bleb capsule. Most surgeons have abandoned the postoperative systemic antifibrosis regimen of Molteno (138,139), consisting of prednisone, colchicine, and flufenamic acid, because of a lack of demonstrated efficacy and the potential for systemic toxicity. More recently, consideration has been given to the application of topical mitomycin C to the episclera and overlying Tenon's capsule and conjunctiva immediately prior to drainage plate installation (140). Local inhibition of fibroblast proliferation might lead to attenuation of the bleb capsule with an attendant decrease in resistance to aqueous flow. Improved intraocular pressure control or less need for postoperative antiglaucoma medications might result. This may be particularly advantageous in young children, given their inherent tendency to exuberant scar tissue formation. Decreased capsular resistance may allow better pressure control with smaller-surface-area implants.

The magnitude and duration of the effect of mitomycin C remain to be substantiated by long-term clinical trials. However, short-term complications related to the use of potent antiproliferative agents must be anticipated and the surgical technique appropriately modified. Prolonged ocular hypotony and its attendant complications (serous or hemorrhagic choroidal detachment, flat anterior chamber, cataract, and maculopathy), conjunctival leak or wound dehiscence, tube erosion, plate extrusion, and endophthalmitis might all result with increased frequency due to attenuation of the bleb capsule and overlying Tenon's capsule and conjunctiva in the presence of a large synthetic explant.

Early tube ligature release should be avoided following the application of mitomycin C. The use of drainage devices with flow-restriction modifications should also be considered, as the time to the development of adequate capsular resistance to prevent hypotony may be unpredictable and may extend beyond the point of spontaneous polyglactin ligature release. A smaller scleral plate might help to minimize the occurrence of ocular hypotony following antimetabolite application (140). A fornix-based conjunctival flap should be used to place the incision as far from the scleral plate and site of mitomycin C application as possible. This should help to prevent wound dehiscence and implant extrusion.

Complications

During or following implantation of a glaucoma drainage device, children are susceptible to any of the numerous complications that occur in adults. There are, however, several postoperative complications that occur with greater frequency in children.

Severe, persistent, anterior uveitis has been found in as many as 13% to 34% of children following drainage device implantation (103–105). In adults, the incidence of this complication has varied between 2% and 6% (108,111, 141–143). The inflammatory reaction is sometimes accompanied by the formation of fibrin in the anterior chamber or white precipitates on the outer surface of the tube, and generally responds to topical corticosteroids. Rarely, the inflammatory reaction is recalcitrant to prolonged, aggressive medical therapy, and removal of the tube is necessary.

The etiology of this pathologic inflammatory response is unclear. It may represent a response to the silicone tube, the episcleral plate, or surface contaminants on these materials. Damage or mechanical trauma to the iris, ciliary body, or cornea, incarceration of intraocular tissues in the tube ostium, and recurrent intraocular bleeding are not evident. Successful implantation of a second drainage implant following removal of the first because of persistent, severe inflammation has been accomplished without recurrence of a similar inflammatory response.

Dystrophic calcification of the outer surface of a silicone rubber drainage tube is a rare occurrence; it developed in two children following Molteno implantation (Fig. 37-9) (144). Youth and the presence of the implant for many years were implicated as risk factors for the occurrence of calcification in these children. The small, white, calcific plaques can mimic inflammatory deposits, although the anterior chamber will be quiet.

Despite a relative paucity of clinical data, the risk of retinal detachment following glaucoma drainage implantation in young children appears to be significantly higher

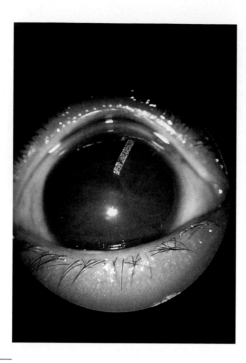

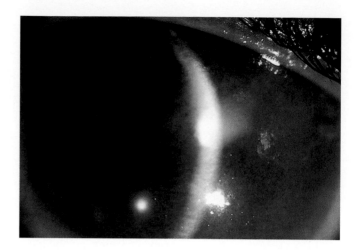

FIGURE 37-10. *Corneal stromal thickening and opacification secondary to endothelial compromise due to tube-cornea touch in a 9-year-old child.*

FIGURE 37-9. *Calcific deposits on the external surface of the anterior-chamber portion of a Molteno tube in a 7-year-old child. The Molteno implant was initially placed at age 11 months. A segment of the tube was removed at the time of surgical revision because of uncontrolled intraocular pressure. There was no evidence of intraocular inflammation. Energy dispersive spectroscopy confirmed the presence of calcium and phosphorus in the plaques. (Courtesy of Paul S. Fellenbaum, MD.)*

than the risk in adults. The incidence of retinal detachment in several large series of adult patients after drainage implant surgery has varied between 0% and 8% (107,108,145,146). Hill et al (105) identified this complication in 11 (16%) of 70 patients younger than 21 years following Molteno implantation for nonneovascular glaucoma. Waterhouse et al (147) reviewed 350 consecutive patients who underwent Molteno implant surgery and identified 16 patients who developed subsequent rhegmatogenous retinal detachment, for an incidence of 5%. Although the ages of each patient who developed a retinal detachment are not given, a higher incidence of this complication among younger patients is suggested by the demographic information presented. The median age of the 16 patients with retinal detachment was 9 years. Moreover, the most common glaucoma diagnoses were infantile glaucoma (4 patients) and pediatric glaucoma after congenital cataract surgery (4 patients). One additional patient had glaucoma associated with Peter's anomaly.

The reasons for a higher incidence of retinal detachment among children following drainage tube implantation are not entirely clear. In the series of Waterhouse et al (147), retinal detachment was not directly related to the Molteno surgery in some patients. Most patients in this study had undergone multiple surgical procedures (median = 3) prior to the development of retinal detachment. It is likely, therefore, that surgical manipulation other than Molteno implantation played some role in the pathogenesis of the retinal detachments. The presence of firm vitreoretinal adhesions in children may predispose them to retinal tear formation following posterior vitreous detachment after surgery.

Early identification of a retinal detachment is crucial, given the rapid development of proliferative vitreoretinopathy in young children who have undergone multiple surgeries. Clinical signs of retinal detachment, such as an unexplained increase in anterior-chamber reaction or a reduction in intraocular pressure, must be carefully assessed at each postoperative visit, especially within the first 4 to 6 months after surgery. Reliance on a subjective or objective decrease in visual acuity should be avoided. Young children may be incapable of reporting such a change or may not notice a difference in vision owing to poor baseline visual function. This is especially true if the visual function in the fellow eye is normal. Dilated fundus examination should be performed frequently.

As discussed previously, tube-related complications occur with greater frequency in young children as compared with adults. These include forward migration of the anterior-chamber portion of the tube with corneal endothelial contact and decompensation (Fig. 37-10), transscleral or transcorneal erosion of the anterior portion of the tube, and retraction of the tube out of the anterior chamber. The incidence of tube-cornea touch ranged from 13% to 20% in several series of children following drainage implantation (103–105). This is significantly higher than the 0% to 2% incidence reported in multiple series of adult patients (108,113,141). The thinness and greater elasticity of the sclera and peripheral cornea in young children (especially those with enlarged globes) compared with adults likely contribute to this difference. Retraction of the proximal tube tip from the anterior chamber is a rare complication in adult patients (107). This was noted in 1 (4%) of 23 children in the series of Netland and Walton (103) and 3 (4%) of 70 patients in the series of Hill et al (105).

POSTOPERATIVE MANAGEMENT

Trabeculectomy

The postoperative medical regimen in children following trabeculectomy is similar to that used in adults, with several modifications to enhance compliance and practicality. A postoperative subconjunctival injection of an antibiotic and a steroid is generally recommended. A cephalosporin such as cefazolin (25–50 mg) may provide better gram-positive coverage as a single agent than an aminoglycoside provides. Dexamethasone or prednisolone should be used as the corticosteroid. In children between the ages of 2 and 5 years, who may present particular difficulty with postoperative eyedrop administration, consideration should be given to administering a sub-Tenon's injection of a longer-acting steroid preparation, such as triamcinolone acetonide (20–40 mg). This should be injected deep in the inferior conjunctival fornix through a 25-gauge needle. The use of oil-based depot steroids should be avoided, as this may make certain postoperative complications requiring the discontinuation of steroids more difficult to manage.

A topical antibiotic and corticosteroid should be started on the first postoperative day. Consideration may be given to the use of ointments for children in whom eyedrop administration is particularly difficult. Use of a combination antibiotic-corticosteroid preparation such as tobramycin-dexamethasone may also facilitate medication administration. Topical antibiotics should be continued for the first 2 to 3 postoperative weeks, and corticosteroids for 1 to 3 months, in tapering doses depending on the degree of conjunctival and intraocular inflammation. Trimethoprim sulfate–polymyxin B sulfate or the fluoroquinolone agents (ciprofloxacin, norfloxacin) provide excellent, broad-spectrum coverage and are not irritating to the ocular surface. However, these antibiotics are not available in combination with a topical steroid. Prednisolone acetate 1% or prednisolone sodium phosphate 1%, given initially every 1 to 2 hours while awake, provides good anti-inflammatory coverage. Fluorometholone acetate 0.1% and rimexolone acetate 1% are also potent steroids with good corneal penetration. Their main advantage of extending the time interval to the development of a steroid-induced intraocular pressure elevation is not particularly advantageous following filtering surgery. A topical cycloplegic agent such as atropine sulfate 1% or scopolamine hydrobromide 0.25% should also be used for the first 4 weeks post-

operatively and sometimes longer, depending on the clinical situation.

In cooperative children, laser suture lysis should be performed, as in adults, based on the intraocular pressure, bleb appearance, response to digital ocular massage, and time interval from surgery (148). The time between surgery and suture lysis may be significantly shorter in children because of the more rapid and extensive wound healing in comparison with adults. Releasable scleral flap sutures may require removal within the first 1 to 2 weeks after surgery. This is particularly true in very young children in whom the sutures have been tied tightly to restrict aqueous flow in the early postoperative period.

Drainage Implants

The postoperative medical management of glaucoma drainage devices is similar to that of trabeculectomy. The major difference lies in the decreased need for topical steroids, as fibroblast proliferation and encapsulation of the drainage plate are desirable prior to initiation of aqueous flow through the system. A subconjunctival injection of an antibiotic and corticosteroid is generally given at the conclusion of the operative procedure, as described already. Injections should not be given in the quadrant into which the drainage device has been installed.

Postoperative treatment with a topical antibiotic and corticosteroid is begun on the first postoperative day. Initially, each eyedrop or ointment can be given four times per day. A combination antibiotic-steroid preparation may be used exclusively, at a dosing interval of every 4 to 6 hours. Following spontaneous or planned ligature release an increase in intraocular inflammation generally occurs. Increasing the frequency of topical steroid administration to every 1 to 2 hours for 1 to 2 weeks is recommended at this point. The topical antibiotic should be continued for 2 to 3 weeks. The topical steroid should be tapered gradually over 6 to 12 weeks, depending on the degree of inflammation. A topical cycloplegic agent such as atropine sulfate 1% or scopolamine hydrobromide 0.25% should also be used for the first 4 weeks postoperatively.

The use of antibiotic, corticosteroid, and cycloplegic ointments is an acceptable alternative to eyedrops in very young children who may cooperate poorly with eyedrop administration. The use of aqueous suppressant medications may be required for the management of elevated intraocular pressure during the first 1 to 2 weeks after installation of a nonvalved drainage device with an occlusive tube ligature. It is advisable to avoid the use of aqueous suppressants, if possible, in order to minimize the occurrence or duration of hypotony following spontaneous or planned ligature release. Ligature release, rather than medical therapy, should be considered after the second postoperative week for intraocular pressure elevations beyond a tolerable level for the degree of optic nerve head damage.

SPECIAL CONSIDERATIONS

Alterations in the normal ocular anatomy and physiology specific to several conditions associated with congenital or developmental glaucoma necessitate special precautions and procedural modifications during trabeculectomy or glaucoma drainage implantation.

Sturge-Weber Syndrome

Elevated episcleral venous pressure associated with orbital and ocular hemangiomas in the Sturge-Weber syndrome predisposes to choroidal and suprachoroidal effusion intraoperatively and during the early postoperative period. This is most common in children with a diffuse choroidal hemangioma. In such patients, prophylactic posterior sclerotomies in one or both inferior quadrants are recommended, prior to entering the anterior chamber during trabeculectomy. The sclerotomies should be radially oriented, approximately 3 mm in length, centered 5 to 8 mm posterior to the limbus, and performed through small, radial incisions in the conjunctiva and Tenon's capsule. These are left open to drain any suprachoroidal fluid that may accumulate during or after the procedure. A Kelly Descemet's membrane punch or Gass sclerotomy punch may be used to excise a small piece of sclera from one side of the incision, thereby enlarging the opening and facilitating fluid outflow. Alternatively, cautery may be applied to the edges of the scleral incision to gape the sclerotomy. At the conclusion of the case, the conjunctiva and Tenon's capsule can be closed in a single layer using a running 9-0 polyglactin suture on a vascular needle.

Choroidal effusion may be more likely in the presence of Sturge-Weber syndrome, with sudden and severe decompression of the globe. Therefore, if the preoperative intraocular pressure is extremely high (i.e., ≥40 mm Hg), efforts should be made to medically lower the intraocular pressure prior to incising the eye. During trabeculectomy, rapid closure of the scleral flap and repressurization of the globe will also limit the occurrence and extent of choroidal effusion. Preplacement of two scleral flap sutures prior to performing the internal block excision will help to expedite flap closure.

Maintaining a relatively high intraocular pressure and, certainly, avoiding hypotony in the early postoperative period will also help to limit the development of choroidal effusion and its sequelae, such as shallow or flat anterior chamber. Tight flap closure with postoperative laser suture lysis is the optimal approach in older, cooperative children. When this is not possible, consideration should be given to the use of one or more 10-0 polyglactin flap sutures, which will allow for tight flap closure early and enhanced aqueous outflow following spontaneous dissolution. Releasable flap sutures of 10-0 nylon provide another means of achieving tight flap closure in the early postoperative period in very young children. General anesthesia may be required in the first 1 to 2 postoperative weeks to allow suture removal.

Drainage implant surgery should also be approached with the intention of maintaining a relatively high intraocular pressure in the early postoperative period. Valved devices should be avoided because of their unpredictability and the frequency of early postoperative pressures in the subphysiologic range. Use of a nonvalved device with an occlusive ligature or a two-stage insertion is the safest approach. The use of aqueous suppressants prior to ligature release should be minimized. Consideration should be given to planned ligature release in a setting where augmentation of the anterior-chamber volume using balanced salt solution or a viscoelastic substance is possible should transient hypotony occur.

Aniridia

The complete or partial absence of the iris in this condition makes trabeculectomy or tube insertion technically more difficult, especially in phakic eyes. Care must be exercised to avoid damage to the lens and zonule intraoperatively, and to avoid postoperative shallowing of the anterior chamber. Damage to the corneal endothelium is more likely with incomplete degrees of chamber shallowing, owing to the absence of the protective cushion normally afforded by the iris.

During trabeculectomy, it is advisable to fill the anterior chamber with viscoelastic substance prior to performing the internal block excision. After the scleral flap is partially secured, residual viscoelastic substance can be irrigated from the anterior chamber. Unless there is complete absence of iridial tissue in the meridian of the trabeculectomy fistula, an iridectomy should be performed to prevent postoperative occlusion of the ostium by the rudimentary iris stump. Relatively tight scleral flap closure is desirable in the early postoperative period to avoid hypotony and anterior-chamber flattening.

Scleral fistulization for drainage tube implantation is also most safely performed after anterior-chamber injection of a viscoelastic agent. Care should be taken to avoid overdeepening the anterior chamber as this will make estimation of proper tube positioning difficult and may result in tube-lens contact postoperatively. The use of a nonvalved drainage device with an occlusive ligature or a two-stage insertion to minimize the occurrence of postoperative hypotony is advised.

Peter's Anomaly

The extent of anterior-segment malformation in patients with Peter's anomaly must be considered in determining the optimal surgical procedure. In the presence of a relatively deep anterior chamber with no corneolenticular adhesion, trabeculectomy or drainage tube insertion may be performed with limited technical difficulty, despite the presence of a central corneal opacity. Extreme shallowing or flattening of the anterior chamber, especially in the presence of a corneolenticular adhesion, usually necessitates more extensive anterior-segment reconstruction if the glaucoma surgery is to be effective.

Penetrating keratoplasty, lensectomy, and often pars plana or anterior vitrectomy are generally required to decompress the anterior chamber sufficiently to allow drainage tube insertion or trabeculectomy. Without a more extensive anterior reconstruction, persistent anterior-segment shallowing with anterior movement of the lens, iris, and vitreous is likely to result in obstruction of a trabeculectomy fistula with eventual surgical failure. Excessive anterior-chamber crowding would also preclude limbal insertion of a drainage tube. Anterior-chamber deepening following lens extraction provides space for limbal tube placement. If complete pars plana vitrectomy is performed concurrently, the tube should be inserted through a pars plana scleral fistula, thereby minimizing the chance of anterior-segment complications.

Retinopathy of Prematurity

The management of chronic angle-closure glaucoma secondary to retinopathy of prematurity varies depending on the prior surgical history and the extent of anterior-segment abnormality. In patients who have undergone prior vitrectomy and scleral buckling surgery, conjunctival scarring may limit the technical feasibility of trabeculectomy.

In the presence of a scleral buckle, installation of a glaucoma drainage implant may be complicated by extensive scar tissue formation around the encircling element and the anterior aspect of the rectus muscles. The scleral plate must be positioned over the encircling band or tire. The low profile (i.e., 0.9-mm thickness) of the Baerveldt Glaucoma Implant is advantageous in such patients. The implant may be sutured directly to the silicone encircling band if necessary to allow proper anteroposterior positioning. Alternatively, in patients who have undergone prior scleral buckling surgery with a large encircling element, a silicone tube can be used to shunt aqueous from the anterior or posterior chamber to the fibrous capsule surrounding the scleral explant (122).

In patients who previously underwent surgical repair of a complicated retinal detachment, the possible need for further vitreoretinal surgery should be anticipated. Placement of a glaucoma drainage device in one of the inferior quadrants and insertion of the tube through a scleral fistula at the level of the limbus rather than the pars plana will obviate the need for repositioning should intravitreal silicone oil be required in the future.

REFERENCES

1. Skuta GL, Parrish RK. Wound healing in glaucoma filtering surgery. *Surv Ophthalmol* 1987;32:149–170.
2. Addicks EM, Quigley JA, Green WR, Robin AL. Histologic characteristics of filtering blebs in glaucomatous eyes. *Arch Ophthalmol* 1983;101:795–798.
3. Jampel HD, McGuigan LJB, Dunkelberger GR, et al. Cellular proliferation after experimental glaucoma filtration surgery. *Arch Ophthalmol* 1988;106:89–94.
4. Joseph JP, Miller MH, Hitchings RA. Wound healing as a barrier to successful filtration surgery. *Eye* 1988;2(suppl):S113–S123.
5. Desjardins DC, Parrish RK II, Folberg R, et al. Wound healing after filtering surgery in owl monkeys. *Arch Ophthalmol* 1986;104:1835–1839.
6. Minckler DS, Shammas A, Wilcox M, Ogden TE. Experimental studies of aqueous filtration using the Molteno implant. *Trans Am Ophthalmol Soc* 1987;85:368–389.
7. Wilcox MJ, Minckler DS, Ogden TE. Pathophysiology of artificial aqueous drainage in primate eyes with Molteno implants. *J Glaucoma* 1994;3:140–151.
8. Holm-Pedersen P, Zederfeldt B. Strength development of skin incisions in young and old rats. *Scand J Plast Reconstr Surg* 1971;5:7–12.
9. Holm-Pedersen P, Nilsson K, Branemark PI. The microvascular system of healing wounds in young and old rats. *Adv Microcirc* 1973;5:80–106.
10. Sussman MD. Aging of connective tissue: physical properties of healing wounds in young and old rats. *Am J Physiol* 1973;224:1167–1171.
11. Uitto J. A method for studying collagen biosynthesis in human skin biopsies in vitro. *Biochim Biophys Acta* 1970;201:438–445.
12. Gressel MG, Heuer DK, Parrish RK II. Trabeculectomy in young patients. *Ophthalmology* 1984;91:1242–1246.
13. Mills KB. Trabeculectomy: a retrospective long-term follow-up of 444 cases. *Br J Ophthalmol* 1981;65:790–795.
14. Jerndal T, Lundstrom M. 330 trabeculectomies—a follow-up study through 1/2–3 years. *Acta Ophthalmol Scand* 1977;55:52–62.
15. Wilson P. Trabeculectomy: long-term follow-up. *Br J Ophthalmol* 1977;61:535–538.
16. Ridgway AEA. Trabeculectomy. A follow-up study. *Br J Ophthalmol* 1974;58:680–686.
17. Inaba Z. Long-term results of trabeculectomy in the Japanese: an analysis by life-table method. *Jpn J Ophthalmol* 1982;26:361–373.
18. Susanna R, Oltrogge EW, Carani JCE, Nicolela MT. Mitomycin as adjunct chemotherapy with trabeculectomy in congenital and developmental glaucomas. *J Glaucoma* 1995;4:151–157.
19. Miller MH, Rice NSC. Trabeculectomy combined with β-irridiation for congenital glaucoma. *Br J Ophthalmol* 1991;75:584–590.
20. Smith RM. Mortality in pediatric surgery and anesthesia. In: Smith RM, ed. *Anesthesia for infants and children.* 4th ed. St. Louis: Mosby, 1980:653–661.
21. Tiret L, Mivoche Y, Hatton F, et al. Complications related to anesthesia in infants and children: a prospective survey of 40240 anesthetics. *Br J Anaesth* 1988;61:263–269.
22. SaintMaurice C. Paediatric anesthesia. *Curr Opin Anaesth* 1994;7:249–250.
23. Zwaan J. Simultaneous surgery for bilateral pediatric cataracts. *Ophthalmic Surg Lasers* 1996;27:15–20.
24. Phelan MJ, Higginbotham EJ. Contact transscleral Nd:YAG cyclophotocoagulation for the treatment of refractory pediatric glaucoma. *Ophthalmic Surg Lasers* 1995;26:401–403.
25. Bechrakis NE, Muller-Stolzenburg NW, Helbig H, Foerster MH. Sympathetic ophthalmia following laser cyclocoagulation. *Arch Ophthalmol* 1994;112:80–84.
26. Lam S, Tessler HH, Lam BL, Wilensky JT. High incidence of sympathetic ophthalmia after contact and noncontact neodymium:YAG cyclotherapy. *Ophthalmology* 1992;99:1818–1822.
27. Pastor SA, Iwach A, Nozik RA, et al. Presumed sympathetic ophthalmia following Nd:YAG transscleral cyclophotocoagulation. *J Glaucoma* 1993;2:30–31.
28. Sidoti PA, Lopez PF, Michon J, Heuer DK. Delayed-onset pneumococcal endophthalmitis after mitomycin-C trabeculectomy: association with cryptic nasolacrimal obstruction. *J Glaucoma* 1995;4:11–15.
29. Greenfield DS, Suner IJ, Miller MP, et al. Endophthalmitis after filtering surgery with mitomycin. *Arch Ophthalmol* 1996;114:943–949.
30. Shields MB, Scroggs MW, Sloop CM, Simmons RB. Clinical and histopathologic observations concerning hypotony after trabeculectomy with adjunctive mitomycin C. *Am J Ophthalmol* 1993;116:673–683.
31. Zacharia PT, Deppermann SR, Schuman JS. Ocular hypotony after trabeculectomy with mitomycin C. *Am J Ophthalmol* 1993;116:314–326.
32. Yo C, Sidoti PA, Morinelli E, Heuer DK. Trabeculectomy with mitomycin-C in pediatric patients. *Invest Ophthalmol Vis Sci* 1995;36(suppl):87.
33. Mockovak ME, Erzurum SA, Goldenfeld M, et al. Trabeculectomy with intraoperative mitomycin-C in pediatric patients. *Invest Ophthalmol Vis Sci* 1995;36(suppl):87.

34. Hutchinson AK, Grossniklaus HE, Brown RH, et al. Clinicopathologic features of excised mitomycin filtering blebs. *Arch Ophthalmol* 1994;112: 74–79.

35. Nuyts RMMA, Felten PC, Pels E, et al. Histopathologic effects of mitomycin C after trabeculectomy in human glaucomatous eyes with persistent hypotony. *Am J Ophthalmol* 1994;118:225–237.

36. Beauchamp GR, Parks MM. Filtering surgery in children: barriers to success. *Ophthalmology* 1979;86:170–180.

37. Burke JP, Bowell R. Primary trabeculectomy in congenital glaucoma. *Br J Ophthalmol* 1989;73:186–190.

38. Fulcher T, Chan J, Lanigan B, et al. Long term follow up of primary trabeculectomy for infantile glaucoma. *Br J Ophthalmol* 1996;80:499–502.

39. Debnath SC, Teichmann KD, Salamah K. Trabeculectomy versus trabeculotomy in congenital glaucoma. *Br J Ophthalmol* 1989;73:608–611.

40. Cadera W, Pachtman MA, Cantor LB, et al. Filtering surgery in childhood glaucoma. *Ophthalmic Surg* 1984;15:319–322.

41. Sturmer J, Broadway DC, Hitchings RA. Young patient trabeculectomy. *Ophthalmology* 1993;100:928–939.

42. Costa VP, Katz LJ, Spaeth GL, et al. Primary trabeculectomy in young adults. *Ophthalmology* 1993;100:1071–1076.

43. Heuer DK, Gressel MG, Parrish RK II, et al. Trabeculectomy in aphakic eyes. *Ophthalmology* 1984;91:1045–1051.

44. Heuer DK, Parrish RK II, Gressel MG, et al. 5-Fluorouracil and glaucoma filtering surgery. II. A pilot study. *Ophthalmology* 1984;91:384–394.

45. Heuer DK, Parrish RK II, Gressel MG, et al. 5-Fluorouracil and glaucoma filtering surgry. III. Intermediate follow-up of a pilot study. *Ophthalmology* 1986;93:1537–1546.

46. Rockwood EJ, Parrish RK II, Heuer DK, et al. Glaucoma filtering surgery with 5-fluorouracil. *Ophthalmology* 1987;94:1071–1078.

47. Fluorouracil Filtering Surgery Study Group. Three-year follow-up of the Fluorouracil Filtering Surgery Study. *Am J Ophthalmol* 1993;115:82–92.

48. Liebmann JM, Ritch R, Marmor M, et al. Initial 5-fluorouracil trabeculectomy in uncomplicated glaucoma. *Ophthalmology* 1991;98:1036–1041.

49. Chen CW. Enhanced intraocular pressure controlling effectiveness of trabeculectomy by local application of mitomycin-C. *Trans Asia Pacific Acad Ophthalmol* 1983;9:172–177.

50. Chen CW, Huang HT, Bair JS, Lee CC. Trabeculectomy with simultaneous topical application of mitomycin-C in refractory glaucoma. *J Ocul Pharmacol* 1990;6:175–182.

51. Palmer SS. Mitomycin as adjunct chemotherapy with trabeculectomy. *Ophthalmology* 1991;98:317–321.

52. Kupin TH, Juzych MS, Shin DH, et al. Adjunctive mitomycin C in primary trabeculectomy in phakic eyes. *Am J Ophthalmol* 1995;119:30–39.

53. Mermoud A, Salmon JF, Murray ADN. Trabeculectomy with mitomycin C for refractory glaucoma in blacks. *Am J Ophthalmol* 1993;116:72–78.

54. Khaw PT, Sherwood MB, MacKay SLD, et al. Five-minute treatments with fluorouracil, floxuridine, and mitomycin have long-term effects on human Tenon's capsule fibroblasts. *Arch Ophthalmol* 1992;110:1150–1154.

55. Jampel HD. Effect of brief exposure to mitomycin C on viability and proliferation of cultured human Tenon's capsule fibroblasts. *Ophthalmology* 1992;99:1471–1476.

56. Khaw PT, Doyle JW, Sherwood MB, et al. Prolonged localized tissue effects from 5-minute exposures to fluorouracil and mitomycin-C. *Arch Ophthalmol* 1993;111:263–267.

57. Yaldo MK, Stamper RL. Long-term effects of mitomycin on filtering blebs: lack of fibrovascular proliferative response following severe inflammation. *Arch Ophthalmol* 1993;111:824–826.

58. Madhavan HN, Rao SB, Vijaya L, Neelakantan A. In vitro sensitivity of human Tenon's capsule fibroblasts to mitomycin C and its correlation with outcome of glaucoma filtration surgery. *Ophthalmic Surg* 1995;26:61–67.

59. Wolner B, Liebmann JM, Sassani JW, et al. Late bleb-related endophthalmitis after trabeculectomy with adjunctive 5-fluorouracil. *Ophthalmology* 1991;98:1053–1060.

60. Ticho U, Ophir A. Late complications after glaucoma filtering surgery with adjunctive 5-fluorouracil. *Am J Ophthalmol* 1993;115:506–510.

61. Whiteside-Michel J, Liebmann JM, Ritch R. Initial 5-fluorouracil trabeculectomy in young patients. *Ophthalmology* 1992;99:7–13.

62. Zalish M, Leiba H, Oliver M. Subconjunctival injections of 5-fluorouracil following trabeculectomy for congenital and infantile glaucoma. *Ophthalmic Surg* 1992;23:203–205.

63. Herschler J. Commentary. In: Zalish M, Leiva H, Oliver M. Subconjunctival injection of 5-fluorouracil following trabeculectomy for congenital and infantile glaucoma. *Ophthalmic Surg* 1992;23:203–205.

64. Dietze PJ, Feldman RM, Gross RL. Intraoperative application of 5-fluorouracil during trabeculectomy. *Ophthalmic Surg* 1992;23:662–665.

65. Smith MF, Sherwood MB, Doyle JW, Khaw PT. Results of intraoperative 5-fluorouracil supplementation on trabeculectomy for open-angle glaucoma. *Am J Ophthalmol* 1992;114:737–741.

66. Egbert PR, Williams AS, Singh K, et al. A prospective trial of intraoperative fluorouracil during trabeculectomy in a black population. *Am J Ophthalmol* 1993;116:612–616.

67. Feldman RM, Dietze PJ, Gross RL, Oram O. Intraoperative 5-fluorouracil administration in trabeculectomy. *J Glaucoma* 1994;3:302–307.

68. Skuta GL, Beeson CC, Higginbotham EJ, et al. Intraoperative mitomycin versus postoperative 5-fluorouracil in high-risk glaucoma filtering surgery. *Ophthalmology* 1992;99:438–444.

69. Prata JA, Minckler DS, Baerveldt G, et al. Trabeculectomy in pseudophakic patients: postoperative 5-fluorouracil versus intraoperative mitomycin C antiproliferative therapy. *Ophthalmic Surg* 1995;26:73–77.

70. Lamping KA, Belkin JK. 5-Fluorouracil and mitomycin C in pseudophakic patients. *Ophthalmology* 1995;102:70–75.

71. Kitazawa Y, Kawase K, Matsushita H, Minobe M. Trabeculectomy with mitomycin: a comparative study with fluorouracil. *Arch Ophthalmol* 1991;109:1693–1698.

72. Khaw PT, Doyle JW, Sherwood MB, et al. Effects of intraoperative 5-fluorouracil or mitomycin C on glaucoma filtration surgery in the rabbit. *Ophthalmology* 1993;100:367–372.

73. Katz GJ, Higginbotham EJ, Lichter PR, et al. Mitomycin C versus 5-fluorouracil in high-risk glaucoma filtering surgery. *Ophthalmology* 1995;102:1263–1269.

74. Kushner BJ. Congenital nasolacrimal system obstruction. *Arch Ophthalmol* 1982;100:597–600.

75. Wolner B, Liebmann JM, Sassani JW, et al. Late bleb-related endophthalmitis after trabeculectomy with adjunctive 5-fluorouracil. *Ophthalmology* 1991;98:1053–1060.

76. Higginbotham EJ, Stevens RK, Musch DC, et al. Bleb-related endophthalmitis after trabeculectomy with mitomycin C. *Ophthalmology* 1996;103:650–656.

77. Caronia RM, Liebmann JM, Friedman R, et al. Trabeculectomy at the inferior limbus. *Arch Ophthalmol* 1996;114:387–391.

78. Fourman S. Scleritis after glaucoma filtering surgery with mitomycin-C. *Ophthalmology* 1995;102:1569–1571.

79. Shuster JN, Krupin T, Kolker AE, Becker B. Limbus- v fornix-based conjunctival flap in trabeculectomy. A long-term randomized study. *Arch Ophthalmol* 1984;102:361–362.

80. Murchison JF, Shields MB. Limbal-based vs fornix-based conjunctival flaps in combined extracapsular cataract surgery and glaucoma filtering procedure. *Am J Ophthalmol* 1990;109:709–715.

81. Tahery MM, Lee DA. Review: pharmacologic control of wound healing in glaucoma filtration surgery. *J Ocul Pharmacol* 1989;5:155–179.

82. Blok MDW, Kok JHC, van Mil C, et al. Use of the megasoft bandage lens for treatment of complications after trabeculectomy. *Am J Ophthalmol* 1990;110:264–268.

83. Fourman S, Wiley L. Use of a collagen shield to treat a glaucoma filter bleb leak. *Am J Ophthalmol* 1989;107:673–674. Letter.

84. Grady FJ, Forbes M. Tissue adhesive for repair of conjunctival buttonhole in glaucoma surgery. *Am J Ophthalmol* 1969;68:656–658.

85. Awan KJ, Spaeth PG. Use of isobutyl-2-cyanoacrylate tissue adhesive in the repair of conjunctival fistula in filtering procedures for glaucoma. *Ann Ophthalmol* 1974;6:851–853.

86. Hill RA, Aminlari A, Sassani JW, Michalski M. Use of a symblepharon ring for treatment of over-filtration and leaking blebs after glaucoma filtration surgery. *Ophthalmic Surg* 1990;21:707–710.

87. Ruderman JM, Allen RC. Simmons' tamponade shell for leaking filtration blebs. *Arch Ophthalmol* 1985;103:1708–1710.

88. Melamed S, Hersh P, Kersten D, et al. The use of glaucoma shell tamponade in leaking filtration blebs. *Ophthalmology* 1986;93:839–842.

89. Riley SF, Smith TJ, Simmons RJ. Repair of a disinserted scleral flap in trabeculectomy. *Ophthalmic Surg* 1993;24:349–350.

90. Brown SVL. Management of a partial-thickness scleral-flap buttonhole during trabeculectomy. *Ophthalmic Surg* 1994;25:732–733.

91. Derick RJ, Pasquale L, Quigley HA, Jampel H. Potential toxicity of mitomycin C. *Arch Ophthalmol* 1991;109:1635. Letter.

92. Seah SKL, Prata JA Jr, Minckler DS, et al. Mitomycin-C concentration in human aqueous humor following trabeculectomy. *Eye* 1993;7:652–655.

93. Prata JA Jr, Minckler DS, Koda RT. Effects of external irrigation on mitomycin-C concentration in rabbit aqueous and vitreous humor. *J Glaucoma* 1995;4:32–35.

94. Gandolfi SA, Vecchi M, Braccio L. Decrease of intraocular pressure after subconjunctival injection of mitomycin in human glaucoma. *Arch Ophthalmol* 1995;113:582–585.

95. Kee C, Pelzek CD, Kaufman PL. Mitomycin C suppresses aqueous humor flow in cynomolgus monkeys. *Arch Ophthalmol* 1995;113:239–242.

96. Stamper RL, McMenemy MF, Lieberman MF. Hypotonous maculopathy after trabeculectomy with subconjunctival 5-fluorouracil. *Am J Ophthalmol* 1992;114:544–553.

97. Beck AD, Lynch MG, Noe R, et al. The use of a new laser lens holder for performing suture lysis in children. *Arch Ophthalmol* 1995;113:140–141.

98. Shin DH. Removable-suture closure of the lamellar scleral flap in trabeculectomy. *Ann Ophthalmol* 1987;19:51–55.

99. Cohen JS, Osher RH. Releasable scleral flap suture. *Ophthalmol Clin North Am* 1988;1:187–197.

100. Kolker AE, Kass MA, Rait JL. Trabeculectomy with releasable sutures. *Arch Ophthalmol* 1994;112:62–66.

101. Wise JB. Mitomycin-compatible suture technique for fornix-based conjunctival flaps in glaucoma filtration surgery. *Arch Ophthalmol* 1993;111:992–997.

102. Miller KN, Blasini M, Shields MB, Ho CH. A comparison of total and partial tenonectomy with trabeculectomy. *Am J Ophthalmol* 1991;111:323–326.

103. Netland PA, Walton DS. Glaucoma drainage implants in pediatric patients. *Ophthalmic Surg* 1993;24:723–729.

104. Fellenbaum PS, Sidoti PA, Heuer DK, et al. Experience with the Baerveldt implant in young patients with complicated glaucomas. *J Glaucoma* 1995;4:91–97.

105. Hill RA, Heuer DK, Baerveldt G, et al. Molteno implantation for glaucoma in young patients. *Ophthalmology* 1991;98:1042–1046.

106. Nesher R, Sherwood MB, Kass MA, et al. Molteno implants in children. *J Glaucoma* 1992;1:228–232.

107. Lloyd MA, Baerveldt G, Fellenbaum PS, et al. Intermediate-term results of a randomized clinical trial of the 350- versus the 500-mm² Baerveldt implant. *Ophthalmology* 1994;101:1456–1564.

108. Heuer DK, Lloyd MA, Abrams D, et al. Which is better? One or two? A randomized clinical trial of single-plate versus double-plate Molteno implantation for glaucomas in aphakia and pseudophakia. *Ophthalmology* 1992;99:1512–1519.

109. Siegner SW, Netland PA, Urban RC Jr, et al. Clinical experience with the Baerveldt glaucoma drainage implant. *Ophthalmology* 1995;102:1298–1307.

110. Minckler DS, Heuer DK, Hasty B, et al. Clinical experience with the single-plate Molteno implant in complicated glaucomas. *Ophthalmology* 1988;95:1181–1188.

111. Lloyd MA, Sedlak T, Heuer DK, et al. Clinical experience with the single-plate Molteno implant in complicated glaucomas. Update of a pilot study. *Ophthalmology* 1992;99:679–687.

112. Prata JA Jr, Mermoud A, LaBree L, Minckler DS. In vitro and in vivo flow characteristics of glaucoma drainage implants. *Ophthalmology* 1995;102:894–904.

113. The Krupin Eye Valve Filtering Surgery Study Group. Krupin eye valve with disk for filtration surgery. *Ophthalmology* 1994;101:651–658.

114. Fellenbaum PS, Almeida AR, Minckler DS, et al. Krupin disk implantation for complicated glaucomas. *Ophthalmology* 1994;101:1178–1182.

115. Coleman AL, Hill R, Wilson MR, et al. Initial clinical experience with the Ahmed Glaucoma Valve implant. *Am J Ophthalmol* 1995;120:23–31.

116. Krawitz PL. Treatment of distal occlusion of Krupin eye valve with disk using cannular flush. *Ophthalmic Surg* 1994;25:102–104.

117. Sidoti PA, Morinelli EN, Heuer DK, et al. Tissue plasminogen activator and glaucoma drainage implants. *J Glaucoma* 1995;4:258–262.

118. Lundy DC, Sidoti P, Winarko T, et al. Intracameral tissue plasminogen activator following glaucoma surgery: indications, effectiveness, and complications. *Ophthalmology* 1996;103:274–282.

119. Ball S, Ellis GS, Herrington RG, Liang K. Brown's superior oblique tendon syndrome after Baerveldt Glaucoma Implant. *Arch Ophthalmol* 1992;110:1368.

120. Smith SL, Starita RJ, Fellman RL, Lynn JR. Early clinical experience with the Baerveldt 350-mm² glaucoma implant and associated extraocular muscle imbalance. *Ophthalmology* 1993;100:914–918.

121. Prata JA, Minckler DS, Green RL. Pseudo-Brown's syndrome as a complication of glaucoma drainage implant surgery. *Ophthalmic Surg* 1993;24:608–611.

122. Sidoti PA, Minckler DS, Baerveldt G, et al. Aqueous tube shunt to a preexisting episcleral encircling element in the treatment of complicated glaucomas. *Ophthalmology* 1994;101:1036–1043.

123. Hoare Nairne JEA, Sherwood D, Jacob JSH, Rich WJCC. Single stage insertion of the Molteno tube for glaucoma and modifications to reduce postoperative hypotony. *Br J Ophthalmol* 1988;72:846–851.

124. Molteno ACB, Polkinghorne PJ, Boebyes JA. The Vicryl tie technique for inserting a draining implant in the treatment of secondary glaucoma. *Aust N Z J Ophthalmol* 1986;14:343–354.

125. Price FW Jr, Whitson WE. Polypropylene ligatures as a means of controlling intraocular pressure with Molteno implants. *Ophthalmic Surg* 1989;20:781–783.

126. Liebmann J, Ritch R. Intraocular suture ligature to reduce hypotony following Molteno seton implantation. *Ophthalmic Surg* 1992;23:51–52.

127. Egbert PR, Lieberman MF. Internal suture occlusion of the Molteno glaucoma implant for the prevention of postoperative hypotony. *Ophthalmic Surg* 1989;20:53–56.

128. Kooner KS, Goode SM. Removable ligature during Molteno implant procedure. *Am J Ophthalmol* 1992;114:102–103.

129. Latina MA. Single stage Molteno implant with combination internal occlusion and external ligature. *Ophthalmic Surg* 1990;21:444–446.

130. Sherwood MB, Smith MF. Prevention of early hypotony associated with Molteno implants by a new occluding stent technique. *Ophthalmology* 1993;100:85–90.

131. Gandham SB, Costa VP, Katz JL, et al. Aqueous tube-shunt implantation and pars plana vitrectomy in eyes with refractory glaucoma. *Am J Ophthalmol* 1993;116:189–195.

132. Sheppard JD, Shrum KR. Pars plana Molteno implantation in complicated inflammatory glaucoma. *Ophthalmic Surg* 1995;26:218–222.

133. Varma R, Heuer DK, Lundy DC, et al. Pars plana Baerveldt tube insertion with vitrectomy in glaucomas associated with pseudophakia and aphakia. *Am J Ophthalmol* 1995;119:401–407.

134. Freedman J. Scleral patch grafts with Molteno setons. *Ophthalmic Surg* 1987;18:532–534.

135. Brandt JD. Patch grafts of dehydrated cadaveric dura mater for tube-shunt glaucoma surgery. *Arch Ophthalmol* 1993;111:1436–1439.

136. Tanji TM, Lundy DC, Minckler DS, et al. Fascia lata patch graft in glaucoma tube surgery. *Ophthalmology* 1996;103:1309–1312.

137. Sidoti PA, Minckler DS, Baerveldt G, et al. Epithelial ingrowth and glaucoma drainage implants. *Ophthalmology* 1994;101:872–875.

138. Molteno ACB, Straughan JL, Ancker E. Control of bleb fibrosis after glaucoma surgery by anti-inflammatory agents. *S Afr Med J* 1976;50:881–885.

139. Molteno ACB. Mechanisms of intraocular inflammation. *Trans Ophthalmol Soc NZ* 1980;32:69–72.

140. Perkins TW, Cardakli UF, Eisele JR, et al. Adjunctive mitomycin-C in Molteno implant surgery. *Ophthalmology* 1995;102:91–97.

141. Wilson RP, Cantor L, Katz JL, et al. Aqueous shunts. Molteno versus Schocket. *Ophthalmology* 1992;99:672–678.

142. Schocket SS, Nirankari VS, Lakhanpal V, et al. Anterior chamber tube shunt to an encircling band in the treatment of neovascular glaucoma and other refractory glaucomas. A long-term study. *Ophthalmology* 1985;92:553–562.

143. Heher KL, Lim JI, Haller JA, Jampel HD. Late-onset sterile endophthalmitis after Molteno tube implantation. *Am J Ophthalmol* 1992;114:771–772. Letter.

144. Fellenbaum PS, Baerveldt G, Minckler DS. Calcification of a Molteno implant. *J Glaucoma* 1994;3:81–83.

145. Fellenbaum PS, Almeida AR, Minckler DS, et al. Krupin disk implantation for complicated glaucomas. *Ophthalmology* 1994;101:1178–1182.

146. Smith MF, Sherwood MB, McGorray SP. Comparison of the double-plate Molteno drainage implant with the Schocket procedure. *Arch Ophthalmol* 1992;110:1246–1250.

147. Waterhouse WJ, Lloyd MAE, Dugel PU, et al. Rhegmatogenous retinal detachment after Molteno glaucoma implant surgery. *Ophthalmology* 1994;101:665–671.

148. Morinelli EN, Sidoti PA, Heuer DK, et al. Laser suture lysis after mitomycin-C trabeculectomy. *Ophthalmology* 1996;103:306–314.

Aqueous Misdirection: Malignant Glaucoma

David K. Dueker

Historically the term *malignant glaucoma* was used to describe extreme shallowing of the anterior chamber with marked pressure elevation in an eye undergoing surgery, usually peripheral iridectomy, for angle-closure glaucoma. And while other causes for the clinical syndrome have been identified (1–4), it is still most commonly seen as a postoperative complication of surgery in an eye with some degree of angle closure, although currently the surgery is more apt to be a filtering operation or cataract extraction. The search for effective treatment of this condition, which is notoriously resistant to traditional glaucoma therapy, has required original thinking and imaginative, unconventional approaches to therapy.

Although still widely known as *malignant glaucoma*, with good reason, several attempts have been made to provide a name that would be more indicative of the pathogenic mechanism. The term *aqueous misdirection* has been incorporated in the title of this chapter because it identifies a key malfunction in this form of glaucoma, which is helpful in guiding therapy. Posterior aqueous misdirection results from blockade to the normal flow pathway of aqueous. Names based on the potential sites of blockage have been suggested, and these remind us appropriately that blockade precedes misdirection, at least initially. But since the potential sites of blockage are multiple, and all result in a similar clinical picture, the term *aqueous misdirection* has a unifying appeal. This does not remove the recognized value of the arresting and time-honored term *malignant glaucoma*, which now has the further advantage of being perhaps the most productive term for modern computer-aided literature searches (5).

The normal flow of aqueous humor proceeds initially from the ciliary processes into the posterior chamber, through the pupil, and into the anterior chamber. Pupillary block glaucoma is an angle-closure glaucoma in which aqueous is secreted normally into the posterior chamber, but is then blocked, relatively or absolutely, from flowing into the anterior chamber. The resulting pressure forces the iris forward over the chamber angle, occluding the normal outflow pathways there. This blockage is relieved by making a full-thickness opening in the iris.

In contrast, aqueous misdirection is an angle-closure glaucoma in which aqueous is abnormally secreted behind the posterior chamber into the vitreous space, where it causes a buildup of volume leading to a generalized forward movement of the anterior hyaloid, lens (or capsule and intraocular lens) if present, and iris. Clinically this may resemble angle closure caused by pupillary block, but it will not be relieved by an iridotomy or iridectomy. Successful treatment must either redirect the aqueous to its normal pathway or provide an alternative pathway for the posteriorly misdirected aqueous humor to reach the anterior chamber.

PREDISPOSING FACTORS

The normal eye (Fig. 38-1) has adequate space between the lens and the ciliary processes so that direct physical contact will not occur, even with the small shifts in lens position produced by accommodation or with the increase in lens size that occurs with normal aging. It is difficult to postulate a mechanism by which lens movement would produce aqueous blockade at the ciliary body in the normally proportioned eye. However, in a smaller eye (Fig. 38-2) the lens may be large relative to the space it occupies, in which case the eye is predisposed to both relative pupillary block as well as to more posterior blockage leading to aqueous misdirection. It is not surprising, then, that relative pupillary

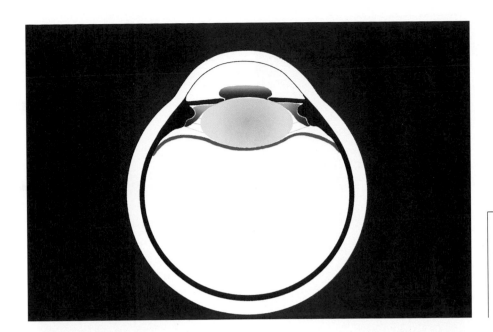

FIGURE 38-1.   *In a normally proportioned eye, small forward movements of the lens, or small inward movements of the ciliary body, such as those produced by accommodation, would still not compromise the normal forward progression of aqueous flow.*

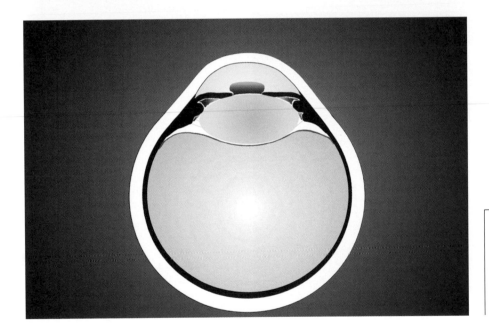

FIGURE 38-2.   *Eyes predisposed to aqueous misdirection tend to be shorter than normal, and therefore hyperopic, with a large lens resting in a relatively cramped anterior segment. These are the same anatomic features that predispose to angle closure by relative pupillary block.*

block and aqueous misdirection can occur sequentially in the same eye.

Given the anatomic predisposition of a small anterior segment, other factors may act to trigger an attack of aqueous misdirection. These include increases in lens size, forward movement of the lens, inward movement of the ciliary body, increases in vitreous volume, and inflammatory changes in the aqueous humor. These same factors may also develop or increase during an attack of malignant glaucoma, acting to prolong and worsen the attack and rendering the eye increasingly resistant to therapy.

Therefore, one must recognize the eye that is predisposed to this problem, and when it occurs, act decisively to initiate a progressively more intense therapeutic intervention,

recognizing that progressive worsening and resistance to treatment are the natural course of this disease.

STAGES IN DEVELOPMENT

Given an eye predisposed by a lens–anterior chamber disproportion, the most likely instigator of aqueous misdirection is forward movement of the lens (Fig. 38-3). In the classic case of acute angle closure treated by surgical iridectomy, forward movement of the lens is a natural result of opening an eye at high pressure. The sudden decompression of the anterior chamber causes the lens to move forward into contact with the ciliary processes, diverting aqueous humor posteriorly, thus creating a situation that tends to

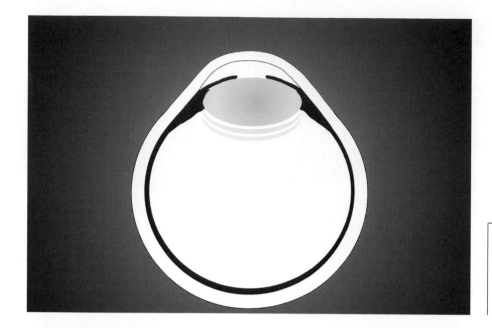

FIGURE 38-3.   *As the lens moves forward, under the influence of various possible events (e.g., ciliary muscle contraction, ciliary body swelling, decompression of the anterior chamber), the chance for lens–ciliary body touch is high.*

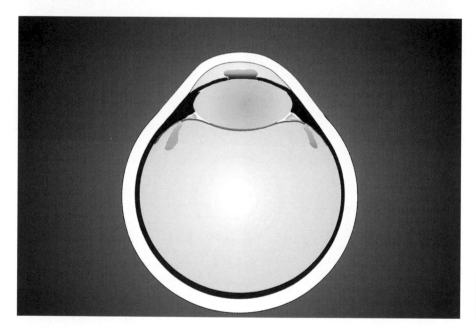

FIGURE 38-4.   *The anterior hyaloid moves anteriorly along with the lens, and aqueous humor, which is blocked from forward flow, is diverted into the vitreous.*

hold the lens in an anterior position (Fig. 38-4). In such cases, an iridectomy does not produce the expected peripheral chamber deepening and relief from elevated pressure, but instead, a further loss of chamber depth and a persistence or worsening of pressure elevation occur. Furthermore, since both lens and iris are now pushed forward, the anterior chamber is characterized by profound central as well as peripheral shallowing.

Much of what is known about the mechanism of aqueous misdirection is derived from clinical observations regarding the effects of various treatments. For example, the contributing role of anterior-chamber decompression to the cycle of forward lens movement and subsequent malignant glaucoma is supported by the relative rare occurrence of malignant glaucoma after iridotomy by laser (6), in which

no sudden anterior-chamber decompression is caused. The importance of reversing forward lens position is also emphasized by the success of mydriatic-cycloplegic therapy (7), which tends to pull the lens posteriorly. Conversely, the ability of miotic therapy to initiate or worsen malignant glaucoma can be attributed to forward lens movement (8). Considering the disease from this frame of reference, it is quite logical to select a name emphasizing the central role of the lens (direct lens block) (2,9) or of lens–ciliary body contact (ciliary block) (10,11). But further changes involving alterations in the vitreous and hyaloid face may occur in an affected eye. These require the clinician to shift the focus of treatment posteriorly, and help to explain why treatments directed at lens position, or even lens removal, become ineffective.

The key elements in the more advanced stages are the secretion of aqueous into the vitreous and importantly, an induced alteration in the anterior hyaloid face and anterior vitreous which tends to trap the aqueous posteriorly. Grant (12) and Epstein et al (13) showed that the resistance to aqueous flow across the normal vitreous and hyaloid is low and would not lead to sequestration of aqueous posteriorly. However, under conditions of increased pressure or flow, the impedance rises markedly. They also pointed out that as the hyaloid face is forced forward into increased contact with the lens and ciliary body, its surface area for fluid exchange is reduced. Thus, malignant glaucoma seems to be best understood as a cascade of self-reinforcing effects that maintain and worsen the glaucoma while continuously shifting the pathologic changes posteriorly (Figs. 38-5 to 38-7) (12–14).

DIFFERENTIAL DIAGNOSIS

Several conditions present with clinical signs similar to aqueous misdirection. Pupillary block potentially may be confused, and the diagnosis of malignant glaucoma cannot be seriously entertained unless the opening created by iridectomy or iridotomy is confirmed to be patent. Other clinical conditions that mimic aqueous misdirection do so by causing a posterior volume expansion that leads to clinical findings similar to those produced by aqueous misdirection. In the postoperative setting, with confirmed patent iridotomy sites, the two most important causes of a malig-

nant glaucoma-like picture are suprachoroidal hemorrhage and serous choroidal detachment.

A suprachoroidal hemorrhage usually occurs as a sudden event in the early postoperative period, whereas aqueous misdirection can occur in the early postoperative period, or even months or years later. The acute onset of severe pain with suprachoroidal hemorrhage helps to differentiate it from the mild to moderate aching pain of pupillary block or aqueous misdirection. The anterior chamber is markedly and diffusely shallow and the intraocular pressure is moderately to highly elevated. Clinical examination will reveal choroidal elevations that are dark brown. If the fundus view is poor, ultrasound examination is extremely helpful.

Serous choroidal detachment occurs postoperatively, usually in association with some degree of overfiltration. Profound hypotony and absence of pain help to differentiate this condition. Clinical examination reveals a diffusely shallow chamber and light-brown choroidal elevations. Ultrasound can be helpful in detecting this finding when the fundus view is poor or when the elevations are low and quite anterior.

Numerous other clinical conditions can cause the clinical findings of diffuse shallowing of the anterior chamber and elevated intraocular pressure characteristic of malignant glaucoma. These primarily include lesions that either expand the vitreous volume directly (e.g., infectious or inflammatory swelling of the vitreous) or reduce the space available to the normal vitreous (e.g., retinal/choroidal swelling,

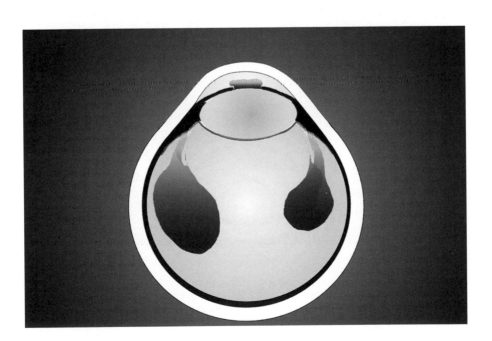

FIGURE 38-5. *If the shallow chamber and aqueous diversion persist, the vitreous face moves into further apposition with the posterior surface of the lens and ciliary body. Up to this point, the condition probably remains reversible through repositioning of the lens posteriorly (e.g., with mydriatic-cycloplegic therapy, coupled with vitreous dehydration and aqueous suppression), which would allow the aqueous to resume its normal path.*

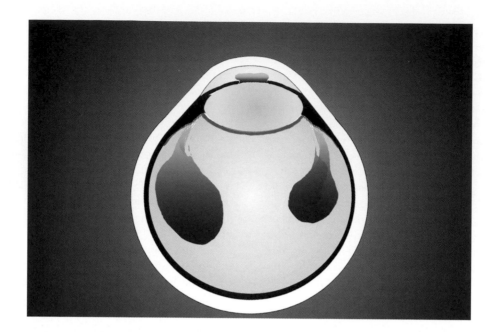

FIGURE 38-6. *With a continued unbroken attack, inflammation in the anterior segment leads to firm attachment of the hyaloid to the ciliary body (as has been confirmed by pathologic examination), and thus an irreversible diversion of aqueous into the vitreous space. In addition, this diverted aqueous is now "trapped" in the vitreous by increased flow resistance in the anterior hyaloid membrane and anterior vitreous induced by inflammation, tissue compaction, and loss of free surface area (12–14). At this point, the condition is no longer reversible by lens repositioning (or even lens removal), since the misdirection of aqueous is no longer dependent on ciliary block.*

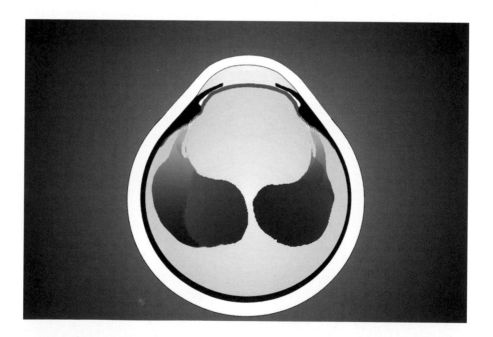

FIGURE 38-7. *Aqueous misdirection in an aphakic eye. Treatment will require release of the entrapped aqueous through disruption of the relatively impermeable structure of the anterior vitreous. Though the lens may have been crucial in instigating aqueous misdirection, the misdirection now persists through direct secretion of aqueous into the peripheral anterior vitreous.*

scleral buckling) (2). Conditions that cause swelling or forward rotation of the ciliary body can also produce a clinical picture similar to aqueous misdirection (15). Often these conditions are not confused with aqueous misdirection because the clinical setting and associated findings clearly suggest the true underlying disease from the outset. Fortunately for the clinician, even when these other disorders are not initially obvious, careful stepwise application of the recommended protocol for managing malignant glaucoma and its more common mimics will also prove appropriate for diagnosis and initial treatment of these more rare conditions.

MANAGEMENT

Medical

The initial therapy of malignant glaucoma is medical. Many of the accepted elements are common to the urgent care of most types of severe glaucoma: aqueous suppressants and osmotics to reduce intraocular pressure, and corticosteroids to reduce inflammation. Relaxation of the ciliary muscle results in tightening of the zonules and posterior movement of the lens. On this basis, Chandler and Grant (7) suggested mydriatic-cycloplegic therapy for malignant glaucoma, and this is now recognized as a standard part of therapy for this disorder. As a corollary, miotic therapy is strictly avoided because it has the opposite effect on the lens and may precipitate or exacerbate an attack.

In general, therapy is begun using all useful elements in combination—aqueous suppression, osmotics, cortico-steroids, and mydriatic-cycloplegics—because they act in a complementary fashion. The primary exception is glaucoma with a possible element of pupillary block. In this instance, dilatation of the pupil should be avoided initially as it may compromise the performance of a laser iridotomy, and in fact, short-term use of a miotic may be needed for this purpose. Once pupillary block has been ruled out with an adequate iridotomy, mydriatic-cycloplegic therapy is immediately begun. Other diseases in the differential diagnosis may not be ruled out yet, but this is not crucial because the initial medical therapy for malignant glaucoma is appropriate for the others as well.

Overall, approximately 50% of eyes with malignant glaucoma will respond to medical therapy alone. In eyes that are responsive to medical therapy, the intensive regimen outlined below should be slowly tapered under continued close monitoring of chamber depth, intraocular pressure, and inflammation. Cycloplegic therapy should be continued for months or years, and some patients will require it indefinitely. Mydriatic-cycloplegic treatment is most effective in phakic eyes; it is less effective (16) although worth trying in pseudophakic eyes (17), and tends to be least effective in aphakic eyes, although there may be some benefit from relaxing the ciliary musculature (18).

Table 38-1 provides specific guidelines for medical treatment.

Laser

Laser therapy can be extremely helpful at several stages of the disease. The utility of a laser iridotomy to rule out pupil-lary block has already been noted. In addition, the opposite eye should be routinely assessed for possible laser iridotomy,

Table 38-1.   Specific Guidelines for Medical Treatment

1. Topical β-blocker, 1 gtt bid*
2. Topical α₂-agonist, 1 gtt bid*
3. Carbonic anhydrase inhibitor, initiate with oral or parenteral administration and maintain with oral or topical route: e.g., acetazolamide, 500-mg tablets, followed by dorzolamide, 1 gtt bid*
4. Topical prednisolone acetate 1%, 1 gtt qid to qh depending on severity of inflammation
5. Topical mydriatic-cycloplegic: initiate with 1% cyclopentolate and 2.5% phenylephrine, 1 gtt of each q10 min × 3; maintain with 1% atropine, tid
6. Systemic osmotic: oral glycerol (1.0–1.5 g/kg) or isosorbide (1.5 g/kg), or intravenous mannitol (1–2 g/kg)*

Note: Leave at least 5 min between drop instillation, and have patient leave eyes closed after drop instillation.

* In the specific instance of low or normal intraocular pressure, such as may occur after filtration surgery, it is advisable to delay institution of these drugs aimed at lowering pressure until other causes of postoperative diffusely shallow chamber have been ruled out by clinical examination or ultrasound examination of the posterior segment. It is important to remember that in the presence of a functioning filter, aqueous misdirection may not be accompanied by marked pressure elevation; instead, the pressure may be in the high teens—i.e., higher than expected under the circumstances, and usually higher than seen with postoperative choroidal detachment. In a hypotonous case, if choroidal detachment is found, aqueous suppressants and osmotic agents would not be used, though continued use of mydriatic-cycloplegic therapy and corticosteroids would be advisable. In a normotensive case with a functioning filter and chamber shallowing due to aqueous misdirection, aqueous suppression can be helpful in re-forming the chamber since a reduction in aqueous production also reduces the amount misdirected.

since there is a high probability of a crowded anterior segment and a narrow angle. In fact, if the opposite eye does not have a narrow angle, this should raise suspicion that one is dealing with one of the alternative causes for the clinical findings of malignant glaucoma. Therapeutic laser can also be used to disrupt the elements that entrap the aqueous posteriorly, and this may save the patient from more complex invasive surgery when an eye fails to respond to medical therapy.

Herschler (19) introduced the idea of relieving blockade at the interface between the lens and ciliary body by using a thermal laser to shrink the ciliary processes in order to relieve "ciliary block." He treated the ciliary processes through a surgical iridectomy using an argon laser. This treatment successfully led to chamber deepening in five of six eyes that had not responded to medical treatment up to that point. In discussing this report, Simmons (20) noted several possible explanations for the beneficial effect, in addition to the proposed mode of action. Weber et al (21) also reported success with this technique, and thought that the response of the eyes in their series was most consistent with direct relief of ciliolenticular block, as proposed by Herschler (19).

Herschler's technique requires adequate visualization of the ciliary processes, which is not always present. When applicable, it has the advantage of ease of use and safety, particularly in phakic eyes, and should reasonably be con-sidered for use in eyes that are not responsive to medical therapy, prior to more invasive surgery.

Epstein et al (22) introduced the use of neodymium: yttrium-aluminum-garnet (Nd:YAG) laser photodisruption of the anterior hyaloid in the treatment of malignant glaucoma. This technique can be dramatically effective, and serves to confirm the importance of increased flow resistance in the anterior vitreous for maintaining posterior aqueous entrapment. Originally reported in aphakic eyes, it is now more commonly used in pseudophakic eyes with posterior-chamber intraocular lenses.

Chandler's original procedure for vitreous aspiration in malignant glaucoma (see below) employed an aspirating needle inserted into the vitreous through a peripheral iridectomy. Epstein's technique uses a photodisruptive laser to open the anterior hyaloid membrane and anterior vitreous either in the same location or more centrally, although, of course, the eye is closed and there is no aspiration of vitreous. The success of this maneuver demonstrates that interruption of the anterior barrier is more critical than physical removal of vitreous. On the other hand, not all eyes respond, and some that respond initially have a recurrence and may ultimately require more definitive vitreous removal. A possible explanation for failure is that the thickened anterior vitreous is not adequately opened by laser photodisruption, or as suggested by Shaffer (23), the aqueous has been misdirected posterior to the vitreous. Recurrence after initial success may represent recompaction of the anterior vitreous under the influence of continuing aqueous misdirection.

Table 38-2 provides specific guidelines for laser therapy (19,21,22,24) and Figure 38-8 demonstrates Epstein's method (16,22,24–28).

Surgical

Observations made during surgical intervention for malignant glaucoma have been a rich source of knowledge about this complex condition. In particular, surgery has emphasized the importance of the vitreous in this disorder. Successful surgical protocols have also demonstrated that this disease responds best to a meticulous stepwise approach pursued with an open mind regarding the causative mechanism.

Chandler noted that lens removal was more likely to be associated with cure of malignant glaucoma if it was accompanied by vitreous loss. Shaffer (23) advocated purposeful incisions of the vitreous face at the time of lens removal to release trapped aqueous (Fig. 38-9). To allow preservation of the lens and still decompress the vitreous, Chandler developed a procedure of needle aspiration through a surgical iridectomy. Because of lens complications with this technique, Chandler et al (29) later modified the approach by using a pars plana entry site (Fig. 38-10). This method of deep vitreous aspiration was refined by Simmons et al (18,30) to incorporate advances in instrumentation; it is the final phase of the stepwise surgical protocol "Chandler's confirmation procedure."

Table 38-2. Specific Guidelines for Laser Therapy

1. Continue with all aspects of full medical therapy as outlined in Table 40-1.
2. Consider Herschler's method for thermal laser shrinkage of ciliary processes, particularly in phakic eyes with a large iridectomy. Focus on the ciliary processes through an iridectomy, viewing directly through the cornea or through a gonioscopy lens as needed. Treat 2–4 processes with 30–50 applications. Herschler (19) noted chamber deepening in 2–4 days, but Weber et al (21) noted an immediate effect.

Argon laser settings:	Spot size	100–200 μm
	Power	300–1000 mW
	Duration	0.1 sec
	End point	Visible shrinkage of ciliary processes and/or chamber deepening

3. Use Epstein's method (22) for laser-mediated photodisruption of the anterior hyaloid/anterior vitreous, particularly in aphakic or pseudophakic eyes (see Fig. 38-8). Focus on the anterior hyaloid through an iridectomy using a capsulotomy lens. The central hyaloid may be opened in an aphakic eye if an adequate peripheral access is not available. In a pseudophakic eye, a lens positioning hole is also an effective site if access peripheral to the lens is blocked (24). In pseudophakic eyes, a capsulotomy will almost always be made along with disruption of the anterior hyaloid because of the close approximation of these structures in this condition.

Nd:YAG laser settings:	Power	3–10 mJ
	End point	Visible tissue disruption, sometimes with immediate chamber deepening, but this may be delayed several hours

4. Repeat treatment. If laser therapy is not initially successful, or if initial success is followed by recurrence, a single repeat treatment may be considered. However, multiple repeat treatments are not usually productive, and instead, planning should shift to surgical intervention. Meanwhile, full medical treatment should continue.

The three steps of this procedure are designed both to reveal and to treat, as needed, pupillary block, choroidal separation (serous or hemorrhagic), and malignant glaucoma with posterior aqueous diversion. In recent years, pupillary block usually has been ruled out by performing a laser iridotomy in uncertain cases prior to surgery. However, when this is not possible, the first surgical step should be a surgical iridectomy. If this step confirms pupillary block by producing a deepening of the chamber and softening of the eye, the surgery proceeds no further.

When the chamber remains shallow, the second step is taken. This next step explores the possibility of suprachoroidal fluid using two sclerotomies, usually in the two inferotemporal quadrants. These sclerotomies are purposely made somewhat anteriorly in the pars plana region; Simmons advocates a 3-mm radial incision centered 3 mm posterior to the limbus. If fluid or blood is found, it is drained and the anterior chamber is re-formed. This sequence confirms the diagnosis of choroidal separation and no further surgery is done. Subtle amounts of suprachoroidal fluid may escape ultrasound detection,

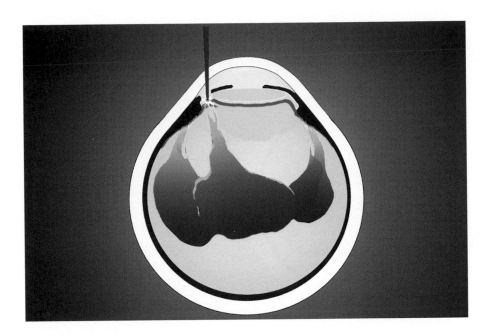

FIGURE 38-8.   *Epstein et al (22) introduced Nd:YAG laser photodisruption as a means to disrupt the anterior hyaloid membrane and compacted anterior vitreous, thus releasing trapped aqueous humor. The laser may be focused on the anterior hyaloid through a peripheral iridectomy, as depicted here. The central hyaloid may be disrupted in an aphakic eye, or in a pseudophakic eye a lens positioning hole (24,25) may be used for access instead of a peripheral iridectomy. Quite often the anterior hyaloid and the lens capsule are in close approximation and therefore both are disrupted simultaneously. Since the capsule, the anterior hyaloid, and the anterior vitreous can contribute to posterior retention of aqueous, this form of treatment should not be abandoned until openings have been attempted in all layers (16,25–28).*

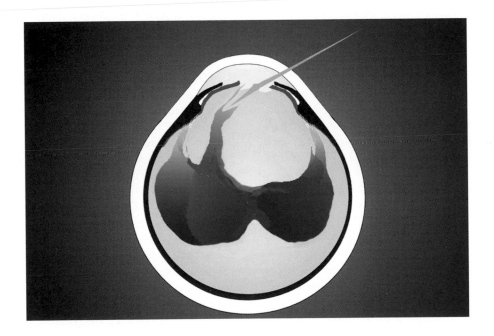

FIGURE 38-9.   *Shaffer (23) noted that deep incisions into the anterior vitreous after lens removal would relieve diverted aqueous and allow the anterior chamber to form.*

or may require sensitive equipment that is not universally available. Thus, this second step is an important one even when suprachoroidal fluid is not suspected by careful preoperative examination.

If the first two steps are not productive, the diagnosis of malignant glaucoma with aqueous misdirection has been confirmed and this signals the need for vitreous aspiration. The traditional method utilizes a sharp 18-gauge needle

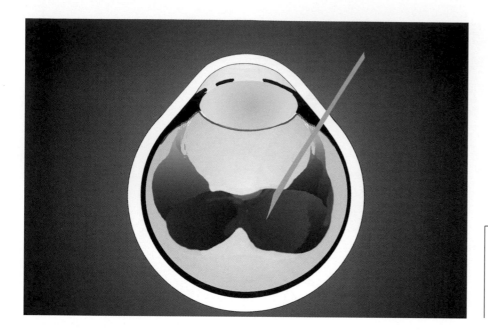

FIGURE 38-10. *Chandler et al (29) introduced vitreous aspiration through the pars plana, which opens the anterior vitreous and relieves pressure in the vitreous. This is step 3 in "Chandler's confirmation procedure" (18).*

introduced into the eye through one of the two sclerotomies to a depth of 12 mm in the direction of the optic nerve. It may be noted that the anterior placement of the sclerotomy helps to ensure that the hyaloid face is disrupted by the needle and may explain why more posterior entry wounds have been associated with lower success rates. Once in the eye, the tip of the needle is slowly moved in an arc of approximately 4 mm, and then 1.0 to 1.5 mL of fluid vitreous is slowly aspirated. The final 0.25 mL of aspirate is reinjected into the eye to reduce the chance of incorporating a vitreous strand in the needle; the needle is then slowly removed from the eye. The now hypotonous globe is reinflated through a previously made paracentesis wound, first with a small amount of saline solution and then with a large air bubble. Simmons et al now advocate an automated vitreous suction-cutting apparatus, when available, for vitreous removal.

If malignant glaucoma recurs after this surgical intervention, the procedure can be repeated. It is important to remember that removal of vitreous alone is likely to be ineffective if the anterior hyaloid is not adequately opened. In case of a recurrence, therefore, Nd:YAG laser hyaloidotomy should be tried once more prior to further surgery, as it may be more effective after vitreous removal. In pseudophakic eyes, at the time of vitrectomy, lasting success is more likely if a deliberate effort is made to surgically open a connection between the anterior and posterior segments (31) (Fig. 38-11). Finally, in phakic eyes, lens removal and subsequent hyaloidotomy is still occasionally required because adequate disruption of the altered hyaloid face may not be possible with the lens present. Lens removal should be a "last resort," however; even if the lens is cataractous, it is better to resolve the attack of malignant glaucoma by other means and remove the lens later under more controlled circumstances (18,30).

CONCLUSIONS

Malignant glaucoma remains a complex and difficult disorder that still fully justifies its original name. A cascade of self-perpetuating fluid and tissue alterations driven by a posterior misdirection and sequestration of aqueous humor seems to explain the difficulties encountered in its management and in the variable response of this disorder to different forms of intervention.

There seems to be an early "reversible" stage in which forward movement of the lens blocks normal aqueous flow at the ciliary body. Such eyes may be treated successfully with mydriatic-cycloplegic therapy, which tightens the zonules and moves the lens posteriorly. Such eyes might also be the ones that would respond to laser shrinkage of a few ciliary processes (if it can be assumed—a guarded assumption—that this treatment has no effect on the adjacent hyaloid face). Other eyes appear to reach an "irreversible" state: resistant to medical therapy and continuing to have aqueous misdirection even after removal of the lens. These eyes require vitreous disruption, by laser or surgery, for resolution. In such eyes, a portion of normally produced aqueous seems to be delivered directly into the vitreous, probably as a result of adhesions of the peripheral hyaloid to the ciliary body. This posteriorly misdirected aqueous becomes entrapped in the vitreous because of abnormal flow resistance developing in the anterior vitreous and hyaloid membrane, and because forward movement of the hyaloid face causes it to lose free surface area.

Although it may be tempting to suppose that all eyes progress through the stage from reversibility to nonreversibility, there is really no basis for this assumption. Some eyes may follow this path and others may immediately enter the nonreversible phase requiring vitreous disruption or removal, or both. The response to therapy does not resolve

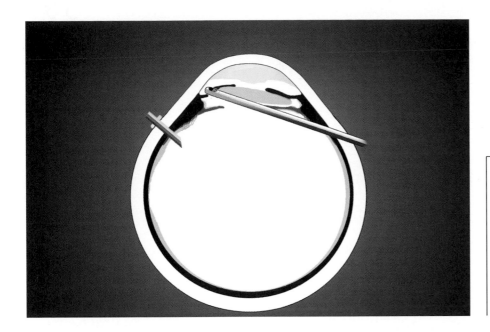

FIGURE 38-11. *Surgical therapy has two goals—to decompress and remove vitreous and to provide a fluid connection between the posterior segment and the anterior segment. The maneuver depicted here—removal of anterior vitreous and lens capsule at an iridectomy site—is a useful way to provide this fluid connection in a pseudophakic eye, though it must be done with care to avoid dislocating the intraocular lens (31).*

the issue: Some eyes show definite reversibility short of vitreous surgery; other eyes are not in the reversible phase and whether they were at some prior point is not known. What is known, through the efforts of observant clinicians, sometimes daring surgeons, and thoughtful research scientists, is a systematic therapeutic approach that has a high probability of offering the most effective, least traumatic treatment for each variant of this complex and challenging disease. The success of treatment is greatly enhanced by early diagnosis and diligent and timely application of the therapeutic steps.

REFERENCES

1. Schwartz AL, Anderson DR. "Malignant glaucoma" in an eye with no antecedent operation or miotics. *Arch Ophthalmol* 1975;93:379–381.
2. Levene RZ. Current concepts of malignant glaucoma. *Ophthalmic Surg* 1986;17:515–520.
3. Epstein DL. The malignant glaucoma syndromes. In: Epstein DC, Allingham RR, Schuman JS, eds. *Chandler and Grant's glaucoma.* 4th ed. Baltimore: Williams & Wilkins 1997:285–303.
4. Cyrlin MN. Malignant glaucoma. In: Albert DN, Jakobiec FA, eds. *Principles and practice of ophthalmology, clinical practice.* Vol. 3. Philadelphia: WB Saunders, 1994:1520–1528.
5. Lieberman MF. Diagnosis and management of malignant glaucoma. In: Higginbotham EJ, Lee DA, eds. *Management of difficult glaucoma: a clinician's guide.* Boston: Blackwell Science, 1994:183–194.
6. Cashwell LF, Martin TJ. Malignant glaucoma after laser iridotomy. *Ophthalmology* 1992;99:651–658.
7. Chandler PA, Grant WM. Mydriatic-cycloplegic treatment in malignant glaucoma. *Arch Ophthalmol* 1962;68:353.
8. Rieser JC, Schwartz B. Miotic induced malignant glaucoma. *Arch Ophthalmol* 1972;87:706.
9. Levene R. A new conception of malignant glaucoma. *Arch Ophthalmol* 1972;87:497–506.
10. Weiss DI, Shaffer RN. Ciliary block (malignant) glaucoma. *Trans Am Acad Ophthalmol* 1972;76:450–461.
11. Shaffer RN, Hoskins HD. Ciliary block (malignant) glaucoma. *Ophthalmology* 1978;85:215–221.
12. Grant WM. Experimental aqueous perfusion in enucleated human eyes. *Arch Ophthalmol* 1963;69:783–801.
13. Epstein DL, Hashimoto JM, Anderson PJ, et al. Experimental perfusions through the anterior and vitreous chambers with possible relationships to malignant glaucoma. *Am J Ophthalmol* 1979;88:1078–1086.
14. Quigley HA. Malignant glaucoma and fluid flow rate. *Am J Ophthalmol* 1980;89:879–880. Letter.
15. Phelps CD. Angle closure glaucoma secondary to ciliary body swelling. *Arch Ophthalmol* 1974;92:287–290.
16. Tomey KF, Senft SH, Antonios SR, et al. Aqueous misdirection and flat chamber after posterior chamber implants with and without trabeculectomy. *Arch Ophthalmol* 1987;105:770–773.
17. Dickens CJ, Shaffer RN. The medical treatment of ciliary block glaucoma after extracapsular cataract extraction. *Am J Ophthalmol* 1987;103:237.
18. Yaqub MK, Simmons RB, Simmons RJ. Malignant glaucoma. In: Sayyad F, Spaeth GL, Sheilds MB, Hitchings RA, eds. *The refractory glaucomas.* New York: Igaku-Shoin, 1995:107–142.
19. Herschler J. Laser shrinkage of the ciliary processes—a treatment for malignant (ciliary block) glaucoma. *Ophthalmology* 1980;87:1155–1158.
20. Simmons RJ. Discussion of Herschler J: Laser shrinkage of the ciliary processes—a treatment for malignant (ciliary block) glaucoma. *Ophthalmology* 1980,87.1158–1159.
21. Weber PA, Henry MA, Kapetansky FM, et al. Argon laser treatment of the ciliary processes in aphakic glaucoma with flat anterior chamber. *Am J Ophthalmol* 1984;97:82–85.
22. Epstein DL, Steinert RF, Puliafito CA. Neodymium-YAG laser therapy to the anterior hyaloid in aphakic malignant (cilio-vitreal block) glaucoma. *Am J Ophthalmol* 1984;98:137–143.
23. Shaffer RN. Role of vitreous detachment in aphakic and malignant glaucoma. *Trans Am Acad Ophthalmol Otolaryngol* 1954;58:217.
24. Risco JM, Tomey KF, Perkins TW. Laser capsulotomy through intraocular lens positioning holes in anterior aqueous misdirection. *Arch Ophthalmol* 1989;107:1569.
25. Little BC, Hitchings RA. Pseudophakic malignant glaucoma: Nd:YAG capsulotomy as a primary treatment. *Eye* 1993;7:102–104.
26. Brown RH, Lynch MG, Tearse JF, et al. Neodymium-YAG vitreous surgery for phakic and pseudophakic malignant glaucoma. *Arch Ophthalmol* 1986;104:1464–1466.
27. Epstein DL. Pseudophakic malignant glaucoma—is it really pseudo-malignant? *Am J Ophthalmol* 1987;103:231–233.
28. Tomey KF, Traverso CE. Neodymium-YAG laser posterior capsulotomy for the treatment of aphakic and pseudophakic papillary block. *Am J Ophthalmol* 1987;104:402–407.
29. Chandler PA, Simmons RJ, Grant WM. Malignant glaucoma: medical and surgical treatment. *Am J Ophthalmol* 1968;66:495–502.
30. Maestre FA, Simmons RJ. Malignant glaucoma. In: Ritch R, Shields MB, Krupin T, eds. *The glaucomas.* St. Louis: Mosby, 1996:841–855.
31. Lynch MG, Brown RH, Michels RG, et al. Surgical vitrectomy for pseudophakic malignant glaucoma. *Am J Ophthalmol* 1986;102:149–153.

Surgery for Complications

Paul Palmberg

The risk-benefit ratio of modern glaucoma filtering surgery is highly dependent on the skill of the surgeon to achieve success and avoid complications with the procedure chosen and on the state of the patient's eye at the time of surgery. The role of skill has been increased successively by the introduction of guarded procedures, laser suture lysis, and the use of the antimetabolites 5-fluorouracil and mitomycin C, each of which can influence the flow of aqueous through the bypass. Having a mastery of these means of manipulating flow and knowing how to adjust their use to account for the state of the eye at the time of surgery and thereafter enables the surgeon to maximize the chance of success and minimize the risk of complications. In short, in this chapter on surgery for complications after glaucoma filtering procedures, the major emphasis is on the means to prevent complications from occurring, because the best way to deal with complications is to prevent them from happening.

The complications to be addressed are the failing bleb, the leaking bleb, the painful bleb, the exuberant bleb, the infected bleb, flat anterior chamber, aqueous misdirection, hypotony maculopathy, choroidal detachment, suprachoroidal hemorrhage, and cataract.

FAILING BLEB

Blebs fail when the conditions necessary for their continued existence cease to exist. A steady supply of aqueous is required to distend blebs and to feed the cells in the hydrated Tenon's capsule tissue within. Blebs are most stable when the aqueous flow maintains sufficient tissue turgor pressure to collapse the blood vessels in the conjunctiva and Tenon's capsule of the bleb, and when the aqueous is free of inflammatory cells or flare. Under such conditions, there is little source of serum-derived growth factors to stimulate fibrosis or vascularization. To reach stable maturity, however, blebs must first get off to a good start as beneficiaries of proper construction and suturing of the scleral flap, and survive the postoperative wound-healing phase.

Immediate bleb failure can be due to the sutures in the scleral flap being too tight, or due to obstruction of the internal filtering ostium by a blood clot, iris, or vitreous. Most such failures can be avoided by intraoperative testing to detect excessive resistance after suturing of the scleral flap. Balanced salt solution is injected into the anterior chamber through a paracentesis using a 30-gauge cannula, and the flow at the scleral flap is observed until it reaches a steady state. The detection of flow is assisted by using a surgical cellulose sponge to absorb aqueous periodically from the wound edge. At equilibrium flow, the intraocular pressure (IOP) then can be estimated by pressing on the center of the cornea with a 30-gauge cannula and noting the force needed to depress it (Fig. 39-1) (1,2). Initially, one can use an electronic hand-held tonometer (Tonopen) to calibrate the estimation technique. At this point, detection of an IOP that is too high should prompt sequential removal of flap sutures until a steady flow of aqueous occurs at an acceptable pressure. The pressure desired at this stage may be 8 to 12 mm Hg for the usual filtration surgery, or perhaps 15 to 20 mm Hg in eyes in which the preoperative IOP was 30 mm Hg or higher, in order to try to reduce the risk of suprachoroidal hemorrhage, but the scleral flap need not be sutured tighter than that. Very tight suturing performed in an overzealous attempt to avoid hypotony will prevent aqueous flow and bleb formation.

In eyes in which mitomycin was used, presumably with injury to the local capillary network in the conjunctiva and Tenon's capsule (3), and in which there was an insufficient flow to produce a bleb elevation, I frequently observed an early ingrowth of vessels, in a radial pattern, entering

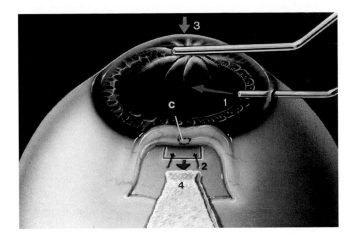

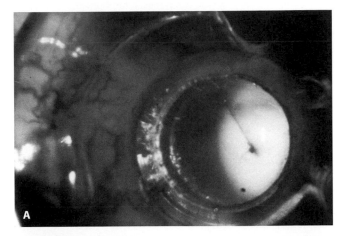

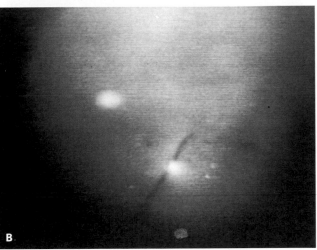

FIGURE 39-1. *Estimation of the intraocular pressure at equilibrium. 1. The anterior chamber is filled with balanced salt solution through a paracentesis, using a 30-gauge cannula. 2. Filtration is monitored to equilibrium flow at the scleral flap by absorbing fluid with a cellulose sponge. 3. The intraocular pressure can then be estimated by pressing on the central cornea with the 30-gauge cannula. A Tonopen with gas-sterilized covers can be used intraoperatively at first when one is learning the technique in order to provide calibration. c = corneal site of internal ostium anterior to the base of the scleral flap. (Reproduced by permission from Palmberg P. Prevention and management of complicated hypotony in trabeculectomy with mitomycin.* Highlights Ophthalmol *1993;21:67–77.)*

FIGURE 39-2. *Argon laser suture lysis. A. A Hoskins laser suture lysis lens is used to compress the bleb overlying a 10-0 nylon suture to be lysed. B. The argon laser cutting a suture.*

an ischemic bleb and leading to fibrosis and failure of the procedure.

To avoid this from happening, at surgery one should obtain a continuous flow of aqueous and an IOP in the chosen range. If removal of all sutures fails to achieve the desired result, the scleral flap should be elevated and the internal ostium explored. If the anterior chamber was entered via a tunnel anterior to the base of the scleral flap ("safety-valve incision"), as a guard against future hypotony after an antimetabolite-augmented procedure (2,4), the valvelike property of the wound may be too good and an additional bite with a punch may be needed to reduce the resistance of the wound. If a blood clot, iris, or vitreous is encountered, it should be removed and testing repeated.

A reduction in bleb size and rise in IOP encountered after 3 to 7 days usually indicate the development of vascularization and scarring of Tenon's capsule and conjunctiva, or fibrosis of the episclera around the scleral flap, or both, due to the effects of postoperative inflammation. Such response is best avoided by either five injections of 5-fluorouracil during the first 2 weeks after primary filtering surgery (5,6) or the intraoperative use of mitomycin in either primary or complex filtering surgery (7–9). Once scarring begins, one must act quickly before it is too late to save the bleb. At this point, laser suture lysis (10) or needle elevation of the scleral flap (11), followed by injections of

5-fluorouracil, might salvage adequate bleb function. Laser suture lysis of 10-0 nylon sutures in the scleral flap is performed with a 50- to 200-μm spot of an argon or 75-μm spot of a diode laser (12), after compression of the overlying bleb with a Hoskins or Ritch suture lysis lens to visualize the suture (Fig. 39-2). An energy of 0.3 to 1.0 W (depending on bleb wall thickness and opacity) for 0.02 to 0.05 second will usually suffice. In very transparent blebs, as obtained after surgery with 5-fluorouracil or mitomycin use, suture lysis with a 100- to 200-μm spot size is preferable to use of a 50-μm spot, to avoid burning the overlying conjunctiva and Tenon's capsule. Such burns can produce buttonholes immediately, or can stimulate adhesions of Tenon's capsule to the episclera that dimple the bleb surface and lead much later to hole formation as the surrounding bleb expands.

The development of a rising IOP and formation of a Tenon's cyst inside the conjunctiva of a bleb, as a "balloon within a balloon," can be treated by temporary reinstitution of medical therapy, to allow time for remodeling of the bleb

(13–15), or by needling. Costa et al (15) reported that in a randomized trial, patients treated with medical therapy did better than those treated by initial needling of the bleb. Medical treatment was successful in 9 of 10 patients, with the mean tension falling from 25 mm Hg before reinstitution of medical therapy to 20 mm Hg at 1 month, 17 mm Hg at 3 months, and 14 mm Hg at 6 months, with the steady fall in pressure correlating with the evolution of the blebs from Tenon's cysts to more functional blebs.

Resort to needling of a bleb is indicated when added medical therapy does not initially lower the pressure to a level at which one would be willing to observe the patient, or does not eventually lower the pressure adequately. Needling is most likely to succeed when both the conjunctiva and Tenon's capsule are relatively avascular and when the conjunctiva is mobile over the Tenon's cyst. It can be performed at the slit lamp after apraclonidine (Iopidine, Alcon, Ft. Worth, TX) is applied for vasoconstriction, proparacaine is given for anesthesia, the lids are cleansed with povidone-iodine soap, and a lid speculum is placed. A 30-gauge needle, placed on a 1-mL syringe and bent at a 45-degree angle with a blade breaker, makes an ideal tool for needling blebs (Fig. 39-3). The needle is passed in under the edge of the bleb along the scleral surface and into an avascular part of a Tenon's cyst. The cyst wall can be punctured with the needle tip and then torn by pulling to the side. The Tenon's capsule within the conjunctiva is then usually seen to hydrate and to lose its encapsulated appearance.

LEAKING BLEB

The flow of aqueous within blebs is a dynamic process. Over time the shape and consistency of blebs frequently change. Preferential flow through one area of a bleb may cause that area to expand and the Tenon's capsule in that area to become more hydrated and transparent. As a result, the overlying conjunctiva may be stretched, leading to rapid transudation through that area or even a frank epithelial defect. Leaks can also result from direct trauma to the eye or even from the rubbing action of the lids on exposed blebs. Leaks may also result directly from laser suture lysis when a laser burn produces an epithelial defect, or indirectly when a laser burn of the Tenon's capsule results in the formation of an adhesion to the episclera that rivets the bleb surface to the sclera, followed later, after bleb expansion, by tractional hole formation in the overlying bleb.

The detection and prompt treatment of significant bleb leaks is important, as leaks considerably increase the risk of bleb infection and endophthalmitis. They can also cause hypotony when the scleral flap resistance to flow is low. Bleb leaks should be suspected whenever hypotony is present, or when patients with thin, transparent blebs complain of an increase in tearing or irritation. While gross leaks may be visible upon slit-lamp inspection, detection is aided markedly by applying fluorescein to the surface of the bleb and viewing with the cobalt blue filter in place. When a single drop of saline solution or anesthetic is used to wet a fluorescein strip, the applied dye will be so dense that it will appear dark on the surface of the bleb. With the lids held away from the bleb to prevent dilution of the dye by tears, any flow of aqueous through the bleb will be detected as an area that becomes green and then yellow as the dye in that area is diluted. A rivulet of color change may flow down from the leak site, constituting a positive result on Seidel's test (Fig. 39-4). When hypotony is present, one may need to apply gentle pressure to the globe to demonstrate the leak site, which may otherwise be intermittent.

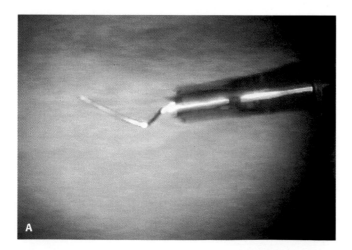 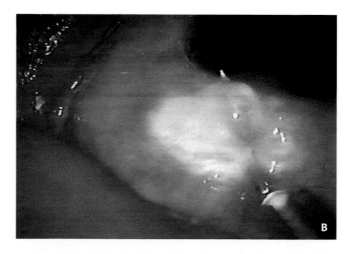

FIGURE 39-3.   *Needling to open the scleral tunnel of a filtering procedure. A. A 30-gauge needle is bent to a bayonet shape. B. The needle is passed under the conjunctiva behind the bleb and then into the bleb, and then passed into the scleral tunnel and into the anterior chamber to reduce the resistance to flow.*

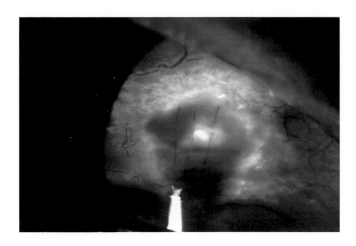

FIGURE 39-4. *Seidel's test for a bleb leak. Concentrated fluorescein is applied with a paper strip to the site of laser suture lysis, revealing a bleb leak.*

There is general agreement that leaks associated with conjunctival epithelial defects should be repaired. In such eyes a rivulet of aqueous flow is detected, and after the eye is rinsed, the Tenon's capsule is seen to be stained with fluorescein. There is less agreement about the management of thin blebs with rapid transudation of aqueous, but no epithelial defect. In these eyes, hypotony is usually not present, the eye is not irritated, and Seidel's test reveals an area that lights up but does not produce a rivulet of flow and, after rinsing, no fluorescein stains the Tenon's capsule, showing that the epithelial barrier is intact. While such blebs are probably at a somewhat increased risk of infection, the risk likely is not great enough to warrant any treatment that would risk loss of bleb function.

There are a number of current treatments for bleb leaks, indicating that none is truly satisfactory. The most conservative treatment is to apply an 18-mm therapeutic soft contact lens for 1 to 2 weeks, tamponading the leak while the conjunctival epithelium has an opportunity to heal over the hole (16). Unfortunately, contact lens tamponade succeeds in only a minority of eyes in which the bleb formed under the influence of an antimetabolite. Direct suturing of the site of leak, using a microvascular needle, is a reasonable option when the tissue of the bleb is not too thin or ischemic, but is likely to create new leaks in very thin blebs. The use of butyryl methacrylate glue and a silicone disk over the hole has not proved very successful for thin blebs, even with a soft lens covering the site, as motion of the eye against the lids usually results in the glue being torn from the site. One popular treatment is the injection of autologous blood into the bleb (17–19). One withdraws 0.1 to 0.5 mL of blood from the arm of the patient into a 1-mL syringe and then exchanges the larger-bore needle used to draw the blood with a 30-gauge needle. The needle is bent, using a blade breaker, at a 45-degree angle to facilitate viewing the tip while the blood is injected into the bleb at

the slip lamp, with the eye under topical anesthesia. After waiting about 4 minutes so as to approach the time at which clotting of the blood will occur, one inserts the needle a few millimeters beyond the outer edge of the bleb, advances the needle under the conjunctiva into the bleb cavity, and brings the tip as close as possible to the inner aspect of the hole in the bleb. The objective is to have a small quantity of blood passing out through the hole in the bleb, so that clotting occurs, with some of the clot inside the bleb and some outside, with the hole occluded by clot. With this method, the bleb leak will be healed in about half of the patients. Merely placing blood within the bleb is much less successful. The use of blood carries some risk of stimulating excessive healing and bleb failure, can result in reflux of blood into the anterior chamber or even the vitreous (20), and can induce corneal graft rejection and reactivation of toxoplasmic chorioretinitis (21). Fibrin glue has also been used to repair a bleb leak (22). Other potential treatments include amputation of the portion of the bleb containing the hole, followed by advancement of conjunctiva from behind or followed by a free conjunctival graft (23,24). While usually a definitive treatment of the bleb leak, such reoperation carries a significant risk of filtration failure.

Recently, colleagues and I (25) reported the use of compression sutures for leaking blebs (Fig. 39-5). With a 9-0 nylon suture on a CU-3 needle (Alcon, Ft. Worth, TX), a 2- to 3-mm horizontal bite is placed in the peripheral part of the cornea next to the bleb. The suture is then draped back over the bleb and a parallel 2- to 4-mm bite taken in the conjunctiva–Tenon's capsule posterior to the bleb. The suture is then tied tightly over the bleb, compressing the area with the hole between the two parallel lengths of suture on top and the underlying sclera. Compression of the Tenon's capsule within the bleb probably reduces its hydraulic conductivity, as has been postulated to occur in the compacted Tenon's capsule in a Tenon's cyst wall (14), resulting in either absent or markedly reduced leakage as disclosed by Seidel's test. The knot is rotated into the cornea and the eye treated with polymyxin B sulfate–trimethoprim sulfate (Polytrim) or ofloxacin (Ocuflox) four times a day and prednisolone acetate 1% four times a day. The eye is inspected at weekly intervals and the stitch removed when no leak is indicated by Seidel's test and, upon rinsing, no stain of Tenon's capsule is seen, indicating that the epithelial hole has healed. This treatment has been successful in 73% of patients. The combined effect of compression sutures and blood injection has yet to be evaluated.

PAINFUL BLEB

Blebs can cause pain in a variety of ways. First, large and thick blebs (Tenon's cysts) can create an impediment to upper eyelid movement and create pain by friction. Second, large and thick blebs can interfere with the smooth passage

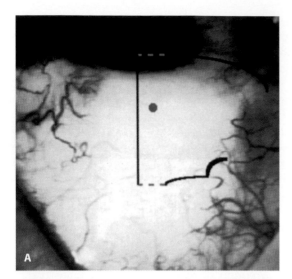

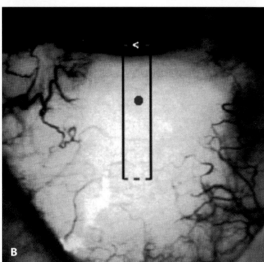

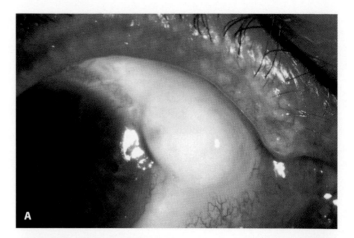

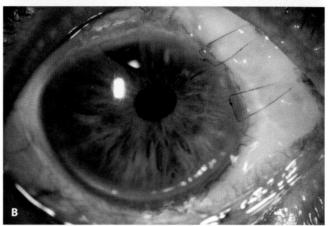

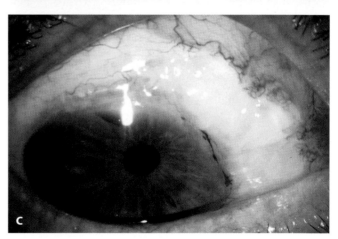

FIGURE 39-5. *Bleb compression stitch. A. A 9-0 nylon suture is passed in the peripheral part of the cornea at half depth and then back over the bleb to one side of the leak, and a bite is taken of conjunctiva and Tenon's capsule behind the bleb. B. The stitch is then passed back over the bleb on the other side of the leak and tied tightly, the knot is trimmed, and the knot is rotated into the peripheral part of the cornea.*

FIGURE 39-6. *Compression stitches for a bleb causing a corneal dellen. A. A nasal filtering bleb with a high profile near the limbus produced a quite painful dellen. B. Two 9-0 nylon compression stitches in place over the bleb, flattening it. C. Final bleb appearance after stitch removal at 2 weeks, with "white suspenders" of apparent connective tissue now present within the bleb, holding it in a lower profile. The dellen had healed and did not recur in the remaining 2 years the patient lived.*

of the upper lid over the cornea which is necessary for the spreading of meibomian gland secretions over the tear film, resulting in areas lacking the oily layer, consequent local tear break up, dry spots, and dellen formation (Fig. 39-6). Third, when high, ischemic blebs have a crescentic shape that parallels the limbus (Fig. 39-7A), the movement of the upper eyelid over them may capture air, forming large bubbles of tear fluid that subsequently pop (Fig. 39-7B), apparently producing a mild local trauma and burning pain, termed *bubble dysesthesia* (26).

Treatment of Tenon's cyst blebs, which are generally associated with elevated IOP, consists of lubrication with

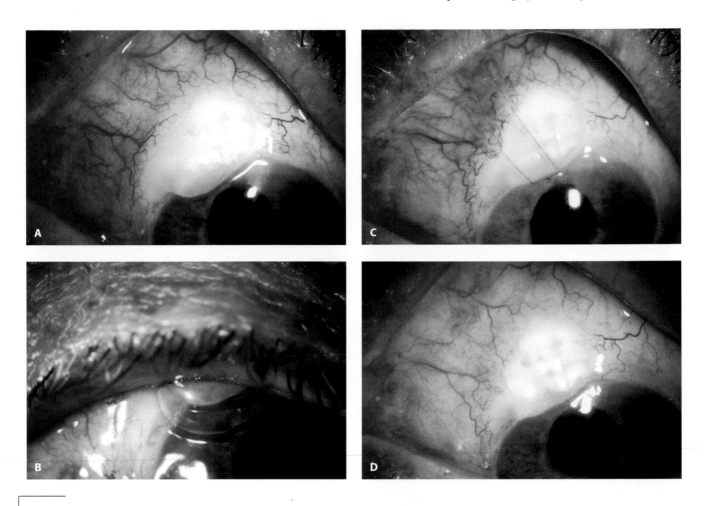

FIGURE 39-7. *Compression stitches for "bubble dysesthesia". A. The kidney-shaped bleb that enabled formation of bubbles from air and tears when the lid passed over the temporal side of the bleb. B. A large bubble of air and tears was formed by passage of the lid over the bleb during normal blinking. C. A 9-0 nylon compression stitch is in place over the bleb. D. After 3 weeks the stitch was removed and the profile of the bleb was reduced in height in the offending region, with marked reduction in bubble formation and an 85% reduction in subjective discomfort.*

artificial tears to reduce friction and improve the stability of the tear film, coupled with supplemental medical therapy to reduce the IOP, which may allow the compressed Tenon's capsule in the bleb wall to hydrate and the bleb to become less tense and lower in profile. If medical therapy for 6 months proves ineffective or the pressure is judged too high to wait, needling, as discussed already, may prove effective. Revision to excise much of the connective tissue in the Tenon's cyst wall can relieve the problem, but recurrence is common.

The blebs that cause bubble dysesthesia are quite different from the Tenon's cyst type of bleb. They are usually ischemic, thin walled, and associated with low-normal pressures. The incidence of such ischemic blebs has increased with the use of antimetabolites in filtering surgery. Treatment with artificial tears is rarely sufficient in alleviating the discomfort. I have found that bleb compression stitches are quite successful in treating this problem. One or more 9-0 nylon sutures are anchored in cornea, passed back over the

portion of the bleb that is capturing air upon blinking, anchored in conjunctiva–Tenon's capsule posterior to the bleb, and passed back over the bleb. The knot is tied tightly and rotated into the cornea (Fig. 39-7C). If the bleb is so thin that the cinching up of the stitches might traumatize the bleb surface, then prior to suture placement one can aspirate a small amount of aqueous from the anterior chamber through the cornea with a 30-gauge needle on a tuberculin syringe to decompress the bleb. Some 1 to 4 weeks after compression suture placement, when the conjunctiva under the mattress compression stitch appears to have contracted, forming "white suspenders," the stitch is removed. The bleb is then reduced in height (Fig. 39-7D) and no longer forms bubbles after blinking. Tenon's cyst blebs can also be reduced in height and dellen resolved with compression stitches (see Figs. 39-6B and 6C). Approximately 83% of patients achieved substantial subjective improvement with one treatment. The pressure control was unaffected by such treatment.

EXUBERANT BLEB

Usually a bleb will not enlarge in such a way as to grow down onto the cornea. Perhaps the Tenon's insertion into the limbal sclera is the barrier that usually prevents herniation of hydrated Tenon's under the corneal epithelium. When a bleb does expand onto the cornea (Fig. 39-8), it can produce several unwanted consequences. First, it can interfere with the proper spread of the surface oily layer of the tears, producing dellen. Second, the bleb and overlying lid can exert a distorting force on the superior aspect of the cornea, producing irregular astigmatism and reduced best-corrected visual acuity. Third, and rarely, the bleb can grow down over the pupil, interfering with vision.

When an exuberant bleb causes symptoms, I either recess it or amputate it. The portion of the bleb that overhangs the cornea is first pushed back to the limbus with a dull spatula. A cleavage plane has always been found under the bleb. If the exuberant portion of the bleb is ischemic and thin, after it is undermined and pushed back up superior

to the limbus one can place a compression stitch, which in a few weeks results in a permanent contraction of that portion of the bleb. However, when the exuberant portion of the bleb is spongy in appearance, one can simply cut it off at the limbus with curved Vannas scissors. The cut edge of the bleb nearly always demonstrates negative results on Seidel's test, and resuturing in such cases is unnecessary. One need not amputate the entire bleb to deal with an exuberant bleb.

INFECTED BLEB

With the advent of antimetabolites in filtering surgery, blebs that are thinner and more subject to infection are being produced (Fig. 39-9). The risk of infection over a several-year period was 0.2% to 0.5% in the era of guarded procedures without antimetabolites (27,28), but has risen to 1% to 4% with the use of either 5-fluorouracil or mitomycin (29–31), similar to the risk in the era of full-thickness filtering procedures, which produced thin and cystic blebs (32,33).

The blebs produced with guarded procedures and without antimetabolites are often quite low in profile. Supplemental medical therapy is required in more than half the patients after several years, suggesting that there is often little, if any, flow through them. Part of the reason for the low rate of infection with such blebs is that many of them were nonfunctional. They also commonly yield pressures that, even with reinstituted medical therapy, are in the upper-normal range, and thus are inadequate to prevent progressive visual field loss in one-third to one-half of patients (34–37). Indeed, in this regard the introduction of guarded procedures was a step backward in glaucoma management, even though they did reduce the incidence of complications. Fortunately, the advent of antimetabolite use

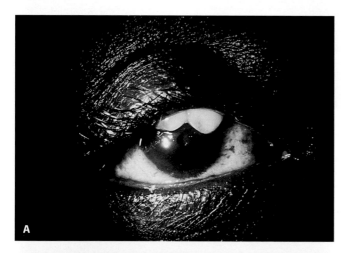

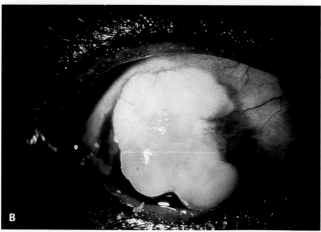

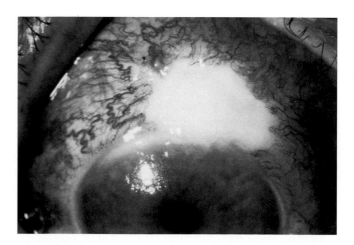

FIGURE 39-8.   *Exuberant bleb. A. An exuberant bleb has extended down over the limbus. B. The same bleb viewed with the lid lifted and the patient looking down.*

FIGURE 39-9.   *Bleb-related endophthalmitis. Infected bleb in a patient with an upper respiratory tract infection with* Hemophilus influenzae.

in guarded filtering surgery may now allow for the better pressure control needed to reduce the risk of glaucoma progression and avoid the early postoperative complications associated with full-thickness procedures.

The finding of an increased risk of infection with antimetabolite-produced blebs is not an adequate argument for a return to filtering surgery without antimetabolites, but rather a reason to seek ways of reducing the risk of such infection. The most important risk factor identified is bleb placement at the inferior limbus. Wolner et al (38) reported that the risk of either blebitis or endophthalmitis was 9% for filters at the inferior limbus and 3% for filters at the superior limbus at a few years after filtering surgery with adjunctive 5-fluorouracil. Higginbotham et al (39) reported a cumulative incidence of 8.9% for filters below and 1.1% above for mitomycin-augmented procedures, Coronia et al (40) reported similar results (11.5% for filters below for procedures with primarily 5-fluorouracil and some with mitomycin), and colleagues and I (41) reported a cumulative incidence of 8% for filters below and 1.3% for filters above—with mitomycin. As a result of these findings, I advocate performing filtering surgery with adjunctive 5-fluorouracil or mitomycin quite close to the 12-o'clock position, where the barrier of the Tenon's capsule is thickest and where the bleb will be protected by the upper eyelid, will not be rubbed by passage of the lid margin over the bleb during blinking, and will not be in contact with the meibomian gland orifices. In patients with posterior blepharitis, I also recommend treatment with warm compresses and oral doxycycline to eliminate obstruction of the gland orifices and infection of the glands. I also noted that laser suture lysis with a 50-μm spot size risks not only immediate hole formation (see Fig. 39-4), but also a more subtle burning of ischemic blebs, which later results in the adhesion of Tenon's capsule to the sclera that dimples the bleb surface, and later produces tractional hole formation. In one such case, a patient presenting with endophthalmitis had a strand of mucopurulent material that was attached to the bleb exactly over the cut in a scleral flap suture. I have found that use of an argon laser with a 100- or 200-μm spot size enables facile cutting of flap sutures at quite low energies, 0.3 to 0.6 W, for 0.02- to 0.05 second, with a much reduced risk of whitening the overlying bleb. The sutures are cut just as easily, despite use of only one-fourth to one-sixteenth the energy density, perhaps because the suture is being heated over a longer length than occurs with a 50-μm spot size. This finding of greater safety with an argon laser and a larger spot size may be analogous to the observation of Lieberman (12) that the 75-μm spot size of the diode laser cuts stitches well, without producing conjunctival burns. One can also use a krypton laser to cut nylon stitches, with a 50-μm spot size and 0.3 to 0.6 W, for 0.02- to 0.10-second, as the wavelength of the krypton laser penetrates conjunctiva and Tenon's capsule well, usually not producing burns, even if some blood is present, and it is well absorbed by nylon sutures.

Blebitis, a condition in which a cellular reaction is noted in the bleb, with surrounding conjunctival hyperemia, but the anterior chamber is clear or nearly so, can be adequately treated with topical and perhaps subconjunctival antibiotics and steroids, without resort to intravitreal injection of antibiotics (42). It is not clear whether this condition actually represents an infection or may represent an immunologic condition in which antigens outside the eye are reaching the anterior chamber, usually a privileged immunologic site (43). Of note, there are very large differences in the relative incidences of blebitis and endophthalmitis in different series, with Wolner et al (38) reporting 7 cases of blebitis and only 2 of endophthalmitis in their series of 5-fluorouracil–augmented procedures, whereas colleagues and I observed only 4 cases of blebitis and 19 cases of endophthalmitis in 1400 eyes treated with mitomycin. I usually maintain patients on one drop of prednisolone acetate daily for a very long time after primary filtering surgery, and usually do not ever stop it in patients who have had complex filtering surgery. I suspect that many cases of blebitis reported by others who do not continue steroid therapy are due not to infections, but to an immunologic phenomenon. I successfully treated cases of blebitis for which there was a low index of suspicion for infection (e.g., no bleb hypopyon, no mucopurulent discharge) by use of steroids alone, or at least with immediate use of steroids along with antibiotics. I especially recommend treatment with steroids alone when blebitis occurs about 3 to 9 days after suspension of the use of postoperative steroids, where the condition is almost surely due to steroid withdrawal iritis (44).

Bleb-associated endophthalmitis, with marked anterior-chamber reaction and vitreal involvement, requires a vitreous tap for culture and intravitreal injection of antibiotics and steroid.

The current therapy at the Bascom Palmer Eye Institute includes vitreous aspiration for culture, and injection of 1 mg of vancomycin, 2.25 mg of ceftazidine, and 400 μg of dexamethasone (each in a volume of 0.1 mL) into the vitreous cavity, along with subconjunctival injection of fortified vancomycin 25 mg and ceftazidine 100 mg. Vitrectomy is performed when the vitreal opacity is great. It is currently not possible to say whether vitrectomy should be reserved for patients with only light perception vision, as has been advocated for postcataract endophthalmitis as the result of the National Eye Institute–sponsored trial (45), as the organisms that most often cause bleb-associated endophthalmitis, β-hemolytic streptococcus and *Hemophilus influenzae*, are far more virulent than are *Staphylococcus epidermidis* and *Staphylococcus aureus* organisms that cause most postcataract infections. The failure of intravenous administration of antibiotic to show any benefit in the postcataract endophthalmitis trial may not have precluded the potential benefit of the use of other antibiotics, especially those that penetrate the eye better when administered intravenously. However, it does appear that intravitreal antibiotics are sufficient to sterilize the eye in most patients.

FLAT ANTERIOR CHAMBER

A flat anterior chamber can occur postoperatively, owing to overfiltration, diversion of aqueous through the uveal-scleral tract due to choroidal detachment or a cyclodialysis cleft, or forward displacement of the lens-iris diaphragm by aqueous misdirection or suprachoroidal hemorrhage. By far the most common cause is overfiltration due to failure to adequately test and adjust the scleral flap resistance during filtration surgery. Such creation of adequate scleral flap resistance is made especially important when either 5-fluorouracil or mitomycin has been employed, as these markedly reduce the formation of resistance to flow through the Tenon's capsule and conjunctiva. Consequently, one must abandon the old strategy of sewing scleral flap sutures just tight enough to hold the anterior chamber at surgery, since antimetabolite use prevents the development of further resistance to flow in the Tenon's capsule–conjunctiva over the next few days that one used to depend on to yield the desired pressure. Without a rise in pressure over the first few days after surgery, an IOP of 2 to 6 mm Hg is likely to result in the accumulation of serous fluid in the suprachoroidal space and a choroidal detachment, which then allows secreted aqueous to exit via the uveal-scleral pathway, causing the hypotony to persist and further contributing to anterior-chamber shallowing by causing an anterior rotation of the ciliary body. The diversion of aqueous flow also deprives the filtering bleb of sufficient flow to maintain it, and vascularization and scarring may occur.

When a truly flat anterior chamber occurs (i.e., with lens-cornea touch), action must be taken immediately to re-form the chamber. Contact between the lens epithelium and corneal endothelium deprives each of these metabolically active tissues of its source of nutrition, the aqueous humor, and persistent touch can result in cataract formation and corneal decompensation within a period of several hours to a day. Re-formation of the chamber can be accomplished by either tamponade or resuturing of the filtration site or by filling the anterior chamber with a viscoelastic agent or air. When no antimetabolite has been used, short-term measures may suffice. A pressure patch of cotton pads, placed to exert pressure over the filtration site, may increase the resistance to aqueous outflow sufficiently to re-form the chamber. However, one would be wise to remove the patch within half an hour to determine that the chamber has indeed re-formed, and then to replace it and see the patient again within a day. The use of a Simmons' shell tamponade (Fig. 39-10), which has a depression in its plastic surface that presses selectively over the filtration site, is a more reliable means of maintaining a chamber. The use of air or a viscoelastic agent should be seen as a very temporary measure, as neither is likely to hold the chamber for more than a few hours. When a flat chamber occurs and antimetabolites were used in the filtration surgery, it is usually necessary to return to the operating room to place additional scleral flap sutures

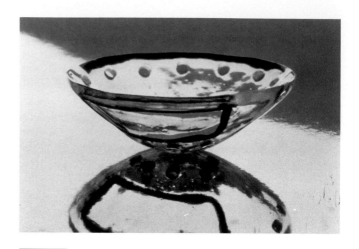

FIGURE 39-10. *Simmons' shell tamponade. The device has a depressed portion, outlined in black, that fits over the bleb to tamponade flow.*

to increase the resistance to outflow. Choroidal detachments may also need to be drained to eliminate excessive uveoscleral outflow (see below).

When an anterior chamber is merely shallow, perhaps with iris-cornea touch but without lens-cornea touch, one may observe as long as the bleb is inflated and any choroidal detachments are not kissing or at least are not likely to become adherent to each other owing to excessive inflammation. When fibrin bridges across touching choroidal detachments, re-formation of the chamber and drainage of the choroidal detachments is indicated. Otherwise, one can observe the situation, and usually the choroidal detachments will resolve spontaneously in several days to a month. Observation is likely the best choice when the pressure is at least 6 mm Hg, the choroidal detachments are small or moderate in size, the choroidal detachments and shallowness of the anterior chamber are not rapidly worsening during the first few days of observation, and a functional bleb is present.

It is generally believed that patients with choroidal detachments or shallow anterior chambers should be treated with intensive topical steroids (i.e., prednisolone acetate 1% every 2 hours) to reduce inflammation, vascular leakage, and synechia formation, and topical atropine (1% twice daily) to deepen the chamber by cycloplegia and to avoid synechia formation by dilation. Deepening the chamber with atropine also reduces the risk of the development of aqueous misdirection. More controversial is the use of oral steroids to treat choroidal detachments. While oral steroids may indeed reduce vascular leakage and speed resolution of the choroidal detachments, they have significant risks of raising blood pressure and blood glucose values, and their use should be determined by the severity of the ocular condition and the risk of side effects in each patient.

AQUEOUS MISDIRECTION

A serious postoperative complication of filtration surgery is the development of aqueous misdirection, also known as *ciliary block glaucoma* or *malignant glaucoma*. In this condition, the flow of aqueous humor from the posterior chamber is diverted to the vitreous cavity, forcing the vitreous body and lens-iris diaphragm forward. The anterior chamber shallows and the IOP rises. Aqueous misdirection occurs after no more than 1% to 2% of filtration surgery procedures, but occurs especially in an eye that is congested owing to an attack of angle-closure glaucoma and in which the anterior chamber was already shallow owing to hyperopia or over-filtration.

The mechanism by which aqueous misdirection develops is uncertain, but initially may involve a forward displacement of the lens and vitreous due to choroidal congestion or overfiltration, resulting in apposition of the lens and ciliary body, with the latter acting like an O ring to seal the passage of aqueous forward. Congestion of the ciliary processes, fibrin deposition, and even the forward movement of the vitreous base due to choroidal congestion may also play roles in obstructing forward aqueous flow. However, pupillary block does not contribute to the mechanism, as attested by the lack of iris bombé and the inability of iridectomy to resolve the blockage.

The initial medical treatment of aqueous misdirection consists of cycloplegia and mydriasis with atropine and phenylephrine; reduction in aqueous flow with β-blockers, carbonic anhydrase inhibitors, and perhaps apraclonidine or brimonidine; and reduction in vitreous volume with osmotic agents (46). When initial medical treatment is successful, use of atropine for at least a few months is advised to reduce the risk of recurrence. Unfortunately, initial medical treatment is not successful in at least half of the patients seen, and I would advise moving on to more definitive treatment within 24 hours if there is no response, not waiting 5 days as is often advocated in textbooks, especially if the pressure is very high. If the patient is pseudophakic and an iridectomy of sufficient size is present and corneal clarity is sufficient, yttrium-aluminum-garnet (YAG) laser treatment to create a hole in the zonular apparatus behind the iridectomy and to disrupt the anterior vitreous face is often successful (47). If medical and laser therapy fail, as they do in the majority of patients, definitive results may be obtained with pars plana vitrectomy to remove the vitreous body (48). To be successful, such vitrectomy may need to include removal of the vitreous quite close to the back of the lens capsule. Testing should be performed intraoperatively at the end of vitrectomy to see if re-formation of the anterior chamber through a paracentesis results in recurrence of aqueous misdirection, with passage of the injected balanced salt solution back through the zonular diaphragm as if through a one-way valve. If this occurs, the treatment has been incomplete and one will need either to perform a lensectomy in phakic patients or to pass a vitreous cutting instrument through the zonular apparatus and peripheral iris into the anterior chamber, creating a direct connection between the vitreous cavity and the anterior chamber and definitively resolving the blockage (48).

HYPOTONY MACULOPATHY

The use of antimetabolites in filtering surgery has increased the incidence of cases in which the visual acuity is reduced because of persistent hypotony. Such reduction in vision occurs in two forms, a milder form in which the vision is reduced by the presence of irregular or variable astigmatism, and a more severe form in which the vision is reduced by the presence of chorioretinal folds, which Gass named *hypotony maculopathy* (49). Although hypotony maculopathy was recognized as early as 1955 by Dellaporta (50), it rarely occurred after even full-thickness filtering surgery, was unheard of after trabeculectomy in the preantimetabolite era, and was rare even after 5-fluorouracil filtering surgery (51). With mitomycin use, however, the incidence of hypotony maculopathy has been reported to be 2% to 24% after primary filtering surgery and 1% to 5% after complex filtering surgery (7–9,17,18,52–56).

The mechanism by which persistent hypotony produces chorioretinal folds is probably scleral contraction. In accord with this idea is the observation of a reduction in axial length as measured by ultrasonography and a corresponding 1- to 2-diopter hyperopic shift that persists even after the eye is redistended. Such scleral contraction and hypotony maculopathy occur more frequently in the young (in whom the sclera is more elastic), in myopes (in whom the sclera is thinner), in patients in whom the preoperative pressure was particularly high (in whom the sclera had been stretched), and in patients in whom the postoperative pressure became 0 to 2 mm Hg (in whom the sclera was under virtually no stretch).

The persistent hypotony in such patients appears to be due to inhibition by mitomycin of the formation of a resistance to aqueous outflow in the Tenon's capsule and episclera, coupled with the loss of scleral flap resistance to aqueous flow caused by laser suture lysis. An alternative mechanism, ciliary body injury from the penetration of mitomycin, has been suggested, but appears unlikely to play a major role because hypotony never occurs in the absence of an ischemic filtering bleb, and the hypotony promptly resolves upon resuturing of the scleral flap. Nevertheless, there is evidence that aqueous humor flow is reduced on average by about 25% in eyes receiving mitomycin that developed especially low pressures (57) (<9 mm Hg).

The best way of dealing with hypotony maculopathy is to prevent its occurrence. I devised a "corneal safety-valve incision" for filtering surgery in which aqueous must flow through a short tunnel in front of the base of the scleral flap

(Fig. 39-11). The incision itself acts as a valve that sets a minimum IOP (usually 4–6 mm Hg) for the eye. Since this base pressure depends only on wound architecture, when successfully constructed the safety-valve effect should prevent the pressure from ever falling below the opening pressure. Sutures in the scleral flap then add additional resistance, adjusting the IOP at equilibrium to the desired level (usually 8–12 mm Hg). With the technique, the incidence of hypotony maculopathy was 3.8% in primary mitomycin filtering procedures, 1.0% in combined procedures, and 0.5% in complex filters (4).

When hypotony maculopathy occurs, it is best treated right away, as it will not go away spontaneously after mitomycin procedures, and Gass (49) noted that the chorioretinal folds can become permanent over a period of weeks to

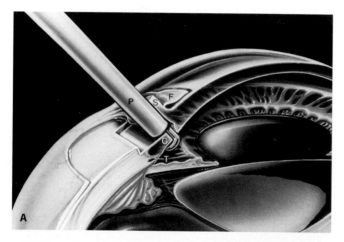

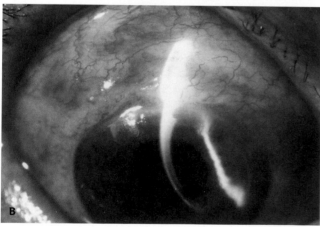

FIGURE 39-11.   *Corneal safety-valve incision. A. A Kelly punch performs a posterior lip sclerectomy at the internal entry of a tunnel incision. The 0.75-mm punch in the 1.0-mm tunnel leaves a 0.25-mm tunnel in front of the base of the scleral flap to act as a valve to prevent hypotony. B. The wound seen from the corneal side. P = Kelly punch; S = scleral flap; F = flap of conjunctiva laid in cornea; C = corneal site to be punched; T = trabecular meshwork. (Reproduced by permission from Palmberg P. Prevention and management of complicated hypotony in trabeculectomy with mitomycin. Highlights Ophthalmol 1993;21:67–77.)*

months. Treatment with an oversized contact lens to tamponade over the bleb or with intrableb blood injection has a low success rate in reversing hypotony maculopathy. Resuturing the scleral flap to adjust the IOP to the mid-normal range has resolved the hypotony, but only restored vision in about half of the patients. However, I devised a surgical treatment that was successful in flattening the chorioretinal folds in the macula and restoring the vision to, or nearly to, the prefilter level in 18 patients (11 of our own and 7 referred), with no failures and two recurrences (subsequently successfully reoperated). The technique is described in detail elsewhere (4). Briefly, it involves reoperating to place two sets of stitches in the scleral flap, one set to adjust the IOP at equilibrium flow to 8 to 12 mm Hg, and a second set of sutures to adjust the IOP to about 20 to 25 mm Hg, in order to temporarily stretch the sclera and thus flatten the chorioretinal folds (Fig. 39-12). The flattening takes a few days to 4 weeks, after which the second set of stitches is cut by laser suture lysis to reduce the IOP to the target pressure set by the first set of stitches, which should be preserved, if possible, to avoid recurrence of hypotony. Recurrence of hypotony maculopathy was observed in 2 relatively young, myopic males at pressures of 6 and 8 mm Hg. This suggests that permanent scleral shrinking (evidenced by a hyperopic shift that remains after restoration of IOP) makes an eye vulnerable to a recurrence of hypotony maculopathy at a low-normal pressure that would not be sufficiently low to produce hypotony maculopathy initially.

CHOROIDAL DETACHMENT AND POSTOPERATIVE (DELAYED) SUPRACHOROIDAL HEMORRHAGE

The occurrence of choroidal detachment and the rationale for its management were detailed earlier. This section deals with the differentiation of choroidal detachment due to accumulation of serous fluid from that due to delayed suprachoroidal hemorrage, and the management of the latter.

For the most part, suprachoroidal hemorrhage occurs during the first week after filtration surgery or after changes in IOP due to laser suture lysis or lysis of a seton ligature. The risk of its occurrence is low, about 1%, when the preoperative IOP is 20 mm Hg or less, but rises steeply for higher preoperative pressures, to 6% for pressures higher than 30 mm Hg and 12% for pressures higher than 40 mm Hg (58). The risk is also higher in the eyes of patients with high myopia, with systemic hypertension, or after a vitrectomy. The hemorrhage often occurs during a Valsalva maneuver, such as coughing, sneezing, or blowing of the nose, or when putting the head lower than the heart, during heavy lifting, or during defecation. In all of these situations, a pressure wave passes along blood vessels in the wall of the eye, and could lead to a vascular rupture. The dependence of the risk of hemorrhage on the preoperative IOP suggests that either reduced vascular tone in arterioles or vascular

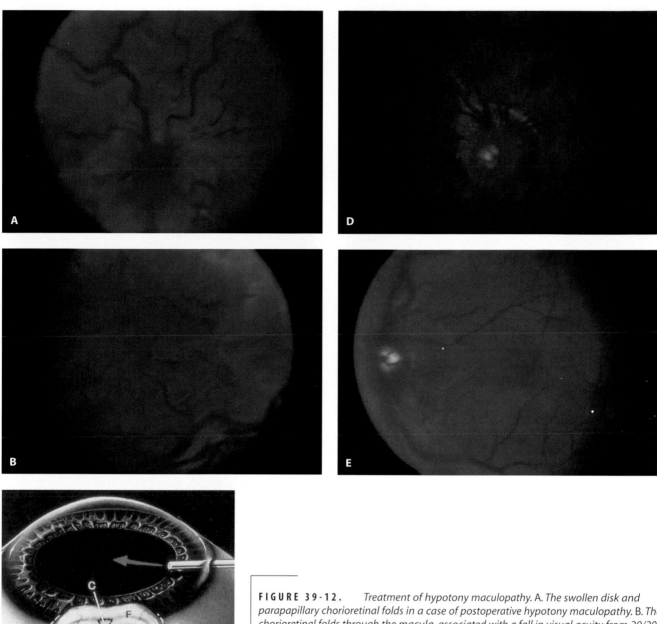

FIGURE 39-12. *Treatment of hypotony maculopathy. A. The swollen disk and parapapillary chorioretinal folds in a case of postoperative hypotony maculopathy. B. The chorioretinal folds through the macula, associated with a fall in visual acuity from 20/20 to 6/200. C. The two-sets-of-stitches technique, with set A (two stitches) applied to adjust the pressure at equilibrium flow to 8 to 12 mm Hg and set B (one stitch) applied to adjust the pressure at equilibrium flow to about 20 to 25 mm Hg. D. The disk after resolution of hypotony maculopathy at 4 weeks. E. The macula after resolution of hypotony maculopathy at 4 weeks, with a visual acuity of 20/20 − 3 and no more symptoms of distortion. C = corneal site of filtering ostium; F = flap of conjunctiva resting on cornea.*

congestion in veins and capillaries, or both, are predisposing factors.

Several surgeon-controlled factors appear to reduce the risk of suprachoroidal hemorrhage. When possible, the IOP should be reduced by intensified medical therapy for a few days preoperatively. It is much safer to operate on an eye with a pressure of 30 mm Hg than one with a pressure of 50 mm Hg. When the preoperative IOP has been 30 mm Hg or more, or the eye has the risk factors of high myopia, systemic hypertension, or a previous vitrectomy, it is probably

wise to use additional scleral flap sutures to adjust the IOP to about 20 mm Hg at equilibrium flow, after using a normal set of stitches to create a resistance to flow that will yield the IOP that one would like to achieve (e.g., 8–12 mm Hg). The latter sutures may then be cut by laser or released after a week when the period of higher risk of hemorrhage has passed. I also observed a reduction in the incidence of suprachoroidal hemorrhage after instructing patients during the first postoperative week to open their mouth when coughing, sneezing, or blowing their nose, in order to relieve the buildup of air pressure, and to first bend their knees, when picking up their shoes or other objects on the floor, in order to keep the head above the heart. They are also instructed to go for walks and to eat fruits and vegetables to avoid constipation.

Despite patients' taking precautions, some suprachoroidal hemorrhages will occur. Depending on the volume and rapidity of bleeding, the patient may either feel the onset of a severe pain in the eye and note a shadow in the vision or, with small and self-limited hemorrhages, feel and note nothing. Severe hemorrhages, presumably from the rupture of short posterior ciliary arteries, will cause severe pain due to distention of the choroid and high IOP, and will expand the suprachoroidal space on one side of the eye until it reaches the opposite wall. Forward expansion will shallow or flatten the anterior chamber. Eyes with recent extracapsular cataract wounds or corneal grafts may rupture. Owing to this risk, patients needing glaucoma surgery for a pressure of 35 mm Hg or more and corneal transplantation may best undergo an operation for glaucoma first, and then transplantation later, and combined procedures for cataract and glaucoma are best done by phacoemulsification with filtration performed in the tunnel incision, as such incisions shut rather than split open when the IOP rises suddenly.

The management of delayed suprachoroidal hemorrhage remains controversial. Some have advocated operating within a few days to evacuate the clot, others have advocated waiting about 2 weeks for the blood to liquefy (with B-scan ultrasonography being the best means of monitoring clot lysis), and others have observed just as good visual results by waiting for the hemorrhage to resorb spontaneously, as it nearly always does within a month. Action clearly is indicated in those few patients in whom breakthrough bleeding into the vitreous cavity occurs and ultrasound indicates the presence of a retinal detachment, or when choroidal expansion covers the filtering ostium and the pressure is very high. In the latter case, iridoplasty may contract the iris and free the filtering ostium, or partial clot evacuation may reduce the suprachoroidal volume sufficiently to uncover the filtering ostium.

One can differentiate serous choroidal detachments from suprachoroidal hemorrhage in several ways. A history of sudden, severe pain and the observation of an elevation of choroid coming from one side of the vitreous cavity suggests delayed suprachoroidal hemorrhage. On the other hand, the painless, gradual increase in size over several days or weeks of dome-shaped choroidal elevations on both the temporal and nasal sides of the vitreous cavity, in a setting of hypotony, suggests serous choroidal detachment. A purple discoloration to the usually brown color of the choroidal surface indicates that hemorrhage is present, but the discoloration is often not present when hemorrhage is. Definitive tests include transillumination of the mass using a Finoff light in a dark room, which will reveal either a transilluminating serous choroidal or a dark suprachoroidal hemor-

rhage, and A- and B-scan ultrasound, which differentiates the structureless serous choroidal detachment from the structure of blood clot.

It is usually unimportant to distinguish a small serous choroidal detachment from a small suprachoroidal hemorrhage, as both will resolve spontaneously with good visual results. With moderate to large elevations of the choroid, however, it may be useful to differentiate the cause in order to determine the management and the likely time to resolution. With a suprachoroidal hemorrhage, the choroidal elevation will likely increase in size for a while, due to imbibition of fluid as the clot lyses. One might consider draining the blood if "kissing" choroidal detachments are present, since the contact of choroid to choroid would likely continue for some time. During such a procedure, however, no action to alter the scleral flap resistance would be indicated. On the other hand, with moderate or serous choroidal detachments and a pressure value in the teens, resolution should occur spontaneously and soon, and no action would be needed. With large serous choroidal detachments and a pressure of 6 mm Hg or less, one might use a shell tamponade to hasten resolution by elevating the IOP, or if the condition showed no sign of resolution after 1 month, one would both drain the choroidals and revise the scleral flap to achieve sufficient resistance to prevent future hypotony and recurrence of choroidal detachments.

The technique for draining serous choroidal detachments may also be used for liquefied blood. A 7-0 Vicryl traction suture in the inferior corneal periphery may be used to supraduct the globe. A paracentesis is placed temporally, if one is not already present from the recent surgery. An inferior limbal peritomy is performed from the 4- to 8-o'clock positions and calipers are used to mark locations 3 mm behind the limbus in the 4:30- and 7:30-o'clock meridians. A half-thickness incision about 2 mm long and parallel to the limbus is then made, and a perpendicular incision is made posteriorly from one end, forming an L-shaped flap in each inferior quadrant (Fig. 39-13A). The apex of the L-shaped flap is then grasped and lifted with a toothed forceps, gaping the incision and giving countertraction, while a small sharp blade is used to deepen the incision little by little until the suprachoroidal space is opened. If the entry of the flaps happens to be over pockets of serous fluid or lysed blood, evacuation of them can be achieved simply by increasing the IOP by lifting the flap with a forceps, rolling a cotton-tipped swab along the scleral surface to milk fluid toward the opening (Fig. 39-13B), and periodically reinflating the eye by injecting balanced salt solution through the paracentesis. It may be helpful to absorb fluid from the opening with cellulose spear sponges. When the incisions do not happen to lie over pockets of fluid and a cotton-tipped swab does not mobilize the fluid, it may be necessary to use a cyclodialysis spatula to very gently separate the choroid from the inner wall of the sclera at the site of entry to obtain communication with an adjacent pocket of fluid. This is done while lifting the flap so that the entry of the spatula

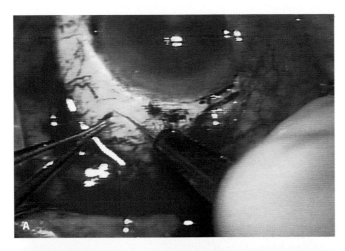

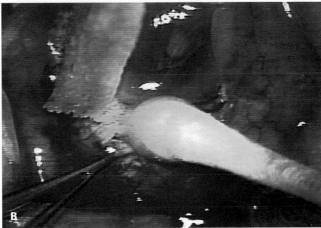

FIGURE 39-13. *Drainage of choroidal detachments. A. Cutting an L-shaped posterior sclerotomy. B. Pressing fluid to the sclerotomy with a rolling action of a cotton-tipped swab.*

is parallel to the inner wall of the sclera, and the passage should be for no more than a few millimeters. After drainage, when the outer surface of the choroid rises to the level of the incision, one can use indirect ophthalmoscopy to judge the adequacy of drainage or the location of additional fluid. Large residual pockets of fluid usually can be brought to the incision by use of the rolling action of a cotton-tipped swab. When all readily accessible fluid has been drained, the scleral incisions are left open (to help prevent reaccumulation of fluid) and the conjunctival peritomy is closed.

I do not advocate trying to evacuate large, formed clots. When very high IOPs with flat chambers require early intervention, drainage of only a small portion of the suprachoroidal blood may be necessary to achieve re-formation of the anterior chamber and to free the choroid from a filtration ostium. This can be done through a single small incision, as detailed already. More extensive procedures with large scleral incisions have been described for evacuation of large clots, but probably risk injury to the choroid

and retina, recurrence of hemorrhage, and extrusion of intraocular contents.

CATARACT

The most common cause of decreased visual function after filtration surgery is cataract. The average of literature values suggests about a 20% greater prevalence of cataract in the filtered eye compared to the opposite eye after a few years (59). Complications that interfere with lens metabolism are especially likely to promote cataract, as in postoperative flat chamber (with contact of the lens epithelium to the corneal endothelium) and choroidal detachment (which reduces aqueous flow over the lens by diversion to uveal-scleral outflow). In addition, the prolonged use of postoperative steroids is associated with posterior subcapsular cataract formation.

Colleagues and I and others developed techniques for filtration surgery that attempt to reduce the risk of cataract formation by avoiding instrumentation of the anterior chamber and the need for iridectomy. Zimmerman et al (60) reported a nonpenetrating trabeculectomy, and we use a corneal safety-valve incision, both of which yield filtration with enough resistance to aqueous flow to maintain a formed anterior chamber prior to placement of scleral flap sutures. Consequently, the iris does not become incarcerated in the site of filtration, even without an iridectomy. Theoretically, the omission of iridectomy should preserve the normal flow of aqueous over the lens equator and anterior epithelium by avoiding the shunting of aqueous from the posterior chamber to the anterior chamber through the iridectomy. However, in comparing consecutive series done with and without an iridectomy, colleagues and I did not observe a significant difference in cataract incidence (61). Further, an iridectomy should be performed whenever the anterior chamber is shallow prior to placement of scleral flap sutures, or in patients likely to squeeze their lids postoperatively (all children and those adults with blepharospasm), as otherwise there is a significant risk of iris incarceration in the ostium at a later date.

The advent of small-incision phacoemulsification has simplified the management of cataract occurring after filtration surgery. One can remove the lens from a temporal approach through the limbus or clear cornea, without injuring a superior limbal bleb. About 10% of blebs will be lost to postcataract surgery inflammation, however.

CONCLUSIONS

The use of guarded filtering procedures and adjunctive antimetabolites, with intraoperative estimation of the IOP at equilibrium flow and adjustment of scleral flap resistance as needed, has greatly increased the predictability and therefore the effectiveness and safety of filtration surgery. Excessive postoperative scarring of the filtration site and overfiltration can be markedly reduced through these means. While the use of antimetabolites has markedly improved the ability to achieve target pressures previously associated with visual field stability, they also result in an increased rate of such complications as hypotony maculopathy and bleb leaks and infections. Improved techniques can reduce the incidence of these complications, and most postoperative complications can be treated successfully.

REFERENCES

1. Palmberg P. Combined cataract and glaucoma surgery with mitomycin. *Ophthalmol Clin North Am* 1995;8:365–381.

2. Palmberg P. Prevention and management of complicated hypotony in trabeculectomy with mitomycin. *Highlights Ophthalmol* 1993;21:67–77.

3. Shields MB, Scroggs MW, Sloop CM, et al. Clinical and histopathological observations concerning hypotony after trabeculectomy with adjunctive mitomycin C. *Am J Ophthalmol* 1993;116:673–683.

4. Suner IJ, Greenfield DS, Miller MP, et al. Hypotony maculopathy following filtering surgery with mitomycin C: incidence and treatment. *Ophthalmology* 1997;104:207–215.

5. Liebmann JM, Ritch R, Marmor M, et al. Initial 5-fluorouracil trabeculectomy in uncomplicated glaucoma. *Ophthalmology* 1991;98:1036–1041.

6. Goldenfeld M, Krupin T, Ruderman JM, et al. 5-Fluorouracil in initial trabeculectomy. A prospective, randomized, multicenter study. *Ophthalmology* 1994;101:1024–1029.

7. Chen C-W. Enhanced intraocular pressure controlling effectiveness of trabeculectomy by local application of mitomycin-C. *Trans Asia Pacific Acad Ophthalmol* 1983;9:172–177.

8. Kitazawa Y, Kawase K, Matsushita H, et al. Trabeculectomy with mitomycin. A comparative study with fluorouracil. *Arch Ophthalmol* 1991;109:1693–1698.

9. Skuta GL, Beeson CC, Higginbotham EJ, et al. Intraoperative mitomycin versus postoperative 5-fluorouracil in high-risk glaucoma filtering surgery. *Ophthalmology* 1992;99:438–444.

10. Hoskins KD, Migliazzo C. Management of failing filtering blebs with the argon laser. *Ophthalmic Surg* 1984;15:731–733.

11. Greenfield DS, Miller MP, Suner IJ, Palmberg P. Needle elevation of the scleral flap for failing filtration blebs after trabeculectomy with mitomycin. *Am J Ophthalmol* 1996;122:195–204.

12. Lieberman MF. Diode laser suture lysis. *Arch Ophthalmol* 1996;114:364.

13. Sherwood MB, Spaeth GL, Simmons ST, et al. Cysts of Tenon's capsule following filtration surgery: medical management. *Arch Ophthalmol* 1987;105:1517–1523.

14. Scott DR, Quigley HA. Medical management of a high bleb phase after trabeculectomies. *Ophthalmology* 1988;1169–1173.

15. Costa VP, Correa MM, Kara-Jose N. Needling versus medical treatment in encapsulated blebs: a randomized, prospective study. *Ophthalmology* 1997;104: 1215–1220.

16. Blok MD, Kok JH, Van Mil C, et al. Use of megasoft bandage lens for treatment of complications after trabeculectomy. *Am J Ophthalmol* 1990;110:264–268.

17. Wise JB. Treatment of chronic postfiltration hypotony by intrableb injection of autologous blood. *Arch Ophthalmol* 1993;111:827–830.

18. Nuyts RM, Greve EL, Geijssen HC, Langerhorst CT. Treatment of hypotonous maculopathy after trabeculectomy with mitomycin C. *Am J Ophthalmol* 1994;118:322–331.

19. Smith ME, Magauran RG, Betchkal J, Doyle JW. Treatment of postfiltration bleb leaks with autologous blood. *Ophthalmology* 1995;102:868–871.

20. Zallas MM, Schuman JS. A serious complication of intrableb injection of autologous blood for the treatment of postfiltration hypotony. *Am J Ophthalmol* 1994;118:251–253.

21. Chen PP, Palmberg PF, David JL, Culbertson WW. Corneal graft rejection and recurrent toxoplasmosis after intrableb autologous blood injection. *Arch Ophthalmol* 1996;114:633. Letter.

22. Kajiwara K. Repair of a leaking bleb with fibrin glue. *Am J Ophthalmol* 1990;109:599–601.

23. Buxton JN, Lavery KT, Liebmann JM, et al. Reconstruction of filtering blebs with free conjunctival autografts. *Ophthalmology* 1994;101:635–639.

24. Wilson MR, Kotas-Neumann R. Free conjunctival patch for repair of persistent bleb leak. *Am J Ophthalmol* 1994;11:569–594.

25. Zacchei AC, Palmberg PF, Mendosa A, Robinson JC. Compression sutures: a new treatment leaking or painful filtering blebs. *Invest Ophthalmol Vis Sci* 1996;37(suppl):444.

26. Grajewski A, Hodapp E, Huang A. Bubble dysesthesia. Presented at the American Glaucoma Society meeting, Key West, FL, February 1995.

27. Katz LJ, Cantor LB, Spaeth GL. Complications of surgery in glaucoma. Early and late bacterial endophthalmitis following glaucoma filtering surgery. *Ophthalmology* 1985;92:959–963.

28. Mills KB. Trabeculectomy: a retrospective long-term follow-up of 444 cases. *Br J Ophthalmol* 1981;65:790–795.

29. Rockwood EJ, Parrish RK II, Heuer KD, et al. Glaucoma filtering surgery with 5-fluorouracil. *Ophthalmology* 1987;94:1071–1078.

30. The Fluorouracil Filtering Surgery Study Group. Three-year follow-up of the Fluorouracil Filtering Surgery Study. *Am J Ophthalmol* 1993;115:82–92.

31. Ticho U, Ophir A. Late complications after glaucoma filtering surgery with adjunctive 5-fluorouracil. *Am J Ophthalmol* 1993;115:506–510.

32. Hattenhauer JM, Lipsich MP. Late endophthalmitis after filtering surgery. *Am J Ophthalmol* 1971;72:1097–1101.

33. Tabara KF. Later infections following filtering procedures. *Ann Ophthalmol* 1976;8:1228–1231.

34. Roth SM, Spaeth GL, Starita RJ, et al. The effects of postoperative corticosteroids on trabeculectomy and the clinical course of glaucoma: five-year follow-up study. *Ophthalmic Surg* 1991;22:724–729.

35. Werner EB, Drance SM, Schulzer M. Trabeculectomy and the progression of glaucomatous field loss. *Arch Ophthalmol* 1977;95:1374–1377.

36. Greve EL, Dake CL. Four-year follow-up of a glaucoma operation. *Int Ophthalmol* 1979;1:139–145.

37. Rollins DR, Drance SM. Five-year follow-up of trabeculectomy in the management of chronic open angle glaucoma. In: New Orleans Acad Ophthalmol, Symposium on Glaucoma, 1981:295–300.

38. Wolner B, Liebmann JM, Sassani JW, et al. Late bleb-associated endophthalmitis after trabeculectomy with adjunctive 5-fluorouracil. *Ophthalmology* 1991;98: 1053–1060.

39. Higginbotham EJ, Stevens RK, Musch DC, et al. Bleb-related endophthalmitis after trabeculectomy with mitomycin C. *Ophthalmology* 1996; 103:650–656.

40. Coronia RM, Liebmann JM, Friedman R, et al. Trabeculectomy at the inferior limbus. *Arch Ophthalmol* 1996;114:387–391.

41. Greenfield DS, Suner IJ, Miller MP, et al. Endophthalmitis following filtering surgery with mitomycin. *Arch Ophthalmol* 1996;114:943–949.

42. Brown RH, Yang LH, Walker SD, et al. Treatment of bleb infection after glaucoma surgery. *Arch Ophthalmol* 1994;112:57–61.

43. Streilein JW, Takeuchi M, Taylor AW. Immune privilege, T-cell tolerance and tissue-restricted autoimmunity. *Hum Immunol* 1997;52:138–143. Review.

44. Krupin T, LeBlanc RP, Becker B, et al. Uveitis in association with topically administered corticosteroids. *Am J Ophthalmol* 1970;70:883–885.

45. Endophthalmitis Vitrectomy Study Group. Results of the Endophthalmitis Vitrectomy Study: a randomized trial of immediate vitrectomy and of intravenous antibiotics for the treatment of postoperative bacterial endophthalmitis. *Arch Ophthalmol* 1995;113:1479–1496.

46. Simmons RJ, Maestre FA. Malignant glaucoma. In: Ritch R, Shields MB, Krupin T, eds. *The glaucomas*. 2nd ed. Vol II. St. Louis: Mosby, 1996: 841–855.

47. Epstein DL, Steinert RF, Puliafito CA. Neodymium-YAG laser therapy to the anterior hyaloid in aphakic malignant (cilio-vitreal block) glaucoma. *Am J Ophthalmol* 1984;98:137–143.

48. Harbour JW, Rubsamen PE, Palmberg P. Pars plana vitrectomy in the management of phakic and pseudophakic malignant glaucoma. *Arch Ophthalmol* 1996;114:943–949.

49. Gass JDM. Hypotony maculopathy. In: Bellows JG, ed. *Contemporary ophthalmology*. Baltimore: Williams & Wilkins, 1972:343–366.

50. Dellaporta A. Fundus changes in postoperative hypotony. *Am J Ophthalmol* 1955;40:781–785.

51. Stamper RL, McMenemy M, Lieberman MF. Hypotonous maculopathy after trabeculectomy with subconjunctival 5-fluorouracil. *Am J Ophthalmol* 1992;114:544–553.

52. Neelakantan A, Rao BS, Vijaya L, et al. Effect of concentration and duration of application of mitomycin C in trabeculectomy. *Ophthalmic Surg* 1994;25: 612–615.

53. Kupin TH, Juzych MS, Shin DH, et al. Adjunctive mitomycin C in primary trabeculectomy in phakic eyes. *Am J Ophthalmol* 1995;119:30–39.

54. Kitazawa Y, Suemori-Matsushita H, Yamamoto T, Kawase K. Low-dose and high-dose mitomycin trabeculectomy as an initial surgery in primary open-angle glaucoma. *Ophthalmology* 1993;100:1624–1628.

55. Costa VP, Wilson RP, Moster MR, et al. Hypotony maculopathy following the use of topical mitomycin C in glaucoma filtration surgery. *Ophthalmic Surg* 1993;24:389–394.

56. Zacharia PT, Deppermann SR, Schuman JS. Ocular hypotony after trabeculectomy with mitomycin C. *Am J Ophthalmol* 1993;116:314–326.

57. Diestelhorst M, Uestuendag C, Kriegelstein GK. The effect of mitomycin C on aqueous humor flow, flare and intraocular pressure in eyes with glaucoma two years after trabeculectomy. Presented at the European Glaucoma Society, 5th Congress, Paris, June 22, 1996.

58. Fluorouracil Filtering Surgery Study Group. Risk factors for suprachoroidal hemorrhage after filtering surgery. *Am J Ophthalmol* 1992;113:501–507.

59. Liebmann JM, Ritch R. Complications of glaucoma filtering surgery. In: Ritch R, Shields MB, Krupin T, eds. *The glaucomas*. 2nd ed. Vol III. St Louis: Mosby, 1996:1703–1736.

60. Zimmerman TJ, Kooner KS, Ford VJ, et al. Trabeculectomy versus nonpenetrating trabeculectomy: a retrospective study of two procedures in phakic patients with glaucoma. *Ophthalmic Surg* 1984;15:734–740.

61. Norris E, Schiffman J, Palmberg P. Does an iridectomy increase the risk of cataract after filtering surgery? Presented at the Brazilian Congress of Ophthalmology, Goiana, Brazil, Sept. 5, 1997.

Surgical Pathology of Glaucoma

M. A. SAORNIL   DANIEL M. ALBERT

The surgery done for the treatment of glaucoma has the objective of decreasing the intraocular pressure by either increasing the outflow or reducing the production of aqueous humor, by modifying the anatomic structures involved in its production (ciliary body) or drainage (anterior-chamber angle). Surgical techniques for glaucoma can be carried out either conventionally or with different types of lasers, the uses of which are expanding. The objective of this chapter is to illustrate and review the bases and effects of the more usual surgical operations and adjuvant treatments on tissues, in both successful and unsuccessful cases.

BASES OF LASER TREATMENTS

Laser energy is very commonly used in glaucoma surgery. The tissue effects produced by the laser energy are of three types: thermal, ionizing, and photochemical (1).

The *thermal effect* consists of tissue heating by absorption of the laser energy at temperatures high enough to induce chemical changes that produce local inflammation and scarring (photocoagulation), or to vaporize intracellular and extracellular fluids (photovaporization). A short exposure time and high energy cause tissue disruption. This reaction can be used to make holes in ocular tissues (laser iridotomy). At lower energy levels, laser can produce contraction of collagen; this effect is the mechanism for pupilloplasty, iridoplasty, and perhaps, trabeculoplasty. When very intense laser energy is focused on a small area for a very short period of time, the *ionizing effect* adds to the thermal one and causes photodisruption. The neodymium:yttrium-aluminum-garnet (Nd:YAG) laser is the most commonly used photodisruptor. In glaucoma, photodisruption is intended to create iridotomies, or to re-establish outflow after filtering procedures failed, by cutting scar tissue. In malignant glau-

coma, photodisruption is used for vitreolysis. The target tissue can also be volatilized by the *photochemical effect* (photoablation, photodynamic therapy).

These tissue interactions with lasers, especially photocoagulation and photodisruption, are used in numerous glaucoma surgical procedures.

PROCEDURES ON THE TRABECULAR MESHWORK: ARGON LASER TRABECULOPLASTY

Procedures involving the trabecular meshwork have the objective of increasing the aqueous outflow by either widening the preexisting ducts or opening new apertures in the meshwork and adjacent structures. In 1961 Zweng and Flocks (2) first described laser application to the trabecular meshwork as glaucoma treatment. With the xenon arc photocoagulator of Meyer-Schwickerath, they coagulated the anterior-chamber angle in cats, dogs, and monkeys and the histopathologic effects revealed fragmentation of the trabecular meshwork and destruction of ciliary processes.

In the 1970s several investigators tried to make holes in the angle to provide direct communication between the anterior chamber and Schlemm's canal (laser trabeculotomy), but the results were very unpredictable and they lasted only weeks or months (3–5). Worthen and Wickham (5) described the histopathologic changes associated with argon laser applications in monkeys (Figs. 40-1, 40-2). They found trabecular perforations, which eventually closed in most eyes as a result of fibrosis, and that the reduction in intraocular pressure was usually temporary. In 1976 Ticho and Zauberman (6) realized that in spite of the lack of permanent openings in the trabecula, intraocular pressure reduction occurred in some patients. This led to a new concept in laser trabecular therapy in which lower energy levels were used to photocoagulate rather than penetrate the trabecular meshwork. Three years later, Wise and Witter (7) described a new method of laser treatment later called

trabeculoplasty. Several authors (8–10) corroborated the results and argon laser trabeculoplasty (ALT) became one of the most common procedures for modern glaucoma treatment. In spite of the clinical demonstration of the efficacy of ALT in increasing aqueous outflow (6,9,11–13), the mechanism of action of this technique is still uncertain.

Wise and Witter (7) postulated that localized burns in the trabecular meshwork caused shrinkage of collagen and trabecular retraction, which would open the meshwork between scars, increasing the aqueous outflow. Studies of laser-treated monkeys noted widened intertrabecular spaces (Fig. 40-3) (14). This "mechanical" theory, perhaps the most popular, is supported by several studies in humans and animals.

Histopathologic examination of the trabecular meshwork in human eyes after trabeculoplasty showed necrosis of the cells and disruption of the trabecular beams, without evidence of penetrating holes in Schlemm's canal (Fig. 40-4) (8,15,16).

Laboratory studies in monkeys indicated alternative or additional mechanisms of action, suggesting that laser treat-

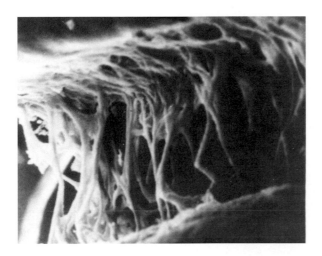

FIGURE 40-1. *Scanning electron photomicrograph illustrating the appearance of normal Cebus monkey angle. Note the smooth beams of the trabecular meshwork (below) and the even transition into the corneal endothelium (above). (×300.) (Reproduced by permission from Worthen DM, Wickam MG. Laser trabeculectomy in monkeys. Invest Ophthalmol Vis Sci 1973;12: 707–711.)*

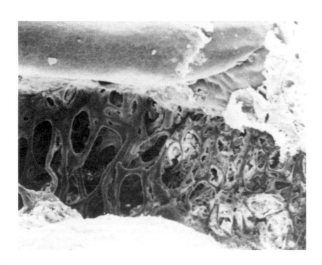

FIGURE 40-2. *Cebus monkey angle that received several bursts of 200 mW laser energy for 0.2 seconds using a 50-μ beam. The differential effect between the denuded corneal endothelium above and the less affected trabeculum below is apparently due to the number of individual bursts delivered in each location. The openings in treated trabeculum actually appear smaller than do those present in untreated area and appear white or "hot." (×500). (Reproduced by permission from Worthen DM, Wickam MG. Laser trabeculectomy in monkeys. Invest Ophthalmol Vis Sci 1973;12:707–711.)*

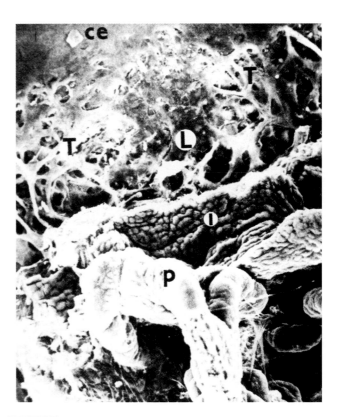

FIGURE 40-3. *Scanning electron micrograph of lasered site. Flattened, scarred laser region (L) covered by cellular extension from corneal endothelium (ce). The label T indicates adjacent, nonlasered trabecular meshwork; I, iris; and P, ciliary process. (×200.) (Reproduced by permission from Melamed S, Pei J, Epstein DL. Delayed response to argon laser trabeculoplasty in monkeys. Arch Ophthalmol 1986;104:1078–1083.)*

ment modifies the physiology in trabecular cells, based on findings such as changes in the glycosaminoglycan turnover and in the cell density, and increases in phagocytic activity or cellular division (Fig. 40-5) (16–21). Van Buskirk et al

(22) studied human autopsy eyes and found that ALT eliminates some trabecular cells, which may stimulate the remaining cells to produce an extracellular matrix of a different composition offering less resistance to aqueous flow.

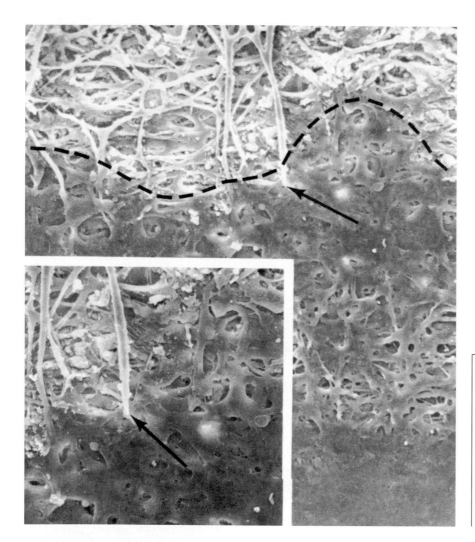

FIGURE 40-4.   *Eighteen hours after argon laser. The burn area showing coagulative necrosis is indicated by the area below the interrupted line. Note the fragmented trabecular beam (arrow) at the edge of the lesion. (SEM ×290.) Inset shows the same fragmented beam at higher magnification (arrow). (SEM ×440.) (Reproduced by permission from Rodrigues MM, Spaeth GL, Donohoo P. Electron microscopy of argon laser therapy is phakic open-angle glaucoma. Ophthalmology 1982;89:198–210.)*

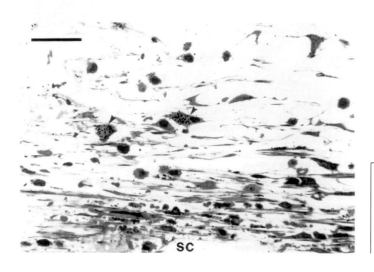

FIGURE 40-5.   *An argon laser burn with dividing cells (arrows) in the corneoscleral meshwork. The label SC indicates Schlemm's canal. Bar = 100 μm. (Reproduced by permission from Dueker DK, Norberg M, Johnson DH, et al. Stimulation of cell division by argon and Nd:YAG laser trabeculoplasty in cynomolgus monkeys. Invest Ophthalmol Vis Sci 1990;31:115–124.)*

All these findings suggest that ALT produces physiologic changes in trabecular cells.

Although laser trabeculoplasty has been performed almost exclusively with the argon blue-green laser, the argon green (23), krypton yellow and red (24), and Nd:YAG lasers (21) have been tested. Recently, the diode laser was tested and shown to accomplish this procedure successfully. McMillan et al (25) compared the effects of applications of the argon and the diode laser in the trabecular meshwork and concluded that the histopathologic changes are comparable at similar energy levels (Figs. 40-6 and 40-7).

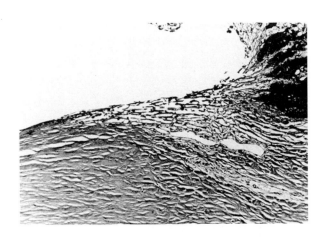

FIGURE 40-6.   *Light microscopic photograph of trabecular meshwork following diode laser trabeculoplasty (1200 mW, 0.1 seconds, 100 μ). No observable changes are visible. (H&E, ×125.) (Reprinted from McMillan TA, Stewart WC, Legler UFC, et al. Comparison of diode and argon laser trabeculoplasty in cadaver eyes.* Invest Ophthalmol Vis Sci *1994;35:706–710.)*

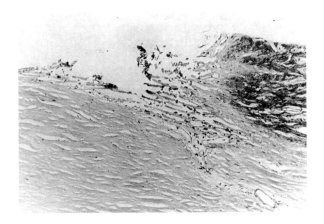

FIGURE 40-7.   *Light microscopic photograph of trabecular meshwork after argon laser trabeculoplasty (700 mW, 0.1 seconds, 50 μ). Trabecular beam fragmentation and coagulation with depression of the trabecular meshwork are visible. (H&E, ×125.) (Reprinted by permission from McMillan TA, Stewart WC, Legler UFC, et al. Comparison of diode and argon laser trabeculoplasty in cadaver eyes.* Invest Ophthalmol Vis Sci *1994;35:706–710.)*

PROCEDURES ON THE CILIARY BODY: CYCLOPHOTOCOAGULATION

Techniques acting on the ciliary body have the objective of reducing the intraocular pressure by decreasing aqueous production. These procedures are seldom the first choice of treatment because the results are difficult to predict, and damage to ocular structures or inflammation often leads to complications. These techniques are useful for patients in whom the more usual procedures have failed or are contraindicated.

Cyclocryotherapy has been the most commonly used cyclodestructive procedure, but laser cyclophotocoagulation is becoming the preferred technique. Other more recently evaluated cyclodestructive elements include ultrasound and microwaves (1). Cyclocryotherapy destroys the ciliary processes by producing intracellular ice crystals that are lethal for the cell and by inducing hemorrhagic infarction, resulting from the obliteration of the microcirculation in the frozen tissue leading to ischemic necrosis (10). Histologic studies of eyes treated with this procedure showed destruction of vascular, stromal, and epithelial elements of ciliary processes and substitution of these elements by a fibrous scar (Figs. 40-8 to 40-10) (26,27).

Photocoagulation of the ciliary body (cyclophotocoagulation) can be applied via a *transscleral* approach, passing through the conjunctiva, sclera, and ciliary muscle before reaching the ciliary processes, or a *transpupillary* route, directly over the ciliary body.

Transscleral cyclophotocoagulation was employed from the 1960s with different sources of light energy (28–31). However, widespread interest in the procedure came with the specially designed Nd:YAG laser (32–34). Other types including argon, krypton, and diode lasers have also been tested (Fig. 40-11) (35–37).

The transscleral route has the advantages of being quick, easy, and noninvasive, but the disadvantages include a lack of visualization of the processes treated and damage to the adjacent tissues, leading to unpredictable results and complications (1).

Histologic studies in rabbits showed that transscleral cyclophotocoagulation with the Nd:YAG laser causes selective destruction of the ciliary epithelium with formation of a blister-like elevation and damage to the vessels, leading to atrophy of the ciliary processes and reduction in intraocular pressure (33,34,38). These effects have been observed in pigmented but not in albino rabbits, suggesting that the laser energy is absorbed by the melanin in the pigmented epithelium (39). Comparison between the noncontact and the contact Nd:YAG laser in enucleated porcine and human eyes showed coagulative lesions in all eyes: Noncontact lesions were larger and more homogeneous and affected primarily the pigment epithelium, and contact lesions had full-thickness thermal effects, involving sclera (Figs. 40-12 and 40-13) (40). A shorter duration of exposure to the

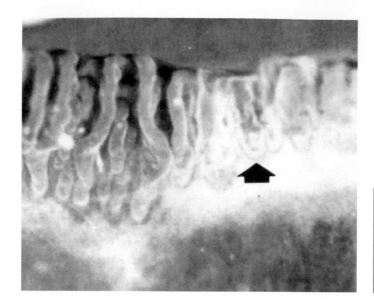

FIGURE 40-8.   *Gross appearance of ciliary pars plicata, one month after cryotherapy (M-5) at junction between treated (right) and untreated (left) areas. In the cryotreated area, the processes are lost with fibrous tissue replacement (arrow). (Reprinted by permission from Quigley HA. Histological and physiological studies of cyclocryotherapy in primate and human eyes. Am J Ophthalmol 1976;82:722–732.)*

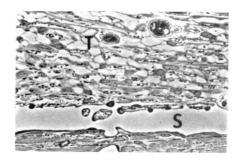 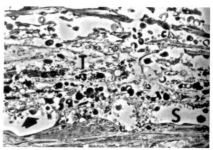

FIGURE 40-9.   *Light micrographs comparing monkey trabecular meshwork (T) and Schlemm's canal (S) in a normal eye (left) and in an eye immediately after cryotherapy with anterior probe placement (right). Note the red and white blood cells (right; arrow) filling the intertrabecular spaces and indistinct inner wall of Schlemm's canal. (Epoxy-embedded, paraphenylenediamine, phase contrast, ×375.) (Reprinted by permission from Quigley HA. Histological and physiological studies of cyclocryotherapy in primate and human eyes. Am J Ophthalmol 1976;82:722–732.)*

Nd:YAG laser is associated with greater tissue disruption and inflammation (41).

Use of the Nd:YAG or the krypton laser in rabbits resulted in similar lesions, with more inflammatory reaction occurring in krypton-induced lesions, in which 70% of the energy is absorbed by pigment epithelium compared to 30% for the Nd:YAG–induced lesions (42). The damage produced by the diode laser appeared more widespread than that created by the Nd:YAG laser, causing coagulative necrosis in the ciliary muscle (37,43).

Studies in human autopsy eyes or eyes enucleated after treatment showed changes similar to those observed in rabbits, with blister-like elevation of the ciliary epithelium with minimal ciliary muscle and scleral damage (44,45), scarce inflammatory cells between the epithelial layers and the stroma (46), and granulomatous inflammation, seen in one isolated eye enucleated 70 days after treatment (47). Examination of the eyes treated 24 hours before enucleation

revealed destruction of ciliary body epithelium, occlusion of the capillaries of the ciliary processes, and stromal necrosis (48). Above all, these findings suggest that the presumable mechanism for the decrease in intraocular pressure from transscleral Nd:YAG cyclophotocoagulation is the destruction of the ciliary epithelium.

Transpupillary cyclophotocoagulation consists of photocoagulation of the ciliary processes with the argon laser in eyes in which a sufficient number of the processes can be visualized gonioscopically (large iridectomy, neovascular glaucoma with retraction of the iris).

Histopathologic studies demonstrated the capability of the technique to selectively destroy ciliary processes (49–51). The effect in lowering intraocular pressure depends on the number of ciliary processes treated and the intensity of the laser burns in each process.

An optional technique in aphakic eyes with glaucoma is *intraocular cyclophotocoagulation*, endophotocoagulation through a pars plana incision with visualization through the pupillary route, usually in the course of a vitrectomy, leading also to the selective destruction of the ciliary processes (52–54).

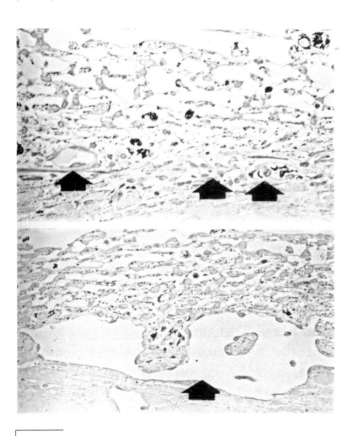

FIGURE 40-10. *Light micrographs of trabecular meshwork and Schlemm's canal from treated (top) and untreated (bottom) areas of the same monkey eye two months after cryotreatment. The meshwork shows no difference between areas, but Schlemm's canal (arrows) consists of three small segments in the treated area, while it has a normal large caliber at the opposite side of the eye. (Epoxy-embedded, paraphenylenediamine, phase contrast, ×250.) (Reprinted by permission from Quigley HA. Histological and physiological studies of cyclocryotherapy in primate and human eyes. Am J Ophthalmol 1976;82:722–732.)*

FILTERING SURGERY PROCEDURES

Laser Sclerostomy: Successful Bleb

Filtering operations are the most common techniques performed in adults with open-angle glaucoma. Whether incisional (the most frequent) or laser, all filtering operations share the same basic mechanism of action. The aim is to create an opening between the anterior chamber and the subconjunctival space through which aqueous humor flows directly (full-thickness fistula, or sclerostomy) or indirectly (partial-thickness fistula, or trabeculectomy) into the subconjunctival space (1).

In the 1980s March et al (55) reported their results using a high-power Q-switched Nd:YAG short-pulse laser in human cadaver eyes, which produces an explosion of tissue at the point of focus (nonthermal process) called *optical breakdown* (Figs. 40-14 to 40-16). In the eyes, with the cornea previously trephined, they demonstrated perforation of the sclera. Using a specially designed goniolens, a study on the eye of a patient scheduled for enucleation because of melanoma demonstrated the histopathologic sclerostomy without complication (56). The same procedure was then tested in cynomolgus monkeys and achieved a significant reduction in intraocular pressure (57). Examination with scanning electron microscopy revealed no significant damage to the iris, lens, or cornea, except in the area adjacent to the sclerostomy where the investigators found a focal rupture of Descemet's membrane and mild endothelial cell loss. The sclerostomy was evident for more than 180 days.

Modifications of the technique have been tested with the objective of enhancing the laser energy absorption of the sclera and introducing the new concept of dye-matched laser ablation using a pulse-dye laser. Scleral perforation is obtained at lower energy levels, diminishing the secondary effects (inflammation, hemorrhages, damage to surrounding structures). Wetzel and Scheu (58) designed an experimental study in rabbits to find an optimal combination of laser parameters with biocompatible dyes. Histologic examinations on the first postoperative day showed smaller thermal

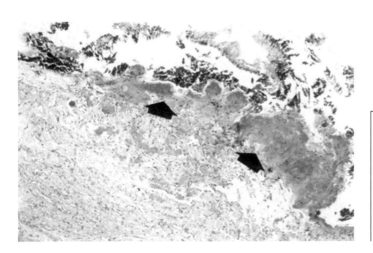

FIGURE 40-11. *Nd:YAG laser lesion at a duration of 2 seconds and 7300 mW showing marked disruption of the ciliary epithelium with pigment clumping. Focal coagulation of the underlying stroma is seen (arrows), but the remainder of the ciliary muscle is relatively undisturbed (H&E, ×125.) (Reprinted by permission from Simmons RB, Prum BE Jr, Shields SR, et al. Videographic and histologic comparison of Nd:YAG and diode laser contact transscleral cyclophotocoagulation. Am J Ophthalmol 1994;117:337–341.)*

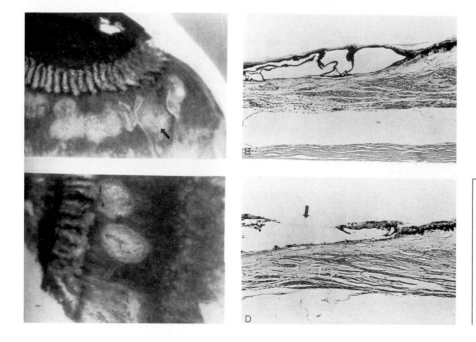

FIGURE 40-12. *Noncontact laser at 3 mm posterior to the limbus in human eyes. Moderate burns (A, arrow; B) and more severe neuroepithelial perforations (D, arrow) are seen in pars plana. (B, D stained with H&E, ×25.) (Reprinted by permission from Schubert HD. Noncontact and contact pars plana transscleral neodymium:YAG laser cyclophotocoagulation in postmortem eyes. Ophthalmology 1989;96:1471–1475.)*

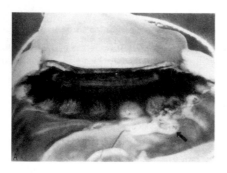 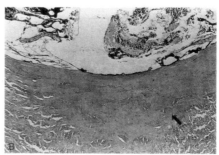

FIGURE 40-13. *Contact laser applied 3 to 5 mm from the limbus in porcine eyes. A. Coagulation of all tissue layers is seen (arrow). B. Arrow shows border of transscleral coagulation. (H&E, ×25.) (Reprinted by permission from Schubert HD. Noncontact and contact pars plana transscleral neodymium:YAG laser cyclophotocoagulation in postmortem eyes. Ophthalmology 1989;96:1471–1475.)*

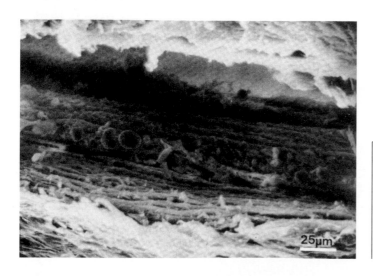

FIGURE 40-14. *Scanning electron micrograph of laser incision. Laser beam path is located in peripheral cornea approximately 500 μm anterior to trabecular meshwork. Laser energy appears to have induced splitting of stroma along natural cleavage planes. Higher magnification of fistula is shown in Figure 15. (Reprinted by permission from Gherezghiher T, March WF, Koss MC, Nordquist RF. Neodymium:YAG laser sclerostomy in primates. Arch Ophthalmol 1985;103:1543–1545.)*

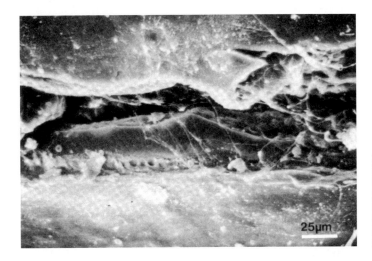

FIGURE 40-15.   *Scanning electron micrograph of lumen of laser incision (Figure 14, arrow). Note clean wall of cleavage path where only a few red blood cells are present. (Reprinted by permission from Gherezghiher T, March WF, Koss MC, Nordquist RF. Neodymium:YAG laser sclerostomy in primates.* Arch Ophthalmol *1985;103:1543–1545.)*

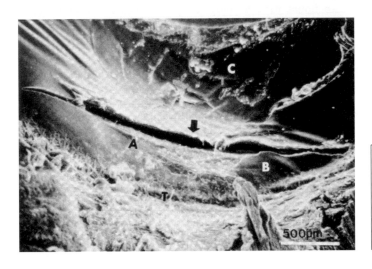

FIGURE 40-16.   *Scanning electron micrograph of conjunctival filtering bleb. Conjunctiva was parted to allow observation of laser-induced fistula. Within lumen, small amount of fibrin and few red blood cells can be seen. (Reprinted by permission from Gherezghiher T, March WF, Koss MC, Nordquist RF. Neodymium:YAG laser sclerostomy in primates.* Arch Ophthalmol *1985;103:1543–1545.)*

necrosis zones, but more often, fibrin reaction, iris adhesions, and circumscribed detachment of Descemet's membrane near the internal ostium without major complications. A human clinical trial with the dye-enhanced ablation and a pulse-dye laser is presently in progress (59).

The application of laser energy using a fiberoptic system permits the delivery of wavelengths of laser light that are usually absorbed by ocular media. The main disadvantage is that a small incision in the eye is required. The procedure has been performed with argon, Nd:YAG, excimer, and holmium lasers (60).

Trabeculectomy: Successful Bleb

Trabeculectomy is a filtering procedure that attempts to minimize the complications of full-thickness procedures (excessive aqueous filtration, flat anterior chamber, synechial formation, endophthalmitis), placing a partial-thickness scleral flap over the fistula. Sugar (61) proposed the procedure in 1961 and Cairns (62) popularized it in 1968, calling the technique *trabeculectomy*.

The routes of aqueous outflow associated with trabeculectomy are not well known yet. Formerly, it was thought that aqueous might flow into the cut ends of Schlemm's canal, but two studies demonstrated fibrosis of the canal at this level in monkey and human eyes (63,64). Aqueous might filter through a cyclodialysis (if tissue is dissected posterior to the scleral spur) or through outlet channels and connective tissue substance of the scleral flap.

Most of the successful filtering procedures produce an elevation of conjunctiva over the surgical area called a *filtering bleb*, which consists of normal conjunctival epithelium. The subconjunctival tissue in successful blebs is loosely arranged with clear spaces, whereas failed blebs have dense collagenous tissue (Figs. 40-17 to 40-19) (65). External filtration through the filtering bleb (through the conjunctiva to the tear film, or to vascular or perivascular spaces, lymphatic vessels, and aqueous veins) is the main means of pressure reduction (1,66–68).

Whether the route of external filtration is primarily through or around the partial-thickness scleral flap is still

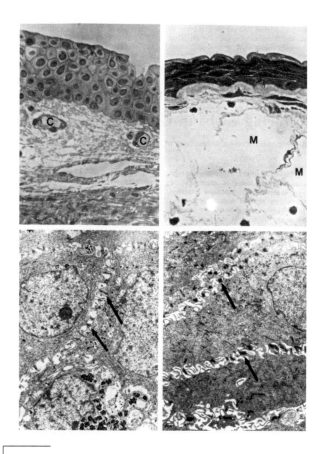

FIGURE 40-17. *Top left: Normal epithelium in tissue from failed bleb. Note capillaries (C) in dense collagenous connective tissues. (Paraphenylenediamine, ×530.) Top right: Normal epithelium in functioning bleb tissue. Note microcystic spaces (M). (Paraphenylenediamine, ×530.) Bottom left and right: Electron micrographs of epithelium in failed (left) and functioning (right) bleb tissue; arrows indicate normal desmosomal junctions found in both instances. (×6600.) (Reprinted by permission from Addicks EM, Quigley HA, Green WR, Robin AL: Histologic characteristics of filtering blebs in glaucomatous eyes. Arch Ophthalmol 1983;101:795–798.)*

controversial. Perfusion studies of human autopsy eyes in which the margins of the trabeculectomy were sealed with adhesive showed significant flow through the scleral flap (69). However, other studies in eyes with successful trabeculectomies showed the primary route of external filtration to be around the margins of the scleral flap (70).

FAILURE OF FILTERING SURGERY

Wound Healing

The incision of any tissue by laser or knife is followed by a process that attempts to heal the wound. Filtering surgery in eyes with glaucoma differs from most surgical procedures in that the success of the procedure depends on the inhibition of wound healing. Thus, modulation of wound healing may be necessary for the surgery to be successful in selected patients. As understanding of the wound-healing process

after filtering surgery has progressed, possible factors responsible for failure of the surgery have been identified and new healing inhibitors have been tested (71–73).

A surgical incision with a clean edge damages one or more layers of tissue and causes minimal damage to the adjacent tissues. This initial wound is the most important factor affecting the final scar; the second most important factor is surgical repair.

Initial Phase: Coagulation and Inflammation

After the incision is made, damaged tissues release substances that stimulate hemostasia and blood clotting. Within seconds, mediators from platelets, vessels, damaged cells, and collagen are released to start the coagulation process. The permeability of adjacent vessels increases, causing edema, and neutrophils appear within 1 hour, their numbers peaking at 48 hours and subsiding in a week. The neutrophils act to prevent infection. Fibronectin, fibrin, plasma factors, matrix proteins, and collagen clot to stabilize the wound, facilitating the movement of other cellular components in the wound (71,73).

Intermediate Phase: Cleanup and Repair

The initial phase is followed by cleanup and preparation for repair. Activated monocytes/macrophages migrate to phagocytose the necrotic tissue, to promote wound debridement and the release of factors that stimulate fibroblast migration and proliferation, and to modulate this phase, which lasts several (6–10) weeks and ends with the reparative phase. Transforming growth factor (TGF)-β is a powerful chemotactic agent for monocytes.

Fibroblasts originating from mesenchymal cells in the blood and in adjacent tissues are attracted to the wound. In animal models of filtering surgery, fibroblasts were observed to come from episcleral and subconjunctival tissue and to proliferate along the walls of the limbal fistula on the sixth day (Figs. 40-20 and 40-21) (74). These cells are essential to the process of scar formation. They secrete procollagen, which is converted into mature collagen and is stabilized by mucopolysaccharides, also secreted by the fibroblasts. Activated monocytes produce substances that activate and organize fibroblasts and vessels during the first week of repair. These fibroblasts and vessels in turn contribute to ending the acute inflammatory response.

Reparative Phase: Healing and Scarring

Angiogenesis immediately follows the movement of fibroblasts into the wound. The endothelial cells begin to migrate toward the angiogenic stimulus [fibroblast growth factors (FGF), TGF-α] producing new vessels. While the tissue is still in an active state of healing, the proliferating fibroblasts, myofibroblasts, and capillaries are referred to as *granulation tissue*, which coming from the sides of the wound joins the edges together. Wound closure is achieved by the combination of two processes: epithelialization (superficial wounds)

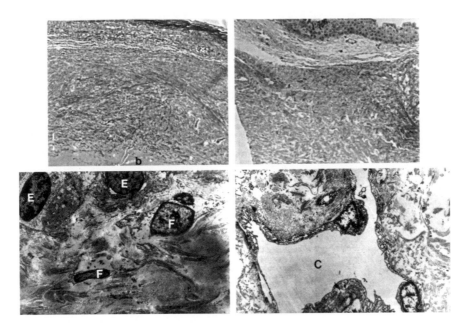

FIGURE 40-18.   *Top left and right: Light micrographs showing density and thickness of collagenous connective tissue in failed blebs; note interior of bleb cavity (b). (Paraphenylenediamine, ×380.) Bottom left and right: electron micrographs of connective tissue from failed blebs showing epithelial cells (E), fibroblasts (F), and small blood vessel (C). (×3000.) (Reprinted by permission from Addicks EM, Quigley HA, Green WR, Robin AL. Histologic characteristics of filtering blebs in glaucomatous eyes. Arch Ophthalmol 1983;101:795–798.)*

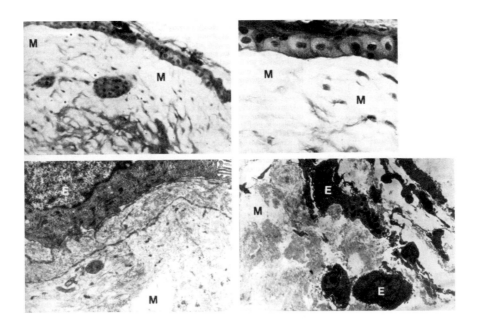

FIGURE 40-19.   *Top left and right: Electron micrographs of collagenous connective tissue from functioning blebs with microcystic spaces (M) in connective tissue; specimens were embedded in paraffin and some amorphous material overlies epithelium. (PAS; left, ×360, right, ×580.) Bottom left and right: Electron micrographs of connective tissue from functioning blebs showing epithelial cells (E) and microcystic spaces (M). (Left, ×1100; right, ×2100.) (Reprinted by permission from Addicks EM, Quigley HA, Green WR, Robin AL. Histologic characteristics of filtering blebs in glaucomatous eyes. Arch Ophthalmol 1983;101:795–798.)*

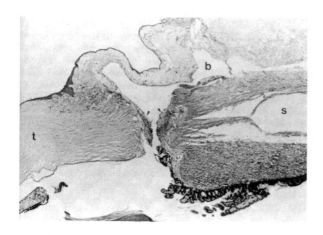

FIGURE 40-20. *Postoperative day 6. Section taken through center of sclerostomy wound. Wound is open but tongues of fibrovascular connective tissue (arrowheads) line edges. The label* t *indicates wound to corneal traction suture; b, subconjunctival bleb; and s, supraciliary space. (H&E, ×8.) (Reprinted by permission from Desjardins DC, Parrish RK II, Folberg R, et al. Wound healing after filtering surgery in owl monkeys.* Arch Ophthalmol *1986;104:1835–1839.)*

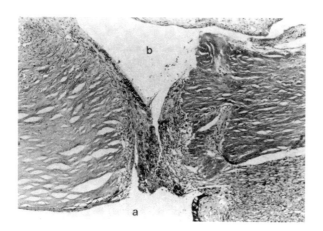

FIGURE 40-21. *Postoperative day 6 (same eye as illustrated in Figure 20). Section here is taken through edge of sclerostomy wound. Note inflamed fibrous tissue that lines wound. The label* a *indicates anterior chamber; b, bleb. (H&E, ×33.) (Reprinted by permission from Desjardins DC, Parrish RK II, Folberg R, et al. Wound healing after filtering surgery in owl monkeys.* Arch Ophthalmol *1986;104:1835–1839.)*

and contraction, which starts at 5 to 7 days and is maximally observed 4 to 5 weeks after the time of incision or injury.

Remodeling

The last part of the wound healing process begins during the fibroblastic phase and may last for more than 1 year. Collagen matures and is transformed into type I, the number of blood vessels and fibroblasts decreases, and a dense scar is formed.

The successive phases described here occur in varying degrees in filtering procedures. There is little information to explain why glaucoma filtration surgery is successful in some patients and fails in others. If the natural tendency of the wound is to heal, there must be some inhibitory mechanisms that allow filtering blebs to remain formed. Inhibitory factors of cell growth in aqueous humor have been suggested to be partially responsible (73,75–77).

Failing Blebs

Failure of filtering surgery may result from obstruction of the fistula by the iris, ciliary body, or vitreous (Fig. 40-22), or failure of the filtering bleb to function (1).

The most common cause of failure of filtering surgery is *scarring of the filtering bleb* by proliferation of fibroblasts with production of collagen and glycosaminoglycans in the subconjunctival space. Addicks et al (65) studied histopathologically failed and successful glaucoma filtrating surgery in humans, and found that the density and thickness of the fibrovascular tissue in unsuccessfully treated eyes were greater than those in normal or successfully treated eyes.

Encapsulated blebs, also called *Tenon's capsule cysts* or *high bleb phase*, are also common, occurring in 10% to 14% of eyes in published series. They are characterized by a highly elevated, smooth-domed bleb with large vessels, avascular spaces, and no microcysts, usually appearing during the first postoperative month. Movement of the conjunctiva reveals a fibrovascular layer of tissue lining the bleb. It is important to distinguish the encapsulated bleb from the typical failing bleb because the prognosis and the treatment vary notably (78–80). Encapsulated blebs have been associated with long-term glaucoma therapy and with argon laser trabeculoplasty, suggesting that they may cause increased inflammation of the conjunctiva and Tenon's capsule following filtering surgery (81).

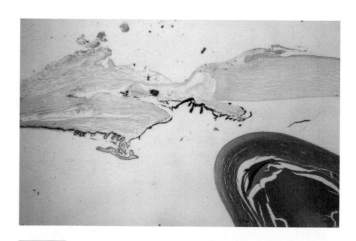

FIGURE 40-22. *Failure of filtering surgery. Obstruction of the fistula by the iris. (H&E, ×5.)*

A histopathologic study of failed blebs showed a marked inflammatory response with abundant fibroblasts and deposition of new collagen in the first months. Later failures exhibited a hypocellular capsule of fibrous tissue lined by a thick layer of fibrin beneath the conjunctiva and Tenon's capsule. Those with late failure had a "microkeloid-appearing" bleb wall. This capsule separates the bleb from the normal conjunctiva and Tenon's capsule (82).

Although it is not well known, aqueous humor can play an important role in the failure or success of the blebs. Aqueous usually slows or stops the growth of conjunctival fibroblasts in culture, perhaps because it contains an inhibitory factor for fibroblast proliferation (75). In 1990 Jampel (77) showed that the high concentration of ascorbic acid present in aqueous humor is cytotoxic to dividing human Tenon's capsule fibroblasts, which may participate in the development of a successful filtering bleb. The lack of endothelialization or epithelialization in surgical coloboma of the iris also supports the hypothesis that aqueous humor may contain a substance that inhibits cell growth in vivo (83). This factor may be altered or reduced in some individuals, accounting for the surgical failures (73). Studying aqueous humor after cataract surgery and comparing it in glaucomatous eyes and also in eyes after failed filtering surgery, several authors (76,84–86) found differences indicating that the aqueous humor composition in glaucomatous patients may be different from that in normal individuals, lacking the inhibitory properties for cell growth and having decreased fibrinolitic activity, suggesting that these changes may be responsible for the surgical failure.

Modulation of Wound Healing

Modulation of wound healing after glaucoma filtration surgery may help to increase the success rate of the procedure in eyes with a poor prognosis. Modulation can be achieved by different therapies, such as drugs or radiation.

Experimental and clinical studies demonstrated the efficacy of *topical corticosteroids* in extending the duration of a functioning filtering bleb (87).

5-Fluorouracil (5-FU) is a fluorinated pyrimidine analogue antimetabolite that inhibits DNA synthesis, and is most effective against cells actively synthesizing DNA during the S phase of the cell cycle. 5-FU inhibits fibroblast proliferation in vivo, reducing collagen synthesis and scar formation (88–91). Several studies showed that 5-FU improves bleb formation and prevents scarring in monkeys (Figs. 40-23 and 40-24) (89), and in patients resistant to the usual treatments (those with neovascular, aphakic, or pseudophakic glaucoma) when it is given by subconjunctival injection after filtrating surgery (92,93).

Drugs interfering with cellular replication have adverse effects on tissues with a rapid turnover rate, such as corneal and conjunctival epithelium. Complications like conjuncti-

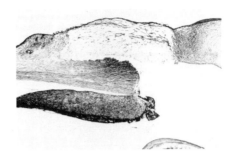

FIGURE 40-23. *Histology of a 5-FU treated eye, showing a patent sclerostomy, basal iridectomy, and filtering bleb. (H&E, ×10.) (Reprinted by permission from Gressel MG, Parrish RK II, Folberg R. 5-Fluorouracil and glacoma filtering surgery. I. An animal model. Ophthalmology 1984;91:378–383.)*

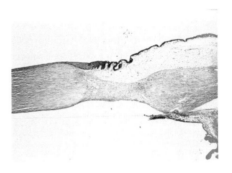

FIGURE 40-24. *Histology of a control eye. A basal iridectomy is present. Fibrovascular connective tissue bridges the surgical site. Neither a bleb nor episcleral scarring is present. (Periodic acid-Schiff, ×10.) (Reprinted by permission from Gressel MG, Parrish RK II, Folberg R. 5-Fluorouracil and glacoma filtering surgery. I. An animal model. Ophthalmology 1984;91:378–383.)*

val wound leaks and corneal epithelial defects are common, and attempts are being made to find lower effective doses and alternative delivery systems to prevent the secondary effects (94–97).

Mitomycin C is an alkylating antitumor antibiotic that selectively interrupts DNA replication, inhibiting mitosis and protein synthesis, and is active against cells, independent of the phase of the cell cycle (98). Mitomycin C inhibits the proliferation of cultured animal and human subconjunctival fibroblasts with a potency 100 times higher than that of 5-FU (91–99).

Experimental studies showed that surgical success increased in eyes treated with mitomycin C, and histopathologic studies revealed well-formed, hypocellular bleb cavities (100–102). Clinical studies comparing the efficacy of mitomycin C and 5-FU showed the former to be more effective. In addition to conjunctival leaks and hypotony, scleral ulcerations are a common complication reported with mitomycin C; the incidence of corneal epithelial defects is lower with mitomycin C than with 5-FU (103–105).

FILTERING SURGERY: IMPLANT DEVICE AND SURROUNDING CYST

To avoid the closure of the drainage fistula in eyes with complicated glaucoma treated by filtering operations, a wide variety of foreign materials have been placed in the fistula. Although these have been consistently unsuccessful over the years, as the experience with this surgery grows, the results are improving and research is still seeking new promising designs (106). There are two types: tubes and valves.

With the implantation of tubes, the objective is to get the aqueous humor to drain through the lumen of the translimbal implant. Experimental studies demonstrated that these devices maintain flow from the anterior chamber to the subconjunctival space 6 months after implantation (107). Different materials (hydrogel, Teflon, silicone) have been used (108–110). To improve the success of these implants, tubes with subconjunctival mechanical reservoirs into which the humor can drain were designed: an acrylic plate (Molteno implant) (111) and an encircling scleral band (112). The most widely published experience has been with the Molteno implant, which is useful for glaucomas resistant to conventional treatments such as neovascular glaucomas, aphakic glaucoma associated with epithelial downgrowth, and developmental glaucomas (113–115). To avoid the complication of excessive drainage causing hypotony, one-way valve tubes that open at a predetermined level of intraocular pressure were designed: Ahmed implant, Krupin eye disk, and Optimed implant (46,116,117).

Tissue responses to these implants vary, although formation of a thick collagenous wall and the presence of metaplastic myoblasts are universal findings (118).

Severe complications have included vitreous hemorrhage, retinal detachment, malignant glaucoma, hyphema, choroidal effusion, endothelial cell loss, and endophthalmitis (119–122); however, postoperative hypotony is the main complication with glaucoma implants, with or without flow regulators. The hypotony may be caused by valve or ligature failure, leakage around the tube, or a decrease in aqueous production due to a decrease in ciliary body function after surgery (116,117).

Although a fibrous capsule commonly develops around the plate and the tube, the devices are constructed to create a sizable filtering bleb in the potential space between the plate and the capsule and to prevent fibrous obstruction of the tube-plate junction, once aqueous flow begins. Nevertheless, in some eyes the implant fails because of excessive fibrosis and impermeability of the capsule (123,124). Experimental studies in monkeys showed a fibrous reaction and fibrovascular ingrowth that ensheathes the entire apparatus and stabilizes the device within 1 to 2 weeks, and demonstrated filtration of aqueous through the capsule surrounding the plate. Occlusion of anterior-chamber tubes (by

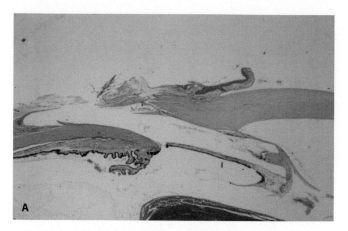

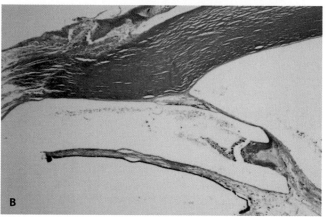

FIGURE 40-25.   *Enucleated eye because of neovascular glaucoma developing after glaucoma surgery with a Molteno valve implant. Fibrous capsule is seen around the tube from the scleral surface to the anterior chamber. The lumen of the tube is obstructed by fibrous proliferation. (A: H&E, ×5; B: Masson trichrome, ×10.)*

vitreous, by the sequelae of postoperative inflammation, by blood or fibrous tissue) in the postoperative period has been reported (Fig. 40-25) (123,125).

Nevertheless these implants are very helpful for the treatment of complicated glaucomas when there are no other therapeutic options.

REFERENCES

1. Shields MB. *Textbook of glaucoma.* Baltimore: Williams & Wilkins, 1992:527–628.
2. Zweng HC, Flocks M. Experimental photocoagulation of the anterior chamber angle. A preliminary report. *Am J Ophthalmol* 1961;52:163.
3. Krasnov MM. Laseropuncture of anterior chamber angle in glaucoma. *Am J Ophthalmol* 1973;75:674–678.
4. Demailly P, Haut J, Bonnet-Boutier M. Trabeculotomie au laser a l'argon. *Bull Soc Ophthalmol Fr* 1973;73:259–264.
5. Worthen DM, Wickham MG. Laser trabeculotomy in monkeys. *Invest Ophthalmol Vis Sci* 1973;12:707–711.
6. Ticho U, Zauberman H. Argon laser application to angle structures in the glaucomas. *Arch Ophthalmol* 1976;94:61–64.

7. Wise JB, Witter SL. Argon laser therapy for open angle glaucoma. A pilot study. *Arch Ophthalmol* 1979;97:319–322.

8. Wise JB. Long-term control of adult open angle glaucoma by argon laser treatment. *Ophthalmology* 1981;88:197–202.

9. Schwartz AL, Whitten ME, Bleiman B, Martin D. Argon laser trabecular surgery in uncontrolled phakic open angle glaucoma. *Ophthalmology* 1981;88:203–212.

10. Wilkes TDI, Fraunfelder FT. Principles of cryosurgery. *Ophthalmic Surg* 1979;10:21–30.

11. Wilensky JT, Jampol LM. Laser therapy for open angle glaucoma. *Ophthalmology* 1981;88:213–217.

12. Lichter PR. Argon laser trabeculoplasty. *Trans Am Ophthalmol Soc* 1983;80:288–301.

13. Brubaker RF, Liesegang TJ. Effect of trabecular photocoagulation on the aqueous humor dynamics of the human eye. *Am J Ophthalmol* 1983;96:139–147.

14. Melamed S, Pei J, Epstein DL. Delayed response to argon laser trabeculoplasty in monkeys. *Arch Ophthalmol* 1986;104:1078–1083.

15. Rodrigues MM, Spaeth GL, Donohoo P. Electron microscopy of argon laser therapy in phakic open-angle glaucoma. *Ophthalmology* 1982;89:198–210.

16. Alexander RA, Grierson I, Church WH. The effect of argon laser trabeculoplasty upon the normal human trabecular meshwork. *Graefes Arch Clin Exp Ophthalmol* 1989;227:72–77.

17. Melamed S, Pei J, Epstein DL. Short-term effect of argon laser trabeculoplasty in monkeys. *Arch Ophthalmol* 1985;103:1546–1552.

18. Van Buskirk EM, Pond V, Rosenquist RC, Acott TS. Argon laser trabeculoplasty. Studies of mechanism of action. *Ophthalmology* 1984;91:1005–1010.

19. Reiss GR, Wilensky JT, Higginbotham EJ. Laser trabeculoplasty. *Surv Ophthalmol* 1991;35:407–428.

20. Bylsma SB, Samples JR, Acott TS, Van Buskirk EM. Trabecular cell division after argon laser trabeculoplasty. *Arch Ophthalmol* 1988;106:544–547.

21. Dueker DK, Norberg M, Johnson DH, et al. Stimulation of cell division by argon and Nd:YAG laser trabeculoplasty in cynomolgus monkeys. *Invest Ophthalmol Vis Sci* 1990;31:115–124.

22. Van Buskirk EM. Pathophysiology of laser trabeculoplasty. *Surv Ophthalmol* 1989;33:264–272.

23. Smith J. Argon laser trabeculoplasty: comparison of bichromatic and monochromatic wavelengths. *Ophthalmology* 1984;91:355–360.

24. Makabe R. Comparison of kripton and argon laser trabeculoplasty. *Klin Monatsbl Augenheilkd* 1986;189:118–120.

25. McMillan TA, Stewart WC, Legler UFC, et al. Comparison of diode and argon laser trabeculoplasty in cadaver eyes. *Invest Ophthalmol Vis Sci* 1994;35:706–710.

26. Quigley HA. Histological and physiological studies of cyclocryotherapy in primate and human eyes. *Am J Ophthalmol* 1976;82:722–732.

27. Ferry AP. Histopathologic observations on human eyes following cyclocryotherapy for glaucoma. *Trans Am Acad Ophthalmol Otolaryngol* 1977;83:90–94.

28. Vucicevic ZM, Tsou KC, Nazarian IH, et al. A cytochemical approach to the laser coagulation of the ciliary body. *Bibl Ophthalmol* 1969;8:467–478.

29. Smith RS, Stein MN. Ocular hazards of transscleral laser radiation: II. Intraocular injury produced by ruby and neodymium lasers. *Am J Ophthalmol* 1969;67:100–110.

30. Beckman H, Sugar HS. Neodymium laser cyclocoagulation. *Arch Ophthalmol* 1973;90:27–28.

31. Beckman H, Waeltermann J. Transscleral ruby laser cyclocoagulation. *Am J Ophthalmol* 1984;98:788–795.

32. Wilensky JT, Welch D, Mirolovich M. Transscleral cyclocoagulation using a neodymium:YAG laser. *Ophthalmic Surg* 1985;16:95–98.

33. Deveyi RG, Trope GE, Hunter WH. Neodymium-YAG transscleral cyclocoagulation in rabbit eyes. *Br J Ophthalmol* 1987;71:441–444.

34. England C, Van der Zypen E, Fankhauser F, Kwasniewska S. Ultrastructure of the rabbit ciliary body following transscleral cyclophotocoagulation with the free-running Nd-YAG laser: preliminary findings. *Lasers Ophthalmol* 1986;1:61.

35. Peyman GA, Conway MD, Raichand M, Lin J. Histopathologic studies on transscleral argon-krypton photocoagulation with an exolaser probe. *Ophthalmic Surg* 1984;15:496–501.

36. Schuman JS, Jacobson JJ, Puliafito CA, et al. Experimental use of semiconductor diode laser in contact transscleral cyclophotocoagulation in rabbits. *Arch Ophthalmol* 1990;108:1152–1157.

37. Simmons RB, Prum BE, Shields SR, et al. Videographic and histologic comparison of Nd:YAG and diode laser contact transscleral cyclophotocoagulation. *Am J Ophthalmol* 1994;117:337–341.

38. Van der Zypen E, England C, Fankhauser F, Kwasniewska S. The effect of transscleral laser cyclophotocoagulation on rabbit ciliary body vascularization. *Graefes Arch Clin Exp Ophthalmol* 1989;227:172–179.

39. Cantor LB, Nichols DA, Katz LJ, et al. Neodymium-YAG transscleral cyclophotocoagulation. *Invest Ophthalmol Vis Sci* 1989;30:1834–1837.

40. Schubert HD. Noncontact and contact pars plana transscleral neodymium: YAG laser cyclophotocoagulation in postmortem eyes. *Ophthalmology* 1989;96:1471–1475.

41. Echelman DA, Nasisse MP, Shields MB, et al. Influence of exposure time on inflammatory response to neodymium:YAG cyclophotocoagulation in rabbits. *Arch Ophthalmol* 1994;112:977–981.

42. Immonen I, Suomalainen V-P, Kivela T, Viherkoski E. Energy levels needed for cyclophotocoagulation: a comparison of transscleral contact cw-YAG and krypton lasers in the rabbit eye. *Ophthalmic Surg* 1993;24:530–533.

43. Brancato R, Trabucchi G, Verdi M, et al. Diode and Nd:YAG laser contact transscleral cyclophotocoagulation in a human eye: a comparative histopathologic study of the lesion produced using a new fiber optic probe. *Ophthalmic Surg* 1994;25:607–611.

44. Hampton C, Shields MB. Transscleral neodymium-YAG cyclophotocoagulation. A histologic study of human autopsy eyes. *Arch Ophthalmol* 1988;106:1121–1123.

45. Allingham RR, de Kater AW, Bellows AR, Hsu J. Probe placement and power levels in contact transscleral neodymium:YAG cyclophotocoagulation. *Arch Ophthalmol* 1990;108:738–742.

46. Blasini M, Shields MB, Hickingbotham D. A temporary glaucoma valve for transient intraocular pressure elevation. *Ophthalmic Surg* 1990;21:199–201.

47. Shields SM, Stevens JL, Kass MA, Smith ME. Histopathologic findings after Nd:YAG transscleral cyclophotocoagulation. *Am J Ophthalmol* 1988;106:100–101.

48. Marsh P, Wilson DJ, Samples JR, Morrison JC. A clinicopathologic study of noncontact transscleral Nd:YAG cyclophotocoagulation. *Am J Ophthalmol* 1993;115:597–602.

49. Lee PF, Pomerantzeff O. Transpupillary cyclophotocoagulation of rabbit eyes. An experimental approach to glaucoma surgery. *Am J Ophthalmol* 1971;71:911–920.

50. Bartl G, Haller BM, Wocheslander E, Hogmann H. Light and electron microscopic observations after argon laser photocoagulation of ciliary processes. *Klin Monatsbl Augenheilkd* 1982;181:414–416.

51. Shields MB. Cyclodestructive surgery for glaucoma: past, present and future. *Trans Am Ophthalmol Soc* 1986;83:285–303.

52. Fleishman JA, Swartz M, Dixon JA. Argon laser endophotocoagulation. An intraoperative trans-pars plana technique. *Arch Ophthalmol* 1981;99:1610–1612.

53. Landers MB, Trese MT, Stefansson E, Bessler M. Argon laser intraocular photocoagulation. *Ophthalmology* 1982;89:785–788.

54. Shields MB, Chandler DB, Hickingbotham D, Klintworth GK. Intraocular cyclophotocoagulation. Histopathologic evaluation in primates. *Arch Ophthalmol* 1985;103:1731–1735.

55. March WF, Gherezghiher T, Koss MC, et al. Histologic study of a neodymium-YAG laser sclerostomy. *Arch Ophthalmol* 1985;103:860–863.

56. March WF, Gherezghiher T, Koss MC, Nordquist RE. Design of a new contact lens for YAG laser filtering procedures. *Ophthalmic Surg* 1985;16:328–330.

57. Gherezghiher T, March MF, Koss MC. Neodymium:YAG laser sclerostomy in primates. *Arch Ophthalmol* 1985;103:1543–1549.

58. Wetzel W, Scheu M. Laser sclerostomy ab interno using continuous wave and pulsed lasers in a rabbit model. *Int Ophthalmol* 1994;18:71–75.

59. Latina MA, Melamed S, March WF, et al. Gonioscopic ab interno laser sclerostomy. A pilot study in glaucoma patients. *Ophthalmology* 1992;99:1736–1744.

60. Lederer CM, Thomas JV. Laser surgery for glaucoma. In: Thomas JV, Belcher CD, Simmons R, eds. *Glaucoma surgery*. St. Louis: Mosby, 1992:157–194.

61. Sugar HS. Experimental trabeculectomy in glaucoma. *Am J Ophthalmol* 1961;51:623.

62. Cairns JE. Trabeculectomy. Preliminary report of a new method. *Am J Ophthalmol* 1968;5:673–679.

63. Rich AM, McPherson SD. Trabeculectomy in the owl monkey. *Ann Ophthalmol* 1973;5:1082–1088.

64. Spencer WH. Histologic evaluation of microsurgical glaucoma techniques. *Trans Am Acad Ophthalmol Otolaryngol* 1972;76:389–397.

65. Addicks EM, Quigley HA, Green WR, Robin AL. Histologic characteristics of filtering blebs in glaucomatous eyes. *Arch Ophthalmol* 1983;101:795–798.

66. Kronfeld PC. The chemical demonstration of transconjunctival passage of aqueous after antiglaucomatous operations. *Am J Ophthalmol* 1952;35:38.

67. Galin MA, Baras I, McLean JM. How does a filtering bleb work? *Trans Am Acad Ophthalmol Otolaryngol* 1965;69:1082–1091.

68. Teng CC, Chi HH, Katzin HM. Histology and mechanism of filtering operations. *Am J Ophthalmol* 1959;47:161.

69. Shields MB, Bradbury MJ, Shelburne JD, Bell SW. The permeability of the outer layers of limbus and anterior sclera. *Invest Ophthalmol Vis Sci* 1977;16:866–869.

70. Shields MB. Trabeculectomy vs full-thickness filtering operation for control of glaucoma. *Ophthalmic Surg* 1980;11:498–505.

71. Skuta GL, Parrish RK. Wound healing in glaucoma filtering surgery. *Surv Ophthalmol* 1987;32:149–170.

72. Tahery MM, Lee DA. Review: pharmacologic control of wound healing in glaucoma filtration surgery. *J Ocul Pharmacol* 1989;5:155–179.

73. Costa VP, Spaeth GL, Eiferman RA, Orengo-Nania S. Wound healing modulation in glaucoma filtration surgery. *Ophthalmic Surg* 1993;24:152–170.

74. Desjardins DC, Parrish RK II, Folberg R, et al. Wound healing after filtering surgery in owl monkeys. *Arch Ophthalmol* 1986;104:1835–1839.

75. Herschler J, Claflin AJ, Fiorentino G. The effect of aqueous humor on the growth of subconjunctival fibroblasts in tissue culture and its implications for glaucoma surgery. *Am J Ophthalmol* 1980;89:245–249.

76. Herschler J. The inhibitory factor in aqueous humour. *Vision Res* 1981;21:163.

77. Jampel HD. Ascorbic acid is cytotoxic to dividing human Tenon's capsule fibroblasts. A possible contributing factor in glaucoma filtration surgery success. *Arch Ophthalmol* 1990;108:1323–1325.

78. Sherwood MB, Spaeth GL, Simmons ST, et al. Cysts of Tenon's capsule following filtration surgery. Medical management. *Arch Ophthalmol* 1987;105:1517–1521.

79. Scott DR, Quigley HA. Medical management of a high bleb phase after trabeculectomies. *Ophthalmology* 1988;95:1169–1173.

80. Richter CU, Shingleton BJ, Bellows AR, et al. The development of encapsulated filtering blebs. *Ophthalmology* 1988;95:1163–1168.

81. Sherwood MB, Grierson I, Millar L, Hitchings RA. Long-term morphologic effects of antiglaucoma drugs on the conjunctiva and Tenon's capsule in glaucomatous patients. *Ophthalmology* 1989;96:327–335.

82. Hitchings RA, Grierson I. Clinico pathological correlation in eyes with failed fistulizing surgery. *Trans Ophthalmol Soc UK* 1983;103:84–88.

83. Snell AC Jr. Wound healing of the iris. *Am J Ophthalmol* 1956;41:499–505.

84. Mehra KS, Dube B, Dube RK. Fibrinolytic activity in blood and aqueous humour in glaucoma. *Indian J Ophthalmol* 1983;31:827–829.

85. Ledbetter SR, Hatchell DL, O'Brien WJ. Secondary aqueous humor stimulates the proliferation of cultured bovine corneal endothelial cells. *Invest Ophthalmol Vis Sci* 1983;24:557–562.

86. Joseph JP, Grierson I, Hitchings RA. Partial characterization of the fibroblast chemotactic constituents of human aqueous humour. *Int Ophthalmol* 1989;13:125–130.

87. Starita RJ, Fellman RL, Spaeth GL, et al. Short- and long-term effects of postoperative corticosteroids on trabeculectomy. *Ophthalmology* 1985;92:938–946.

88. Blumenkranz MS, Hartzer MK, Hajek AS. Selection of therapeutic agents for intraocular proliferative disease. *Arch Ophthalmol* 1987;105:396–399.

89. Gressel MG, Parrish RK, Folberg R. 5-Fluorouracil and glaucoma filtering surgery: I. An animal model. *Ophthalmology* 1984;91:378–383.

90. Lee DA, Shapourifar-Tehrani S, Kitada S. The effect of 5-fluorouracil and cytarabine on human fibroblast from Tenon's capsule. *Invest Ophthalmol Vis Sci* 1990;31:1848–1855.

91. Yamamoto T, Varani J, Soong HK, Lichter PR. Effects of 5-fluorouracil and mitomycin C on cultured rabbit subconjunctival fibroblasts. *Ophthalmology* 1990;97:1204–1210.

92. The Fluorouracil Filtering Surgery Study Group. Fluorouracil Filtering Surgery Study one-year follow-up. *Am J Ophthalmol* 1989;108:625–635.

93. Heuer DK, Parrish RK II, Gressel MG, et al. 5-Fluorouracil and glaucoma filtering surgery: III. Intermediate follow-up of a pilot study. *Ophthalmology* 1986;93:1537–1546.

94. Franks WA, Hitchings RA. Complications of 5-fluorouracil after trabeculectomy. *Eye* 1991;5:385–389.

95. Hasty B, Heuer DK, Minckler DS. Primates trabeculectomies with 5-fluorouracil collagen implants. *Am J Ophthalmol* 1990;109:721–725.

96. Lee DA, Flores RA, Anderson PJ, et al. Glaucoma filtration surgery in rabbits using bioerodible polymers and 5-fluorouracil. *Ophthalmology* 1987;94:1523–1530.

97. Alvarado JA. The use of a liposome-encapsulated 5-fluoorotate for glaucoma surgery: I. Animal studies. *Trans Am Ophthalmol Soc* 1990;87:489–514.

98. Verweij J, Pinedo HM. Mitomycin C: mechanism of action, usefulness and limitations. *Anticancer Drugs* 1990;1:5–13.

99. Jampel HC. Effect of brief exposure to mitomycin-C on viability and proliferation of cultured human Tenon's capsule fibroblasts. *Ophthalmology* 1992;99:1471–1476.

100. Palmer SS. Mitomycin as adjunct chemotherapy with trabeculectomy. *Ophthalmology* 1991;98:317–321.

101. Wilson MR, Lee DA, Baker RS, et al. The effects of topical mitomycin on glaucoma filtration surgery in rabbits. *J Ocul Pharmacol* 1991;7:1–8.

102. Pasquale LR, Thibault D, Dorman-Pease ME, et al. Effect of topical mitomycin-C on glaucoma filtration surgery in monkeys. *Ophthalmology* 1992;99:14–18.

103. Kitazawa Y, Kawase K, Matsushita H, Minobe M. Trabeculectomy with mitomycin. A comparative study with fluorouracil. *Arch Ophthalmol* 1991;109:1693–1698.

104. Skuta GL, Beeson CC, Higginbotham EJ, et al. Intraoperative mitomycin versus postoperative 5-fluorouracil in high risk glaucoma filtering surgery. *Ophthalmology* 1992;99:438–444.

105. Katz GJ, Higginbotham EJ, Lichter PR, et al. Mitomycin C versus 5-fluorouracil in high risk glaucoma filtering surgery. *Ophthalmology* 1995;102:1263–1269.

106. Williams AS. Setons in glaucoma surgery. In: Albert DM, Jakobiec FA, eds. *Principles and practice of ophthalmology.* Vol. 3. Philadelphia: WB Saunders, 1994:1655–1666.

107. Egerer I, Freyler H. Aqueous outflow following seton operations. *Klin Monatsbl Augenheilkd* 1979;174:93–98.

108. Krejci L. Hydrogel capillary drain for glaucoma: nine years' clinical experience. *Glaucoma* 1980;2:259–263.

109. Honrubia FM, Gomez ML, Hernandez A, Grijalbo MP. Long-term results of silicone tube in filtering surgery for eyes with neovascular glaucoma. *Am J Ophthalmol* 1984;97:501–504.

110. Kuljaca Z, Ljubojevic V, Momirov D. Draining implant for neovascular glaucoma. *Am J Ophthalmol* 1983;96:372–376.

111. Molteno ACB. New implant for drainage in glaucoma. Clinical trial. *Br J Ophthalmol* 1969;53:606–615.

112. Schocket SS, Nirankari VS, Lakhanpal V, et al. Anterior chamber tube shunt to an encircling band in the treatment of neovascular glaucoma and other refractory glaucomas. A long-term study. *Ophthalmology* 1985;92:553–562.

113. Ancker E, Molteno ABC. Molteno drainage implant for neovascular glaucoma. *Trans Ophthalmol Soc UK* 1982;102:122–123.

114. Fish LA, Heuer DK, Baerveldt G, et al. Molteno implantation for secondary glaucomas associated with advanced epithelial ingrowth. *Ophthalmology* 1990;97:557–561.

115. Billson F, Thomas R, Aylward W. The use of two stage Molteno implants in developmental glaucoma. *J Pediatr Ophthalmol Strabismus* 1989;26:3–8.

116. Krupin T, Ritch R, Camras CB, et al. A long Krupin-Denver valve implant attached to a 180° scleral explant for glaucoma surgery. *Ophthalmology* 1988;95:1174–1180.

117. Prata JA, Mermoud A, LaBree L, Minckler DS. In vitro and in vivo flow characteristics of glaucoma drainage implants. *Ophthalmology* 1995;102:894–904.

118. Classen L, Kivela T, Tarkkanen A. Histopathologic and immunohistochemical analysis of the filtration bleb after unsuccessful glaucoma seton implantation. *Am J Ophthalmol* 1996;112:205–212.

119. Perkins TW. Endophthalmitis after placement of a Molteno implant. *Ophthalmic Surg* 1990;21:733–734.

120. Huna R, Melamed S, Hirsh A, Treister G. Retinal detachment adherent to posterior chamber IOL after Molteno implant surgery. *Ophthalmic Surg* 1990;21:854–856.

121. Melamed S, Cahane M, Gutman I, Blumental M. Postoperative complications after Molteno implant surgery. *Am J Ophthalmol* 1991;111:319–322.

122. McDermot ML, Swendris RP, Shin DH, et al. Corneal endothelial cell counts after Molteno implantation. *Am J Ophthalmol* 1993;115:93–96.

123. Minckler DS, Shammas A, Wilcox M, Ogden TE. Experimental studies of aqueous filtration using the Molteno implant. *Trans Am Ophthalmol Soc* 1987;85:368–392.

124. Cameron JD, White TC. Clinico-histopathologic correlation of a successful glaucoma pump-shunt implant. *Ophthalmology* 1988;95:1189–1194.

125. Minckler DS, Heuer DK, Hasty B, et al. Clinical experience with the single-plate Molteno implant in complicated glaucomas. *Ophthalmology* 1988;95:1181–1188.

Retina and Vitreous Surgery

WILLIAM F. MIELER, SURESH R. CHANDRA,
FRANK L. MYERS, T. MICHAEL NORK,
AND THOMAS S. STEVENS
Section Editors

Principles of Scleral Buckling and Pneumatic Retinopexy

Timothy W. Olsen

The goals of this chapter are to introduce the basic principles and pertinent anatomy, and to describe some standard techniques of scleral buckling and pneumatic retinopexy. Most primary retinal detachments can be repaired using one or both of these techniques. For a resident in ophthalmology, the surgical principles and complexities of retinal detachment repair may represent one of the more confusing and difficult areas to approach in ophthalmic surgery. While techniques used in scleral buckling surgery vary widely, most retinal specialists agree that certain basic principles are always followed.

CLINICAL EVALUATION

Most of the decision-making process of a primary retinal detachment repair occurs during the office examination. The physician's role as an "educated advisor" serves to inform the patient of possible ways that the retina can be reattached, the risks associated with each, and the likelihood of success. This process involves the patient in the decision making and provides the basis for informed consent.

PATIENT HISTORY

Important historical information related to retinal detachments includes the timing and characteristic of visual symptoms, the area and extent of an existing scotoma, a history of associated trauma, the history of retinal detachment or tears in the opposite eye, associated pain, and a family history of retinal detachment. A particularly concerning history would be that of recent photopsias with a scotoma progressing from the inferior visual field toward the center

of vision. This history implies a recent posterior vitreous separation with a superior retinal detachment progressing toward, but not yet involving, the fovea. Duration of macular involvement by the detachment is prognostic of future vision, reattachment rate, and urgency of repair.

A history of trauma is frequently associated with retinal detachments (1) and should be accurately documented. The use of protective eye wear and its availability is also important for work-related trauma. If trauma is suspected, other intraocular injuries that should be suspected include globe rupture, hyphema, angle recession, dislocated or subluxated lens, iris tears, optic nerve involvement, and choroidal hemorrhages.

Clinical Examination

Anterior-Segment Examination

Visual acuity and confrontational visual field testing may help to identify the extent of the retinal detachment and the degree of macular involvement. The intraocular pressure in nontraumatic eyes with a retinal detachment is commonly low, most likely due to an increase in uveoscleral outflow (2). The intraocular pressure may be elevated, especially in the presence of trauma-related injuries. In a rare condition known as the Schwartz syndrome an elevated intraocular pressure is associated with a retinal detachment and presumably is due to photoreceptor outer segments in the anterior chamber and trabecular meshwork (3). Pigmented cells or "tobacco dust" in the anterior vitreous are also suggestive of a retinal detachment. The presence of iris neovascularization in an individual with no other risk factors may indicate chronic retinal detachment (4). Gonioscopy is recommended for trauma-related detachments to assess for possible angle recession. However, this examination should be postponed in the presence of a hyphema,

Financial support was provided by a Heed/Knapp Ophthalmic Foundation Fellowship Award.

microhyphema, or recent iris trauma, due to the risk of hemorrhage.

Lenticular status is important when the technique of primary retinal detachment repair is considered. Cortical cataracts that may not be visually significant to the patient may impair adequate visualization of the retinal periphery. The presence of pseudophakia or aphakia may also determine the best method of retinal reattachment. Multiple small peripheral retinal holes that are difficult to identify clinically may be present in these eyes. Pseudophakic eyes frequently have the following features that can make visualization of peripheral retinal pathology difficult: a small optic size, peripheral retained cortical material, opacified capsular fibrosis, and peripheral lens distortion (seen particularly with silicone lenses). In eyes with an anterior-chamber lens or a history of capsular rupture, anterior vitreous may be present and should be recognized. Anterior-chamber paracentesis during detachment repair or pneumatic retinopexy may be complicated by vitreous incarceration into the paracentesis.

Posterior-Segment Examination

The Fellow Eye   The examiner and patient will be more comfortable if the patient is placed in a supine position. A careful, depressed, dilated fundus examination should begin with the *uninvolved* fellow eye. Pathology is frequently found and needs to be recognized. If the symptomatic eye is examined first, this pathology is frequently neglected and may go undetected. Asymptomatic tears, lattice degeneration, vitreous separation, and retinoschisis are helpful and significant findings in the fellow eye. Occasionally a subclinical or asymptomatic retinal detachment is discovered. Bilateral involvement is particularly prevalent in the human immunodeficient virus (HIV)–infected population affected by cytomegaloviral (CMV) retinitis and subsequent retinal detachments.

Detachment Configuration   Indirect ophthalmoscopy of the affected eye should begin with an assessment of the extent and configuration of the retinal detachment. A 28- or 30-diopter (D) lens is useful for this part of the examination because it offers a lower-magnification, panoramic view of the posterior pole. A common mistake is to immediately and randomly look for a peripheral retinal tear. Lincoff and Gieser (5) outlined the characteristic contours of subretinal fluid to help find the retinal break. They correctly pointed out that this "awareness" becomes second nature to retinal surgeons; however, ophthalmology residents will benefit from studying the principles of subretinal fluid formation associated with a rhegmatogenous retinal detachment.

Foveal involvement by the detachment may be more easily detected using slit-lamp biomicroscopy. Occasionally, a bullously detached retina from a superior break will "hang" over the fovea. In this situation, central vision may be decreased without the fovea being detached. Supine positioning usually helps to make this distinction. Macular detachment implies a worse visual prognosis while the proximity of the detachment to the fovea also predicts the urgency of repair. A shallow retinal detachment may be difficult to identify, even with binocular ophthalmoscopy. Difficulty visualizing the choroidal vascular pattern through shallowly detached retina is a useful indicator of subretinal fluid.

Scleral Depression   The next step is the localization of the causative retinal break plus any other retinal breaks, including those in attached retina. Because of the higher magnification, a 20-D lens is useful during this part of the examination. Scleral depression requires patience and a cooperative patient. The examiner should be adept at using either hand to depress or hold the lens. A drop of topical anesthetic is particularly useful, especially for depression in the fornices at the 3-o'clock and 9-o'clock positions where direct depression on the globe may be required.

A common cause of failure of primary retinal detachment repair is a new or missed retinal break (6). Frequently, additional breaks are found in the vicinity of the primary break (5). The key to scleral depression is to maximize the alignment between the tip of the scleral depressor and the examiner's view. First, place the depressor in the area to be examined and line up the tip of the depressor with the examiner's view through the pupil and then interpose the lens. The depressor is gently moved in a back-and-forth, anterior-to-posterior direction or a side-to-side motion. The kinetic depressed examination will elevate and obliquely illuminate a torn flap of retina adherent to the vitreous base. Breaks without a flap of torn retina such as a slit tear or a small hole will be stretched open by the indentation of the scleral depressor.

PRINCIPLES OF SCLERAL BUCKLING

Localization

During scleral buckling surgery, the single most important task is to localize the retinal break or breaks. Localization in the operating room is both an intraocular and an extraocular process. Intraocular localization using the indirect ophthalmoscope localizes the actual retinal break. Extraocular localization identifies the location of the retinal break relative to the opaque external surface of the sclera. Scleral depression is the "connection" that transfers internal to external localization. Once all retinal breaks are localized on the sclera, various techniques of "thermotherapy" are available to create a chorioretinal adhesion to seal the break. The sclera is then pushed inward by an externally placed scleral buckle to reappose the retinal pigment epithelium to the edges of the retinal break. Various buckling materials of different shapes and sizes are made for this purpose. The material used and method of attachment to the sclera are less important than the precise external localization of the buckle.

Success or failure of the scleral buckle frequently depends on accurate localization. If the scleral buckle closes the retinal hole, the operation is a success. If an edge of the retinal hole remains unsupported from improper localization or a hole is missed, the operation usually fails. More conservative surgeons tend to use broader, more extensive buckling elements while others use precisely placed smaller elements. Either method is acceptable as long as all retinal breaks are supported. The subsequent risks of proliferative vitreoretinopathy should also be considered.

The Retinal Pigment Epithelial "Pump"

The subretinal space is a potential space between the original layers of the embryonic cup. Under normal conditions, fluid is not present in this space unless a retinal break allows liquid vitreous into this space, or another pathologic condition exists. However, not all retinal breaks lead to a retinal detachment. The balance between two opposing forces will determine the fate of a retinal break. One force is liquid vitreous dissecting through open retinal breaks. Vitreous traction may hold a retinal tear open or extend a small tear into a larger tear, thus increasing the amount of fluid that may enter the subretinal space. The primary opposing force is the retinal pigment epithelial pump (7–10). The retinal pigment epithelium is a polarized monolayer of highly specialized cells that make up the outer blood-retina barrier. These cells have a tremendous capacity to remove fluid from the subretinal space. The balance between the forces results in a retinal detachment when the amount of fluid entering the retinal break exceeds the ability of the pigment epithelial pump to remove this fluid. Factors that would favor detachment include large retinal tears, multiple tears, tears held open by traction, the presence of liquefied vitreous, and aged or dysfunctional retinal pigment epithelium. Factors that favor attachment include small breaks, formed vitreous (i.e., in children), healthy retinal pigment epithelium, and a fibrotic reaction around a break that may "seal" the retinal break to the subjacent pigment epithelium. Often during scleral buckling surgery, a detached retina may require external drainage of this subretinal fluid. Some argue that drainage procedures are not necessary and add unnecessary risk to the surgery. If the retinal break is sealed, the fluid balance may shift toward retinal reattachment and the retinal pigment epithelium effectively pumps out the remaining subretinal fluid. While there is not a clear consensus regarding external drainage, the basic principles of fluid dynamics are widely accepted.

Anatomy

Internal and External Anatomy

An understanding of the anatomy of the vitreous base and ora serrata as they correspond to external structures such as the extraocular muscles and corneoscleral limbus is essential. In other words, one should understand the inside of the eye relative to the outside (Fig. 41-1). The closest anatomic relationship available to establish this connection is the underlying location of the ora serrata relative to the insertion of the extraocular muscles along the spiral of Tillaux (11). The nasal ora serrata is located approximately 5 to 6 mm posterior to the corneoscleral limbus under the rectus medialis insertion while the temporal ora serrata is located approximately 7 mm posterior to the corneoscleral limbus under the rectus lateralis insertion. The vitreous base insertion is approximately 2 to 6 mm wide and begins 5 mm posterior to the limbus circumferentially. The vitreous base therefore extends slightly more posteriorly into the nasal retina (12). Because most retinal tears occur near the posterior aspect of the vitreous base, the area 8 to 12 mm

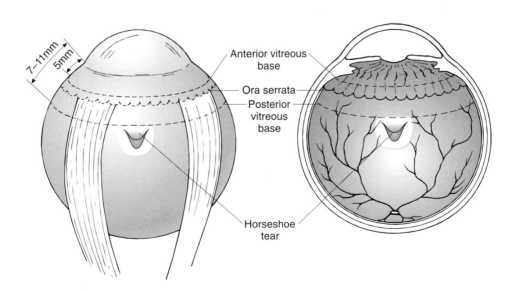

FIGURE 41-1.   *A comparison of the internal anatomy with the external landmarks.*

posterior to the corneoscleral limbus is the most common area for retinal breaks to be localized. These are generalizations and tears may occur anywhere, and each tear should be localized. Anatomic relationships are also affected by globe size and are altered in children, highly myopic eyes, microphthalmic eyes, and other conditions.

Retinal dialyses are breaks that occur in the region under the vitreous base. The posterior edge of the dialysis is therefore supported by the base and prevented from folding posteriorly. This helps to distinguish a dialysis from a giant retinal tear. Dialyses are easily repaired with standard scleral buckling techniques. Superior dialysis may also be treated using pneumatic retinopexy (13).

The Vitreous

The strongest connection between the vitreous and the retina occurs at the vitreous base (12). The second strongest point of vitreous attachment occurs at the optic nerve. Other areas of relative adherence include the parafoveal region and along the retinal vasculature (14). With the aging process, the vitreous becomes more syneretic and liquefied (15). Mechanical and shearing forces play a role in causing a posterior vitreous detachment, which is diagnosed clinically as Weiss's ring. Prior to the vitreous detachment, forces exerted by the vitreous gel are distributed throughout the multiple adhesion sites. However, after vitreous separation, forces generated from eye movements are directed at the remaining site of firm vitreoretinal adherence along the posterior edge of the vitreous base. Additionally, the retina is much thinner in this area and thus more susceptible to tearing.

Timing of Reattachment Surgery

A detached retina that requires a scleral buckle is not an ophthalmic emergency. However, there are situations when surgery is *urgent*. The classic example is a rapidly progressing superior bullous rhegmatogenous retinal detachment that is about to detach the fovea. This should be reattached as soon as it is safely possible. Studies indicated that retinal detachments involving the fovea have a worse visual prognosis than those that do not (16,17). There is some evidence the surgery may be delayed until the following morning when ophthalmic nursing and equipment are more readily available and less expensive than "on-call" teams (18,19). Admitting the patient with bilateral occlusive patching may decrease the saccadic eye movements and slow the rate of flow of liquid vitreous into the subretinal space. Occasionally, this may actually decrease the amount of subretinal fluid. The presence of a demarcation line indicates a chronic detachment. If the macula is detached, the situation is also less urgent. Several studies showed that the longer the macula is detached, the worse the final visual outcome is (17,20). The potential acuity meter may also be useful in predicting the final visual outcome (21) but this will not change the management of the detachment.

SURGICAL TECHNIQUE

Anesthesia

In most patients, the safest method of anesthesia is a standard retrobulbar injection. This method avoids the rare but potentially serious risks of general anesthesia, which include death, cardiac arrest or arrhythmia, airway injury, aspiration, pneumonia, stroke, and brain damage. Faster postoperative recovery and less nausea are also advantages of local anesthesia. Retrobulbar anesthesia is generally given while the patient is temporarily sedated using a short-acting anesthetic agent. Bupivacaine (0.75%; 5–7 mL) with hyaluronidase gives a relatively quick-acting, and long-duration anesthesia. A lid block is optional. If the patient feels some discomfort later in the procedure, additional retrobulbar anesthesia is added with a blunt-tipped cannula. Anesthesiologists may administer sedating agents to help the patient remain comfortable throughout the procedure. The major risks of the retrobulbar injection include globe perforation, optic nerve injury, intrasheath injection with intracranial involvement or contralateral optic nerve involvement, apnea, seizures, and retrobulbar hemorrhage. A retrobulbar anesthetic may be given at the conclusion of the procedure using a blunt-tipped cannula, to help with postoperative pain control.

Draping and Preparation

The operative eye should be examined briefly by the surgeon or a qualified assistant to ensure that preparation is performed on the correct eye. Following the retrobulbar block or induction of general anesthesia, the fellow eye should be protected and shielded to prevent inadvertent pressure by the surgeon or assistant. Some surgeons prefer to trim the eyelashes (optional step) by using scissors coated with an ocular lubricant on each blade. This prevents the lashes from falling into the eye and fornices. Next, the eye is prepared with an ophthalmic povidone-iodine solution (5% Betadine) and draped to occlude the lashes from the surgical field. Occasionally, a lateral canthotomy is helpful to increase the exposure of the globe. After a heavy lid speculum is inserted, corneal exposure becomes important. Frequent application of a methylcellulose solution will serve to improve visualization throughout the procedure. Likewise, if a blood clot forms on the cornea during the surgical procedure, it should be irrigated and methylcellulose reapplied. This simple technique will help to maintain corneal clarity and improve retinal visualization during indirect ophthalmoscopy.

Scleral Buckling Surgery

The Peritomy

A 360-degree conjunctival peritomy is performed. The initial incision is made by grasping both conjunctiva and

Tenon's capsule with a toothed forceps and cutting in a radial fashion using a blunt curved scissors in the sector chosen for the radial relaxing incision (Fig. 41-2). Elevating the conjunctiva and Tenon's capsule, the closed scissors are used to bluntly separate Tenon's capsule from the underlying sclera. Conjunctiva and Tenon's capsule are incised in tandem for 360 degrees adjacent to the limbus while two separate radial relaxing incisions approximately 5 mm in length and 180 degrees apart are recommended to avoid conjunctival tearing. Some recommend that the relaxing incisions be made at the 3-o'clock and 9-o'clock position. The advantage of this location is that the radial incisions overlie the medialis and lateralis recti muscles; therefore, there is less risk of buckle extrusion postoperatively. Another location for the relaxing incisions is superonasal to inferotemporal (i.e., in the right eye, at 4-o'clock and 10-o'clock positions). The advantage to this location is that the radial relaxing incisions are not readily visible in the interpalpebral fissure, and the risk of scarring between conjunctiva and the rectus muscles is less.

Isolating the Rectus Muscles

A curved tenotomy scissors is then used to dissect the quadrants between each of the four rectus muscles. The cut edge of conjunctiva is grasped and elevated using a toothed forceps. Closed curved scissors are inserted between the conjunctiva and bare sclera and spread. This action will create a taut edge of Tenon's capsule. The conjunctiva and Tenon's capsule are elevated together. Closed tenotomy scissors are inserted into each quadrant between the capsule and sclera and opened with a spreading motion (Fig. 41-3).

A muscle hook is used to engage each rectus muscle insertion. With a cotton-tipped applicator, adherent Tenon's capsule is stripped posteriorly from the rectus muscle, and a 2-0 silk tie is passed underneath the insertion with a fenestrated muscle hook or a hemostat. The rectus superior is

the last muscle to be isolated and requires special care to avoid incorporating fibers from the underlying obliquus superior muscle that may result in a postoperative torsional diplopia. Rotating the globe inferiorly, a cotton-tipped applicator is then passed along the lateral border of the rectus superior, stripping Tenon's capsule and exposing the muscle insertion site (Fig. 41-4). A muscle hook is then passed under the muscle insertion site as far anteriorly as possible with direct visualization from a temporal to nasal direction. Passing the hook too far posteriorly may result in the capture of obliquus superior fibers. Additionally, a second muscle hook may be passed in a nasal to temporal fashion. Elevating and spreading the two hooks will allow for visualization of any engaged obliquus fibers. A 2-0 silk suture is passed under the insertion and tied with multiple separate knots. This serves to identify the rectus superior and provide proper globe orientation during the procedure. The final

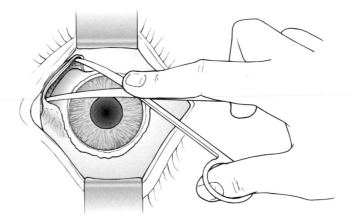

FIGURE 41-3.   *Blunt dissection of the quadrants separating Tenon's capsule from the sclera.*

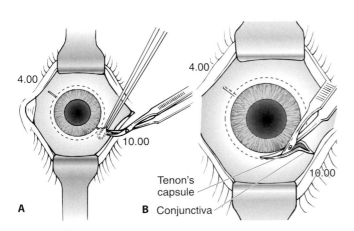

FIGURE 41-2.   *A. The conjunctiva and Tenon's capsule are tented up and cut in a radial fashion. B. A 360-degree peritomy.*

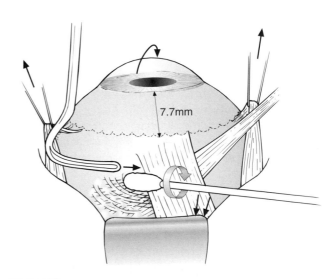

FIGURE 41-4.   *Isolating the rectus superior.*

step is to examine the quadrants for pathology. With a Schepens'-style retractor in place to pull conjunctiva and Tenon's capsule away from the sclera, each quadrant is examined for a staphyloma, areas of scleral ectasia, tumors, or other pathology.

Reoperations

Isolating the rectus muscles during a buckle revision requires careful dissection of the tissue planes. Blunt-tipped scissors are used primarily; however, sharp-tipped scissors, with the potential risk of intrascleral dissection and globe perforation, may occasionally be necessary. After the conjunctiva has been retracted, a capsule surrounding the buckle (explant) is entered, with the scissors over the surface of the buckle. Dissection between the scleral buckle and the sclera is dangerous because scleral tissue may be very thin. After the capsule is opened, the area of revision is cautiously cleared of remaining capsule to expose the sclera. Extensive dissection around scleral *implants* should be avoided because of the risk of globe perforation.

Indirect Ophthalmoscopy

The previously discussed technique of scleral depression and localization techniques are applicable in the operating room. The surgeon has the advantage of controlling the globe and direct exposure of the sclera. The retina must be examined in a systematic fashion in order to identify, localize, and support all breaks with an appropriate scleral buckle. The surgeon begins by examining the posterior pole to re-evaluate the configuration and extent of the retinal detachment and to look for the presence of any posterior holes or tears. The assistant then systematically rotates the eye to provide the surgeon with a view of the peripheral retina. Occasionally, during surgery, the corneal epithelium will become hazy and preclude adequate visualization of the retinal pathology. In these situations, epithelial debridement is performed using a rounded, sharp blade to scrape a central zone of epithelium from the underlying Bowman's layer. Debridement beyond the inner border of the pupil is not necessary. Healing is generally rapid, even in diabetic patients (22).

Localization

When a retinal break is internally localized, a specialized scleral depressor with a small open cylinder at its tip, or "marker-depressor," is used for external localization. With the tip pressed firmly against the sclera for a short period of time, a temporary, blue-gray ring of scleral dehydration is created. This external scleral mark is dried with a cotton-tipped applicator and a water-soluble ink mark is made to designate the location of the break. The marker-depressor is re-placed on the ink mark and the eye is rotated back for the surgeon to verify correct external localization of the retinal break. Small breaks can be localized using a single mark while larger horseshoe-shaped or multiple adjacent tears require a corresponding mark to designate the extent

of the tear or tears. The posterior extent of the tear is the most important mark during encirclement and also the most difficult to accurately localize, especially with a bullously detached retina. The common mistake is to externally localize the retinal break too far posteriorly, owing to an optical effect known as *parallax*. This occurs when a relatively large space separates the wall of the eye from the posterior border of the retinal tear. Viewing the posterior border of the elevated tear from a vertical direction (i.e., through the pupil) creates the impression that the scleral depressor is localizing the posterior border of the tear when in fact the depressor is posterior to the true external localization site (Fig. 41-5). To overcome this problem, two techniques can be used. Deeply indenting the wall of the eye with the scleral depressor to reappose the choroid and the retinal break will eliminate the space between the retina and the eye wall, thus eliminating or minimizing parallax. The second technique is to drain subretinal fluid. While this adds risk, extremely bullous detachments may necessitate drainage for other reasons.

The Chorioretinal Adhesion

Currently, cryotherapy is the most common method of thermotherapy used to create a chorioretinal adhesion during scleral buckling procedures. The cryotherapy probe is protected by a thermal sleeve that allows direct contact of sclera with a small circular knob at the tip of the probe. A separate knob is located on the handle of the cryoprobe 180 degrees away from this cryotip. The knob is used for tactile feedback of the cryotip location. The cryoprobe achieves a −80°C freeze within a few seconds of activation of the foot pedal. Other methods include the use of diathermy, indirect laser, or transscleral diode laser (23). The primary disadvantage of diathermy is that it causes thermal injury to the sclera, and therefore necessitates scleral dissections prior to

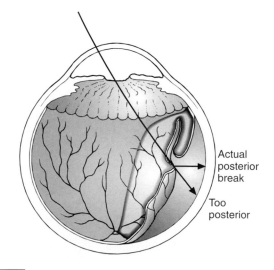

Actual posterior break

Too posterior

FIGURE 41-5. *Inadvertent posterior localization secondary to parallax.*

buckle placement (implants). Cryotherapy does not have an injurious effect on the sclera (24) and facilitates external placement of a scleral buckle (explants). Indirect laser techniques necessitate direct apposition of the retina to the retinal pigment epithelium. Transscleral diode laser utilizes the diode laser delivered externally with an illuminated probe, visualized internally by the surgeon.

After localization, cryotherapy is applied to each break. The softened globe from scleral depression improves the surgeon's ability to approximate the choroid to the retinal breaks. The freeze is applied along the borders of the retinal tear and extended anteriorly to the ora serrata on each side of the tear (Fig. 41-6). Both choroidal and retinal whiten-

ing is the desired end point of cryotherapy that results in a strong chorioretinal adhesion (25,26). Overtreating the choroid or treating bare choroid inside the borders of the retinal tear should be avoided because there is evidence that cryotherapy may liberate or disperse the retinal pigment epithelium and increase the subsequent risk of proliferative retinopathy (27,28). After the foot pedal is released, a firm adhesion ("iceball") is present between the tip of the cryoprobe and the eye wall. Attempting to pull the probe off of the sclera or twist it off should be avoided because this can lead to a fracture of the choroid with subsequent hemorrhage. The patient's body temperature will thaw the freeze in a few seconds.

A common mistake is to use the shaft, rather than the tip, of the cryoprobe to indent the sclera. If one is treating the temporal region of the retina, the actual tip of the cryoprobe may be located under the macula, and activation of the probe could have severe consequences (Fig. 41-7). Therefore, only the tip of the cryoprobe should be used for depression. The probe tip should be directed toward the center of the eye rather than toward the orbital apex. "Suspicious areas" may also be treated to help identify true retinal breaks. Small retinal breaks or discontinuities of retina appear as reddish-orange spots in the center of the white freeze.

The Scleral Buckle

A wide variety of variously sized and shaped scleral buckles are available. Most are made of either solid silicone or a porous silicone sponge material. Some of the more common elements are shown in Figure 41-8.

Techniques of scleral buckle placement include implantation of the buckling materials into the sclera or explanting the buckling elements on the scleral surface using

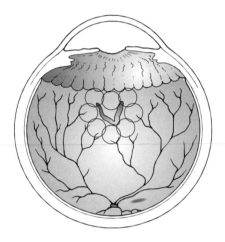

FIGURE 41-6. *Encircling the retinal break with cryotherapy and anterior to the ora serrata.*

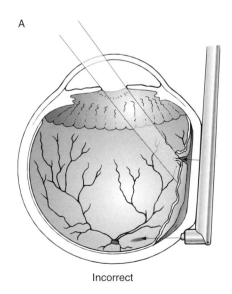

Incorrect

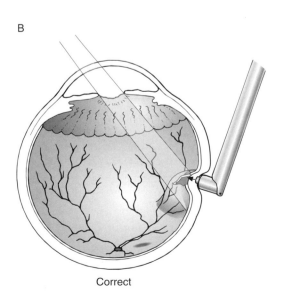

Correct

FIGURE 41-7. A. *Improper cryotherapy depression can lead to posterior treatment.* B. *Proper probe position.*

Bands

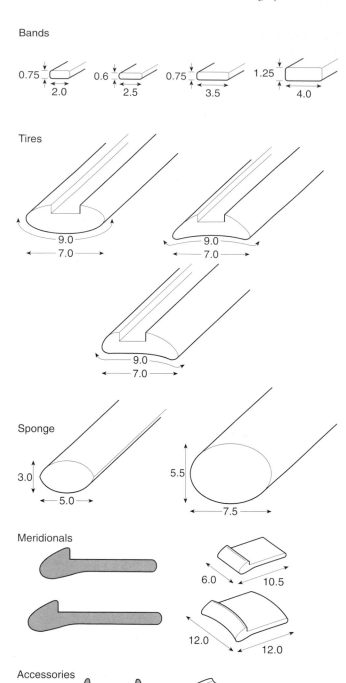

Tires

Sponge

Meridionals

Accessories

FIGURE 41-8.   *Commonly used scleral buckling elements.*

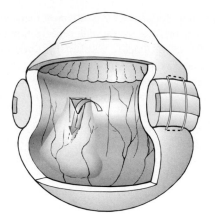

FIGURE 41-9.   *The "fish-mouth" phenomenon from encirclement with radial folds.*

scleral sutures. Techniques of implantation may be required when diathermy is used to create a chorioretinal adhesion but are not necessary following cryotherapy. The most important aspect of buckle placement is the position of the element relative to the site of the retinal tear. The goal is to indent the wall of the eye and bring the retinal pigment epithelium into contact with and support the retinal hole.

Radial Elements   Radial elements can be used alone to close a single retinal break, or they can be used in combination with encircling elements. Larger retinal tears generally require a radial element to decrease the risk of radial folds that may occur with encirclement. The "fish-mouth" phenomenon can occur when a radial fold at the posterior edge of a large retinal break remains folded open, allowing fluid to dissect posteriorly (Fig. 41-9). Radial elements help to alleviate this problem by increasing the internal surface area of the choroid underneath the retinal break and provide a larger surface for the retinal hole to rest on.

Two commonly used radial elements are a radial sponge and a solid silicone meridional element. The difference is the internal contour provided by the element. A sponge provides a sloping indentation while a meridional element has a flat rectangular indentation. Either element is easily cut to conform to the desired size. A meridional element is more commonly used with an encircling tire because it has a ledge that supports the element on the posterior border of the encircling tire and prevents it from extruding anteriorly. The most commonly used sponges are the 5- and 7.5-mm sponges (Nos. 506 and 507 style, respectively) that are elliptical in cross section. The size refers to the sponge's width; they can be cut to any desired length. An elliptical sponge can be cut lengthwise with a straight scissors to decrease the bulk of the sponge.

The size of the sponge should be approximately 2 mm wider than the retinal tear, to ensure that all borders of the tear are supported. Imbrication or "wrapping" the sclera around the borders of the element provides significant internal indentation of the choroid. The sutures are placed in a mattress style, leaving 1 mm of sclera on each side of the sponge for effective imbrication. Too much imbrication can lead to an undesirably steep indentation while too little imbrication will not support the break. The sutures should extend 2 mm anterior to the anterior horns of the retinal tear and 3 mm posterior to the posterior border of the retinal tear to ensure that the edges of the tear are well supported (Fig. 41-10). If too narrow of a posterior border is indented, the posterior edge of the retinal tear may remain open on the posterior slope of indentation, thus allowing fluid to enter the subretinal space.

Meridional elements may also be imbricated into the sclera in conjunction with encirclement. When used with a tire, anterior-to-posterior mattress sutures effectively imbricate the element and the tire. Should a break fall under a rectus muscle insertion, placement of too large of an element can result in a postoperative motility disturbance. For example, small breaks under the rectus superior can be supported using thinner elements, often referred to as *buttons* (i.e., No. 22 style). Pneumatic retinopexy should also be considered for isolated tears under the rectus superior.

A temporary radial element for small retinal detachments that may be used in an outpatient setting is the orbital balloon (29). This device creates a temporary external indentation. Laser photocoagulation may be used to create a chorioretinal adhesion, and the balloon is removed in approximately 1 week, after a chorioretinal adhesion forms. Excellent primary reattachment rates of over 90% have been reported with this device when used with laser photocoagulation (30).

Encirclement The primary goal of encirclement is to support the entire vitreous base. Narrow encircling elements are referred to as bands (2–4mm) while the wider form is a tire (5–12mm). A band is either used alone, with a radial element, or used to hold a tire or sponge in place. Either a 2.5- or 2.0-mm encircling band (No. 240 or 40 style) fits

into the groove (2.5mm) of the tire to secure it to the globe circumferentially. The advantage of a 2-mm band is that it slides more easily in the groove of the tire. The most commonly used tire is 7mm wide and either symmetric (No. 287 or 277 style) or asymmetric (No. 276 style).

Two methods of attachment are commonly used, scleral sutures or belt loops. The preplacement of scleral sutures in each quadrant facilitates the encirclement and prevents the buckle from slipping posteriorly (Fig. 41-11). Two commonly used sutures are a 4-0 white silk suture with an R-7 style needle (Alcon) or a 5-0 nylon with an S-24 style needle (Ethicon). Both are spatulated needles that glide in a parallel fashion with the scleral lamellae. The R-7 needle is shorter and results in a shorter needle pass through the sclera. Because of this, two mattress sutures may be placed in each quadrant when a tire is used. The use of two sutures per quadrant may increase the axial shortening that occurs with broad encircling elements (31). The S-24 needle is longer, resulting in a longer needle track, and usually only requires a single broad mattress suture per quadrant. When scleral sutures are passed, the needle tip should be visualized at all times to avoid scleral perforation. If a scleral bite becomes too shallow, the needle pass is completed and an adjacent scleral bite is taken. Removing the needle, by backing it out, will weaken the sclera. Caution should be exercised in areas of thin sclera such as in a highly myopic eye or an eye with patches of bluish discoloration and areas of scleral ectasia. On average, the sclera is thinnest at the equator or approximately 12 to 14mm posterior to the corneoscleral limbus. The mean thickness at this location is approximately 0.4mm, but the sclera may be as thin as

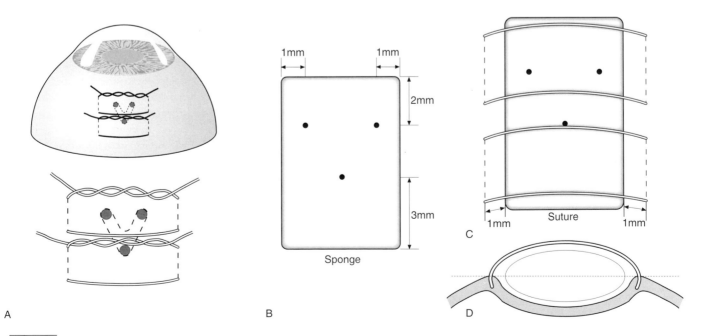

FIGURE 41-10. A. *Suture placement for a radial sponge.* B. *Proper sponge size, extending beyond the borders of the retinal break.* C. *Proper placement of mattress sutures relative to the sponge.* D. *Cross-sectional view of desired imbrication.*

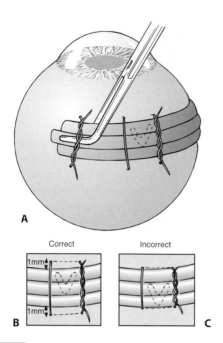

Correct | Incorrect

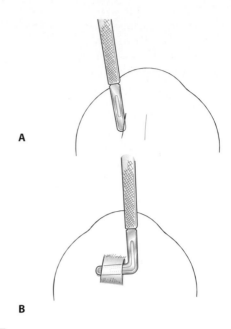

FIGURE 41-11. A. *Passing an encircling element through preplaced mattress sutures. B. Proper location of the break on the anterior slope of the buckle. C. Improper positioning of the break on the posterior slope of the buckle.*

FIGURE 41-12. A. *Vertical incision for belt loops. B. The intrascleral lamellar dissection.*

0.1 mm, albeit rarely (32). Obviously, vortex vessels should be avoided. Belt loops were glued to the sclera in a young child with blue sclera, to avoid passing sutures through extremely thin sclera (33).

Alternatively, belt loops can be used to secure an encircling band in each quadrant. A sharp No. 64 blade is held perpendicular to the sclera, and two partial-thickness, parallel, scleral incisions of the appropriate length to accommodate the band are made perpendicular to the limbus. Next, a curved, sharp, spatulated blade is used to dissect between the two vertical incisions at a midscleral depth. Once the edge of sclera has been engaged at the appropriate depth, the tip of the blade is pushed toward the second incision using a sweeping and elevating motion, thus minimizing the risk of dissection into the globe (Fig. 41-12). To facilitate the passage of the band through the belt loops, the end of the band should be cut in an angled fashion.

The band or tire is passed under each rectus muscle for encirclement and the ends of the band are then joined, usually in the superonasal aspect of the globe, using a silicone sleeve. A "sleeve spreader" is used to stretch the sleeve open and allow access to the ends of the band (Fig. 41-13). The first end of the band is passed through the spread sleeve from the "backdoor." The second end of the band is then passed on top of the first end through the "frontdoor" of the sleeve. Once the band and forceps are in the sleeve, a forceps is then used to push the sleeve off of the sleeve spreader. The band should be examined for twists created during its manipulation.

Indentation of the globe using encircling tires is achieved primarily by imbrication (31). Standard imbrication is achieved by placing the mattress suture bites approximately 2 mm wider than the encircling band or tire (see Fig. 41-11). Suture bites are placed 9 mm apart with the standard 7-mm tire. Bands achieve indentation by tightening the encirclement and decreasing the circumference of the eye (31). The best way to judge the degree of buckle elevation is by visualizing the internal height of indentation. Measuring the amount a band is tightened in millimeters may help to achieve a consistent indentation. It is difficult to determine the amount to tighten a band in eyes with a low intraocular pressure (common during buckling). When an eye is soft, either from drainage, paracentesis, or depression, the band may easily be overtightened. A tight encirclement may lead to radial folds in the retina, ocular ischemia, choroidal detachments, induced myopia, and postoperative pain. Patients with sickle cell anemia may be at greater risk for ocular ischemia if encirclement is employed (34). A history of sickle cell anemia should be inquired of all black patients undergoing scleral buckling surgery. Anterior-segment ischemia occurred in a patient with sickle cell trait associated with scleral buckling surgery (35).

Drainage

Disadvantages Drainage of subretinal fluid can result in significant complications, and performance of this step during buckling surgery is controversial. Studies demonstrated that nondrainage procedures have an equally high success rate as do drainage procedures. Lincoff and Kreissig (36) reported an 89% success rate in 1000 consecutive nondrainage procedures. Potential complications

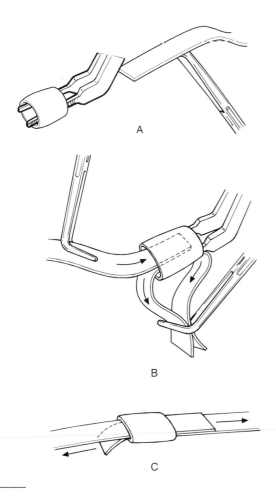

FIGURE 41-13. *Step 1: The band is passed through the "backdoor" of the sleeve. Step 2: The band is passed through the "frontdoor" of the sleeve on top of the secured opposite end. Step 3: The band may be tightened.*

from drainage include subretinal and possibly submacular hemorrhage, retinal incarceration, and retinal hole formation.

Advantages   The two most important reasons to drain subretinal fluid are to reappose the retina and to reduce the volume of the eye. Volume reduction allows for the imbrication of the explant with better control of the intraocular pressure. Immediate, postoperative reattachment of the retina is not an indication to drain subretinal fluid. Drainage does allow for assessment of the adequacy and location of the scleral buckle or the presence of radial folds with the fishmouth phenomenon. Many retinal surgeons believe that the benefits of a cautious drainage procedure in selective patients outweigh the risks.

Bullous Detachments   The retinal break in a bullous retinal detachment may not be reapposed intraoperatively to the choroid by the buckle; however, the "fluid dynamics" may be altered enough to decrease the amount of subretinal fluid

from entering the subretinal space. As discussed earlier, if the balance of subretinal fluid formation is altered, the retinal pigment epithelium may be able to remove more subretinal fluid than what enters through the break and the retina will reattach. If the hole remains open and fluid continues to "overwhelm" the retinal pigment epithelial pump, or the pumping function is compromised, the retina will remain detached. In certain situations, it may be reasonable to drain subretinal fluid and reappose the tear to shift the balance of subretinal fluid dynamics in favor of retinal reattachment. Additionally, the retinal reapposition facilitates cryotherapy and minimizes parallax. The cryotherapy freeze may only need to occur at the level of the retinal pigment epithelium to create an adequate chorioretinal adhesion; however, there is some evidence that extending the freeze to the retina will increase the strength of the adhesion (25,26).

Intraocular Pressure   Drainage is the most useful way to manage intraocular pressure during the placement of the buckling elements and prevent severe ischemic injury to the optic nerve. The intraocular pressure during scleral buckling surgery has been reported to be as high as 210 mm Hg (37). The amount of intraocular volume displacement during the placement of broad buckling elements may be up as much as $1.8\,cm^3$ or 45% of the vitreous volume (38).

Other methods are available to lower the intraocular pressure during the buckling procedure. Scleral depression during the examination and cryotherapy will soften the eye. An anterior-chamber paracentesis will remove 0.2 to 0.4 mL of fluid. For a small circumferential band or a small radial element, these methods alone may be adequate. However, if a circumferential tire is placed, imbrication of the sclera in one or two quadrants may occlude the central retinal artery. For this reason, after each mattress suture is tied, the intraocular pressure should be assessed digitally. Experienced physicians are able to determine digitally when the intraocular pressure is over 30 mm Hg (39). Drainage prior to securing the scleral mattress sutures around the buckling elements will allow for a substantial reduction of intraocular volume. Acetazolamide or mannitol can be used to medically manage the intraocular pressure; however, these techniques are slower in action, offer less effective pressure lowering, and have the uncommon risks of immune-mediated reactions and intracranial hemorrhage.

Paracentesis using a 30-gauge needle on a tuberculin syringe with the plunger removed allows the surgeon to support the globe with one hand, hold the syringe with the other, and keep a constant view of the tip of the needle in the anterior chamber. Aqueous will flow in a slow controlled manner into the empty syringe barrel as long as the intraocular pressure is higher than the atmospheric pressure. A cotton-tipped applicator on the globe may also be used to provide contralateral pressure for the paracentesis. The needle track is made through the peripheral region of the cornea with the tip of the needle held bevel-up between the periphery of the iris and corneal endothelium, and away from the lens. Aphakic eyes or eyes with anterior-chamber intraocular lenses are at risk for vitreous incarceration into the paracentesis drainage site. Careful preoperative examination of the lens and anterior chamber will help to identify eyes at risk.

Timing of Drainage   Drainage is easiest to perform after the mattress sutures have been placed and the buckling elements are in position, but prior to tightening the scleral sutures. Passing scleral mattress sutures in a firm eye is much easier and safer than in a soft eye. Occasionally, during placement of a scleral mattress suture, a deep needle pass in an area of detached retina causes inadvertent drainage of subretinal fluid, thus obviating the need for another drainage site. Following any drainage, planned or unplanned, the retina should be inspected with indirect ophthalmoscopy for choroidal hemorrhage, new retinal holes, or incarceration.

Drainage Technique   Several factors should be considered when selecting the drainage site. First, the retina should be reinspected to ensure that it is detached under the selected area. Drainage sites to avoid include areas adjacent to the vortex veins, areas under large retinal breaks, and areas treated with cryotherapy. Vortex vessels are surrounded by a crowded vascular network that increases the risk of hemorrhage during the puncture of the choroid. Draining directly under a large retinal tear may result in vitreous "runthrough." This occurs when liquid vitreous from the vitreous cavity, rather than subretinal fluid, drains through the retinal tear and out the drainage site. Should the eye continue to drain, become extremely soft, or even collapse during drainage, "runthrough" should be suspected. Drainage should be located away from large retinal tears. Choroid previously treated with cryotherapy may also be more likely to bleed because of vascular engorgement. A good area for drainage is at either the superior or the inferior border of the horizontal rectus muscles. Passing the 2-0 silk rectus muscle suture under the encircling element at the muscle border will lift the element off of the scleral surface and provide excellent exposure for drainage (Fig. 41-14).

The optic nerve may preclude a subretinal hemorrhage from entering the macula if a drainage site is selected in the nasal quadrants. The surgical exposure of the nasal quadrants is more limited by the patient's nose and orbit. Exposure of the temporal quadrants for drainage is much simpler and drainage is safe when the fovea is still attached to preclude a possible subretinal hemorrhage from the macula. If the fovea is detached and a temporal drainage site is selected, a choroidal hemorrhage may pool under the fovea. The drainage should be located under an area that is designated for external support with a buckling element. This will support the scleral opening or potential complications such as an iatrogenic retinal hole or retinal incarceration. If the drainage site does not fall under a supporting element, a lamellar scleral suture can be used to close the sclerotomy after drainage.

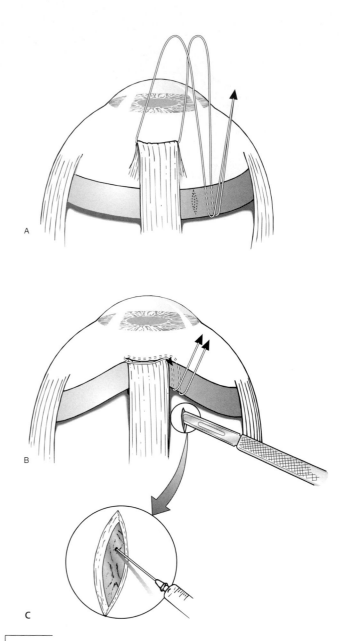

FIGURE 41-14.   A. *The 2-0 silk muscle tie is passed under the band.* B. *Sclera is cut vertically to expose the choroid.* C. *Bare choroid is punctured with a needle.*

The following description represents one of many possible ways to create a drainage site. After the drainage site has been identified, a No. 64 blade is held perpendicular to the globe and a long, partial-thickness, vertical incision is made into the sclera. A broad side-to-side scraping motion pushes the scleral fibers aside and creates a relatively broad exposure to the deeper scleral fibers. Eventually, the dissection will reveal the brown-black color of the choroid. The use of diathermy at this point is optional. Some surgeons will use a diathermy probe to shrink the sclera at the borders of the dissection; however, the side-to-side scraping action of the blade also spreads the scleral fibers and allows for excellent exposure to the choroid. Diathermy may be used to treat the underlying choroid (40,41). The globe should not be too firm during drainage because of the increased risk of retinal incarceration. A rapid gush of subretinal fluid may bring the detached retina quickly into apposition with the drainage site and cause either obstruction to further drainage or retinal incarceration.

Either a 30-gauge needle on a tuberculin syringe or a small-caliber tapered needle held with a needle driver is commonly used to puncture the choroid. Large-bore needles or spatulated needles are contraindicated and risk causing a choroidal hemorrhage. While argon laser has been used to create external drainage, it is unclear that it offers a clear benefit over conventional methods (42,43). The needle is slowly passed through the exposed choroid and slowly withdrawn. Jabbing motions or deep insertion of the needle should be avoided. As the needle is withdrawn, a straw-colored fluid will seep from the drainage site. As the eye softens, the flow will diminish. Cotton-tipped applicators may be placed around the globe in the space between the globe and the orbit to maintain adequate intraocular pressure and thereby maintain adequate flow of subretinal fluid from the drainage site (Fig. 41-15). Avoid depressing the sclera posterior to the drainage site as this will push the small opening in the choroid in toward the retina and potentially occlude the flow. When the flow stops, the retina must be reinspected to assess the drainage site for possible retinal incarceration or other complications. Do not

attempt to redrain from the same site prior to internal inspection.

If no fluid drains during attempted drainage, and proper location of the drainage has been confirmed, the most likely reason is incomplete or inadequate perforation of the choroid. Multiple attempts to perforate the choroid increase the risk of a hemorrhagic complication. A second possibility is that the scleral dissection is inadequate and exposure of the perforated choroid is blocked by scleral fibers. This problem necessitates meticulous dissection and preparation of the scleral bed before needle perforation is attempted. Another possible cause is shifting subretinal fluid. The patient's head and globe should be tilted to allow dependent subretinal fluid to flow toward the drainage site.

If the drain initially worked well and some of the subretinal fluid drained, but then the drain stopped working, the desired goal may have been achieved and further attempts to drain the remaining fluid would add risk without providing additional benefit. One must remember that the goal is to reapproximate the retinal break to the supporting elements and to decrease the intraocular volume of the eye to allow space for the imbricated buckling elements. The decision to make a second drainage site requires an assessment of these surgical goals.

Complications of Drainage An iatrogenic retinal hole or incarcerated retina requires treatment with cryotherapy, and the area should be supported by a buckling element. Iatrogenic retinal tears may result from attempts to manually reduce incarcerated retina. Significant incarceration is avoided by avoiding high intraocular pressures during the drainage procedure. The flow of fluid from the drainage should be slow yet steady. Again, once flow stops through the drainage site, intraocular pressure should remain low and the retina re-examined.

A small subretinal hemorrhage is occasionally seen and is usually self-limiting. However, if a significant amount of subretinal hemorrhage develops under the macula, further management is necessary, and several options are available. First, the patient's head may be tilted to place the macula in a less dependent position. Converting to pars plana vitrectomy to evacuate the submacular hemorrhage may also be considered when a large amount of blood is present (44,45). Another option would be to introduce an intraocular gas bubble and place the patient in a face-down position. This technique may force a fresh subfoveal hemorrhage away from the fovea and into the more peripheral subretinal space. Observation and proper positioning may offer the safest management option for a thin layer of submacular blood.

The Soft Eye Following the drainage procedure, the eye may be extremely soft. During the drainage, cotton-tipped applicators were inserted between the globe and the orbital tissues to maintain adequate intraocular pressure for drainage. Removal of all the cotton-tipped applicators at this point should be avoided. Instead, one or two applicators are

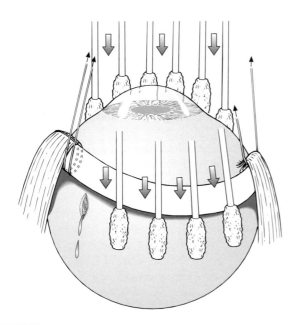

FIGURE 41-15. *Intraocular pressure is maintained by multiple cotton-tipped applicators placed between the globe and the orbit.*

removed at a time to allow for the mattress sutures of the scleral buckling elements to be tightened and secured. If the globe is still too soft, a pars plana injection of a balanced salt solution will re-establish normal intraocular pressure while the remaining cotton-tipped applicators are removed. Avoiding low intraocular pressures with this technique will minimize choroidal hemorrhage from the drainage and potentially decrease the development of postoperative choroidal detachments.

Closing

A final indirect ophthalmoscopic inspection is made of the retina, fovea, optic nerve, retinal tears, location and height of the supporting elements, amount of residual subretinal fluid, and drainage site. Any final adjustments of explant location, buckle height, or tightness of the band should be made at this time. Fish-mouthing of a retinal break can be corrected by either loosening the encircling band or adding an additional radial element. Bands should be pulled to a modest height. A low intraocular pressure at this point may overestimate the buckle height. Using supplemental pneumatic techniques, a pars plana injection of a gas or sterile air is performed following the final retinal inspection. Once air or gas is injected, clear visualization of the posterior pole is often lost. Suture knots on the scleral buckle should be rotated posteriorly, and trimmed. The loose ends of the band should be trimmed and the buckle should be inspected for sharp or jagged edges that may erode through the conjunctiva postoperatively. The quadrants are inspected and irrigated with an antibiotic solution.

Closure of Tenon's capsule and conjunctiva may seem trivial, but when a scleral buckle is in place, a meticulous conjunctival closure is essential for many reasons. Reoperations are relatively common and access to the buckle is highly dependent on previous closure. Scleral buckling elements can become infected if exposed through inadequately closed conjunctiva. Also, a restrictive strabismus can result from improper conjunctival closure. Glaucoma is not uncommon after retinal detachment and future filtering surgery may depend on good conjunctival closure. Obviously, a good cosmetic result is important to the patient.

At the beginning of the procedure, conjunctiva and Tenon's capsule were forced posteriorly into the orbit. Two nontoothed forceps work well to retrieve the previously cut edges of the two layers that should remain in tandem. The relaxing incisions are identified and laid out at the respective positions near the limbus. A 6-0 plain gut suture is first passed through the sclera approximately 1 mm posterior to the limbus. Next, the corners of Tenon's capsule and conjunctiva from the relaxing incision are secured and tied. The short end of the suture is cut, and the long end is used in a running fashion to close the radial relaxing incision (Fig. 41-16). The edges of conjunctiva should be everted to prevent epithelial inclusion cysts. Approximately 2 to 3 mL of bupivacaine is injected into the retrobulbar space using a curved blunt cannula, to provide postoperative pain control

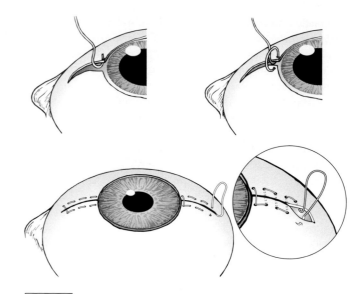

FIGURE 41-16. *Closing the radial relaxing incisions and everting the edges of conjunctiva.*

(46). Finally, the opposite radial relaxing incision is closed in a similar manner. Care is taken not to "hood" or partially cover the cornea with conjunctiva.

Complications Following Scleral Buckling

Failure to Reattach the Retina

Failure to reattach the retina results from an unfavorable balance of subretinal fluid dynamics that favors flow into the subretinal space, overwhelming the retinal pigment epithelial pump. Possible causes include failure to detect and support all retinal breaks, inadequately supported breaks, formation of new retinal breaks, an inadequate chorioretinal adhesion, and proliferative vitreoretinopathy (PVR). PVR is a cellular proliferation on the retinal surface causing contraction and foreshortening of the retina with "rolled edges" around the retinal breaks. PVR may prevent adequate reapposition of the retinal break to the underlying supporting element. Encircling techniques, to some extent, relieve some of this contraction on the retina; however, pars plana vitrectomy procedures allow access for removal of more severe PVR. If PVR formation is suspected preoperatively, a more substantial scleral buckle (i.e., with a 7.0-mm tire) is recommended. The inferior region of the retina is more commonly affected by PVR and should be broadly supported. Features that have been associated with PVR formation include multiple or large retinal breaks, heavy cryotherapy treatment, chronic retinal detachment, associated trauma with vitreous hemorrhage, and others. In one of the largest available series, Rachal and Burton (47) reviewed 1088 consecutive scleral buckling surgeries for primary retinal detachments and reported a 76% initial success rate. PVR was the most common reason for failure. Other preoperative features that may predict failure of scleral buckling include vitreous hemorrhage, previous retinal detachment, a total retinal detachment, and a low intraocular pressure (<10 mm Hg) (48). Augmenting buckle material, modifying existing buckle material, replacing the buckle, and retreatment of inadequate chorioretinal adhesion are the techniques used for secondary buckle repair (49).

Choroidal Detachments

A choroidal detachment results from fluid accumulation between the choroid and the sclera and occurs in approximately 40% of patients after scleral buckling surgery (50,51). It is more commonly associated with the use of larger scleral buckling elements and detachments in older individuals. The mechanism probably relates to the impaired outflow of blood via the choroidal circulation. Time and observation comprise the treatment of limited choroidal detachment; however, massive choroidal detachments or choroidal detachments causing angle-closure glaucoma should be surgically drained.

Angle Closure

Angle-closure glaucoma either with or without pupillary block can occur following scleral buckling procedures. Swelling or congestion of fluid near the ciliary body can cause anterior rotation of the periphery of the iris and occlude the angle. Such patients should be treated medically to provide control of elevated intraocular pressure while the swelling subsides. If the condition persists, the angle is at risk of permanent synechial closure. Peripheral laser iridoplasty (52) utilizes the argon laser to induce contraction of the periphery of the iris away from the chamber angle. If angle closure persists, drainage of anteriorly located suprachoroidal fluid may alleviate the pressure on the periphery of the iris. Rarely, the scleral buckle may need to be removed.

Other Complications

Anterior-segment ischemia is uncommon but should be suspected in cases of encirclement with highly elevated buckles. Disinsertion of a rectus muscle to facilitate buckle placement is also a risk factor. Signs and symptoms include postoperative corneal edema, elevated intraocular pressure, pain, and an anterior-chamber reaction. Treatment should initially be symptomatic with topical corticosteroids and cycloplegia. Buckle removal may be required.

Postoperative diplopia is very common in extreme fields of gaze after scleral buckling surgery (53). It is less common in primary gaze, and only 3% to 5% of patients complain of diplopia postoperatively (54,55). Other studies indicated that the risk of diplopia increases with larger buckles, and occurs in approximately 30% of patients with high encircling buckles (56). Radial elements alone are less likely to cause extraocular muscle imbalances postoperatively (57).

Monocular diplopia may also be a sign of macular pucker formation. Most eyes with retinal detachment also have an accompanying posterior vitreous separation that can lead to epiretinal membrane formation. Additionally, proliferative cellular material from a retinal break or hole plus the use of cryotherapy may contribute to macular pucker formation. Some degree of epiretinal membrane formation or macular pucker is present in approximately 10% to 50% of all retinal detachments repaired with scleral buckling (58–61).

Encirclement may induce a significant amount of induced myopia from axial lengthening of the globe. Smiddy et al (62) noted a mean induced myopia of 2.75 D in eyes with encircling buckles.

As with most forms of ophthalmic surgery, endophthalmitis can occur after scleral buckling surgery (in approximately 0.02% of patients) (63,64). The incidence of infected scleral buckles is low (1.1%–1.5%) (65,66). Infected buckles are associated with buckle exposure, and removal of the infected buckle is recommended.

Postoperative inflammation can lead to the formation of cystoid macular edema (60), which is more common in aphakic eyes and in older patients (67). Angiographic edema occurs in up to 25% of phakic eyes (67). Standard treatment with topical nonsteroidal agents or periocular corticosteroids is indicated.

Acquired peripheral retinal telangiectasia is also a rare complication of scleral buckling surgery (68).

PRINCIPLES OF PNEUMATIC RETINOPEXY

The basic principles of pneumatic retinopexy are the same as those described for scleral buckling. Instead of depressing the wall of the eye inward, the retinal break is pushed toward the wall of the eye (Fig. 41-17). The technique of pneumatic retinopexy shifts the balance of subretinal fluid dynamics in favor of fluid resorption by taking advantage of the surface tension and buoyancy of an intraocular gas bubble. A decision to use pneumatic techniques instead of scleral buckling or vitrectomy depends on many factors and is best made by the patient and surgeon together.

Advantages and Disadvantages

Some retinal surgeons may argue that pneumatic retinopexy techniques should represent first-line treatment for primary retinal detachments in selected patients. The main advantage of pneumatic retinopexy is that hospital admission and the risks and costs associated with surgery may be avoided. In today's medical environment of cost containment and managed care, a less expensive, equally efficacious procedure is preferable.

In a multicentered randomized controlled clinical trial (69), a comparison of the success rates after a single operation using either pneumatic retinopexy or scleral buckling surgery demonstrated that the reattachment rate

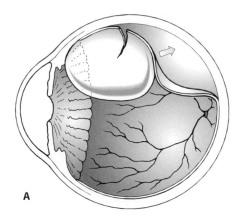

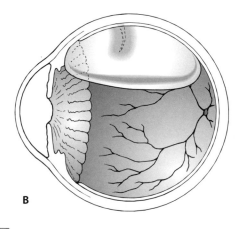

FIGURE 41-17.   A. *Intraocular gas bubble occluding the retinal break.* B. *After the retinal pigment epithelium has pumped out the fluid, and cryotherapy is applied.*

was approximately 80% to 85% for either technique. After a second procedure (either pneumatic retinopexy or scleral buckling surgery), the overall success rate was approximately 98% and not significantly different for either group. Therefore, pneumatic retinopexy offers a viable option for primary retinal reattachment in selected patients and does not seem to jeopardize the reattachment rate of a second procedure. Two-year follow-up available on 90% of these patients confirmed the previous conclusions (70).

The major disadvantage of pneumatic retinopexy is that not all patients with primary retinal detachment qualify as good candidates for pneumatic retinopexy. For the randomized trial comparing pneumatic retinopexy to scleral buckling (69), the exclusion criteria were as follows: 1) breaks larger than one clock hour or multiple breaks extending over more than one clock hour of the retina, 2) breaks in the inferior four clock hours, 3) the presence of PVR grade C or D, 4) physical disability or mental incompetence precluding maintenance of the required position, 5) severe or uncontrolled glaucoma, and 6) cloudy media precluding full assessment of the retina. Caution should be used when

interpreting results of this study to the clinical setting for a patient who would be ineligible for the study. A recent study (6) that included some eyes with "additional pathology" showed lower initial success rates (69%) for single-procedure pneumatic retinopexy. With reoperations (pneumatic retinopexy, scleral buckling, and/or vitrectomy), the reattachment rates approached 98%. Other potential complications include new retinal breaks (13%) and PVR (4%), subretinal gas (71), chronic macular detachment (72), and others.

Larger retinal breaks have been successfully repaired using pneumatic techniques; even giant retinal tears have been successfully treated with pneumatic retinopexy (73). However, treatment of large breaks with the subsequent risk of PVR needs to be addressed before such techniques are recommended.

PNEUMATIC TECHNIQUES

Steps of the preoperative evaluation discussed for scleral buckling surgery should be performed before pneumatic retinopexy, including obtaining detailed informed consent.

Preparation

One of the more cumbersome tasks of pneumatic retinopexy is to have all of the available equipment in a single location and readily available during the procedure. First, the eye should be anesthetized using either sequential local infiltration or a retrobulbar block. Sequential local infiltration provides pain control without the associated risks of a retrobulbar anesthetic. A topical drop of local anesthetic agent is applied followed by a drop of 5% ophthalmic povidone-iodine. Cotton-tipped applicators are soaked with sterile lidocaine and held as a pledgette over the site designated for the gas injection and in the area of the retinal break. A lid speculum is inserted, a 30-gauge needle on a tuberculin syringe with 2% lidocaine is then used to engage conjunctiva, and a subconjunctival bleb is raised.

Sterile gas is filtered with two 0.22-μm Millipore filters and infused into a 5-mL syringe with a three-way stopcock and a tuberculin syringe on the third port. The plunger will slowly retract as pressure from the gas tank fills the 5-mL syringe. Pulling back on the plunger to fill the syringe should be avoided because a leak in the tubing could dilute the gas. The initial syringe of gas should be discarded and then refilled to prevent dilution. The stopcock is closed to the gas tubing and opened to the tuberculin syringe until it is ready to be used. The tuberculin syringe is filled by using pressure on the plunger of the 5-mL syringe. The remaining gas serves as a readily available, reserve supply. The stopcock is placed in a midposition between the two syringes and a 30-gauge needle is quickly transferred to the tuberculin syringe.

The Chorioretinal Adhesion

Techniques of cryotherapy have been discussed previously. Cryotherapy for pneumatic retinopexy necessitates the transconjunctival approach. If a tear is too posterior, the conjunctival fornix may obstruct the necessary placement of the cryotherapy probe. Posterior breaks or bullously detached retinas can be treated with either slit-lamp, indirect laser photocoagulation or cryotherapy on the following day.

Paracentesis

At this point, the globe is generally soft owing to scleral depression and possibly cryotherapy. However, some believe that paracentesis lowers the elevated pressure spike that occurs following the gas injection. Pseudophakic eyes should have a paracentesis prior to injection of the gas. A paracentesis following gas injection, especially with the patient in the supine position, may result in migration of gas into the anterior chamber.

Gas Volume and Expansion

Two fluorinated hydrocarbon gases are available for pneumatic techniques. Pure sulfur hexafluoride (SF_6) will double in size while C_3F_8 will expand four times its initial volume. The geometry of gas bubbles in eyes of different sizes was described by Parver and Lincoff (74). In a 21-mm-axial-length eye, to cover a 90-degree arc or three clock hours of retina, 0.28 mL of gas is required. In order to cover a 120-degree arc or four clock hours, 0.75 mL of gas is required. However, retinal detachments commonly occur in larger myopic eyes. Therefore, in a 24-mm-axial-length eye, three clock hours requires 0.42 mL of gas while four clock hours requires 1.13 mL of gas. The advantage of SF_6 gas is its short duration in the eye (2 weeks), but it also requires a larger initial injection of approximately 0.5 mL (expands to 1.0 mL) (75) to adequately cover most retinal breaks. C_3F_8 gas has the advantage of fourfold expansion (75) in the eye and thus requires a smaller volume of approximately 0.3 mL (expands to 1.2 mL) to tamponade a similar area. However, C_3F_8 also remains in the eye for 4 to 6 weeks. Use of either gas is acceptable as long as the respective physical properties of each are understood. The use of intraocular air has the advantage of being nonexpansible and may therefore decrease the risk of new breaks (76,77). Injecting a larger volume requires more aggressive management of the intraocular pressure.

Injecting the Gas

The patient is placed in a supine position with the head tilted at approximately a 45-degree angle to allow for exposure of the fornix on the side opposite the break. Approximately 3.5 mm is measured posterior to the corneoscleral limbus. A useful tool for measurement is the uncapped end of a tuberculin syringe, which is generally 4 mm wide (this should be confirmed as width may vary by manufacturer). The blunt tip of the tuberculin syringe is gently depressed onto the anesthetized conjunctiva, forming a ring-shaped impression. The plunger on the gas-filled tuberculin syringe is then advanced until the desired volume of gas to be injected remains. The needle is passed through the pars plana and visualized by the surgeon in the vitreous cavity. The needle is slightly withdrawn so that the tip of the needle has just passed into the vitreous. Gas is then injected in a "brisk" manner. As the needle is withdrawn, a cotton-tipped applicator is rolled over the puncture site, and the patient's head is rotated to move the bubble away from the puncture site to prevent gas from escaping. An inspection is made of the central retinal artery to ensure that it is still patent. If a paracentesis was not done before the injection of gas, it may be necessary at this point. The patient's intraocular pressure should be monitored and treated as necessary. Gas expansion should not cause significant elevation of intraocular pressure; however, this should be monitored postoperatively.

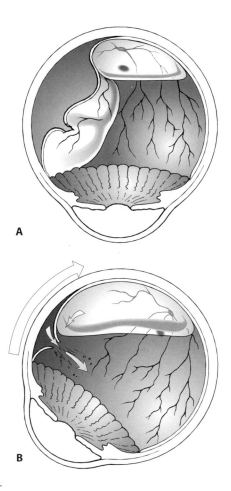

FIGURE 41-18. *A. Intraocular gas tamponades the macula. B. The "steamroller" maneuver forces subretinal fluid into the vitreous as the patient slowly sits upright.*

During the gas injection, multiple small gas bubbles, or "fish eggs," may form and may preclude adequate visualization of the posterior pole or of retinal breaks. The danger of fish eggs is that a bubble may pass through a retinal break and expand subretinally. Fish eggs are prevented by 1) brisk injection of the gas (not a jet stream and not slow), 2) shallow needle placement in the vitreous, and 3) injection in the uppermost site of the globe. Simply thumping the anesthetized globe with a cotton-tipped applicator may coalesce the bubbles. Alternatively, the patient can be placed in a face-down position to keep the bubbles away from the break, until they coalesce. This generally occurs by the next day, and positioning to occlude the break may resume.

If gas is inadvertently injected anterior to the vitreous face, the bubble may become entrapped. One can either remove the gas and reinject a second gas bubble, or position the patient face-down overnight. Passive aspiration of the entrapped gas can be performed with the plunger removed from the tuberculin syringe and a 30-gauge needle.

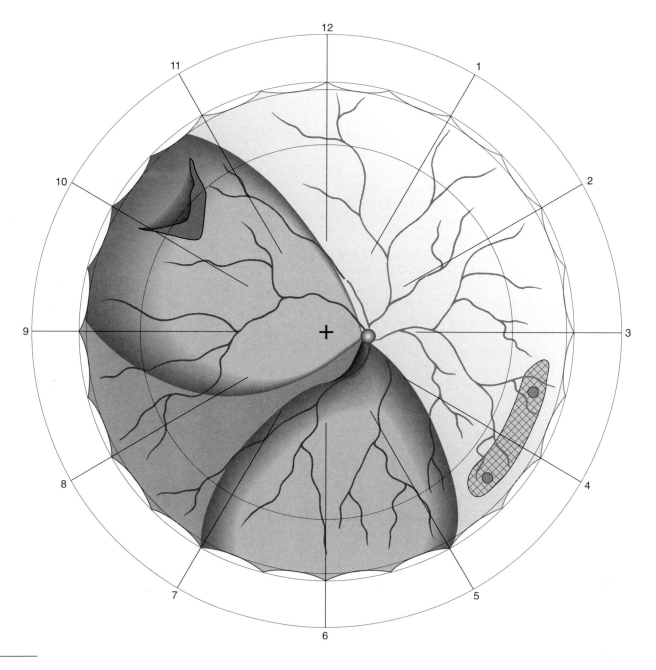

FIGURE 41-19.   *A temporal retinal detachment in a pseudophakic eye, a horseshoe tear, and inferonasal lattice with holes.*

"Steamrolling"

One configuration of retinal detachment that requires special consideration is a relatively bullous detachment that is approaching, but not yet involving the fovea. Positioning the patient so the break is occluded by the bubble can "steamroll" fluid posteriorly and actually detach the fovea. Therefore, after the gas has been injected, and the patient is still in a supine position, he or she is asked to roll from the supine to the prone position in a direction that will cause the bubble to cross attached retina. The patient remains prone for approximately 5 to 10 minutes. This will place the bubble's buoyant force toward the fovea. Assuming the bullous detachment is superior, the patient is assisted off the table, instructed to remain face-down, and allowed to sit in an examination chair. Over the next 10 to 15 minutes, the patient is asked to *very slowly* lift the head to an upright position. This allows the bubble to "steamroll" the subretinal fluid anteriorly and out the superior retinal break (Fig. 41-18). Steamrolling the retina flat may liberate retinal pigment epithelial cells into the vitreous and increase the risk of PVR. Likewise, there is evidence that cryotherapy will cause increased dispersion of retinal pigment epithelium into the vitreous (27,28). Therefore, cryotherapy should be avoided prior to the steamroller maneuver and postponed to the following day when the retina is reapposed. After pneumatic retinopexy, patients should be followed closely in the perioperative period because most failures occur soon after the procedure (6).

Education

The ultimate success or failure of pneumatic retinopexy depends on numerous factors, but educating the patient about positioning is essential. Placing a patch over the eye with a positioning arrow indicating the location of the retinal break is helpful. If a longer-acting gas is used, the patient should be instructed to avoid the supine position until the bubble is gone, to prevent gas-induced cataract formation.

CASE PRESENTATION

How would you approach retinal detachment (Fig. 41-19) in a 55-year-old pseudophakic patient's eye? A horseshoe tear found at the 10- to 11-o'clock position should be supported, but should the area of lattice degeneration in an area of attached retina with atrophic holes at the 4-o'clock position also be supported? Such a case may be handled differently by different retinal surgeons. Some would simply place a radial element to support the causative horseshoe tear. This would not cause a significant refractive change and would be fairly easy to address surgically. Other surgeons would perform a pneumatic retinopexy by injecting an intraocular gas bubble to reappose the torn tissue and recommend proper positioning. Neither of these techniques address the accompanying lattice degeneration. Still others might select an encircling band or a broad encircling tire to support the tear, lattice, and entire vitreous base. The confusing part of retinal detachment repair is that all of the above-mentioned methods may succeed in repairing the detached retina, but any of these methods may also fail. Therefore, the goal of choosing the proper scleral buckling plan is to choose the method that is *most* likely to succeed. For this patient, a reasonable plan would be to place a radial element under the horseshoe tear and encircle the eye with a 4.0-mm band (42 style). The rationale for the radial element is to decrease the risk of the "fish-mouth" phenomenon while the band supports the area of lattice degeneration and the vitreous base. In this patient drainage was not performed because the retina was reapposed by the sponge and the macula was detached. Temporal drainage would have the risk of a submacular hemorrhage. Also, adequate intraocular pressure control was achieved by a paracentesis.

REFERENCES

1. Olsen TW, Chang T, Sternberg P Jr. Retinal detachments associated with blunt trauma. *Semin Ophthalmol* 1995;10:17–27.
2. Pederson JE. Experimental retinal detachment. IV. Aqueous humor dynamics in rhegmatogenous detachments. *Arch Ophthalmol* 1982;100:1814–1816.
3. Schwartz A. Chronic open-angle glaucoma secondary to rhegmatogenous retinal detachment. *Am J Ophthalmol* 1973;75:205–211.
4. Tanaka S, Ideta H, Yonemoto J, et al. Neovascularization of the iris in rhegmatogenous retinal detachment. *Am J Ophthalmol* 1991;112:632–634.
5. Lincoff H, Gieser R. Finding the retinal hole. *Arch Ophthalmol* 1971;85:565–569.
6. Grizzard WS, Hilton GF, Hammer ME, et al. Pneumatic retinopexy failures: cause, prevention, timing, and management. *Ophthalmology* 1995;102:929–936.
7. Frambach DA, Marmor MF. The rate and route of fluid resorption from the subretinal space of the rabbit. *Invest Ophthalmol Vis Sci* 1982;22:292–302.
8. Miller SS, Hughes BA, Machen TE. Fluid transport across retinal pigment epithelium is inhibited by cyclic AMP. *Proc Natl Acad Sci USA* 1982;79:2111–2115.
9. Negi A, Marmor MF. The resorption of subretinal fluid after diffuse damage to the retinal pigment epithelium. *Invest Ophthalmol Vis Sci* 1983;24:1475–1479.
10. Negi A, Marmor MF. Mechanisms of subretinal fluid resorption in the cat eye. *Invest Ophthalmol Vis Sci* 1986;27:1560–1563.
11. White MH, Lambert HM, Kincaid MC, et al. The ora serrata and the spiral of Tillaux. Anatomic relationship and clinical correlation. *Ophthalmology* 1989;96:508–511.
12. Anatomy and physiology. In: Michels RG, Wilkinson CP, Rice TA, eds. *Retinal detachment*. St. Louis: CV Mosby, 1990:1–27.
13. Melgen SE, Michels M. Pneumatic retinopexy for the treatment of giant retinal dialyses. *Am J Ophthalmol* 1994;118:762–765.
14. Grignolo A. Fibrous components of the vitreous body. *Arch Ophthalmol* 1952;47:760–774.
15. Foos RY, Wheeler NC. Vitreoretinal juncture. Synchysis senilis and posterior vitreous detachment. *Ophthalmology* 1982;89:1502–1512.
16. Burton TC, Lambert RW Jr. A predictive model for visual recovery following retinal detachment surgery. *Ophthalmology* 1978;85:619–625.
17. Burton TC. Recovery of visual acuity after retinal detachment involving the macula. *Trans Am Ophthalmol Soc* 1982;80:475–497.
18. Hartz AJ, Burton TC, Gottlieb MS, et al. Outcome and cost analysis of scheduled versus emergency scleral buckling surgery. *Ophthalmology* 1992;99:1358–1363.
19. Lichter PR. The timing of retinal detachment surgery: patient and physician considerations. *Ophthalmology* 1992;99:1349–1350.
20. Tani P, Robertson DM, Langworthy A. Prognosis for central vision with anatomic reattachment in rhegmatogenous retinal detachment with macula detached. *Am J Ophthalmol* 1981;92:611–620.
21. Friberg TR, Eller AW. Prediction of visual recovery after scleral buckling of macula-off retinal detachments. *Am J Ophthalmol* 1992;114:715–722.

22. Snip RC, Thoft RA, Tolentino FA. Similar epithelial healing rates of the corneas of diabetic and nondiabetic patients. *Am J Ophthalmol* 1980;90:463–468.

23. Haller JA, Lim JI, Goldberg MF. Pilot trial of transscleral diode laser retinopexy in retinal detachment surgery. *Arch Ophthalmol* 1993;111:952–956.

24. Olsen TW, Edelhauser HF, Lim JI, Geroski DH. Human scleral permeability: effects of age, cryotherapy, transscleral diode laser, and surgical thinning. *Invest Ophthalmol Vis Sci* 1995;36:1893–1903.

25. Laqua H, Machemer R. Repair and adhesion mechanisms of the cryotherapy lesion in experimental retinal detachment. *Am J Ophthalmol* 1977;81:833–846.

26. Lincoff H, Kreissig I, Jakobiec F, Iwamoto T. Remodeling of cryosurgical adhesion. *Arch Ophthalmol* 1981;99:1845–1849.

27. Campochiaro PA, Kaden IH, Vidaurri-Leal J, Glaser BM. Cryotherapy enhances intravitreal dispersion of viable retinal pigment epithelial cells. *Arch Ophthalmol* 1985;103:434–436.

28. Glaser BM, Vidaurri-Leal J, Michels RG, Campachiaro PA. Cryotherapy during surgery for giant retinal tears and intravitreal dispersion of viable retinal pigment epithelial cells. *Ophthalmology* 1993;100:466–470.

29. Lincoff H, Kreissig I, Han YS. A temporary balloon buckle for the treatment of small retinal detachments. *Ophthalmology* 1979;86:586–592.

30. Kreissig I, Failer J, Lincoff H, Ferrari F. Results of a temporary balloon buckle in the treatment of 500 retinal detachments and a comparison with pneumatic retinopexy. *Am J Ophthalmol* 1989;107:381–389.

31. Harris MJ, Blumenkranz MS, Wittpenn J, et al. Geometric alterations produced by encircling scleral buckles: biometric and clinical considerations. *Retina* 1987;7:14–19.

32. Olsen TW, Auberg SY, Geroski DH, Edelhauser HF. Human sclera: Thickness and surface area. *Am J Ophthalmol* 1998;25:237–241.

33. Sternberg P Jr, Teideman J, Prensky JG. Sutureless scleral buckle for retinal detachment with thin sclera. *Retina* 1988;8:247–249.

34. Cohen SB, Fletcher ME, Goldberg MF, Jednock NJ. Diagnosis and management of ocular complications of sickle hemoglobinopathies: Part V. *Ophthalmic Surg* 1986;17:369–374.

35. Cartwright MJ, Blair CJ, Combs JL, Stratford TP. Anterior segment ischemia: a complication of retinal detachment repair in a patient with sickle cell trait. *Ann Ophthalmol* 1990;22:333–334.

36. Lincoff H, Kreissig I. The treatment of retinal detachment without drainage of subretinal fluid (modification of the Custodis procedure: part VI). *Trans Am Acad Ophthalmol Otol* 1972;76:1221–1233.

37. Gardner TW, Quillen DA, Blankenship GW, Marshall WK. Intraocular pressure fluctuations during scleral buckling surgery. *Ophthalmology* 1993;100:1050–1054.

38. Thompson JT, Michels RG. Volume displacement of scleral buckles. *Arch Ophthalmol* 1985;103:1822–1824.

39. Baum J, Chaturvedi N, Netland PA, Dreyer EB. Assessment of intraocular pressure by palpation. *Am J Ophthalmol* 1995;119:650–651.

40. Saran BR, Brucker AJ, Maguire AM. Drainage of subretinal fluid in retinal detachment surgery with the EI-Mofty insulated diathermy electrode. *Retina* 1994;14:344–347.

41. Girard P, Bodard E, Pasticier A, et al. Drainage of subretinal fluid: technic and results. *J Fr Ophtalmol* 1978;1:649–654.

42. Ibanez HE, Bloom SM, Olk RJ, et al. External argon laser choroidotomy versus needle drainage technique in primary scleral buckle procedures. A prospective randomized study. *Retina* 1994;14:348–350.

43. Aylward GW, Orr G, Schwartz SD, Leaver PK. Prospective randomised, controlled trial comparing suture needle drainage and argon laser drainage of subretinal fluid. *Br J Ophthalmol* 1995;79:724–727.

44. Wade EC, Flynn HW Jr, Olsen KR, et al. Subretinal hemorrhage management by pars plana vitrectomy and internal drainage. *Arch Ophthalmol* 1990;108:973–978.

45. Rubsamen PE, Flynn HW Jr, Civantos JM, et al. Treatment of massive subretinal hemorrhage from complications of scleral buckling procedures. *Am J Ophthalmol* 1994;118:299–303.

46. Duker JS, Nielsen J, Vander JF, et al. Retrobulbar bupivacaine irrigation for postoperative pain after scleral buckling surgery. A prospective study. *Ophthalmology* 1991;98:514–518.

47. Rachal WF, Burton TC. Changing concepts of failures after retinal detachment surgery. *Arch Ophthalmol* 1979;94:480–483.

48. Grizzard WS, Hilton GF, Hammer ME, Taren D. A multivariate analysis of anatomic success of retinal detachments treated with scleral buckling. *Graefes Arch Clin Exp Ophthalmol* 1994;232:1–7.

49. Smiddy WE, Glaser BM, Michels RG, deBustros S. Scleral buckle revision to treat recurrent rhegmatogenous retinal detachment. *Ophthalmic Surg* 1990;21:716–720.

50. Packer AJ, Maggiano JM, Aaberg TM, et al. Serous choroidal detachment after retinal detachment surgery. *Arch Ophthalmol* 1983;101:1221–1224.

51. Valone J Jr, Moser D. Management of rhegmatogenous retinal detachment with macula detached: steroids, choroidal detachment and acuity. *Ophthalmology* 1986;93:1413–1417.

52. Burton TC, Folk JC. Laser iris retraction for angle closure glaucoma following retinal detachment. *Ophthalmology* 1988;95:742–748.

53. Spencer AF, Newton C, Vernon SA. Incidence of ocular motility problems following scleral buckling surgery. *Eye* 1993;7:751–756.

54. Kanski JJ, Elkington AR, Davies MS. Diplopia after retinal detachment surgery. *Am J Ophthalmol* 1973;76:38–40.

55. Fison PN, Chignell AH. Diplopia after retinal detachment surgery. *Br J Ophthalmol* 1987;71:521–525.

56. Kalman A, Heinrich T, Balogh T, Messmer EP. Results of conventional retinal detachment surgery. III. Orthotoptic results. *Klin Monatsbl Augenheilkd* 1992;200:458–460.

57. Smiddy WE, Loupe D, Michels RG, et al. Extraocular muscle imbalance after scleral buckling surgery. *Ophthalmology* 1989;96:1485–1489.

58. Lobes LA Jr, Burton TC. The incidence of macular pucker after retinal detachment surgery. *Am J Ophthalmol* 1978;85:72–77.

59. Kraushar MF, Morse PH. The relationship between retina surgery and preretinal macular fibrosis. *Ophthalmic Surg* 1988;19:843–848.

60. Barr CC. The histopathology of successful retinal reattachment. *Retina* 1990;10:189–194.

61. Uemura A. Preretinal membrane in the macular area before and after the scleral buckling procedure. *Nippon Ganka Gakkai Zasshi* 1992;96:1022–1025.

62. Smiddy WE, Loupe DN, Michels RG, et al. Refractive changes after scleral buckling surgery. *Arch Ophthalmol* 1989;107:1469–1471.

63. Ho PC, McMeel JW. Bacterial endophthalmitis after retinal sugery. *Retina* 1983;3:99–102.

64. Duker JS, Belmont JB. Late bacterial endophthalmitis following retinal detachment surgery. *Retina* 1989;9:263–266.

65. Hagler WS, Jarrett WH II, Smith JA. Infections after retinal detachment surgery. *South Med J* 1975;68:1564–1569.

66. Smiddy WE, Miller D, Flynn HW. Scleral buckle removal following retinal reattachment surgery: clinical and microbiologic aspects. *Ophthalmic Surg* 1993;24:440–445.

67. Meredith TA, Reeser FH, Topping TM, Aaberg TM. Cystoid macular edema after retinal detachment surgery. *Ophthalmology* 1980;87:1090–1095.

68. Gray RH, Gregor ZJ. Acquired peripheral retinal telangiectasia after retinal surgery. *Retina* 1994;14:10–13.

69. Tornambe PE, Hilton GF. Pneumatic retinopexy, a multicenter randomized controlled clinical trial comparing pneumatic retinopexy with scleral buckling. The Retinal Detachment Study Group. *Ophthalmology* 1989;96:772–783.

70. Tornambe PE, Hilton GF, Brinton DA, et al. Pneumatic retinopexy. A two-year follow-up study of the multicenter clinical trial comparing pneumatic retinopexy with scleral buckling. *Ophthalmology* 1991;98:1115–1123.

71. Hilton GF, Tronambe PE. Pneumatic retinopexy. An analysis of intraoperative and postoperative complications. The Retinal Detachment Study Group. *Retina* 1991;11:285–294.

72. Ambler JS, Zegarra H, Meyers SM. Chronic macular detachment following pneumatic retinopexy. *Retina* 1990;10:125–130.

73. Irvine AR, Lahey JM. Pneumatic retinopexy for giant retinal tears. *Ophthalmology* 1994;101:524–528.

74. Parver LM, Lincoff H. Geometry of intraocular gas used in retinal surgery. *Mod Probl Ophthalmol* 1977;18:338–343.

75. Crittenden JJ, deJuan E Jr, Tiedeman J. Expansion of long-acting gas bubbles for intraocular use. Principles and practice. *Arch Ophthalmol* 1985;103:831–834.

76. Algvere PV, Gjotterberg M, Olivestedt G, Fituri S. Results of pneumatic retinopexy with air. *Acta Ophthalmol (Copenh)* 1992;70:632–636.

77. Sebag J, Tang M. Pneumatic retinopexy using only air. *Retina* 1993;13:8–12.

Management of Complicated Retinal Detachment

John M. Lewis   Gary W. Abrams   Jane C. Werner

Retinal detachments are considered "complicated" when reparation requires more than a scleral buckle. Complicated retinal detachments may be associated with vitreous hemorrhage, proliferative vitreoretinopathy (PVR), giant tears, posterior holes or tears, choroidal detachments, ocular inflammatory diseases, trauma, and tractional retinal detachments. Complicated retinal detachments associated with giant retinal tears, ocular inflammatory diseases, trauma, and proliferative retinopathies such as diabetic retinopathy will be discussed elsewhere.

RETINAL DETACHMENT WITH PROLIFERATIVE VITREORETINOPATHY

Overview

PVR is the leading cause of failure in retinal detachment surgery, occurring in approximately 7% of all retinal detachments (1). During the past two decades, major advances have been made both in the understanding of the pathogenesis of PVR and in the surgical treatment of the disease (2–8).

PVR is characterized by the formation of cellular membranes on the retinal surface, the retinal undersurface, and in the vitreous cavity (Fig. 42-1) (9). Cells within the membranes are derived from the retinal pigment epithelium (10,11) and from retinal glial tissue (12,13). These cells enter the vitreous cavity or subretinal space via breaks in the retina, undergo transformation to take on characteristics of fibroblasts or macrophages, and proliferate in a sheet-like configuration. Fibroblast-like transformed cells have contractile properties, with the ability to pull collagen fibers in a "hand-over-hand" manner (2). Thus the proliferative cellular membrane can insert into the vitreous and exert forces leading to tractional retinal detachment. Involvement is often most severe inferiorly; this finding is consistent with

the idea that dispersed retinal pigment epithelium cells that settle on the inferior retina due to gravitational effects play a prominent role in PVR formation.

Primary PVR can occur in a long-standing rhegmatogenous retinal detachment. More commonly, it occurs secondarily after scleral buckling, vitreous surgery, or pneumatic retinopexy treatment for rhegmatogenous retinal detachment, and is the leading cause of surgical failure and redetachment of the retina. Experimental study has shown that various factors associated with surgery, such as extensive application of cryotherapy (14), fibrin formation (15), and blood–retinal barrier breakdown may increase PVR formation.

Surgical Anatomy

The severity and extent of PVR can be described according to a classification system developed by the Retina Society in 1983 (Table 42-1) (5) and updated in 1991 (Tables 42-2 and 42-3) (6). Posterior PVR (posterior to the equator) consists of focal and diffuse retinal contractions and subretinal membranes, while anterior PVR (at or anterior to the equator) consists of focal, diffuse, or circumferential full-thickness folds, anterior retinal displacement, and subretinal membranes. Focal contractions are "star folds," which are caused by contraction of a localized epiretinal membrane. Diffuse contractions involve four or more disk areas and are induced by larger membranes (Fig. 42-2). Folds without epiretinal membranes usually indicate the presence of subretinal membranes.

Anterior PVR may result from deposition and proliferation of pigment epithelial cells on the inferior peripheral retina along with contraction at the posterior edge of the vitreous base (Fig. 42-3). These membranes induce circumferential contraction, shortening the circumference of the

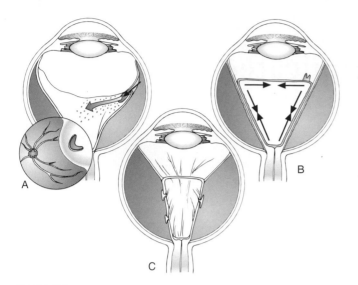

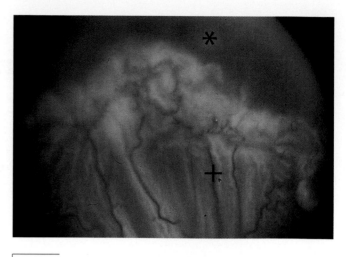

FIGURE 42-1.   A. *Migration of pigment epithelial and other cells into vitreous cavity and subretinal space. B. Proliferation and contraction of cells on retinal and vitreous interfaces. C. Fixed folds due to contraction of cellular membranes. (Adapted from Abrams GW, Aaberg TM. Posterior segment vitrectomy. In: Waltman SR (ed.). Surgery of the eye. New York: Churchill-Livingstone, 1988: 903–1012.)*

FIGURE 42-3.   *Contraction along posterior edge of vitreous base with central displacement of retina. Peripheral retina stretched(*); posterior retina in radial folds(+) (anterior type 4). (Reprinted courtesy of Ophthalmic Publishing Company, from Machemer R, Aaberg TM, Freeman HM, et al. An updated classification of retinal detachment with proliferative vitreoretinopathy. Am J Ophthalmol 1991;112:159–165.)*

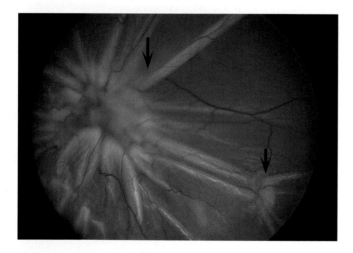

FIGURE 42-2.   *Posterior PVR: Starfold (small arrow) (posterior type 1), diffuse contraction (large arrow) (posterior type 2). Classification is CP12. (Reprinted by permission from Abrams GW, Aaberg TM. Posterior segment vitrectomy. In Waltman SR (ed.). Surgery of the eye. New York: Churchill-Livingstone, 1988:903–1012.)*

Table 42-1.   The Retina Society Classification of Retinal Detachment with PVR

Grade	Clinical Signs
A	Minimal vitreous haze
	Vitreous pigment clumps
B	Moderate wrinkling of the inner retinal surface
	Rolled edge of retinal break
	Retinal stiffness
	Vessel tortuosity
C	Marked full-thickness fixed retinal folds
C1	One quadrant
C2	Two quadrants
C3	Three quadrants
D	Massive fixed retinal folds in four quadrants
D1	Wide funnel shape
D2	Narrow funnel shape*
D3	Closed funnel (optic nervehead not visible)

* Narrow funnel shape exists when the anterior end of the funnel can be seen by indirect ophthalmoscope within the 45-degree field of a +20 D condensing lens (Nikon or equivalent).

retina at the posterior vitreous base, which is pulled centrally. The retina posterior to the vitreous base develops radial folds, while retina anterior to the posterior edge of the vitreous base is smooth and pulled centrally (Fig. 42-4). With chronicity, there may be contraction of the vitreous base, which pulls the retina posterior to it anteriorly toward the pars plana, thus resulting in anterior retinal displacement. However, anterior retinal displacement is more commonly seen in eyes that have

previously had a vitrectomy (Fig. 42-5). In these eyes, proliferating cells form a membrane on the surface of the remaining peripheral vitreous, which contracts, pulling the retina posterior to the vitreous base anteriorly toward the pars plana (Fig. 42-6A), the pars ciliaris (Fig. 42-6B), or even the posterior surface of the iris (Fig. 42-6C). In the most extreme instances, the membranes can pull the retina to the edge of the retracted pupil (Fig. 42-6D).

Table 42-2. Updated Classification of PVR Described by Grade

Grade	Features
A	Vitreous haze
	Vitreous pigment clumps
	Pigment clusters on inferior retina
B	Wrinkling of inner retinal surface
	Retinal stiffness
	Vessel tortuosity
	Rolled and irregular edges of retinal break
	Decreased mobility of vitreous
C	
CP1–12*	Posterior to equator:
	Focal, diffuse, or circumferential full-thickness folds
	Subretinal strands
CA1–12	Anterior to equator:
	Focal, diffuse, or circumferential full-thickness folds
	Anterior displacement
	Subretinal strands
	Condensed vitreous with strands

* Expressed in the number of clock hours involved.

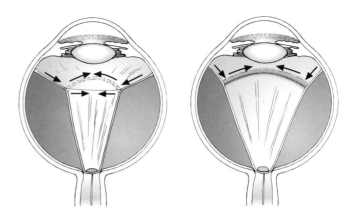

FIGURE 42-4. *Proliferative vitreoretinopathy grade C. Type 4: circumferential contraction with proliferation immediately behind insertion of the posterior hyaloid pulling retina centrally, stretching the retina anterior to it, and creating radial folds posteriorly. Schematic drawing of situation in nonvitrectomized eye (left) and vitrectomized eye (right). Arrows show direction of pull. (Adapted courtesy of Ophthalmic Publishing Company, from Machemer R, Aaberg TM, Freeman HM, et al. An updated classification of retinal detachment with proliferative vitreoretinopathy. Am J Ophthalmol 1991;112:159–165.)*

Table 42-3. Updated Classification of PVR: Grade C PVR Described by Contraction Type

Type	Location	Features
1 Focal	Posterior	Starfold posterior to vitreous base
2 Diffuse	Posterior	Confluent starfolds posterior to vitreous base
		Optic disk may not be visible
3 Subretinal	Posterior or Anterior	Proliferations under retina:
		"Napkin-ring" around disk
		"Clothesline" moth-eaten-appearing sheets
4 Circumferential	Anterior	Contraction along posterior edge of vitreous base with central displacement of the retina
		Peripheral retina stretched
		Posterior retina in radial folds
5 Anterior displacement	Anterior	Vitreous base pulled anteriorly by proliferative tissue
		Peripheral retinal trough
		Ciliary processes may be stretched or may be covered by membrane
		Iris may be retracted

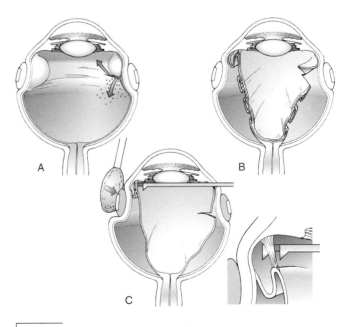

FIGURE 42-5. *Anterior retinal displacement in PVR. A. Proliferation of cells on vitreous base and retina following vitrectomy and scleral buckle. B. Contraction of cellular membranes pulls retina at posterior vitreous base anteriorly. C. Vitreous base depressed into view. Membrane exerting anterior–posterior traction is sectioned with vertically cutting scissors. (Adapted from Abrams GW, Aaberg TM. Posterior segment vitrectomy. In: Waltman SR (ed.). Surgery of the eye. New York: Churchill-Livingstone, 1988:903–1012.)*

Surgical Technique

Scleral Buckle vs. Vitrectomy

Primary retinal detachment associated with low-grade PVR (grade A or B and limited grade C) can usually be managed by retinal reattachment surgery with a scleral buckle (16). In cases where retinal detachment is associated with higher grades of PVR and in recurrent retinal detachment with significant PVR, or anytime when it is not anticipated that a scleral buckle will adequately relieve traction to reattach the retina, vitreous surgery is usually indicated to relieve tractional membranes and successfully reattach the retina.

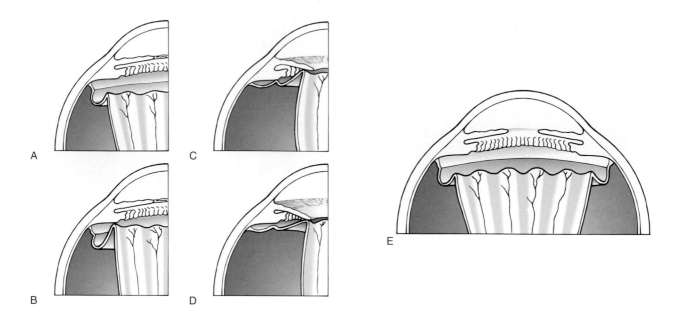

FIGURE 42-6.   *Anterior PVR: Anterior retinal displacement. Retina at posterior aspect of vitreous base is drawn to anterior vitreous base (A), to ciliary processes (B), to posterior iris (C), and to pupil with iris retraction (D). (E). Posterior insertion of the vitreous base drawn anteriorly creating retinal trough. Folds that radiate posteriorly are caused by circumferential contraction. (Adapted from Lewis H, Aaberg TM. Anterior proliferative vitreoretinopathy. Am J Ophthalmol 1988;105:277.)*

Management with Scleral Buckle Only

When scleral buckling alone is judged adequate to treat a retinal detachment associated with PVR, the general goals of retinal reattachment surgery must be achieved, including closure of all breaks and relief of vitreoretinal traction. The techniques required are discussed in detail in Chapter 41, but special considerations must be made in the presence of PVR. With few exceptions, it is necessary to support the vitreous base for 360 degrees by placing an encircling element. Sometimes a fairly high degree of indentation is necessary to relieve anterior traction adequately. The recommended width of the buckling element may vary with the location of retinal breaks and the width of the vitreous base. A narrower element will suffice if retinal breaks are relatively anteriorly located and the vitreous base is not excessively broad; however, a broader silicone tire or sponge might be preferable if the vitreous base extends more posteriorly. We use silicone tires or sponges varying from 5 to 7 mm in width. Scleral sutures are usually placed 2 mm wider than the buckle, to increase scleral indentation and buckle height. In general, placement of the buckle with its anterior edge 2 mm posterior to the muscle insertion ring provides support for the posterior vitreous base and anterior insertion of hyaloidal traction. Obviously, specific conditions require modifications of these general rules of thumb, such as long myopic eyes with altered anatomic relationships. If a silicone tire and encircling band are used in an eye with PVR, it is important that the tire be extended throughout the inferior 180 degrees of the vitreous base, and a conscious effort may be made to achieve greater buckle height inferiorly by varying the width of the scleral bites, since the inferior fundus is usually the most severely involved with tractional membranes.

As in any retinal detachment repair, all retinal breaks must be carefully identified and localized. Additional radial buckling elements sutured in place beneath the encircling element may sometimes be helpful in rhegmatogenous retinal detachment with PVR that is treated by scleral buckling alone. Breaks associated with traction can sometimes be supported sufficiently to relieve tractional forces.

Opening for Pars Plana Vitrectomy

When a vitrectomy is done for an eye with PVR, if no scleral buckle is present, we recommend encircling the eye with a scleral buckle to support the vitreous base and the retina just posterior to the vitreous base. If the eye already has an encircling scleral buckle, we usually do not revise or replace that element. Sometimes it is necessary to supplement an existing scleral buckle, especially inferiorly, if there is not adequate inferior support of the vitreous base. If the eye has previously had only a radial scleral buckle, the radial element is usually removed and an encircling scleral buckle placed.

If the decision is made to perform a pars plana vitrectomy, eyes with significant PVR still require an encircling element to support the vitreous base and relieve anterior traction. Therefore, in eyes that do not have a preexisting encircling element, a 360-degree conjunctival peritomy is made just posterior to the limbus and the rectus muscles isolated with 2-0 silk sutures. We often place the sutures for the scleral buckle prior to vitrectomy. At this time, the eye is firmer and easier to place the sutures. We usually wait until after the vitrectomy is completed to place the buckling element around the eye. In most cases, we use a 4.5-mm-wide encircling band to create a moderate buckle. Some surgeons prefer to preplace scleral "belt-loop" incisions, which may be technically easier prior to vitrectomy when the eye is firmer. The disadvantage of preplacing sutures or belt loops is that the surgeon loses the ability to choose the type and placement of the buckle based on the intraoperative findings; however, in our experience we rarely have to change the location or type of scleral buckle following the vitrectomy. We feel that the 4.5-mm encircling band will adequately support the vitreous base in most cases of PVR following vitrectomy and that the reduced volume of the band and reduced compression of vortex veins by the narrower element reduce complications related to the scleral buckle in comparison with broader, bulkier elements.

If the eye has an encircling element in place, it can be left unaltered in most cases and conjunctival incisions made in the usual fashion for a vitrectomy, exposing the temporal and superonasal sclera. Occasionally, modification of the previous buckle is desirable. The buckling element is located by dissecting through its fibrous capsule. Then the band can be tightened, the buckle can be repositioned, additional sutures can be placed to increase the height or location of the buckle, or an additional scleral buckling element can be placed. If, however, only a radial or segmental circumferential element was placed at the time of previous surgery, it is usually best removed and replaced by an encircling element.

Vitrectomy is most often performed via a 3-port pars plana approach. Sclerotomy incisions are made 3.0 mm from the limbus in aphakic and pseudophakic eyes, or when pars plana lensectomy is planned. In the somewhat uncommon circumstance in which the eye is to be left phakic (see below), the incision is made 3.5 mm from the limbus. These distances must be modified if significant anterior displacement of the retina exists, in which case entry into the vitreous cavity is made more anteriorly.

Incisions for the infusion and instruments are generally made parallel to the limbus. When performing repeat vitrectomy, parallel incisions intended for the instruments should be separated by at least 1 mm from previous incisions so the sclerotomies do not extend into the old sclerotomy sites during vitrectomy and create large scleral defects. If the sclera is thinned and macerated at the sites of the previous sclerotomies, it may be advantageous to make radial incisions, as these are less likely to extend into previous incisions. The actual entry into the vitreous cavity must be controlled, especially if the retina is bullous, to avoid retinal perforation. In aphakic or pseudophakic eyes, the microvitreoretinal (MVR) blade should be inserted iris-parallel, and the tip visualized in the pupil before it is withdrawn. The infusion cannula is then inserted and tied permanently in

place. A 4-mm cannula is preferred in most cases, but in cases with severe anterior proliferative membranes and poor visualization, a 6-mm cannula may facilitate entry into the vitreous cavity. Before infusion to the eye is initiated, the tip of the cannula must be visualized through the pupil to prevent subretinal infusion of fluid. This can be done through the operating microscope by grasping the base of the cannula with nontoothed forceps and rotating the eye until the tip comes into view, or by using a fiberoptic light probe externally and looking at the eye from an acute angle (17). Once it has been positively ascertained that the tip of the cannula is in the vitreous cavity and is free of any membranes or tissue, the infusion is turned on.

If the pupil will not dilate adequately, we dilate the pupil using mechanical pupillary stretching (Fig. 42-7). Our preferred pupillary stretching devices are small plastic hooks placed through the limbus in four quadrants (18) (Flexible Iris Retractors, Grieshaber, Inc., Kennesaw, GA). We lyse synechiae and remove residual capsular material as much as possible prior to placing the stretching hooks in order to minimize iris trauma. Limbal openings are made parallel with and just anterior to the iris plane with a Ziegler-type blade. The small hooks are secured externally at the limbus with a small locking device.

Lensectomy

The crystalline lens, if present, should be removed in most cases with significant PVR, even if clear. Visual rehabilitation is most critically related to the status of the retina, and therefore refractive concerns must be secondary. It is not possible to do an adequate vitreous base dissection in the phakic eye. Removal of the lens allows more complete dissection of the vitreous base and anterior membranes, and removal of all capsular material may decrease the likelihood

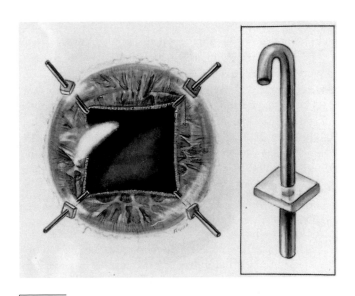

FIGURE 42-7. *Pupillary stretching using flexible iris retractors.*

of recurrent anterior PVR. In addition, with prolonged gas tamponade, the lens will almost always develop a cataract. Management in the postoperative period, including the ability to do a fluid–gas exchange and to administer postoperative laser photocoagulation, is facilitated by removing the lens. If, on the other hand, a posterior chamber intraocular lens (IOL) is already in place, it can usually be left in place, as, in most cases, it does not hinder dissection of the vitreous base and anterior membranes. Occasionally, proliferative tissue adherent to the residual lens capsule must be trimmed or removed with the vitreous cutter to facilitate adequate visualization and surgical manipulations in the periphery. If it appears excessive membranes are adherent to the peripheral lens capsule, or if the posterior chamber IOL is unstable, we remove the IOL through the limbus.

Anterior chamber IOLs are somewhat more problematic. The optic may come in contact with and damage the corneal endothelium if the lens is pushed forward by a gas bubble postoperatively. Gas or silicone oil can easily prolapse around the lens into the anterior chamber, degrading visualization of the retina intraoperatively as well as postoperatively. For these reasons, many surgeons prefer to remove anterior chamber IOLs. This step is completed via a limbal incision after infusion has been established to the eye, but with the infusion in a closed position. Sodium hyaluronate or another viscoelastic material is used to maintain the volume of the anterior chamber as well as to protect the corneal endothelium during this procedure.

The crystalline lens is removed through the pars plana, except in cases with extremely hard nuclei, in which case the nucleus is removed through the limbus. Following ultrasonic fragmentation of the nucleus and removal of the cortical material, we recommend complete removal of the lens capsule (19). An opening is made in the anterior capsule with the vitrectomy instrument. One can then grasp the peripheral capsule with vitreous forceps and exert enough traction to expose the zonules in the pupil. While retracting the capsule, the zonules can then be cut with a vertically cutting scissor (we prefer the MPC scissor, Grieshaber, Inc., Kennesaw, GA) placed through the opposite sclerotomy site (Fig. 42-8). We feel complete removal of the lens capsule will reduce the likelihood of recurrent anterior PVR that can sometimes present with membranes adherent to the peripheral lens capsule. In addition, removal of the capsule will prevent synechiae of the iris to the lens capsule, which can leave a distorted, retracted, fixed pupil.

Vitrectomy

A lens ring to hold the contact lens can be placed following placement of the pupillary stretching devices. We suture a lens ring in place and utilize several lenses as necessary to visualize the posterior and peripheral retina. We peel most posterior membranes using a plano-concave lens, while prism lenses are used in the periphery. A wide-angle lens system with image inverter is also used in selected situations

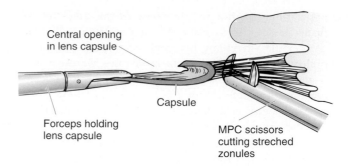

FIGURE 42-8. *En bloc removal of the lens capsule following phacofragmentation and removal of the nucleus and cortex of the lens. After opening is made in the anterior lens capsule in the pupillary area with the vitrectomy cutter, the edge of the central capsulotomy is grasped with vitreoretinal forceps, and the capsule is retracted to expose the zonules in the pupil. The zonules are sectioned with automated, vertically cutting vitreoretinal scissors, and the capsule is removed through the sclerotomy site or with the vitreous cutter.*

(20,21). The wide-angle lens is especially useful if there is a constricted view due to a posterior chamber lens with opacified peripheral capsule.

We remove the central vitreous with the vitreous cutting instrument, then remove gross peripheral vitreous. In most cases a posterior vitreous detachment will already be present in cases of PVR. Rarely, in eyes with high myopia or vitreoretinal degenerations, there is incomplete or no posterior vitreous separation. In those cases, after the core vitrectomy is completed, the posterior cortical vitreous should be separated from the disk with the vitreous cutter, suction catheter, or membrane pick, then peeled from the retinal surface. If the vitreous is tightly adherent to the posterior retina such as seen in Stickler syndrome, vitreous should be trimmed close to the adhesions and sectioned as much as possible with automated vertically cutting scissors.

If there is significant anterior PVR, we delay extensive shaving of the vitreous base and peripheral membrane dissection until after posterior membranes have been removed, because access to and removal of these membranes are easier once posterior membranes and midperipheral membranes with adherent vitreous have been removed. In the absence of anterior PVR, it is best to excise or "shave" the vitreous to the surface of the retina and pars plana at the vitreous base area at this stage of the case. The posterior membranes fixate the retina and reduce mobility of the anterior retina, which makes peripheral viteous removal safer with less risk of anterior retinal breaks. If at any point the retina is excessively mobile during peripheral vitrectomy and there is danger of peripheral retinal damage, peripheral vitrectomy can be delayed until posterior membranes have been removed. Then perfluorocarbon liquid (PFCL) can be used to stabilize the retina during peripheral vitreous removal.

The vitreous base can be visualized with a standard lens system (either hand held or with a sutured lens ring) using scleral depression, or by using a wide-angle system without scleral depression. Using a standard lens system, we perform anterior vitrectomy by two methods. In the first method, the vitreous cutter and the fiberoptic endoillumination probe are both placed in the eye. An assistant depresses the peripheral retina and vitreous base into view as the vitreous is excised (Fig. 42-9). This method is especially useful for removing vitreous in the inferior 140 degrees and the superior 100 degrees. Using this method, it is difficult to excise all of the peripheral vitreous in the horizontal meridians. The second method, especially useful in the horizontal meridians, utilizes external illumination (22). The vitrectomy cutter is placed through a sclerotomy site. A plug is placed

in the opposite sclerotomy site, and the surgeon depresses the retina and vitreous base in the area 180 degrees from where the vitreous cutter has entered the eye. The assistant holds the fiberoptic light probe in contact with the contact lens, directing the light toward the area to be cut (Fig. 42-10). Because the light probe actually touches the contact lens, there is no light reflection, and the visualization is similar to that seen with endoillumination. We have found this method superior to that in which the microscope light is used for peripheral visualization.

Scleral depression is not always required to visualize and shave the vitreous base when using the 125-degree wide-angle lens with an image inversion system. A "bullet" light probe is used to disperse the light over a broad area when using the wide-angle lens system. The vitreous structure is more easily seen when using a standard light probe held close to the vitreous, so we have found the standard lens system with scleral depression most useful for PVR.

Membrane Peeling

Posterior Membranes We begin epiretinal membrane dissection at the posterior pole. All membranes that can be located are meticulously stripped from the retinal surface. Posterior membranes are peeled from the surface of the retina in a posterior-to-anterior fashion, so that greater force is applied to the thicker posterior retina. The technique of bimanual dissection, using an illuminated pick (Fig. 42-11)

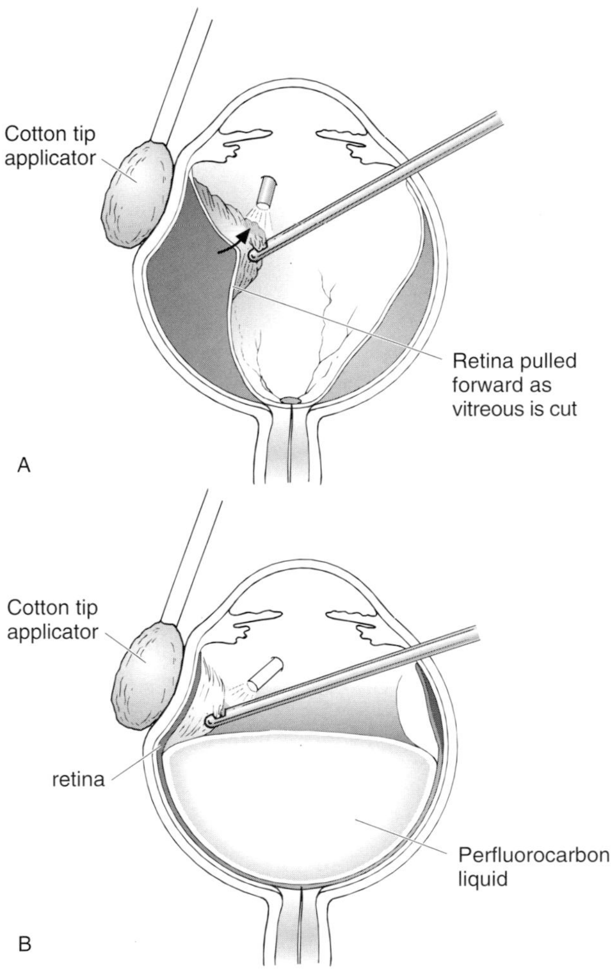

Cotton tip applicator

Retina pulled forward as vitreous is cut

A

Cotton tip applicator

retina

Perfluorocarbon liquid

B

FIGURE 42-9. *Vitrectomy removal of anterior vitreous in an eye with bullous retinal detachment. A. Retina is extremely mobile and is pulled toward the vitreous cutter as vitreous is excised, risking anterior retinal breaks. B. PFCL is injected to flatten and stabilize the posterior retina. PFCL is injected to the posterior edge of remaining vitreous, holds retina in place, and reduces retinal mobility during peripheral vitrectomy.*

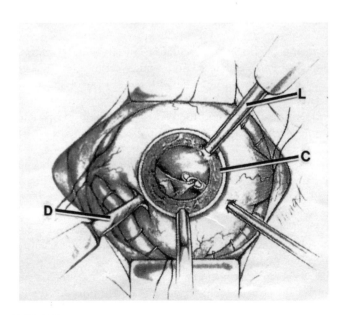

FIGURE 42-10. *Lightpipe (L) held in contact with contact lens (C) illuminates vitreous base pushed into view by scleral depressor (D). (Reprinted courtesy of the American Medical Association, Chicago, IL, from Murray TG, Boldt HC, Lewis H, et al. A technique for facilitated visualization of the vitreous base, pars plana, and pars plicata. Arch Ophthalmol 1991;109:1458–1459.)*

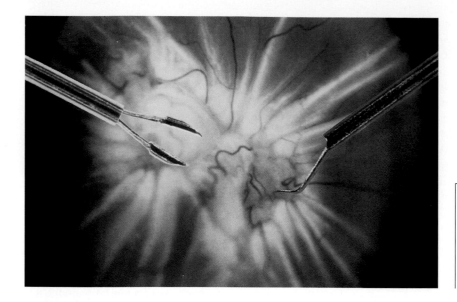

FIGURE 42-11. *Instruments for membrane removal in PVR. Left: Diamond-dusted vitreoretinal forceps (Grieshaber and Company, Fallsington, PA). Right: Illuminated pick (Escalon, Mukwanago, WI). Bending shaft of pick 30 degrees away from the light axis gives a broader field of illumination and reduces the shadow cast by the pick.*

and vitreous forceps, is the most effective for this purpose. There are several types of forceps that can be used to grasp membranes, but we have found that diamond-dusted forceps (see Fig. 42-11) most reliably hold the membrane during bimanual dissection.

Membrane peeling can be initiated by either of two methods, depending on the characteristics of the membrane: thicker membranes with prominent edges can be directly grasped with the forceps (Fig. 42-12), and flatter, less distinct membranes are best elevated with the illuminated pick prior to grasping with the forceps. Membranes can usually be easily seen, but sometimes with extensive confluent membranes, no edges can be identified. Signs of this type of membrane include obscuration of portions of retinal vessels by the membrane and a stiff, smooth, gray appearance of the retina. Large retinal folds can be obscured by the membranes. In this situation, the pick is placed in a fold and gently pulled toward the center of the fold in order to engage the membrane (Fig. 42-13A). Once the membrane is engaged and the edge elevated, it is grasped with the forceps for stripping (Fig. 42-13B). Some tightly adherent membranes can be more easily engaged with a sharp-barbed blade such as the MVR blade (Fig. 42-14).

When an edge of the membrane has been partially elevated, it can be grasped with forceps and stripped anteriorly, with the pick used to separate adhesions and stabilize the retina (see Fig. 42-13B). During removal of midperipheral membranes, the membrane is often pulled centrally with the forceps, and the blunt edge of the pick is placed between the membrane and the peripheral retina (Fig. 42-15). As the membrane is pulled centrally, the blunt edge of the pick separates the membrane from the retina. When a tight adhesion is encountered, excessive force should not be applied, as a retinal tear is likely to occur. Rather, vertically cutting automated scissors should be introduced to segment the membrane from the retina at the adherent site. If any retinal

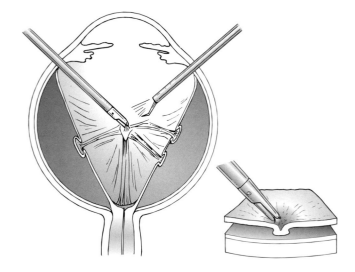

FIGURE 42-12. *Grasping epiretinal membrane with vitreoretinal forceps. The forceps grasp the body of the membrane by "pinching" the surface or edge of the membrane. While the diamond-dusted vitreoretinal forceps (see Fig. 42-11) will engage membranes with thickened edges, newer, finer, pointed end-grabbing forceps are superior for this maneuver. Once the membrane is grasped with the forceps, the illuminated pick is used to apply counter-traction on the retina as the membrane is peeled.*

breaks do occur, they should immediately be marked with intraocular diathermy.

Often, large membranes can be peeled in a single sheet from the retinal surface. This is especially true in so-called "mature PVR," in which several weeks have passed and the membranes have become fairly thick. In the past, some experts recommended waiting for this point in the disease process before intervening, allowing the proliferation to "mature" to facilitate membrane removal. Thin "immature"

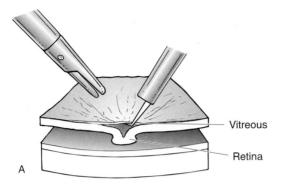

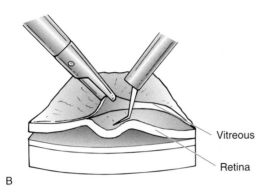

FIGURE 42-13. *Bimanual membrane-peeling using an illuminated pick and vitreoretinal forceps. A. The edge of the membrane is elevated with the illuminated pick. If an edge is not apparent, the tip of the pick is placed in the trough of a retinal fold and stripped toward the center of a star fold until the membrane is engaged. The membrane is usually engaged in the center of the star fold. B. After the edge of the membrane is elevated with the illuminated pick, the edge is grasped with the diamond-dusted vitreoretinal forceps and pulled anteriorly. The blunt, posterior edge of the illuminated pick is placed against the retina adjacent to the membrane to hold the retina in place as the membrane is peeled from the retina.*

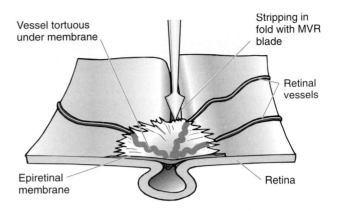

FIGURE 42-14. *Thinner, "tight" membranes may be difficult to engage with the blunt illuminated pick, so these membranes are sometimes best engaged for peeling with a sharp blade. We prefer the microvitreoretinal (MVR) blade. We barb the tip of the blade prior to membrane peeling. The barbed MVR blade is placed in a fold adjacent to the membrane and stripped toward the membrane. Most membranes can be elevated in this fashion.*

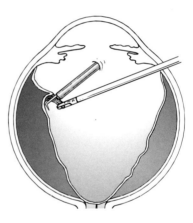

FIGURE 42-15. *Separation of peripheral membranes and vitreous from the retina. The membrane or vitreous is grasped with diamond-dusted vitreoretinal forceps and pulled centrally. The blunt edge of the illuminated pick is placed at the junction of the vitreous or membrane with the retina and the tissue is pulled over the pick. The membrane will usually separate, and vitreous will usually separate anteriorly to the posterior edge of the vitreous base.*

membranes are friable and more likely to fragment, leaving residual islands of tissue that are difficult to remove and a potential source of reproliferation. However, the disadvantage of waiting for membranes to mature is potential progression of photoreceptor degeneration, and most authorities no longer delay surgery for this reason. A helpful technique for very immature membranes is to stroke them with a silicone "brush" found on the tip of the backflush brush. Zivojnovic has found the "retinal scratcher" useful for this technique. A new instrument, a diamond-dusted silicone cannula, is now available that is useful for the removal of small patches of thin epiretinal membranes (Fig. 42-16) (23).

The posterior cortical vitreous is often adherent to peripheral membranes posterior to the vitreous base. This probably occurs because of incorporation of the posterior hyaloid into membranes formed at the junction of the separated posterior vitreous and the vitreous base (Fig. 42-17A). With increasing and more posterior membrane formation, we suspect that the vitreous is gradually pulled in by the contracting membranes to give a relatively posterior adherence of the posterior hyaloid, well posterior to the vitreous base (Fig. 42-17B). It is important to strip the posterior hyaloid anteriorly to its insertion into the vitreous base. We

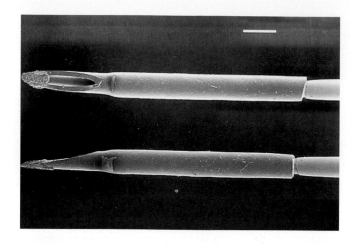

FIGURE 42-16. *Diamond-dusted membrane cannula. The tapered silicone tip has been dusted with diamonds to create a surface that will engage and peel diaphanous, immature membranes.*

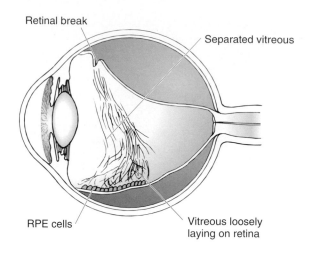

A

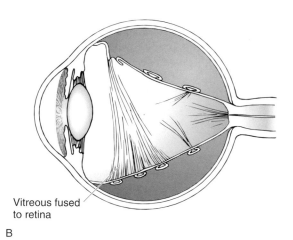

B

FIGURE 42-17. *Reattachment of peripheral separated vitreous to the retina posterior to the vitreous base in PVR. A. Rhegmatogenous retinal detachment with posterior vitreous separation and large retinal break. Released pigment epithelial cells in the vitreous cavity settle on the inferior retina between the detached retina and the vitreous. As membranes form, the vitreous attaches to the membranes that are attached to the retina. B. PVR with vitreous now fused with the peripheral retina posterior to the vitreous base. As membranes are peeled, the vitreous should be separated anteriorly to the posterior aspect of the vitreous base.*

have found it useful to grasp the edge of the posterior hyaloid with the vitreous forceps, place the blunt portion of the illuminated pick at the junction between the hyaloid and the peripheral retina, and pull the hyaloid centrally to allow the pick to separate the hyaloid from the retina (similar to the method described in Fig. 42-15). This technique also identifies the point of permanent adherence of the hyaloid to the posterior border of the vitreous base. Once the peripheral hyaloid is separated to the vitreous base, it is excised with the vitrectomy instrument. If the retina becomes excessively mobile, PFCL can be injected over the posterior pole to stabilize the retina during vitrectomy (see Fig. 42-9; see also below) (24).

Anterior Membranes   If anterior PVR is present, peripheral membranes must be dissected. Membranes may be focal, diffuse, or subretinal (see Tables 42-1 and 42-2; Figs. 42-3–42-6). Focal and diffuse membranes are peeled in a fashion similar to posterior membrane peeling, although vitreous is often adherent to the membranes. Subretinal membranes may not be apparent until after epiretinal membranes have been removed. The most difficult form of anterior PVR to manage is anterior retinal displacement, in which the retina at the posterior vitreous base or even more posteriorly is pulled anteriorly by contracting anterior vitreous and membranes (see Fig. 42-6) (4,25). A circumferential "trough" of variable depth and area may be present at the vitreous base formed between the anteriorly displaced retina and the anterior retina and pars plana. Initially, the type of anterior PVR must be identified.

Sometimes, in advanced forms of anterior PVR, it is difficult to see a peripheral trough, and the surgeon might erroneously believe that no anterior retinal displacement is present. The only sign of anterior retinal displacement may be obscuration of the ora serrata and the finding of a fibrous circumferential membrane adherent to the pars plana or

ciliary processes. Usually, however, a peripheral trough can be seen peripheral to a circumferential fold of anteriorly displaced retina. The membrane that bridges from the anteriorly displaced retina toward the anterior structures must be cut (Fig. 42-18). It is often easiest to initially open this membrane with the sharp tip of the MVR blade (Fig. 42-18A). Then vertically cutting vitreoretinal scissors can be inserted to section the membrane circumferentially (Fig. 42-18B). The membrane should be circumferentially sectioned throughout the extent of anterior displacement of the retina.

When the membrane is sectioned, the anterior-posterior element of traction is relieved, and the anteriorly displaced retina will fall posteriorly. Remnants of the membrane can exert circumferential traction and sometimes can be excised with the vitrectomy instrument. If membrane remnants are tightly adherent, then a bimanual technique is used in which the membrane is fixated with an illuminated pick or illuminated forceps as it is cut with the vertically cutting scissors (Fig. 42-18C). If possible, the whole extent of the membrane should be eliminated, but if this is not possible, remnants should be sectioned vertically in multiple areas along its circumference in order to eliminate circumferential traction. Vitreous in the trough should be trimmed back to the surface of the pars plana and peripheral retina with the vitreous cutter.

The techniques of peripheral vitreous removal utilizing scleral depression or a wide angle viewing system are described above. Retinal breaks are sometimes created during the dissection process. Breaks should be identified, and all traction relieved around the area of these breaks. In some cases, it is not possible to relieve anterior contraction adequately with dissection so a peripheral relaxing retinotomy is necessary (see below). Because it is difficult to remove posterior and peripheral membranes after an extensive retinotomy, we wait until all of the posterior and peripheral membranes have been removed before proceeding with retinectomy.

Once the posterior and peripheral membranes have been removed, the retina becomes quite mobile. The pars plana is often detached, and any remaining vitreous is easily incarcerated in the sclerotomy sites. There is risk of peripheral retinal incarceration in the sclerotomy sites. The retina can

be stabilized and further peripheral vitreous removal and membrane dissection can be facilitated by the use of PFCL (Fig. 42-19; see also Fig. 42-9). An initially small volume of PFCL (usually about 1 mL) is injected over the optic nerve. We usually wait until posterior membranes have been completely removed before injecting the PFCL. While a small posterior retinal break is not a contraindication to the use of PFCL, we usually do not use PFCL in the presence of large breaks. Excessive traction on the retina in the presence of even a small retinal break may also cause PFCL to go through the break. It is important not to inject the PFCL directly over a break as the stream of PFCL will go beneath the retina. Initially, only enough PFCL is injected to stabilize the posterior retina and improve the ability to remove peripheral vitreous and membranes. Injection of too much PFCL may cover and compress the remaining vitreous. Additional PFCL can be injected to further flatten the retina as the dissection is carried anteriorly.

Subretinal Membranes

Subretinal membranes are less common in PVR than epiretinal membranes, and even when present, often do not interfere with successful retinal reattachment (26). In these cases they can be left in place. In some cases, subretinal membranes that appear to be elevating the retina will break or stretch during fluid–gas exchange or after injection of PFCL, leading to release of traction (see below).

In cases in which subretinal membranes prevent retinal reattachment after fluid–gas exchange or injection of PFCL, of if they are felt by an experienced surgeon to be significant, the traction from these membranes must be relieved (27). If a single subretinal strand is tenting the

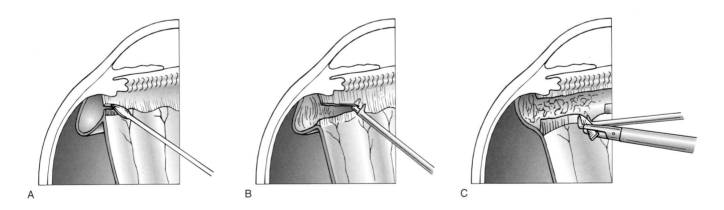

A   B   C

FIGURE 42-18. *Management of anterior retinal displacement in PVR. A circumferential membrane has formed on the peripheral vitreous and, with contraction, has pulled the retina at the posterior aspect of the vitreous base anteriorly to the anterior pars plana. The membrane obscures a "trough" of redundant retina created by the anterior displacement of the retina. A. The membrane is sectioned circumferentially with an MVR blade. B. Once an opening is made in the membrane with the MVR blade, the automated, vertically cutting vitreoretinal scissors use used to section the membrane throughout its extent. Anterior retinal displacement is most commonly found in the inferior 180 degrees of the retina. C. The "trough" has opened up and the retina has relaxed posteriorly. If a circumferential membrane remains on the posterior aspect of the vitreous base, it should be removed or radially sectioned. An illuminated pick or illuminated forceps can be used to fixate the membrane for removal or sectioning with automated, vertically cutting vitreoretinal scissors. The arrow points at an area that has been radially sectioned, while the forceps holds the edge of the membrane and exposes it for dissection with the scissors.*

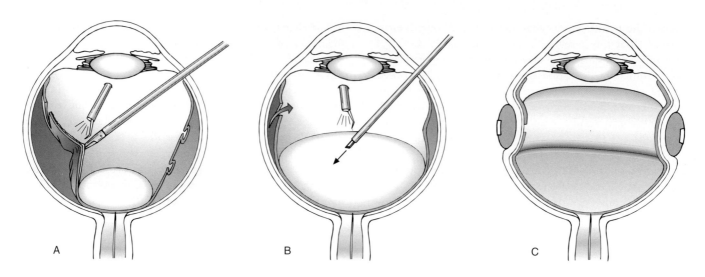

FIGURE 42-19. *Use of PFCL for PVR. A. Following removal of posterior membranes, a small volume of PFCL is injected over the posterior retina. The PFCL reduces retinal mobility during removal of peripheral membranes. B. After the membranes have been removed, the retina is reattached by injecting more PFCL. Subretinal fluid drains into the vitreous cavity from the anterior retinal break. C. More PFCL has been injected to reattach the retina. Sometimes a small amount of subretinal fluid will remain anterior to the PFCL. Try to avoid immersing the infusion cannula in the PFCL, because bubbles will obstruct the view and small bubbles can go through large open breaks.*

retina, it can be cut with scissors after creating an adjacent retinotomy with diathermy and will often retract back, allowing the retina to settle (Fig. 42-20). If not, or if multiple subretinal strands or a large sheet is present, the retinotomy is enlarged to allow the insertion of microforceps. The membrane should be grasped and gentle traction applied in a back and forth motion, breaking adhesions and attachments, while both ends are observed to ensure that the retina is not torn at a remote site (Fig. 42-20C). In rare cases of extensive subretinal fibrosis with a so-called napkin ring configuration, where the membranes completely encircle the optic nerve in the subretinal space, a large peripheral retinotomy must be made (see below), usually on the order of 90 degrees or more, and the retina folded over to allow complete removal of the membrane. A bimanual technique is required, with a lighted pick or similar instrument used to elevate and hold the inverted retina, while scissors are used to section the membrane. Then microforceps are used to grasp, tease, and regrasp the membrane until it is completely free (Fig. 42-21).

Scleral Buckle

When all membranes have been removed from the surface of the retina, it should be mobile and ready to be reattached. In eyes that do not already have an encircling band, this is an appropriate time to place a scleral buckle. Determination of the appropriate position of the scleral buckle follows many of the same considerations discussed previously. If removal of all anterior membranes and most of the anterior vitreous was accomplished, a 3.5- or 4.5-mm encircling element is usually adequate to support the vitreous base. If continued peripheral vitreoretinal traction is present, espe-

cially if this traction extends postequatorially, a broader buckle is required. A 7-mm-wide solid silicone element will provide broad support in this situation.

One disadvantage of placing a buckle at this stage in the procedure is that the subretinal fluid makes it difficult to assess buckle height. However, after retinal reattachment with PFCL injection or fluid–gas exchange, buckle height can be reassessed and adjusted if need be.

Relaxing Retinotomies and Retinectomies

Some eyes with severe PVR, particularly those undergoing reoperation and those with anterior PVR, have areas of retinal shortening that make reattachment impossible, despite meticulous removal of membranes. In such instances, raising the height of the scleral buckle can sometimes adequately relieve persistent traction. If this maneuver is not successful, or if the surgeon decides against revising the scleral buckle, retinotomy with or without retinectomy is necessary to reattach the retina (28,29). Sometimes this determination is not made until air or PFCL is injected into the eye (see below) and is noted to go subretinally through a break associated with elevated retina.

Relaxing retinotomy is usually done because of retinal contraction due to anterior PVR, with anterior retinal displacement being the most common indication. However, any type of contraction, especially when chronic, can sometimes require retinotomy to relieve traction. Rarely, a focal area of posterior contraction cannot be relieved by removal of membranes, and a focal retinotomy must be performed.

For anterior contraction, after all other membranes have been removed, diathermy is applied posterior to the area of

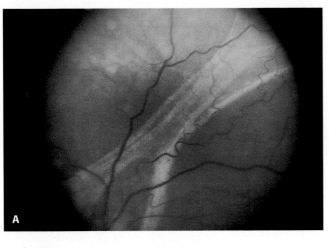

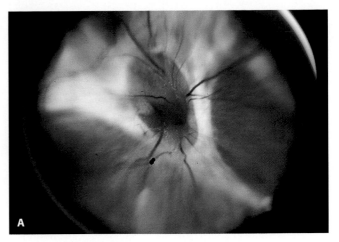

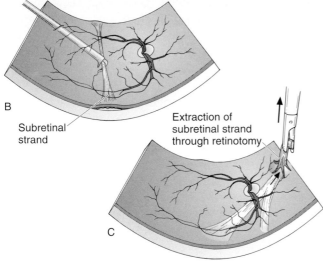

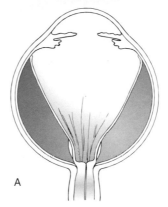

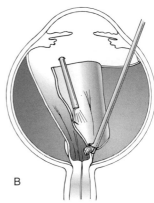

FIGURE 42-21. A, B. *Subretinal "napkin ring" membrane (posterior type 3). C. Membrane sectioned and removed through peripheral retinotomy. (A. Courtesy of Hilel Lewis, MD, Cleveland Clinic Fandation, Cleveland, OH; B, C. Adapted from Abrams GW. Retinotomies and retinectomies. In Ryan SJ (ed.).* Retina. *vol. 3. St. Louis: CV Mosby, 1989:317–346.)*

FIGURE 42-20. A. *Branching subretinal strand. B. Sectioning of subretinal strand through peripheral retinotomy. Scissors are placed through a small retinotomy created adjacent to the membrane with diathermy. If the membrane is not adherent to the retina or choroid, the ends of the membrane should retract after sectioning. C. Extraction of subretinal strand through retinotomy. The membrane is grasped with forceps and removed with a gentle, side-to-side motion. If the membrane is strongly adherent to retina or choroid, it should be sectioned. (A. Courtesy of Hilel Lewis, MD, Cleveland Clinic Fandation, Cleveland, OH; B, C. Adapted from Abrams GW. Retinotomies and retinectomies. In: Ryan SJ (ed.).* Retina. *vol. 3. St. Louis: CV Mosby, 1989:317–346.)*

contraction (Fig. 42-22). For focal contraction, diathermy is used to encircle the area to be excised. It is important to treat all vessels with heavy diathermy to prevent hemorrhage. The retinotomy should extend beyond the area of contraction into normal retina. The actual retinotomy is usually made with automated vertically cutting vitreous scissors (see Fig. 42-22A). Cutting the retina with the vitreous cutter is less controlled and can lead to hemorrhage and inadvertent excision of larger areas of the retina than desired. For anterior retinal contractions, circumferential

retinotomies are usually performed. Radial retinotomies are rarely indicated. Radial retinotomies tend to extend posteriorly into the posterior pole and often inadequately relieve traction. Retinotomies in the posterior pole, which involve more functionally important retina, should also be avoided. Use of a partial fill of PFCL will stabilize the retina during performance of the retinotomy and prevent folding and inversion of the flap of the now giant tear after the retina is cut. If the retinotomy extends into attached retina, the retina should be carefully separated from the underlying retinal pigment epithelium with the tip of the scissors or a membrane pick before cutting, to avoid damage to the choroid. The ends of the retinotomy may be angled toward the ora serrata to relieve residual traction present in these regions (Fig. 42-22B). In most cases, we prefer to remove the anterior flap of devascularized retina to decrease the

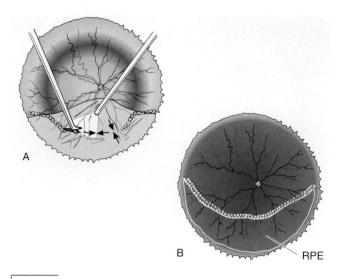

FIGURE 42-22.   A. *Inferior relaxing retinotomy to relieve traction in contracted retina. The retina to be cut is diathermized, primarily by diathermizing blood vessels, extending into normal retina on each end of contracted retina. Cut is made with vertically cutting scissors along the posterior edge of contracted retina. B. Retina reattached following relaxing retinotomy. Retinotomy is extended anteriorly to ora serrata or ciliary body (if pars plana is involved). The anterior retina is excised. (Adapted from Abrams GW. Retinotomies and retinectomies. In: Ryan SJ (ed.). Retina. vol. 3. St. Louis: CV Mosby, 1989:317–346.)*

likelihood of reproliferation and possibly lower the risk of rubeosis. This procedure is accomplished with the vitreous cutter, again with care taken to avoid damage to the choroid.

A retinotomy greater than 90 degrees in circumference creates the problem of management of a giant retinal tear. The best method for reattaching the retina in the presence of a giant tear is the use of a PFCL (discussed below) (30). PFCLs have the advantage of ease of use and do not require manipulation of the flap under gas or silicone oil.

If a large relaxing retinotomy (>90 degrees) is performed to treat an eye with PVR, careful consideration should be made of the type of retinal tamponade to use. Eyes undergoing retinotomy and retinectomy are more likely to have postoperative hypotony, which suggests that silicone oil may be preferred in such eyes (31).

Reattachment of the Retina with PFCL

If PFCL was used to stabilize the retina during membrane removal or retinotomy, additional PFCL is injected to reattach the retina (24). If PFCL was not used, the retina can be reattached pneumatically with air or with PFCL, according to the characteristics of the retina. If a large retinotomy has created a giant tear, PFCL should be used to reattach the retina (30). If there is no giant break and a posterior break exists, pneumatic reattachment can be performed, using the posterior break to simultaneously drain subretinal fluid. More often, however, breaks will be fairly anterior, and

reattachment of the retina is performed with PFCL prior to fluid–air exchange.

When PFCL is to be used, the surgeon should make quite sure that all traction has been removed from around retinal breaks. If breaks with elevated edges are present, the PFCL can pass through the break and move subretinally, requiring further manipulations to remove it, even including a retinotomy.

We prefer a PFCL with an index of refraction allowing good visibility such as perfluoro-n-octane (32). The PFCL can be injected manually with a syringe or with a surgeon-controlled automated fluid injector. We inject the PFCL through a silicone-tipped cannula and start injection over the optic disk. Once a large enough bubble of PFCL is present over the optic nerve, the tip of the silicone cannula can be inserted into the PFCL during subsequent injection to ensure that a single bubble is produced (see Fig. 42-19A). During injection, fluid is allowed to escape from the sclerotomy site. As the bubble of PFCL slowly increases in size, the posterior pole should be noted to flatten, and the choroidal pattern should become apparent. The PFCL is injected slowly and the peripheral retina assessed during injection. This procedure is particularly important if a giant retinotomy has been created, because the edge can become folded beneath the perfluorocarbon.

In addition, it is important to observe if the peripheral retina flattens during PFCL injection. If the retina remains elevated, injection should be stopped. PFCL should be removed to at least the posterior aspect of the remaining traction and the traction relieved. A wide-angle viewing system is ideal for observation of the entire fundus during this process. Injection is continued until the PFCL extends well onto the scleral buckle anteriorly (see Fig. 42-19C). Try to avoid immersing the tip of the infusion port in the PFCL, because multiple bubbles of PFCL are created by the fluid flow. These bubbles may obstruct the view and go beneath the edge of a large break. In most cases, fluid will drain from known or unrecognized anterior retinal breaks, and the contour of the buckle will be apparent. Occasionally, fluid will accumulate anteriorly, obscuring the outline of the buckle (Fig. 42-23A). In such cases, tipping the eye so that the PFCL forces the fluid toward a known retinal break will sometimes flatten the retina (Fig. 42-23B). Occasionally, however, intraocular diathermy must be used to create an anterior drainage retinotomy over the buckle in an area of nonvascular retina. This retinotomy should be made as anteriorly as possible to avoid trapping subretinal fluid anterior to the retinotomy (Fig. 42-23C).

At this point, the entire posterior retina should be reattached. Areas of persistent retinal elevation beneath the PFCL indicate persistent traction, which must be relieved if surgery is to be successful. Most remaining epiretinal membranes can be removed beneath the PFCL. If it is necessary to remove the PFCL, it should be carefully aspirated into a syringe for reuse later in the case. Further membrane peeling can then be performed, or retinotomy and retinectomy can

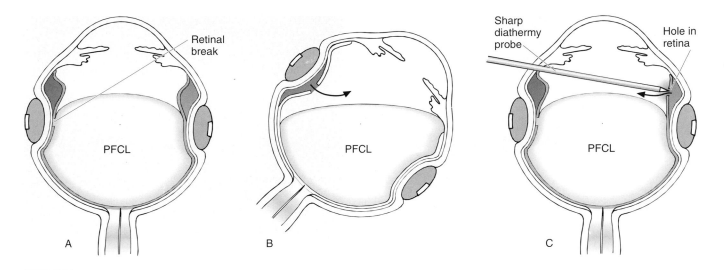

FIGURE 42-23. A. *Fluid trapped anterior to retinal break following retinal reattachment with PFCL. B. Eye tilted so PFCL will force subretinal fluid out of retinal break. C. If unable to force subretinal fluid out by tilting the eye, an anterior drainage retinotomy is made with endodiathermy to allow drainage of subretinal fluid (arrow). Injection of more PFCL will now attach the anterior retina.*

be carried out as discussed above if separation of membranes is not possible.

Occasionally, retinal reattachment under PFCL is prevented by subretinal strands or membranes. In many cases, the retina will reattach despite such tissues. Sometimes the weight of the PFCL acting over time will relax the traction applied by subretinal membranes, and the surgeon may wish to wait for several minutes to reassess the retinal status. If there appears to be less retinal elevation, more PFCL can be injected and further observation for retinal flattening carried out. If the PFCL does not overcome the traction from the subretinal membranes, the PFCL should be removed by aspirating it back into the same syringe, for reuse later in the case, and the subretinal membranes dealt with as discussed above.

Laser Endophotocoagulation

The PFCL affords an excellent view for application of laser endophotocoagulation to the now reattached retina, although the field of view is less than with a gas-filled eye. All retinal breaks, previously marked with diathermy, are surrounded with confluent laser spots (Fig. 42-24). Laser can then be applied over the scleral buckle for 360 degrees, using the prism fundus contact lens or a wide-angle viewing system (Fig. 42-25). Peripheral laser is facilitated by raising the level of the PFCL well onto the buckle, to ensure that no subretinal fluid is present. An angled laser probe is also helpful for treating superior retina. Laser burns should be of moderate intensity and placed for two to three rows, with a separation between spots of approximately one burn width (Fig. 42-26). Confluent and overly intense peripheral photocoagulation (Fig. 42-27) can occasionally lead to stasis of venous return from the ciliary body to the vortex system.

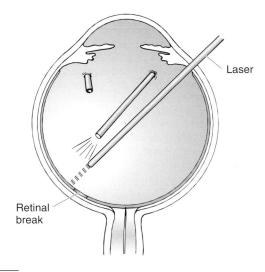

FIGURE 42-24. *Laser endophotocoagulation. Treated retinal breaks with one or two rows of confluent laser. (Adapted from Abrams GW. Retinotomies and retinectomies. In: Ryan SJ (ed.). Retina. vol. 3. St. Louis: CV Mosby, 1989:317–346.)*

Occasionally, visualization of the periphery is difficult, and photocoagulation of this region is delayed until the eye is filled with air. We treat any posterior retinal breaks with laser, but do not perform scatter treatment posterior to the scleral buckle.

Removal of PFCL

On completion of laser endophotocoagulation, an inferior peripheral iridectomy is made if silicone oil is to be used in an aphakic eye (see below) (33). Then, fluid/PFCL–air exchange is carried out. We prefer active suction with an

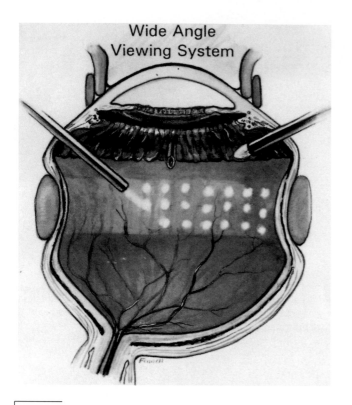

FIGURE 42-25.   *Laser endophotocoagulation using a wide-angle system. The wide-angle view allows visualization of the peripheral retina during endophotocoagulation. Treatment is applied using a scatter technique on the retina supported by the scleral buckle. The bullet light probe is used with the wide-angle viewing system to give wide field illumination. (Adapted from Abrams GW, Glazer LC. Proliferative vitreoretinopathy. In: Freeman WR (ed.). Practical atlas of retinal disease and therapy. 2nd ed. Philadelphia: Lippincott-Raven, 1997:303–323.)*

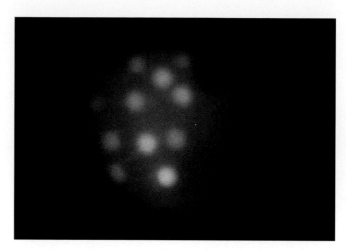

FIGURE 42-26.   *One burn width between laser applications during scatter treatment. (Adapted from Abrams GW, Glazer LC. Proliferative vitreoretinopathy. In: Freeman WR (ed.). Practical atlas of retinal disease and therapy. 2nd ed. Philadelphia: Lippincott-Raven, 1997:303–323.)*

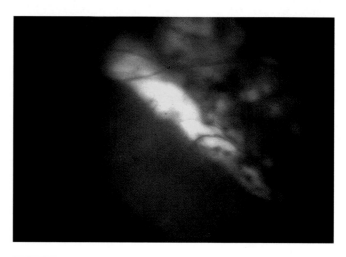

FIGURE 42-27.   *Excessive laser treatment to peripheral retina on scleral buckle.*

aspiration silicone-tipped cannula for this purpose. Alternative instruments preferred by some surgeons are backflush brushes or extrusion needles, providing passive egress of PFCL and intraocular fluid from the eye. In the phakic or pseudophakic eye, a biconcave contact lens is placed on the cornea to overcome the higher refractive power of the air-filled eye. With the aspiration cannula and fiberoptic light probe in the eye, the infusion line is switched from fluid to air, with the pressure of the air pump typically set at approximately 40 mm Hg. Preliminary aspiration is performed just behind the iris plane, until air fills the anterior vitreous cavity. Then the silicone cannula tip is placed near the peripheral retina at the level of the PFCL–fluid interface, so that an air–PFCL interface is achieved and there is minimal risk of reaccumulation of subretinal fluid. Next the cannula is positioned over the optic nerve, and the remainder of the PFCL is aspirated. As the eye fills with air, the fluid level can be safely determined by the "dipping" maneuver. The silicone cannula is inserted toward the optic nerve head until the bright reflex disappears, indicating that the tip of the cannula has reached the fluid (Fig. 42-28). Aspiration is initiated and continued until the reflex

reappears. This process is continued until all the fluid is removed from the eye.

In the presence of a giant retinotomy (usually 180 degrees or more), there is a risk of retinal slippage during the exchange of PFCL for air. This can be prevented by adequate "drying" of the edge of the retinotomy during the air exchange (24), accomplished by filling the vitreous cavity anterior to the flap of the giant retinotomy with air, then aspirating fluid from beneath the anterior edge of the retinotomy before removing the PFCL (Fig. 42-29). The anterior edge of the retina can be visualized during fluid–air exchange with a wide-angle viewing system or, alternatively, with an indirect ophthalmoscope. If fluid is left behind the edge of the retinotomy, as PFCL–air exchange proceeds, fluid forced posteriorly during the exchange will allow posterior slippage of the edge of the tear. If PFCL goes beneath the retina, it must be removed, which may require refilling the eye with fluid. Once fluid is removed from behind the anterior edge of the retina, PFCL–air exchange is completed and all PFCL is removed from the eye.

Perfluoro-n-octane is easily seen and removed, and because of the high vapor pressure, remaining small bubbles will evaporate in air at body temperature. However, perfluorodecalin and perfluorophenanthrene, two other commonly used liquid PFCLs, are less easily seen, have a lower vapor pressure, and will not evaporate in air (32), so we recommend dripping approximately 0.1 to 0.3 mL of balanced saline onto the posterior retina to identify any remaining PFCL (which will coalesce into more easily seen bubbles in the balanced saline) to facilitate removal.

The optical properties of a gas-filled eye allow a wider field of view than those of liquid, and usually a more complete view of the periphery is obtained after fluid–air exchange. If inadequate laser treatment of the periphery was accomplished under PFCL, particularly laser treatment of retina overlying the scleral buckle, more complete endophotocoagulation can now be performed in many cases. In pseudophakic eyes, condensation of fluid on the IOL can impede visualization, as discussed below.

Reattachment of the Retina Without PFCL

If PFCL is not used, we reattach the retina with a fluid–air exchange. All retinal breaks should be marked with endodiathermy prior to fluid–air exchange so they can be seen

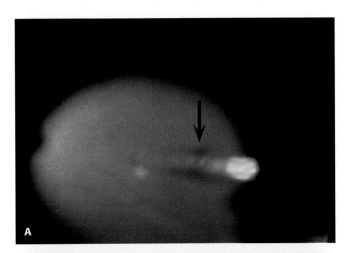
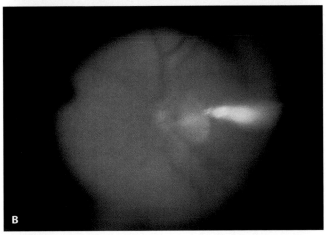

FIGURE 42-28. A. *Fluid–air exchange. The tip of the suction needle is held just anterior to the break. Note the fluid meniscus (arrow) on shaft of drainage needle. B. Removing final bit of fluid over optic nerve. The needle tip is repeatedly "dipped" into fluid at the retinal break and over the optic disk. A light reflex is seen to disappear as the needle tip contacts the fluid meniscus. (Adapted from Abrams GW, Aaberg TM. Posterior segment vitrectomy. In: Waltman SR (ed.). Surgery of the eye.* New York: Churchill-Livingstone, 1988:903–1012.)

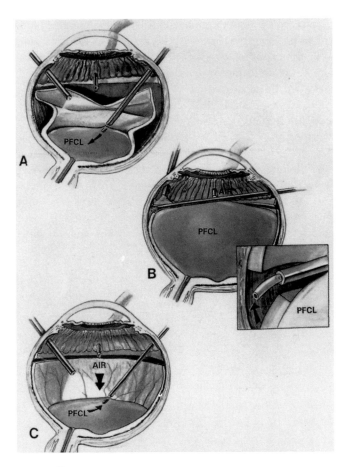

FIGURE 42-29. *Unfolding flap of giant tear or large retinotomy with PFCL. A. PFCL is injected over the posterior pole to unfold flap of giant tear. With retina stabilized with PFCL, removal of anterior vitreous and anterior dissection are made easier. PFCL can be injected to the level of the anterior edge of the giant tear after all membranes are removed. B. PFCL–air exchange. The space anterior to the PFCL is filled with air. The edge of the tear is "dried" to prevent slippage. Fluid behind the edge is aspirated with the soft-tip needle until the edge is completely flat. C. PFCL–air exchange is completed. All PFCL is removed with the soft-tip needle. (Adapted from Abrams GW, Glazer LC. Proliferative vitreoretinopathy. In: Freeman WR (ed.). Practical atlas of retinal disease and therapy. 2nd ed.* Philadelphia: Lippincott-Raven, 1997:303–323.)

and treated through the air bubble. Before switching from fluid to air, the decision of whether to use gas or silicone oil tamponade must be made, because if silicone oil is to be used, it is preferable to create an inferior peripheral iridectomy in a fluid-filled eye (see below). Air is supplied by the air pump and fluid is usually removed with an aspiration soft silicone–tipped needle, just as described above for removal of PFCL. There is usually a posterior or peripheral retinal break available for removal of subretinal fluid. If a posterior break is present, then it is used for subretinal fluid drainage (Fig. 42-30). If no posterior break is present, we do not usually make a posterior drainage retinotomy. Drainage through a peripheral break is facilitated by the use of the extendable cannulated extrusion needle in which the soft-silicone tube can be extended through the peripheral break into the subretinal space posteriorly (Fig. 42-31) (34). In most cases, a simple nonextendable, soft-tipped cannula will suffice for the same purpose. If there is no accessible break for drainage, we usually make a drainage retinotomy with the endodiathermy probe in the peripheral retina in an area to be supported by the scleral buckle.

Once the retina is reattached under air, confluent laser endophotocoagulation is applied to surround all breaks, identification of which is facilitated by previous labeling with diathermy as discussed above. If a retinal burn is not noted despite adequate power and laser application interval, residual subretinal fluid is likely present at the margin of the break, and further aspiration should be performed. Treatment of all breaks is followed by peripheral laser treatment over the scleral buckle as described above in conjunction with PFCL.

Not uncommonly, visibility will deteriorate after fluid–air exchange due to the appearance of corneal striae, or due to condensation of fluid on the IOL in pseudophakic eyes, occasionally to the point where completion of endolaser treatment becomes difficult or impossible. Use of a wide-angle viewing system can often improve fundus visualization. The posterior surface of the IOL can be more evenly wetted by application of a soft-tipped cannula in a sweeping fashion. Another maneuver that is often helpful is the application of sodium hyaluronate to the corneal endothelium. A small amount of viscoelastic injected onto the endothelial surface often dramatically improves visibility.

Silicone IOLs may create significant problems during fluid–air exchange (35). Because of the hydrophobic nature of the silicone, condensation will reoccur during fluid–air exchange, even if it is wiped away with a silicone-tipped cannula, obscuring the view of the retina in the air-filled eye. It may be possible to dry the posterior surface with a steady stream of air from the air pump via a needle held against the posterior surface of the IOL during fluid–air exchange (36).

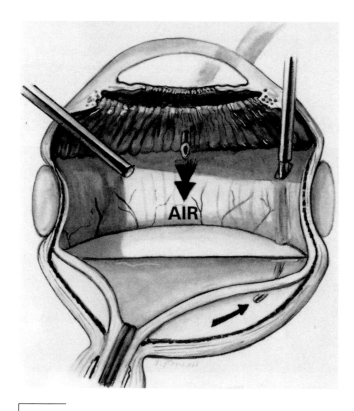

FIGURE 42-31.   *Fluid–air exchange using a peripheral retinal break. Drainage retinotomy is created anteriorly over the scleral buckle. Extendable soft silicone tubing of the cannulated extrusion needle is passed through the retinotomy into the posterior subretinal space for fluid–air exchange. (Adapted from Abrams GW, Glazer LC. Proliferative vitreoretinopathy. In: Freeman WR (ed.). Practical atlas of retinal disease and therapy. 2nd ed. Philadelphia: Lippincott-Raven, 1997:303–323.)*

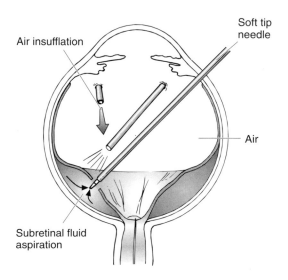

FIGURE 42-30.   *Fluid–air exchange. Subretinal fluid is aspirated through the posterior retinal break as the eye is simultaneously filled by the air pump. (Adapted from Abrams GW. Retinotomies and retinectomies. In: Ryan SJ (ed.). Retina. vol. 3. St. Louis: CV Mosby, 1989:317–346.)*

Air–Gas Exchange

Following laser treatment, two sclerotomy sites are closed, usually with 7-0 polyglycolic acid sutures. At least 25 mL of a nonexpansile mixture of C_3F_8 gas (12% to 14%) are flushed through the eye (37). We have shown experimentally that a predictable gas concentration can be obtained using this method. The gas mixture is insufflated through the infusion port and allowed to egress through a 27-gauge, $\frac{1}{2}$-inch-length needle inserted through the pars plana and vented to atmosphere. A tuberculin syringe with the plunger removed can be used as a handle for the needle. Following the gas flush, the needle is removed, then the infusion port is removed and that site closed. We then reform the eye to a normal pressure with the gas mixture via a 30-gauge needle through the pars plana. We try to leave the intraocular pressure at approximately 10 mm Hg at the completion of surgery.

The conjunctiva can be closed with absorbable suture such as 6-0 plain gut, bringing the flap of conjunctiva to the limbus and assuring that all sclerotomies are well covered. In eyes that have undergone multiple prior surgical procedures, this can be quite difficult and time consuming, but must be done in careful fashion. If the conjunctiva is retracted, it can sometimes be released by making multiple small circumferential cuts in the undersurface of Tenon's capsule with a sharp, rounded blade, and drawn closer to the limbus. Subconjunctival injection of an antibiotic, while of unproven value, is standard practice, as is subconjunctival corticosteroid injection, usually with dexamethasone. Placement of ointment in the palpebral fissure and an eye patch completes the procedure.

Silicone Oil

The Silicone Study found that visual and anatomic results in eyes with PVR were similar in most analyses regardless of whether silicone oil or C_3F_8 gas was used as the intraocular tamponade and both modalities were superior to SF_6 gas (38–40). While the surgeon and patient will jointly decide on the tamponade to use in most cases, some factors will contribute to the decision. Gas may be preferred over silicone oil if it is likely that silicone oil will herniate into the anterior chamber and contact the cornea, such as when the iris diaphragm is not intact or when an IOL is present without an intact iris-capsular-IOL diaphragm. Oil may be preferred for patients unable to maintain prone positioning such as children or mentally or physically impaired patients. Silicone oil is associated with a lower incidence of postoperative hypotony and is preferred in certain cases, including eyes with preoperative hypotony and eyes with rubeosis or requiring extensive anterior dissection of membranes, as these eyes are at greater risk of postoperative hypotony. Silicone oil may be preferred in the face of a giant tear or retinotomy, which will also more likely have postoperative hypotony. Silicone oil is preferred if the patient must travel by air or if the patient must travel to a higher elevation. Silicone oil is preferred over gas in the presence of residual vitreous or choroidal or large subretinal hemorrhage. An obvious disadvantage of silicone oil as a means of intraocular tamponae is the need for a second operation if silicone oil is eventually removed.

When silicone oil is to be used, an inferior iridectomy should be created in the aphakic eye (Fig. 42-32) (33). The vitreous cutter is inserted behind the inferior peripheral iris at its base, with the vitrectomy instrument facing the iris, then the iris is engaged. Excision of iris tissue must be controlled, and care must be taken to confine the iridectomy to near the iris base and not to extend it to the pupillary margin. As partial thickness iris is removed,

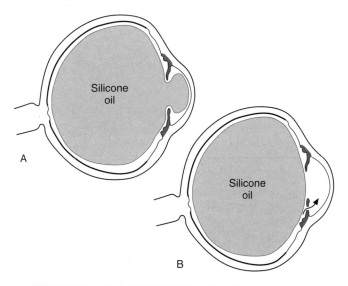

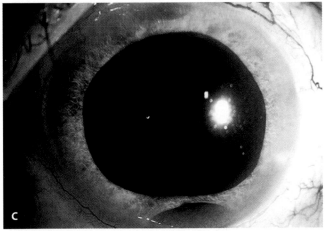

FIGURE 42-32.   *Inferior iridectomy. A. Without inferior iridectomy, silicone oil herniates into the anterior chamber due to pupillary block mechanism. B. Inferior iridectomy allows access of aqueous into the anterior chamber, relieving pupillary block so that aqueous no longer forces silicone oil into the anterior chamber. C. Inferior iridectomy. (Adapted from Abrams GW, Glazer LC. Proliferative vitreoretinopathy. In: Freeman WR (ed.). Practical atlas of retinal disease and therapy. 2nd ed. Philadelphia: Lippincott-Raven, 1997:303–323.)*

the surgeon begins to see the tip of the vitreous cutter through the thin residual anterior iris stroma and can in this manner guide placement of the instrument to complete the process.

If the retina has been reattached with air, then silicone oil can be infused into the air-filled eye at the end of the case. Alternatively, a fluid–silicone exchange or PFCL–silicone oil exchange can be performed. When infusing silicone oil into the air-filled eye, the 5000-centistoke oil that is most commonly used has high viscosity and requires high pressure tubing if injected through the infusion port. We usually inject silicone oil into the air-filled eye in the following manner. With the infusion port in place and the air pump engaged to the infusion port tubing, we close one sclerotomy site and preplace a suture in the other site. We inject the silicone oil through an 18- or 20-gauge angiocath that has been trimmed to approximately 10 mm in length. As the silicone oil is injected, the pressure is adjusted and maintained at the present pressure by the air pump, which remains attached to the infusion tubing. In phakic or pseudophakic eyes, injection of silicone oil is continued until the oil just reaches the posterior lens. The syringe is removed and the preplaced sclerotomy suture closed. The infusion cannula can then be removed and the final sclerotomy closed. A small amount of oil will escape during suturing of the final sclerotomy, helping to ensure that the eye is not overfilled with silicone oil.

In aphakic eyes, injection is continued until the oil level is at the level of the infusion cannula. The silicone syringe is removed from the eye, and the preplaced superotemporal sclerotomy suture is closed. Then, after clamping the air line, the infusion cannula can be removed from the eye and the tip of the silicone oil syringe inserted into the infusion sclerotomy. To maintain the appropriate intraocular pressure and allow the escape of air from the eye, a 30-gauge needle can be attached to the air pump (still set at 15 mm Hg) and inserted into the anterior chamber through the limbus. Injection is continued until the silicone oil just reaches the iris plane. Then the silicone oil syringe and needle are removed from the eye, and the final sclerotomy is closed. Again, a small amount of oil will escape, helping to prevent an overfill of silicone oil. Regardless of the phakia status of the eye, it may be prudent to place a plug in the sclerotomy before closing it and measure the intraocular pressure. A pressure reading of above 20 mm Hg may indicate an overfill, and a small amount of silicone oil should be removed through the open sclerotomy and the pressure remeasured. We try to leave the closing pressure at approximately 10 mm Hg. The anterior chamber is left at normal depth. If the anterior chamber shallows, a small amount of oil is removed and the anterior chamber is reformed with air injected through the limbus. It is important that the intraocular pressure be left at a low–normal level so as not to inadvertently overfill or underfill the eye with silicone oil.

If a posterior chamber IOL is present with an intact iris-capsular-IOL diaphragm, we do not make an inferior iridectomy. If the diaphragm is not intact and/or silicone oil herniates around the IOL into the anterior chamber, an inferior iridectomy will sometimes keep the silicone oil out of the anterior chamber; however, sometimes the oil will go into the anterior chamber in spite of the iridectomy. Residual capsular material can obstruct an iridectomy, so patency should be confirmed at surgery. If the iridectomy is open and oil has gone into the anterior chamber, the oil can be pushed posteriorly with viscoelastic material injected into the anterior chamber. If the eye is making adequate aqueous, it may be necessary to remove the IOL and capsule and reopen the iridectomy in order to keep the silicone oil out of the anterior chamber. A stable anterior chamber lens can be left in place if an adequate inferior iridectomy is made. Unstable anterior chamber lenses should be removed.

After all sclerotomies are closed, the eye is irrigated copiously with saline solution to remove residual silicone oil, and the conjunctiva is closed as described above.

If the pressure is within a normal range and the retina is stable, the silicone oil can be removed 2 months or more following surgery. It is often possible to remove recurrent epiretinal membranes at the time of silicone oil removal. The Silicone Study found that approximately 20% of retinas detach following silicone oil removal (41).

In the presence of hypotony, it is probably best to leave the silicone oil in the eye. Hypotonous eyes usually end up with corneal decompensation in the presence of silicone oil, because the silicone oil herniates forward and touches the corneal endothelium. Unfortunately, with silicone oil removal, these eyes often become phthisical. Whereas the visual prognosis is poor in either situation, the eye will probably remain more stable with silicone oil remaining in the eye than otherwise.

Early Postoperative Management

Eyes with PVR require significant postoperative management. Early postoperative management is directed toward 1) careful control of the intraocular pressure (IOP), 2) adequate retinal tamponade, 3) control of inflammation, 4) elimination of hemorrhage and fibrin, and 5) detection and management of recurrent retinal detachment.

Han et al (42) found that 36% of patients developed an intraocular pressure of 30 mm Hg or more following vitrectomy. Patients undergoing surgery for PVR have many of the risk factors for elevation of IOP: scleral buckle, lensectomy, scatter endophotocoagulation, and sometimes a fibrin pupillary membrane postoperatively. We monitor IOP carefully in the postoperative period. We normalize IOP at the end of the case, and if the patient has preexisting glaucoma or other factors indicating high risk for elevation of the IOP (e.g., scleral buckle and scatter photocoagulation), we give topical ocular antihypertensive medications. We check the IOP approximately 2 to 4 hours following surgery, then recheck as needed. We treat elevated IOP medically in most cases, but extreme elevation of pressure sometimes requires paracentesis of fluid or gas.

We ensure that the gas bubble is adequate to tamponade all retinal breaks and laser treatment postoperatively. We prefer to have the eye at least 80% filled with gas in the postoperative period. If the gas bubble is inadequate postoperatively, as sometimes occurs, we do a fluid–gas exchange to "top up" the gas bubble. For fluid–gas exchange in the aphakic eye, we prepare the eye with 5% povidine-iodine solution to the lids and the conjunctival cul-de-sac. We make a limbal incision with a disposable Ziegler-type blade. Then, with the patient prone, we inject gas into the eye through a 30-gauge needle inserted through the limbal incision (Fig. 42-33). As gas is injected, fluid will run out around the shaft of the needle through the limbal opening. The limbal incision is self-sealing and usually leaves a relatively normal IOP. We usually use a 15% mixture of C_3F_8 for the postoperative fluid–gas exchange.

In a phakic eye or in an eye with a posterior chamber implant, we perform the fluid–gas exchange through the pars plana. We use a two-needle technique. With the patient placed on his or her side, we insert a 30-gauge needle attached to a 10-cc syringe filled with the selected gas mixture (usually 14% C_3F_8 gas) through the pars plana in the most superior position and into the vitreous cavity. We then insert a 27-gauge needle attached to a 10-cc syringe through the pars plana at the most dependent position. We usually place the needle for air insufflation (which is now superior) nasally, and the needle for fluid

aspiration (which is now dependent, inferiorly) temporally (Fig. 42-34).

We aspirate fluid from the dependent syringe as we simultaneously fill the eye with air from the superior syringe. We sequentially equalize the volume of fluid aspirated through the dependent syringe with the amount of gas injected through the superior syringe. Usually, we sequentially aspirate 0.5 mL of fluid then inject 0.5 mL of gas, until the fluid is replaced with gas. As we fill the eye with air, we turn the head toward a more prone position so we can aspirate more fluid. We aspirate as the needle is slowly withdrawn to remove as much fluid as possible.

To control inflammation, we give subconjunctival Decadron (5–10 mg) at the conclusion of surgery. We also treat with frequent topical corticosteroids postoperatively. We usually give the topical corticosteroids every hour while awake for the first few days of the postoperative period. We usually do not give systemic corticosteroids because of the potential systemic risks involved and because the benefit has not been clearly demonstrated.

If significant postoperative fibrin formation causes pupillary block, interferes with postoperative fluid–gas exchange, or interferes with the view to the extent that it complicates postoperative evaluation and management, we lyse the fibrin

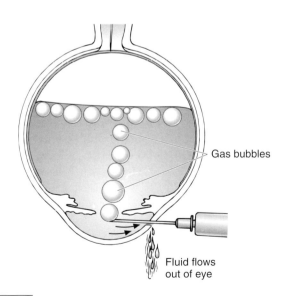

Gas bubbles

Fluid flows out of eye

FIGURE 42-33. *Postoperative fluid–gas exchange in the aphakic eye. A selected gas mixture (5 to 10 mL) is insufflated into the eye through a 30-gauge needle placed through a limbal incision made with a Ziegler-type blade. Because the self-sealing limbal incision is larger than the diameter of the needle, fluid will drain out of the incision as the gas is injected. Small bubbles will coalesce in the first hours after the exchange.*

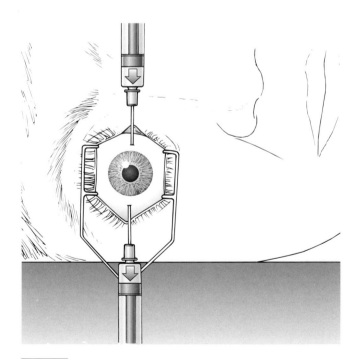

FIGURE 42-34. *Postoperative fluid–gas exchange in the phakic or pseudophakic eye. The superior (nasal) syringe contains air or gas mixture. The inferior (temporal) syringe is for aspiration of fluid in the vitreous cavity. Exchange is done by sequentially injecting 0.5 mL of air or gas and aspirating the same volume of fluid until the fluid in the vitreous cavity is exchanged for the air or gas. We use a 30-gauge needle for injection and 27-gauge needle for aspiration.*

with tissue plasminogen activator (tPA) (43–45). We usually wait 48 to 72 hours following surgery to administer tPA in order to minimize the possibility of intraocular hemorrhage. We recommend injecting 3 μg of tPA in 0.1 mL of balanced saline with a 30-gauge needle through the limbus. In the presence of severe fibrin formation and/or hemorrhage, we usually do a fluid–gas exchange to clear the fibrin products and/or hemorrhage after lysis with the tPA.

We closely monitor patients for the development of recurrent retinal detachment. Retinal detachment is most easily seen by looking around (not through) a gas bubble. We usually examine the patients every 1 to 2 weeks until the gas bubble has resolved. If retinal detachment is detected, we look for the cause. Usually retinal detachment indicates the presence of an untreated retinal break and/or excessive retinal traction. The most common cause of recurrent retinal detachment is residual anterior traction that opens an anterior break. Eyes with anterior contraction can sometimes be reattached successfully with a repeat fluid–gas exchange.

After the retina is flattened, laser treatment is applied in several rows to the retina over the scleral buckle and sometimes 360-degrees posterior to the scleral buckle. We have found that postoperative laser photocoagulation in the air-filled eye is most easily administered using a laser with a long wavelength, such as krypton red or diode laser, and a panfunduscopic contact lens.

Although some degree of retinal detachment anterior to the scleal buckle may remain, often fluid can be demarcated, and the posterior retina will remain attached. This is compatible with long-term stability and recovery of functional visual acuity in some cases; however, some cases with anterior retinal detachment will become hypotonus. If there is significant retinal contraction posterior to the scleral buckle, we do not recommend doing a fluid–air exchange because of the risk of further contraction and posterior tear formation. With posterior contraction, we recommend reoperation.

Eyes with silicone oil can have unique postoperative considerations, including herniation of the silicone oil into the anterior chamber and pupillary block glaucoma due to the silicone oil. Both problems usually result from closure of the peripheral iridectomy. Sometimes, however, the oil will be in the anterior chamber in the first few days following surgery in spite of an open iridectomy. If the eye is producing adequate aqueous, the silicone oil will recede behind the pupil as flow of aqueous is established through the peripheral iridectomy. Keeping the patient in an upright position with the face tilted forward will help establish the proper aqueous flow. If the eye is not making adequate aqueous, the oil will continue to herniate forward. Usually, if the silicone oil has pushed the iris forward with shallowing of the anterior chamber following surgery, simply positioning the patient upright with the face tilted forward or having the patient lie prone will cause it to recede to its normal position.

Fibrin can close a peripheral iridectomy and cause pupillary block with shallowing of the anterior chamber and glaucoma or herniation of the silicone oil into the anterior chamber. Sometimes the fibrin will resolve with topical corticosteroids, but if it persists more than 48 to 72 hours, we inject tPA (3 μg) to lyse the fibrin. If postoperative fibrin formation has caused adherence of the peripheral iris to the cornea, surgically reforming the anterior chamber may be necessary. In the surgical suite, we inject viscoelastic to reform the anterior chamber. Removing a small amount of silicone oil may occasionally be necessary.

Results

There has been slow, steady improvement in the surgical results of PVR management in the past 25 years. Grizzard and Hilton (16) used a high encircling scleral buckle technique and reported a 35% retinal reattachment rate in eyes with the equivalent of C1 to D2 PVR (Retina Society classification). Machemer and Norton (46) found vitrectomy alone was not successful for PVR, but Machemer and Laqua (3) combined membrane peeling techniques with vitrectomy and their retinal reattachment rate at 6 months increased to 36%.

Early surgical techniques of vitrectomy and membrane peeling were effective in managing posterior membranes in PVR. The major cause of failure was anterior retinal proliferation and contraction. Charles (47) first described anterior displacement of the retina in PVR. Lewis and Aaberg (4) described the pathoanatomy, and Elner and colleagues (25) showed the histopathology of anterior PVR. Aaberg (48) correlated the chronology of surgical advances and understanding of the pathoanatomy of PVR with improvement in results and management of PVR.

There has been continued improvement in both anatomic and visual results in management of PVR. Lewis, Aaberg, and Abrams (7) reported complete retinal reattachment in 73 (90%) of 81 eyes that had not undergone a previous vitrectomy. Of the eyes that were completely reattached, 85% (62/73) obtained a visual acuity of 5/200 or better. Lewis and Aaberg (8) reported complete anatomic reattachment in 27 (73%) of 37 eyes that had undergone a previous vitrectomy for PVR, with visual acuity of 5/200 or better in 67% (18/27) of eyes with complete attachment. The IOP was less than 5 mm Hg in 4 of their 5 cases with recurrent anterior retinal detachment. The cause of surgical failure was cellular reproliferation and traction with anterior PVR present in 9 of 12 cases that developed a recurrent retinal detachment.

The Silicone Study was a multicenter, randomized, controlled clinical trial funded by the National Eye Institute comparing silicone oil and gases in the management of PVR. The surgical method included vitrectomy, removal of posterior membranes, dissection for anterior PVR if present, and reattachment of the retina with air, followed by randomization to 1000-centistoke silicone oil or gas. An inferior iridectomy was created in silicone oil eyes. There were two groups of eyes: group 1 eyes had not undergone a previous vitrectomy; group 2 eyes had undergone a previous unsuccessful vitrectomy with gas for retinal detachment. The study involved a 36-month follow-up on most eyes randomized to silicone oil or C_3F_8 gas, and long-term follow-up, up to 72 months, on many of the eyes with attached maculas at 36 months.

Eyes were randomized to silicone oil or 20% SF_6 gas in the initial portion of the study and silicone oil or 14% C_3F_8 gas in the major portion of the study. While results with silicone oil were superior to SF_6 (38), there was little difference between silicone oil and C_3F_8 gas (2). Thus, both silicone oil and C_3F_8 gas produced better results than SF_6 gas.

At 36 months, C_3F_8 eyes had a higher rate of complete retinal attachment posterior to the scleral buckle than silicone oil eyes (approximately 80% versus 60%, $p < 0.05$) in group 1 (no previous vitrectomy) (40). No such difference was found in group 2 (previous vitrectomy) eyes. Between 55% and 65% of oil and gas eyes with complete posterior attachment in both group 1 and group 2 had visual acuity of 5/200 or better (no significant difference). Although hypotony was more common in gas eyes than oil eyes, the difference was not significant among eyes with complete posterior attachment in either group 1 or group 2. There was no difference in keratopathy in eyes with complete posterior attachment.

On long-term follow-up (up to 72 months) of all eyes with attached maculas at 36 months, regardless of gas used or previous vitrectomy status, there was no significant difference between gas and oil in anatomic or visual outcome or in the incidence of keratopathy. In contrast, significantly more gas eyes had hypotony than did oil eyes (approximately 18% versus 5%, $p < 0.001$). Further analyses compared gas-treated, oil-retained, and oil-removed eyes.

1. *Oil-retained versus oil-removed eyes:* Oil-removed eyes had a higher rate of complete posterior retinal attachment, a higher percentage of eyes with visual acuity of 5/200 or better, and a lower rate of keratopathy. There was no difference in hypotony.
2. *Gas-treated versus oil-removed eyes:* There was no difference in complete posterior retinal attachment, but oil-removed eyes had a higher percentage of eyes with visual acuity of 5/200 or better at 60 months, less keratopathy at 48 months, and a lower rate of hypotony.
3. *Gas-treated versus oil-retained eyes:* Gas-treated eyes had a higher rate of complete posterior attachment and visual acuity of 5/200 or better. There was no difference in hypotony, but oil-retained eyes showed a trend toward more keratopathy (not significant).

Oil-removed eyes had a better outcome than oil-retained and gas-treated eyes in this study. However, silicone oil removal was at the surgeon's discretion, and oil was more likely to be removed in eyes with attached retinas, better visual acuities, and fewer complications. Oil-removed eyes also had fewer reoperations than oil-retained eyes, so surgeon bias makes it difficult to determine if it is better to remove or retain oil. An earlier Silicone Study report attempted to remove surgeon bias from the analysis (41). Silicone oil was removed from 100 (45%) of 222 eyes that received silicone oil in the study. In a matched-pairs analysis, eyes with silicone oil removed were more likely to experience improvement in visual acuity and suffer retinal detachment than eyes with silicone oil retained.

A number of subgroup analyses were reported in the Silicone Study. There was no difference in retinal reattachment or visual acuity between group 1 and group 2 eyes (49). Though uncommon, elevated IOP (>25 mm Hg) was more prevalent in silicone oil eyes (8%) than in C_3F_8 eyes (2%) ($p < 0.05$) (50). Chronic hypotony (IOP $\leq$ 5 mm Hg) was 1) more prevalent in eyes randomized to C_3F_8 gas than in those randomized to silicone oil (31% versus 18%; $p < 0.05$), 2) more prevalent in eyes with anatomic failure (48% versus 16%; $p < 0.01$), and 3) correlated with poor postoperative vision ($p < 0.001$) and retinal detachment ($p < 0.001$). Diffuse contraction of the retina anterior to the equator was an independent factor prognostic of chronic hypotony.

Relaxing retinotomies were more commonly done in group 2 eyes (42%) than in group 1 eyes (20%) ($p < 0.0001$) (31). The incidence of hypotony (IOP $\leq$ 5 mm Hg) was greater in gas eyes than silicone oil eyes undergoing relaxing retinotomies. Relaxing retinotomies were done more commonly in eyes with anterior PVR than in eyes without anterior PVR. Visual acuity and the retinal reattachment rate were better in eyes without relaxing retinotomies than in eyes with relaxing retinotomies.

Eyes with posterior PVR had a better outcome at 6 months than eyes with anterior PVR (51). For eyes with anterior PVR, significant predictors of poor (<5/200) visual acuity were a preoperative PVR grade of D1 or worse (Retina Society Classification) and the use of C_3F_8 gas as the intraocular tamponade. Eyes with anterior PVR and clinically significant posterior PVR changes had a better visual prognosis if silicone oil was used instead of gas.

In eyes with attached maculae, the incidence of corneal abnormalities at 24 months was 27% and did not differ significantly between silicone oil and gas groups (52). Corneal abnormalities were correlated with poor visual acuity and hypotony. Factors predictive of corneal abnormalities were iris neovascularization, aphakia or pseudophakia, postoperative aqueous flare, and reoperations.

The overall prevalence of macular pucker among eyes with attached maculae was 15% (53). There was no difference in the prevalence of postoperative macular pucker in eyes randomized to gas versus silicone oil or between group 1 and group 2 eyes. Postoperative macular pucker was three times as likely to develop in eyes that were preoperatively aphakic or pseudophakic than in eyes preoperatively phakic.

Recent improvements such as PFCL and wide-angle viewing were not available for the Silicone Study. The impact of these advances on the results of the study are unknown. We expect further technical advances to improve our ability to manage PVR. In spite of the excellent surgical results in PVR management, many problems with recurrent proliferation remain. Whereas an increased percentage of cases can be reattached with surgery, inhibition of reproliferation with pharmacologic agents to prevent subsequent retinal detachment has been sought by many investigators for over 20 years and counting. There are five major areas of investigation into reducing cellular proliferation in PVR: anti-inflammatory therapy (54), direct inhibition of cellular proliferation (55–60), prevention of attachment of proliferating cells to collagen (61), immunotoxin therapy (62), and gene therapy (involving the "suicide gene") (63). Additionally, there are new modalities under development, such as sustained release devices, to better deliver drug therapy to the eye. These avenues of research offer hope that PVR can be prevented from occurring in most cases, and cured if it does occur.

RETINAL DETACHMENT ASSOCIATED WITH VITREOUS HEMORRHAGE

Overview

Vitreous hemorrhage most commonly occurs due to retinal tears associated with posterior vitreous separation. The patient frequently has photopsia and floaters followed by visual loss. Retinal detachment may also be associated with postsurgical hemorrhage, or hemorrhage may be present following a failed retinal reattachment procedure.

Vitreous hemorrhage can obscure the retina. However, peripheral tears and retinal detachment can sometimes be visualized with the indirect ophthalmoscope in spite of a dense vitreous hemorrhage because the area of the vitreous base may not be obscured. Visualization is sometimes obtained following bed rest and head elevation.

Ultrasound may reveal a retinal detachment. Areas of vitreoretinal adhesion may be identified, and larger flaps of horseshoe tears may be seen with ultrasound. Mapping the extent and degree of elevation of the retinal detachment is usually possible with ultrasound.

If vitreous hemorrhage prevents adequate visualization for a scleral buckling procedure, vitrectomy is indicated. Sometimes peripheral visualization is adequate to permit a scleral buckling procedure, and visualization may be improved by bed rest, bilateral patching, and head elevation. We proceed to vitrectomy if a retinal detachment is present; the risk of PVR may be increased by delaying surgery in the presence of vitreous hemorrhage.

If a definite acute retinal tear without retinal detachment is detected by ultrasound, and visualization is not adequate for treatment, vitrectomy is indicated. However, a trial of bed rest with head elevation and bilateral patching is indicated for 48 to 72 hours to see whether the hemorrhage will settle enough to permit visualization and treatment without vitrectomy.

Surgical Anatomy

Posterior vitreous separation is present in most cases. Retinal tears are usually located at the posterior edge of the vitreous base that is the anterior extent of the posterior vitreous separation. The retinal detachment may be quite bullous; sometimes there is little separation between the posterior hyaloid and the retina.

Surgical Technique

The eye is prepared for vitrectomy in the usual manner. If a scleral buckle is planned, a 360-degree conjunctival incision is made, and the muscles are isolated with sutures. If a preexisting buckle is not to be revised, transconjunctival sutures are placed through the rectus muscles and a limited conjunctival approach is used. Entrance into the eye is in the usual manner. If the pars plana is detached, openings should be made more anteriorly than usual. We use a 4-mm infusion port. Care must be taken if a longer infusion port is used, so that it does not impact the equator of the lens or the retina over the scleral buckle. For this reason, we rarely use the long infusion ports in phakic eyes or in eyes with anteriorly located scleral buckles.

The central vitreous is removed, then the posterior hyaloid is incised over attached retina if possible. If the retina is completely detached, then a less bullous area is selected. Preoperative ultrasound is helpful, but the configuration of the retinal detachment may change at surgery. The hyaloid is incised posteriorly over the optic nerve if the retina is totally detached, because the retina is flat at the edge of the optic disk. If the posterior hyaloid is separated from the retina and the vitreous is collapsed anteriorly, the cutting port is directed anteriorly and the vitreous and posterior hyaloid face may curl around the instrument tip into the port during vitrectomy. It is usually necessary to face the cutting port parallel with a collapsed hyaloid, or directly toward a thickened or taut hyaloid, in order to incise the hyaloid.

Once the hyaloid is incised, the instrument tip is placed through the opening and the cutting port is directed away from the detached retina toward the edge of the hyaloid. Low suction is applied, and the retina is kept in view during vitrectomy. Vitreous is cut in a centrifugal fashion, eventually excising the vitreous to the surface of the vitreous base. In the periphery, there is danger of suctioning bullous retina into the cutting tip. The vitreous should be cut over detached retina with lower levels of suction and with the vitreous cutter facing away from the detached retina. PFCL (see above) injected over the posterior retina will stabilize the retina during excision of peripheral vitreous and reduce the likelihood of retinal damage. The PFCL should be injected so the meniscus remains posterior to the vitreous in the periphery, thus avoiding compression of the vitreous and allowing it to be engaged with the vitreous cutter. Vitreous is cut back to the periphery as far as can be safely done.

The posterior retina should be examined closely for the presence of epiretinal membranes. Membranes should be removed in the same manner done for PVR. If the retina is mobile, without any folds or membranes, then the retina can be reattached. Prior to reattaching the retina, plugs should be placed in the sclerotomy sites and the peripheral retina thoroughly examined with the indirect ophthalmoscope. All retinal breaks should be identified and localized. Peripheral retinal breaks can be treated with either laser or cryotherapy. Cryotherapy can be performed at this time or after reattachment of the retina with air or PFCL, but breaks should be marked with diathermy if possible so they can be identified when the retina is reattached. Laser is performed after the retina is reattached.

If peripheral retinal breaks are present, an appropriate encircling scleral buckle is usually placed to support the breaks and vitreous base area. The sutures and scleral buckle are usually placed at this time, although some surgeons place the buckle after reattachment of the retina. If scatter treatment on the buckle is anticipated, it is best to have the buckle in place prior to insufflating air, because sometimes the pupil will become miotic in the aphakic eye or with fluctuation of IOP in the air-filled eye. If a posterior retinal break is present, fluid–air exchange is performed as described above for PVR. If a posterior break is not accessible for endodrainage, we usually reattach the retina with PFCL as described above.

When the retina is reattached, laser endophotocoagulation is applied to all accessible retinal breaks. Laser is most easily applied through PFCL, but can also be done through air. Breaks should be surrounded with confluent laser. In aphakic and pseudophakic eyes, laser endophotocoagulation can be used to treat both posterior and anterior breaks, but in phakic eyes, there is a risk of damage to the lens with the endoprobe when treating peripheral breaks. Delivery of the laser by the indirect ophthalmoscope (indirect laser photocoagulation) is often preferred for peripheral breaks. In the absence of PVR, if vitreous traction has been satisfactorily relieved, only the retinal breaks are treated with laser or cryoretinopexy. However, if there is significant traction, laser scatter treatment should be placed on the peripheral retina supported by the scleral buckle in two to three rows, with at least one burn width between laser spots. If PFCL is in the eye, it should be exchanged for air as described above. An air–gas exchange is done if a long-acting gas is to be used.

Results

Ratner et al (64) reported retinal reattachment in 21 (50%) of 42 eyes with retinal detachment and vitreous hemorrhage. Of the 42 eyes, 18 (43%) obtained visual acuity of 5/200 or better. A more recent study using more modern techniques reported retinal reattachment in 55 (89%) of 62 eyes with preoperative vitreous hemorrhage (65). The authors found no difference in the incidence of postoperative PVR between eyes with and without preoperative vitreous hemorrhage.

Surgical failure in these eyes may result from complications of the vitrectomy. Eyes with preexisting rhegmatogenous retinal detachment have a higher incidence of entrance site problems, including dialysis, subretinal infusion, and retinal incarceration. Iatrogenic tears are easily created in detached retina. Other causes of failure to reattach the retina include failure to identify tears and PVR. Tears may be hidden in the hemorrhagic vitreous base. A broad buckle covering the area from the ora serrata to near the equator will close most peripheral tears. PVR probably occurs more rapidly in eyes with vitreous hemorrhage. For that reason, we recommend surgery soon after the onset of hemorrhage if retinal detachment occurs. Eyes with vitreous hemorrhage should be followed closely with ultrasound to detect retinal detachment at an early stage. Poor visual function following retinal reattachment may be due to macular dysfunction from longstanding retinal detachment, PVR, or epiretinal membrane formation.

POSTERIOR RETINAL BREAKS

Overview

Posterior breaks may lead to retinal detachment in a variety of conditions. Macular holes may be idiopathic or associated with high myopia, or may follow trauma (66–70). Most do not lead to retinal detachment beyond the immediate margin of the macular hole, and management of macular holes without extensive retinal detachment is described in Chapter 52. Posterior breaks may be associated with proliferative retinopathies (diabetic retinopathy or branch vein occlusion), posterior lattice degeneration, or uveal colobomas. Retinal detachments due to posterior breaks usually do not extend to the ora serrata, and peripheral breaks are usually not present.

A scleral buckle may reattach the retina in some eyes with breaks well posterior to the equator. Various procedures using slings, straps, scleral pockets, or permanent or temporary radial scleral buckling elements have been reported (71–74). However, there is risk of damage to the optic nerve, macula, vortex veins, and posterior ciliary vessels in the treatment of far posterior tears, and a scleral buckling procedure carries the risk of scleral perforation or rupture or choroidal hemorrhage in highly myopic eyes. Those eyes not easily and safely managed by a scleral buckling procedure are candidates for vitrectomy.

Surgical Anatomy

Macular holes usually do not lead to extensive retinal detachment. The incidence is extremely low in nonmyopic eyes with macular holes but is not uncommon if myopia of 6.00 diopters (D) or greater is present (Fig. 42-35A, B) (75–76). Retinal detachment is usually associated with vitreoretinal adhesion and traction. Gass believes that macular holes are the result of tangential retinal traction, and that the vitreous remains attached to the retina surrounding the hole in most cases. It is the combination of the macular hole and the associated vitreous traction that leads to both the common localized and the less common extensive retinal detachment. In cases of proliferative retinopathy, posterior lattice degeneration, and uveal coloboma, traction is nearly always present. These breaks are usually the result of partial posterior vitreous separation, with vitreous traction on the flap of the tear and often on the adjacent retina. In most retinal detachments associated with posterior holes, vitreous traction is necessary for the retinal detachment to occur. Exceptions are highly myopic eyes with posterior staphylomas in which the retina may detach even though a complete posterior vitreous separation occurs. In these eyes, the retina is probably relatively shortened in comparison to the configuration of the deep staphyloma, and the retinal pigment epithelium may function inadequately to pump out subretinal fluid.

Surgical Technique

A scleral buckle is usually not performed. Preparation and vitrectomy are the same as described above. Frequently,

vitreous adhesions not identified preoperatively are recognized at surgery. Adhesions are initially recognized when the retina moves and is pulled toward the vitreous as the adherent vitreous is cut. Sometimes it is necessary to strip vitreous and/or associated epiretinal membranes from the retinal surface. We use an illuminated pick or barbed needle or a blade to strip the vitreous. Sometimes the vitreous is best grasped near the retina with vitreous forceps, then in a bimanual technique, the retina is held back with the blunt side of the illuminated pick and the vitreous is stripped free. Alternatively, the pick can be used to bluntly separate adhesions as the vitreous is held under traction. If vitreous is tightly adherent and will not strip free, it is cut near the retinal surface, then adhesions are cut with automated vertically cutting scissors. All adhesions are cut, and remaining vitreous is trimmed back toward the vitreous base.

Macular Hole Without Staphyloma

After all vitreous adhesions have been released and vitrectomy is completed, we inspect the peripheral retina for retinal breaks. If no breaks are seen, the retina is reattached with a fluid–air exchange. Fluid can be drained through the macular hole to reattach the retina. The subretinal fluid is aspirated with gentle suction with a soft-tipped needle. Alternatively, a backflush brush can be used if care is taken that the air pressure is somewhat lower than for a routine fluid–gas exchange, so the extrusion pressure is not too high. It is important not to suction the retina into the orifice of the aspirating needle. Usually, the subretinal fluid will stream out of the hole when low suction is applied while the soft-tipped needle is held just anterior to the hole. Too much suction will sometimes enlarge the hole by stretching the edges as the fluid traverses the hole. If chronic subretinal fluid has become proteinaceous, the fluid is easily

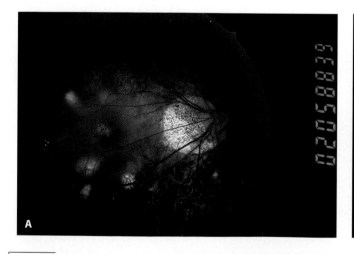

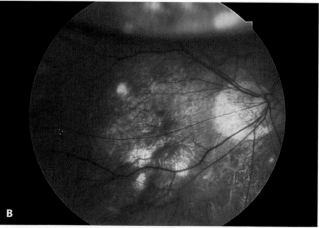

FIGURE 42-35. *The right eye of a patient with high myopia who had a localized rhegmatogenous retinal detachment due to a macular hole. A. Preoperative fundus photograph. B. Appearance of the macula 10 days after pars plana vitrectomy and fluid–gas exchange, with no direct treatment applied to the macular hole. There is still a partial gas fill in the vitreous cavity. The retina is reattached.*

visualized as it streams out of the hole into the aspirating needle.

At the end of the fluid–air exchange, we do not aggressively aspirate fluid at the hole when the retina is flat. We remove as much intraocular fluid as possible by waiting approximately 15 minutes to let more fluid accumulate in the posterior pole, then aspirate the accumulated fluid. We do not treat the macular hole with laser or other adhesive modality. The air is exchanged for a nonexpansile gas (12% to 14% C_3F_8). We ask the patient to stay in the prone position for the first two weeks following surgery. If retinal detachment recurs postoperatively, a repeat fluid–gas exchange is performed (77). Then, when the macula is flat, the hole is treated with external laser.

Macular Hole with Posterior Staphyloma

Initial management is the same as for macular hole without posterior staphyloma. Most macular holes associated with staphylomas will require treatment; nevertheless, we generally do not treat these tears initially. If retinal detachment recurs postoperatively, we flatten these tears with repeat fluid–gas exchange and treat with laser.

Posterior (Nonmacular) Break

After vitrectomy and release of all traction from the break, the margins of the break are marked by whitening with endodiathermy. Fluid–air exchange is performed with drainage through the posterior break by an aspirating soft-tipped needle. The break is treated with two rows of surrounding laser endophotocoagulation. The patient is in a prone position postoperatively for approximately 1 week to keep the tear closed while air or gas remains in the eye.

Results

Binder and Riss (78) compared 27 eyes with macular holes and retinal detachments treated with nonvitrectomy techniques from 1972 until 1977 with 18 eyes treated with vitrectomy and gas insufflation from 1978 until 1981 at the same eye clinic. The anatomic reattachment rate was higher in the vitrectomy group (17 of 18) than in the nonvitrectomy group (16 of 27). No eyes in the nonvitrectomy group had better than 6/60 vision, while one-third of eyes that underwent vitrectomy had visual acuity of 6/12 to 6/48. Poorer vision in the nonvitrectomy group was due to buckling of the macula or sometimes repeated treatment of the macula. In 3 cases treated with vitrectomy, no treatment was applied to the macular hole.

Gonvers and Machemer (79) treated 6 cases of retinal detachment due to macular holes with vitrectomy and fluid–gas exchange and positioning. No treatment was applied to the breaks. Of the 6 eyes, 5 remained attached, but one required a repeat fluid–air exchange. Also, 5 of 6 eyes were highly myopic. Final vision ranged from 3/200 to 20/100.

Several authors have also attempted treatment of retinal detachment due to macular hole by performing gas injection without pars plana vitrectomy. Blankenship and Ibanez-Langlois exchanged liquid vitreous with an intravitreal gas bubble and achieved successful reattachment in 15 of 19 eyes (80). One patient required repeated exchange and 3 required vitrectomy. Visual acuity of 20/400 was obtained in 9 patients. Miyake reported successful reattachment after gas injection in 15 of 18 eyes, with follow-up from 4 to 32 months (81). Another study compared vitrectomy and gas injection with gas injection alone in 43 eyes, and found similar final attachment rates (82).

Complications are the same as for vitrectomy surgery in general. Because the intraocular maneuvers are limited and the procedures short, a low incidence of complications is found in this group of eyes. However, redetachment rates are high, and the need for reoperation is not uncommon. Residual epiretinal tissue over the posterior retina causing tangential traction is thought to be the cause of recurrent detachment in some cases (83,84). Complications may be less with vitrectomy than with scleral buckling for some highly myopic eyes.

NONDIABETIC TRACTION RETINAL DETACHMENT

Most retinal detachments result from vitreous traction. However, we differentiate traction retinal detachments from other retinal detachments by the presence of either direct vitreous traction that prevents the retina from contacting the retinal pigment epithelium, or direct vitreous traction that prevents a retinal break from settling on an adequately positioned scleral buckle. Traction retinal detachment requires pars plana vitrectomy to adequately relieve vitreoretinal traction and reattach the retina. Common etiologies of traction retinal detachment such as proliferative diabetic retinopathy, advanced proliferative vitreoretinopathy, retinopathy of prematurity, and penetrating trauma are discussed elsewhere in the text. Other etiologies include vitreous incarceration in a surgical wound, lower grades of PVR, vitreomacular traction syndrome, and complicated branch retinal vein occlusion and associated diseases. While other conditions can also cause traction retinal detachments, the principles of treatment of the above conditions can be used for most other etiologies.

Vitreous Incarceration in a Surgical Wound

Overview

Vitreous incarcerated in a cataract wound can cause direct vitreous traction on the retina. Incarceration may result from vitreous loss from a broken posterior capsule during phacoemulsification or from a limited choroidal hemorrhage in which vitreous is extruded from the wound (Fig. 42-36A). This may result in traction retinal detachment with vitreous strands bridging between the wound and the retina (Fig. 42-36B). These detachments may occur soon after surgery if a great deal of vitreous was lost at surgery or if a retinal break occurred at the time of cataract surgery. Alternatively, the retinal detachment may occur weeks to months after surgery if fibrous proliferation at the wound caused additional traction. A similar picture can sometimes be seen following vitrectomy if inadequate vitreous was removed and vitreous traction from the sclerotomy wound is transmitted to the retina (Fig. 42-37A). In addition, vitreous incarceration in a scleral drain site during a scleral buckling procedure can lead to significant vitreous traction. We have seen traction retinal detachment following resolution of a postoperative, nonexpulsive choroidal hemorrhage following glaucoma filtration surgery. In this case, vitreous was extruded through the filter site into the subconjunctival space.

Surgical Anatomy

Characteristically, these retinal detachments are rhegmatogenous and have horseshoe retinal breaks with highly elevated retinal flaps, though occasionally the retinal detachments are purely tractional. Vitreous can usually be seen bridging between the wound and the retina.

Surgical Technique

We initiate pars plana vitrectomy as described above. Vitreous traction is usually directed toward the vitreous base, and the posterior vitreous is often separated. If posterior vitreous separation has not occurred, then vitreous is separated from the optic disk and retina with suction, picks, and/or vitreous forceps as necessary. Vitreous strands from the wound to the retina are severed with the vitrectomy cutter (Fig. 42-37B). If the vitreous is organized, it may be neces-

sary to cut the membranes with scissors, though this is rare. We remove vitreous attached to flaps of retinal breaks and strip any epiretinal membranes present. The vitreous is shaved to the surface of the peripheral retina at the vitreous base using scleral depression or a wide-angle viewing system.

If the retina becomes bullous as traction is released, then PFCL can be used to stabilize the retina as peripheral vitreous or membranes are removed. If a posterior break is present, a fluid–air exchange will reattach the retina. If breaks are only peripheral, the retina can be reattached with PFCL. We usually treat retinal breaks with laser endophotocoagulation, although indirect laser photocoagulation or cryotherapy can be used alternatively. No gas tamponade or scleral buckle is required if there are no retinal breaks and traction has been released. We usually place an encircling scleral buckle to support peripheral retinal breaks.

Results

Kreiger (85) reported on 4 patients who developed retinal detachments secondary to tears caused by traction from incarcerated vitreous at a sclerotomy site, and who underwent reoperation. All detachments were successfully repaired, although visual outcome was poor in 1 eye in which silicone oil was required because of severe PVR.

Vitreous Traction on Retinal Breaks Following Scleral Buckle

Overview

Most retinal detachments with lower grades of PVR are managed with a scleral buckle. With grades A and B (see Table 42-1), there can be vitreous contraction induced by

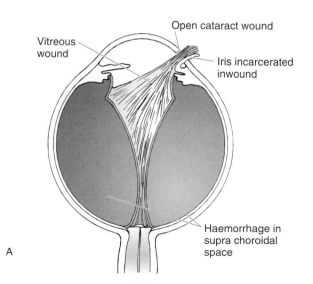
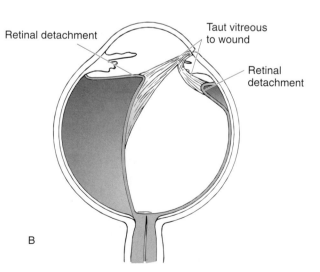

FIGURE 42-36.   *An intraoperative choroidal hemorrhage leading to a tractional retinal detachment. A. An eye with an intraoperative choroidal hemorrhage during cataract surgery. The mass effect of the choroidal hemorrhage displaces vitreous into the open cataract wound. B. With resolution of the choroidal hemorrhage, the band of incarcerated vitreous applies tractional force to the retina, leading to tractional retinal detachment.*

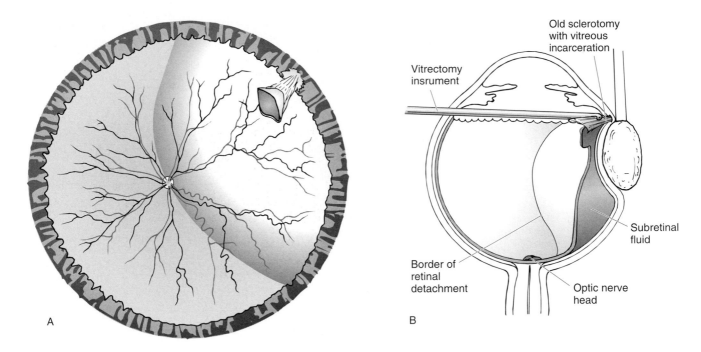

FIGURE 42-37.   *Vitreous incarceration in a sclerotomy wound after pars plana vitrectomy leads to a retinal detachment. A. Vitreous streams from the sclerotomy site in the pars plana to the vitreous base, producing peripheral traction on the retina, with a resultant retinal break formation and a traction/rhegmatogenous retinal detachment. B. Release of vitreous traction with vitrectomy.*

proliferative cells. Vitreous traction on a retinal break can sometimes prevent the retinal break from making contact with the retinal pigment epithelium on a scleral buckle and prevent reattachment of the retina (Fig. 42-38A). In addition, some large posterior retinal breaks, even in the absence of PVR, can "fish-mouth" and not close on a scleral buckle. If the retinal break is in the superior 180 degrees, injection of an air or gas bubble will usually tamponade the break, except for extreme levels of traction. Inferior retinal breaks are problematic because of the difficulty of tamponading with air or gas. Sometimes elevating the height of a scleral buckle or adding a radial element will close the retinal break, but it is less traumatic to the eye to directly relieve traction with a vitrectomy in some cases.

Surgical Anatomy

In PVR, findings include pigmented vitreous cells and reduced mobility of the vitreous on eye movement. Breaks are often large, and vitreous can be seen tenting the flap of the tear.

Surgical Technique

The central vitreous is removed with the vitreous cutter. Vitreous attachments to the flap of the retinal tear should be cut (Fig. 42-38B). Scleral depression or a wide-angle viewing system may be necessary to visualize the retinal break. We recommend shaving the peripheral vitreous to the surface of the anterior retina. If there is significant mobility of the anterior retina, PFCL can be used to

stabilize the retina. We usually reattach the retina with PFCL, then apply laser photocoagulation to the retinal breaks. We use laser endophotocoagulation in aphakic and pseudophakic eyes and indirect laser photocoagulation in phakic eyes. In reoperation of eyes with early PVR, we recommend scatter laser photocoagulation 360 degrees to the retina supported by the scleral buckle, because of the risk of anterior retinal traction in the postoperative period. We leave air or gas in the eye for postoperative tamponade of the retinal breaks.

Results

Friedman and D'Amico treated 9 patients who had recurrent retinal detachents due to persistent vitreous traction on retinal breaks after scleral buckle surgery (86). All patients were treated with vitrectomy, relief of traction on the retinal break, and gas tamponade. Long-term reattachment was achieved with 7 of the 9 patients with a single operation, and in 1 additional patient after two vitrectomies.

Vitreomacular Traction Syndrome

Overview

Vitreomacular traction syndrome classically has vitreoretinal traction on the posterior pole causing visual loss. While most cases do not have retinal detachment, sometimes traction retinal detachment of the macula and even a larger area of the posterior pole evolves when vitreous separates from the retina, except at the macula and optic disk area.

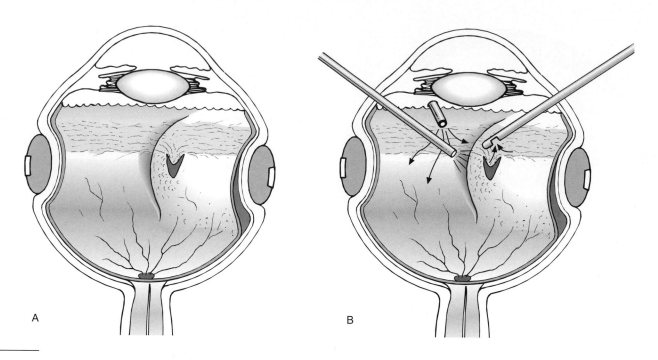

A

B

FIGURE 42-38.   *Recurrent rhegmatogenous retinal detachment after scleral buckle surgery due to vitreous traction on a preexisting retinal break. A. A band of vitreous elevates the inferior retinal break, leading to subretinal fluid overlying the buckle and extending posteriorly to involve the macula. B. Release of vitreous traction with vitrectomy allows the retina to be reattached.*

Surgical Anatomy

On examination, the vitreous is seen to bridge in a taut fashion from the posterior pole adherence to the vitreous base, separated from the midperipheral retina. There is epiretinal membrane that fuses the posterior cortical vitreous to the retina in the posterior pole, and there is often fibrous tissue at the optic disk where the vitreous remains attached (Fig. 42-39). The contractile elements in the epiretinal and epipapillary fibrous tissue may be the cause of the taut antero-posterior traction between the vitreous base and the posterior pole that results in traction retinal detachment.

Surgical Technique

At vitrectomy, the vitreous attachments to the posterior pole are cut, relieving antero-posterior traction. Then the epiretinal membranes are stripped with a membrane pick and forceps. If no retinal breaks are discovered after the vitreous is removed to the vitreous base area, air or gas tamponade is not necessary.

Results

Melberg and colleagues (87) reported on the results of vitrectomy in 9 patients who had vitreomacular traction syndrome with macular detachment (87). Macula reattachment was achieved in 7 eyes (78%), and visual acuity was improved in 4 eyes and stable in 4 eyes. Visual acuity was thought to be limited in some cases by chronic macular detachment, premacular fibrosis, cystoid macular edema, and

macular schisis. These results are not as favorable as for eyes undergoing vitrectomy for vitreomacular traction without macular detachment, a condition for which one series found vision improvement of two or more lines in 12 (80%) of 15 eyes (88).

Retinal Branch Vein Occlusion and Associated Diseases

Overview

Traction retinal detachments arising from other causes are fairly rare. However, retinal branch vein occlusion can be complicated by retinal neovascularization occasionally leading to traction retinal detachment (Fig. 42-40) (89,90).

Other rare causes of traction or combined tractional-rhegmatogenous retinal detachments include sickle cell disease (91), Coat's disease (92), and angiomatosis retinae (92), which are managed in a fashion similar to that for venous occlusive disease.

Surgical Anatomy

As in proliferative diabetic retinopathy, traction retinal detachment is associated with both anterior-posterior traction due to vitreous adherence to epiretinal fibrovascular membranes, and tangential traction caused by contraction of these membranes. If retinal breaks are present, the detachment is termed a combined traction-rhegmatogenous detachment.

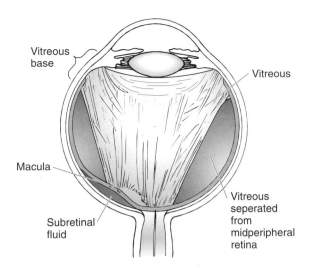

FIGURE 42-39.   *The vitreomacular traction syndrome associated with detachment of the macula. The vitreous is separated from the midperipheral retina, and partially separated from the posterior pole, but remains attached at the disk and the macula. The vitreous has become taut and exerts anterior–posterior traction between the posterior pole and the vitreous base, leading to elevation of the macula and subretinal fluid. A fibrous ring and intraretinal edema are often present in the macula.*

Surgical Technique

The usual indication for vitrectomy in traction retinal detachment due to venous occlusive disease is detachment involving or threatening the macula, or a progressive extramacular traction-rhegmatogenous retinal detachment. The technique is similar to that used in vitrectomy for diabetic-related retinal detachments, detailed above.

To summarize briefly, a three-port pars plana vitrectomy is performed, starting with a core vitrectomy and removal of vitreous opacities, which are often significant. Starting at the optic nerve head, fibrovascular membranes are segmented or delaminated with intraocular scissors and forceps. Vitreous is separated from the retinal surface as far anteriorly as possible, with particular care taken to make sure all vitreous traction is relieved from around any retinal breaks. Then, pneumatic reattachment is performed, with simultaneous aspiration of subretinal fluid via a silicone-tipped cannula through a pre-existing or iatrogenic posterior retinal break. If no posterior break is present, PFCL can be used to reattach the retina in a manner similar to that described for PVR. Then, all retinal breaks are treated with endophotocoagulation. Scatter laser endophotocoagulation is also applied to the peripheral retinal areas drained by obstructed vessels. An encircling band is placed in selected cases to decrease traction from the anterior vitreous, and pars plana lensectomy is performed when cataract obscures visualization of the fundus.

Results

A recent study of pars plana vitrectomy for traction retinal detachment after retinal branch vein occlusion revealed a

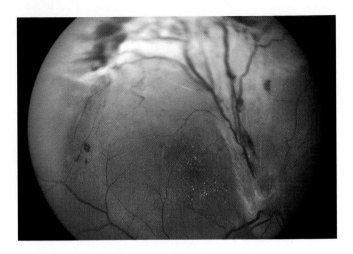

FIGURE 42-40.   *Fundus photograph of a tractional retinal detachment secondary to a branch retinal vein occlusion. Fibrovascular membranes run from the optic disk along the superior temporal vascular arcades, arising from NVE and NVD. As these membranes proliferate and contract, traction is exerted on the retina, leading to a detachment involving the macula.*

final anatomic success rate of approximately 86%, with 59% of eyes achieving visual acuity of 20/200 or better (93). Complications in this study included iatrogenic retinal breaks in 23% of eyes, and recurrent retinal detachment requiring additional surgery occurred in 36%.

Less frequent complications include recurrent vitreous hemorrhage, cataract progression, epimacular membrane formation, corneal opacification, and neovascular glaucoma.

COMBINED RHEGMATOGENOUS RETINAL DETACHMENT AND CHOROIDAL DETACHMENT

Overview

Rhegmatogenous retinal detachment presenting with simultaneous choroidal detachment in the absence of trauma and recent eye surgery is considered rare (94). In one series of 1000 consecutive retinal detachments, simultaneous choroidal detachment was present preoperatively in only 4 cases (95). The condition is seen most commonly in highly myopic individuals with chronic rhegmatogenous detachments. There appears to be an increased incidence among Asians, which may be related to the preponderance of high myopia among these individuals. The presence of a choroidal detachment has been associated with an increased incidence of postoperative PVR formation and redetachment (96) [although there is conflicting evidence in the literature regarding this assertion (97)], leading to a poorer prognosis than for simple rhegmatogenous retinal detachment.

The pathogenesis of combined retinal and choroidal detachment is theorized to be related to hypotony. A rhegmatogenous retinal detachment occurs first, and it may be initially unnoticed or ignored by the patient. Eyes harboring retinal detachments are known to be subject to hypotony, which may be due to decreased aqueous production and/or increased activity of the retinal pigment epithelium pump. Highly myopic, hypotonous eyes may be predisposed to development of a choroidal effusion, because of anatomic and physiologic features such as the poor support of the anterior uveal veins. With time, a significant choroidal detachment develops, which may be associated with significant anterior chamber reaction. Laser flare-cell meter measurements have shown the aqueous protein level to be 70 times higher in eyes with combined retinal and choroidal detachment than in eyes with simple retinal detachment (98).

Surgical Anatomy

Fundus examination often reveals a fair degree of vitreous haze and debris. Because of its chronic nature, the detachment is usually quite bullous, and multiple breaks are common. PVR may be present.

Surgical Technique

Traditionally, combined retinal and choroidal detachment has been treated with scleral buckling and external drainage of subretinal fluid, sometimes combined with drainage of suprachoroidal fluid. If there is significant ocular inflammation, some authorities recommend treatment with topical and/or systemic anti-inflammatory medications, delaying surgery until anterior chamber reaction is reduced in the hope of decreasing the risk of postoperative PVR.

More recently, initial repair of combined retinal and choroidal detachment using pars plana vitrectomy combined with scleral buckling has been reported (99). One potential advantage with this technique is drainage of suprachoroidal fluid via the instrument and infusion sclerotomies, eliminating the need for a separate scleral cut-down. A possible disadvantage of vitrectomy would be the potentially increased risk of postoperative PVR formation.

Prior to performing surgery, the severity of the choroidal detachment should be evaluated with indirect ophthalmoscopy and possibly echography. From this information, an area with a lower choroidal elevation can be chosen for the infusion cannula site. There is risk of retinal damage and hemorrhage during creation of the sclerotomy sites, so the tip of the blade should not contact the elevated retina and choroid. There is also risk of suprachoroidal infusion, so it is important to visualize the tip of the infusion port within the eye prior to opening the infusion. As noted, suprachoroidal fluid will usually drain when sclerotomies are made for the instrument ports. Surgery then proceeds in a fashion similar to that for retinal detachment with PVR, with removal of the vitreous, membrane peeling, encircling

scleral buckle placement, endolaser treatment, and gas or silicone oil tamponade.

Results

Results in the literature are limited, but in a recent small series of patients with rhegmatogenous retinal detachment and choroidal detachment treated with pars plana vitrectomy, 90% achieved retinal reattachment without reoperation after 6 months of follow-up (99).

RETINAL DETACHMENT IN OCULAR INFLAMMATORY DISEASE

Overview

Patients with uveitis may develop retinal detachments due to several mechanisms. Retinal detachments can be exudative, tractional, or rhegmatogenous. There are often tractional elements to the rhegmatogenous retinal detachments. Exudative retinal detachments are treated medically, while tractional and rhegmatogenous retinal detachments usually require surgery.

Fibrous proliferation secondary to intraocular inflammation may cause abnormally strong vitreoretinal adhesions posterior to the vitreous base, resulting in retinal breaks when a posterior vitreous separation occurs. Surgical repair often requires vitrectomy as well as a scleral buckle. There is a significant risk of recurrent retinal detachment with PVR following repair of retinal detachments in uveitis. Factors linked to a high propensity to develop PVR, such as breakdown of the blood-ocular barrier, influx of inflammatory cells and macrophages, and stimulation of growth factors, are present in active ocular inflammatory disease. Cataracts and hypotony are often found in patients with uveitis and further complicate surgical management.

Certain forms of uveitis are more prone to retinal detachment than others. In an older series of 44 eyes with rhegmatogenous retinal detachments (1.7% of a large series of consecutive retinal detachments), the causes of the inflammatory disease were classified as follows: toxoplasmosis, 36%; pars planitis, 25%; and ocular toxocariasis, 7%. In 32% of the eyes, no cause could be established (100). Retinal detachments are common following viral retinitis, and these retinal detachments are covered elsewhere.

Surgical Anatomy

Foci of retinal inflammation and inflammation-induced neovascularization may cause scarring and vitreoretinal adhesions. In nonrhegmatogenous traction retinal detachment, there is vitreous traction on areas of vitreoretinal adhesion, which causes the retinal detachment. When a retinal break occurs in an area of adhesion, a traction-rhegmatogenous retinal detachment may occur. Retinal breaks at the vitreous base due to posterior vitreous separation may cause retinal detachments in patients with uveitis. These may be complicated and difficult to repair because of vitreous haze and cataract. Epiretinal membranes seen before surgery can lead to fixed folds and recurrent retinal detachment with PVR. Even without preexisting epiretinal membranes, retinal detachments in uveitis are more likely to develop recurrent retinal detachment and PVR. In pars planitis, retinal breaks associated with peripheral fibrovascular proliferation at the vitreous base may cause complicated retinal detachments. The peripheral retinal traction creates a picture similar to anterior PVR. In toxocariasis, there may be extensive vitreous, retinal, and subretinal proliferation that leads to retinal breaks and detachment.

Additional anatomic problems these patients develop include cyclitic membranes with anterior retinal displacement and ciliary body traction. Hypotony may lead to phthisis bulbi even in the face of successful retinal reattachment.

Surgical Techniques

Eyes with uveitis and retinal detachment are prone to develop severe inflammation postoperatively. Preoperative treatment with periocular or systemic corticosteroids may reduce inflammation. Machemer has shown that administration of corticosteroids prior to surgery is more effective than postoperative administration (54). Pretreatment with corticosteroids may induce synthesis of intracellular effector proteins that inhibit the inflammatory cascade. While treatment with corticosteroids for 5 to 7 days prior to surgery will best inhibit inflammation, it is not always best to wait that long to repair a recent rhegmatogenous retinal detachment. In that case, pretreatment the day prior to surgery may still help to reduce the postoperative inflammatory reaction. Patients with toxoplasmosis should be treated with the full regimen for toxoplasmosis in addition to corticosteroids.

In eyes with peripheral retinal breaks without PVR, and in which the media are clear enough to permit adequate peripheral retinal examination, the retinal detachment can usually be repaired using a scleral buckle without vitrectomy. Cryotherapy should be minimized, because it may incite further inflammation.

Eyes with cataract or media hazy enough to prevent adequate peripheral retinal examination will require a vitrectomy, as will eyes with significant retinal traction or PVR. The entrance sites for vitrectomy should be well planned preoperatively. Sclerotomy sites should be moved more anteriorly in eyes with the anterior retinal displacement sometimes found in pars planitis and PVR. Sclerotomy sites should be moved away from peripheral granulomas and areas of fibrosis. Preoperative ultrasound is sometimes useful in planning sclerotomy placement.

Eyes with cataracts will require lensectomy. Extensive posterior synechiae are often present and complicate lensec-

tomy. After placing the infusion port, sclerotomies are created nasally and temporally. If the cataract prevents inspection of the infusion port to see if it has penetrated the pars plana epithelium, the port should not be opened to fluid infusion until penetration is visually confirmed. During lensectomy and the initial posterior vitrectomy procedure, infusion can be with a handheld 20-gauge infusion needle as described above. We usually break posterior synechiae prior to lensectomy by sweeping the synechiae with a small blunt cannula on a syringe of viscoelastic. The viscoelastic will maintain anterior chamber depth, clear the anterior surface of the lens, and partially dilate the pupil after sweeping the synechiae. Iris retractors may be necessary to dilate the pupil, but should be avoided if possible because they can potentially incite more inflammation. The lens should be removed with ultrasound phacofragmentation, and the lens capsule removed, as described above, to reduce the likelihood of anterior fibrosis and traction.

Vitrectomy techniques are similar to those described above for traction retinal detachment, vitreous hemorrhage, and PVR. Membranes can be extremely thick and tenacious, and it is sometimes best to section membranes if they do not readily peel from the retina. Extensive fibrosis associated with toxocariasis may require sectioning as well as membrane peeling. Retinal traction should be released and the vitreous shaved to the surface of the peripheral retina at the vitreous base, using scleral depression. We apply only enough laser to treat retinal breaks, except for PVR cases, where we recommend peripheral scatter treatment on the retina, supported by a scleral buckle. We utilize gas for most retinal detachments; however, when the eye is hypotonous, silicone oil may be preferred. Postoperative periocular and/or systemic corticosteroids should be administered in most cases. We give subconjunctival Decadron (5–10 mg) at the end of all cases, and posterior subtenons (posterior to the equator) triamcinolone acetonide in some cases.

Results

Hagler and colleagues reported the results of surgery for 44 retinal detachments associated with uveitis (100). In this 1978 study, 38 eyes were treated with scleral buckle and cryotherapy and only 2 eyes were treated with vitrectomy. The retina was reattached in 91% of eyes, and vision improved in 57%. Compared to a large series of retinal detachments in eyes without uveitis, retinal detachments following ocular inflammatory disease had a longer duration of the retinal detachment, fewer observable retinal breaks, a higher incidence of visible vitreous membranes and preoperative macular puckers, a younger age distribution, and a higher incidence of phakic patients. No significant difference in the presence or types of retinal folds, the rate of operative complications, or the rate of reattachment at six months was shown.

Thumann and colleagues reported the results of vitrectomy in 50 eyes with uveitis (101). The indications for surgery were opaque media, retinal detachment, and cyclitic or preretinal membranes. Eyes with preoperative retinal detachment had a worse visual outcome (mean visual acuity of 0.2) than those without preoperative retinal detachment (mean visual acuity of 0.5). Persistent hypotony following surgery was found in 7 eyes.

Retinal detachment follows pars planitis in 22% (102) to 51% (103) of eyes. In mild to moderate forms of the disease, retinal breaks may form on the posterior edge of the organized peripheral fibrosis. Most of these detachments can be managed with a scleral buckle. However, severe forms of pars planitis have extensive neovascularization and fibrous proliferation with vitreoretinal traction and fixed folds, and a picture similar to anterior PVR. These eyes usually require vitrectomy (104).

Small et al (105) reported the results of vitrectomy for 12 eyes with tractional macular detachment due to *Toxocara canis*. Traction retinal detachments were found in 10 eyes, and 2 eyes had combined traction-rhegmatogenous retinal detachments. Granulomas were located peripherally in 9 eyes and in the posterior pole in 3 eyes. One eye had a central macular granuloma. The authors found that membranes were difficult to peel from the retina and were best sectioned or delaminated from their retinal and optic nerve attachments. With a minimum of 6 months' follow-up, the retina was completely attached in 10 eyes (83%). Visual acuity improved in 7 eyes. Poor postoperative visual acuity correlated with large folds through the macula identified preoperatively.

Morse and McCuen (106) used vitrectomy and silicone oil injection to treat 5 eyes with profound hypotony associated with loss of vision complicating bilateral chronic uveitis. Uveitis was due to toxoplasmosis in 2 eyes, psoriatic arthritis in 1 eye, Vogt-Koyanagi-Harada disease in 1 eye, and an undetermined cause in 1 eye. Visual acuity and IOP improved in 3 of the 5 eyes at 6 months, but vision declined later in 2 of the 3 with initial improvement.

REFERENCES

1. Rachel WF, Burton TC. Changing concepts of failures after retinal detachment surgery. *Arch Ophthalmol* 1979;97:480–483.
2. Glaser BM, Cardin A, Biscoe B. Proliferative vitreoretinopathy: the mechanism of development of vitreoretinal traction. *Ophthalmology* 1987;94:327–332.
3. Machemer R, Laqua H. A logical approach to the treatment of massive periretinal proliferation. *Ophthalmology* 1978;85:584–593.
4. Lewis H, Aaberg TM. Anterior proliferative vitreoretinopathy. *Am J Ophthalmol* 1988;105:277–284.
5. Retina Society Terminology Committee. The classification of retinal detachment with proliferative vitreoretinopathy. *Ophthalmology* 1983;90:121–125.
6. Machemer R, Aaberg TM, Freeman HM, et al. An updated classification of retinal detachment with proliferative vitreoretinopathy. *Am J Ophthalmol* 1991;112:159–165.
7. Lewis H, Aaberg TM, Abrams GW. Causes of failure after initial vitreoretinal surgery for severe proliferative vitreoretinopathy. *Am J Ophthalmol* 1991;111:8–14.
8. Lewis H, Aaberg TM. Causes of failure after repeat vitreoretinal surgery for recurrent proliferative vitreoretinopathy. *Am J Ophthalmol* 1991;111:15–19.
9. Machemer R, Laqua H. Pigment epithelial proliferation in retinal detachment (massive periretinal proliferation). *Am J Ophthalmol* 1975;80: 1–23.
10. Machemer R, van Horn D, Aaberg TM. Pigment epithelial proliferation in human retinal detachment with massive periretinal proliferation. *Am J Ophthalmol* 1978;85:181–191.
11. Mueller-Jensen K, Machemer R, Azarnia R. Autotransplantation of retinal pigment epithelium in intravitreal diffusion chambers. *Am J Ophthalmol* 1975;80:530–537.
12. Laqua H, Machemer R. Glial cell proliferation in retinal detachment (massive periretinal proliferation). *Am J Ophthalmol* 1975;80:1–23.
13. van Horn DL, Aaberg TM, Machemer R, Fenzl R. Glial cell proliferation in human retinal detachment with massive periretinal proliferation. *Am J Ophthalmol* 1977;84:383–393.
14. Glaser BM, Vidaurri-Leal J, Michels RG, Campochiaro PA. Cryotherapy during surgery for giant retinal tears and intravitreal dispersion of viable retinal epithelial cells. *Ophthalmology* 1993;100:466–470.
15. Vidaurri-Leal J, Glaser BM. Effect of fibrin on morphologic characteristics of retinal pigment epithelial cells. *Arch Ophthalmol* 1984;102:1376–1379.
16. Grizzard WS, Hilton GF. Scleral buckling for retinal detachment complicated by periretinal proliferation. *Arch Ophthalmol* 1982;100:419–422.
17. de Juan ED Jr, Landers MB III. New techniques for visualization of infusion cannula during vitreous surgery. *Am J Ophthalmol* 1984;97:657.
18. de Juan E Jr, Hickingbotham D. Flexible iris retractor. *Am J Ophthalmol* 1991;111:776.
19. Lewis H, Aaberg TM, Abrams GW, Han DP, Kreiger AE. Management of the lens capsule during pars plana lensectomy. *Am J Ophthalmol* 1987;103: 109–110.
20. Spitznas M. A binocular indirect ophthalmomicroscope (BIOM) for non-contact wide-angle vitreous surgery. *Graefes Arch Clin Exp Ophthalmol* 1987;225:13–15.
21. Spitznas M, Reiner J. A stereoscopic diagonal inverter (SDI) for wide-angle vitreous surgery. *Graefes Arch Clin Exp Ophthalmol* 1987;225: 9–12.
22. Murray TG, Boldt HC, Lewis H, et al. A technique for facilitated visualization of the vitreous base, pars plana, and pars plicata. *Arch Ophthalmol* 1991;109:1458–1459.
23. Lewis JM, Park I, Ohji M, et al. Diamond-dusted silicone cannula for epiretinal membrane separation during vitreous surgery. *Am J Ophthalmol* 1997;124:552–554.
24. Chang S, Ozmert E, Zimmerman NJ. Intraoperative perfluorocarbon liquids in the management of proliferative vitreoretinopathy. *Am J Ophthalmol* 1988;106:668–674.
25. Elner SG, Elner VM, Diaz-Rohena R, et al. Anterior proliferative vitreoretinopathy. Clinicopathologic, light microscopic and ultrastructural findings. *Ophthalmology* 1988;95:1349–1357.
26. Lewis H, Aaberg TM, Abrams GW, et al. Subretinal membranes in proliferative vitreoretinopathy. *Ophthalmology* 1989;96:1403–1415.
27. Machemer R. Surgical approaches to subretinal strands. *Am J Ophthalmol* 1980;90:81–85.
28. Machemer R, McCuen BW, de Juan E. Relaxing retinotomies and retinectomies. *Am J Ophthalmol* 1986;102:7–12.
29. Abrams GW. Retinotomies and retinectomies. In: Ryan SJ, ed. *Retina*. 2nd ed., vol. 3. St. Louis: CV Mosby, 1994:2203–2237.
30. Chang S, Lincoff H, Zimmerman NJ, Fuchs W. Giant retinal tears. Surgical techniques and results using perfluorocarbon liquids. *Arch Ophthalmol* 1989;107:761–766.
31. Blumenkranz MS, Azen SP, Aaberg TM, et al. Silicone Study Group: relaxing retinotomy with silicone oil or long-acting gas in eyes with severe proliferative vitreoretinopathy (Silicone Study Report 5). *Am J Ophthalmol* 1993;116:557–564.
32. Nabih M, Peyman GA, Clark LC, et al. Experimental evaluation of perfluorophenanthrene as a high specific gravity vitreous substitute: a preliminary report. *Ophthalmic Surg* 1985;20:286–293.
33. Ando F. Intraocular hypertension resulting from pupillary block by silicone oil. *Am J Ophthalmol* 1985;99:87–88.
34. Flynn HW Jr, Lee WG, Parel JM. A simple extrusion needle with flexible cannula tip for vitreoretinal microsurgery. *Am J Ophthalmol* 1988;105(2):215–216.
35. Eaton AM, Jaffe GJ, McCuen BW II, Mincery GJ. Condensation on the posterior surface of silicone intraocular lenses during fluid-air exchange. *Ophthalmology* 1995;102:733–736.
36. Sternberg P. Personal Communication, Vail Vitrectomy Symposium, March 14, 1996, Vail, Colorado.

37. Williams DF, Peters MA, Abrams GW, et al. A two-stage technique for intraoperative fluid–gas exchange following pars plana vitrectomy. *Arch Ophthalmol* 1990;108:1484–1486.

38. Silicone Study Group. Vitrectomy with silicone oil or sulfur hexafluoride gas in eyes with severe proliferative vitreoretinopathy: results of a randomized clinical trial (Silicone Study Report 1). *Arch Ophthalmol* 1992;110:770–779.

39. Silicone Study Group. Vitrectomy with silicone oil or perfluoropropane gas in eyes with severe proliferative vitreoretinopathy: results of a randomized clinical trial (Silicone Study Report 2). *Arch Ophthalmol* 1992; 110:780–792.

40. Abrams GW, Azen SP, McCuen BW II, et al. Vitrectomy with silicone oil or long-acting gas in eyes with severe proliferative vitreoretinopathy: results of additional and long-term follow-up (Silicone Study Report 11). *Arch Ophthalmol* 1997;115:335–344.

41. Hutton WL, Azen SP, Blumenkranz MS, et al. Silicone Study Group: the effects of silicone oil removal (Silicone Study Report 6). *Arch Ophthalmol* 1994;112:778–785.

42. Han DP, Lewis H, Lambrou FH Jr, et al. Mechanisms of intraocular pressure elevation after pars plana vitrectomy. *Ophthalmology* 1989;96:1357–1362.

43. Williams GA, Lambrou FH, Jaffe GJ, et al. Treatment of postvitrectomy fibrin formation with intraocular tissue plasminogen activator. *Arch Ophthalmol* 1988;106:1055–1058.

44. Jaffe GJ, Green GDJ, Abrams GW. Stability of recombinant tissue plasminogen activator. *Am J Ophthalmol* 1989;108:90–91.

45. Boldt GC, Abrams GW, Murray TG, et al. The lowest effective dose of tissue plasminogen activator for fibrinolysis of postvitrectomy fibrin. In: Stirpe M, ed, *Advances in Vitreoretinal Surgery*. New York: Ophthalmic Communications Society, Inc., 1992;353–357.

46. Machemer R, Norton EWD. A new concept for vitreous surgery: III. Indications and results. *Am J Ophthalmol* 1972;74:1034.

47. Charles S. Vitreous microsurgery. 2nd ed. Baltimore: Williams & Wilkins, 1987:137–138.

48. Aaberg TM. Management of anterior and posterior proliferative vitreoretinopathy. XLV. Edward Jackson memorial lecture. *Am J Ophthalmol* 1988;106:519–32.

49. McCuen BW, Axen SP, Stern W, et al. Vitrectomy with silicone oil or perfluoropropane gas in eyes with severe proliferative vitreoretinopathy: results in group 1 versus group 2 (Silicone Study Report 3). *Retina* 1993;13:279–284.

50. Barr CC, Lai MY, Lean JS, et al. Postoperative intraocular pressure abnormalities in the Silicone Study (Silicone Study Report 4). *Ophthalmology* 1993;100:1629–1635.

51. Diddie KR, Azen SP, Freeman GM, et al. Anterior proliferative vitreoretinopathy in the Silicone Study (Silicone Study Report 10). *Ophthalmology* 1996;103:1092–1099.

52. Abrams GW, Azen SP, Barr CC, et al. The incidence of corneal abnormalities in the Silicone Study (Silicone Study Report 7). *Arch Ophthalmol* 1995;113:764–769.

53. Cox MS, Azen SP, Barr CC, et al. Macular pucker after successful surgery for proliferative vitreoretinopathy (Silicone Study Report 8). *Ophthalmology* 1995;102:1884–1891.

54. Machemer R. Proliferative vitreoretinopathy (PVR): a personal account of its pathogenesis and treatment. Proctor lecture. *Invest Ophthalmol Vis Sci* 1988;12:1771–83.

55. Wiedemann P, Sorgente N, Bekhor C, et al. Daunomycin in the treatment of experimental proliferative vitreoretinopathy. Effective doses in vitro and in vivo. *Invest Ophthalmol Vis Sci* 1985;26:719–725.

56. Heath TD, Lopez NG, Lewis GP, Stern WH. Fluoropyrimidine treatment of ocular cicatricial disease. *Invest Ophthalmol Vis Sci* 1986;27:940–945.

57. Innocenzi R, Glazer L, Stec L, et al. Treatment of experimental PVR in the rabbit with low molecular weight heparin. *Invest Ophthalmol Vis Sci* 1993;34:950.

58. William RG, Chang S, Comaratta MR, Simoni G. Does the presence of heparin and dexamethasone in the vitrectomy infusate reduce reproliferation in proliferative vitreoretinopathy? *Graefes Arch Clin Exp Ophthalmol* 1996;234:496–503.

59. Yang CS, Khawly JA, Hainsworth DP, et al. An intravitreal sustained release triamcinolone and 5-fluorouracil codrug in the treatment of experimental proliferative vitreoretinopathy. *Arch Ophthalmol* 1998;116:69–77.

60. Fekrat S, de Juan E, Campochiaro R. The effect of oral 13-cis retinoic acid on retinal redetachment after surgical repair in eyes with proliferative vitreoretinopathy. *Ophthalmology* 1995;102:412–418.

61. Avery RL, Glaser BM. Inhibition of retinal pigment epithelial cell attachment by a synthetic peptide derived from the cell-binding domain of fibronectin. *Arch Ophthalmol* 1986;104:1220–1222.

62. Jaffe GJ, et al. Antitransferrin receptor immunotoxin inhibits proliferating human retinal pigment epithelial cells. *Arch Ophthalmol* 1990;108:1163–1168.

63. Sakamoto T, Kimura H, Scuric Z, et al. Inhibition of experimental proliferative vitreoretinopathy by retroviral vector-mediated transfer of suicide gene. Can proliferative vitreoretinopathy be a target of gene therapy? *Ophthalmology* 1995;102:1417–1424.

64. Ratner CM, Michels RG, Auer C, Rice TA. Pars plana vitrectomy for complicated retinal detachments. *Ophthalmology* 1983;90:1323.

65. Duquesne N, Bonnet M, Adeleine P. Preoperative vitreous hemorrhage associated with rhegmatogenous retinal detachment: a risk factor for postoperative proliferative vitreoretinopathy? *Graefes Arch Clin Exp Ophthalmol* 1996;234:677–682.

66. Aaberg TM. Macular holes: a review. *Surv Ophthalmol* 1970;15:139.

67. Aaberg TM, Blair CJ, Gass JDM. Macular holes. *Am J Ophthalmol* 1970;69:555.

68. Yaoeda H. Clinical observations on macular hole. *Acta Soc Ophthalmol Jpn* 1967;71:1723.

69. Mikuni M, Kobayashi S, Yaoeda H. Treatment of retinal detachment with macular hole. *Folia Ophthalmol Jpn* 1967;18:659.

70. Margherio RR, Schepens CL. Macular breaks. I. Diagnosis, etiology, and observations. *Am J Ophthalmol* 1972;74:219.

71. Kloti R. Silver clip for central retinal detachments with macular hole. *Mod Prob Ophthalmol* 1974;12:330.

72. Muinos A, Mateus F, Heredia CD. Retinal detachment with holes in the posterior pole. *Mod Prob Ophthalmol* 1974;12:315.

73. Oliver GL. Retinal detachments caused by macular and perimacular breaks. *Can J Ophthalmol* 1969;4:24.

74. Rosengren B. Indentation of the sclera by means of a silver ball in the surgical treatment of retinal detachment. *Acta Ophthalmol* 1960;38:109.

75. Meyer-Schwickerath G. Macular holes and retinal detachment. In: McPherson A, ed. *New and controversial aspects of retinal detachment*. Hoeber: New York, 1968:443.

76. Howard GM, Campbell CJ. Surgical repair of retinal detachments caused by macular holes. *Arch Ophthalmol* 1969;81:317.

77. Stern WH, Blumkranz MI. Fluid-gas exchange after vitrectomy. *Am J Ophthalmol* 1983;96:400.

78. Binder S, Riss B. Advances in intraocular techniques in the treatment of retinal detachments arising from holes of the posterior pole. *Br J Ophthalmol* 1983;67:147.

79. Gonvers M, Machemer R. A new approach to treating retinal detachment with macular hole. *Am J Ophthalmol* 1983;94:468.

80. Blankenship GW, Ibanez-Langlois S. Treatment of myopic macular hole and detachment. Intravitreal gas exchange. *Ophthalmology* 1987;94:333–336.

81. Miyake Y. A simplified method of treating retinal detachment with macular hole. Long-term follow-up. *Arch Ophthalmol* 1986;104:1234–1236.

82. Garcia-Arumi J, Correa CA, Corcostegui B. Comparative study of different techniques of intraocular gas tamponade in the treatment of retinal detachment due to macular hole. *Ophthalmologica* 1990;201:83–91.

83. Stirpe M, Michels RG. Retinal detachment in highly myopic eyes due to macular holes and epiretinal traction. *Retina* 1990;10:113–114.

84. Seike C, Kusaka S, Sakagami K, et al. Reopening of macular holes in highly myopic eyes with retinal detachments. *Retina* 1997;17:2–6.

85. Kreiger AE. Wound complications in pars plana vitrectomy. *Retina* 1993;13:335–344.

86. Friedman ES, D'Amico DJ. Vitrectomy alone for the management of uncomplicated recurrent retinal detachments. *Retina* 1995;15:469–474.

87. Melberg NS, Williams DF, Balles MW, et al. Vitrectomy for vitreomacular traction syndrome with macular detachment. *Retina* 1995;15:192–197.

88. McDonald HR, Johnson RN, Schatz H. Surgical results in the vitreomacular traction syndrome. *Ophthalmology* 1994;101:1397–1402.

89. Murakami K, Ho PC, Trempe CL, Pruett RC. Tractional detachment of the macula following branch retinal vein occlusion. *Ann Ophthalmol* 1983;15:760–765.

90. Berger BB. Branch vein occlusion: traction macular detachment. *Ann Ophthalmol* 1984;16:623–624.

91. Jampol LM, Green JL Jr, Goldberg MF, Peyman GA. An update on vitrectomy surgery for retinal detachment repair in sickle cell disease. *Arch Ophthalmol* 1982;100:591–593.

92. Machemer R, Williams JM Sr. Pathogenesis and therapy of traction detachment in various retinal vascular diseases. *Am J Ophthalmol* 1988;105:170–181.

93. Ikuno Y, Ikeda T, Sato Y, Tano Y. Tractional retinal detachment after branch retinal vein occlusion: influence of disc neovascularization on the outcome of vitreous surgery. *Ophthalmology* 1998;105:417–423.

94. Rahman N, Harris GS. Choroidal detachment associated with retinal detachment as a presenting finding. *Can J Ophthalmol* 1992;27:245–248.

95. Mester U, Volker B. Pre- and postoperative choroidal detachment in retinal surgery. *Klin Monatsbl Augenheilkd* 1982;180:35–36.

96. Girard P, Mimoun G, Karpouzas I, Montefiore G. Clinical risk factors for proliferative vitreoretinopathy after retinal detachment surgery. *Retina* 1994;14:417–424.

97. Dumas C, Bonnet M. Choroidal detachment associated with rhegmatogenous retinal detachment: a risk factor for postoperative PVR? *J Fr Ophthalmol* 1996;19:455–463.

98. Tanaka F, Emi K, Danjo S. Choroidal detachment associated with rhegmatogenous retinal detachment and aqueous flare. *Nippon Ganka Gakkai Zasshi* 1991;95:1129–1134.

99. Yang CM. Pars plana vitrectomy in the treatment of combined rhegmatogenous retinal detachment and choroidal detachment in aphakic or pseudophakic patients. *Ophthalmic Surg Lasers* 1997;28:288–293.

100. Hagler WS, Jarrett WH III, Chang M. Rhegmatogenous retinal detachment following chorioretinal inflammatory disease. *Am J Ophthalmol* 1978;86:373–379.

101. Thumann G, Bartz-Schmidt KU, Esser P, et al. Vitrectomy in treatment of eyes with complicated uveitis. *Klin Monatsbl Augenheilkd* 1997;211:241–244.

102. Smith RE, Godfrey WA, Kimura SJ. Complications of chronic cyclitis. *Am J Ophthalmol* 1976;82:277–282.

103. Brockhurst RJ, Schepens CL. Uveitis. IV. Peripheral uveitis: the complication of retinal detachment. *Arch Ophthalmolol* 1968;80:747–753.

104. Michelson JB. Inflammatory retinal detachment. In: Michelson JB, Nozik RA, eds. *Surgical treatment of ocular inflammatory disease*. Philadelphia: Lippincott, 1988.

105. Small KW, McCuen BW II, de Juan E Jr, Machemer R. Surgical management of retinal traction caused by toxocariasis. *Am J Ophthalmol* 1989;108:10–14.

106. Morse LS, McCuen BW II. The use of silicone oil in uveitis and hypotony. *Retina* 1991;11:399–404.

Basic Vitreoretinal Surgical Techniques

Michael Humayun   Hilel Lewis

Vitreoretinal surgical techniques have revolutionized the management of complicated retinal detachments. Since the advent of vitreous surgery, surgeons have implemented these techniques in managing a variety of patients. Along with vitreous surgery also came the development of various surgical instruments to help surgeons manage a wide spectrum of surgical disorders.

Initially, Kasner (1) advocated the removal of vitreous gel through a large wound. This technique was modified and utilized in the management of patients with amyloidosis (2). Thereafter, Machemer et al (3) employed a pars plana approach to excise vitreous. This technique allowed for a controlled and watertight management of posterior-segment surgical disorders. Along with pars plana vitrectomy came the surgical instrumentation necessary to implement the procedures (4–8). Since then, many authors have added to the instrumentation and techniques initially described by Machemer and Kasner.

With vitrectomy, surgeons are now able to manage a wide variety of disorders that could not have been managed with scleral buckling alone. A combination of vitrectomy and scleral buckling can now be utilized to manage complicated retinal detachments. In order to understand vitreous surgery, one needs to understand the basic surgical techniques and instrumentation necessary to perform successful vitrectomy.

INSTRUMENTATION AND EQUIPMENT

Instrumentation and equipment are an integral part of successful pars plana vitrectomy. The operating room microscope, wrist rests, and infusion systems along with various instruments for different surgical scenarios are discussed.

Operating Microscope

Vitreous surgery is commonly performed using an operating room microscope. In rare instances, indirect ophthalmoscopy with vitrectomy can be utilized. However, for the majority of procedures, binocular viewing while seated at an operating room microscope is the standard. The microscope has advantages in that stereo viewing along with a bimanual technique can be employed. A ceiling-mounted microscope with both stereo viewing for the surgeon and assistant can be utilized. A plastic drape allows for manipulation of the oculars, for various microscopic functions, and also for the assistant's focus. The surgeon directly controls both XY and up and down maneuvering with a foot pedal. Microscopic illumination is also controlled with the foot pedal.

In addition to the binocular viewing system of the operating room microscope, a panoramic viewing system utilizing contact lenses that offer a 68- and 130-degree panoramic angle of observation can be employed. An image inverter is directly placed on the operating room microscope, allowing the surgeon to view the image directly. However, the assistant views an indirect yet panoramic image.

Operating Room Table

The operating room table has wrist rests at its head, allowing the surgeon to set up for a localized trough and field and also for resting his or her wrists and arms. Added stability can also be achieved by resting one's hands on a patient's forehead. The table also has functions of raising and lowering the bed and up and down tilting of the head to keep patients comfortable who either have degenerative neck disorders or have difficulty lying completely flat on their backs.

Vitrectomy Instrumentation

Vitrectomy instrumentation involves both aspiration and cutting systems to safely remove vitreous gel. At the same time, an irrigating system maintaining a constant intraocular infusion and pressure maintains the volume. Thus, an infusion system and cutting and aspiration equipment, coupled with an illuminating source, are the basic and integral components of a surgical setup. A combined infusion-illumination system utilizing the lighted infusion cannula can be employed (9–13). However, separate-function instrumentation provides excellent control and visibility and currently is utilized most commonly.

Vitrectomy probes using guillotine-like movements to cut vitreous also are used most commonly. Thus, both cutting and aspiration are provided by the vitreous cutter. The separate fiberoptic probe serves as a light source (14). The infusion cannula serves to primarily infuse balanced salt solution to maintain ocular volume. This cannula is usually sutured to the sclera. Hilton (15) described the use of cannulas that did not require suturing. However, when there is excess manipulation as during scleral depression, a sutured infusion cannula provides optimal stability.

As for the light source, a fiberoptic probe provides excellent illumination and the surgeon can switch from one sclerotomy to another to achieve different angles of illumination. Also during vitrectomy, the fiberoptic probe can be positioned to illuminate the vitreous for more efficient removal. A fixed light source, either to the cannula or at various sclerotomy sites, may provide adequate illumination, but is limited in its function of tilting the probe or in adjusting its intensity by bringing it closer or farther from the site where illumination is required.

Infusion System

The infusion system utilizing a sutured cannula is usually placed inferotemporally. We place a 4-mm infusion cannula, sutured with 6-0 polyglactin 910 (Vicryl) suture in a mattress fashion. The infusion system is usually under hydrostatic control and is connected to a hanging bottle, which is kept at a desired height. The hydrostatic pressure can be increased, for example, to tamponade bleeding, by raising the bottle temporarily. Some surgeons may add epinephrine to the infusion bottle to maintain pupillary dilatation. We have been adding 3 mL of 50% dextrose to prevent intraoperative lenticular opacities in diabetic patients (16).

It is important to note that the intraocular pressure is dependent on the hydrostatic pressure generated by the infusion bottle and also by the egress of fluid through the sclerotomies or at the time of aspiration with various instruments. Vitrectomy cutting functions are directly controlled by the foot pedal. The aspiration is also variably controlled by the surgeon's foot pedal. A certain maximum, however, can be set directly on the machine's monitor. This maximum can be adjusted only when the surgeon desires and instructs the technician to directly adjust it on the monitor.

With the panoramic viewing systems, the infusion cannulas and vitrectomy aspiration and cutting equipment are easily viewed. However, to achieve a wider field of illumination during panoramic viewing, a bullet, fiberoptic light source can be employed.

Contact Lens

Viewing during vitreous surgery is integral in helping to achieve surgical success. In addition to the panoramic viewing systems discussed earlier, vitrectomy and surface work is conducted using a plano concave contact lens system. Various types of contact lens systems have been described (17–24). Some of these lenses contain an infusion system to irrigate fluid while the assistant holds the lens. Others can be placed within a surgical ring that is sutured to the sclera. Thereafter, prism lenses may be utilized to view various quadrants. This lens ring can also hold a panoramic viewing lens, though more commonly an assistant needs to hold these lenses with the designated handle. Lenses with an infusion system generally provide optimum visualization and can be maneuvered by the assistant during vitrectomy. The balanced salt solution is ideal for irrigation with this system.

In lenses placed within the lens ring and with the panoramic viewing systems, either sodium hyaluronate or hydroxypropyl methylcellulose (Goniosol) can be effectively utilized. During fluid-air exchange, either the panoramic viewing lenses or a biconcave lens of −100 diopters can be employed in phakic patients (25). The image is minified; however, the view is adequate for completing the surgical objective. In aphakic patients a lens system for viewing during fluid-air exchange is not necessary.

Aspiration Systems

Commonly the vitreous surgeon is confronted with patients with vitreous and preretinal hemorrhage. The vitreous cutter using both aspiration and cutting is highly effective in cutting vitreous gel. Subhyaloid hemorrhage or layered preretinal hemorrhage can be evacuated with various aspirating equipment. A tapered- or blunt-tip instrument with a channel or side port that is vented externally can be employed to evacuate such hemorrhage (26,27). The atmospheric pressure in relation to the intraocular pressure allows controlled egress of the hemorrhage.

Soft silicone-tipped cannulas can also be utilized for aspiration. This instrument can be directly connected to the monitor to adjust the degree of aspiration. The surgeon then can control aspiration with the foot pedal. This latter technique may allow for more controlled aspiration, especially when a highly mobile retina during a retinal detachment case is present.

Forceps

Various forceps have been designed to allow for differing vitreoretinal maneuvers and procedures. Finer forceps such as the mini-diamond-tipped forceps are excellent for membrane peeling. The PIC-forceps can also be utilized for membrane peeling and are excellent to remove the remaining anterior or posterior capsule after lensectomy. Intraocular foreign bodies can be removed with diamond-coated forceps (28–30). Nonmagnetic foreign bodies are grasped well with these forceps, allowing for controlled removal. Magnetic foreign bodies can also be grasped with these forceps; however, an intraocular magnet may allow for greater control and less trauma to the surrounding tissues during removal.

Membrane Peeling Instruments

Some membranes do not have a readily available edge to allow grasping and removal with forceps. In these cases, the surgeon must create an edge. Instruments such as Michel's pick are excellent in creating an edge. In other cases the myringotomy tip can be bent by the surgeon to create an edge. Some surgeons have also advocated the use of a 25-gauge needle with a bent tip to create an edge. Once an edge is created, the mini-diamond-tipped or equivalent forceps can be utilized to grasp the membrane and peel tangentially and slightly anteroposteriorly. A new instrument, the Lewis PIC-forceps, is excellent for creating an edge and then removing epiretinal membranes.

Intraocular Scissors

When membrane dissection is necessary, intraocular scissors can be employed. Both vertical and horizontal scissors can be utilized to initially segment and then delaminate tractional membranes. More commonly, the membrane peeler cutter scissors, which are activated by a foot pedal, can be utilized both for segmentation and for delamination of tractional membranes. These scissors are also excellent for creating retinectomies in shallowly detached retinas. A vitreous cutter can also be utilized for more bullous detachments. However, to avoid possible damage to the underlying retinal pigment epithelium in shallowly detached retinas requiring retinectomy, the membrane peeler cutter is an excellent tool.

Diathermy

To control bleeding or to mark breaks or other vitreoretinal anatomy, the intraocular diathermy can be an excellent tool. We have also found diathermy to be useful in cauterizing focal areas of surface episcleral vessels.

Various types of diathermy have been described (31–33). The most common use for diathermy remains the control of bleeding. Diabetic patients with fibrovascular stalks can have significant bleeding during dissection. Even after the infusion bottle is elevated, persistent bleeding can be present. Intraocular diathermy can be an excellent tool to control such bleeding. However, some shrinkage of retinal tissues is commonly noted when diathermy is applied. Also, caution must be exercised when heating fibrovascular tissue close to the optic nerve. The current can damage the optic nerve.

Another use of diathermy involves creating a drainage retinotomy. The diathermy serves as an excellent source through which a retinotomy can be created with little if any bleeding. Thereafter, a tapered flute needle or a soft silicone-tipped cannula can be utilized to drain subretinal fluid. This retinotomy is also marked so that laser photocoagulation can be placed around the retinectomy site after the subretinal fluid is aspirated.

Similarly intraocular diathermy can be used to mark preexisting retinal breaks prior to retinal reattachment. These breaks are sometimes difficult to identify once the retina is completely reattached. The marks of the intraocular diathermy can be readily identified and the breaks can then be surrounded with laser photocoagulation to create a seal.

The intraocular diathermy is also excellent for marking the margins of a retinectomy. Either a single or a double row of diathermy marks can be placed along the margins of the retinectomy site. Thereafter, either the vitreous cutter in more bullous detachments or a membrane peeler cutter in more shallow retinal detachments can be employed to create the retinectomy edge with very little, if any bleeding. Bleeding at the edges of the retinectomy site can also be controlled either by elevating the infusion bottle or by utilizing intraocular diathermy directly at the bleeding sites. Similarly, if elevation of the infusion bottle is unsuccessful, intraocular diathermy can be applied.

FRAGMENTATION AND LENS REMOVAL

In certain patients, lens removal is necessary either to obtain an adequate view or to achieve the surgical objective of complete retinal reattachment. Various fragmentation techniques have been described (34–37). Either a pars plana, scleral tunnel, or even clear corneal approach can be utilized.

The scleral tunnel approach requires a phacofragmentation hand piece. This approach has the advantage of controlled lens removal, thereby leaving the posterior capsule intact to allow insertion of an intraocular lens (IOL). We have utilized this technique effectively, especially when a macular hole and cataract are present and in patients undergoing diabetic vitrectomy with preexisting cataract. Also, it is successful in patients after failed macular hole surgery or with open macular holes whose lenticular opacities worsened after the initial vitrectomy. In placing a lens, we recommend a polymethylmethacrylate (PMMA) lens with a 7-mm optic, to avoid iris IOL capture in cases of gas tamponade. It is also recommended to place the IOL prior to the fluid-air exchange, to avoid capsule becoming forwardly displaced prior to IOL implantation. We do not recommend leaving the patient aphakic and then reinserting the IOL at a later date, as the gas tamponade may cause chronic iridocapsular adhesions, making it difficult to implant an IOL later.

Clear corneal lens removal is commonly utilized in a patient with a functioning bleb. A similar phacofragmentation hand piece as used for the scleral tunnel approach is utilized. A diamond blade or keratome can be utilized to create a clear corneal wound. After a continuous tear capsulorrhexis is performed utilizing a bent cystotome needle or the Utratta forceps, a standard phacoemulsification can be performed. The phacoemulsification hand piece has combined irrigation, aspiration, and fragmentation functions. Either a pulse or continuous mode of fragmentation can be employed. The surgeon is readily able to control these functions with a foot pedal. Lens placement through the clear corneal incision can then be performed. A posterior infusion cannula can be placed prior to either a scleral tunnel or clear corneal approach but need not be turned on as the phacofragmentation hand piece has irrigation capability.

We generally prefer the scleral tunnel approach in such cases, allowing for a larger optic IOL to be placed, not only to prevent iris IOL capture but also to allow easier visibility of the retinal periphery during postoperative follow-up. The scleral tunnel approach allows enlarging the wound more readily without compromising visual function. We have also been performing pars plana vitrectomy after lens removal and before IOL placement. The scleral tunnel wound is commonly sutured and then a pars plana vitrectomy is performed. This allows for easier maneuverability as during scleral depressed vitrectomy, without having to be concerned about the stability of the IOL. Care must be taken not to create a rent in the posterior capsule during such maneuvers. A small air bubble introduced into the vitreous cavity may help delineate the margins of the posterior capsule. After the vitrectomy is completed, and prior to fluid-air exchange, the IOL is placed directly in the bag. Thereafter the scleral tunnel wound is closed and the fluid-air exchange is performed. It is important to mention that we have not been using silicone-oil IOLs because of the difficulty of viewing during fluid-air exchange. We also do not use them in patients who are at high risk for having complicated retinal detachments requiring possible future silicone-oil tamponade. Either PMMA or acrylic IOLs can be successfully utilized. When the posterior capsule has a rent, the IOL can still be placed within the bag or in the sulcus. In these cases, condensations on the IOL may form during fluid-air exchange. A soft-tipped cannula can be used to coalesce the condensations, allowing for a brief period of adequate viewing. However, if longer periods of viewing are necessary, sodium hyaluronate can be placed on the lens through the pars plana incisions.

Anterior-segment lens removal approaches, such as the scleral tunnel and the clear cornea approach, have their advantages and disadvantages. They can be excellent in visually rehabilitating certain select patients, by placing air in the capsular-bag IOL. However, these approaches can lead to intraoperative corneal edema, especially when the lens nucleus is hard and longer phacoemulsification times are necessary to achieve removal. Thereafter, during pars plana vitrectomy, the view posteriorly can be compromised, especially when fine membrane peeling is to be performed.

Management of small pupils and posterior synechiae during lens removal can pose certain problems. Synechiae can sometimes be gently broken with the cyclodialysis spatula or with sodium hyaluronate. If this is unsuccessful, flexible iris retractors have been an excellent tool for managing both miotic pupils and pupils with synechiae. All four iris retractors can be positioned and a continuous tear capsulorrhexis can be performed prior to lens removal.

A pars plana approach for lens removal is utilized commonly when an IOL will not be placed. A myringotomy blade is introduced through the lens to soften the nucleus. In young patients with soft lenses, the vitreous cutter can be utilized to remove the lens. A combination of cutting and aspirating will allow for controlled removal. In general, both the anterior and the posterior capsule are left intact. If the anterior capsule is violated, the anterior chamber may shallow at the time of lens removal, especially during aspiration. If the posterior capsule is violated, lens material will fall back into the vitreous cavity.

When the lens nucleus is harder, fragmentation techniques can be employed. A myringotomy blade is utilized to soften the central nucleus. The fragmentation probe can then be introduced through one side and a 21-gauge bent needle through the other side for secondary irrigation. The primary infusion cannula is turned off to prevent the posterior capsule from coming forward. Care is taken not to disrupt either the anterior or the posterior capsule during lens fragmentation. After the lens nucleus and cortex are completely removed, the lens capsule can be removed either with the vitreous cutter or with the PIC-forceps (38). Simultaneous scleral depression will allow for complete removal of both the peripheral cortex and the capsule. If left, the cortex and capsule can be a nidus for chronic inflammation and can sometimes even contribute to the epiciliary proliferation resulting in possible hypotony.

The advantage of a pars plana technique is that virtually no corneal edema occurs, thus allowing for enhanced visualization during vitrectomy. The disadvantages are that in-the-bag IOL placement is not possible. Only a sulcus-situated IOL can be placed if the anterior capsule is left intact.

Patients with posteriorly dislocated lenses are commonly managed with a lens fragmentation technique through the pars plana. When the dislocated lens causes excess inflammation or elevated intraocular pressure, visual dysfunction from cystoid macular edema, or anatomic disruption such as retinal detachment, removal is warranted (39). Commonly these lens fragments are removed via pars plana lens fragmentation (40). For this technique, vitrectomy is performed and the lens material is removed off the surface of the retina with aspiration and then fragmented with the ultrasonic lens fragmentation device. The endoilluminator is utilized to secure the lens fragments and at times can be used to crush the fragments into the fragmenter port. In certain cases, the lens pieces may fall back, causing either macular injury or retinal breaks elsewhere. To prevent such an occurrence, we use perfluorocarbon liquid to float lens fragments and then with the lens fragmentation device we aspirate the lens material off the surface of the perfluorocarbon bubble, and perform fragmentation. Commonly, lens fragmentation is performed on the nasal side to ensure that both the orientation of the lens fragments and the added liquid perfluorocarbon serve as safety measures against large fragments of lens material dislodging and causing iatrogenic trauma.

This technique has also been used successfully when there are dislocated lens fragments and coincident retinal detachment (39). The liquid perfluorocarbon will serve not only to provide a cushion against the sharp lens fragments but also to displace any subretinal fluid from the preexisting retinal break resulting in simultaneous retinal reattachment. The liquid perfluorocarbon can then be aspirated or a perfluorocarbon liquid–air exchange can be performed.

When these techniques are used, it is important to maintain the lens fragments on the perfluorocarbon bubble. If liquid perfluorocarbon is added without monitoring the lens fragments, the fragments can become embedded into the basal vitreous gel or against the inner eye wall. Thus, we recommend removing as much of the basal vitreous gel as possible and then maintaining the lens fragments on top of and in the middle of the perfluorocarbon bubble. It is also important to use low ultrasonic fragmentation and higher aspiration so that the lens fragment will not propulse backward.

PHOTOCOAGULATION

To seal retinal breaks or to implement panretinal photocoagulation after diabetic vitrectomy or to treat the edge of a retinectomy, photocoagulating can be employed. Various authors have described techniques for endophotocoagulation (41–45). Endophotocoagulation can be performed either with an illuminated endolaser or with an endolaser probe that requires separate endoillumination from a fiberoptic light source. In the cases of diabetic vitrectomy, an endolaser is introduced through one sclerotomy and an endoilluminator

through the other. We have been successful in achieving excellent visibility for panretinal endophotocoagulation treatment through the panoramic viewing system. The endoillumination from the bullet light source provides a field of light of excellent intensity, coupled with a panoramic view for panretinal laser placement.

A similar approach can be utilized by treating around retinal breaks, retinotomy sites, and at the edge of the retinectomy site. The laser trigger is controlled by a foot pedal while the power and duration can be adjusted by the circulating technicians. The surgeon can also control the intensity of the burn and its size, usually varying between 500 to 800 μm, by the distance he or she keeps the endolaser probe laser during activation. We have been successful in utilizing both the argon and the diode system for endophotocoagulation. A filter system incorporated into the operating room microscope allows for safety to the surgeon during endolaser treatment (45). The assistant must wear protective goggles to achieve similar protection. The filter remains in position throughout endophotocoagulation. The panoramic viewing system allows us to reach the retinal periphery during treatment. Surgeons who do not have access to panoramic viewing systems may use the coaxial illumination of the operating room microscope or the illuminated endolaser probe with simultaneous scleral depression to reach the retinal periphery.

Some surgeons prefer using indirect laser ophthalmoscopy to treat anterior pathology. Simultaneous scleral depression with indirect laser application can be performed. A protective filter for the surgeon is built within the indirect ophthalmoscope. However, all operating room personnel must wear protective goggles. Though equally as effective, focal laser treatment around an isolated break, retinotomy, or along a retinectomy edge is difficult, especially after fluid–air exchange when the view can be limited. Thus, the indirect laser delivery system is best for anterior pathology and scatter laser treatment. Rarely, corneal or lens injury occurs while utilizing this system.

Now that the principles of technique and instrumentation necessary for vitrectomy have been introduced, we present our surgical technique for a basic three-port pars plana vitrectomy.

BASIC VITRECTOMY

It is important to establish a systematic approach in managing patients with vitreoretinal disorders. All patients must have a complete history and ophthalmic examination performed. Careful drawings of the anatomy and preoperative photographs where necessary should be obtained. A preoperative surgical plan should be established. An assessment of whether a vitrectomy or combined scleral buckling with vitrectomy is appropriate should be performed. The risks, benefits, and alternatives should be reviewed with the patient. A discussion of general versus retrobulbar anesthesia should ensue. We perform the majority of our vitreoretinal procedures with retrobulbar anesthesia and use general anesthesia in children or in patients who cannot cooperate or have undergone multiple reoperations.

Vitrectomy is now employed for various types of vitreoretinal disorders. Cases ranging from macular holes, macular pucker, vitreous hemorrhage, to diabetic tractional retinal detachments and complicated retinal detachments with proliferative vitreoretinopathy are managed differently. Various instruments and methods of tamponade can be employed depending on the severity of the differing disorders. However, the basic concepts of vitreous surgery are similar.

The pupil is dilated preoperatively. Intravenous sedation by the anesthesiologist is initiated and then a retrobulbar block is given. Various lid blocks such as the Van Lint, modified Van Lint, O'Brien, and Nadbath blocks can be given. The area is prepared with povidone-iodine (Betadine) solution. A protective shield is placed over the fellow eye. When general anesthesia is used, we also pack the nose with gauze to prevent nasal secretions from coming into the surgical field. The surgical field is also composed of wrist rests, which allow for an excellent trough to be created so that all fluids can be safely confined and suctioned by the aspirating drain. Various types of lid speculums that are available can be effective in maintaining adequate exposure. We use the heavy wire lid speculum in the majority of our vitreoretinal procedures.

The operating microscope, which is already draped, is then placed in position. The surgeon and assistant adjust their oculars. The surgeon via foot pedal control is able to raise and lower the microscope to achieve excellent focus and centration. In procedures combining scleral buckling with pars plana vitrectomy, a 360-degree circumferential conjunctival peritomy is performed with the 0.12 forceps and Westcott scissors. Care is taken to stay close to the limbus without creating buttonholes in the conjunctiva. Complete identification and removal of Tenon's layer is performed. Relaxing radial conjunctival incisions are created at the 3- and 9-o'clock positions. If a prior functioning bleb is present, the conjunctival peritomy can extend posteriorly behind the bleb. When vitrectomy alone is to be performed, a conjunctival peritomy involving a radial temporal incision is performed, extending circumferentially adjacent to the limbus inferiorly and superiorly. Thereafter, a nasal conjunctival peritomy, starting radially first and extending circumferentially along the limbus and superiorly, is created. All Tenon's layers are removed, especially in the areas where there will be placement of the infusion line and sclerotomies.

Surface wet field cautery is performed with the diathermy tip while the assistant irrigates the ocular surface. We have been cauterizing inferotemporally, superotemporally, and superonasally in our patients. In patients undergoing primary vitrectomy who are phakic, two double armed 6-0 polyglactin 910 sutures are placed in a mattress fashion 3.5 mm back from the limbus in the inferotemporal quadrant below the meridian of the lateral rectus muscle. The needles are cut and three throws are placed to ensure that the mattress suture will not come undone during vitrectomy. A 4-mm infusion line connected to the vitrectomy instrumentation and bottle of balanced salt solution is then turned on to assess for adequate flow and to evacuate any air bubbles that may have been introduced at the time of setup. The myringotomy blade is utilized to create a circumferential sclerotomy between the mattress sutures inferotemporally 3.5 mm from the limbus. The blade tip is viewed to ensure that one has adequately penetrated into the vitreous cavity. When there is a choroidal detachment, anterior proliferative vitreoretinopathy, or other conditions that may limit viewing of the infusion cannula, a 6-mm infusion cannula can be placed. However, in the majority of patients, a 4-mm infusion cannula is placed. With the assistant holding the infusion cannula flat, the surgeon ties the 6-0 polyglactin 910 suture with a loop knot to secure the infusion cannula. The assistant must take care not to tilt the infusion cannula, thereby avoiding iatrogenic lens injury. After the infusion cannula is secured, it is important to ensure that its tip is easily viewed in the posterior chamber. This can be confirmed by using a light pipe in the fellow hand to view the infusion cannula. The infusion line is only turned on if the cannula is well viewed. Premature turning on of the infusion cannula can result in infusion into the suprachoroidal space. Also in eyes with anterior proliferative vitreoretinopathy with anterior retinal detachment, the infusion line can be accidentally placed subretinally and can transfix the retina. If the infusion line is not viewed, it should not be turned on and then assessment of why it is not viewed should be performed.

In eyes with choroidal detachments limiting view of the infusion line, an anterior-chamber infusion line with a 25-gauge butterfly needle can be placed to provide irrigation and chamber maintenance until a posterior-chamber infusion line can be safely placed and adequately viewed. Only then is it safe to turn on the posterior infusion line.

To prevent transfixing the retina or placing the infusion line subretinally in patients with anterior proliferative retinopathy and retinal detachment, we have been placing the sclerotomies 1.5 to 2.0 mm posterior to the limbus in a meridian where there is no anterior proliferative vitreoretinopathy (46–48). In these cases, use of a larger infusion cannula (e.g., 6 mm) is advised. Removal of the peripheral lens capsule may also be warranted, to adequately view the infusion line and prevent further incorporation of the capsule into the anterior tractional membranes (38).

When choroidal detachment occurs from a suprachoroidal placement of the infusion line, the irrigation must be stopped. A separate sclerotomy for the infusion line must be created in a quadrant where there is no choroidal detachment. Only after ensuring that this second infusion cannula is already visible should the infusion be turned on. The first infusion line in the suprachoroidal space should then be removed. The choroidal detachment may lessen or disappear at the time of removal and also when the second properly placed infusion line is turned on.

In the majority of patients, the infusion line is well viewed and is turned on. Steri-Strips are placed to secure the tubing leading to the infusion line. Attention is given to the superonasal quadrant where the myringotomy blade is used to create a circumferential sclerotomy 4.0 mm back from the limbus. One must ensure that the myringotomy blade is clearly viewed. The endoilluminator is placed in the superonasal sclerotomy. The myringotomy blade is used to create circumferential superotemporal sclerotomy 4.0 mm back, through which a vitreous cutter is introduced. In general, the sclerotomies are placed about 160 to 170 degrees apart, to achieve adequate bimanual maneuverability during surgery.

During phakic vitrectomy, care is taken not to cross or to come anteriorly, to avoid iatrogenic lens trauma. Vitrectomy is conducted by illuminating the vitreous with the endoilluminator and then cutting along the edge of the vitreous gel. Care is taken not to perform sudden movements away from the retina, to avoid iatrogenic breaks. A central core vitrectomy in addition to peripheral vitrectomy is performed. The peripheral vitreous gel is removed as safely as possible without compromising the lens or periphery of the retina.

Next, the posterior hyaloid is identified and it is determined whether it is separated or not. Usually in eyes with vitreous hemorrhage and rhegmatogenous retinal detachments, the posterior hyaloid is separated. In these cases the posterior hyaloid is then removed. When hemorrhage is lying on the anterior surface of the retina, it is best to create a small opening in the posterior hyaloid and then with either a flute needle or silicone-tip cannula, the blood is aspirated. If one enters the posterior hyaloid prematurely and creates a large opening, the hemorrhage may become dispersed and limit the surgeon's view.

In the setting of rhegmatogenous retinal detachments, careful, low-suction high-cutting-speed vitrectomy is performed, especially when the retina is mobile. Iatrogenic breaks can be common in these situations if caution is not exercised. In diabetic tractional retinal detachments, the vitreous may serve as a third arm to allow for delamination via an en bloc technique. Another approach is to remove the fibrovascular tissue with a tissue manipulator and membrane peeler cutter by performing delamination.

If the posterior hyaloid is not separated, we have used a vitreous cutter set at about 300 mm Hg of aspiration. The cutter is placed close to the optic nerve and the posterior hyaloid is engaged. With gentle tangential movement and slight posterior movement, the posterior hyaloid is separated. Care is taken not to pull rapidly or immediately anteriorly or posteriorly, to prevent iatrogenic breaks. The silicone-tip cannula can be utilized to ensure that the posterior-chamber hyaloid has been completely removed, and if not, it can also be utilized to separate the posterior hyaloid. For

example, in patients with stage 3 macular holes, we perform an initial vitrectomy to create a pocket for our surgical instruments to reach posteriorly. Thereafter, we separate the posterior hyaloid. Then, we complete our core and peripheral vitrectomy. If one performs a core vitrectomy and then separates the posterior hyaloid, further vitrectomy to remove the posterior cortical vitreous will need to be performed.

After the posterior hyaloid is separated and a complete vitrectomy is performed, we close the sclerotomies with scleral plugs and examine the retinal periphery with scleral depression and indirect ophthalmoscopy. It is important to examine the entire retinal periphery, as iatrogenic breaks can be associated with separation of the posterior hyaloid. Careful attention should be given to the meridians of the sclerotomies, as breaks posterior to the site of the sclerotomies are most common. This may be related to traction induced by passing instruments in and out of the sclerotomies. If retinal breaks are noted, cryotherapy or laser photocoagulation can be used. After vitrectomy, gas tamponade is also necessary in these patients. If an associated retinal detachment is present, placement of a scleral buckle may also be indicated.

The majority of vitreoretinal surgery patients require gas tamponade, which is discussed later. However, in the majority of patients who do not have retinal breaks, vitrectomy without fluid-air exchange or gas tamponade is commonly performed. In such or similar cases, one may close the sclerotomies directly after vitrectomy. The sclerotomies may be closed either with 7-0 polyglycolic acid (Dexon) or polyglactin 910 suture in a figure-eight pattern. It is important to take partial-thickness scleral bites. If a deep bite is performed, pigment along the suture may be noted. If this occurs, it is prudent to remove the suture and place a new partial-thickness suture. We have been closing the nasal sclerotomy first, especially in eyes requiring gas tamponade. After closing the nasal sclerotomy, we close the temporal sclerotomy in similar fashion. If surface bleeding is encountered, cautery may be applied directly to the bleeding site. Care must be taken not to overcauterize the sclerotomy site, as scleral tissue can shrink, thereby affecting subsequent closure.

After the sclerotomy is closed, the 6-0 polyglactin suture anchoring the infusion cannula is loosened to allow the surgeon to manipulate the infusion cannula out while simultaneously tightening the 6-0 suture. This technique avoids possible hypotony from occurring from escape of the intraocular fluid or gas. The intraocular pressure may be checked afterward with the Schiøtz tonometer.

The conjunctiva is approximated with 7-0 polyglactin 910 suture either in an interrupted fashion or in a continuous pattern. If a scleral buckle is present, we close Tenon's layer with 7-0 polyglycolic acid sutures to the insertion muscles first, and then close the conjunctiva with 7-0 polyglactin 910. Attention must be given to careful conjunctival closure, as inadequate closure may result in the sclerotomies being exposed postoperatively. If a scleral buckle is present, the buckle may become exposed or infected, requiring possible removal. Other complications associated with scleral conjunctival closure are inclusion cysts and granulation tissue. It is important not to imbricate the epithelial surfaces against one another. Also care must be taken not to incorporate the plica semilunaris into the conjunctival closure.

After conjunctival closure, we inject gentamicin and dexamethasone subconjunctivally. Atropine ointment, a patch, and a metal shield are placed. Postoperative positioning is instituted immediately if necessary and the patient is taken to the recovery room.

Vitrectomy in phakic and pseudophakic patients varies somewhat. It is important to determine the type of IOL and whether the posterior capsule is open or not. Condensations on the IOL during fluid-air exchange or air–silicone oil exchange are more common with silicone IOLs. A posterior capsulotomy may also allow for condensation on the IOL. Thus, if the surgical goal can be achieved with adequate visualization, we do not recommend performing a primary surgical capsulectomy.

Placing the infusion line in pseudophakic or aphakic patients requires the surgeon to measure 3 mm posterior to the limbus where the myringotomy blade can be used to enter. Sclerotomies superonasally and superotemporally can also be placed 3 mm posterior to the limbus. The remainder of the vitrectomy can be performed in a similar manner to that described earlier. Care must be taken not to come too anteriorly in patients in whom an intact posterior capsule is present. A small air bubble can be placed during vitrectomy to delineate the margins of the posterior capsule, to avoid iatrogenic capsular trauma. In the majority of patients, the IOLs are stable and will not dislocate or decenter during vitrectomy. Only in recently operated patients after cataract surgery is it best to be careful to avoid dislocating or decentering the IOL.

Many vitreoretinal procedures are reoperations. Whether they are expected reoperations such as silicone-oil removal or reoperations because of recurrent retinal detachment with proliferative vitreoretinopathy, the surgeon must take care in evaluating the surface sclera and assessing the location of the prior sclerotomy sites. Reoperation through prior sclerotomy sites risks not only leakage from the sclerotomy site during surgery but also inadequate closure of the sclerotomy sites. Thus, in reoperations we make sclerotomies radial and anterior to the previous sclerotomy sites. This technique provides added protection from the joining and enlarging and leaking of sclerotomy sites during surgery. The closure of the sclerotomy sites is performed utilizing the same technique as described previously.

FLUID-AIR EXCHANGE

When fluid-air exchange is anticipated, both the surgeon and the operating staff must establish the surgical plans and goals. The air allows tamponade of either retinal breaks or macular holes or other vitreoretinal pathology. An automated pump or injection of air can be utilized (49–51). The air is infused through the infusion cannula at a pressure of 30 mm Hg while either the silicone-tipped cannula or flute needle can be employed to aspirate the intraocular fluid. The view during fluid-air exchange can deteriorate and requires using either the panoramic viewing system or a biconcave lens of −100 diopters (50). With the latter lens, the image is minified and the view is not as wide as with the panoramic viewing system. In aphakic patients, no lens is necessary for viewing as the air bubble enters the anterior chamber, providing the refractive power necessary for adequate viewing. However, long-term contact with air against the corneal endothelium can cause corneal striae and limit a surgeon's view. To improve viewing, one can coat the corneal endothelium with sodium hyaluronate (49).

Fluid-air exchange in pseudophakic patients with intact posterior capsules may result in adequate viewing. However, if the posterior capsule is open, condensations can form during fluid-air exchange, limiting a surgeon's view. A temporary solution is to use a silicone-tipped cannula to gently brush the back surface of the IOL to remove the condensations. Invariably, however, condensations re-form, limiting the view. Thus, the temporary solution is used when the fluid-air exchange is nearly completed and only minor steps need to be performed prior to completion of the surgery. When a longer viewing time is necessary to complete the procedures, sodium hyaluronate can be used to coat the back surface of the IOL to improve visualization. Excellent visualization can be achieved utilizing this technique, allowing drainage through either the macular hole or retinal break sites. If endophotocoagulation is to be applied at this time, the surgeon must be facile in doing so. If too much time is allowed to elapse, fluid may reaccumulate, making laser placement difficult.

AIR-GAS EXCHANGE

After the fluid-air exchange, the surgeon must determine whether gas tamponade is necessary (52,53). Two commonly used gases in vitreous surgery are sulfur hexafluoride and perfluoropropane. The surgeon must also discern what concentration of gas must be employed. If the patient is under general anesthesia, nitrous oxide must be turned off approximately 20 minutes prior to the exchange; otherwise, unwanted expansion of the gas can occur. The concentration of gas is withdrawn from the tank using filters and a three-way stopcock. Initial samples of gas are flushed out of the 60-mL syringe. After several flushes, a sample of gas is drawn into the 60-mL syringe. Depending on the concentration desired, the remainder of the syringe is filled with air through a filter. Attention is directed toward the surgical field. We first close the nasal sclerotomy and place the closing suture on the temporal sclerotomy. Thereafter, the air infusion line is clamped and the 60-mL syringe with the desired concentration of gas for tamponade is connected directly to it. Slow injection of the gas with simultaneous expression of air through the temporal sclerotomy site is performed. We have been flushing with up to 50 mL of gas mixture prior to closing the temporal sclerotomy site. A 35-mL flush would be adequate. Thereafter, the intraocular pressures are evaluated and if soft, more gas can be injected. The infusion line is removed and the sclerotomy is closed with the preplaced mattress 6-0 polyglactin 910 suture. If the eye becomes soft as the gas is expressed out of the sclerotomy site, a 30-gauge needle can be placed on the 60-mL syringe and gas injected through the pars plana to achieve adequate intraocular pressure. We most commonly use a nonexpansile concentration of gas to achieve tamponade. The patient is positioned postoperatively, depending on the locations of the vitreoretinal pathology requiring tamponade.

SILICONE-OIL TAMPONADE

For longer tamponade, silicone oil has been advocated (54–61). More commonly, in the United States silicone oil is used for complicated retinal detachments and for detachments with multiple breaks in necrotic retina as in cytomegalovirus (CMV) retinitis or acute retinal necrosis. Silicone oil is lighter than water and thus can support superior retinal pathology much better than inferior pathology. Use of silicone oil can result in complications such as cataract formation, glaucoma, and corneal toxicity (62–64). Thus, the surgeon and patient must discuss the risks and benefits of utilizing silicone oil, including that additional surgery will be necessary to remove the oil. The advantages of longer-term tamponade, allowing for air travel and obviating the need for a prone position except during the first 12 hours, are also discussed. However, patients must understand that they cannot lie on their back while silicone oil is in the eye. If they do, the oil will come forward, touching the lens or cornea, resulting in cataract development and corneal toxicity.

We commonly perform air–silicone oil exchange. The fluid-air exchange allows us to visualize whether further traction is present. If excessive traction is still present, subretinal air migration will occur. In these cases, further membrane peeling or possible relaxing retinectomies may be necessary to reattach the retina. Meticulous control of intraocular bleeding is advised, as hemorrhage under silicone oil can result in reproliferation. Prior to the fluid-air exchange, we perform an inferior peripheral iridectomy in aphakic and pseudophakic patients with an open posterior capsule. If the patient is pseudophakic with a closed posterior capsule, consideration for an inferior iridectomy can be given, as silicone oil can still migrate into the anterior chamber through areas where there is loss of zonular integrity. The inferior iridectomy allows for aqueous humor to pass underneath the silicone oil into the anterior chamber (65,66).

AIR–SILICONE OIL EXCHANGE

Our technique for silicone-oil injection utilizes a silicone-oil pump controlled by a foot pedal with both vacuum and aspiration modes. Similarly a short infusion tube can be utilized to inject silicone oil by hand (58). After fluid-air exchange and laser photocoagulation where necessary, we inject silicone oil through a superior sclerotomy. The air pressure is turned down as the silicone oil increases. The amount of oil injected is considered adequate when the oil interphase is posterior to the iris plane in aphakic eyes or the oil reaches the posterior lens or IOL surface. In addition, as the infusion air pressure is turned off during silicone-oil injection, the surgeon may also see oil rise up the infusion line tubing, signaling adequate filling. The oil infusion syringe is withdrawn and the sclerotomies are closed. The air infusion line is also withdrawn and closed with the preplaced 6-0 polyglactin 910 suture. Prior to closure of the sclerotomies, the intraocular pressure is measured; if it is low, further silicone oil can be injected and if it is high, silicone oil can be partially removed. Copious irrigation of the surface sclera, cornea, and conjunctiva is performed to remove any surface silicone oil.

INJECTION OF PERFLUOROCARBON LIQUIDS

Since the advent of vitreous surgery, newer instruments and methods of tamponade have been developed to improve current vitreoretinal techniques. Perfluorocarbon liquids have greatly aided vitreoretinal surgeons in managing various ocular disorders (67–71). Their heavier-than-water properties have allowed them to function as a tool for tamponade in many patients. Viewing through the liquids is also facilitated in many procedures.

The decision on when to utilize perfluorocarbon liquids must be made by surgeon. Once the decision to use perfluorocarbon liquids has been reached, the technical staff must coordinate and arrange for the necessary equipment. We have been using the panoramic viewing system, and the Chang cannula to inject the liquid perfluorocarbon while allowing simultaneous egress of balanced salt solution. The liquid perfluorocarbon bubble is initially injected over the optic nerve slowly so as to allow for the formation of one bubble. Care must be taken to inject slowly over larger breaks or tears, to avoid possible subretinal migration. Generally, this is not a problem as long as traction off the break or tear is relieved prior to injection.

We commonly fill the eye with perfluorocarbon, as in the case of retinal detachment, allowing egress of subretinal fluid through an anterior preexisting break. The perfluorocarbon liquids can also be used to partially fill the eye when lens fragments or IOLs need to be floated up (70,71). The added cushioning of the perfluorocarbon liquids not only protects the retina from iatrogenic trauma during lens fragmentation, but also can allow for complete reattachment of the coincident rhegmatogenously detached retina. Perfluorocarbon liquids are also excellent for unfolding giant tears. We have also utilized them to secure the posterior part of the retina so that either anterior-membrane peeling or vitrectomy can be performed in areas of detached retina. Once the perfluorocarbon liquid injection is completed, we commonly place laser directly to the vitreoretinal pathology or relaxing retinectomy sites. The view is superior to that with air and thus photocoagulation is easier to perform through perfluorocarbon liquids than through air.

If subsequent gas tamponade is necessary, we simultaneously aspirate perfluorocarbon liquids while sterile air is injected through the infusion line. Perfluorocarbon liquid aspiration can be performed with either the silicone-tipped cannula or the flute needle. It is important to try to remove all of the perfluorocarbon because long-term contact can result in corneal and retinal toxicity. In patients with giant retinal tears, care must be taken to dry the edge of the giant tear first during perfluorocarbon liquid–air exchange, to prevent slippage. When a scleral buckle is also going to be placed, we place the scleral buckle first, then perform vitrectomy and secure the retina with perfluorocarbon liquids, then tighten up the buckle, and finally perform endolaser photocoagulation followed by perfluorocarbon liquid–air exchange. If gas tamponade is necessary, an air-gas exchange can be performed as described previously.

PERFLUOROCARBON LIQUID–SILICONE OIL EXCHANGE

In some settings such as giant retinal tears of 270 degrees or more with continual slippage, as the surgeon goes from perfluorocarbon to air, a perfluorocarbon liquid–silicone oil exchange can be performed without first going to air. The technique utilizes the placement of the perfluorocarbon as already described. The exchange is performed as silicone oil is injected with an automated infusion pump while the perfluorocarbon liquid is simultaneously aspirated with the silicone-tipped cannula or the flute needle. It is important to aspirate the saline anterior to the perfluorocarbon first. When the silicone-oil bubble makes contact with the perfluorocarbon, the interface is visible so that the perfluorocarbon can be aspirated. Small bubbles of perfluorocarbon and small bubbles of air may limit adequate aspiration of all of the perfluorocarbon during silicone-oil injection. However, perfluorocarbon liquid bubbles will settle onto the surface of the retina, allowing easier recognition and removal. The silicone oil is injected and the adequate amount of fill is determined in a similar manner as described before.

REMOVAL OF SILICONE OIL

Silicone oil is effective in providing long-term tamponade and has been more popular in the European countries. Its use in the United States is still limited to complicated forms of retinal detachment and in rare instances when a patient cannot position for tamponade or needs to travel by air emergently. Silicone oil over a long term can result in complications such as corneal toxicity, cataract, and glaucoma. Thus after a period of adequate tamponade, vitreoretinal surgeons have been removing the oil. The risk-benefit ratio for removing the oil should be discussed with the patient. Although removing the oil may obviate any possible future complications, there is always a risk of recurrent retinal detachment after the oil is removed. Some authors (72) reported a risk of recurrent retinal detachment as high as 25%. Others were successful in maintaining retinal reattachment after silicone-oil removal (73). Some surgeons have left silicone oil for permanent tamponade in certain patients.

Removal of silicone oil involves placing an infusion cannula and then making a single, usually superotemporal sclerotomy. Either a lavage technique or active suction can be employed to effectively remove oil. The lavage technique involves making a superotemporal sclerotomy and leaving it open while balance salt saline solution is infused through the inferotemporal infusion line. This technique will allow the balanced salt solution to displace the silicone oil out of the superotemporal sclerotomy site. The globe can be manipulated so that adequate egress of silicone oil can be achieved. Sometimes, opening the sclerotomy with either the 0.12 or Calibri forceps allows for expedited silicone-oil removal. However, this technique lets silicone oil extrude and cover all external surfaces and instruments, making them difficult to work with. Copious irrigation with balanced salt solution can help clear these surfaces.

We have been utilizing the active suction technique, which obviates this problem. A standard inferotemporal infusion cannula is placed and a superotemporal sclerotomy is created. The infusion cannula is turned on while active suction through an 18-gauge angiocath connected to a syringe is employed. Care must be taken not to injure the lens or other internal structures during oil removal, as direct visualization of the needle tip is sometimes limited. In the majority of such cases, the patients are aphakic and the needle tip is well viewed during removal. As the oil bubble becomes smaller, the eye may be rotated, allowing the silicone oil to float toward the tip of the needle. At the end of oil removal, care must be taken not to continue active suction because sudden hypotony can occur. Sometimes the remainder of minimal residual silicone oil can be removed by the lavage technique, as described earlier.

Small bubbles of silicone oil that become trapped in the anterior chamber in aphakic patients can be removed with the flute needle. However, in phakic or pseudophakic patients with an intact capsule but zonular weakness that allowed silicone oil to migrate into the anterior chamber, removal can be more difficult. In such or similar patients, an anterior-chamber paracentesis with a super-sharp blade can be created. Simultaneous anterior-chamber infusion of balanced salt solution through another paracentesis site with a 30-gauge needle while keeping posterior pressure on the larger paracentesis site can allow for controlled egress of the anterior-chamber silicone oil. Afterward, the larger paracentesis site used for egress of silicone oil can be closed with 10-0 nylon. The anterior-chamber balanced salt solution infusion site utilizing the 30-gauge needle does not require suturing.

After the silicone oil is completely removed, the superotemporal sclerotomy is closed, the inferotemporal infusion cannula is turned off and removed, and the inferotemporal sclerotomy site is sutured with the preplaced 6-0 polyglactin 910 suture. We irrigate the ocular surfaces with balanced salt solution in order to completely remove any residual surface silicone oil. The conjunctiva is then sutured in the standard fashion with 7-0 polyglactin 910 as described before.

COMPLICATIONS

Any type of ophthalmic surgery involves risks of bleeding and infection. However, vitreous surgery usually involves certain common complications that are more specific (74).

Globe Perforation and Retrobulbar Hemorrhage

Complications arising from retrobulbar anesthesia resulting in globe perforation or retrobulbar hemorrhage cause significant vision loss. Care must be taken, especially in highly myopic eyes with encircling scleral buckles. We utilize a blunt or special 25-gauge needle to induce retrobulbar block. An inferotemporal site is selected and a needle is used to perforate the skin. Gentle horizontal manipulation can ensure that the globe has not been perforated. If the eye moves during this manipulation, the needle should be immediately withdrawn without injection of any anesthetic. When an adequate entry has been performed, we commonly aspirate to ensure that no vessel has been perforated. If blood is aspirated, no anesthetic is injected and the needle is withdrawn and external pressure tamponade is instituted. If subconjunctival hemorrhage or highly elevated intraocular pressure is noted during retrobulbar injection, no further anesthetic should be injected. The needle should be withdrawn and immediate pressure tamponade should be placed. The intraocular pressure should be measured and patency of the central retinal artery assessed by visualizing pulsations with the indirect ophthalmoscope. In the majority of patients, digital compression can result in limiting the pressure elevation and degree of retrobulbar hemorrhage. We also administer intravenous mannitol. If the central retinal artery is closed, a lateral canthotomy can be performed. The goal of such a procedure is to reduce the intraocular pressure so that the central retinal artery remains patent.

If a globe perforation is suspected during retrobulbar injection, from either immediate hypotony or movement of the globe during injection, immediate indirect ophthalmoscopy should be performed. Choroidal, intraretinal, or vitreous hemorrhage may be seen. A retinal tear can sometimes be obscured by this hemorrhage. Small tears can be managed with either cryotherapy or indirect laser photocoagulation. However, larger tears with associated retinal detachment may need vitreous surgery. If a severe vitreous hemorrhage forms and obscures the view, an immediate pars plana vitrectomy to clear the hemorrhage and treat possible retinal tears needs to be instituted.

Surgical Sclerotomy Complications

Complications of sclerotomy sites can occur. Care must be taken to ensure that the sclera will allow for adequate closure, especially with reoperations. During placement of the infusion line, the cannula must be viewed prior to turning on the infusion or a choroidal detachment can occur. After the sclerotomy is created, it is important to excise any prolapsed vitreous with either the vitreous cutter or Westcott scissors. The surgeon must be careful not to pull on the prolapsed vitreous, which could result in iatrogenic retinal breaks. We turn off the infusion line while the sclerotomy site is unprotected, with either an instrument or a plug. This decreases the likelihood of incarcerating a detached retina or of prolapsing vitreous. It is important to view the retinal periphery after vitrectomy to ensure that no iatrogenic breaks, especially in the areas of the sclerotomy sites, have occurred. We commonly perform this step prior to the fluid-air exchange while the view is good. If iatrogenic breaks are encountered, either cryotherapy or indirect laser photocoagulation combined with possible gas tamponade can be employed. Fibrous ingrowth through sclerotomy sites can occur postoperatively (75,76). Resulting traction can cause recurrent vitreous hemorrhage and possible retinal detachment. In contrast, diabetic patients can also have recurrent vitreous hemorrhages from fibrovascular proliferation that involves the peripheral retina and anterior hyaloid, resulting in retinal detachment and hypotony (77,78). Thus, one must differentiate anterior hyaloidal fibrovascular proliferation from fibrous ingrowth from sclerotomy sites resulting in recurrent vitreous hemorrhage.

Meticulous closure of the sclerotomy site also obviates any complications such as leakage. If the sclera is severely damaged from reoperations, thereby limiting adequate closure, a scleral patch graft can be employed.

Vitrectomy Complications

Complications during pars plana vitrectomy can occur (74). Tugging on the vitreous base during the vitrectomy or iatrogenic trauma to the retina while working through a poor view secondary to media opacity can result in such an occurrence. These iatrogenic breaks may commonly occur along the vitreous base and posterior to the sclerotomy sites either during vitrectomy or while introducing various surgical instruments through the sclerotomy (79,80). Care must be taken not to rapidly move the vitreous cutter. The presented vitreous should be cut and then aspirated. Iatrogenic breaks in highly mobile detached retina can also be avoided by increasing the cutting speed and decreasing the aspiration. Sometimes perfluorocarbon liquids can stabilize the posterior retina while the anterior vitreous is safely removed. Retinal tears can be treated with either cryotherapy or laser photocoagulation and possible gas tamponade. It is important, however, to recognize and manage these breaks intraoperatively.

Lens trauma during a pars plana vitrectomy can occur, especially during anterior or peripheral vitreous removal. Combined scleral depression along with vitrectomy can also result in iatrogenic lenticular trauma. Only peripheral vitreous gel that can be safely removed is excised. In phakic patients, it is important not to cross instruments. Instead, the instruments should be removed and switched in order to remove the vitreous in the opposite quadrant.

Intraoperative lens opacities, not resulting from direct iatrogenic trauma, can also occur. In diabetic patients, we add 3 mL of 50% dextrose irrigating balanced salt solution to prevent intraoperative lenticular opacities (16). Diabetic patients may also have continued progression of their lenticular opacity, even postoperatively. Nondiabetic patients can also develop a cataract after vitrectomy (81). Some of these changes can be associated with continuous air or gas contact against the posterior lens. Thus, a proficient technique of minimizing an intraoperative supine position may decrease the development of a cataract. The use of perfluorocarbon liquids allows photocoagulation to be placed proficiently, thereby minimizing the time air is in contact with the posterior lens surface. Prone positioning postoperatively is instituted for tamponade and may minimize direct lenticular contact.

If, however, significant lenticular opacity does develop and limits the view to complete a surgeon's objective, a lensectomy needs to be performed. In certain settings such as some giant retinal tears or proliferating vitreoretinopathy, clear lens removal may also be necessary to achieve the surgical goal.

Finally, when the view is not clear, the surgeon must determine the cause. A common occurrence is epithelial corneal edema during vitrectomy. The corneal epithelial edema can be lessened by directly rolling a wet cotton tip on the corneal surface. If the edema persists, the epithelium can be scraped gently with a blade. Care must be taken to remove all of the epithelium off the surgical field. Corneal edema can also occur, especially in aphakic eyes, with air or gas contact against the endothelium. In these cases, visualization can be improved by using sodium hyaluronate to coat the endothelium (49).

Intraocular Hemorrhage

Intraocular hemorrhage can be mild or severe and can sometimes result in a poor view, limiting surgical repair. Spontaneous hyphema from either iris or angle neovascularization or hypotony can also limit a surgeon's view. Diathermy can be readily applied at the bleeding sites. In cases of spontaneous hypotony in phakic patients with a resulting mild hyphema, we have also been successful in irrigating the anterior chamber with a 30-gauge needle and balanced salt solution. This technique greatly clears the central hemorrhage, allowing adequate visualization.

Intraoperative vitreous hemorrhage occurs more commonly while performing relaxing retinectomies and while dissecting fibrovascular tissue in diabetic patients (80). Diathermy to prominent vessels in the fibrovascular tissue or to the edges of the retinectomy site prior to dissection can limit intraoperative hemorrhage. If intraoperative hemorrhage is noted, the intraocular pressure can be elevated by raising the infusion bottle. Sometimes thrombin can be added to the infusion bottle to limit bleeding (82,83). It is important to meticulously remove all hemorrhages, especially in eyes where silicone oil is employed. Hemorrhage under oil can lead to membrane reproliferation.

However, even with meticulous control of intraoperative hemorrhage, postoperative bleeding is relatively common after diabetic vitrectomy (84). Usually the hemorrhage is mild and clears in several weeks. If the hemorrhage is dense, an ultrasound examination should be performed to ensure that a concurrent retinal detachment is not also present.

The hemorrhage usually clears more rapidly after vitrectomy and thus fluid-gas exchange or repeat vitrectomy is not necessary. However, if a retinal detachment is present, or the patient is monocular, or has bilateral vitreous hemorrhage, or has iris neovascularization requiring panretinal photocoagulation, fluid-air or gas exchange can be performed. In the majority of our patients, we have not found this to be necessary.

Elevated Intraocular Pressure

Complications from elevated intraocular pressure are routinely encountered postoperatively. The majority of these complications are mild and can be managed with pressure-lowering medications.

Postoperative inflammation can also result in elevated intraocular pressure. Aggressive use of topical steroids and close follow-up are instituted. A postoperative hyphema may also result in fibrin formation and elevated intraocular pressure, requiring frequent administration of topical steroids. In some patients, pupillary block can occur from either choroidal effusions or closure of the inferior iridectomy by fibrin in patients with silicone oil. We have been successful in lysing fibrin by injecting tissue plasminogen activator, 3 μg/0.1 mL of balanced salt solution, into the anterior chamber. We have not been utilizing this technique in patients with iris neovascularization, diabetic patients, or patients who have had a retinectomy. We generally wait at least 7 days before injecting tissue plasminogen activator in patients with relaxing retinectomies, to prevent any bleeding from the edge of the retinectomy sites. If the pressure is still elevated, an anterior-chamber paracentesis can be performed.

Gas tamponade can also result in elevated intraocular pressure. Care must be taken to ensure that the correct concentration of gas is injected for tamponade. Also nitrous oxide must be turned off prior to gas tamponade. Postoperatively, the surgeon must judge the percent gas fill. If the intraocular pressure is significantly elevated and the gas fill is high, pars plana tap can be performed to remove a portion of the gas.

Elevated intraocular pressure 4 to 8 weeks after surgery can be related either to a steroid response or to recurrent vitreous hemorrhage or dispersed vitreous hemorrhage with the blood cells obstructing trabecular meshwork (84). Steroid responders can be managed by tapering the topical steroids. Lavage of the vitreous cavity can be performed in patients with persistently elevated intraocular pressure from blood cells obstructing the trabecular meshwork. Close follow-up with repeated intraocular pressure checks should be performed.

Endophthalmitis

Postoperative infection resulting in endophthalmitis can result in significant visual loss. Postoperative pain warrants immediate examination by the surgeon. Sometimes it is difficult to discern whether the patient has postoperative inflammation versus early endophthalmitis. If a hypopyon is present, the diagnosis can be more readily apparent.

Though endophthalmitis after pars plana vitrectomy is rare, it has occurred (85,86). In such or similar patients, immediate vitreous and anterior-chamber tap should be performed and intravitreal antibiotics injected. The response to the intravitreal antibiotics should be followed closely. Sometimes a repeat tap and injection of intravitreal antibiotics may need to be performed.

Retinal Detachment

Retinal detachment may occur either from an iatrogenic break occurring during surgery or from recurrent proliferative membranes forming after surgery. Careful examination of the retinal periphery with treatment of any intraoperative iatrogenic retinal breaks may circumvent the development of postoperative retinal detachment.

However, the most common cause of failure of retinal detachment after vitreoretinal surgery is the occurrence of proliferative vitreoretinopathy (46–48). This requires extensive membrane dissection, scleral buckling, and possibly relaxing retinectomies to achieve retinal reattachment. Many of these patients also require a longer-term tamponade with silicone oil. Management requires identifying the anatomic cause of recurrent retinal detachment and establishing a surgical plan to achieve retinal reattachment.

REFERENCES

1. Kasner D. Vitrectomy: a new approach to the management of vitreous. *Highlights Ophthalmol* 1969;11:304.
2. Kasner D, Miller GR, Taylor WH, et al. Surgical treatment of amyloidosis of the vitreous. *Trans Am Acad Ophthalmol Otolaryngol* 1968;72:410.
3. Machemer R, Buettner H, Norton EWD, Parel JM. Vitrectomy: a pars plana approach. *Trans Am Acad Ophthalmol Otolaryngol* 1971;75:813.
4. Machemer R. A new concept for vitreous surgery: two instrument techniques in pars plana vitrectomy. *Arch Ophthalmol* 1974;92:407.
5. Machemer R, Parel JM, Buettner H. A new concept for vitreous surgery: instrumentation. *Am J Ophthalmol* 1972;73:1.
6. Machemer R. *Vitrectomy: a pars plana approach.* New York: Grune & Stratton, 1975.
7. Parel JM, Machemer R, Aumayr W. A new concept for vitreous surgery: an automated operating microscope. *Am J Ophthalmol* 1974;77:161.
8. Charles S, McCarthy C, Eichenbaum D. A chin-operated switch for motorized three-axis microscopic movement. *Am J Ophthalmol* 1975;80:150.
9. Meyers SM, Bonner RF, Leighton SB. Combined illumination-irrigation 20-gauge probes for vitrectomy. *Arch Ophthalmol* 1982;100:622.
10. May DR, Dignam BJ. A 19-gauge illuminating infusion probe. *Arch Ophthalmol* 1983;101:1288.
11. Coleman DJ, Orcutt D. A lighted irrigator for vitrectomy. *Am J Ophthalmol* 1983;95:565. Letter.
12. Zinn KM, Grinblat A, Katzin HM, et al. A new endoillumination infusion cannula for pars plana vitrectomy. *Ophthalmic Surg* 1980;11:850.
13. Edelhauser HF, VanHorn DL, Hyndiuk RA, Schultz RO. Intraocular irrigating solutions. Their effect on the corneal endothelium. *Arch Ophthalmol* 1975;93:648.
14. Zinn KM, Grinblat A, Katzin HM, et al. An improved endoillumination probe for pars plana vitrectomy. *Ophthalmic Surg* 1980;11:698.
15. Hilton GF. A sutureless self-retaining infusion cannula for pars plana vitrectomy. *Am J Ophthalmol* 1985;99:612.
16. Haimann MH, Abrams GW. Prevention of lens pacification during diabetic vitrectomy. *Ophthalmology* 1984;91:116.
17. Parel JM, Machemer R. Steam-sterilizable fundus contact lenses. *Arch Ophthalmol* 1988;99:151.
18. Huamonte FU, Liang JC. Lens holder and modified contact lens for pars plana vitrectomy. *Arch Ophthalmol* 1981;99:154.
19. Schirmer KE, Kloeti R. Contact lenses for fundus examination and vitreous surgery with focal illumination. *Can J Ophthalmol* 1973;8:416.
20. Stenkula S. A new type of contact lens for vitrectomy. *Am J Ophthalmol* 1979;87:575.
21. Tolentino FI, Freeman HM. A new lens for closed pars plana vitrectomy. *Arch Ophthalmol* 1979;97:2197.
22. Sebestyen JG. Biconcave contact lens for vitreous surgery. *Am J Ophthalmol* 1979;87:719.
23. De Juan E. Landers MB III, Hickingbotham D. An improved contact-lens holder for vitreous surgery. *Am J Ophthalmol* 1985;99:213.
24. Federman JL, Decker WL, Grabowski WM. Coverslip lens. *Am J Ophthalmol* 1983;95:848.
25. Landers MB III, Stefansson E, Wolbarsht ML. The optics of vitreous surgery. *Am J Ophthalmol* 1981;991:611.
26. Escoffery RF, Grand MG. A flute syringe for vitreous surgery. *Arch Ophthalmol* 1980;98:2059.
27. Zivojnovic R, Vijfvinkel GJ. A modified flute needle. *Am J Ophthalmol* 1983;96:548.
28. Hutton WL. Vitreous foreign body forceps. *Am J Ophthalmol* 1977;84:430.
29. Hickingbotham D, Parel JM, Machemer R. Diamond-coated all-purpose foreign-body forceps. *Am J Ophthalmol* 1981;91:267.
30. Charles S. Illuminated intraocular foreign-body forceps for vitreous surgery. *Arch Ophthalmol* 1981;99:1399.
31. Tate GW Jr, Hutton WL, Vaiser A, Snyder WB. A coaxial electrode for intraocular diathermy. *Am J Ophthalmol* 1975;79:691.
32. Schepens CL, Delori F, Rogers FJ, Constable IJ. Optimized underwater diathermy for vitreous surgery. *Ophthalmic Surg* 1975;6:82.
33. Parel JM, Machemer R, O'Grady GE, et al. Intraocular diathermy coagulation. *Graefes Arch Clin Exp Ophthalmol* 1983;221:31.
34. Shock JP. Phacofragmentation and irrigation of cataracts: a preliminary report. *Am J Ophthalmol* 1972;74:187.
35. Girard LJ. Lensectomy through the pars plana by ultrasonic fragmentation. *Ophthalmology* 1979;86:1985.
36. Girard LJ. Pars plana lensectomy by ultrasonic fragmentation. Results of a retrospective study. *Ophthalmology* 1981;88:434.

37. Benson WE, Blankenship GW, Machemer R. Pars plana lens removal with vitrectomy. *Am J Ophthalmol* 1977;84:150.

38. Lewis H, Aaberg TM, Abrams GW, et al. Management of the lens capsule during pars plana lensectomy. *Am J Ophthalmol* 1987;103:109.

39. Lewis H, Blumenkranz JS, Chang S. Treatment of dislocated crystalline lens and retinal detachment with perfluorocarbon liquids. *Retina* 1992;12:299.

40. Hutton WL, Snyder WD, Vaiser A. Management of surgically dislocated intravitreal lens fragments by pars plana vitrectomy. *Ophthalmology* 1978;85:173.

41. Charles S. Endophotocoagulation. *Retina* 1981;1:117.

42. Fleishman JA, Swartz M, Dixon JA. Argon laser endophotocoagulation. An intraoperative trans-pars plana technique. *Arch Ophthalmol* 1981;99:1610.

43. Landers MB III, Trese MT, Stefansson E, Bessler M. Argon laser intraocular photocoagulation. *Ophthalmology* 1982;89:785.

44. Peyman GA, Salzano TC, Green JL Jr. Argon endolaser. *Arch Ophthalmol* 1981;99:2037.

45. Carroll CP, Peyman GA. A microscope filter for endophotocoagulation. *Arch Ophthalmol* 1981;99:327.

46. Lewis H, Aaberg TM. Anterior proliferative vitreoretinopathy. *Am J Ophthalmol* 1988;105:277.

47. Lewis H, Aaberg TM. Causes of failure after repeat vitreoretinal surgery for severe proliferative vitreoretinopathy. *Am J Ophthalmol* 1991;111:15.

48. Lewis H, Aaberg TM, Abrams GW. Causes of failure after initial vitreoretinal surgery for severe proliferative and vitreoretinopathy. *Am J Ophthalmol* 1991;111:8.

49. Landers MB III. Sodium hyaluronate as an aid to internal fluid-gas exchange. *Am J Ophthalmol* 1982;94:557.

50. Landers AM. Pars plana vitrectomy techniques: air-fluid exchange in the phakic eye. *Ocular Ther Surg* 1982;1:56.

51. Stern WH, Blumenkranz MS. Fluid-gas exchange after vitrectomy. *Am J Ophthalmol* 1983;96:400.

52. Norton EWD. Intraocular gas in the management of selected retinal detachments. *Trans Am Acad Ophthalmol Otolaryngol* 1973;77:85.

53. Abrams GW, Edelhauser HF, Aaberg TM, Hamilton LH. Dynamics of intravitreal sulfur hexafluoride gas. *Invest Ophthalmol* 1974;13:863.

54. Peterson J. The physical and surgical aspects of silicone oil in the vitreous cavity. *Graefes Arch Clin Exp Ophthalmol* 1987;225:452.

55. Cibis PA. Vitreous transfer and silicone injections. *Trans Am Acad Ophthalmol Otolaryngol* 1964;68:983.

56. Scott J. A rationale for the use of liquid silicone. *Trans Ophthalmol Soc UK* 1977;97:235.

57. McCuen BW, De Juan E Jr, Machemer R. Silicone oil in vitreoretinal surgery. Part 1. Surgical techniques. *Retina* 1985;5:189.

58. Scott J. The use of viscoelastic materials in the posterior segment. *Trans Ophthalmol Soc UK* 1983;103:280.

59. Fastenberg DM, Diddie KR, Delmage JM, Dorey K. Intraocular injection of silicone oil for experimental proliferative vitreoretinopathy. *Am J Ophthalmol* 1983;95:663.

60. Billington BM, Leaver PK. Vitrectomy and fluid/silicone oil exchange for giant retinal tears: results at 18 months. *Graefes Arch Clin Exp Ophthalmol* 1986;224:7.

61. Lambrou FH, Burke JM, Aaberg TM. Effect of silicone oil on experimental tractional retinal detachment. *Arch Ophthalmol* 1987;105:1269.

62. Casswell AG, Gregor ZJ. Silicone oil removal. The effect on the complications of silicone oil. *Br J Ophthalmol* 1987;71:893.

63. Pang MP, Peyman GA, Kao GW. Early anterior segment complications after silicone oil injection. *Can J Ophthalmol* 1986;21:271.

64. Casswell AG, Gregor ZJ. Silicone oil removal. Operative and postoperative complications. *Br J Ophthalmol* 1987;71:898.

65. Beekhuis WH, Ando F, Zivojnovic R, et al. Basal iridectomy at 6 o'clock in the aphakic eye treated with silicone oil: prevention of keratopathy and secondary glaucoma. *Br J Ophthalmol* 1987;71:197.

66. Ando F. Intraocular hypertension resulting from pupillary block by silicone oil. *Am J Ophthalmol* 1985;99:87.

67. Change S. Low viscosity liquid fluorochemicals in vitreous surgery. *Am J Ophthalmol* 1987;103:38.

68. Chang S, Sparrow JR, Iwamoto T, et al. Experimental studies of tolerance to intravitreal perfluoro-octane liquid. *Retina* 1991;11:367.

69. Chang S, Lincoff H, Zimmerman NJ, Fuchs W. Giant tears: surgical techniques and results using perfluorocarbon liquids. *Arch Ophthalmol* 1989;107:761.

70. Lewis H, Blumenkranz MS, Chang S. Treatment of dislocated crystalline lens and retinal detachment with perfluorocarbon liquids. *Retina* 1992;12:299.

71. Lewis H, Sanchez G. The use of perfluorocarbon liquids in the repositioning of posteriorly dislocated intraocular lenses. *Ophthalmology* 1993;100:1055.

72. Ando F, Miyake Y, Oshima K, Yamanaka A. Temporary use of intraocular silicone oil in the treatment of complicated retinal detachment. *Graefes Arch Clin Exp Ophthalmol* 1986;224:32.

73. Gonnvers M. Temporary silicone oil tamponade in the management of retinal detachment with proliferative vitreoretinopathy. *Am J Ophthalmol* 1985;100:239.

74. Lewis H, Lehmer JM. Complications of vitreoretinal surgery. In: Charlton JF, Weinstein GW, eds. *Ophthalmic surgery complications—prevention and management.* Philadelphia: JB Lippincott, 1995:215–251.

75. Pulhorn G, Teichmann KD, Teichmann I. Intraocular fibrous proliferation as an incisional complication in pars plana vitrectomy. *Am J Ophthalmol* 1977;83:810.

76. Buettner H, Machemer R. Histopathologic findings in human eyes after pars plana vitrectomy and lensectomy. *Arch Ophthalmol* 1977;95:2029.

77. Lewis H, Abrams GW, Foos RY. Clinicopathologic findings in anterior hyaloidal fibrovascular proliferation after diabetic vitrectomy. *Am J Ophthalmol* 1987;104:614.

78. Lewis H, Abrams GW, Williams GA. Anterior hyaloidal fibrovascular proliferation after diabetic vitrectomy. *Am J Ophthalmol* 1987;104:607.

79. Faulborn J, Conway BP, Machemer R. Surgical complications of pars plana vitreous surgery. *Ophthalmology* 1978;85:116.

80. Oyakawa RT, Schachat AP, Michels RG, Rice TA. Complications of vitreous surgery for diabetic retinopathy. Intraoperative complications. *Ophthalmology* 1983;90:517.

81. deBustros S, Thompson JT, Michels RG, et al. Surgical management of epiretinal membranes. *Ophthalmology* 1986;93:978.

82. deBustros S, Glaser BM, Johnson MA. Thrombin infusion for the control of intraocular bleeding during vitreous surgery. *Arch Ophthalmol* 1985;103:837.

83. Thompson JT, Glaser BM, Michels RG, deBustros S. The use of intravitreal thrombin to control hemorrhage during vitrectomy. *Ophthalmology* 1986;93:279.

84. Novak MA, Rice TA, Michels RG, Auer C. Vitreous hemorrhage after vitrectomy for diabetic retinopathy. *Ophthalmology* 1984;91:1485.

85. May DR, Peyman GA. Endophthalmitis after vitrectomy. *Am J Ophthalmol* 1976;81:520.

86. Ho PC, Tolentino FI. Bacterial endophthalmitis after closed vitrectomy. *Arch Ophthalmol* 1984;102:207.

Adjuncts to Vitreoretinal Surgery

JANET R. SPARROW   STANLEY CHANG

The introduction of intravitreally injected gaseous and liquid materials as adjuncts to vitreoretinal surgery has played a vital role in improving surgical outcomes. In the management of complicated retinal detachment these materials serve as intraoperative tools to reestablish intraocular volume and to aid in the removal of epiretinal membranes. Importantly, these materials can substitute for microsurgical instruments to manipulate and mechanically flatten the detached retina. Postoperatively, intravitreal gases and silicone liquid are used to tamponade a retinal tear and to maintain the retina in apposition to the pigment epithelium.

VISCOELASTICS

The viscoelastic properties of sodium hyaluronate (Healon; 1%) make it a valuable intraoperative aid to ocular surgery. The molecular weight of sodium hyaluronate is approximately 4,000,000 and it has a viscosity greater than 400,000 centistokes at near zero shear (steady state). At high shear, however, when the polymer is made to flow, it undergoes a reversible deformation such that the viscosity decreases to approximately 110 centistokes. It is this change in viscosity that renders the material injectable through small-gauge cannulas and yet ensures that the material will regain its shape in the eye. These viscoelastic properties can also be utilized in the separation of epiretinal membranes in cases of proliferative diabetic retinopathy (1). During viscodissection, epiretinal membranes are hydraulically lifted as the fluid is injected between retina and proliferative tissue. In this way, the membranes are separated from the retinal surface without trauma and the remaining attachments can be more easily cut. Any blood is also displaced so that the epiretinal membranes can be more easily distinguished from retina. The material should be injected carefully, however, since if the retina is atrophic and thus fragile, iatrogenic

retinal tears can be caused by an injection force that is too great.

During repair of a trauma-related corneal laceration, sodium hyaluronate can facilitate the repositioning uveal tissue and can be used to reform the anterior chamber. For the removal of intraocular foreign bodies in cases of penetrating trauma, sodium hyaluronate can be employed to gently lift a foreign body from the retinal surface or choroid.

During the repair of giant retinal tears, sodium hyaluronate has been used to unfold the retina and to contain hemorrhage (2–5). Having a specific gravity only slightly greater than saline (1.0084 at 20°C) (3), however, sodium hyaluronate does not exert the force that is possible with the use of a liquid of high density such as perfluorocarbon liquid. Sodium hyaluronate is also miscible with water and therefore does not segregate in a phase distinct from intraocular fluid. Furthermore, intraocular pressure may become elevated postoperatively if large volumes of sodium hyaluronate are left in the vitreous cavity at surgery.

PERFLUOROCARBON LIQUIDS

Properties of Perfluorocarbon Liquids

Perfluorocarbon liquids (PFCLs) have several features that make them especially favorable adjuncts to vitreoretinal surgery. For instance, since the density of PFCL (ranging from 1.76 to 2.0) is almost twice that of water, the force that can be exerted by PFCLs against the retina is 10 times greater than that exerted by the same volume of silicone or fluorosilicone oil (6). The high density of PFCL makes it a useful tool to manipulate retina in conjunction with vitrectomy. PFCLs are also immiscible with water and their interfacial tension with water is sufficient to ensure that in the environment of the eye, the liquid will remain as a single confluent globule. In addition, the surface tension, although less than that of gas, provides some resistance to passage of the PFCL through a retinal break.

PFCLs can be obtained as low-viscosity fluids (2 to 3 centistokes at 25°C), allowing easy injection and aspiration through small-gauge microsurgical instruments. The liquid is also optically clear, and since the index of refraction of PFCL is slightly different from that of saline and silicone liquid, PFCL forms an easily visible interface with these other liquids. On the other hand, the difference in refractive index is not sufficient to create significant optical aberrations during membrane dissection, permitting the use of conventional contact lenses. PFCLs also do not absorb radiation at wavelengths used for laser photocoagulation of retina (488 to 810 nm), therefore laser treatment can be delivered through the liquid (7,8).

Several low-viscosity PFCLs have been studied for their potential intraoperative use, including perfluorotributylamine ($C_{12}F_{27}N$) (9–12), perfluorodecalin ($C_{10}F_{18}$) (10–13), perfluorophenanthrene ($C_{14}F_{24}$) (14,15), perfluoroethylcyclohexane (C_8F_{16}) (16), foralkyl Ac-6 (17), perfluorooctylbromide (18,19), perfluoro-n-octane (C_8F_{18}) (10–12,20,21), and perfluoro-tri-n-propylamine (22). Compared with fluorocompounds containing heteroatoms such as nitrogen or oxygen, those composed only of carbon and fluorine atoms are more suited to a biological environment, since the high stability of the carbon–fluorine bond rends the liquid virtually nonreactive (23). Hydrogen-containing impurities, which can be present in PFCLs if the hydrocarbon precursor is not fully fluorinated (24), are also not desirable since they probably exhibit tissue reactivity (25). Perfluoro-n-octane, in particular, is most suitable for intravitreal use since it is obtainable as a highly purified compound. Indeed, analysis of perfluoro-n-octane by nuclear magnetic resonance spectroscopy has shown that the compound does not contain protonated impurities (i.e., hydrogen) (20). Unlike some other PFCLs, perfluoro-n-octane is also nonpolar, a feature contributing to its chemical nonreactivity. Importantly, also, when perfluoro-n-octane is exposed to argon and YAG laser, endodiathermy, and endoillumination, its chemical structure remains unchanged, and insignificant (parts per million) deposition of dissolved contaminants is observed (26). Another favorable characteristic of perfluoro-n-octane is that it has a relatively low boiling point and higher vapor pressure than other PFCLs. Consequently, small amounts of perfluoro-n-octane that remain after removal of the liquid will vaporize during fluid–air exchange.

Indications for Use, Techniques, and Complications

An intraoperative device, low-viscosity PFCLs have proved to be of value in a wide range of cases. For instance, the use of PFCL offers significant advantages in the management of severe degrees of proliferative vitreoretinopathy (Retina Society classification, grade C-3 and D) (Fig. 44-1).

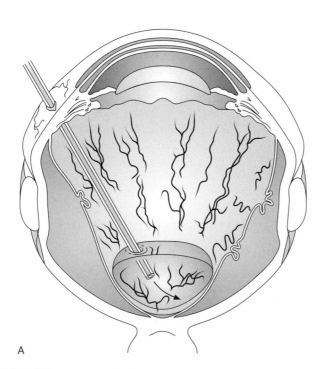 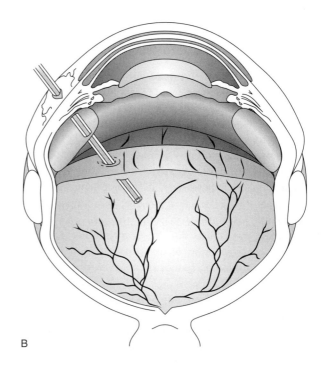

FIGURE 44-1. *Total retinal detachment with proliferative vitreoretinopathy. A. Perfluorocarbon liquid is used to open the funnel of the detachment and flatten the retina. B. As epiretinal membranes are removed in a posterior-to-anterior direction, additional perfluorocarbon liquid can be injected with the tip of the cannula positioned within the liquid.*

Not only does injection of the liquid (0.5–1.0) over the optic disk aid in opening the funnel of the detachment and flattening the retina, it also serves to reveal sites of residual traction and mechanically braces the retina during membrane dissection. As epiretinal membranes are removed beginning posteriorly and progressing anteriorly above the liquid, additional PFCL can be added. In this way, the removal of anterior proliferation is greatly facilitated. Subretinal membranes may undergo sufficient flattening under the PFCL that their removal is not necessary. Moreover, the need for posterior drainage retinotomy is obviated since the PFCL displaces the subretinal fluid anteriorly where it can exit through preexisting retinal breaks. If relaxing retinotomies (circumferential or radial) are required to remove persistent traction at the vitreous bases, the size of retinotomy can be kept to a minimum by observing the retina flatten under the PFCL as retinotomy is performed (10,11,27). The PFCL is of particular benefit in positioning the large retinal flap (10,11,27). When perfluorocarbon gas is to be used for postoperative tamponade, the PFCL is removed by fluid–air exchange (Fig. 44-2), with aspiration of liquid beginning anteriorly. If PFCLs with lower vapor pressure are used (e.g., perfluorodecalin, perfluorophenanthrene), lavage with balanced salt solution may be required to remove residual PFCL from the retinal surface (6). A perfluorocarbon gas–air mixture is then flushed through the vitreous cavity. If silicone liquid is to be injected, it can either be delivered directly by automated infusion as PFCL is aspirated (fluid–fluid exchange), or it can be injected after complete fluid–air exchange.

Overall, the intraoperative use of PFCL in cases of severe proliferative vitreoretinopathy minimizes retinal trauma, permits more thorough membrane removal, facilitates the stabilization of macula, and reduces the duration of surgery (27). All these factors contribute to the excellent rates of final anatomical attachment (28–30) (85% and 78%), improved visual outcomes, and the reduction in postoperative reproliferation (31).

In proliferative diabetic retinopathy, PFCLs have been used intraoperatively to flatten the rhegmatogenous component of a retinal detachment so that adequate endophotocoagulation can be applied (32,33). PFCLs do not, however, facilitate the control of intraoperative hemorrhage in these cases, and indeed extra care must be taken to ensure entire removal of the PFCL when significant intraocular bleeding is present.

Excellent results are also obtained when PFCL is used to facilitate the surgical management of giant retinal tears (Fig. 44-3). In these cases, anatomical success rates of 66% to 100% are achieved (12,34–42). The PFCL can be used to manipulate the flap of the tear, thereby minimizing the retinal trauma that can occur from the use of microsurgical tools and eliminating the need for prone positioning. As in cases with severe proliferative vitreoretinopathy, posterior retinotomy to remove subretinal fluid is not necessary since the PFCL drives the fluid anteriorly. The PFCL also serves to stabilize the tear against the retinal pigment epithelium

while endophotocoagulation or transscleral cryotherapy is applied to the posterior edge of the tear through the liquid. Additionally, some cases of giant retinal tears can be managed without scleral buckling or lens removal (12,35,43).

The repair of retinal detachment in conjunction with a macular hole can also be managed by injection of a small amount of PFCL over the posterior pole. The macula will then flatten against the pigment epithelium so that

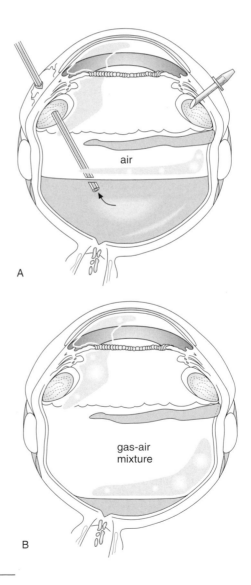

FIGURE 44-2. *Upon completion of vitrectomy, fluid–air exchange is performed. Fluid is aspired as air enters through the infusion line. At the end of surgery, air is substituted with the desired gas–air mixture.*

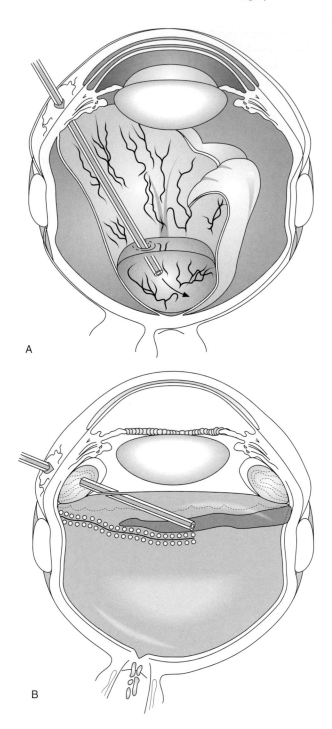

A

B

FIGURE 44-3. *Giant retina tear with proliferative vitreoretinopathy. A. The perfluorocarbon liquid serves to unfold the tear and stabilizes the retina during membrane dissection. B. The perfluorocarbon liquid supports the repositioned retina while endophotocoagulation is applied through the liquid.*

endophotocoagulation can be applied. The PFCL can also be helpful in detecting peripheral retinal breaks. These tears become apparent, due to the difference in refractive indices of subretinal fluid and PFCL, as the subretinal fluid is forced through them. The use of PFCL together with tissue plasminogen activator for the surgical removal of submacular blood in eyes with age-related macular degeneration has been reported to diminish surgically induced retinal trauma (44).

With retinal detachment due to penetrating trauma, PFCL can be injected after the hemorrhagic vitreous is removed by core vitrectomy. The PFCL serves to flatten the retina without posterior retinotomy and facilitates separation of the hemorrhage from the vitreous base (11,45). If blood has pooled subretinally, the PFCL will also displace the blood anteriorly, from where it can be aspirated internally through an existing retinal tear. In traumatic retinal detachments complicated by subretinal membranes or when proliferation has occurred around an injury site, the PFCL will help flatten retinal folds and permit visualization. When removing foreign bodies, such as wood or plastic, the fragments can be floated anteriorly on the surface of the PFCL. Although heavier bodies made of glass or metal will sink in the PFCL, the latter can be used to stabilize the fragment as it is grasped with forceps.

The placement of PFCL over the posterior pole of the retina during intravitreal ultrasonic lens phacofragmentation to remove displaced crystalline lens fragments prevents trauma to the retina from falling lens fragments. The PFCL also acts as a protective surface, reflecting the ultrasonic stream (15,46–50). Injected PFCL can assist in the removal of a dislocated hard crystalline lens or intraocular lens by lifting it away from the retinal surface and into the anterior vitreous cavity where it can be managed (46–50).

Care must be taken to avoid passage of the PFCL into the subretinal space through a retinal break (10,12,39) or retinotomy (27). In a report of 223 patients, this was a problem in 0.9% of cases (51). Because the PFCL droplet can cause a focal detachment of overlying retina and because the possibility exists of adverse effects on adjacent photoreceptor cells (52,53), subretinal PFCL should be removed intraoperatively.

Retention of the PFCL within the vitreous cavity after surgery has been reported with incidences of 1.3% to 3.5% (28,54), although residual droplets of PFCL have not been known to cause adverse effects in either patients (10,12) or animal models (20,55). On the other hand, large volumes (50% of vitreous volume) of PFCL (perfluorophenanthrene) inadvertently remaining after surgery have been reported to cause secondary glaucoma due to angle closure (56). If ophthalmoscopic visualization of the retained PFCL is not possible, ultrasonographic (51,57) or ^{19}F-nuclear magnetic resonance imaging (58–60) can be used.

INTRAOCULAR GAS

Functional Role of Gas

An intraocular gas bubble can serve effectively in the post-operative repair of a retinal detachment in two ways (61). First, the surface tension formed between the gas bubble and the surrounding aqueous serves to tamponade a retinal break, thereby preventing a subretinal accumulation of fluid. Second, the gas bubble, having a specific gravity lower than that of water, exerts a buoyant force that flattens the retina and displaces subretinal fluid. Optimal use of this buoyant force provided by the gas bubble necessitates sustained head positioning such that the bubble is positioned over the retinal break until chorioretinal adhesion provided by diathermy or cryotherapy is established. Moreover, since a gas bubble rises to the uppermost part of the eye and the buoyant force is greatest at the apex of the arc of contact of the gas bubble with the retinal surface, intraocular gas is most useful for superior retina breaks. It is at a disadvantage, however, when a retinal tear is located at the inferior pole, since the lower meniscus of the bubble exerts little or no contact with retina. Ultimately, tamponading an inferior retinal break adequately requires a disproportionately larger increase in bubble volume (62–64).

Since intravitreally used high-molecular-weight gases such as sulfur hexafluoride and perfluorocarbon are less soluble in water than the low-molecular-weight blood gases nitrogen, oxygen, and carbon dioxide, the latter gases, which are normally dissolved in tissue fluids, diffuse into the intra-vitreally injected gas and the total gas volume increases. Following an injection of pure expanding gas into the eye, the most rapid expansion occurs within the first 6 to 8 hours, with the rate being determined by the properties of the gas and the presence of the convection currents in the adjacent vitreous (65). The gas bubble then continues to expand until the partial pressures of the gases in the bubble equilibrate with that in the surrounding tissue fluid. Sulfur hexafluoride (SF_6) reaches its maximum expanded volume by 24 to 48 hours after injection (66). With perfluoropropane (C_3F_8), the maximum expanded volume is reached after 72 to 96 hours (67–69). After the expansion phase, all of the gases diffuse out of the vitreous cavity, and the gas bubble diminishes in volume by first order exponential decay (70,71). It is, however, the time interval before the bubble is reduced to half its size that is of greatest clinical importance, because a small gas bubble exerts insufficient buoyant force. Consequently, a gas bubble may be of therapeutic value for only 30% of its lifetime in the eye. Ideally, a gas bubble should be present at therapeutic volume until the chorioretinal adhesion induced by photocoagulation or cryotherapy becomes maximal [estimated to be 8 to 14 days (72,73)] or until the active phase of reproliferation has subsided in cases complicated by proliferative vitreoretinopathy. It is in the treatment of inferior retinal breaks of course that gas bubble size and longevity are most critical. The half-lives of gases vary with the volume and concentration of gas injected and with the presence/absence of lens and vitreous, diffusion barriers, blood flow, aqueous production, and outflow and ocular elasticity, contour, and size (71,74–76). For perfluoro-propane–air mixtures the half-life is commonly 20 to 30 days (69,74,77).

Clinical Applications of Intraocular Gas

The use of intraocular gases is considered standard care by vitreoretinal surgeons in North America (78). While air can be used as a nonexpanding gas, high-molecular-weight gases such as sulfur hexafluoride (79) and those in the perfluorocarbon family have low water solubility and thus greater intraocular longevity without having adverse effects on the retina (80). Consequently, they have been associated with higher rates of retinal reattachment (81,82). Gases in the perfluorocarbon family that have been investigated for use include perfluoromethane (CF_4) (67,70, 76,83), perfluoroethane (C_2F_6) (67,70,76,83), perfluoropropane (C_3F_8) (65,67,68,70,71,83–87), octofluorocyclobutane (C_4F_8) (88,89), and perfluoro-n-butane (C_4F_{10}) (67,83,90). The features of some gases which are empolyed intraocularly are presented in Table 44-1.

Nevertheless, since the final volume reached by an intra-vitreal gas bubble can vary, and with it the potential for a postoperative rise in intraocular pressure, the use of gas–air mixtures with reduced expansile capability is favored. Minimally expanding gas concentrations are beneficial compared with nonexpanding concentrations, because complete filling of the vitreous cavity with a nonexpansile gas–air mixture requires that the patient be placed in the prone position with the surgeon facing the patient from below. Conversely, intravitreal injection of a gas–air mixture that undergoes a small increase in size postoperatively avoids the hazards associated with prone positioning (91,92). Minimal expansion can be achieved with gas–air concentrations of 20% to 25%, for perfluoroethane and 17% to 20% for perfluoropropane. With sulfur hexafluoride a gas concentration of 40% in air can be used without a rise in intraocular pressure (93). Concentrations of approximately 16% for perfluoroethane, 14% for perfluoropropane, and 18% for sulfur hexafluoride are nonexpanding (68,94). Expansile mixtures are contraindicated in patients with preexisting glaucoma. Similarly, if by

Table 44-1.   Features of Some Intraocular Gases Used in Vitreoretinal Surgery

	Fold Expansion	Nonexpanding Concentration	Minimally Expanding Concentration
Sulfur hexafluoride	1.9–2.0	18%	20–25%
Perfluoromethane	1.9	—	—
Perfluoroethane	3.3	16%	20%
Perfluoropropane	4	12%	17%

preoperative gonioscopic examination outflow is suspected of being compromised by neovascularization or anterior synechiae, nonexpanding gas–air mixtures should be used. In nonglaucomatous eyes, 12% and 20% concentrations of C_3F_8 gas in air are reported to increase intraocular pressure with similar frequency, while the 20% concentration had the advantage of longer duration tamponade (69). While complete filling of the vitreous cavity by fluid–gas exchange, with either minimally expanding or nonexpansile gas, may be the objective under conditions such as an inferior retinal break, it is not necessarily indicated in the treatment of superior retinal breaks. Partially filling can also be used to diagnosis occult retinal breaks in the presence of retinal detachment (95).

To achieve an adequate-sized intravitreal gas bubble, thorough evacuation of intravitreal fluid is necessary. Accordingly, it is recommended that, 10 minutes after the initial fluid–air exchange, fluid aspiration be repeated (96). Similarly, to attain the desired intraocular gas concentration, intraocular air must be completely flushed from the eye by using a sufficient volume of the gas–air mixture (this volume is estimated to be 25 ml) (97). The gas–air mixture should be prepared immediately before injection so that the gas-to-air ratio is not changed by efflux of gas from the plastic syringe (98).

The choice of gas to be used for a given clinical condition is based on clinical experience. The issues to be considered include the type and location of the retinal problem and the duration of therapy required. Air and sulfur hexafluoride are the most commonly used agents for scleral buckling procedures (80,99) since only short-duration tamponade is required. Sulfur hexafluoride can also be used to treat superior retinal breaks above the horizontal meridian (94), proliferative diabetic retinopathy (81,94), milder forms of proliferative vitreoretinopathy (94), and pneumatic retinopexy (100). Serial injections of sulfur hexafluoride can also be used to achieve an adequate-size gas bubble of shorter duration (94). On the other hand, perfluorocarbon gases, because of their greater longevity, are preferred for complicated forms of retinal detachment (83,91) such as giant retinal tears, penetrating trauma, or retinal detachment from macular holes in highly myopic eyes. Perfluoropropane (C_3F_8) is the most commonly used perfluorocarbon gas (99,101,102). Nevertheless, perfluoroethane can be used for pneumatic retinopexy, for internal tamponade of rhegmatogenous retinal detachments associated with posterior retinal breaks, and for proliferative diabetic retinopathy, traction retinal detachment, and penetrating trauma. For giant retinal tears not complicated by proliferative vitreoretinopathy and highly myopic eyes with retinal detachment from macular holes, perfluoroethane can provide a therapeutic volume of gas until the chorioretinal adhesion resulting from photocoagulation or cryotherapy is established (36). Milder forms of proliferative vitreoretinopathy may also be managed using perfluoroethane. In addition, perfluoroethane is preferred for postoperative

fluid–gas exchange. Perfluoroethane, because it is retained for a shorter duration, allows more rapid rehabilitation of the patient compared with perfluoropropane. It is also a desirable gas since it is less frequently associated with cataract formation.

Conversely, for the management of giant retinal tears complicated by proliferative vitreoretinopathy or retinal detachments with severe forms of proliferative vitreoretinopathy (Retina Society classification, grades C-3 and D), perfluoropropane gas is preferred (65,103–105). In fact, a multicenter randomized, prospective clinical trial (the Silicone Study) concluded that C_3F_8 gas is superior to SF_6 gas for intraocular tamponade after vitrectomy for rhegmatogenous retinal detachment complicated by severe proliferative vitreoretinopathy (106,107). In these cases perfluoropropane has the advantage of being able to provide more than a 50% fill for 3 weeks after surgery. Perfluoropropane (16%) has also been used together with vitrectomy and TGF-b2 for the closure of macular holes (108). While perfluoropropane is routinely used in some centers for pneumatic retinopexy (78,109) and for the management of giant retinal tears (92), shorter lasting gases, such as perfluoroethane, may be equally effective (36).

Postoperative Management and Complications

Patients with intraocular gas bubbles must maintain the head in a prone position to prevent contact between the bubble and anterior structures. Especially for children, the elderly, or the debilitated, this positioning can be problematic, as can the need for postoperative indirect ophthalmoscopic examination. Scattering of light at the interface between the gas bubble and intraocular fluid also obscures the patient's vision and complicates fundus examination and postoperative application of laser photocoagulation.

If expanding concentrations of gas are used, careful monitoring of gas bubble size and intraocular pressure is particularly important. Disproportionate bubble expansion can cause shallowing of the anterior chamber, pupillary block glaucoma, and central retinal artery occlusion. Intraocular pressure should be measured 6 to 8 hours following surgery (89) by using applanation tonometry, because Schiotz tonometry, under these conditions, underestimates pressure measurements (110–112). The incidence of elevated intraocular pressure in the immediate postoperative period ranges between 26% and 59% (80,81,83,113). In most cases, intraocular pressure can be controlled by administering timolol and acetazolamide during the initial 24 hours (94,113), and once complete expansion is achieved, intraocular pressure should stabilize. Intraocular pressure can be more difficult to manage in cases of compromised outflow, and in patients suspected of having occluded angles from neovascularization or peripheral anterior synechiae, expanding concentrations of gas should be avoided. Permanent glaucoma secondary to gas use is infrequent. Very occasionally, increased intraocular pressure occurs when the volume of the fully expanded gas bubble exceeds the vitreous volume (91,103). In this case, gas must be aspirated.

Lens opacities, pupillary block glaucoma, and, in aphakic eyes, corneal endothelial decompensation (113) are potential complications of intravitreal gas, not as a result of chemical toxicity (80,82,91,94,114) but because of mechanical barriers to diffusion. Gases with greater longevity are more likely to cause these changes (86,91). Lens opacities occur most often when the gas bubble occupies more than two-thirds of the vitreous volume (80,82,83) and are first visualized as feathery posterior subcapsular changes or as posterior subcapsular vacuoles, most often in superior lens. The opacity can be transient and can disappear if a layer of aqueous is retained between the gas bubble and the posterior lens surface. The incidence of keratopathy in eyes receiving perfluoropropane gas has been reported as 6% to 33% (113,115,116). Because of the possibility of prolonged contact between the gas bubble and the corneal endothelium, the occurrence of corneal abnormalities is related to lens status (aphakia and pseudophakia versus phakic eyes) (117,118). Previous vitrectomy is also a factor. The Silicone Study has found that the frequency of keratopathy was similar in the gas-injected (28%) and silicone liquid–filled (26%) eyes following surgery for severe proliferative vitreoretinopathy (116).

Air travel, and other situations involving rapid changes in atmospheric pressure, can cause expansion of a gas bubble (119,120). During a rapid change in bubble size the eye has little time to compensate by outflow of aqueous humor (121), thus elevated intraocular pressure can occur, which in turn compromises blood flow through the central retinal artery. From measurements made in animal experiments, it is estimated that an intraocular gas volume of 0.6 mL or 10% of the volume of the eye may be safe for air travel (122). Clinical experience (94,122) and the findings of Lincoff et al (122) indicate, however, that volumes of intraocular gas of up to 1.0 mL can be tolerated. Judicious use of the inhalation anesthetic, nitrous oxide, is also indicated in patients with intraocular gas bubbles, since the highly soluble nitrous oxide gas rapidly diffuses into the intraocular gas bubble and can cause bubble expansion and elevated intraocular pressure (123,124).

Aqueous flare has been observed both by slit-lamp examination and by flaremetry following intraocular injection of gas in both humans and rabbits (65,83,114,125). Consistent with this observation, anterior chamber fluorophotometry in rabbits has revealed a short-term breakdown in the blood–ocular barrier following intravitreal injection of gas (126,127), while studies of leakage across the blood–retinal barrier are conflicting (128,129). Although the issue of whether intravitreal gas can augment proliferative processes is not resolved (130,131), it is commonly suggested that an intravitreal gas bubble should be designed to persist only as long as is therapeutically necessary (130).

It is important to visualize the tip of the needle during gas injection so as to avoid injecting the gas under the nonpigmented ciliary epithelium (132). During pneumatic retinopexy, small gas bubbles may pass through existing retinal tears and expand in the subretinal space. With this complication, scleral buckling can be used to close the retinal breaks and displace the subretinal gas bubble (133); otherwise vitrectomy and air–fluid exchange may be necessary. Gas may also pass into the subretinal space when fluid–gas exchange is performed in eyes with large tears induced by recurrent proliferation (102). In these eyes, vitrectomy revision is indicated.

SILICONE LIQUID

Properties of Silicone Liquid

Since silicone liquid is lighter than water (specific gravity of 0.97), a silicone globule contacts retina with an upward buoyant force. The force exerted in this way is estimated to be $1/30$ of the pressure exerted by a gas bubble (134). The surface tension of silicone liquid with water (40 mN/m) is also less than that of a gas bubble. Consequently, while a gas bubble can apply tamponading forces both superiorly and posteriorly (135), a silicone globule can effectively support a surgically reattached retina above the horizontal meridian but provides little tamponade to posterior retina with the patient sitting upright (136) and is unable to resist radially directed tractional forces on retina (135,137–139). On the other hand, it is postulated that a silicone globule positioned contiguous with the surface of the retina may induce a tangential realignment of tractional forces that become less effective than radially transmitted traction (137). A large silicone globule within the vitreous cavity may also reduce the fluid currents that otherwise contribute to retinal redetachment (135,136,140).

Since the refractive index of silicone (1.404) is greater than that of vitreous, in phakic eyes the concavity of the silicone globule's anterior surface (conforming to lens curvature) can induce hyperopic changes (to about +5) (137,141). Conversely, in aphakic eyes the convexity of the silicone globule increases the refractive power of the eye, an advantage for many aphakic patients (137,141).

Indications and Clinical Considerations

The use of silicone liquid is most frequently indicated when long-term or permanent support and tamponade are needed in cases complicated by proliferative vitreoretinopathy (82,142–152), giant retinal tears (145,147,150,153–156), retinal detachment due to proliferative diabetic retinopathy (136,145,148,150,157,158), or ocular trauma (141,150). In the United States, silicone liquid has been used in the primary surgery if the patient is unable to comply with the postoperative positioning and fluid–gas exchange requirements of gas (159). While this is a factor in recommending silicone liquid rather than gas for children, the surgical results in children have been less rewarding because of a greater tendency for reproliferation (160). Silicone liquid may also be chosen over gas in the primary procedure, if the patient must travel by air. It has also been used after an unsuccessful primary procedure in cases of severe ocular trauma (161), and after the failure of previous scleral buckling, vitrectomy, membrane dissection, and intraocular gas injection for the treatment of proliferative vitreoretinopathy. Conversely, in Europe, silicone liquid has been more frequently used in conjunction with primary reattachment surgery for the management of giant retinal tears, proliferative diabetic retinopathy, and ocular trauma (141,150). Nevertheless, the Silicone Study concluded that whereas silicone liquid was superior to sulfur hexafluoride gas in the management of retinal detachment complicated by severe (grade C3 or worse) proliferative vitreoretinopathy, no difference was observed between silicone liquid and perfluoropropane gas in terms of reattachment, visual results, and complications (106). Whether employed in the primary or secondary procedure, silicone liquid is commonly used with one or more other surgical techniques, including extensive membrane peeling, the use of a broad scleral buckle, retinal photocoagulation, and/or retinotomy (136,144,158,159, 162–164). Scleral buckling of an inferior tear, in conjunction with intravitreally placed silicone liquid, is advocated to promote contact between the silicone globule and the tear (165). While silicone liquid has frequently been chosen over gas in cases of extensive relaxing retinotomies and retinectomy, particularly when large areas of exposed retinal pigment epithelium must be covered (158,166–169), the Silicone Study confirmed that silicone liquid and perfluoropropane (C_3F_8) gas are equally effective adjuncts in the presence of a retinotomy. With silicone liquid, however, hypotony was less frequently observed (170). When complete endolaser photocoagulation is not possible intraoperatively, intravitreal silicone liquid permits excellent visualization of the fundus so that retinal tears or retinotomies can be treated postoperatively (171). Its use, of course, also eliminates the need for repeated postoperative fluid–gas exchange.

Intravitreal silicone liquid is reported to reduce preexistent iris neovascularization or to prevent the postoperative development of iris neovascularization (136,137,157,163, 169,172), a serious complication of proliferative diabetic retinopathy or persistent retinal detachment (173). While silicone liquid may modulate neovascularization by serving as a barrier to diffusion/convection (174), an effect on anterior segment neovascularization is not always realized (158,175) and may vary with the degree of fill and other factors (141). The incidence of silicone liquid–induced band keratopathy is less in cases of proliferative diabetic retinopathy than of proliferative vitreoretinopathy, possibly because of already elevated glucose levels in the blood and aqueous humor (10).

In advanced human immunodeficiency virus (HIV) infection with retinal detachment secondary to cytomegalovirus, silicone liquid is used to tamponade present and impending retinal holes caused by the progressive necrotizing retinitis (176–178). For these patients, silicone liquid is preferred over gas since the latter impairs vision and necessitates prolonged face-down positioning. In a study of 350 AIDS patients treated with vitrectomy and silicone liquid, the macula remained attached in 94% of patients; 68% of patients had ambulatory vision and 56% retained visual acuity for a median survival time of 7 months (177). Indeed, it has been suggested that approval by the Food and Drug Administration of silicone liquid use in humans was influenced by the potential importance of the liquid in the treatment of HIV-associated retinal detachment (179).

Notwithstanding the benefits of silicone liquid, because of its low specific gravity, it is most efficacious when a retinal tear/detachment is located superiorly. Conversely, the inferior quadrants—where proliferative vitreoretinopathy, the most common cause of failed reattachment surgery (180–182), also tends to be most pronounced (175,180)—are commonly the site of persistent or recurrent detachments following the use of silicone liquid (155,165,183,184). Redetachment, while having an obvious impact on visual rehabilitation, also precipitates lens and corneal damage by forcing the silicone globule anteriorly (185). Solutions to the problems encountered with inferior retinal breaks await the development of devices such as high specific gravity liquids (e.g., high-viscosity PFCLs), perhaps for use in conjunction with silicone liquid (186–188). Antiproliferative drugs, whether infused after vitrectomy (189) or delivered within the silicone globule itself (retinoic acid and BCNU) (190–192) are also under investigation for use in conjunction with silicone liquid.

Important issues concerning the removal of silicone liquid remain (139,146,149,151,183,193,194). The Silicone Study reported that silicone liquid was removed in 40% to 57% of eyes but that removal was commonly performed only on those eyes exhibiting good anatomical and functional results (106,108,115,194). In another study, the liquid was removed in 81% of patients with proliferative vitreoretinopathy (195). In the case of retinas that are reattached at the time of removal, visual acuity tends to improve (194). Recovery from secondary glaucoma has also been realized in 68% of patients after removal (196). Other reasons for removal can include cataract formation and emulsification. In some instances the patient refuses to consent to the removal procedure. Silicone liquid is removed as early as 3 to 8 weeks (145,149,153,155,197) after surgery in some cases. In the Silicone Study with severe proliferative vitreoretinopathy, the liquid was required to remain intravitreally for a minimum of 8 weeks (194). Usually it is preferred that removal be performed at 3 to 6 months postoperatively (162,197,198) but periods of up to a year and longer have also been reported (115,194,195,197). In the case of proliferative diabetic retinopathy, the surgical success rate is considered to have no relationship to the duration of silicone liquid treatment (196). While this was also the conclusion of one study of the use of silicone liquid for management of proliferative vitreoretinopathy (194), another has reported better results after a longer period of intravitreal silicone liquid (up to 22 months) (196). Redetachment after removal occurs at a rate of 9% to 50% (137,146,193,195,196, 199–201); in the Silicone Study the frequency was 20% (14% after reoperation) (194). Methods of removal employ techniques of passive drainage, designated cannulas, and vacuum aspiration pumps (137,141,197,202,203); however, residual silicone liquid droplets can still be a problem (203) despite careful lavage.

Ocular Tolerance and Complications

Silicone liquids are linear synthetic polymers made of repetitive [—Si—O—] units. The differences among silicone liquid species are a feature of the length of the polymer, which affects the viscosity, and the hydrocarbon radicals, which constitute the side groups of the polymer. Clinically used silicone liquids are generally polydimethylsiloxanes. The importance of using only highly purified high viscosity silicone liquid of homogeneous polymer length cannot be overstated. Low molecular weight constituents are probably responsible for infiltrating surrounding tissues and inciting macrophage reactions (204) and also increase the tendency of the liquid to emulsify (205), a situation conducive to angle block glaucoma and keratopathy. Adverse tissue reactions may also be the result of a high content of hydroxyl-end groups and of catalytic remnants of the polymerization process (primarily heavy metal ions) (205). The high-viscosity materials (5000 cs) are more resistant to emulsification than the 1000-cs material and are associated with a lower incidence of glaucoma (205–208). Indeed, only the 5000-cs liquid is currently approved by the Food and Drug Administration for noninvestigational use in humans.

Some complications of silicone filling, particularly those involving the anterior segment, arise from mechanical rather than chemical factors. For instance, corneal complications, reported in 10% to 28% of patients (106,115), are precipitated by the presence of silicone liquid in the anterior chamber (207,209), and lodging of a silicone globule in the iris diaphragm can cause pupillary block glaucoma. To reduce the risk of the latter and to keep the anterior chamber free of silicone in aphakic eyes, avoidance of overfilling (134) and the use of an inferior basal iridectomy (106,210) are advocated. While the inferior iridectomy allows the silicone globule to return to the vitreous cavity when the patient is prone, in a significant proportion of patients spontaneous postoperative closure of the iridectomy occurs (211) with resulting corneal abnormalities (116). YAG laser (116) and tissue plasminogen activator have both been used to restore the patency of the iridectomy (212), and an artificial iris diaphragm with imitation inferior iridectomy has been developed (213).

Lens opacifications most frequently arise between 6 and 18 months after surgery (214), and cataracts can appear or worsen even after silicone removal (136,149). To prevent prolonged contact between the silicone globule and the posterior lens capsule in phakic patients, avoidance of the supine position should be stressed. To facilitate the surgical approach and to preempt cataract formation, some surgeons prefer lensectomy during the primary procedure. The alternative is to retain the lens for protection of anterior segment structures, with lens extraction and intraocular lens implant being options at the time of silicone removal, should a cataract develop (137,214).

Besides the risk of pupillary block glaucoma in the aphakic eye, angle block glaucoma can occur at rates of 6% to 25% (151,152,195,215,216) in both phakic and aphakic eyes secondary to emulsification of the liquid. Emulsification, reported to occur at rates of up to 56% (216), becomes a more significant factor with time (135,217,218), and, as noted above, occurs less readily with high-viscosity liquids. Despite obstruction of the angle, glaucoma may not be manifest if aqueous production is abnormally decreased or if the retina is detached (136). Moreover, intraocular pressure will return to normal once silicone liquid is removed (136).

SUMMARY

The use of intraocular gases, viscoelastics, PFCLs, and silicone oil has had a major impact on the progress of vitreoretinal surgery. Our understanding of the chemical and physical properties that contribute to the efficacy of these materials has been expanded and much work has been done to ensure that high-quality materials are used. Future investigations will continue to address the proliferative processes that confound surgical efforts and will provide alternatives for long-term vitreous substitution.

REFERENCES

1. Michels RG, Stark WJ, Stirpe M, eds. *Sodium hyaluronate in anterior and posterior segment surgery.* Padova, Italy: Liviana Press, 1989.
2. Schepens CL. *Retinal detachment and allied diseases.* Philadelphia: W.B. Saunders, 1983.
3. Fitzgerald CR. The use of Healon® in a case of rolled-over retina. *Retina* 1981;1:227.
4. Brown GC, Benson WE. Use of sodium hyaluronate for the repair of giant retinal tears. *Arch Ophthalmol* 1989;107:1246.
5. Folk JC, Weingeist TA, Packer AJ. Sodium hyaluronate (Healon) in closed vitrectomy. *Ophthalmic Surg* 1986;17:299.
6. Chang S. Low viscosity liquid fluorochemicals in vitreous surgery. *Am J Ophthalmol* 1987;103:38.
7. Azzolini C, Docchio F, Brancata R, Trabucchi G. Interactions between light and vitreous fluid substitutes. *Arch Ophthalmol* 1992;110:1468.
8. Azzolini C, Brancato R, Trabucchi G, et al. Endophotocoagulation through perfluorodecalin in rabbit eyes. *Int Ophthalmol* 1994;18:33.
9. Chang S, Zimmerman NJ, Iwamoto T, et al. Experimental vitreous replacement with perfluorotributylamine. *Am J Ophthalmol* 1987;103:29.
10. Chang S, Ozmert E, Zimmerman NJ. Intraoperative perfluorocarbon liquids in the management of proliferative vitreoretinopathy. *Am J Ophthalmol* 1988;106:668.
11. Chang S, Reppucci V, Zimmerman NJ, et al. Perfluorocarbon liquids in the management of traumatic retinal detachments. *Ophthalmology* 1989;96:785.
12. Chang S, Lincoff H, Zimmerman NJ, Fuchs W. Giant retinal tears: surgical techniques and results using perfluorocarbon liquids. *Arch Ophthalmol* 1989;107:761.

13. Hammer ME, Rinder DF, Hicks EL, et al. Tolerance of perfluorocarbons, fluorosilicone and silicone liquids in the vitreous. In: Freeman HM, Tolentino FI, eds. *Proliferative vitreoretinopathy.* New York: Springer-Verlag, 1988:156–161.

14. Nabib M, Peyman GA, Clark LC. Experimental evaluation of perfluorophenanthrene as a high specific gravity vitreous substitute: a preliminary report. *Ophthalmic Surg* 1989;20:286.

15. Liu K-R, Peyman GA, Chen M-S. Use of high density vitreous substitutes in the removal of posteriorly dislocated lenses or intraocular lenses. *Ophthalmic Surg* 1991;22:503.

16. Sparrow JR, Matthews P, Iwamoto T, et al. Retinal tolerance to intravitreal perfluoroethylcyclohexane liquid in the rabbit. *Retina* 1993;13:56–62.

17. Marin J, Manzanas L, Refojo MF, Tolentino FI. Foralkyl AC-6, a perfluorocarbon liquid intravitreous tamponade agent with diminished dispersion tendency. *Invest Ophthalmol Vis Sci* 1990;31(Suppl):24.

18. Flores-Aguilar M, Munguia D, Loeb E, et al. Intraocular tolerance of perfluorooctylbromide (Perflubron). *Retina* 1995;15:3.

19. Conway MD, Peyman GA, Karacorlu M, et al. Perfluorooctylbromide (PFOB) as a vitreous substitute in non-human primates. *Int Ophthalmol* 1993;17:259.

20. Chang S, Sparrow JR, Iwamoto T, et al. Experimental studies of tolerance to intravitreal perfluoro-n-octane liquid. *Retina* 1991;11:367.

21. Chang S, Sparrow JR, Iwamoto T, et al. Experimental studies of tolerance to intravitreal perfluoro-N-octane liquid. *Retina* 1991;11:367–374.

22. Bryan JS, Friedman SM, Mames RN, Margo CE. Experimental vitreous replacement with perfluorotri-n-propylamine. *Arch Ophthalmol* 1994;112:1098.

23. Sargent JW, Seffl RJ. Properties of perfluorinated liquids. *Fed Proc* 1970;29:1699.

24. Grafstein D. Detection, estimation and removal of impurities in fluorocarbon liquids. *Anal Chem* 1954;26:523.

25. Sparrow JR, Ortiz R, MacLeish PR, et al. Fibroblast behavior at aqueous interfaces with perfluorocarbon, silicone and fluorosilicone liquids. *Invest Ophthalmol Vis Sci* 1990;31:638.

26. Bourke RD, Simpson RN, Cooling RJ, Sparrow JR. The stability of perfluoro-n-octane during vitreoretinal procedures. *Arch Ophthalmol* 1996;114:537.

27. Han DP, Rychwalski PJ, Mieler WF, Abrams GW. Management of complex retinal detachment with combined relaxing retinotomy and intravitreal perfluoro-n-octane injection. *Am J Ophthalmol* 1994;118:24.

28. Coll GE, Chang S, Sun J, et al. Perfluorocarbon liquid in the management of retinal detachment with proliferative vitreoretinopathy. *Ophthalmology* 1995;102:630.

29. Carroll BF, Peyman GA, Mehta NJ, et al. Repair of retinal detachment associated with proliferative vitreoretinopathy using perfluoroperhydrophenanthrene (Vitreon). Vitreon Study Group. *Can J Ophthalmol* 1994;29:66.

30. Banker AS, Freeman WR, Vander JF, et al. Use of perflubron as a new temporary vitreous substitute and manipulation agent for vitreoretinal surgery. *Retina* 1996;16:285.

31. Stolba U, Binder S, Velikay M, et al. Use of perfluorocarbon liquids in proliferative vitreoretinopathy: results and complications. *Br J Ophthalmol* 1995;79:1106.

32. Mathis A, Pagot V, David J-L. The use of perfluorodecalin in diabetic vitrectomy. *Forstschr Ophthalmol* 1991;88:148.

33. Mathis A, Pagot V, Idder A, Maleze F. Use of perfluorodecalin during vitrectomy in diabetics. *J Fr Ophthalmol* 1993;16:584.

34. Freeman HM. Current management of giant retinal breaks and fellow eyes. In: Ryan SJ, ed. *Retina.* St. Louis: CV Mosby, 1989:431.

35. Kreiger AE, Lewis H. Management of giant retinal tears without scleral buckling. Use of radical dissection of the vitreous base and perfluoro-octane and intraocular tamponade. *Ophthalmology* 1992;99:491.

36. Chang S. Giant retinal tears: surgical management with perfluorocarbon liquids. In: Lewis H, Ryan SJ, eds. *Medical and surgical retina.* St. Louis: CV Mosby, 1994.

37. Le Mer Y, Haut J. Use of perfluoro-octane liquid in the treatment of giant tears with inversion of the retina: preliminary results. *J Fr Ophthalmol* 1990;13:247.

38. Le Mer Y, Kroll P. Die anwendung von flussigen perfluorocarbon bei Riesenrissen. *Klin Monatsbl Augenheilkd* 1991;198:264.

39. Glaser BM, Carter JB, Kuppermann BD, Michels RG. Perfluoro-octane in the treatment of giant retinal tears with proliferative vitreoretinopathy. *Ophthalmology* 1991;98:1613.

40. Millsap CM, Peyman GA, Mehta NJ, et al. Perfluoroperhydrophenanthrene (Vitreon) in the management of giant retinal tears: results of a collaborative study. *Ophthalmic Surg* 1993;24:759.

41. Mathis A, Pagot V, Gazagne C, Malecaze F. Giant retinal tears: surgical techniques and results using perfluorodecalin and silicone oil tamponade. *Retina* 1992;12:S7–S10.

42. Darmakusuma IE, Glaser BM, Sjaarda RN, et al. The use of perfluoro-octane in the management of giant retinal tears without proliferative vitreoretinopathy. *Retina* 1994;14:323.

43. Verstraeten T, Williams GA, Chang S, et al. Lens-sparing vitrectomy with perfluorocarbon liquid for the primary treatment of giant retinal tears. *Ophthalmology* 1995;102:17.

44. Kamei M, Tano Y, Maeno T, et al. Surgical removal of submacular hemorrhage using tissue plasminogen activator and perfluorocarbon liquid. *Am J Ophthalmol* 1996;121:267.

45. Desai UR, Peyman GA, Harper CA. Perfluorocarbon liquid in traumatic vitreous hemorrhage and retinal detachment. *Ophthalmic Surg* 1993;24:537.

46. Shapiro MJ, Resnick KI, Kim SH, Weinberg A. Management of dislocated crystalline lens with a perfluorocarbon liquid. *Am J Ophthalmol* 1991;112:401–405.

47. Movshovich A, Berrocal M, Chang S. The protective properties of liquid perfluorocarbons in phacofragmentation of dislocated lenses. *Retina* 1994;14:457–462.

48. Lewis H, Blumenkranz MS, Chang S. Treatment of dislocated crystalline lens and retinal detachment with perfluorocarbon liquids. *Retina* 1992;12:299.

49. Lewis H, Sanchez G. The use of perfluorocarbon liquids in the repositioning of posteriorly dislocated intraocular lenses. *Ophthalmology* 1993;100:1055.

50. Greve MD, Peyman GA, Mehta NJ, Millsap CM. Use of perfluoroperhydrophenanthrene in the management of posteriorly dislocated crystalline and intraocular lenses. *Ophthalmic Surg* 1993;24:593.

51. Manfre L, Fabbri G, Avitabile T, et al. MRI and intraocular tamponade media. *Neuroradiology (Germ)* 1993;35:359.

52. Berglin L, Ren J, Algvere PV. Retinal detachment and degeneration in response to subretinal perfluorodecalin in rabbit eyes. *Graefes Arch Clin Exp Ophthalmol* 1993;231:233.

53. de Queiroz JM, Blanks JC, Ozler SA, et al. Subretinal perfluorocarbon liquids. An experimental study. *Retina* 1992;12:S33.

54. Verma LK, Peyman GA, Wafapoor H, et al. An analysis of posterior segment complications after vitrectomy using the perfluorocarbon perfluoroperhydrophenanthrene (Vitreon). Vitreon Collaborative Study. *Ophthalmic Surg* 1995;26:29.

55. Sparrow JR, Matthews P, Iwamoto T, et al. Retinal tolerance to intravitreal perfluoroethylcyclohexane liquid in the rabbit. *Retina* 1993;13:56–62.

56. Foster RE, Smiddy WS, Alfonso EC, Parrish RK. Secondary glaucoma associated with retained perfluorophenanthrene. *Am J Ophthalmol* 1994;118:253.

57. Hasenfratz G, De La Torre M, Haigis W. Evaluation of eyes harbouring perfluorocarbon liquid with standardized ophthalmic echography. *Ger J Ophthalmol* 1994;3:19.

58. Wilson CA, Berkowitz BA, Hatchell DL. Oxygen kinetics in preretinal perfluorotributylamine. *Exp Eye Res* 1992;55:119.

59. Noske W, Gewiese B, Schilling A, et al. Detection and localization of perfluorodecalin in the human eye by fluorine 19 magnetic resonance. *Ger J Ophthalmol* 1993;2:207–211.

60. Gewiese BKO, Noske W, Schilling AM, et al. Human eye: visualization of perfluorodecalin with F-19 MR imaging. *Radiology* 1992;185:131.

61. De Juan E, McCuen B, Tiedeman J. Intraocular tamponade and surface tension. *Surv Ophthalmol* 1985;30:47.

62. Parver LM, Lincoff H. Geometry of intraocular gas used in retinal surgery. *Mod Probl Ophthalmol (Basel)* 1977;18:338.

63. Parver LM, Lincoff H. Mechanics of intraocular gas. *Invest Ophthalmol* 1978;17:77.

64. Hilton GF, Grizzard WS. Pneumatic retinopexy: a two-step outpatient operation without conjunctival incision. *Ophthalmology* 1986;93:626.

65. Chang S, Coleman JD, Lincoff H, Wilcox LM. Perfluoropropane gas in the management of proliferative vitreoretinopathy. *Am J Ophthalmol* 1984;98: 180.

66. Abrams GW, Edelhauser HF, Aaberg TM, Hamilton LH. Dynamics of intravitreal sulfur hexafluoride gas. *Invest Ophthalmol* 1974;13:863.

67. Lincoff A, Haft D, Liggett P, et al. Intravitreal expansion of perfluorocarbon bubbles. *Arch Ophthalmol* 1980;98:1646.

68. Peters MA, Abrams GW, Hamilton LH. The nonexpansile, equilibrated concentration of perfluoropropane gas in the eye. *Am J Ophthalmol* 1985;100:831.

69. Han DP, Abrams GW, Bennett SR, Williams DF. Perfluoropropane 12% versus 20%. Effect on intraocular pressure and gas tamponade after pars plana vitrectomy. *Retina* 1993;13:302.

70. Lincoff H, Maisel JM, Lincoff A. Intravitreal disappearance rates of four perfluorocarbon gases. *Arch Ophthalmol* 1984;102:928.

71. Thompson JT. Kinetics of intraocular gases. Disappearance of air, sulfur hexafluoride and perfluoropropane after pars plana vitrectomy. *Arch Ophthalmol* 1989;107:687.

72. Bloch D, O'Connor P, Lincoff H. The mechanism of cryosurgical adhesion. III. Statistical analysis. *Am J Ophthalmol* 1971;71:666.

73. Lincoff H, Kreissig I, Jakobiec F, Iwamoto T. Remodeling of the cryosurgical adhesion. *Arch Ophthalmol* 1981;99:1845.

74. Meyers SM, Ambler JS, Tan M, et al. Variation of perfluoropropane disappearance after vitrectomy. *Retina* 1992;12:359.

75. Wong RF, Thompson JT. Prediction of the kinetics of disappearance of sulfur hexafluoride and perfluoropropane. *Ophthalmology* 1988;95:609.

76. Lincoff H, Stergiu P, Smith R, Movshovich A. Longevity of expanding gases in vitrectomized eyes. *Retina* 1992;12:364.

77. Jacobs PM, Twomey JM, Leaver PK. Behavior of intraocular gases. *Eye* 1988;2:660.

78. Ai E, Gardner TW. Current patterns of intraocular gas use in North America. *Arch Ophthalmol* 1993;111:331.

79. Norton EWD. Intraocular gases in the management of selected retinal detachments. *Trans Am Acad Ophthalmol Otolaryngol* 1973;77:OP-85.

80. Fineberg E, Machemer R, Sullivan P, et al. Sulfur hexafluoride in owl monkey vitreous cavity. *Am J Ophthalmol* 1975;79:67.

81. Sabates WI, Abrams GW, Swanson DE, et al. The use of intraocular gases. The results of sulfur hexafluoride gas in retinal detachment surgery. *Ophthalmology* 1981;88:447.

82. Abrams GW, Swanson DE, Sabates WI. The results of sulful hexafluoride gas in vitreous surgery. *Am J Ophthalmol* 1982;94:165.

83. Lincoff H, Coleman J, Kreissig I, et al. The perfluorocarbon gases in the treatment of retinal detachment. *Ophthalmology* 1983;90:546.

84. Crittenden JJ, De Juan E Jr, Tiedeman J. Expansion of long-acting gas bubbles for intraocular use. Principles and practice. *Arch Ophthalmol* 1985;103:831.

85. Miller B, Lean J, Miller H, et al. Intravitreal expanding gas bubble: a morphologic study in the rabbit eye. *Arch Ophthalmol* 1984;102:1708.

86. Foulks GN, de Juan E, Hatchell DL. The effect of perfluoropropane on the cornea in rabbits and cats. *Arch Ophthalmol* 1987;105:256.

87. Lee DA, Wilson MR, Yoshizumi MO, Hall M. The ocular effects of gases when injected into the anterior chamber of rabbit eyes. *Arch Ophthalmol* 1991;109:571.

88. Vygantas CM, Peyman GA, Daily MJ, Ericson ES. Octafluorocyclobutane and other gases for vitreous replacement. *Arch Ophthalmol* 1973;90:235.

89. Killey FP, Edelhauser HF, Aaberg TM. Intraocular sulfur hexafluoride and octofluorocyclobutane. Effects on intraocular pressure and vitreous volume. *Arch Ophthalmol* 1978;96:511.

90. Lincoff A, Lincoff H, Iwamoto I, et al. Perfluoro-*n*-butane. A gas for a maximum duration retinal tamponade. *Arch Ophthalmol* 1983;101:460.

91. Chang S, Lincoff HA, Coleman DJ, et al. Perfluorocarbon gases in vitreous surgery. *Ophthalmology* 1985;92:651.

92. Hoffman ME, Sorr EM. Management of giant retinal tears without scleral buckling. *Retina* 1986;6:197.

93. Machemer R, Allen AW. Retinal tears 180° and greater: management with vitrectomy and intravitreal gas. *Arch Ophthalmol* 1976;94:1340.

94. Chang S. Intraocular gases. In: Ryan SJ, ed. *Retina*. Vol. 3. St. Louis: CV Mosby, 1989;245.

95. Lincoff H, Kreissig I, Coleman DJ, Chang S. Use of an intraocular gas tamponade to find retinal breaks. *Am J Ophthalmol* 1983;96:510.

96. Rubin JS, Thompson JT, Sjaarda RN, et al. Efficacy of fluid-air exchange during pars plana vitrectomy. *Retina* 1995;15:291.

97. Williams DF, Peter MA, Abrams GW, et al. A two-stage technique for intraoperative fluid-gas exchange following pars plana vitrectomy. *Arch Ophthalmol* 1990;108:1484.

98. Humayun MS, Yeo JH, Koski WS, et al. The rate of sulfur hexafluoride escape from a plastic syringe. *Arch Ophthalmol* 1989;107:853.

99. Gardner TW, Norris JL, Zakov ZN. A survey of intraocular gas use in North America. *Arch Ophthalmol* 1988;106:1188.

100. Trillo M, Facino M, Terrile R, et al. Treatment of uncomplicated cases of rhegmatogenous retinal detachment with an expanding gas bubble. *Ophthalmologica* 1993;207:140.

101. Duerksen JS, Oyakawa RT, Lemor M. A nationwide survey of the use of perfluoropropane and sulfur hexafluoride. *Am J Ophthalmol* 1989;108:195.

102. Blumenkranz M, Gardner T, Blankenship G. Fluid-gas exchange and photocoagulation after vitrectomy. *Arch Ophthalmol* 1986;104:291.

103. Bonnet M, Santamaria E, Mouche J. Intraoperative use of pure perfluoropropane gas in the management of proliferative vitreoretinopathy. *Graefes Arch Clin Exp Ophthalmol* 1987;225:299.

104. Aaberg TM. Management of anterior and posterior proliferative vitreoretinopathy. *Am J Ophthalmol* 1988;106:519.

105. Fisher YL, Shakin JL, Slakter JS, et al. Perfluoropropane gas, modified panretinal photocoagulation, and vitrectomy in the management of severe proliferative vitreoretinopathy. *Arch Ophthalmol* 1988;106:1255.

106. The Silicone Study Group. Vitrectomy with silicone oil or sulfur hexafluoride gas in eyes with severe proliferative vitreoretinopathy: results of a randomized clinical trial. Silicone Study Report 1. *Arch Ophthalmol* 1992;110:770.

107. McCuen BW, Azen SP, Stern W, et al. The Silicone Study Group: vitrectomy with silicone oil or perfluoropropane gas in eyes with severe proliferative vitreoretinopathy. Silicone Study Report 3. *Retina* 1993;13:279.

108. Thompson JT, Glaser BM, Sjaarda RN, et al. Effects of intraocular bubble duration in the treatment of macular holes by vitrectomy and transforming growth factor-beta 2. *Ophthalmology* 1994;101:1195.

109. Hilton GF. Pneumatic retinopexy and alternative techniques. In: Ryan SJ, ed. *Retina*. St. Louis: CV Mosby, 1989;225.

110. Aronowitz JD, Brubaker RF. Effect of intraocular gas on intraocular pressure. *Arch Ophthalmol* 1976;94:1191.

111. Poliner LS, Schoch LH. Intraocular pressure assessment in gas-filled eyes following vitrectomy. *Arch Ophthalmol* 1987;105:200.

112. Moses RA. Schiotz tonometry with an air bubble in the eye. *Am J Ophthalmol* 1966;62:281.

113. Sabates NR, Tolentino FI, Arroyo M, Freeman HM. The complications of perfluoropropane gas use in complex retinal detachments. *Retina* 1996;16:7.

114. Lincoff H, Mardirossian J, Lincoff A, et al. Intravitreal longevity of three perfluorocarbon gases. *Arch Ophthalmol* 1980;98:1610.

115. The Silicone Study Group. Vitrectomy with silicone oil or perfluoropropane gas in eyes with severe proliferative vitreoretinopathy: results of a randomized clinical trial. Silicone Study Report 2. *Arch Ophthalmol* 1992;110:780.

116. Abrams GW, Azen SP, Barr CC, et al. The Silicone Study Group: the incidence of corneal abnormalities in the Silicone Study. Silicone Study Report 7. *Arch Ophthalmol* 1995;113:764.

117. Lee DA, Wilson R, Yoshizumi MO, Hall M. The ocular effects of gases when injected into the anterior chamber of rabbit eyes. *Arch Ophthalmol* 1991;109:571.

118. Foulks GN, de Juan E, Hatchell DL, et al. The effect of perfluoropropane on the cornea in rabbits and cats. *Arch Ophthalmol* 1987;105:256.

119. Dieckert JP, O'Connor PS, Schacklett DE, et al. Air travel and intraocular gas. *Ophthalmology* 1986;93:L642.

120. Jackman SV, Thompson JT. Effects of hyperbaric exposure on eyes with intraocular gas bubbles. *Retina* 1995;15:160.

121. Lincoff H, Weinberger D, Reppucci V. Air travel with intraocular gas. I. The mechanisms for compensation. *Arch Ophthalmol* 1989;107:902.

122. Lincoff H, Weinberger D, Stergiu P. Air travel with intraocular gas. II. Clinical considerations. *Arch Ophthalmol* 1989;107:907.

123. Smith RB, Swartz M, Carl B. Effect of nitrous oxide on air in vitreous. *Am J Ophthalmol* 1974;78:314.

124. Wolf GL, Capuano C, Hartung J. Nitrous oxide increases intraocular pressure after intravitreal sulfur hexafluoride injection. *Anesthesiology* 1983;59:547.

125. Yamamoto K, Iwasaki T, Juzoji H, et al. Aqueous laser flaremetry following intravitreous gas injection in rabbits. *Invest Ophthalmol Vis Sci* 1990;31(Suppl):439.

126. Sparrow JR, Chang S, Vinals AF. Evaluation of the blood-aqueous barrier after vitreous replacement with perfluoropropane gas and liquid silicone. *Retina* 1992;12:370.

127. Ogura Y, Tsukada T, Negi A, et al. Integrity of the blood-ocular barrier after intravitreal gas injection. *Retina* 1989;9:199–202.

128. Constable IJ, Swann DA. Vitreous substitution with gases. *Arch Ophthalmol* 1975;93:416.

129. Wong RF, Liggett PE. Intraocular inflammation following intravitreal gas injection. *Invest Ophthalmol Vis Sci* 1990;31(Suppl):438.

130. Chang S, Lincoff H, Ozmert E, et al. Management of retinal detachment with moderate PVR. In: Freeman HM, Tolentino FI, eds. *Proliferative vitreoretinopathy*. New York: Springer-Verlag, 1988;54.

131. Lambrou FH, Burke JM, Aaberg MD. Effect of silicone oil on experimental traction retinal detachment. *Arch Ophthalmol* 1987;105:1269.

132. Lincoff H, Kreissig I, Jakobiec F. The inadvertent injection of gas beneath the retina in a pseudophakic eye. *Ophthalmology* 1986;93:408.

133. O'Connor PR. Intravitreous air injection and the custodis procedure. *Ophthalmol Surg* 1976;7:86.

134. Petersen J. The physical and surgical aspects of silicone oil in the vitreous cavity. *Graefes Arch Clin Exp Ophthalmol* 1987;225:452.

135. Parel J-M. Silicone oils: physicochemical properties. In: Ryan SJ, ed. *Retina*. St. Louis: CV Mosby, 1989:261.

136. Gonvers M. Temporary silicone oil tamponade in the treatment of complicated diabetic retinal detachments. *Graefes Arch Clin Exp Ophthalmol* 1990;228:415.

137. Lucke K, Laqua H. *Silicone oil in the treatment of complicated retinal detachments*. Berlin: Springer-Verlag, 1990.

138. Glaser BM, de Bustros S, Michels RG. Postoperative retinal breaks occurring after intravitreal silicone oil injection. *Retina* 1984;4:246.

139. Lewis H, Burke JM, Abrams GW. Perisilicone proliferation after vitrectomy for proliferative vitreoretinopathy. *Ophthalmology* 1988;95:583.

140. Machemer R. The importance of fluid absorption, traction, intraocular currents, and chorioretinal scars in the therapy of rhegmatogenous retinal detachments. *Am J Ophthalmol* 1984;98:681.

141. Lean JS. Use of silicone oil as an additional technique in vitreoretinal surgery. In: Ryan SJ, ed. *Retina*. St. Louis: CV Mosby, 1989:279–292.

142. Grey RHB, Leaver PK. Results of silicone oil injection in massive preretinal retraction. *Trans Ophthal Soc UK* 1977;97:238.

143. Grey RHB, Leaver PK. Silicone oil in the treatment of massive preretinal retraction. I. Results in 105 eyes. *Br J Ophthalmol* 1979;63:355.

144. Cairns JD, Anand N. Combined vitrectomy, intraocular microsurgery and liquid silicone in the treatment of proliferative vitreoretinopathy. *Aust J Ophthalmol* 1984;12:133.

145. Ando F, Miyake Y, Oshima K, et al. Temporary use of intraocular silicone in the treatment of complicated retinal detachment. *Graefes Arch Clin Exp Ophthalmol* 1985;224:32.

146. Cox MS, Trese MT, Murphy PL. Silicone oil for advanced proliferative vitreoretinopathy. *Ophthalmology* 1986;93:636.

147. Lean JS, Leaver PK, Cooling RJ. Management of complex retinal detachments by vitrectomy and fluid/silicone exchange. *Trans Ophthal Soc UK* 1982;102:203.

148. Lean JS, Van der Zee WAM, Ryan SJ. Experimental model of proliferative vitreoretinopathy (PVR) in the vitrectomised eye: effect of silicone oil. *Br J Ophthalmol* 1984;68:332.

149. Gonvers M. Temporary silicone oil tamponade in the management of retinal detachment with proliferative vitreoretinopathy. *Am J Ophthalmol* 1985;100:239.

150. Lucke KH, Foerster MH, Laqua H. Long-term results of vitrectomy and silicone oil in 500 cases of complicated retinal detachments. *Am J Ophthalmol* 1987;104:624.

151. Yeo JH, Glaser BM, Michels RG. Silicone oil in the treatment of complicated retinal detachment. *Ophthalmology* 1987;94:1109.

152. Sell CH, McCuen MW, Landers MB. Long-term results of successful vitrectomy with silicone oil for advanced proliferative vitreoretinopathy. *Am J Ophthalmol* 1987;103:24.

153. Leaver PK, Lean JS. Management of giant retinal tears using vitrectomy and silicone oil/fluid exchange. *Trans Ophthal Soc UK* 1981;101:189.

154. Billington BM, Leaver PK. Vitrectomy and fluid/silicone-oil exchange for giant retinal tears: results at 18 months. *Graefes Arch Clin Exp Ophthalmol* 1986;224:7.

155. Leaver PK, Cooling RJ, Feretis EB. Vitrectomy and fluid/silicone-oil exchange for giant retinal tears: results at six months. *Br J Ophthalmol* 1984;68:432.

156. Glaser BM. Treatment of giant retinal tears combined with proliferative vitreoretinopathy. *Ophthalmology* 1986;93:1193.

157. McLeod D. Silicone-oil injection during closed microsurgery for diabetic retinal detachment. *Graefes Arch Clin Exp Ophthalmol* 1986;224:55.

158. Rinkoff JS, de Juan E Jr, McCuen BW. Silicone oil for retinal detachment with advanced proliferative vitreoretinopathy following failed vitrectomy for proliferative diabetic retinopathy. *Am J Ophthalmol* 1986;101:181.

159. Iverson DA, Ward TG, Blumenkranz MS. Indications and results of relaxing retinotomy. *Ophthalmology* 1990;97:1298.

160. Ferrone PJ, McCuen BW, de Juan E, Machemer R. The efficacy of silicone oil for complicated retinal detachments in the pediatric population. *Arch Ophthalmol* 1994;112:773.

161. Antoszyk AN, McCuen BW, de Juan E Jr, et al. Silicone oil injection after failed primary vitreous surgery in severe ocular trauma. *Am J Ophthalmol* 1989;107:537.

162. McCuen BW, de Juan E, Machemer R. Silicone oil in vitreoretinal surgery. I. Surgical techniques. *Retina* 1985;5:189.

163. Heimann K, Dahl B, Dimopoulos S, et al. Pars plana vitrectomy and silicone oil injection in proliferative diabetic retinopathy. *Graefes Arch Clin Exp Ophthalmol* 1989;227:152.

164. Cockerham WD, Schepens CL, Freeman HM. Silicone injection in retinal detachment. *Arch Ophthalmol* 1970;83:704.

165. Haut J, Larricart JP, Van Effenterre G, Pinon-Pignero FL. Some of the most important properties of silicone oil to explain its action. *Ophthalmology (Basel)* 1985;191:150.

166. Abrams GW. Retinotomies and retinectomies. In: Ryan SJ, ed. *Retina*. St. Louis: CV Mosby, 1989:317.

167. Han DP, Lewis MT, Kuhn EM, et al. Relaxing retinotomies and retinectomies. Surgical results and predictors of visual outcome. *Arch Ophthalmol* 1990;108:694.

168. Morse LS, McCuen BW, Machemer R. Relaxing retinotomies: analysis of anatomic and visual results. *Ophthalmology* 1990;97:642.

169. Federman JL, Eagle RC. Extensive peripheral retinectomy combined with posterior 360° retinotomy for retinal reattachment in advanced proliferative vitreoretinopathy cases. *Ophthalmology* 1990;97:1305.

170. Blumenkranz MS, Azen SP, Aaberg T, et al. The Silicone Study Group: relaxing retinotomy with silicone oil or long-acting gas in eyes with severe proliferative vitreoretinopathy. Silicone Study Report 5. *Am J Ophthalmol* 1993;116:557.

171. Zauberman H, Hemo I. Silicone oil tamponade for retinal detachment and delayed treatment of retinal tears. *Ophthalmic Surg* 1993;24:600.

172. Scott JD. Use of liquid silicone in vitrectomized eyes. *Dev Ophthal* 1981;2:185.

173. Comaratta MR, Sparrow JS, Chang S. Iris neovascularization in proliferative vitreoretinopathy. *Ophthalmology* 1992;99:898.

174. De Juan E, Hardy M, Hatchell DL, Hatchell MC. The effect of intraocular silicone oil on anterior chamber oxygen pressure in cats. *Arch Ophthalmol* 1986;104:1063.

175. DeCorral LR, Peyman GA. Pars plana vitrectomy and intravitreal silicone oil injection in eyes with rubeosis iridis. *Can J Ophthalmol* 1986; 21:10.

176. Freeman WR, Henderly DE, Wan WL. Prevalence, pathophysiology and treatment of rhegmatogenous retinal detachment in treated cytomegalovirus retinitis. *Am J Ophthalmol* 1987;103:527.

177. Davis JL, Serfass MS, Lai M-Y, et al. Silicone oil in repair of retinal detachments caused by necrotizing retinitis in HIV infection. *Arch Ophthalmol* 1995;113:1401.

178. Nasemann JE, Mutsch A, Wiltfang R, Klauss V. Early pars plana vitrectomy without buckling procedure in cytomegalovirus retinitis-induced retinal detachment. *Retina* 1995;15:111.

179. Blumenkranz MS. The use of silicone oil for HIV-related retinal detachment. *Arch Ophthalmol* 1995;113:1366.

180. Machemer R. Massive periretinal proliferation: A logical approach to therapy. *Trans Am Ophth Soc* 1977;75:556.

181. Rachal WF, Burton TC. Changing concepts of failures after retinal detachment surgery. *Arch Ophthalmol* 1979;97:480.

182. Michels R. Surgery for retinal detachment with proliferative vitreoretinopathy. *Retina* 1984;4:63.

183. Watzke RC. Silicone retinopoiesis for retinal detachment. *Arch Ophthalmol* 1967;77:185.

184. Chan C, Okun E. The question of ocular tolerance to intravitreal liquid silicone. *Ophthalmology* 1986;93:651.

185. McCuen BW, de Juan E, Landers MB, et al. Silicone oil in vitreoretinal surgery. II. Results and complications. *Retina* 1985;5:198.

186. Tanji TM, Peyman GA, Mehta NJ, Millsap CM. Perfluoroperhydro-phenanthrene (Vitreon) as a short-term vitreous substitute after complex vitreoretinal surgery. *Ophthalmic Surg* 1993;24:681.

187. Sparrow JR, Jayakumar A, Berrocal M, et al. Experimental studies of the combined use of vitreous substitute materials of high and low specific gravity. *Retina* 1992;12:134–140.

188. Peyman GA, Conway MD, Soike KF, Clark LC. Long-term vitreous replacement in primates with intravitreal vitreon or vitreon plus silicone. *Ophthalmic Surg* 1991;22:657.

189. Wiedemann P, Leinung C, Hilgers R-D, Heimann K. Daunomycin and silicone oil for the treatment of proliferative vitreoretinopathy. *Graefes Arch Clin Exp Ophthalmol* 1991;229:150.

190. Arroyo MH, Refojo MF, Araiz JJ, et al. Silicone oil as a delivery vehicle for BCNU in rabbit proliferative vitreoretinopathy. *Retina* 1993;13:245.

191. Nakagawa M, Refojo MF, Marin JF, et al. Retinoic acid in silicone and silicone-fluorosilicone copolymer oils in a rabbit model of proliferative vitreoretinopathy. *Invest Ophthalmol Vis Sci* 1995;36:2388.

192. Araiz JJ, Refojo MF, Arroyo MH, et al. Antiproliferative effect of retinoic acid in intravitreal silicone oil in an animal model of proliferative vitreoretinopathy. *Invest Ophthalmol Vis Sci* 1993;34:522.

193. Zilis JD, McCuen BW, de Juan E Jr, et al. Results of silicone oil removal in advanced proliferative vitreoretinopathy. *Am J Ophthalmol* 1989;108:15.

194. Hutton WL, Azen SP, Blumenkranz MS, et al. The Silicone Study Group: the effects of silicone oil removal. Silicone Study Report 6. *Arch Ophthalmol* 1994;112:778.

195. Van Meurs JC, Mertens DAE, Peperkamp E, Post J. Five-year results of vitrectomy and silicone oil in patients with proliferative vitreoretinopathy. *Retina* 1993;13:285.

196. Kampik A, Hoing C, Heidenkummer H-P. Problems and timing in the removal of silicone oil. *Retina* 1992;12:S11.

197. Zivojnovic R. *Silicone oil in vitreoretinal surgery*. Dordrecht, The Netherlands: Martinus Nihjoff/Dr W. Junk Publishers, 1987.

198. McCuen BW, Landers MB, Machemer R. The use of silicone oil following failed vitrectomy for retinal detachment with advanced proliferative vitreoretinopathy. *Ophthalmology* 1985;92:1029.

199. Hutton WL, Fuller DW, Snyder WB. Silicone oil for management of PVR: comparison of six-month and two-year results. In: Freeman HM, Tolentino FI, eds. *Proliferative vitreoretinopathy*. New York: Springer-Verlag, 1988:166.

200. Ando F. Usefulness and limit of silicone oil in the management of complicated retinal detachment. *Jpn J Ophthalmol* 1987;31:138.

201. Federman JL, Schubert HD. Complications associated with the use of silicone oil in 150 eyes after retina-vitreous surgery. *Ophthalmology* 1988;95:870.

202. Fletcher ME, Peyman GA. A simplified technique for the removal of liquid silicone from vitrectomized eyes. *Retina* 1985;5:168.

203. Fan RFT, Chung H, Tolentino FI, et al. Effectiveness of silicone oil removal from rabbit eyes. *Graefes Arch Clin Exp Ophthalmol* 1987;225:338.

204. Gabel V-P, Kampik A, Burkhardt J. Analysis of intraocularly applied silicone oils of various origins. *Graefes Arch Clin Exp Ophthalmol* 1987;225:160.

205. Crisp A, de Juan E, Tiedeman J. Effect of silicone oil viscosity on emulsification. *Arch Ophthalmol* 1987;105:546.

206. Kreiner CF. Chemical and physical aspects of clinically applied silicones. *Dev Ophthalmol* 1987;14:11.

207. Heidenkummer H-P, Kampik A, Thierfelder S. Emulsification of silicone oils with specific physicochemical characteristics. *Graefes Arch Clin Exp Ophthalmol* 1991;229:88.

208. Petersen J, Ritzau-Tondrow U. Chronisches Glaukom nach Silikonolimplantation: Zwei Ole verschiedener viskositat im vergleich. *Fortschr Ophthalmol* 1988;85:632.

209. Sternberg P, Hatchell DL, Foulks GN. The effect of silicone oil on the cornea. *Arch Ophthalmol* 1985;103:90.

210. Ando F. Intraocular hypertension resulting from pupillary block by silicone oil. *Am J Ophthalmol* 1985;99:87.

211. Madreperla SA, McCuen BW. Inferior peripheral iridectomy in patients receiving silicone oil. Rates of postoperative closure and effect on oil position. *Retina* 1995;15:87.

212. MacCumber MW, McCuen BW, Toth CA, et al. Tissue plasminogen activator for preserving inferior peripheral iridectomy patency in eyes with silicone oil. *Ophthalmology* 1996;103:269.

213. Heimann K, Konen W. Artificial iris diaphragm and silicone oil surgery. *Retina* 1992;12:S90.

214. Leaver PK. Complications of intraocular silicone oil. In: Ryan SJ, ed. *Retina*. St. Louis: CV Mosby, 1989:293–306.

215. Barr CC, Lai MY, Lean JS, et al. The Silicone Study Group: postoperative intraocular pressure abnormalities in the silicone study. Silicone Study Report 4. *Ophthalmology* 1993;100:1629.

216. Valone J Jr, McCarthy M. Emulsified anterior chamber silicone oil and glaucoma. *Ophthalmology* 1994;101:1908.

217. Savion N, Alhalel A, Treister G, Bartov E. Role of blood components in ocular silicone oil emulsification. Studies on an in vitro model. *Invest Ophthalmol Vis Sci* 1996;37:2694.

218. Bartov E, Pennarola F, Savion N, et al. A quantitative *in vitro* model for silicone oil emulsification. Role of blood constituents. *Retina* 1992;12:S23–S27.

Principles of Giant Retinal Tears and Treatment

Timothy W. Olsen   T. Michael Nork

ETIOLOGY AND PATHOPHYSIOLOGY

Definition of a Giant Retinal Tear

A giant retinal tear is defined as a retinal break that extends 90 degrees or more around the circumference of the fundus (1,2). Scott (3) proposed that tears extending more than 180 degrees with the vitreous gel detached from the posterior lip of the torn retina may be a more accurate definition. This latter definition emphasizes mobility of the posterior retinal edge independent of the anterior edge. Traditionally, such a large size and mobility placed these tears in a distinct category of those that were particularly difficult to treat. However, with modern treatment methods, the more inclusive definition of any tear extending more than 90 degrees seems most appropriate.

A giant retinal tear posterior to the insertion of the vitreous base will result in an unsupported torn posterior edge. In eyes with media opacities or vitreous hemorrhage, echography may be useful to diagnose a giant retinal tear. Because there is no vitreous support of the posterior edge, the retina can fold over, as shown in Figure 45-1. This folding or retinal apposition is often evident on ultrasound scans (4), and sometimes involves only the anterior edge of the posterior flap, an effect seen with early proliferative vitreoretinopathy (PVR). This has also been termed a *rolled edge*.

Dialysis

A retinal dialysis (Fig. 45-2) is a subcategory of giant retinal tears. Tractional forces at the vitreous base can result in a dialysis or a tearing of the retina at the ora serrata. Smiddy and Green (5) examined the histopathology of 103 eyes with retinal dialysis. They reported that a dialysis generally consists of an avulsion of the vitreous base with a retinal tear at or very near the ora serrata, with a smooth-edged termination of retina visibly attached to the vitreous base (6). The break may occur in the ciliary epithelium, which histopathologically can be seen to be adherent to the detached edge of retina. Spontaneous healing may occur, as hyperplasia of the retinal pigment epithelium or of the ciliary epithelium is able to create some degree of chorioretinal adhesion. Retinal macrocysts are a secondary feature of chronic detachments and are occasionally seen in areas of detached retina separated from the edge of the dialysis. Marcus and Aaberg (7) recommended the occasional need to drain these cysts while Hagler (8) believed that they will disappear on their own following reattachment.

Specific Causes of Giant Retinal Tears

Giant retinal tears are commonly associated with blunt trauma. In a review of 100 giant retinal tears (94 patients) (9), 22 eyes had a history of nonsurgical trauma consisting of either ocular contusion (20) or ocular penetration (2). Most traumatic giant retinal tears (74%) occurred in young males (median age, 17 years) and none of the traumatic tears were bilateral, as compared to 8% that were bilateral in the nontraumatic group. In addition, traumatic giant retinal tears were not as highly associated with myopia as were nontraumatic giant retinal tears (30% versus 71%, respectively). Also, a higher percentage of traumatic giant retinal tears compared to the nontraumatic tears (30% versus 13%, respectively) extended more than 180 degrees.

Aylward et al (10) described their results in the surgical management of traumatically induced retinal detachments associated with giant retinal tears. In a retrospective review of 38 patients over a 10-year period seen at Moorfield's Eye Hospital, approximately 25% of the giant retinal tears were associated with trauma, and these generally occurred in

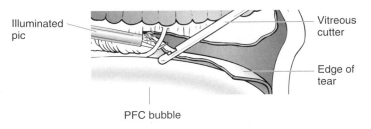

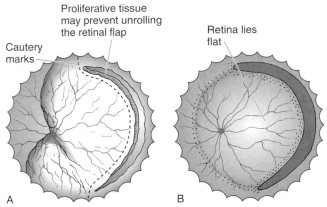

FIGURE 45-12. *Bimanual dissection technique of the vitreous base. An illuminated pick and the vitrectomy cutter are used to dissect the vitreous from the torn edge of retina. PFC = perfluorocarbon liquid.*

FIGURE 45-14. A. *If the edges of the tear cannot be unfolded and do not lie flat because of proliferative vitreoretinopathy, a retinectomy may be performed. This will also provide a more stable configuration to the apices of the tear. A border of normal retina just posterior to the rolled edge is cauterized as shown. The vitrectomy cutter or intraocular scissors are then used to excise the demarcated retina. B. Postretinectomy diagram with laser at the border is shown. The posterior edge of the tear is supported by an encircling scleral buckle.*

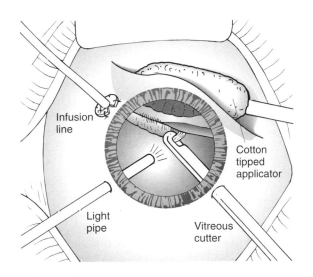

FIGURE 45-13. *External depression by either the assistant or the surgeon facilitates maximal vitreous dissection. The vitreous base is "shaved" as closely as possible to prevent future contraction with extension of the tear.*

vitrectomy cutter. Intraocular cautery is unnecessary because this tissue has been separated from the retinal circulation and will not bleed unless neovascularization is present. Failure to remove the anterior flap of retina may complicate the postoperative course. This tissue remains firmly adherent to the vitreous base and may serve as scaffolding for anterior PVR. The anterior flap may fold anteriorly over the ciliary processes and even to the posterior iris. Additionally, traction may be exerted toward the apices of the retinal tear, resulting in its extension. Such anterior proliferation may subsequently lead to ciliary body detachment and postoperative hypotony.

The configuration of the torn posterior retinal edge needs to be assessed. Retinectomy of the posterior part of the retina should be performed if the configuration of the tear appears unstable. The best configuration is when the ends of the tear extend toward the ora serrata in a gradual

arc or a "smile" appearance with a smooth posterior edge (Fig. 45-14). This profile will decrease the stress at the apices of the tear and minimizes the potential for future contraction to extend the tear. Another indication for retinectomy of the posterior edge of a giant retinal tear includes the presence of proliferative tissue at the torn retina that retinal reapposition to the choroid. After removal of as much of the proliferative tissue as possible, the remaining edge of the tear is delineated with intraocular cautery and carefully excised with the vitrectomy cutter. Again, low vacuum and a high cutting rate will minimize the risk of engaging viable retinal tissue posterior to the cauterized demarcation line. Alternatively, retinal scissors can be used to excise the demarcated anterior retina. Injecting PFC liquid to elevate the meniscal edge to the line of retinal cautery will stabilize the posterior part of the retina. Filling the eye with PFC liquid at this point is unnecessary and may cause difficulties with visualization during the fluid-air exchange.

Establishing a Chorioretinal Adhesion
The PFC liquid should be instilled with the eye rotated so that the posterior extent of the giant tear is in a nondependent position (Fig. 45-15). This will ensure that much of the anterior subretinal fluid is forced through the tear. Caution should be used to prevent excursion of PFC liquid into the subretinal space. Slow infusion of the liquid and slow deliberate rotations of the globe should minimize this complication. If the PFC level is elevated to the infusion cannula, multiple smaller PFC bubbles may form and are more likely to pass into the subretinal space or become

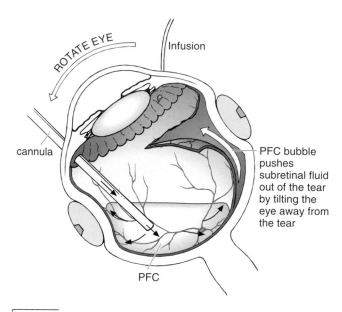

FIGURE 45-15. *Additional perfluorocarbon (PFC) liquid is added with the tear in the nondependent (uppermost) position. This forces subretinal fluid anteriorly, with a majority of the fluid through the tear. Some subretinal fluid still remains anterior to the PFC liquid away from the retinal tear.*

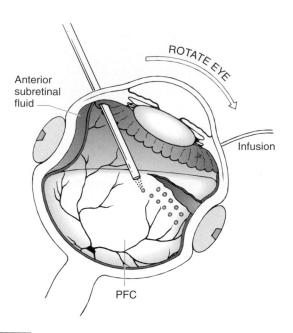

FIGURE 45-16. *The globe is then rotated so that the tear is covered by perfluorocarbon (PFC) liquid. This allows for retinal apposition to the retinal pigment epithelium and endophotocoagulation along the borders of the tear. The treatment is usually extended for 360 degrees along the scleral buckle. Several rows of laser are usually sufficient.*

trapped within more anterior structures. The tear is then rotated to a dependent position and endophotocoagulation is performed using the argon or diode laser under the tamponade of the PFC (Fig. 45-16). The main risk during endophotocoagulation is "lens touch" if a lens-sparing technique is employed. Either gently bending a straight endophotocoagulator probe or using a curved probe will lessen the chance of lens touch. Endophotocoagulation is extended 360 degrees along the scleral buckle, three to five rows wide, and spaced approximately one burn width apart. This effectively creates a symmetric, circumferential, chorioretinal adhesion. Alternatively, indirect photocoagulation or even cryotherapy may be employed to create a chorioretinal adhesion. The disadvantages of cryotherapy include the difficulty of application when a large scleral buckle has been sewn into place, and the increased risk of PVR. During peripheral retinal maneuvers, slow and deliberate scleral depression should be employed to prevent the generation of small PFC droplets that may migrate into the subretinal space. Another option would be to proceed with the fluid-gas exchange and create the chorioretinal adhesion in a gas- or silicone oil–filled eye. Visualization during endophotocoagulation may become more difficult in this situation, especially in a phakic or pseudophakic eye; therefore, most of the laser treatment or cryotherapy should be performed prior to the air-fluid exchange. Endophotocoagulation under the PFC liquid may also decrease the chance of posterior retinal slippage during the fluid-air exchange.

Silicone intraocular lenses create a unique adhesion with silicone oil that can limit vision as well as surgical visual-

ization (46). Condensation can also dramatically interfere with the intraoperative visualization during air-fluid exchanges in eyes with silicone lenses (47,48). Removal of these lenses is occasionally required to allow adequate visualization.

Fluid-Gas Exchange

Some residual subretinal fluid located anterior to the PFC liquid is still present at this point in the eye unless a complete (360-degree) giant retinal tear is present. This fluid becomes trapped under the retina and may dissect anteriorly, detaching the pars plana. Anterior fluid needs to be carefully addressed or it will result in posterior "slippage" of the attached retina. The fluid-gas exchange requires patience and meticulous attention toward the eye position, the fluid meniscus, and the PFC level.

Two alternative forms of secondary tamponade may be used. Silicone oil or air both "float" and will tamponade from an anterior to posterior direction. A fluid-air exchange is the most commonly used secondary tamponade. Alternatively, silicone oil may be infused using specialized silicone-oil infusion tubing that should be sutured in place at the beginning of the procedure. With a trochar cannula infusion system, silicone-oil tubing may be exchanged for the standard fluid infusion.

Infusion of the secondary tamponade should begin with the posterior-most edge of the retinal tear in a dependent position (Fig. 45-17). The surgeon uses passive or gentle-

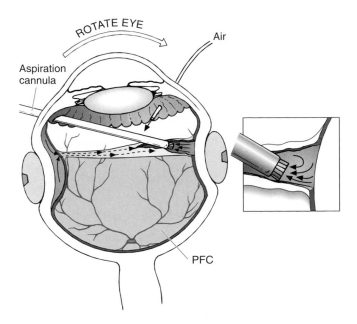

ROTATE EYE

Air

Aspiration cannula

PFC

FIGURE 45-17. *An air-fluid exchange will force the anterior subretinal fluid posterior in a circumferential manner. The fluid is removed at the posterior edge of the giant tear. Perfluorocarbon (PFC) liquid restricts the fluid from the posterior subretinal space. The PFC liquid and air-menisci create a triangular area of fluid. This is slowly and meticulously aspirated using a soft-tip extrusion cannula.*

active aspiration with a soft, silicone-tipped extrusion needle to remove anterior fluid and PFC liquid until the interface rests at the level of the posterior-most edge of the retinal tear. Subretinal fluid is forced out of the subretinal space anteriorly but is still restricted from progressing posteriorly by the remaining PFC. The fluid must then settle in the most dependent region, which is at a level circumferential with the PFC meniscus. Rotating the globe in any direction other than that maintaining the posterior edge of the tear in the most dependent position may trap fluid in a subretinal location. The tamponade provided by the PFC liquid prevents slippage at this point. The surgeon should patiently wait and aspirate the subretinal fluid meniscus from the edge of the retinal tear as it slowly pools in this location. A silicone-tipped extrusion cannula can be used for this maneuver (see Fig. 45-17). If one proceeds too quickly to a complete air-fluid exchange, the residual subretinal fluid will migrate toward the optic nerve in the subretinal space, and the entire retina will slip posteriorly. When the surgeon no longer sees a meniscus of fluid at the air-PFC interface (usually requires approximately 15 minutes of patient aspiration), a complete fluid-air or fluid-oil exchange may be performed.

If fluid dissects posteriorly causing slippage of the retina, the surgeon should reassess the anatomy of the tear and ensure that the subretinal fluid is aspirated at the posterior-most aspect of the tear. To address slippage, several options are available. If there is a minimal amount of posterior fluid

with minimal slippage, postoperative prone positioning with internal tamponade may be sufficient. Should a substantial amount of fluid dissect posteriorly, a posterior drainage retinotomy may be created to remove the fluid. A soft-tipped silicone cannula may be used to gently manipulate the slipped posterior edge of the giant tear anteriorly. Another option would be to return to a fluid-filled eye, reinject PFC liquid, and repeat the fluid-gas exchange procedure. Additional endophotocoagulation may be required after a complete air-fluid exchange.

After the PFC liquid is removed from over the optic nerve, several drops of balanced salt solution should be gently instilled and aspirated to rinse residual PFC liquid droplets. This can be repeated as necessary. A blunt cannula should be used to instill the balanced salt solution. Simply opening the infusion line to the balanced salt solution from an elevated infusion bottle to rinse the PFC is extremely dangerous. A "jet stream" of fluid can easily dislodge a delicately replaced edge of the giant retinal tear.

Retinal Tamponade

The choice of postoperative retinal tamponade in a giant retinal tear depends on several factors. While both perfluoropropane (C_3F_8) gas and silicone oil are equally efficacious for this purpose (49), there are advantages and disadvantages to each. A nonexpansile concentration of C_3F_8 gas (16%) will provide effective short-term tamponade that does not require a secondary procedure for removal. Situations when silicone oil is the preferred tamponade include the following: 1) when prompt visual rehabilitation is necessary such as in a monocular patient, 2) for reoperations, 3) for extensive PVR, 4) when high-altitude travel is necessary, 5) for small children or patients who have difficulty with positioning, 6) for large inferior tears, or 7) when postoperative hypotony is a concern.

If the patient is left aphakic, the surgeon should always remember to perform an inferior peripheral iridectomy to prevent oil-induced pupillary block. If the pupil is widely dilated, end-grasping forceps are used to grasp the inferior iris border and gently pull it centrally. The vitrectomy cutter is then placed in aspiration mode, and a circular section of peripheral iris is engaged into the port. Briefly engaging the vitreous cutter will form a circular inferior iridectomy.

Lenticular Status

As mentioned already, meticulous dissection of the anterior vitreous base necessitates good peripheral visualization and instrumentation. Under no circumstances should a "lens-sparing" technique be employed if the result is failure to relieve traction along the giant retinal tear and anterior vitreous base. The primary surgical goal of giant retinal tear repair is to reappose the retina in a single procedure and minimize the subsequent risk of recurrence. Lenticular status is secondary and the risk of postvitrectomy cataract formation is high.

If the lens is removed prior to the vitrectomy using a pars plana fragmatome, caution should be exercised to avoid dropping lens fragments posteriorly. With an unsupported giant retinal tear, posterior lens fragments may fall into the subretinal space. For this reason, it is safest to perform the initial core vitrectomy with instillation of PFC liquid prior to lens fragmentation. Lens particles falling posteriorly are then less likely to become trapped subretinally. Use of the fragmatome in the posterior segment of an eye with a giant retinal tear, prior to instillation of the PFC, should be avoided. Mobile retina may be engaged by the unprotected tip of the fragmatome. An anterior-approach phacoemulsification procedure through a small incision is preferable. Extracapsular techniques may also be used as long as the wound is adequately sealed for the vitrectomy. A shelved, self-sealing wound construction and proper closure with 10-0 nylon will avoid leakage from the anterior wound during the vitrectomy. Anterior extracapsular techniques may allow for preservation of the capsular bag for ideal lens placement.

CONCLUSIONS

Innovation in vitreoretinal surgery is exemplified in the repair of the giant retinal tear. In the not-so-distant past, repair of this entity was largely unsuccessful, frought with complications, and confined to only a few centers. Today, this still represents a challenging surgical situation, but ophthalmologists are better equipped to deal with the complex technical situations that arise during the repair of a giant retinal tear. Thanks to the innovative technical advancements made by the investigators in the field of vitreoretinal surgery, the prognosis for this condition has dramatically improved.

ACKNOWLEDGMENT

Financial support was provided by the Heed/Knapp Ophthalmic Foundation Fellowship Award (to Dr Olsen).

REFERENCES

1. Fung WE, Norton EW. The use of intravitreal air for the therapy of giant retinal tears. *Trans Pacif Coast Otoophthalmol Soc* 1969;50:59–65.
2. Freeman HM, Schepens CL, Couvillion GC. Current management of giant retinal breaks. II. *Trans Am Acad Ophthalmol Otolaryngol* 1970;74:59–74.
3. Scott JD. Giant retinal tears. *Mod Probl Ophthalmol* 1979;20:275–278.
4. Jalkh AE, Jabbour N, Avila MP, et al. Ultrasonographic findings in eyes with giant retinal tears and opaque media. *Retina* 1983;3:154–158.
5. Smiddy WE, Green WR. Retinal dialysis: pathology and pathogenesis. *Retina* 1982;2:94–116.
6. Green WR. Retina. In: Spencer WH, ed. *Ophthalmic pathology. An atlas and textbook*. Vol. 2. Philadelphia: WB Saunders, 1996.
7. Marcus DF, Aaberg TM. Intraretinal macrocysts in retinal detachment. *Arch Ophthalmol* 1979;97:1273–1275.
8. Hagler WS. Retinal dialysis; a statistical and genetic study to determine pathogenic factors. *Trans Am Ophthalmol Soc* 1980;78:686–733.
9. Kanski JJ. Giant retinal tears. *Am J Ophthalmol* 1975;79:846–852.
10. Aylward GW, Cooling RJ, Leaver PK. Trauma-induced retinal detachment associated with giant retinal tears. *Retina* 1993;13:136–141.
11. McLeod D. Giant retinal tears after central vitrectomy. *Br J Ophthalmol* 1985;69:96–98.
12. Freeman HM. Fellow eyes of giant retinal breaks. *Mod Probl Ophthalmol* 1979;20:267–274.
13. Norton EW, Aaberg T, Fung W, Curtin VT. Giant retinal tears. I. Clinical management with intravitreal air. *Am J Ophthalmol* 1969;68:1011–1021.
14. Scott JD. Congenital myopia and retinal detachment. *Trans Ophthalmol Soc UK* 1980;100:69–71.
15. Dowler JG, Lyons CJ, Cooling RJ. Retinal detachment and giant retinal tears in aniridia. *Eye* 1995;9:268–270.
16. Topilow HW, Nussbaum JJ, Freeman HM, et al. Bilateral acute retinal necrosis. Clinical and ultrastructural study. *Arch Ophthalmol* 1982;100:1901–1908.
17. Hovland KR, Schepens CL, Freeman HM. Developmental giant retinal tears associated with lens coloboma. *Arch Ophthalmol* 1968;80:325–331.
18. Johnston ME, Gonder JR. Giant retinal tears, retinal detachment and retinitis pigmentosa. *Can J Ophthalmol* 1985;20:16–18.
19. Witmer R. Giant retinal tears in retrolental fibroplasia and Marfan's syndrome. *Mod Probl Ophthalmol* 1979;20:279–281.
20. Trevor-Roper PD. Transvitreal diathermy. *Trans Ophthalmol Soc UK* 1960;80:543–550.
21. Ando F, Kondo J. A plastic tack for the treatment of retinal detachment with giant tear. *Am J Ophthalmol* 1983;95:260–261.
22. Usui M, Hamazaki S, Takano S, Matsu H. A new surgical treatment of retinal detachment with giant tear: transvitreoretinal fixation. *Am J Ophthalmol* 1979;95:206–215.
23. Hirose T, Schepens CL, Lopansri C. Subtotal open-sky vitrectomy for severe retinal detachment occurring as a late complication of ocular trauma. *Ophthalmology* 1981;88:1–9.
24. Nishi O, Ideta H. A new suturing method for the treatment of giant retinal tear. *Ophthalmic Surg* 1987;18:359–362.
25. Federman JL, Shakin JL, Lanning RC. The microsurgical management of giant retinal tears with trans-scleral retinal sutures. *Ophthalmology* 1982;89:832–839.
26. Faulborn J. Treatment of giant retinal tears after perforating injuries with vitrectomy and a cyanoacrylate tissue adhesive. *Adv Ophthalmol* 1976;33:204–207.
27. Lobel D, Hale JR, Montgomery DB. A new magnetic technique for the treatment of giant retinal tears. *Am J Ophthalmol* 1978;85:699–703.
28. Trese MT. An inexpensive bed for giant retinal tear surgery. *Am J Ophthalmol* 1982;1982:525.
29. Meyers SM, Cassen JH, Orlowski JP, Krupp NE. Postoperative positioning with a circular electric bed for a giant retinal tear in a retarded patient. *Am J Ophthalmol* 1984;98:816–817.
30. Peyman GA, Rednam KR, Seetner AA. Retinal microincarceration with penetrating diathermy in the management of giant retinal tears. *Arch Ophthalmol* 1984;102:562–565.
31. Irvine AR, Lahey JM. Pneumatic retinopexy for giant retinal tears. *Ophthalmology* 1994;101:524–528.
32. Joondeph BC, Flynn HW Jr, Blankenship GW, et al. The surgical management of giant retinal tears with the cannulated extrusion needle. *Am J Ophthalmol* 1989;108:548–553.
33. Machemer R, Allen AW. Retinal tears 180 degrees and greater. Management with vitrectomy and intravitreal gas. *Arch Ophthalmol* 1976;94:1340–1346.
34. Vidaurri-Leal J, de Bustros S, Michels RG. Surgical treatment of giant retinal tears with inverted posterior retinal flaps. *Am J Ophthalmol* 1984;98:463–466.
35. Leaver PK, Cooling RJ, Feretis EB, et al. Vitrectomy and fluid/silicone-oil exchange for giant retinal tears: results at six months. *Br J Ophthalmol* 1984;68:432–438.
36. Glaser BM. Treatment of giant retinal tears combined with proliferative vitreoretinopathy. *Ophthalmology* 1986;93:1193–1197.
37. Brown GC, Benson WE. Use of sodium hyaluronate for the repair of giant retinal tears. *Arch Ophthalmol* 1989;107:1246–1249.
38. Chang S, Lincoff H, Zimmerman NJ, Fuchs W. Giant retinal tears. Surgical techniques and results using perfluorocarbon liquids. *Arch Ophthalmol* 1989;107:761–766.
39. Verstraeten T, Williams GA, Chang S, et al. Lens-sparing vitrectomy with perfluorocarbon liquid for the primary treatment of giant retinal tears. *Ophthalmology* 1995;102:17–20.
40. Chang S. Low viscosity liquid fluorochemicals in vitreous surgery. *Am J Ophthalmol* 1987;103:38–43.
41. Nabih M, Peyman GA, Clark LC Jr, et al. Experimental evaluation of perfluorophenanthrene as a high specific gravity vitreous substitute: a preliminary report. *Ophthalmic Surg* 1989;20:286–293.

42. Campochiaro PA, Kaden IH, Vidaurri-Leal J, Glaser BM. Cryotherapy enhances intravitreal dispersion of viable retinal pigment epithelial cells. *Arch Ophthalmol* 1985;103:434–436.

43. Glaser BM, Vidaurri-Leal J, Michels RG, Campochiaro PA. Cryotherapy during surgery for giant retinal tears and intravitreal dispersion of viable retinal pigment epithelial cells. *Ophthalmology* 1993;100:466–470.

44. Kreiger AE, Lewis H. Management of giant retinal tears without scleral buckling. Use of radical dissection of the vitreous base and perfluoro-octane and intraocular tamponade. *Ophthalmology* 1992;99:491–497.

45. Mathis A, Pagot V, Heldenbergh O, et al. Treatment of giant retinal tears in phakic patients without lens removal or scleral buckling. *XIXth meeting of the Club Jules Gonin* 1994;51. Abstract.

46. Apple DJ, Federman JL, Krolicki TJ, et al. Irreversible silicone oil adhesion to silicone intraocular lenses. *Ophthalmology* 1996;103:1555–1561.

47. Slusher MM, Seaton AD. Loss of visibility caused by moisture condensation on the posterior surface of a silicone intraocular lens during fluid/gas exchange after posterior vitrectomy. *Am J Ophthalmol* 1994;118:667. Letter.

48. Eaton AM, Jaffe GJ, McCuen BW II, Mincey GJ. Condensation on the posterior surface of silicone intraocular lenses during fluid-air exchange. *Ophthalmology* 1995;102:733–736.

49. Group TSOS. Vitrectomy with silicone oil or perfluoropropane gas in eyes with severe proliferative vitreoretinopathy: results of a randomized clinical trial. Silicone Study Report 2. *Arch Ophthalmol* 1992;110:780–792.

Diabetic Retinopathy

SURESH R. CHANDRA   PIK SHA T. CHAN

Diabetic retinopathy is a retinovascular occlusive disease resulting in abnormal retinal vascular permeability, non-perfusion, new-vessel formation, and fibrous proliferation. It is the leading cause of blindness in the 20- to 74-year age group in the United States. Diabetes mellitus currently affects over 7 million Americans, with an additional 7 million remaining undiagnosed.

EPIDEMIOLOGY

Population-based studies have shown that macular edema and proliferative diabetic retinopathy (PDR) are the primary causes for visual loss in type II (adult-onset) and type I (juvenile-onset) diabetics, respectively. Klein et al (1) reported that the prevalence of retinopathy in juvenile-onset diabetic patients rose from 2% in those with diabetes of less than 2 years' duration to 97.5% in those with diabetes for 15 years or longer. In the adult-onset non-insulin-taking diabetic group, the prevalence of retinopathy rose from 23% in persons who had diabetes for less than 2 years to 57.5% in persons with the disease for 15 years or more. In the adult-onset insulin-taking group, the prevalence of retinopathy rose from 30% for those with diabetes of less than 2 years to 84.5% in those who had it for 15 years or more (2). The prevalence of PDR in the juvenile-onset diabetic group varied from 0% in those who had the disease for fewer than 5 years to 4% in those with the disease for 10 years, 25% with diabetes for 15 years, and 56% in persons with the disease for 20 years (1). The prevalence of PDR in the adult-onset non-insulin-taking group rose from 3% in persons with diabetes for 2 years or less to 4.3% in persons with diabetes for 15 years or more, and in the adult-onset insulin-taking group, the prevalence of PDR was 4% in

those with diabetes for 3 or 4 years and 20.1% in those with diabetes for 15 years or more (2).

Klein et al (3) also reported an increasing frequency of macular edema with increasing duration of diabetes in both juvenile-onset and adult-onset diabetic patients. The prevalence of macular edema in the juvenile-onset diabetic group was 0% in those with diabetes for less than 5 years and 29% in those with diabetes for more than 20 years. The prevalence of macular edema in the adult-onset non-insulin-taking group rose from 3% for those with diabetes for less than 5 years to 28% for those with the disease for more than 20 years. In the adult-onset insulin-taking group, the prevalence of macular edema was 4% in those with diabetes less than 5 years and 35% in those with the disease for more than 20 years.

CLINICAL FEATURES

The two stages of diabetic retinopathy are non-PDR (NPDR) and PDR. Mild NPDR presents with micro-aneurysms, retinal hemorrhages, hard exudates, and soft exudates. Abnormal vascular permeability of serous fluid and lipoproteins from microaneurysms and microvascular abnormalities results in retinal thickening and hard exudates. Hard exudates may be confluent and form circinate rings around leaking microaneurysms and can encroach on the center of the macula, resulting in a decrease in central vision. Any retinal thickening alone or together with hard exudates that involves or threatens the center of the macula is termed *clinically significant macular edema* (CSME). The Early Treatment Diabetic Retinopathy Study (ETDRS) defined CSME as 1) retinal thickening at or within 500 μm of the foveal center, 2) hard exudates within 500 μm of the foveal center when accompanied by retinal thickening, or 3) an area of thickening of at least one disk area located within one disk diameter of the foveal center (4). Fluorescein angiography provides useful information regarding the retinal circulation and vasculature and is beneficial in the diagnosis and management of diabetic retinopathy. Fluorescein angiography shows microaneurysms that are causing retinal edema. Small microaneurysms may not be visible clinically but will be seen as hyperfluorescent dots on fluorescein angiography.

Moderate NPDR presents with microaneurysms, intraretinal dot and blot hemorrhages, microinfarctions of the nerve fiber layer (soft exudates), intraretinal microvascular abnormalities (IRMAs), and venous beading. Severe NPDR is characterized by significant retinal hemorrhages in four quadrants, or significant venous beading in two quadrants, or significant IRMAs in one quadrant, known as the *ETDRS 4, 2, 1 rule*. Very severe NPDR is defined as the presence of two or more of the above criteria (5). Venous beading, IRMAs, and widespread capillary nonperfusion are important markers of significant retinal ischemia. Occlusion of retinal arterioles seen clinically as white threads of retinal arterioles can cause extensive areas of retinal nonperfusion described as "featureless" retina.

PDR is characterized by the formation of new vessels and proliferation of fibrous tissue. Neovascularization may be present at the optic disk or elsewhere. High-risk PDR is defined by the Diabetic Retinopathy Study (DRS) as the presence of three or four of the following risk factors: 1) presence of vitreous or preretinal hemorrhage, 2) presence of new vessels, 3) presence of new vessels on or within one disk diameter of the disk, and 4) presence of new vessels on the disk $\frac{1}{4}$ disk diameter or larger or neovascularization elsewhere $\frac{1}{2}$ disk area or larger in at least one photographic field (6).

Advanced PDR involves contraction of fibrovascular complexes, progressive vitreoretinal traction, and detachment of the retina. Neovascular complexes use vitreous as a scaffold. With posterior vitreous detachment, which occurs at an earlier age in diabetic patients, traction over the retinal neovascular complexes results in subhyaloid or vitreous hemorrhage. Contracting fibrovascular complexes with firm adhesions to the retina may cause anteroposterior traction resulting in traction retinal detachment, or tangential traction resulting in striae or a displacement of the macula called *macular heterotropia*. Tractional forces can even create retinal breaks, causing rhegmatogenous and combined traction-rhegmatogenous retinal detachments. Severe PDR may involve neovascularization of the chamber angle, iris, and ciliary body progressing to neovascular glaucoma, severe visual loss, and phthisis bulbi. In certain patients, diabetic retinopathy may involute spontaneously as a natural time course of the disease process and visual outcome will depend on the severity of the damage in the macular area.

MANAGEMENT

Medical Management

The Diabetes Control and Complications Trial (DCCT) showed tight blood glucose control to be beneficial in preventing and retarding the progression of diabetic retinopathy in patients with type I diabetes with none or mild to moderate NPDR. For patients who had diabetes for 1 to 5 years, the retinopathy progression rates were reduced from 54.1% for those receiving conventional therapy (1–2 injections/day) to 11.5% for those receiving an intensive ($\geq$3 injections/day or pump) insulin regimen. For those with diabetes for 1 to 15 years, the rates dropped from 49.2% for those under conventional therapy to 17.1% for those under intensive insulin therapy (7). Better systemic control of lipids and blood pressure in these patients may also have been a factor in retarding the progression of retinopathy. Isolated case reports showed that in patients with severe NPDR or PDR, the retinopathy may progress once the patients are put on tighter hyperglycemic control (8–10). Other studies (11–13) also showed that tight blood glucose control may cause deterioration of retinopathy in some patients with mild to moderate NPDR, although this generally stabilizes with time. Therefore, it must be remembered that patients with long-standing poor blood glucose control with severe NPDR or PDR would still benefit from good gradual glycemic control.

Surgical Management

The principal goal of the surgical management of diabetic retinopathy is to prevent visual loss by preserving central macular function and arresting the neovascular process. Current treatment modalities consist of panretinal photocoagulation for PDR, focal or grid laser for CSME, and vitreous surgery for proliferative retinopathy with nonclearing vitreous hemorrhage, fibrous proliferation with traction retinal detachment involving the macula, combined rhegmatogenous-traction retinal detachment, advanced progressive traction retinal detachment, and vitreous hemorrhage with progressive iris neovascularization. Since laser photocoagulation and vitreous surgery are not without risks, these measures must be used judiciously to protect central vision as best as possible until the disease process is under control.

Photocoagulation

Indications The indications for laser photocoagulation include focal or grid treatment for CSME and panretinal photocoagulation for high-risk PDR, levels of retinopathy approaching high-risk PDR, severe or very severe NPDR, and extensive anterior-segment neovascularization with or without glaucoma.

The ETDRS showed the beneficial effect of focal or grid photocoagulation for CSME in patients with

NPDR, reducing the risk of severe visual loss (5/200) by 50% (4), whereas the DRS showed that panretinal photocoagulation reduces the risk of severe visual loss (5/200) in eyes with PDR and severe NPDR by 50% to 60% (14,15).

Technique Topical anesthetic is the usual form of anesthesia used when doing laser photocoagulation on the macular area. A fundus contact lens is placed on the eye to be treated. A recent fluorescein angiogram showing microaneurysms and areas of leakage may be viewed to guide in the treatment. Focal treatment or grid treatment is recommended for diabetic macular edema. The ETDRS recommendation (16,17) for treatment of focal diabetic macular edema consists of treatment specifically directed at the microaneurysms, short capillary segments, and intraretinal microvascular abnormalities that leak during fluorescein angiography, located between 500 and 3000 μm from the center of the fovea. The photocoagulation parameters are argon green, 50- to 100-μm spot size, 0.1-second duration, and an initial power setting of 100 mW. The power can be titrated until whitening or darkening of the microaneurysm is achieved, indicating coagulation of the microaneurysm. Treatment of lesions more than 3000 μm from the center of the fovea is recommended if there are hard exudates or retinal thickening that extend closer to the center of the fovea. Follow-up examination is performed at 3 to 4 months following the initial treatment. If there is persistent clinically significant macular edema, retreatment is performed according to the initial treatment protocol (Fig. 46-1).

Patients with diffuse macular edema are treated with grid photocoagulation. Mild-intensity burns of 100-μm spot size, at least one burn width apart, are placed in the area of diffuse leakage, sparing the central 500 μm of the fovea and not closer than 500 μm from the disk margin. If additional grid treatment is needed on follow-up after 3 to 4 months, more lesions can be placed in between the old ones and treatment can be extended up to 300 μm from the center

of the fovea. Extensive macular edema should be treated in divided sessions at 3- to 4-month intervals.

In patients with PDR and severe NPDR, panretinal photocoagulation is performed using topical anesthetic. Retrobulbar or peribulbar anesthesia is used for patients who cannot tolerate the procedure. The DRS recommendation (14,15) for scatter treatment consists of 800 to 1200 moderately white intensity burns using argon green laser, one burn width apart, 500-μm burn lesions, and 0.1-second duration. Treatment is performed in two sessions, approximately 2 weeks apart. The burns are placed outside the temporal vascular arcades, 2 disk diameters temporal to the fovea and 1 disk diameter away from the nasal disk margin, extending to the equator. Goldmann, Rodenstock, or wide-angle lenses may be used to perform the treatment. With the Rodenstock lens, a spot size of 250 μm would give a 500-μm burn size. Retreatment following completion of the initial scatter photocoagulation may be considered if active new vessels persist or if there is recurrent vitreous hemorrhage. Repeat scatter treatment consists of burns to be placed in between or anterior to previous scars (Fig. 46-2).

The DRS, ETDRS and other studies showed that macular edema can develop or get worse after scatter photocoagulation (18–21). The ETDRS recommendation was to do focal treatment for CSME first before performing scatter treatment. In patients with clinically significant macular edema and active proliferative retinopathy, a focal treatment of macular edema combined with scatter treatment to the nasal quadrants may be initiated at the first treatment session, followed by scatter treatment in the temporal quadrants in subsequent sessions (22).

Complications Photocoagulation can cause heating of anterior-segment structures, vitreous, and fibrovascular membranes along the optical path of laser delivery. Lens uptake can be minimized by avoiding blue wavelengths or by using krypton red wavelengths in the treatment. Heavy

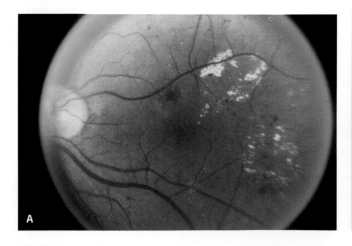
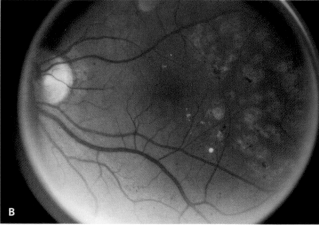

FIGURE 46-1. *Pretreatment (A) and posttreatment (B) photographs of clinically significant macular edema.*

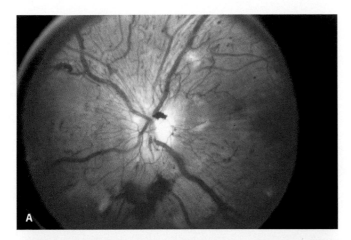

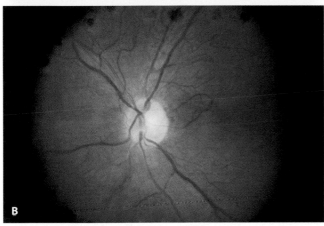

FIGURE 46-2. *Pretreatment (A) and posttreatment (B) photographs of proliferative diabetic retinopathy showing regression of NID after panretinal photocoagulation.*

treatment in the horizontal meridians should be avoided, as ciliary nerves serving pupillary constriction and accommodation can be damaged. Blue wavelengths should be avoided for macular treatment because blue wavelength is absorbed by the xanthophyll pigment in the macula, resulting in damage to the inner layers of the retina.

The side effects associated with macular laser treatment include microscotomas, while those associated with scatter treatment include a decrease in light sensitivity, a loss of peripheral visual field, a loss of accommodation, and some nyctalopia. Excessive and strong-intensity treatment in a single session may give rise to transient mild serous retinal elevation and choroidal detachment. Intense treatment with a small spot size can result in choroidal hemorrhage. The complications of macular laser photocoagulation include inadvertent photocoagulation of the fovea resulting in a central scotoma, break in Bruch's membrane, and choriovitreal and choroidal neovascularization (23–26) and submacular fibrosis (27). Laser scars in the macular region also can enlarge with time and in some patients may threaten central vision (28). Treatment in the macular may exacerbate ischemic visual loss, as in the case of

juxtafoveal treatment in the presence of an already enlarged foveal avascular zone.

Vitreous Surgery

Indications   The main goal of vitreous surgery for PDR is clearance of the optical pathway, removal of the scaffold for neovascularization, and retinal reattachment. This is achieved by complete removal of the vitreous, relief of traction, closure of retinal breaks, removal of proliferative tissues, and hemostasis. Indications of vitreous surgery for diabetic retinopathy include nonresolving vitreous hemorrhage, neovascular glaucoma with vitreous hemorrhage, traction retinal detachment threatening the macula, combined traction-rhegmatogenous retinal detachment, advanced progressive traction retinal detachment, significant premacular hemorrhage, neovascular proliferation unresponsive to photocoagulation, and macular edema due to vitreous traction in selected patients.

The Diabetic Retinopathy Vitrectomy Study (DRVS) was undertaken to evaluate the role of early vitrectomy for severe vitreous hemorrhage and for severe proliferative retinopathy (29–31). Patients with severe vitreous hemorrhage of less than 6 months' duration reducing the visual acuity to 5/200 or less were randomized to receive early vitrectomy or to have vitrectomy deferred for 1 year. The study concluded that early removal of vitreous hemorrhage and the posterior hyaloid face along with any fibrovascular tissue is beneficial in preventing late neovascular complications and providing prompt visual rehabilitation in type I diabetic patients. In the study, 35.6% of those who had early vitrectomy achieved visual acuity of 10/20 or better, compared to 11.7% of those who had vitrectomy deferred. In type II diabetic patients, there was no significant difference in the visual recovery between the early vitrectomy group and the deferral group. For type II diabetic patients, visual acuity of 10/20 or better was achieved in 18.6% of the early vitrectomy group compared to 17.4% of the deferral group. However, there was a slightly higher incidence of no light perception (NLP) in the early vitrectomy group in general, compared to the deferral group. The incidence of NLP in type I diabetics in the early vitrectomy group was 27.7%, compared to 26.2% in the deferral group. In type II diabetics, the difference was more pronounced, 22% in the early vitrectomy group and 12.5% in the deferral group.

For patients with severe PDR who had extensive active neovascular or fibrovascular proliferation and a visual acuity of 10/200 or better, the study concluded that early vitrectomy was beneficial for those with moderately severe PDR: 50% of those in the early vitrectomy group achieved a visual acuity of 10/20 or better, compared to 36.1% in the deferral group. However, there was a small increase in the risk of NLP. In patients with severe and very severe PDR, there was a significant benefit from early vitrectomy. In patients with severe PDR, 43.6% of the early vitrectomy group achieved a visual acuity of 10/20 or better, compared to 20.4% of the deferral group. In diabetics with very severe PDR, the respective percentages were 36% for the early vitrectomy group compared to 10.5% for the deferral group. There was little change in the risk of NLP.

Technique   Diabetic vitrectomy employs a standard three-port technique using an inferotemporal sclerotomy for the infusion cannula and superotemporal and superonasal instrument ports placed 4 mm posterior to the limbus in phakic eyes and 3.5 mm posterior to the limbus in pseudophakic eyes. Standard vitrectomy contact lenses or a panoramic wide-field viewing system together with a stereoscopic image inverter may be used. In the presence of significant cataract, phacoemulsification with posterior-chamber intra-ocular lens implantation followed by vitrectomy, or pars plana lensectomy and vitrectomy followed by posterior-chamber intraocular lens implantation may be performed (32–34). Pars plana lensectomy can be carried out with ultrasonic emulsification. After insertion of the infusion cannula into the inferotemporal sclerotomy, the microvitreal blade is introduced through a superotemporal sclerotomy into the center of the lens nucleus. The blade is then rotated 360 degrees to break up the nucleus. Infusion can be provided using the inferotemporal infusion cannula or via a separate 20-gauge infusion cannula inserted into the lens through the superonasal sclerotomy. A separate 20-gauge infusion cannula has the advantage of a second instrument for manipulation of the lens during ultrasonic emulsification. Flexible iris retractors can be used to enlarge the pupillary opening for viewing in cases of miosis. Hyphema can be lavaged via an anterior-chamber paracentesis with simultaneous infusion via an anterior-chamber cannula until a view is obtained. Lens clarity can be preserved in phakic patients with the addition of dextrose (3 mL of 50% dextrose/500 mL) into the infusion cannula. After placement of the ports and verification of the proper position of the infusion cannula, a vitreous cutter is used to clear vitreous near the ports. A core vitrectomy is performed. The posterior hyaloid face is incised preferably nasally and the posterior hyaloid is then excised 360 degrees and any vitreoretinal adhesions are excised. If a subhyaloid hemorrhage is present, it is removed with an extrusion needle to obtain a view of the retina. If a localized traction retinal detachment is seen on preoperative ultrasound scans, it should be avoided during incision of the posterior hyaloid face. The posterior hyaloid and fibrovascular tissue can be removed using an en bloc technique (35–37) (Fig. 46-3). In this technique, after limited removal of the vitreous, horizontal scissors are used to separate epicenters of fibrovascular tissue from the retinal surface. The remaining vitreous maintains the anteroposterior traction over the posterior hyaloid and the fibrovascular tissue pulling it away from the retinal surface, thus allowing insertion of the horizontal scissors in between the fibrovascular tissue and the retinal surface. After all the fibrovascular tissue attachments have been excised, removal of the vitreous and the fibrovascular tissue is then carried out en bloc with the vitreous cutter.

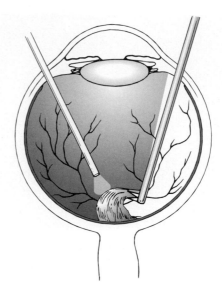

FIGURE 46-3.   *En bloc technique. After limited core vitrectomy, horizontal scissors are inserted under the fibrovascular tissue and epicenters are cut with the vitreous maintaining anteroposterior traction.*

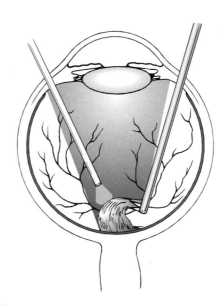

FIGURE 46-4.   *Modified en bloc technique. The posterior hyaloid is removed except in areas where it is attached to fibrovascular tissue. Horizontal scissors are used to cut the epicenters of the fibrovascular tissues.*

In the modified en bloc technique (38) (Fig. 46-4), the posterior hyaloid is circumcised except in areas where it is attached to the fibrovascular proliferations. Horizontal scissors can then be inserted under the posterior hyaloid to dissect the neovascular membranes from the retina. Frequently, there are extensive membranes over the surface of the retina causing horizontal traction. In such cases, segmentation (39) (Fig. 46-5) of membranes is carried out using a vitreoretinal pick to undermine the membrane, creating a space or bridge between the membrane and the retina. Vertical scissors are then used to cut across the membranes and the membranes are trimmed down with the vitreous cutter. Some of the membrane may be peeled if minimally adherent to retina. Delamination (40) (Fig. 46-6) may be carried out to remove some of the membranes by using a bimanual technique in which the membranes are held with a lighted pick or forceps at their attachments to the retina and are excised with horizontal scissors. Minimally adherent epiretinal membranes in the macular area may be incised with a microvitreoretinal blade and peeled from the retina with tissue forceps. The fibrovascular attachment to the optic nerve head can be trimmed with the vitreous cutter and treated with unimanual bipolar diathermy or alternatively, be peeled by using tissue forceps. Hemostasis is maintained throughout the procedure by elevating the infusion bottle to increase the intraocular pressure and using unimanual bipolar diathermy. Elevations in intraocular pressure to control bleeding should be minimized to prevent macular or optic nerve damage in an already vascularly compromised eye. Finally, the remaining peripheral vitreous at the vitreous base is removed with the aid of scleral depression. Instruments are removed from the eye and scleral plugs are placed. The periphery of the retina is carefully examined

for retinal breaks, retinal dialysis, hemorrhage, or other complications using indirect ophthalmoscopy. Peripheral retinal breaks are treated with cryopexy. If there is a retinal detachment, a scleral buckle is placed and the eye is re-entered and all breaks are marked with unimanual bipolar diathermy, an air-fluid exchange is performed, and an internal drainage of subretinal fluid is carried out using a silicone-tip extrusion needle placed at the retinal break or through a retinotomy. Endophotocoagulation or indirect laser can then be used to surround retinal breaks and to apply additional panretinal photocoagulation with argon green or diode lasers. One sclerotomy site is closed with suture, a metal extrusion cannula is inserted into the other sclerotomy site, and a gas-air exchange is performed with 40 to 50 mL of the desired concentration of intraocular gas. The two more common intraocular gases used are sulfur hexafluoride (SF_6) and perfluoropropane (C_3F_8). Sulfur hexafluoride expands twice its size and lasts for about 10 to 14 days while perfluoropropane expands four times its size and lasts for about 55 to 60 days. If a full gas-air exchange is to be done, a non-expanding concentration of the gas would be preferable. For sulfur hexafluoride, the nonexpanding concentration is 18% and for perfluoropropane, 14%. Perfluoropropane may be used in eyes that would require a long internal tamponade. If general anesthesia is used, inhalational nitrous oxide should be turned off to ensure proper gas bubble stability. Silicone oil has occasionally been used in severe cases with extensive diabetic traction retinal detachment. If silicone oil is used instead of gas, an inferior iridotomy should be performed in aphakic patients to prevent pupillary block glaucoma. The remaining sclerotomy site is closed and the infusion cannula removed and the port closed with the preplaced suture. A final adjustment of the intraocular pressure should be made. The patient is positioned face down if gas-air exchange was performed; otherwise head elevation is encouraged. Postoperatively, the patient should be monitored closely for a rise in intraocular pressure (Fig. 46-7).

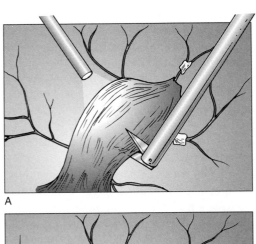

A

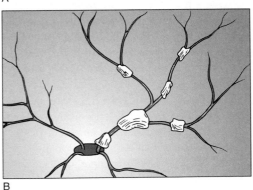

B

FIGURE 46-5.   *Segmentation of fibrovascular tissues using vertical scissors.*

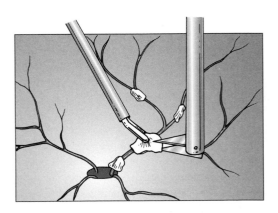

FIGURE 46-6.   *Delamination using tissue forceps and horizontal scissors.*

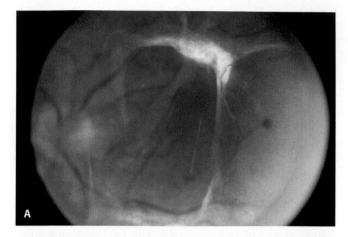

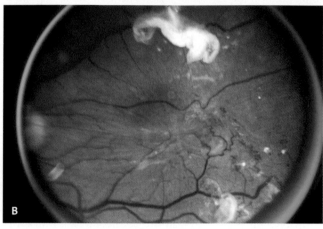

FIGURE 46-7.   *Previtrectomy* (A) *and postvitrectomy* (B) *photographs of proliferative diabetic retinopathy with extensive fibrovascular proliferation.*

Complications   Several intraoperative and postoperative complications can occur during vitrectomy. Diabetic eyes usually have corneal epithelial basement membrane abnormalities (41–43) predisposing them to development of corneal edema. Because of a compromised corneal anatomy, it may take longer for corneal epithelial defects to heal in diabetic eyes. An effort should be made to preserve the corneal epithelium as much as possible during surgery. If corneal edema and Descemet's folds develop during surgery and result in poor visibility, a thin layer of sodium hyaluronate can be injected to coat the corneal endothelium.

Feather-like changes in the posterior lens capsule, which usually are temporary, can occur during or after surgery owing to a difference in glucose concentration between the patient's blood and the irrigating fluid. This can be avoided by adding glucose into the irrigating fluid prior to the surgery (3 mL of 50% dextrose in 500 mL of infusion fluid) (44). Other complications include cataract formation, which may be secondary to instrument touch, prolonged surgery, or contact with intraocular gas bubble.

Vitreous hemorrhage can occur intraoperatively or postoperatively. Intraoperative bleeding can be prevented during surgery with adequate diathermy of fibrovascular tissue before excision. If bleeding occurs during surgery, it can be stopped by elevating the intraocular pressure by adjusting the infusion bottle height, and diathermy of the bleeding site. It is important that the infusion fluid height be brought back to a normal level before the end of the procedure to identify potential bleeders. Addition of thrombin into the infusion fluid can also aid in the control of bleeding (45,46). Postoperative hemorrhage can occur secondary to dispersed blood from retained blood clots, residual neovascular tissue, sclerotomy wound complications, anterior hyaloidal fibrovascular proliferation, or iris new vessels. Postoperative hemorrhage usually clears spontaneously (47,48). If it does not clear, an outpatient air-fluid exchange can be performed. In recurrent vitreous hemorrhage, a vitreous washout is performed in the operating room and the source of the bleeding identified and treated. Reoperation should also be considered if there is rhegmatogenous retinal detachment.

Another complication common in diabetic eyes is severe fibrin formation, which can occur after extensive dissection of neovascular membranes (49). Mild fibrin reaction may be treated with high doses of topical steroids. With severe fibrin reaction, intracameral or intravitreal injection of 3 g of tissue plasminogen activator (tPA) may help clear the fibrin and prevent further fibrin reaction (50).

Retinal detachment can occur secondary to retinal breaks or traction from residual fibrovascular tissue. Therefore, it is important to check the retinal periphery, especially the area of the sclerotomies, at the end of each procedure. A localized area of traction retinal detachment not involving the macula may be observed but surgery is indicated for rhegmatogenous retinal detachment.

Diabetic eyes with extensive ischemia undergoing multiple surgeries may develop anterior hyaloidal neovascular proliferation (51,52). This condition is characterized by fibrovascular proliferation involving the anterior peripheral retina and the anterior hyaloid surface behind the lens. It usually presents with vitreous hemorrhage and if unrecognized and untreated, may lead to hypotony and eventual pthisis bulbi. Aggressive treatment is recommended once this condition is suspected. This consists of lensectomy, resection of anterior vitreous and proliferative tissues, and extensive photocoagulation.

In patients who have had cataract extraction, acceleration of exudative maculopathy can occur weeks following the surgery. There may be an increase in retinal hemorrhages, hard exudates, and macular edema, especially in patients who have not had any laser treatment for exudates in the macula (53).

Anterior-segment neovascularization was also observed to be more common in aphakic eyes than in phakic eyes following vitrectomy (54–58). Cataract extraction and posterior capsulotomy can cause diffusion of angiogenic factors from the posterior to the anterior segment, causing anterior-segment neovascularization (59,60). Neovascular glaucoma can also develop following chronic retinal detachment (61,62), owing to retinal hypoxia inducing neovascular proliferation.

Complications associated with intraocular gas use are elevated intraocular pressure, lens changes, and corneal endothelial decompensation. Increased intraocular pressure usually can be controlled medically but in some instances, removal of some of the intraocular gas may be necessary. Lens changes can be seen as feathering opacities or vacuoles in the posterior lens surface. These changes may still be reversible as long as correct head-down positioning is followed to minimize contact of the intraocular gas to the lens. Bullous keratopathy can occur if the gas bubble is in the anterior chamber, leading to endothelial decompensation. Various complications associated with the use of silicone oil include pupillary block glaucoma, anterior migration of silicone oil, keratopathy, emulsification, and perisilicone proliferation.

These complications underscore the importance of meticulous technique, avoidance of lensectomy, and efficiency in surgical technique to reduce the surgical time in optimizing visual outcome for these patients.

NEOVASCULAR GLAUCOMA

Neovascular glaucoma is a dreaded complication of PDR. Retinal ischemia can induce neovascularization of the anterior segment, leading to rubeosis iridis and angle neovascularization. This can be detected early by routine gonioscopy and undilated pupil examination of the iris of all diabetic patients. In patients with good vision and clear media progressing to neovascular glaucoma, immediate panretinal photocoagulation should be done. If the media is not clear secondary to vitreous hemorrhage, vitrectomy with endophotocoagulation should be performed. This is essential prior to, and in some patients may avoid the need for, definitive filtration and seton procedures. In blind eyes, conservative treatment with topical atropine and steroids can keep the eye comfortable. Cyclodestructive procedures and rarely, enucleation can be performed in patients with a painful blind eye.

CONCLUSIONS

The ETDRS and DRS showed the beneficial effect of focal or grid treatment for clinically significant macular edema and panretinal photocoagulation for high-risk PDR and severe NPDR. The DRVS also showed the benefit of early vitrectomy for severe vitreous hemorrhage in type I diabetic patients and in diabetics with moderatedly severe to very severe PDR. Future developments in diabetic retinopathy management will involve the preservation of macula by prevention of capillary occlusion, inhibition of angiogenesis, and induction of posterior vitreous detachment, all via pharmacologic means. Visual prognosis will also improve with better systemic control of serum glucose levels, hypertension, and serum lipid levels. While the pathogenesis of diabetic retinopathy is unclear, vasoproliferative factors such as vascular endothelial growth factor mediate the proliferative process. The mechanism by which hyperglycemia affects such mediators is unknown. The focus of current research and pharmacologic intervention in diabetes may provide a better understanding of the factors that control these mediators, and subsequently newer methods of therapy.

REFERENCES

1. Klein R, Klein B, et al. The Wisconsin Epidemiologic Study of Diabetic Retinopathy II. Prevalence and risk of diabetic retinopathy when age at diagnosis is less than 30 years. *Arch Ophthalmol* 1984;102:520–526.
2. Klein R, Klein B, et al. The Wisconsin Epidemiologic Study of Diabetic Retinopathy III. Prevalence and risk of diabetic retinopathy when age at diagnosis is 30 years or more. *Arch Ophthalmol* 1984;102:527–532.
3. Klein R, Klein B, et al. The Wisconsin Epidemiologic Study of Diabetic Retinopathy IV. Diabetic macular edema. *Ophthalmology* 1984;91:1464–1474.
4. The Early Treatment Diabetic Retinopathy Study research group report no. 1. Photocoagulation of diabetic macular edema. *Arch Ophthalmol* 1985;103:1796–1806.
5. The Early Treatment Diabetic Retinopathy Study research group report no. 10. Fundus photographic risk factors for progression of diabetic retinopathy. *Ophthalmology* 1991;98:823–833.
6. The Diabetic Retinopathy Study research group report no 3. Four risk factors for severe visual loss in diabetic retinopathy. *Arch Ophthalmol* 1979;97:654–655.
7. The Diabetes Control and Complications Trial research group. The effect of intensive treatment on the progression of diabetic retinopathy in insulin-dependent diabetes mellitus. *Arch Ophthalmol* 1995;113:36–51.
8. Lawson PM, Champion MC, Canny C, et al. Continuous subcutaneous insulin infusion does not prevent progression of proliferative and preproliferative retinopathy. *Br J Ophthalmol* 1982;66:762–766.
9. Puklin JE, Tamborlane WV, Felig P, et al. Influence of long-term insulin infusion pump treatment of type 1 diabetes on diabetic retinopathy. *Ophthalmology* 1982;89:735–747.
10. Van Ballegooie E, Hooymans JM, Timmerman Z. Rapid deterioration of diabetic retinopathy during treatment with continuous subcutaneous insulin infusion. *Diabetes Care* 1984;7:236–242.
11. Dahl-Jorgensen K, Burchmann-Hansen O, Hanssen KF, et al. Rapid tightening of blood glucose control leads to transient deterioration of retinopathy in insulin dependent diabetes mellitus: the Oslo study. *BMJ* 1985;290:811–815.
12. The Kroc Collaborative Study Group. Blood glucose control and the evolution of diabetic retinopathy and albuminuria: a preliminary multicenter trial. *N Engl J Med* 1984;311:365–372.
13. Lauritzer T, Frost-Larsen K, Larsen HW, et al. Effect of one year of near-normal blood glucose levels on retinopathy in insulin dependent diabetics. *Lancet* 1983;1:200–204.
14. The Diabetic Retinopathy Study research group. Preliminary report on effects of photocoagulation therapy. *Am J Ophthalmol* 1976;81:383–396.
15. The Diabetic Retinopathy Study research group report no. 8. Photocoagulation treatment of proliferative diabetic retinopathy: clinical applications of diabetic retinopathy study findings. *Ophthalmology* 1981;88:583–600.
16. The Early Treatment Diabetic Retinopathy study group report no. 4. Photocoagulation for diabetic macular edema. *Int Ophthalmol Clin* 1987;27:265–272.
17. The Early Treatment Diabetic Retinopathy study group report no. 2. Treatment techniques and clinical guidelines for photocoagulation of diabetic macular edema. *Ophthalmology* 1987;94:761–774.
18. The Early Treatment Diabetic Retinopathy Study research group report no. 9. Early photocoagulation for diabetic retinopathy. *Ophthalmology* 1991;98:766–785.
19. Meyers SM. Macular edema after scatter laser photocoagulation for proliferative diabetic retinopathy. *Am J Ophthalmol* 1980;90:210–216.
20. McDonald HR, Schatz H. Macular edema following scatter photocoagulation. *Retina* 1985;5:5–10.

21. The Diabetic Retinopathy Study research group report no. 12. Macular edema in diabetic retinopathy study patients. *Ophthalmology* 1987;94: 754–760.

22. The Early Treatment Diabetic Retinopathy Study group report no. 3. Techniques for scatter and local photocoagulation treatment of diabetic retinopathy. *Int Ophthalmol Clin* 1987;27:254–264.

23. Benson WE, Townsend RE, Pheasant TR. Choriovitreal and subretinal proliferations. Complications of photocoagulation. *Ophthalmology* 1979;86:283–289.

24. Varley MP, Frank E, Purnell EW. Subretinal neovascularization after focal argon laser for diabetic macular edema. *Ophthalmology* 1988;95:567–573.

25. Lewis H, Schachat AP, Haimann MH, et al. Choroidal neovascularization after laser photocoagulation of diabetic macular edema. *Ophthalmology* 1990;97:503–511.

26. Chandra SR, Bresnick GH, Davis MD, et al. Choroidovitreal neovascular ingrowth after photocoagulation for proliferative diabetic retinopathy. *Arch Ophthalmol* 1980;98:1593–1599.

27. Han DP, Mieler WF, Burton TC. Submacular fibrosis after photocoagulation for diabetic macular edema. *Am J Ophthalmol* 1992;113:513–521.

28. Schatz H, Madeira D, McDonald HR, Johnson RN. Progressive enlargement of laser scars following grid laser photocoagulation for diffuse macular edema. *Arch Ophthalmol* 1991;109:1549–1551.

29. The Diabetic Retinopathy Vitrectomy Study research group report no. 2. Early treatment for severe vitreous hemorrhage in diabetic retinopathy. Two-year results of a randomized trial. *Arch Ophthalmol* 1985;103:1644–1652.

30. The Diabetic Retinopathy Vitrectomy Study research group report no. 3. Early vitrectomy for severe proliferative diabetic retinopathy in eyes with useful vision. Results of a randomized trial. *Ophthalmology* 1988;95:1307–1320.

31. The Diabetic Retinopathy Vitrectomy Study research group report no. 5. Early vitrectomy for severe vitreous hemorrhage in diabetic retinopathy. Four-year results of a randomized trial. *Arch Ophthalmol* 1990;108:958–964.

32. Benson WE, Brown GC, Tasman W, et al. Extracapsular cataract extraction, posterior chamber lens insertion and pars plana vitrectomy in one operation. *Ophthalmology* 1990;97:918.

33. Koenig SB, Han DP, Mieler WF, et al. Combined phacoemulsification and pars plana vitrectomy. *Arch Ophthalmol* 1990;108:362.

34. Blankenship GW, Flynn HW, Kokame GT. Posterior chamber intraocular lens insertion during pars plana lensectomy and vitrectomy for complications of proliferative diabetic retinopathy. *Am J Ophthalmol* 1989;108:1.

35. Abrams GW, Williams GA. "En bloc" excision of diabetic membranes. *Am J Ophthalmol* 1987;103:302.

36. Williams DF, Williams GA, Hartz A, et al. Results of vitrectomy for diabetic traction retinal detachments using the en bloc excision technique. *Ophthalmology* 1989;96:752.

37. Abrams GW. En bloc dissection techniques in vitrectomy for diabetic retinopathy. In: Lewis H, Ryan SJ, eds. *Medical and surgical retina*. St. Louis: Mosby–Year Book, 1994:304.

38. Han DP, Murphy ML, Mieler WF. A modified en bloc excision technique during vitrectomy for diabetic traction retinal detachment. Results and complications. *Ophthalmology* 1994;101:803.

39. Meredith TA, Kaplan HJ, Aaberg TM. Pars plana vitrectomy techniques for relief of epiretinal traction by membrane segmentation. *Am J Ophthalmol* 1980;89:408.

40. Charles S. *Vitreous microsurgery*. 2nd ed. Baltimore: Williams & Wilkins, 1987:121.

41. Brightbill FS, Myers FL, Bresnick GH. Postvitrectomy keratopathy. *Am J Ophthalmol* 1978;85:651.

42. Foulks GN, Thoft RA, Perry HD, Tolentino FI. Factors related to corneal epithelial complications after closed vitrectomy in diabetics. *Arch Ophthalmol* 1979;97:1076.

43. Oyakawa RT, Schachat AP, Michels RG, Rice TA. Complications of vitreous surgery for diabetic retinopathy. I. Intraoperative complications. *Ophthalmology* 1983;90:517.

44. Haimann MH, Abrams GW. Prevention of lens opacification during diabetic vitrectomy. *Ophthalmology* 1984;91:116.

45. de Bustros S, Glaser BM, Johnson MA. Thrombin infusion for the control of intraocular bleeding during vitreous surgery. *Arch Ophthalmol* 1985;103:837.

46. Thompson JT, Glaser BM, Michels RG, de Bustros S. The use of intravitreal thrombin to control of hemorrhage during vitrectomy. *Ophthalmology* 1986;93:279.

47. Kerman BM, Kreiger AE, Straatsma BR. Resorption of intravitreal blood following vitrectomy. *Am J Ophthalmol* 1976;82:915.

48. Novak MA, Rice TA, Michels RG, Auer C. Vitreous hemorrhage after vitrectomy for diabetic retinopathy. *Ophthalmology* 1984;91:1485.

49. Jaffe GJ, Schwartz D, Han DP, et al. Risk factors for postvitrectomy fibrin formation. *Am J Ophthalmol* 1990;109:661.

50. Williams DF, Bennett SR, Abrams GW, et al. Low dose intraocular tissue plasminogen activator for treatment of postvitrectomy fibrin formation. *Am J Ophthalmol* 1990;109:606.

51. Lewis H, Abrams GW, Foos RY. Clinicopathologic findings in anterior hyaloidal fibrovascular proliferation after diabetic vitrectomy. *Am J Ophthalmol* 1987;104:614.

52. Lewis H, Abrams GW, Williams GA. Anterior hyaloidal fibrovascular proliferation after diabetic retinopathy. *Am J Ophthalmol* 1987;104:607.

53. Stevens TS, Castrovinci RV, de Venecia G. Aphakia-exacerbated exudative diabetic retinopathy. Presented at the annual meeting of the Association for Research in Vision and Ophthalmology, Sarasota, FL, May 1976.

54. Rice TA, Michels RG, Maguire MG, Rice EF. The effect of lensectomy on the incidence of iris neovascularization and neovascular glaucoma after vitrectomy for diabetic retinopathy. *Am J Ophthalmol* 1983;95:1.

55. Blackenship G, Cortez R, Machemer R. The lens and pars plana vitrectomy for diabetic retinopathy complications. *Arch Ophthalmol* 1979;97:1263.

56. Blackenship GW. The lens influence on diabetic vitrectomy results. Report of a prospective randomized study. *Arch Ophthalmol* 1980;98:2196.

57. Michels RG. Vitrectomy for complications of diabetic retinopathy. *Arch Ophthalmol* 1978;96:237.

58. Schachat AP, Oyakawa RT, Michels RG, Rice TA. Complications of vitreous surgery for diabetic retinopathy. II. Postoperative complications. *Ophthalmology* 1983;90:522.

59. Aiello LM, Wand M, Liang G. Neovascular glaucoma and vitreous hemorrhage following cataract surgery in patients with diabetes mellitus. *Ophthalmology* 1983;90:814.

60. Poliner LS, Christianson DJ, Escoffery RE, et al. Neovascular glaucoma after intracapsular and extracapsular cataract extraction in diabetic patients. *Am J Ophthalmol* 1985;100:637.

61. Aaberg TM, Van Horn DL. Late complications of pars plana vitreous surgery. *Ophthalmology* 1978;85:126.

62. Scuderi JJ, Blumenkratz MS, Blakenship G. Regression of diabetic rubeosis iridis following successful surgical reattachment of the retina by vitrectomy. *Retina* 1982;2:193.

Surgical Management of Open Globe Injuries

ERIC A. POSTEL   WILLIAM F. MIELER

Ocular trauma is a major cause of visual impairment in the United States (1) and levies a tremendous penalty in both direct and indirect costs (2). There are approximately 2.4 million ocular injuries annually. Males are affected approximately nine times more often than females (2–8) and most victims are under the age of 40 (2,4,5,7,8). The devastating effects of blunt trauma are more commonly encountered than those of open globe injury (2–4,8) but open globe (penetrating, perforating, and retained intraocular foreign body (IOFB)) injuries represent a major cause of ocular morbidity (9). Visual impairment can occur through a variety of processes after a traumatic injury. Vision limiting factors may include corneal scarring or decompensation; hyphema formation with glaucomatous complications; cataract formation or subluxation of the lens; vitreous hemorrhage; retinal tear, dialysis, and detachment; choroidal hemorrhage; macular and optic nerve contusive damage; and phthisis bulbi formation. Many of these conditions can be surgically corrected. The personal impact of the injuries is difficult to define, though millions of dollars are spent in hospitalization costs, treatment, and in lost working revenue.

Over the last several decades, the prognosis for patients with open globe injuries has significantly improved. This has been attributed to the advent of enhanced microsurgical techniques and instrumentation, along with an improved understanding of the pathophysiology of ocular trauma and the wound-healing response in injured eyes (9–10).

HISTOPATHOLOGY OF PENETRATING AND PERFORATING INJURY

Winthrop et al (11) reviewed the histopathological findings in 34 eyes after severe penetrating trauma. Thirty-two of thirty-four eyes had retinal detachment, and twenty-seven

had evidence of traction on the retina. Intraocular cellular proliferation was noted within 1 week of injury and typically resulted in formation of a cyclitic membrane by 6 weeks after injury. In eyes with limbal or scleral wounds associated with incarceration of the lens, vitreous, or blood, such membranes were present as early as 2 weeks after injury. Factors associated with a vigorous proliferative response were the site of the wound, adequacy of wound closure, incarceration of tissues in the wound, the extent of involvement of intraocular tissues including the iris, lens, and vitreous, and the presence of massive vitreous hemorrhage.

A similarly high incidence of retinal detachment was noted by Freitag et al (12), who found retinal detachment in 96% of eyes enucleated after traumatic rupture. They also noted hemorrhagic choroidal detachment in 92% of cases, and avulsion or loss of the ciliary body in 76% of eyes. Punnonen (13) noted a similar proliferative response in 48 eyes enucleated after penetrating injury.

PATHOPHYSIOLOGY OF PENETRATING AND PERFORATING INJURY

The wound healing response in the eye is the same as elsewhere in the body and often leads to traction retinal detachment after penetrating ocular injury (10). There is an initial inflammatory response with breakdown of the blood-retinal barrier and an influx, migration, and proliferation of cells, including polymorphonuclear lymphocytes, macrophages, fibroblasts, and myofibroblasts. These cells contract and produce collagen. This contraction on the vitreous scaffold ultimately produces tractional retinal detachment (10).

Animal models have allowed study of the mechanisms that develop after penetrating trauma. Beginning in the late

1970s, Cleary, Ryan, and others studied the pathophysiology of traction retinal detachment occurring after penetrating trauma in animal models (14–21). An 8-mm wound was made through the sclera at the pars plana, resulting in prolapse of the vitreous gel, though there was no damage to the retina or crystalline lens. The wound was then closed with microsurgical techniques. Injection of saline or ground lens material from another monkey into the vitreous cavity of these monkeys did not lead to retinal detachment. However, 73% of the injured eyes developed traction retinal detachment after injection of 0.5 mL of blood into the vitreous cavity (19).

In these animal models, the location of the penetrating injury did play a role in the development of retinal detachment (22). A full-thickness eye wall wound, 8 mm in length, involving the sclera, choroid, and retina, was made at various posterior sites. When the injury was located at the equator, retinal detachment occurred in only 16% of eyes. Similarly, injury through the peripheral retina, and/or ciliary body, resulted in a rate of retinal detachment of 14%. However, when the injury was located at the ora serrata, the rate of retinal detachment was 78%, presumably because of involvement of the vitreous base and different tractional forces on the edge of the induced retinal break.

In another study (22), a wound was made through the sclera, choroid, and retina in monkey eyes. In eyes that did not receive an intravitreal injection of blood, no posterior vitreous detachment (PVD) or retinal detachment developed. However, after injection of intravitreal blood, 91% developed a PVD and 50% went on to develop a traction retinal detachment. These detachments developed by at least eight weeks after the initial injury.

A similar study was performed to determine the effect of perforating injury in rabbit eyes (23). A sharp probe was inserted into the vitreous cavity 7.5 mm posterior to the limbus, and passed out the posterior eye wall inferior to the optic disk. In an effort to simulate the human situation, where it is often impossible to close posterior wounds, the wounds were not closed. Results identical to that mentioned above was noted. In addition, cellular proliferations originating in the wounds crossed the vitreous cavity, following the injury tract.

PREOPERATIVE EVALUATION

Before the ocular examination for an eye injury is performed, it is imperative to obtain a detailed history from the patient, family, or witnesses, as this may give important clues as to the type and extent of ocular damage. In addition to serving medicolegal purposes, the history may raise suspicions regarding the presence of penetrating injury and retained IOFBs, as well as identifying any preexisting ocular conditions. Many patients will be limited historians, due to shock, intoxication, or possibly due to neurological problems associated with the injury. In addition, during these early stages of evaluation it is critical to determine if any

systemic injuries exist, particularly life-threatening injuries, as these take precedence over the immediate management of ocular disorders. Although ophthalmologists are most often called to examine these patients after they have been evaluated systemically, this is not always the case, and an alert ophthalmologist may be the first to identify a life-threatening situation.

As with any ocular examination, the initial step is to document visual function. This can be performed either at distance or near. Vision at presentation is a very important determinant of final visual outcome, as patients with initial vision of 5/200 or better have a 28 times greater chance of salvaging acuity at this level (24). Similarly, patients presenting with vision of 20/200 or better maintained a final level of vision of 20/200 or better in 94% of cases (25). Occasionally ancillary tests such as the flash visual evoked potential (VEP) is utilized in the preoperative assessment of the patient. Patients with a normal VEP had a mean visual outcome of 20/100, while those with an absent response showed a mean final vision of hand motions (26).

Conversely, documentation of no light perception is an extemely poor prognostic finding, with only rare isolated cases recovering functional vision. If the patient at presentation has no light perception in the injured globe, and it is so badly damaged that the ocular integrity cannot be restored, then primary enucleation is recommended. If there is any question regarding possible perception of light, or if the patient has an altered mental status, the globe should be repaired the best that it can be, and then in the early postoperative period, if the patient remains no light perception, enucleation surgery can be performed.

After documentation of vision, it is imperative to assess the full extent of the injury without causing any further damage to the injured eye. Pressure placed on the globe that could cause prolapse of intraocular contents must be avoided. If one is unable to fully assess the extent of injury due to lack of patient cooperation, the examination can be completed in the operating room under anesthesia.

While in many cases the diagnosis is obvious (Fig. 47-1), in some cases a scleral rupture may be hidden under conjunctiva (Fig. 47-2). The first step in diagnosing and treating penetrating or perforating ocular injury is to suspect its presence. Even after mild blunt trauma, the integrity of the globe may be violated. Clues to the presence of a ruptured globe in the setting of blunt trauma include moderate to severe intraocular or periocular hemorrhage (see Fig. 47-2) often associated with limited visual acuity of hand motions or worse, conjunctival hemorrhage and chemosis, media opacification, vitreous strands pointing toward a possible scleral defect, abnormal chamber depth, or low intraocular pressure (27). It must be kept in mind, however, that even in the setting of a scleral rupture, the intraocular pressure may be normal or even elevated. Echography may be helpful to detect a scleral rupture (Fig. 47-3), although a negative examination does not rule out the possibility of an occult rupture. In a similar fashion, computed tomography (CT)

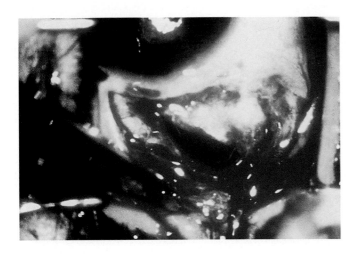

FIGURE 47-1.   *Open globe injury sustained via sharp object with approximately 6-mm scleral laceration with prolapse of uveal tissue.*

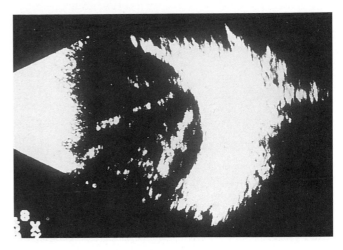

FIGURE 47-3.   *High-resolution B-scan echography documenting vitreous incarceration, pointing toward scleral rupture site.*

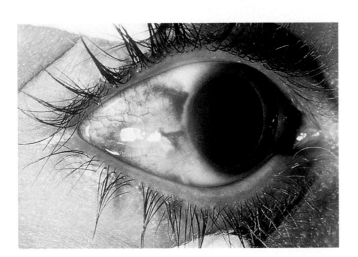

FIGURE 47-2.   *Subconjunctival hemorrhage and chemosis following blunt ocular injury. Ocular examination revealed mild hypotony and vitreous hemorrhage. Exploration of globe revealed scleral laceration beneath lateral rectus muscle insertion.*

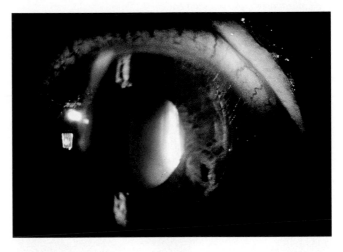

FIGURE 47-4.   *Nasal iridotomy created by intraocular foreign body that lodged in lens behind iris.*

scanning has also been reported to show occult ruptures, with flattening of the posterior contour of the sclera (28). The role of ancillary studies—including echography, magnetic resonance imaging, and x-ray studies—are further discussed in the next section.

In cases with possible retained IOFBs, particular attention should be paid to the identification of entrance and exit wounds (Fig. 47-4), to the path of a suspected IOFB, and to prompt assessment of the posterior segment. Often the initial examination provides the only clear view of the extent of posterior segment injury (Fig. 47-5), and it may also provide the most accurate identification and localization of the retained IOFB. This view may rapidly be lost

by corneal clouding, hyphema formation, development of cataract, or the dispersion of vitreous hemorrhage. Again, the use of ancillary imaging studies in these cases is discussed in the next section.

IMAGING STUDIES

Radiologic studies or echography should be obtained in all cases of penetrating or perforating trauma, in the presence of a retained IOFB, or whenever a ruptured globe is suspected, particularly when opaque media precludes a view of the posterior segment. Conventional x-rays are perhaps the simplest and most readily available method for IOFB identification, but they are of limited use. For many years, the standard technique of localizing foreign bodies involved special applications of conventional x-ray imaging. Plain

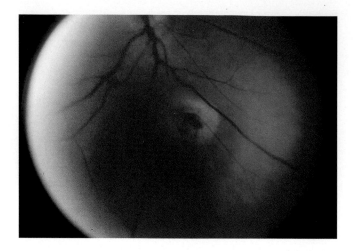

FIGURE 47-5.   *Mild vitreous hemorrhage and retinal foreign body impact site inferior to optic disk. Foreign body was noted to be lying on retinal surface further inferiorly. Within hours after presentation, vitreous hemorrhage became more diffuse, precluding visualization of posterior segment.*

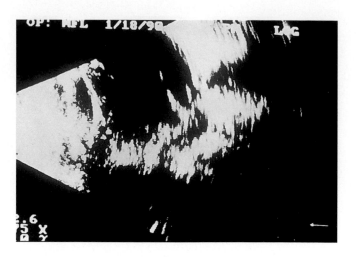

FIGURE 47-7.   *High-resolution B-scan echography documenting posterior scleral laceration, with localized retinal detachment, and overlying vitreous hemorrhage in eye that sustained knife-induced perforating injury.*

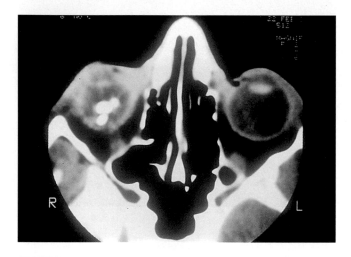

FIGURE 47-6.   *Axial CT scan through orbits, demonstrating multiple intraocular foreign bodies in right eye.*

films of the orbit, including Caldwell or Waters views, could identify a radiopaque foreign body, although localization was difficult at best. Comberg's contact lens and Sweet's external localizer provided better localization, but the techniques involved were cumbersome, and could lead to iatrogenic damage to the eye. Thus, while radiopaque materials can often be imaged with conventional x-ray techniques (29,30), they are difficult to localize.

Computerized tomography (CT) scanning has become the standard method for imaging ruptured globes and detecting and localizing IOFBs because of its sensitivity and other inherent advantages (Fig. 47-6). By assembling many consecutive orbital slices, and reconstructing them in three dimension, the ocular anatomy can be readily demonstrated

and one can determine IOFB presence and location. No manipulation of the globe is necessary, multiple IOFBs may be identified and localized, anteriorly located IOFBs may be discovered, and little patient cooperation is required (31–33). Scanning in two planes is necessary for accurate localization (34).

CT scanning allows detection of IOFBs with diameters of 0.5 mm or more, can distinguish metallic from nonmetallic foreign bodies, and may identify the composition of many nonmetallic IOFBs. CT scanning does have limitations, however. It does not allow differentiation of various types of metallic IOFBs (35) and can miss wooden IOFBs (36), and it is not as helpful as ultrasound in defining various soft-tissue findings such as retinal detachment and vitreous hemorrhage (Fig. 47-7) (37). Recent data suggest that, with modern techniques 3-mm CT scan cuts are as effective as smaller cuts at identifying some IOFBs, at least in an experimental setting (38).

Magnetic resonance imaging (MRI) has also been used to identify and localize IOFBs (39,40), but magnetic IOFBs have been shown to move on exposure to the magnetic field (41,42) and visual loss and vitreous hemorrhage have been attributed to the movement of an occult IOFB and MRI (43).

In most cases of suspected penetrating or perforating trauma, and especially in the setting of a retained IOFB, we suggest routine CT scanning with thin (<1.5 mm) axial and direct coronal cuts when possible. MRI is contraindicated with suspected magnetic IOFBs.

Echography, particularly high-frequency echography (44), is more effective than plain films in the detection of IOFBs (30) and, depending on the echographer's skill, may be as effective as CT scanning (see Fig. 47-7). Rubsamen et al (45) suggested that although CT scanning is still the standard method for IOFB imaging, echography was extremely effective, even through closed lids. Echographic examination accurately identified and localized IOFBs in 46 eyes (Fig. 47-8), including one eye in which the IOFB was a cilium. In addition, echography identified all choroidal hemorrhages, posterior exit sites, retinal detachment, 89% of subretinal hemorrhages, and correctly identified the status of the lens in 82% of cases. Echography can be performed quickly in the office, but in this study, patients with moderate or large corneoscleral lacerations underwent primary wound closure prior to imaging. Echography was then performed either intraoperatively or following closure of the corneal or corneoscleral laceration. Care must be taken to prevent prolapse of intraocular contents if the study is performed on an open globe.

MANAGEMENT OF PENETRATING AND PERFORATING OCULAR INJURY

Mechanism of Injury

Penetrating and perforating injuries, with or without retained IOFBs, have multiple etiologies including work-related injury, especially hammering metal on metal (46,47), assault (48–50), unintentional intraocular injection or perforation particularly during anesthetic administration (51–56), animal bites (57), elastic cords (58), fishhook injuries (59,60), steel wire or suture (61), amniocentesis (62), motor vehicle accidents (63), lawnmower accidents (64), and insect stings (65). Interestingly, wartime ocular injuries have increased in frequency, from about 0.57% of all wartime casualties during the Civil War (45) to 13% during the Desert Shield and Desert Storm operations (66).

In a study examining how the shape of an object affects its ability to penetrate the cornea, Potts and Distler (67)

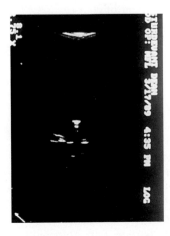
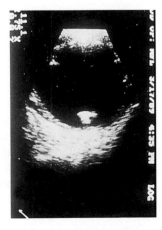

FIGURE 47-8. *Left, high-resolution B-scan echography documenting retained intraocular foreign body (pencil tip) overlying retinal surface. Right, with decreased attenuation, relationship of foreign body to retinal surface can be better appreciated.*

found knife-edged particles, typical of industrial processes, to be the most effective. Such a 20-gauge missile required only 17 mg-msec for penetration, compared to the no-penetration value of 24,840 mg-msec for a BB (68).

Eyes with penetrating or perforating trauma, with or without IOFBs, sustain damage via several mechanisms. The trauma directly affects the tissues that are violated by the penetrating or perforating injury, and there may also be concussive damage to remote sites. Additionally cataract formation or lens subluxation; hyphema; vitreous hemorrhage; retinal tears, detachment, and dialysis; choroidal detachment; endophthalmitis; and, if an IOFB is present, possible metallosis are also seen.

General Principles of Management

The emergent management of penetrating or perforating trauma is guided by a few simple tenets. After a complete ocular examination confirming the diagnosis, and pending surgical repair, the eye should be shielded to avoid any further damage. Infection prophylaxis should be considered especially if there will be a delay in repairing the globe, and the patient's tetanus status should be checked. While most open globe injuries are repaired as soon as the patient is medically cleared for surgery, it appears that in the absence of infection even a delay of up to 36 hours may not adversely affect the outcome (69).

The first goal of surgery is to restore the integrity of the globe. This is accomplished by meticulous wound identification and closure. After the ocular integrity has been restored, attention can be focused on associated ocular problems. Often, these abnormalities are repaired at a later date in a staged approach. Timing of repair is discussed in greater detail in the subsection entitled Timing of Surgery.

It is critical to determine the full extent of the injury. If a corneal laceration extends to the limbus (Fig. 47-9), a conjunctival peritomy should be performed to identify the lesion in its entirety. If no obvious ocular laceration or rupture is noted but the examination is suspicious for rupture (see Fig. 47-2), then a careful exploration of the globe under anesthesia must be performed, with particular attention paid to the regions near the limbus and recti muscle insertions.

Corneal, Corneoscleral, and Scleral Lacerations

Principles guiding repair of lacerations or ruptures of the globe are in general the same, whether in the form of a straightforward corneal laceration or a complex rupture with prolapse of intraocular contents. The primary goal is restoration of the integrity of the globe, with return of the intraocular pressure into the normal range. As noted previously, it is imperative to determine the extent of injury prior to repair of any laceration, and care must be taken not to exacerbate the extent of any injury.

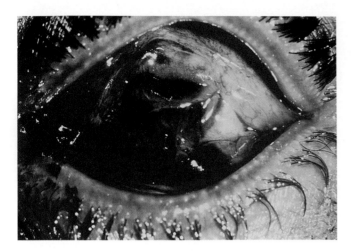

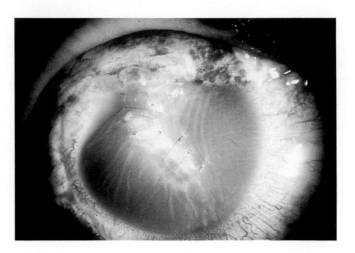

FIGURE 47-9. *Ruptured globe sustained via blunt trauma. Limbus to limbus horizontally aligned corneal laceration, with prolapse of intraocular contents. The full posterior extent of injury could not be appreciated until the patient underwent exploration of the globe. The laceration extended an additional 12 mm posteriorly in the superotemporal direction.*

FIGURE 47-11. *Jagged, vertically aligned corneal laceration, repaired with 10-0 nylon sutures. Note the surrounding corneal stromal edema. The wound extended to limbus superiorly, though did not involve sclera.*

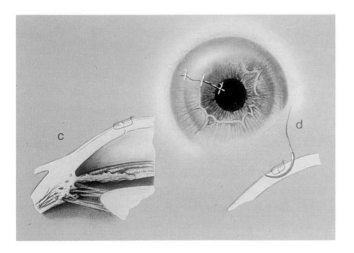

FIGURE 47-10. *Schematic diagram of clean, straight corneal laceration. The initial 10-0 nylon suture is placed in center of wound. All sutures should be approximately two-thirds corneal depth and roughly 1 mm apart. Once wound is reapproximated, it should be checked for possible leakage with Seidel test.*

A simple corneal laceration without tissue loss can be closed with interrupted 10-0 nylon sutures (Figs. 47-10 and 47-11). In general, closure is accomplished by starting in the middle of the laceration site, continually bisecting the wound, and proceeding toward the margins. This allows for a controlled closure. While other approaches can be utilized, the goal of any approach is to ensure that the laceration is watertight. Starting at the midpoint of the lacertion allows for easier maintenance of the anterior chamber, which may also be facilitated by the use of either a viscoelastic sub-

stance or an infusion cannula. Corneal suture bites should be placed approximately one-half to two-thirds tissue thickness, with equal depths on both sides of the laceration. Occasionally, as the repair is in progress, one of the initial sutures needs to be replaced, as it may become loosened as the wound is better reapproximated. If a corneal wound is gaping, a cardinal suture may be placed to reapproximate the wound and to take pressure off subsequent suture placement. This suture is then removed prior to completion of the wound repair. Once all of the sutures have been placed and the wound is watertight, the knots should be buried to limit postoperative irritation. Prolapsed iris/uvea or other intraocular contents should be reposited unless necrotic or obviously infected (Figs. 47-12 and 47-13). Incarcerated tissues may be swept from the wound with the aid of a cyclodialysis spatula (Fig. 47-14).

Stellate corneal lacerations are often difficult to close and may require a temporary cardinal suture to reapproximate the wound. If after suture closure there is persistent leakage, a purse-string suture may be required. This type of suture is placed in a circle configuration through the various portions of the laceration, tied to itself, and the knot buried. When this technique does not work, tissue adhesive may be placed over the laceration site (70). Corneal tissue adhesives may limit the view of the posterior segment at least on a temporary basis. In the setting of significant tissue loss, a corneal patch graft may be necessary.

If a corneal laceration extends to or past the limbus, the first suture should reapproximate the limbus (Fig. 47-15A), as this is a well-defined anatomic site where one knows that the tissue planes are realigned appropriately. After closure of the corneal wound (Fig. 47-15B), the scleral laceration should be carefully explored and closed in a "zipper" fashion from anterior to posterior, with heavier 8-0 or 9-0 nylon (Fig. 47-15C). A lid speculum or lid sutures may facilitate

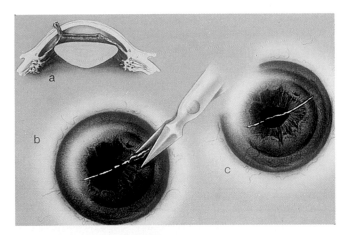

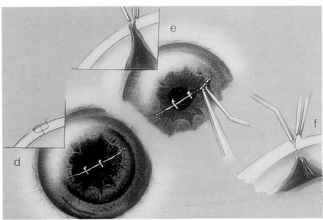

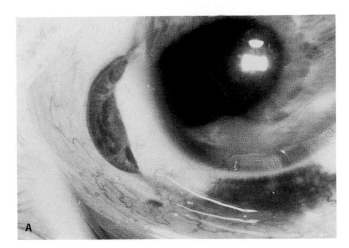

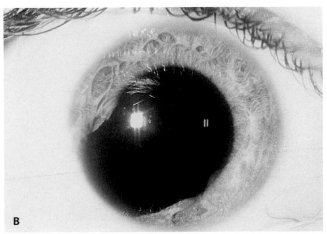

FIGURE 47-12. (A) *Schematic diagram depicting corneal laceration with incarcerated uveal tissue. (B) Tissue is trimmed with scissors at plane of corneal surface. (C) Majority of uveal tissue has been freed from corneal laceration site, though incarcerated tissue may remain at inner surface of wound. (D) Residual prolapsed tissue is reposited with spatula, utilized directly through wound site. (E) Following freeing of residual incarcerated tissue, 10-0 nylon sutures are placed through corneal laceration restoring integrity of the globe.*

FIGURE 47-13. (A) *Anterior scleral laceration with prolapsed uveal tissue sustained with sharp object. (B) Wound was repaired, excising the majority of incarcerated uveal tissue, and lens was also removed at time of initial surgical repair.*

exposure, and a complete peritomy should be performed with gentle dissection to expose all quadrants of the globe. Again, special attention should be paid to the region of the muscle insertions, and traction sutures placed as needed after the primary wound is closed. Occasionally it is necessary to disinsert a muscle to facilitate exploration and closure of a scleral laceration.

While corneal or corneoscleral lacerations are generally quite obvious, detection of scleral lacerations may require exploration. Good exposure of the globe is essential; and, as previously noted, lid sutures or careful placement of a lid speculum will aid in exposure, while minimizing prolapse of ocular contents. The conjunctiva should be opened in all four quadrants. Scleral lacerations are generally repaired with a nonresorbable suture, such as 7-0 to 9-0 nylon. Spatulated needles are generally used, similar to the type of needle employed during placement of a scleral buckle. The wound

is closed with interrupted sutures, starting from anterior to posterior (see Fig. 47-15C), with the end point being a watertight closure.

If a scleral laceration extends toward or beneath a muscle insertion, the muscle may be gently lifted upward away from the surface of the globe with a muscle hook. Occasionally, the muscle will need to be temporarily disinserted to provide adequate visualization and repair. The muscle is placed on a double-armed 6-0 resorbable suture, and cut away from the surface of the globe. Following repair of the scleral laceration, the muscle is placed back at its anatomic location. If a scleral defect is very extensive, on rare occasion a scleral patch graft may need to be employed.

Uveal tissue that prolapsed through the scleral laceration site is generally reposited as the laceration site is being closed, unless it appears necrotic or infected. If uveal tissue is excised, it may be associated with extensive hemorrhage,

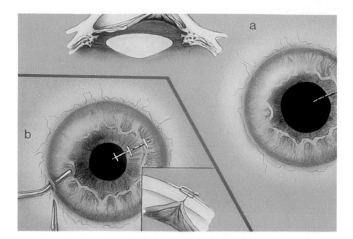

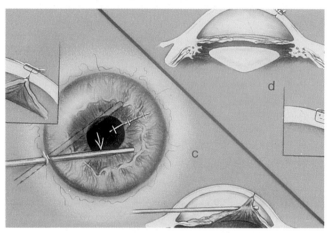

FIGURE 47-14.   (A) *Schematic diagram showing corneal laceration with prolapse of uveal tissue into inner aspect of corneal wound. (B) Infusion cannula is placed in anterior chamber through limbus (or viscoelastics are employed), and wound is sutured. (C) Through previous infusion cannula site, cyclydialysis spatula is ulitilzed to sweep incarcerated tissue out of wound. (D) Inner aspect of corneal wound is now free of incarcerated uveal tissue.*

thus care must be taken to avoid this complication. When there is extruded vitreous, it is generally cut flush with the scleral surface with a sharp scissors. Instruments should never be blindly inserted into the vitreous cavity. If there is apparent prolapse of retina, every attempt should be made to reposit the tissue back into the eye. If a retinal laceration is documented, subsequent repair will be indicated. Cryotherapy is generally not recommended as it may cause increased intraocular inflammation with breakdown of the blood-retinal barrier and possible development of late traction retina detachment (71). Similarly, placement of a prophylactic scleral buckle is generally not recommended. Both of these issues are discussed in greater detail later in the subsections entitled Prophylactic Retinopexy and Retinal Detachment.

Once the integrity of the globe has been restored, we generally recommend deferral of further manipulation unless extenuating circumstances dictate immediate treatment. If endophthalmitis and/or an IOFB are present, then these situations must be addressed and treated primarily. In the absence of these findings, however, we generally recommend delaying further surgery for approximately 7 to 14 days. Numerous findings will require vitrectomy repair, including retinal detachment, disrupted or subluxated lenses, nonclearing vitreous hemorrhage, and hemorrhagic choroidal detachment. By delaying surgery 7 to 14 days, the ocular tissues are less congested, there is a lessened risk of intraoperative hemorrhage, and generally a posterior vitreous separation has developed making further surgery easier to perform. On the converse side, delaying surgical repair may allow for development of fibrovascular proliferation with traction retinal detachment. This timing issue is discussed in greater detail in the next subsection.

Timing of Surgery

Some surgeons advocate immediate or early vitrectomy in cases of penetrating or perforating ocular trauma (72–75) in

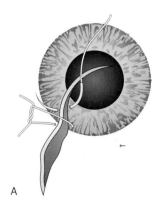
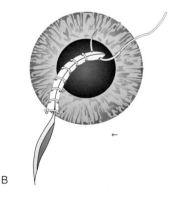
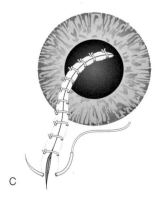

FIGURE 47-15.   (A) *Schematic diagram showing corneoscleral laceration. The initial suture is placed at the limbus, where one can precisely reapproximate the proper alignment of the tissue. (B) Corneal portion of wound is then closed with interrupted 10-0 nylon sutures. (C) Slceral portion of wound is then closed, generally with either 8-0 or 9-0 nylon sutures, making certain to fully explore most posterior extent of laceration.*

an effort to prevent severe inflammatory changes that may occur after injury, to allow immediate visualization and repair of posterior segment injury, and to prevent intraocular proliferation that may lead to retinal detachment. In addition, performing all surgical procedures in one setting eliminates the need for further anesthesia (1).

DeJuan et al (76) noted a trend toward better visual acuity in patients undergoing early vitrectomy, although this may have been due to certain characteristics in the group of eyes undergoing early vitrectomy. These patients had better initial visual acuity, more anteriorly located lacerations, less vitreous hemorrhage, and a higher incidence of IOFBs, each of which has been correlated with a more favorable visual prognosis (76).

There are advantages to delaying vitreous surgery. It allows for further diagnostic evaluation and permits repair in a more controlled atmosphere (1). Delay may also improve visualization by allowing the media to clear. In addition, there is a risk of severe intraoperative hemorrhage when early vitrectomy is performed (77–79), and delaying the surgery may decrease this risk (1,10). Most importantly, delaying vitreous surgery may allow for spontaneous separation of the posterior hyaloid from the retina, thus facilitating more complete and less hazardous vitreous removal (1,10).

Following a penetrating ocular injury in a controlled trial in monkeys, vitrectomy was performed either immediately, at day 14, or 70 days later. There was no difference in outcome between the groups that had vitrectomy either immediately or 14 days after injury (80). A clinical study also supports the conclusion that early vitrectomy does not improve the prognosis (81). In addition, with perforating wounds, the posterior exit site may not be watertight for at least a week after the injury (1), requiring a delay to facilitate vitrectomy in a closed system.

Unfortunately, no prospective study has been performed regarding the timing of surgical intervention after penetrating or perforating trauma. A proposed clinical trial, the Vitrectomy for Trauma Study (VTS), was never funded, and a similar study has never been performed on a prospective basis. It is therefore up to the individual surgeon to determine the optimum time for intervention on a case-by-case basis. In general, we recommend that vitreous surgery be performed 7 to 10 days after the initial injury, unless mitigating circumstances are present, such as the presence of endophthalmitis or a retained IOFB. These recommendations are further reviewed in an editorial by Mieler (82). Delaying repair beyond 14 days is not recommended due to the risk of sympathetic ophthalmia.

Cataract, Subluxed, and Dislocated Lenses

A contusive injury to the eye can impart enough energy to the lens to cause opacification, or it may lead to subluxation or dislocation. In a similar fashion, a penetrating injury that violates the lens capsule will generally also lead to either cataract formation or lens subluxation. By definition, a lens is subluxated when the zonular fibers are broken and it is no longer held securely in place, even though it remains in the pupillary aperture. It is dislocated when all of the zonules are disrupted, allowing the lens to fall into the vitreous cavity.

When assessing a patient following either blunt or penetrating trauma, one must carefully check for the presence of phacodenesis. A sign of lens subluxation is prolapse of vitreous around the lens into the anterior chamber. Surgical extraction of a subluxated or cataractous lens should be considered when the cataract leads to significant visual impairment, or if removal will aid in the visualization and management of associated posterior segment damage. In children, the possibility of amblyopia must also be considered.

When surgery is planned for a subluxated lens, vitreous loss is anticipated. While the surgery can be performed through a limbal approach, a pars plana approach offers significant advantages. In the previtrectomy era, numerous techniques were utilized to prevent the lens from falling posteriorly into the vitreous cavity. Even if the lens position can be stabilized, there are also significant concerns regarding possible aspiration of vitreous into the anterior chamber. This leads to an increased risk of postoperative cystoid macular edema and retinal detachment formation. A pars plana approach avoids many of these concerns and allows for significantly more flexibility when dealing with intraoperative complications.

With a three-port pars plana vitrectomy setup, an infusion cannula is placed through the pars plana 3.0 mm posterior to the limbus in the inferotemporal quadrant and is sutured in place. A second instrument employed in the superonasal quadrant, such as a myringotomy blade or a secondary infusion cannula, is directed into the lens through the equator, helping to hold the lens in place. The third instrument, a phacofragmentor, is then inserted through the opposite pole of the lens (Fig. 47-16A). The lens is then slowly digested. Vitreous should be removed around the margins of the lens prior to phacofragmentation. Soft lenses, such as in children, may be removed solely with aspiration.

If lens remnants fall posteriorly, the secondary infusion cannula can be replaced with an illumination probe (Fig. 47-16B). A vitrectomy is then performed, and the lens remnants are removed with the phacofragmentor. If the lens remnants have fallen onto the retinal surface, they are gently aspirated into the midvitreous cavity prior to removal via phacofragmentation. Remnants of the peripheral lens capsule can also be excised (Fig. 47-16C), though on occasion they are left in place with the intent that they help to secure placement of an intraocular lens, depending on the extent of associated ocular damage. Following removal of the lens, the peripheral retina should be carefully inspected, as should all sclerotomy sites, checking for retinal tears, dialyses, and/or detachment.

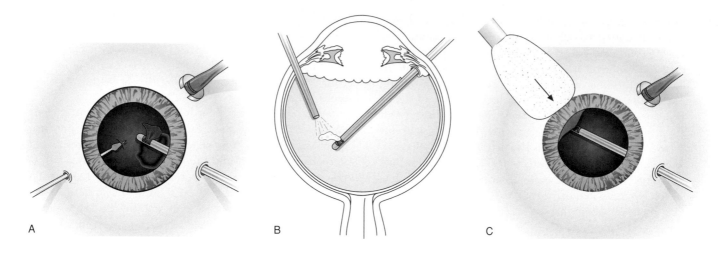

FIGURE 47-16. (A) *Schematic diagram showing three-port pars plana vitrectomy setup. A secondary irrigation needle has been placed into subluxated lens to help secure its position, and irrigation may also help to soften lens.* (B) *If lens remnants fall posteriorly, they may be removed with combination vitrectomy and phacofragmentation.* (C) *Remnants of lens capsule can be removed with vitrectomy cutter. Mild scleral indentation aids in removal of peripheral capsular remnants.*

Management of the patient's monocular aphakic status is controversial, especially in children (83,84). Several intraoperative options exist, and these are discussed in the next subsection. Postoperative contact lens correction is always an option. Posterior chamber intraocular lens placement may be difficult due to compromised zonular support, though lenses can be sutured in the ciliary sulcus utilizing a variety of techniques (85–92). Anterior chamber lens implants may be utilized, as long as there is no significant compromise of angle structures from the effects of the injury (93). Even epikeratophakia may be considered. The method of rehabilitation that is best for the patient must be determined on a case-by-case basis. Unfortunately, long-term follow-up is lacking for all of the lens replacement options, especially in the setting of trauma.

Lens Implantation

In an effort to speed visual rehabilitation after penetrating injury with or without IOFB, posterior-chamber intraocular lenses (PC IOLs) have been implanted during primary repair in selected cases (94,95). Slusher et al (94) reported two patients who underwent concurrent placement of PC IOLs after removal of intraretinal foreign bodies. One patient had a postoperative visual acuity of 20/20, and the other 20/30, with minimal spectacle correction. Chan et al (95) reported that 10 of 11 patients who received primary PC IOL implantation had a final visual acuity of 20/60 or better. Other authors have also described successful lens implantation in association with simultaneous repair of penetrating ocular injuries (96–98). In selected cases where there is a low risk of endophthalmitis, this approach seems reasonable, as long as the patient understands the risks involved. However, given the relatively high incidence of

infection and the propensity for the need for further surgery due to scar tissue formation and retinal detachment, we do not routinely recommend placement of an intraocular lens at the time of initial repair.

Vitreous Hemorrhage and Proliferation

Vitreous hemorrhage may develop secondary to damage to the ciliary body, retinal, or choroidal vessels. The hemorrhage is often limited to the immediate posttraumatic period, thus the initial fundus examination may allow the best visualization of any retinal abnormalities. Subsequent diffusion of the hemorrhage or additional hemorrhage may compromise later examinations. In the presence of a penetrating or perforating ocular injury, scleral indentation should be avoided. If the view of the posterior segment is not adequate, echography should be performed but must be done cautiously so as to avoid possible prolapse of intraocular tissues. As indicated earlier in this chapter, echography is quite sensitive in detecting the presence of posterior vitreous separation, retinal tear, detachment, and dialysis, choroidal hemorrhages, giant retinal tears, subluxated lenses, and occult scleral ruptures (45). These findings will play a significant role in the determination of the need for further surgery, and findings such as hemorrhagic suprachoroidals will not only influence the timing of repair, but also the surgical approach that is eventually employed.

Despite advances in the management of eyes with trauma, a number of patients with posterior penetrating ocular injuries still have a guarded prognosis, especially those with posterior segment involvement. The presence of a pupillary afferent defect, wounds involving the sclera or extending posterior to the insertion of the recti muscles, wounds greater than 10mm in extent, and the presence of vitreous hemorrhage are all associated with a worsened outcome (76,99). The prognosis after a penetrating injury is greatly influenced by the initial damage. When functional loss of the eye occurs, it is generally due to inoperable retinal detachment or loss of ciliary body function secondary to fibrovascular proliferation.

In the setting of vitreous hemorrhage following blunt ocular injury, and in the absence of associated ocular abnormalities, a period of observation for a month or two is warranted to allow for spontaneous clearing of the hemorrhage. In contrast, hemorrhage occurring in association with a penetrating or perforating ocular injury is generally removed much earlier because of the close link between an open-globe injury, hemorrhage, and the fibrovascular proliferative response. Surgery is generally performed within 7 to 10 days following such an injury. The goals of surgery are to clear the ocular media through removal of cataractous lens (if present) and/or vitreous hemorrhage, to remove the vitreous scaffold from the scleral laceration site, to remove the posterior hyaloid to limit epiretinal membrane formation and vitreoretinal traction, and to identify and treat retinal breaks and detachment.

When surgery is performed to clear vitreous hemorrhage, numerous decisions must be made at the onset of surgery. The presence of hemorrhagic choroidals must be ruled out, which is generally done through the use of preoperative echography. This issue is discussed later in the subsection *Suprachoroidal Hemorrhage*. It must also be decided if surgery can be performed initially through the pars plana or through the limbus. If there is hyphema, or difficulty visualizing the tip of the vitreous infusion cannula, then the surgery may need to be started through the limbus. A decision must also be made regarding the status of the lens, if it is still present. In most cases, it is removed to facilitate completion of the vitrectomy procedure. Leaving the lens in place often limits visualization of the anterior retinal periphery and does not allow for meticulous inspection of the vitreous base and peripheral retina. The surgery itself will also generally cause further lens opacification.

For the vitrectomy surgery itself, a standard three-port pars plana vitrectomy is employed. After placement of an infusion cannula 3.0 to 3.5 mm posterior to the limbus in the inferotemporal quadrant, the tip of the cannula is visualized to be certain of its proper placement. If it cannot be seen, a temporary anterior segment infusion cannula may be placed (Fig. 47-17), though this requires removal of the lens as noted previously. Once the tip of the cannula has been visualized, an illumination probe is placed through a second sclerotomy site superonasally and a vitreous cutter is placed through the third site superotemporally. A core vitrectomy is performed, working from anterior to posterior, attempting to visualize the retina as soon as possible in order to avoid an inadvertent encounter with it. The illumination probe and the vitreous cutter are frequently interchanged between the two superior sclerotomy

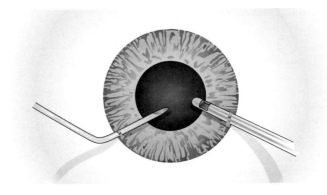

FIGURE 47-17. *Schematic diagram depicting temporary placement of infusion cannula in anterior segment through limbus, following inadequate visualization of pars plana infusion cannula.*

sites, especially if the patient is phakic, in order to avoid striking the posterior surface of the lens and causing a cataract. The posterior hyaloid is removed, along with any tractional proliferation. If there is hemorrhage on the retinal surface, it is aspirated with a soft-tipped extrusion needle or cannula. Tractional proliferation is removed via membrane peeling with delamination or segmentation techniques, employing a variety of intraocular scissors, forceps, and picks. The peripheral retina is then carefully inspected for evidence of possible retinal tear, dialysis, or detachment formation. If abnormalities are found, retinopexy is applied and a scleral buckle is also placed. Additional modalites may be required including the temporary use of liquid perfluorocarbon liquids, long-acting gases, or silicone oil. These areas are further discussed later in the subsections entitled Retinopexy and Retinal Detachment.

If the posterior hyaloid is not spontaneously separated, an attempt should be made to separate it. Generally this can be accomplished by engaging it with either a soft-tipped extrusion cannula or with a sharp myringotomy blade. This process is generally started near the margins of the optic nerve and carried out toward the periphery.

If intraocular hemorrhage occurs during surgery, it is most commonly controlled by temporary elevation of the infusion bottles and/or with intraocular diathermy. Other methods of control have also been suggested, including fluid-gas exchange, silicone oil injection, sodium hyaluronate injection, and the use of irrigation solution additives such as thrombin (100).

The overall prognosis for eyes with vitreous hemorrhage is associated primarily with concurrent retinal abnormalities that may have occurred as part of the initial injury (76,99). Vision limiting factors include macular damage from contusive effects of the injury, including commotio retinae, macular hole formation, and choroidal rupture. Impaired vision also results from retinal tears, detachment, and dialyses, along with choroidal hemorrhages.

Retinal Detachment

It is relatively uncommon for a patient to develop an acute rhegmatogenous retinal detachment following blunt ocular trauma. Most trauma patients are quite young, with more solid vitreous, which tends to provide internal tamponade even in the setting of a retinal tear or dialysis. When problems do arise however, atypical retinal tears tend to be quite large and more posterior in location. Giant retinal tears and dialyses may also be seen. Treatment of these abnormalities is usually quite complex, requiring an array of retinopexy, scleral buckling techniques, vitrectomy surgery, and the use of temporary or permanent internal tamponade agents.

In the setting of a penetrating or perforating ocular injury, the situation is even more complex. In general, detachments occurring after penetrating or perforating injury portend a worsened prognosis. The method of treatment of retinal detachment in cases of penetrating trauma once again includes vitrectomy surgery with relief of any tractional proliferation, creation of a posterior vitreous separation, use of retinotomy and/or retinectomy, possible placement of a scleral buckle, use of retinopexy, fluid-gas exchange, and internal tamponade with either a long-acting

gas or silicone oil. Postoperative positioning may be required.

A particular problem seen with posterior segment penetrating ocular injuries is retinal or vitreous incarceration in the scleral laceration site (Figs. 47-3 and 47-18A). This can make management of a retinal detachment more difficult. If occurring anteriorly, the incarceration site can be treated with retinopexy, the tissue cleared from the incarceration site generally with retinotomy techniques, and the region supported on a scleral buckle (Figs. 47-18A, B, C). More posteriorly located sites generally require creation of a retinotomy (Fig. 47-18D), with the site then demarcated with laser and supported with either a long-acting gas or silicone oil tamponade. With these techniques, Han et al (101) achieved anatomic stability in 11 of 15 eyes (73%), although only six eyes regained vision of 5/200 or better.

In cases of penetrating or perforating trauma where it is not certain if retinal damage has occurred, it is unclear if placement of a prophylactic scleral buckle is warranted. Such a buckle may support the vitreous base and guard against later contraction. It may also provide support of a scleral laceration site where vitreous and/or retina may be incarcerated. A buckle further may provide a sense of security for the surgeon, especially when visualization of the

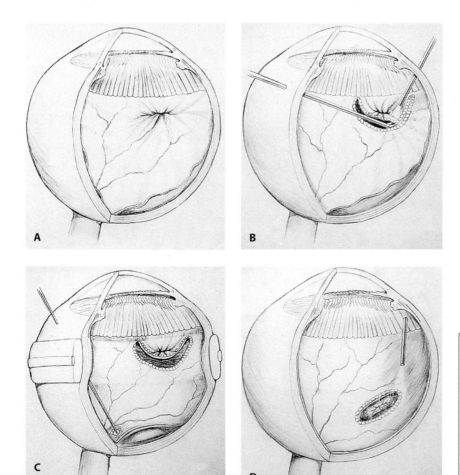

A   **B**   **C**   **D**

FIGURE 47-18.   (A) *Schematic diagram of anterior retinal incarceration site.* (B) *Vitrectomy surgery has been performed and photocoagulation placed along margins of incarceration site. A retinotomy is now being performed to excise incarcerated tissue.* (C) *The region is then supported by scleral buckle.* (D) *Posterior retinal incarceration site. Retinotomy has been performed, to be followed by placement of either long-acting gas or silicone oil to provide tamponade of this region.*

retinal periphery is difficult. Several studies have suggested a beneficial effect from prophylactic scleral buckling (26,102-104), while one study has suggested a possible harmful effect (105). No randomized, controlled clinical trial has proven the efficacy of prophylactic scleral buckling. The authors generally do not recommend routinely placing a prophylactic scleral buckle. In contrast, if definite peripheral retinal tears are documented, they are treated with retinopexy and generally supported with a scleral buckle.

Retinopexy

Retinopexy must be considered whenever retinal injury has occurred after penetrating or perforating trauma. In the setting of a scleral laceration without definite evidence of retinal tear formation, the intent of retinopexy treatment is to form a retinal adhesion at the site of injury in an effort to limit or prevent possible retinal detachment formation. Numerous reports have suggested, however, that in the absence of a functional retinal tear or hole (10), cryotherapy may be contraindicated because it stimulates the dispersion of retinal pigment epithelium (71), causes increased breakdown of the blood-retinal barrier (106,107), and leads to an increased risk of traction retinal detachment (108). In general, we recommend laser retinopexy or cryotherapy when retinal holes or tears are documented and otherwise do not perform prophylactic retinopexy.

Retinal Tamponade

Management of complex retinal detachment after penetrating or perforating trauma often requires either long-acting intraocular gas or silicone oil tamponade. If retinal breaks, retinotomy, or retinectomy are inferiorly located, then silicone oil is particularly useful, although its use generally necessitates at least one additional surgical procedure to remove the oil three to six months after placement. The Silicone Oil Study has shown the effectiveness of either silicone oil or perfluoropropane (C_3F_8) gas as a retinal tamponade for eyes with nontraumatic retinal detachments and severe proliferative vitreoretinopathy (PVR), with some mild differences in postoperative complications (109–114).

Silicone oil has also been used as a successful tamponade for complicated traumatic retinal detachments after failed vitrectomy, with functional success (5/200 or better) in about 50% to 60% of eyes (115,116). However, there has been no randomized, controlled study comparing intraocular gas (C_3F_8) and silicone oil in traumatic retinal detachment with PVR. Given previous reports, however, we generally reserve the use of silicone oil for cases when inferior pathology is present (such as retinotomy or retinectomy) or when the patient is unable to position properly.

Suprachoroidal Hemorrhage

Suprachoroidal hemorrhage is an occasional complication of severe penetrating or perforating ocular trauma. Appositional or "kissing" choroidals may cause angle closure with flattening of the anterior chamber and elevated uncontrolled intraocular pressure. They are often associated with concurrent overlying retinal detachment. Successful treatment of massive posttraumatic suprachoroidal hemorrhage has been reported (117). Surgical drainage is often required, generally after the hemorrhagic choroidal detachment has liquefied sufficiently to allow for easier removal (Fig. 47-19). This usually occurs at an average of 10 to 14 days after occurrence. If there is an associated retinal detachment, successful reattachment can often be achieved with pars plana vitrectomy techniques. Visual recovery is generally in the 20/200 range. A significant number of eyes will have no light perception, however, or have persistent postoperative hypotony (118).

When confronted with massive suprachoroidal hemorrhage with controlled intraocular pressure, we perform serial echographic examinations to monitor for liquefaction of the hemorrhage. As noted previously, this usually occurs within 10 to 14 days. Once that occurs, drainage can proceed. Radial scleral incisions are made at or anterior to the equator in the quadrants with the greatest extent of hemorrhage. The incisions are generally 4 mm in length. The suprachoroidal space is entered with a sharp myringotomy blade, and gentle pressure is placed on the globe. An anterior chamber infusion with either fluid or air (dependent upon the status of the lens) is used to maintain intraocular pressure, and help push the hemorrhage out of the suprachoroidal space, through the sclerotomy site, and out of the eye. In conjunction with the drainage of the hemorrhagic choroidals, pars plana vitrectomy is generally

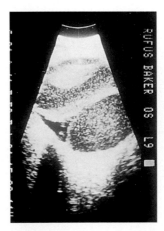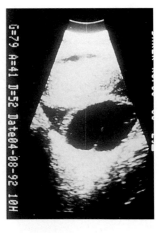

FIGURE 47-19. *High-resolution B-scan echogram (left) showing liquefaction of hemorrhagic choroidal 10 days following development of appositional hemorrhagic choroidal (right) following penetrating ocular injury.*

performed, especially in the setting of an associated retinal detachment.

Endophthalmitis

Trauma accounts for approximately 25% of cases of culture-proven endophthalmitis, with infection occurring in 2% to 7% of penetrating ocular injuries (119). A high index of suspicion must always be maintained for infection in the setting of trauma, as the usual signs and symptoms may be masked by the effects of the trauma. All cases of suspected infection should be dealt with promptly, especially since a delay beyond 24 hours is associated with a worsened outcome. The signs of infection are generally very similar to those occurring in the postoperative setting and include aqueous cell and flare, hypopyon formation (Fig. 47-20), and vitreous cell and flare exceeding that expected from the injury itself. Retinal periphlebitis may also be a sign of early infection.

Cases of suspected infection should have an aqueous paracentesis performed, followed by a vitreous tap for culture purposes. The vitreous specimen is best obtained through the vitrectomy cutter, because then there is no traction placed on the vitreous. Approximately 0.3 cc of undiluted vitreous provides an adequate sample for culture purposes, and then the entire vitreous washings can also be collected at the end of the case and sent for culture purposes. The issue of a vitreous tap versus a full vitrectomy is usually not a concern because most trauma cases require vitrectomy for repair of damage associated with the injury. Centrifugation or passing the material through a membrane filter system may increase the rate of positive cultures (120).

Trauma-related endophthalmitis has a spectrum of causative organisms similar to other types of exogenous endophthalmitis (121), although the incidence of *Bacillus* species infection is much higher, ranging between 25% and 50%. *Staphylococcus* coagulase negative organisms account for approximately 24% of infections, followed by *Streptococcal* species in 13%, *Staphylococcus aureus* in 8%, and gram-negative organisms in 7%. The setting of trauma also carries the risk of polymicrobial infections. The antibiotics employed in the management of endophthalmitis are outlined in Table 47-1. Antibiotic selection is very important, yet in most cases broad-spectrum coverage readily handles the infection (122). In the majority of cases, the intravitreal injections include vancomycin (1.0 mg/0.1 cc), with either ceftazidime (2.25 mg/0.1 cc) or amikacin (200–400 µg/0.1 cc). While antibiotics can be added to the infusion solution, the authors prefer to inject a known amount of antibiotic directly into the vitreous cavity at the completion of the operation, in the doses outlined above. Subjunctival, topical, and systemic antibiotics are also generally employed, with the usual medications and dosages also outlined in Table 47-1.

The mechanism of action of the various antibiotics varies as does their effectiveness against different organisms. Vancomycin acts by inhibition of cell wall assembly, damages protoplasts, and inhibits RNA synthesis. It is the antibiotic of choice for gram-positive coverage, including *Bacillus* species, and *Proprionibacterium acnes*. Cephalosporins, including cefazolin and ceftazidime, are synthetic penicillins active against the bacterial cell wall. They provide good broad-spectrum coverage for gram-positive and some gram-negative organisms, although they are relatively ineffective against enterococcus and methicillin-resistant *Staphylococcal* organisms. The aminoglycosides, including gentamicin and amikacin, act by inhibition of protein synthesis. When utilized, they are chosen for gram-negative coverage. The intraocular therapeutic ratio is a source of concern, as there is a definite risk of retinal toxicity. Ciprofloxacin, a quinolone,

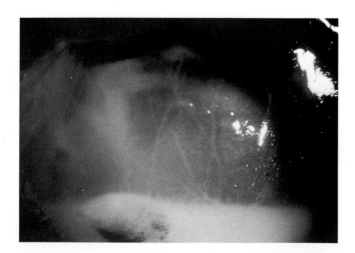

FIGURE 47-20. *Layered hypopyon with corneal clouding and anterior segment fibrin formation in eye following a penetrating ocular injury occurring two days previously.*

Table 47-1. Antibiotics and Corticosteroids Employed in the Management of Acute Bacterial Endophthalmitis

Intravitreal
Vancomycin (1.0 mg) with ceftazidime (2.25 mg) or amikacin (200–400 µg)
Dexamethasone (400 µg) (controversial)
Periocular (Subconjunctival)
Vancomycin (25–50 mg) with ceftazidime (100 mg)
Dexamethasone (4–12 mg)
Topical
Vancomycin (50 mg/cc), or ceftazidime (50 mg/cc)
Topical corticosteroid and cycloplegic
Systemic
Vancomycin (1 gram q 12 hrs IV), or ceftazidime (1 gram q 8 hrs IV), or cefazolin (1 gram q 8 hrs IV), or ciprofloxacin (400 mg q 12 hrs IV), or ciprofloxacin (750 mg q 12 hrs orally)
Prednisone (0.7–1.0 mg/kg/day)

acts by inhibition of DNA synthesis. It provides good coverage against gram-negative aerobes but has limited effectiveness against *Streptococci* and anaerobes. As can be seen, the combination of intravitreal vancomycin with either ceftazidime or amikacin provides broad-spectrum coverage against the majority of organisms that are associated with traumatic endophthalmitis.

The issue of endophthalmitis and the employment of antibiotics, along with the route of administration, are discussed in greater detail in the following section Surgical Management of Retained IOFBs, under Endophthalmitis. Prophylaxis against the risk of infection is also discussed in greater detail in the following section.

Prognosis and Outcome

About 3000 penetrating ocular injuries are recorded each year, approximately 20% of which are assault-related (49,50,123). In a prospective study of 91 patients with penetrating ocular trauma (124), domestic accidents and assult each accounted for about one third of the injuries. Eyes injured by sharp objects with lacerations less than 10 mm in length and with initial visual acuity better than 20/200 fared better than those eyes that suffered blunt trauma, had larger lacerations, or whose initial visual acuity was worse than 20/200 (76,99). Groessl et al (50), in a series of assault-related injuries, found similarly that eyes injured by sharp objects and sustaining lacerations of 10 mm or less tended to fare better than eyes with blunt injury or larger lacerations. In addition, it was noted that eyes with lacerations limited to the anterior segment and not extending posterior to the equator had a better visual prognosis. Other investigators have reported a similar relation between prognosis and laceration location (124,125). Sternberg et al (126) used multivariate analysis to determine prognostic factors in 281 eyes with penetrating ocular injuries. An initial visual acuity of 20/800 or better was the most important predictor of a final acuity of 20/800 or better. Other important prognostic factors in eyes with initial acuities worse than 20/800 included a laceration limited to the cornea, the absence of a subluxed or expelled lens, and lacerations located anterior to the rectus muscle insertions. In patients older than 18, the presence of an IOFB was favorable, although in patients less than 18 the presence of an IOFB strongly correlated with a poor outcome. This discrepancy is likely due to the relatively high proportion of BB injuries in young patients.

The prognosis for eyes with penetrating and perforating trauma has improved over the last 50 years, but it still remains a significant and sometimes devastating cause of ocular morbidity. Cherry (127) performed a large, retrospective study of penetrating ocular trauma between 1952 and 1970 and found only 6% of the injured eyes had a visual acuity of 5/200 or better. A later study in 1984 by deJuan et al (76) from the same institution found that 31% obtained a visual acuity of 5/200 or better, while a 1996 report by

Pieramici et al (99) docmented that 57% of patients achieved a final level of vision at 5/200 or better. Meredith and Gordon (128) reported the results of treatment of 50 eyes with severe posterior penetrating injury and noted that 50% were "visual successes." In the group that suffered sharp injury, visual acuity was 20/400 or better in 62%, while in the blunt injury group 31% had a visual acuity of 20/400 or better. Macular changes were the most common cause of limited visual acuity and were more likely in the blunt trauma group. As noted above, the visual results continue to slowly improve over the years.

Liggett et al (129) retrospectively reported a decreased rate of phthisis and enucleation, and improved anatomic and visual outcomes in vitrectomized versus nonvitrectomized eyes with retinal detachment after penetrating trauma. The differences between the two groups, however, was less significant when controlled for the type of trauma. Bonnet and Fleury (130) reported retinal reattachment in 82% of eyes with retinal detachment after penetrating trauma. Final visual acuity was 20/40 or better in 46% of eyes. Factors found to have an adverse influence were blunt trauma and anterior PVR.

Several authors have reported results of treatment of perforating injury (81,131–133). Vatne and Syrdale (81) and Ramsay et al (131) treated 22 eyes after perforating injury from shotgun pellets, and also found 50% attained 5/200 or better final visual acuity. Preoperative posterior vitreous detachment was associated with a more favorable outcome. In addition, patients with exit wounds outside of the arcades were more likely to have final visual acuities of 20/70 or better.

SURGICAL MANAGEMENT OF RETAINED IOFB

The advent of vitreous microsurgical techniques has revolutionized the treatment of severe ocular injuries, including those with IOFBs. While the majority of eyes can be salvaged and vision restored, in a number of cases the visual prognosis remains guarded (134). In cases where there is trauma to the optic nerve or macula, even with currently available microsurgical techniques, visual recovery may still be limited. Vitrectomy allows for controlled removal of IOFBs and repair of the concurrent intraocular damage, and possibly reduces the risk of endophthalmitis by irrigating fluid through the eye (135). External magnets can also readily remove magnetic IOFBs in select situations (134). The role of the various routes of IOFB extraction will be discussed and reviewed in this section, along with the surgical outcomes. General guidelines for management of IOFBs are listed in Table 47-2.

Mechanism of Injury and Type of Foreign Body

In a series of 105 eyes with intraocular foreign bodies (134), 76 eyes (72%) were injured as a result of hammering

Table 47-2. Management of Intraocular Foreign Bodies

Location and Type	Clear Media	Poorly Visualized
Intravitreal		
Magnetic	External magnet	Vitrectomy, with either rare earth magnet or forceps
Nonmagnetic	Vitrectomy with forceps	Vitrectomy with forceps
Intraretinal		
Magnetic	Scleral cutdown (anterior) or vitrectomy with rare earth magnet or forceps	Vitrectomy with either rare earth magnet or forceps
Nonmagnetic	Scleral cutdown (anterior) or vitrectomy with forceps	Vitrectomy with forceps
Intraocular		
Large size (>5 mm)	Vitrectomy with forceps delivery either through pars plana or limbus	Vitrectomy with forceps delivery either through the pars plana or limbus

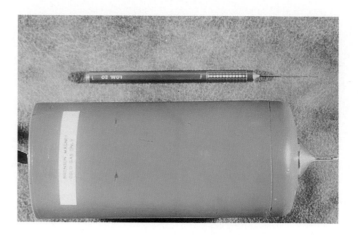

FIGURE 47-21. *Bronson electromagnet and intraocular rare earth magnet.*

metal on metal. Eleven eyes (10%) were injured by shot or BBs, 7 (7%) by an explosion, and 11 (10%) by other mechanisms. In other studies, 70% to 80% of IOFBs occurred in relationship with hammering metal on metal (136,137).

Eighty to ninety percent of IOFBs are metallic (134,138). The most commonly encountered metals are iron (138) and lead, although IOFBs composed of copper, zinc, silver, gold, platinum, and nickel have been noted (139). From 55% to 80% of metallic IOFBs are magnetic (138). Other types of foreign bodies include cilia (140), caterpillar hairs (141), nylon line (142), pencil lead (143), PVC plastic (144), gunpowder (145), bone (146), and iatrogenically introduced materials such as lint, rubber, cotton, and suture material (147).

Wound location may vary depending on the mechanism of injury. Williams et al (134) in their report on retained IOFBs found corneal entrance wounds in 65% of eyes, scleral wounds in 25%, and corneoscleral wounds in 10%. Wound size varied from less than 1 mm to 12 mm in length. Most eyes contained only one foreign body; however, about 8% of eyes harbored at least two. Sixty-one percent of IOFBs were located in the vitreous, 14% were intraretinal, and 5% were subretinal. The remainder were located in the anterior chamber (15%) or lens (8%). Other studies support this data (136–138).

Methods of IOFB Extraction

Magnetic Extraction

External electromagnets and internal rare earth magnets (Fig. 47-21) can be used to remove magnetic foreign bodies from the posterior segment via a direct or indirect approach (148). The direct approach is to place the electromagnet over a scleral cutdown adjacent to the magnetic IOFB (Fig. 47-22). The IOFB should be situated at or anterior to the

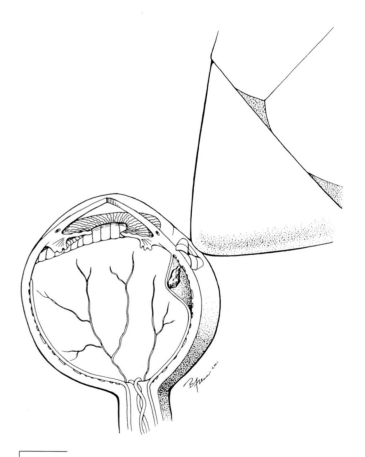

FIGURE 47-22. *Schematic diagram depicting removal of anteriorly located subretinal magnetic IOFB via scleral cutdown with external electromagnet.*

equator of the eye and be either intraretinal or subretinal in location. Visualization and localization by indirect ophthalmoscopy are essential. A scleral cutdown is made over the site of the IOFB, generally in a T-shaped configuration, and diathermy is applied to the uveal bed. In all cases, the scleral incision must be large enough to accommodate the IOFB, which generally means the incision should be at least 1 or 2 mm larger than the greatest dimension of the IOFB. The external electromagnet is then utilized to bring the IOFB through the uvea, where it is either removed directly or grasped with a forceps. The sclerotomy site is then sutured closed. In select situations, especially in the presence of a retinal tear, the IOFB site is treated with either cryotherapy or photocoagulation and is supported with a scleral buckle.

The indirect approach is to place the electromagnet at an extraction site on the pars plana, as close as possible to the location of the IOFB (148). The sclerotomy site is opened with a myringotomy blade and diathermy is also applied to the uveal bed. The magnet should be directed so that as the IOFB is removed, it does not damage any intraocular structure inadvertently. With the external electromagnet, there may be arcing of the magnetic field, thus as the IOFB is extracted from the eye it could strike either the anterior retina or the posterior surface of the lens. The indirect approach is used primarily for small, magnetic, intravitreal IOFBs (Fig. 47-23) or even for IOFBs on the retinal surface that are not encapsulated. Good surgical results have been reported with these methods (149,150). The main disadvantage of electromagnets stems from their

incorrect use or inaccurate foreign body localization, which once again may result in retinal, vitreous base, or lenticular damage (150).

Intraocular rare earth magnets are also available (see Fig. 47-21) and are utilized in conjunction with pars plana vitrectomy when there is evidence of tissue incarceration, associated intraocular damage, or media opacities precluding adequate initial visualization of a magnetic IOFB (Fig. 47-24A). The rare earth magnets have a more unidirectional field but are not as powerful as the external electromagnets. Thus, when an IOFB is removed with a rare earth magnet, it generally needs to be passed off to an intraocular forceps prior to removal from the eye (Fig. 47-24B).

Extraction with Vitrectomy

There is no statistically significant difference in visual outcome between the different routes of extraction

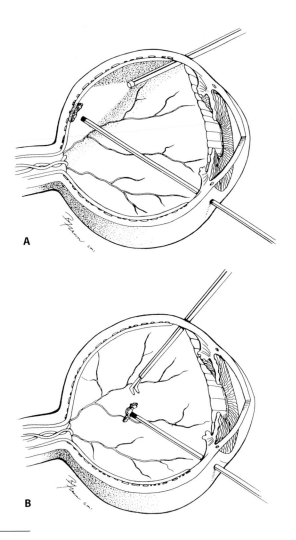

A

B

FIGURE 47-24. (A) *Schematic diagram showing magnetic IOFB lying on retinal surface. Vitrectomy has been performed. The IOFB is then freed of any encapsulated tissue and finally raised off retinal surface with intraocular rare earth magnet.* (B) *Prior to removing IOFB from eye, it is passed off to intraocular forceps in midvitreous cavity.*

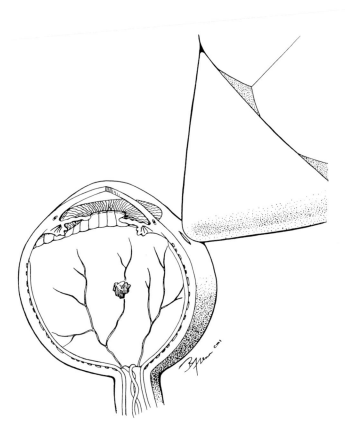

FIGURE 47-23. *Schematic diagram showing removal of magnetic intravitreal foreign body through sclerotomy site at pars plana with external electromagnet.*

(134,149,151) when the method chosen is appropriate for the type of IOFB and associated ocular abnormalities. As noted in the previous section, we suggest that primary external magnet extraction be reserved for cases in which a small intravitreal magnetic foreign body can be visualized and is free from tissue incarceration or encapsulation (see Fig. 47-23). In addition, for relatively anteriorly located magnetic foreign bodies embedded in the retina or choroid that are not encapsulated, removal through a scleral cutdown is appropriate (see Fig. 49-22). However, pars plana vitrectomy with forceps removal of the IOFB should be used in all cases with nonmagnetic foreign bodies (Fig. 47-25), posterior, incarcerated foreign bodies (Fig. 47-26), media opacities precluding view of the IOFB or fundus, associated ocular injuries requiring vitrectomy, lensectomy, or other

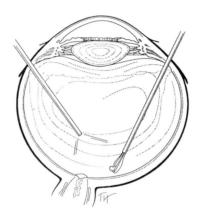

FIGURE 47-25. *Schematic diagram depicting nonmagnetic IOFB lying near retinal surface. Following pars plana vitrectomy to clear any media opacities, the IOFB is grasped with intraocular forceps and removed from eye.*

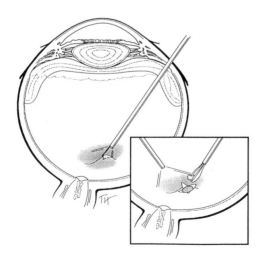

FIGURE 47-26. *Schematic diagram showing incarcerated intraretinal foreign body. The foreign body is freed of all incarcerated tissue and any encapsulated material prior to removal with intraocular forceps. Endophotocoagulation may be applied around base of foreign body either before or following removal.*

manipulations, and in cases with signs and symptoms of endophthalmitis. Even with clear media and an adequate view of the IOFB, a pars plana vitrectomy approach may be beneficial by irrigating fluid through the eye and thus diluting any possible bacterial load and reducing the risk of endophthalmitis (135).

When the IOFB is poorly visualized due to cataract or vitreous hemorrhage, vitrectomy and lensectomy are necessary. If the IOFB is not incarcerated or encapsulated, an intraocular rare earth magnet may be used to secure a magnetic foreign body and either pass it off to a forceps in the midvitreous cavity or, in the case of a large IOFB (>5 mm), possibly bring it into the anterior chamber for removal through a limbal incision. Several such rare earth magnets are available (see Fig. 47-21), some with retractible sleeves to facilitate transfer of foreign bodies to forceps (152). If the IOFB is nonmagnetic, intraocular forceps or gentle aspiration (153) with a soft-tipped instrument may be used to secure the IOFB. Once again, if the IOFB is felt to be too large to be safely removed through the pars plana, it may be brought into the anterior chamber and removed via a limbal wound (Fig. 47-27). If the foreign body is too large to grasp with conventional microsurgical forceps, a ureter stone forceps may be effective in select cases (Fig. 47-28) (154). Special care must be taken when removing the foreign body from the eye. It should be grasped firmly, exposing its narrowest dimension to the sclerotomy site. When it is exposed externally, careful and firm fixation with heavier forceps can facilitate its removal (see Fig. 47-27). If it is dropped from a pars plana extraction site, it can strike the macula and limit visual recovery (1). Injection of perfluorocarbon has been suggested as a means to protect the macula during this maneuver (1). However, perfluorocarbon liquids will not support metallic foreign bodies, though they may dampen impact. In addition, lighter foreign bodies may drop to the edge of the meniscus of the liquid perfluorocarbon, complicating their removal and increasing the risk of iatrogenic retinal damage.

Removal of intraretinal foreign bodies is more difficult and may require careful dissection of a fibrous capsule and segmentation of any adhesions that might induce retinal traction (see Fig. 47-25). As for other types of IOFBs, both external and internal approaches may be used successfully (155) depending on the location of the IOFB. Consideration of retinopexy at the impaction site is appropriate (Fig. 47-29A, B), though of unclear benefit (155–158). The visual prognosis depends largely on the site of impaction, with macular involvement portending a poorer visual prognosis. Nevertheless, up to 49% of cases can attain a visual acuity of 20/40 or better (155).

Comparison of the Treatment Methods

Accurate comparison of the treatment methods is difficult because no controlled, prospective, randomized study has been performed. Comparisons between different patient

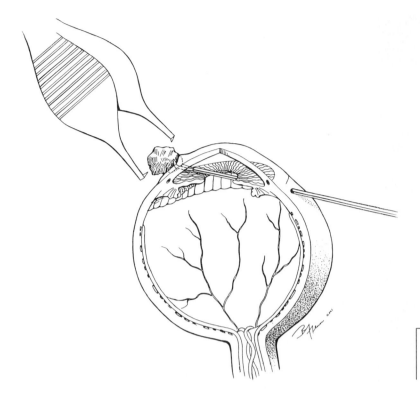

FIGURE 47-27. *Schematic diagram showing removal of large intraocular foreign body through limbal incision.*

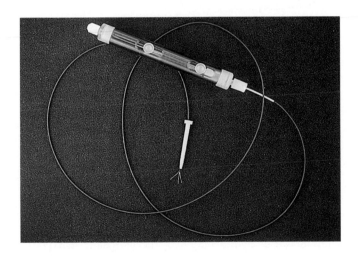

FIGURE 47-28. *Ureteral forceps that may be employed to remove very large IOFB.*

populations are difficult, and case selection plays an important role in deciding the outcome of a given procedure. With these limitations in mind, however, some general conclusions can be made. When used appropriately, either primary magnetic extraction or vitrectomy can provide excellent results, with at least 60% of patients achieving a final visual acuity of 20/40 or better (134). Ross and Tasman (149) reported 20/50 or better vision in 77% of patients in whom magnetic IOFB extraction was performed. Coleman et al (150) reported 35 cases of intraocular foreign bodies, 71% of which were magnetic. In 22 cases, pars plana vit-

rectomy was performed in combination with magnetic extraction using an intraocular electromagnet. Sixty-three percent of patients retained a visual acuity of 20/300 or better after surgery. The researchers prefer such magnetic extraction whenever possible primarily because it minimizes manipulation and wound size, and simplifies the surgical procedure in general.

This favorable outcome for magnetic extraction of IOFBs is due somewhat to the selection criteria. These IOFBs are generally small, magnetic, in eyes with clear media, and in an easily accessible location. These eyes may have little or no associated ocular damage (148). In contrast, cases selected for vitrectomy are often more heterogeneous and associated with more prominent ocular damage. These include eyes with opaque media, retinal detachment, endophthalmitis, non-magnetic IOFBs, encapsulated IOFBs or foreign bodies in the retina or subretinal space, and eyes in which magnetic extraction has failed (148,157,158). DeJuan et al (159) have shown that vitrectomy was beneficial in cases of air-rifle and perforating injuries, and in cases where initial visual acuity was worse than 5/200. Peyman et al (160) reported a small series of 11 eyes with IOFBs treated with primary vitrectomy, 91% of which obtained a final visual acuity of 20/50 or better. In addition, vitrectomy has been associated with a lowered incidence of enucleation after penetrating trauma (134,161).

Retinal Detachment and Retinopexy

If a retinal detachment is present preoperatively, it is managed with either pars plana vitrectomy, scleral buckling,

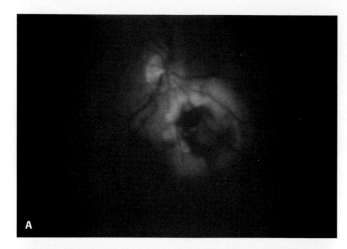

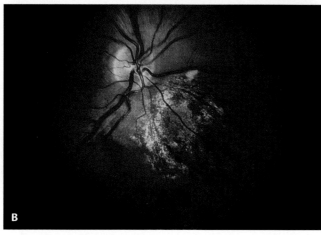

FIGURE 47-29.   (A) *Several rows of endophotocoagulation have been placed around IOFB impaction site adjacent to optic nerve.* (B) *Appearance of eye two months following surgical removal of IOFB.*

retinopexy, gas tamponade, silicone oil, or any combination thereof, depending on the method of IOFB removal, the clarity of the media, or other mitigating circumstances. If no retinal break or detachment is present, however, it is unclear whether prophylactic scleral buckling is essential or beneficial. Although several studies have shown a beneficial effect from prophylactic scleral buckling (26,102–104), no randomized, controlled trial has proven its efficacy.

Controversy exists regarding retinopexy at the site of an intraretinal foreign body. Slusher (156,157) and Ahmadieh (155) used photocoagulation or cryotherapy preoperatively to create an adhesion at the retinal impaction site. However, Ambler (158) treated five patients with intraretinal foreign bodies with vitrectomy but did not perform retinopexy nor separate the posterior hyaloid. Additionally, in only one eye was a fluid-gas exchange performed. Four of the five eyes obtained a visual acuity of 20/20 or better. It was felt that spontaneous retinopexy occurred at the foreign body impact

site and that further treatment with either laser photocoagulation or cryotherapy may stimulate fibrous proliferation, retinal breaks, or hemorrhage, thus potentially worsening the situation. Sternberg (1) has made similar observations, though has noted that retinopexy, complete removal of the posterior hyaloid, and scleral buckling may be necessary if a retinal detachment occurs at the time of foreign body extraction.

Endophthalmitis

The clinical signs and symptoms of endophthalmitis may be masked in the acute phase after severe ocular injury, thereby making diagnosis difficult in some cases. The incidence of endophthalmitis after penetrating injury ranges from 2% to 7% (119) and with retained IOFBs typically ranges from 6% to 13% (134,162), though may be as high as 30% with organic matter contamination (163). The development of endophthalmitis with retained IOFBs is not necessarily predictive of a poor visual outcome, however, if the patient is treated within 24 hours of injury with intravitreal antibiotics (134,164). The association of retinal breaks or detachment with endophthalmitis is also not necessarily a harbinger of a poor visual outcome (165,166).

In a series of retained IOFBs (135), bacterial cultures of removed IOFBs or vitreous were positive in 7 of 25 cases (28%). Prompt surgical intervention with vitrectomy and injection of intravitreal antibiotics in high-risk cases, such as those with organic matter contamination, resulted in all patients recovering 20/70 or better vision, despite potentially virulent growth of organisms including *Bacillus* species. Other earlier studies have also supported the beneficial effect of vitrectomy surgery in the management of endophthalmitis (167–169). A delay in primary repair of more than 24 hours, however, caused a fourfold increased risk (from 3.5% to 13.4%) for the development of infectious endophthalmitis (162). Another factor that may increase the risk of infectious endophthalmitis after penetrating trauma with or without IOFBs is disruption of the crystalline lens (170). Thompson et al (170) reported that lens disruption was present in 24 of 28 eyes with culture-proven endophthalmitis. Distinguishing infection from lens-induced inflammation may be very difficult at times.

As part of the National Eye Trauma System (NETS), Thompson et al (162) reported a series of 34 eyes with infectious endophthalmitis after penetrating injury with retained IOFBs. They found that infectious endophthalmitis was more likely to develop in eyes with home or occupational injuries (9.2%) than in eyes injured in other settings such as recreational, assult, self-inflicted, or motor-vehicle-related injuries. Positive cultures were obtained in 22 of 34 eyes (65%). *Staphylococcus* species accounted for 45% of positive cultures, while *Bacillus* species grew in 36%. Though the difference was not statistically significant, eyes with

Staphylococcus isolated from culture had a much better visual outcome than eyes with *Bacillus*. Surprisingly, the composition of the IOFB had no significant effect on the risk of endophthalmitis developing. Endophthalmitis developed in 7.2% of eyes with metallic IOFBs and in 5.9% of eyes with organic foreign bodies. Boldt et al (163) reported, however, that the incidence of endophthalmitis occurring after contamination with organic matter may be as high as 30%, with *Bacillus* accounting for 46% of cases.

The role of prophylactic intravitreal antibiotics is unclear, especially given reports of antibiotic toxicity (171–173). However, when signs of endophthalmitis are present at the time of surgical repair or IOFB removal, or the nature of the injury suggests a high risk for the development of endophthalmitis, then intravitreal antibiotics such as vancomycin (1.0 mg) with either ceftazidime (2.25 mg) or amikacin (200–400 μg) are indicated (see Table 47-1). This is combined with subconjunctival and fortified topical antibiotic administration and, in most cases, with at least a short course of systemic antibiotics as well. Commonly employed systemic regimens include intravenous vancomycin (1.0 g every 12 hours), a cephalosporin such as ceftazidime (1.0 g every 8 hours), or intravenous or oral ciprofloxacin (750 mg every 12 hours) for one to three days. The use of systemic antibiotics is discussed in greater detail in the next paragraph. Table 49.1 lists antibiotics and dosage levels that are commonly employed in the setting of endophthalmitis.

The results of the Endophthalmitis Vitrectomy Study (EVS) (174) suggest that intravenous antibiotics do not play a significant role in the treatment of postoperative endophthalmitis. It is impossible to extrapolate these results into the setting of penetrating ocular trauma, however, because of the different spectrum of organisms that are encountered. These organisms, especially *Bacillus* species, often have a much greater virulence and are often associated with toxins (175). Therefore, it is presently recommended that patients suffering penetrating ocular trauma with or without retained IOFBs receive prophylactic systemic antibiotics for one to three days. While this is the current standard of care, it should be noted that there is an ongoing trend toward outpatient management, increased use of oral medications, and shorter overall duration of treatment. Past rationale for use of systemic antibiotics was to enhance the level of intravitreal antibiotic. However, few antibiotics readily cross the blood-ocular barrier well enough to obtain bactericidal levels within the vitreous. One antibiotic that does enter the eye quite readily is ciprofloxacin, a quinolone that can achieve an intravitreal therapeutic level with repeated oral administration (176). Intravenous aminoglycosides are not recommended because of concerns with toxicity and with the fact that they do not consistently achieve intravitreal therapeutic levels (177). Once again, the rationale for systemic antibiotic use is based more on the accepted standard of care than upon the evidence of efficacy.

Corticosteroids

The proper use of corticosteroids in the setting of endophthalmitis remains unknown and controversial. One postoperative clinical study has suggested a beneficial effect of intravitreal corticosteroids in the setting of *Staphylococcus aureus* (178), though in an experimental rabbit model similarly involving the same organism (179) there was a worsened outcome and corticosteroids administered systemically offered no apparent advantage (180). While corticosteroids may be beneficial for suppressing inflammation and potentially limiting ocular damage, they can also potentiate an infection. If employed, the following doses are commonly utilized: intravitreal (dexamethasone 400 μg/0.1 cc), periocular (Decadron 4–12 mg), and systemic (prednisone 0.7 to 1.0 mg/kg/d).

Because of the high risk of endophthalmitis and the need for timely repair of ruptured globes, we recommended prompt removal and culture of IOFBs, along with culture of the vitreous and aqueous. Thompson et al (162) have shown that infectious endophthalmitis was much less likely to develop in eyes with primary repair performed within 24 hours of injury than in eyes repaired at a later time. In addition, rapid intervention may allow removal of IOFBs before inflammation stimulates the formation of a fibrous capsule that can make extraction more difficult (162), and it also decreases the risk of metallosis. With chronic and inert IOFBs, a more conservative approach may be taken, particularly if the IOFB is encapsulated. Close observation with serial electroretinography may be sufficient (181). If any worsening of ocular status ensues, then the IOFB can be removed.

Metallosis

Siderosis

Siderosis can occur with any retained iron-contaning IOFB. It results from the accumulation of iron ions in intraocular epithelial structures and can lead to cataract, glaucoma, uveitis, and retinal degeneration. Pupillary mydriasis, heterochromia, and unreactivity can occur (182,183), and these findings may signal an occult IOFB (184). Electroretinography (ERG) is a sensitive test for siderosis and may reveal changes before the visual acuity is affected. The ERG abnormalities are characterized by an initial superonormality followed by a decrease in the beta-wave amplitude, with a normal implicit time (148,185,186). In addition, abnormalities in dark adaptation (148) and electro-oculography (186) have been noted.

Sneed and Weingeist (181) and others (187) have reported encouraging results in the management of siderosis. In a series of 14 eyes, the IOFB was removed in 12, and cataract extraction was necessary in 11 eyes, all of which obtained a final visual acuity of 20/40 or better (181). The location of the foreign body may play a role in the visual outcome: Eyes with a foreign body located posteriorly or in the retina fare worse than those with intralenticular or anterior segment IOFBs (181,186).

Chalcosis

Pure copper IOFBs can cause a severe, purulent inflammatory reaction simulating infectious endophthalmitis. Such a reaction mandates immediate removal of the IOFB in an effort to prevent severe ocular damage and phthisis. Alloys of copper such as bronze or brass may incite a less severe reaction called *chalcosis*. The clinical findings are similar to those associated with endogenous chalcosis from hepatolenticular degeneration (148), and tend to occur if the copper content of the foreign body is at least 85% (188). These include a Kayser-Fleischer ring; an anterior subcapsular, sunflower cataract; a greenish discoloration of the iris and vitreous; and refractile deposits in the internal limiting membrane sometimes associated with a greenish sheen (148,189). Foreign bodies with a copper content of less than 85% have been tolerated in the eye for many years without serious sequelae (188). Rosenthal et al (189) reported that 9 of 10 eyes with retained copper IOFBs had a visual acuity of 20/60 or better.

Prognosis and Outcome

Findings predictive of a final visual acuity of 20/40 or better after penetrating injury with retained IOFBs are an initial visual acuity of 20/40 or better and the need for only one or two operations for the treatment of the injury and its complications (119). Several factors have been associated with a final visual acuity of worse than 5/200 after penetrating injury with retained IOFBs. These are an initial visual acuity worse than 5/200 and a wound of 4 mm or greater in length, independent of location (134). In addition, association of vitreous hemorrhage with IOFBs, and IOFB location within the retina have been associated with a worsened prognosis (190).

Eyes with IOFBs carry a relatively good prognosis when compared to eyes that have suffered other serious penetrating ocular trauma (76,99). DeJuan et al (76) reported a series of 453 patients that suffered penetrating trauma. Final visual acuity was better than or equal to 5/200 in 65% of cases in which there was a retained IOFB compared to 58% of cases without an IOFB. Seventy-nine percent of patients with an IOFB obtained a visual acuity of 5/200 or better in the study by Williams et al (134), and 60% had a final visual acuity of 20/40 or better.

The notable exception to these findings is BB injury, which has a uniformly poor prognosis (76,134,191,192). Of 22 patients with penetrating injuries from BBs in one series, 19 eyes were enucleated and final vision in the remaining eyes was worse than 5/200 (192). We are aware of only one case where good visual acuity (20/30) was salvaged after penetrating BB injury (193). The poor prognosis of BB injury is likely due to the combination of blunt and penetrating trauma that a BB may cause because of its relatively large size and low speed. The most marked pathology after BB injury is located posteriorly and includes tears and hemorrhagic necrosis of the ciliary body; hemorrhagic and serous choroidal detachment; vitreous incarceration and hemorrhage; retinal tears, dialyses, and hemorrhagic detachment; choroidal rupture; and evulsion of the optic nerve (192).

Intraretinal or subretinal foreign bodies are also associated with a more guarded prognosis. Slusher et al (156) reported 14 cases of intraretinal foreign bodies that required vitrectomy for removal. Only 40% obtained a final visual acuity of 20/400 or better, and macular pucker and retinal detachment with proliferative vitreoretinopathy (PVR) developed in 90% of patients. A later report by Slusher (157) involving 16 patients with intraretinal foreign bodies removed via vitrectomy after failed magnetic extraction showed a 60% rate of macular pucker formation postoperatively.

Ahmadieh et al (155) reviewed the records of 75 patients (76 eyes) with intraretinal foreign bodies obtained primarily during wartime. All eyes underwent vitrectomy, including removal of the posterior hyaloid. Eighty-five percent of these patients underwent vitrectomy and foreign body removal more than 30 days after injury. Electromagnetic extraction through the sclera was employed when the foreign body was anterior to the equator (the number of cases is not reported), while intraocular forceps or internal magnetic extraction were used in the other cases. Macular pucker occurred in about 10% of cases. Forty-nine percent achieved a visual acuity of 20/40 or better, and 62% were better than 20/200. Most failures were attributed to retinal detachment with PVR, which was present in 25% of the eyes. Despite the delayed intervention in many of these cases, the rate of retinal detachment postoperatively compares favorably with that reported by Percival (151), where about 30% of eyes that underwent extraction of intraretinal foreign bodies without vitrectomy suffered retinal detachment.

LATE COMPLICATIONS

Despite excellent repair of penetrating and perforating ocular trauma, and appropriate vitreoretinal surgery, numerous late complications can arise. Many of these complications are amenable to further surgical repair. The complications can involve all aspects of the eye.

Corneal decompensation can arise due to direct corneal opacification from a laceration, or there may be gradual corneal thickening if significant endothelial cell loss occurs from the trauma itself or secondary to the surgical repair. Penetrating keratoplasty surgery is often indicated.

Numerous glaucoma complications can arise, once again as a direct result of the trauma, or secondary to the subsequent surgery or adjuncts employed in the course of surgical repair. Pupillary membranes can arise from either proliferation from an anterior scleral laceration that grows into the pupillary space or from proliferation of tissues secondary to inflammation associated with the ocular injury. If a pupillary membrane is extensive, it can cause ciliary body detachment with subsequent hypotony.

Late posterior segment complications include macular epiretinal membrane formation (Fig. 47-30), which is quite common. Tractional and rhegmatogenous retinal detachment may also occur, especially since most scleral lacerations have at least some degree of vitreous (and possible retinal) incarceration. This alters the normal vitreoretinal relationship, increasing traction on the vitreous base. The majority of these complications are amenable to further vitrectomy surgery, though some eyes will succumb to uncontrolled intraocular proliferation with recurrent retinal detachment or to hypotony from ciliary body shutdown.

SYMPATHETIC OPHTHALMIA

Sympathetic ophthalmia is a bilateral inflammatory condition of the uveal tract and is characterized by nodular or diffuse infiltration with epithelioid cells and lymphocytes. It may have a very insidious onset, and its course may vary extensively, with periods of remission and exacerbation. Although the precise cause is unknown, the majority of cases follow open globe injuries or less commonly following intraocular surgery. The inflammation appears in the injured (excited) eye usually within one to two months and is then followed shortly thereafter by similar inflammation in the sympathizing eye. Sympathetic ophthalmia has been reported following penetrating and perforating injuries as well as following pars plana vitrectomy alone [194]. The majority of cases, however, are associated with ocular trauma.

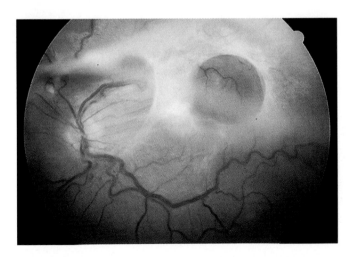

FIGURE 47-30. *Patient developed dense epiretinal membrane six months following removal of intraretinal metallic foreign body. Vision fell to count fingers. Further pars plana vitrectomy surgery was performed and, with removal of membrane, vision returned to 20/50.*

The injured eye exhibits low-grade uveitis and iris thickening, is unresponsive to light, and may develop iris nodules at the pupillary margin and corneal endothelial precipitates. The sympathizing eye generally develops a low-grade uveitis with keratic precipitates, photophobia, and ocular pain. The iris may become thickened and unresponsive, leading to a vascularized pupillary membrane and possible secondary glaucoma. The posterior segment will have retinal and choroidal swelling, whitish spots indicative of Dalen-Fuchs' nodules, and possibly an exudative retinal detachment (Fig. 47-31A) (195).

Evidence points toward an extremely small risk of sympathetic ophthalmia if the injured eye is enucleated within two weeks of the date of the injury (196). Therefore, all surgical repair attempts should be planned within this time frame. However, isolated cases of sympathetic ophthalmia have been reported as early as five days following trauma (195).

Once the diagnosis of sympathetic ophthalmia has been established, enucleation of the exciting eye is generally not recommended as it will not arrest the process, and the exciting eye could end up offering the better vision of the two eyes. However, if there is little or no vision, enucleation may still be recommended (197).

Corticosteroids are the mainstay of therapy for sympathetic ophthalmia. The sympathizing eye has an approximate 60% chance of recovering 20/50 or better vision (Fig. 47-31B) (195,197). High-dose corticosteroids may need to be employed initially, along with a tapering dose of medication for a year or two. On occasion, cytotoxic agents are also utilized if the response to corticosteroids is not adequate. Using corticosteroids from the time of injury does not prevent the development of sympathetic ophthalmia (198).

PREVENTION

Ocular trauma causes tremendous morbidity, especially among young and otherwise healthy individuals. A significant portion of ocular injury could be avoided with the proper use of eye protection and education. Dannenberg et al (199) reported on 635 work-related penetrating eye injuries. The median age of the injured workers was 30 years, 97% were male, and only 6% of the injured workers were wearing safety glasses. Patel and Morgan (200) found that only 1 of 36 (3%) patients with work-related penetrating eye injuries was wearing eye protection when injured.

CONCLUSIONS

Ocular trauma leads to visual loss in a variety of ways. The prognosis most often relates to the severity of the initial injury. There have been significant advances in vitreoretinal surgical techniques and instrumentation over the past 20 years, and we understand the pathophysiology of eye trauma much better. Still, not every eye can be salvaged from

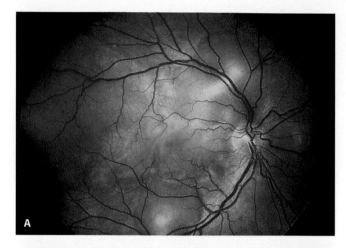

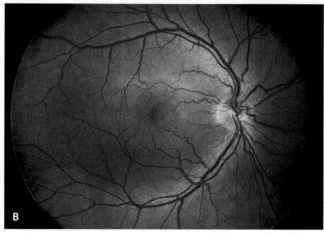

FIGURE 47-31.   (A) *Fellow eye of patient two months following a penetrating ocular injury. The patient developed sympathetic ophthalmia, with extensive intraocular inflammation, and diffuse chorioretinal swelling with multiple pigment epithelial detachments. The visual acuity is 20/80. (B) Follow-up of the patient three months later, following institution of systemic corticosteroids. Vision has returned to 20/20, with resolution of posterior segment abnormalities.*

the effects of trauma, as recurrent intraocular proliferation and ciliary body shutdown cannot be prevented nor adequately treated. Additionally, numerous questions remain regarding optimal management of these injuries, ranging from timing of vitrectomy intervention to proper use and administration of antibiotics. However, if we can experience the same degree of improvement over the next 20 years, we should be able to offer even better management of these challenging injuries.

REFERENCES

1. Sternberg P Jr. Trauma: principles and techniques of treatment. In: Ryan SJ, ed. *Retina.* Vol. 3; ch. 148. St. Louis: CV Mosby, 1994:2351–2378.
2. Schein OD, Hibberd PL, Shingleton BJ, et al. The spectrum and burden of ocular injury. *Ophthalmology* 1988;95:300–305.
3. LaRoche GR, McIntyre L, Schertzer RM. Epidemiology of severe eye injuries in childhood. *Ophthalmology* 1988;95:1603–1607.
4. Liggett PE, Pince KJ, Barlow W, et al. Ocular trauma in an urban population: review of 1132 cases. *Ophthalmology* 1990;97:581–584.
5. Karlson TA, Klein EK: The incidence of acute hospital-treated eye injuries. *Arch Ophthalmology* 1986;104:1473–1476.
6. Strahlman E, Elman M, Daub E, Baker S. Causes of pediatric eye injuries: a population-based study. *Arch Ophthalmol* 1990;108:603–606.
7. Appiah AP. The nature, causes, and visual outcome of ocular trauma requiring posterior segment surgery at a country hospital. *Ann Ophthalmol* 1991;23:430–433.
8. Atmaca LS, Yilmaz M. Changes in the fundus caused by blunt ocular trauma. *Ann Ophthalmol* 1993;25:447–452.
9. Ryan SJ, Stout JT, Dugel PU. Posterior penetrating ocular trauma. In: Ryan SJ, ed. *Retina.* Vol. 3; ch. 147. St. Louis: CV Mosby, 1994:2335–2349.
10. Ryan SJ. Traction retinal detachment. XLIX Edward Jackson Memorial Lecture. *Am J Ophthalmol* 1993;115:1–20.
11. Winthrop SR, Cleary PE, Minckler DS, Ryan SJ. Penetrating eye injuries: a histopathological review. *Br J Ophthalmol* 1980;64:809–817.
12. Freitag SK, Eagle RC, Jaeger EA, et al. An epidemiologic and pathologic study of globes enucleated following trauma. *Ophthalmic Surg* 1992;23:409–423.
13. Punnonen E. Pathological findings in eyes enucleated because of perforating injury. *Acta Ophthalmologica* 1990;68:265–269.
14. Cleary PE, Ryan SJ. Experimental posterior penetrating eye injury in the rabbit. I. Method of production and natural history. *Br J Ophthalmol* 1979;63:306–311.
15. Cleary PE, Ryan SJ. Experimental posterior penetrating eye injury in the rabbit. II. Histology of wound, vitreous and retina. *Br J Ophthalmol* 1979;63:312–321.
16. Cleary PE, Ryan SJ. Histology of wound, vitreous and retina in experimental posterior penetrating eye injury in the rhesus monkey. *Am J Ophthalmol* 1979;88:221–231.
17. Cleary PE, Ryan SJ. Method of production and natural history of experimental posterior penetrating eye injury in the rhesus monkey. *Am J Ophthalmol* 1979;88:212–220.
18. Hsu HT, Ryan SJ. Lens trauma in experimental penetrating eye injury. In: Henking P, ed. *ACTA XXIV International Congress of Ophthalmology.* Philadelphia: JB Lippincott, 1983:1075–1080.
19. Cleary PE, Jarus G, Ryan SJ. Mechanisms in traction retinal detachment. *Br J Ophthalmol* 1980;64:801–808.
20. Cleary PE, Ryan SJ. Mechanisms in traction retinal detachment. *Dev Ophthalmol* 1981;2:228–233.
21. Hsu-Tao H, Ryan SJ. Experimental retinal detachment in the rabbit: penetrating ocular injury with retinal laceration. *Retina* 1986;6:66–69.
22. Hsu-Tao H, Ryan SJ. Natural history of penetrating ocular injury with retinal laceration in the monkey. *Greafes Arch Clin Exp Ophthalmol* 1986;224:1–6.
23. Topping TM, Abrams GW, Machemer R. Experimental double-perforating injury of the posterior segment in rabbit eyes; the natural history of intraocular proliferation. *Arch Ophthalmol* 1979;97:735–742.
24. Sternberg P, deJuan E, Michels RG. Multivariate analysis of prognostic factors in penetrating ocular injuries. *Am J Ophthalmol* 1984;98:467–472.
25. Gilbert CM, Soong HK, Hirst LW. A two year prospective study of penetrating ocular trauma at the Wilmer Ophthalmological Institute. *Ann Ophthalmol* 1987;19:104–106.
26. Hutton WL, Fuller DG. Factors influencing final visual results in severely injured eyes. *Am J Ophthalmol* 1984;97:715–722.
27. Kylstra JA, Lamkin JC, Runyun DK. Clinical predictors of scleral rupture after blunt ocular trauma. *Am J Ophthalmol* 1993;115:530–535.
28. Sevel D, Krausz H, Ponder T, Centeno R. Value of computed tomography for the diagnosis of a ruptured eye. *J Comput Assist Tomogr* 1983;7:870–875.
29. Watson A, Hartley DE. Alternative method of intraocular foreign body localization. *Am J Roentgen* 1984;142:789–790.
30. Bryden FM, Pyott AA, Bailey M, McGhee NJ. Real time ultrasound in the assessment of intraocular foreign bodies. *Eye* 1990;4:727–731.
31. Lobes L Jr. Computed tomography in the detection of intraocular foreign bodies. *Int Ophthalmol Clin* 1982;22:219–234.
32. Lobes LA, Grand MG, Reece J, Penkrot RJ. Computerized axial tomography in the detection of intraocular foreign bodies. *Ophthalmology* 1981;88:26–29.
33. Kollarits CR, DiChior G, Christiansen J, et al. Detection of orbital and intraocular foreign bodies by computerized tomography. *Ophthalmic Surg* 1977;8:45–53.
34. Speirer A, Tadmor R, Treister G, et al. Diagnosis and localization of intraocular foreign bodies by computed tomography. *Ophthalmic Surg* 1985;16:571–575.

35. Zinreich SJ, Miller NR, Aguayo JB, et al. Computed tomographic three-dimensional localization and compositional evaluation of intraocular and orbital foreign bodies *Arch Ophthalmol* 1986;104:515–519.

36. Topilow HW, Ackerman AL, Zimmerman RD. Limitation of computerized tomography in the localization of intaocular foreign bodies. *Ophthalmology* 1984;91:1086–1091.

37. Wilhelm JL, Zakov ZN, Weinstein MA, et al. Localization of suspected intraocular foreign bodies with a modified Delta 2020 scanner. *Ophthalmic Surg* 1981;12:633–641.

38. Dass AB. Personal communication.

39. Williamson TH, Smith FW, Forrester JV. Magnetic resonance imaging of intraocular foreign bodies. *Br J Ophthalmol* 1989;73:555–558.

40. LoBue TD, Deutsch TA, Lobick J, Turner DA. Detection and localization of nonmetallic intraocular foreign bodies by magnetic resonance imaging. *Arch Ophthalmol* 1988;106:260–261.

41. Williams S, Char DH, Dillom WP, et al. Ferrous intraocular foreign bodies and magnetic resonance imaging. *Am J Ophthalmol* 1988;105:398–401.

42. Lagouros PA, Langer BG, Peyman GA, et al. Magnetic resonance imaging and intraocular foreign bodies. *Arch Ophthalmol* 1987;105:551–553.

43. Kelley WM, Paglen PG, Pearson JA, et al. Ferromagnetism of intraocular foreign body causes unilateral blindness after MR study. *Am J Neuroradiology* 1986;7:243–245.

44. Mouby-Mahmoud G, Silverman RH, Coleman DJ. Using high-frequency ultrasound to characterize intraocular foreign bodies. *Ophthalmic Surg* 1993;24:94–99.

45. Rubsamen PE, Cousins SW, Winward KE, Byrne SF. Diagnostic ultrasound and pars plana vitrectomy in penetrating ocular trauma. *Ophthalmology* 1994;101:809–814.

46. Behrens-Baumann W, Praetorius G. Intraocular foreign bodies: 297 consecutive cases. *Ophthalmologica* 1989;198:84–89.

47. Armstrong MF. A review of intraocular foreign body injuries and complications in N. Ireland from 1978–1986. *Intl Ophthalmol* 1988;12:113–117.

48. Vinger PF. Eye injury resulting from violence: research and prevention. *Arch Ophthalmol* 1992;110:765–766.

49. Dannenburg AL, Parver LM, Fowler CJ. Penetrating eye injuries related to assault: the National Eye Trauma System Registry. *Arch Ophthalmol* 1992;110:849–852.

50. Groessl S, Nanda SK, Mieler WF. Assault-related penetrating ocular injury. *Am J Ophthalmol* 1993;116:26–33.

51. Gomez-Ulla F, Gonzalez F, Ruiz-Fraga C. Unintentional intraocular injection of corticosteroids. *Acta Ophthalmologica* 1993;71:419–421.

52. Schneider ME, Milstein DE, Oyakawa RT, et al. Ocular perforation from a retrobulbar injection. *Am J Ophthalmol* 1988;106:35–40.

53. Yanoff M, Redovan EG. Anterior eyewall perforation during subconjunctival block. *Ophthalmic Surg* 1990;21:362–363.

54. Duker JS, Belmont JB, Benson WE, et al. Inadvertent globe perforation during retrobulbar and peribulbar anesthesia: patient characteristics, surgical management, and visual outcome. *Ophthalmology* 1991;98:519–526.

55. Hay A, Flynn HW Jr, Hoffman JI, Rivera AH. Needle penetration of the globe during retrobulbar and peribulbar injections. *Ophthalmology* 1991;98:1017–1024.

56. Grizzard WS, Kirk NM, Pavan PR, et al. Perforating ocular injuries caused by anesthesia personnnel. *Ophthalmology* 1991;98:1011–1016.

57. Jones NP. Perforating eye injuries caused by dog bites. *J Roy Soc Med* 1990;83:332–333.

58. Nichols CJ, Boldt HC, Mieler WF, et al. Ocular injuries caused by elastic cords. *Arch Ophthalmol* 1991;109:371–372.

59. Aiello LP, Iwamoto M, Taylor H. Perforating ocular fishhook injury. *Arch Ophthalmol* 1992;110:1316–1317.

60. Aiello LP, Iwamoto M, Fuyer DR. Penetrating ocular fishhook injuries: surgical management and long-term visual outcome. *Ophthalmology* 1992;99:862–866.

61. Yeatts RP, Harvey J, Bartley GB, Nerney JJ. Ocular injury secondary to periorbital use of stainless-steel wire and suture. *Arch Ophthalmol* 1994;112:213–216.

62. Rummelt V, Rummelt C, Naumann GOH. Congenital nonpigmented epithelial iris cyst after aminocentesis: clinicopathological report on two children. *Ophthalmology* 1993;100:776–781.

63. Nanda SK, Mieler WF, Murphy ML. Penetrating ocular injuries secondary to motor vehicle accidents. *Ophthalmology* 1993;100:201–207.

64. John G, Witherspoon CD, Feist RM, Morris R. Ocular lawnmower injuries. *Ophthalmology* 1988;95:1367–1370.

65. Gilboa M, Gdal-on M, Zonis S. Bee and wasp stings of the eye. Retained intralenticular wasp sting; a case report. *Br J Ophthalmol* 1977;61:662–664.

66. Heier JS, Enzenauer RW, Wintermeyer SF, et al. Ocular injuries and diseases at a combat hospital in support of Operations Desert Shield and Desert Storm. *Arch Ophthalmol* 1993;111:795–798.

67. Potts AM, Distler JA. Shape factor in the penetration of intraocular foreign bodies. *Am J Ophthalmol* 1985;100:183–187.

68. Delori F, Pomerantzeff O, Cox MS. Deformation of the globe under high speed contact. Its relation to contusion injuries. *Invest Ophthalmol Vis Sci* 1969;8:290–301.

69. Barr CC. Prognostic factors in corneoscleral lacerations. *Arch Ophthalmol* 1983;101:919–924.

70. Erdey RA, Lindahl KJ, Temnycky GO, Aquavella JV. Techniques for application of tissue adhesive for corneal perforations. *Ophthalmic Surg* 1991;22:352–354.

71. Campochiaro PA, Kaden IH, Vidaruui-Leal J, Glaser BM. Cryotherapy enhances intravitreal dispersion of viable retinal pigment epithelial cells. *Arch Ophthalmol* 1985;103:434–436.

72. DeJuan E Jr, Sternberg P Jr, Michels RG. Timing of vitrectomy after penetrating ocular injuries. *Ophthalmology* 1976;81:728–732.

73. Coleman DJ. Early vitrectomy in the management of the severely traumatized eye. *Am J Ophthalmol* 1982;93:543–551.

74. Faulborn J, Atkinson A, Oliver C. Primary vitrectomy as a preventive surgical procedure in the treatment of severely injured eyes. *Br J Ophthalmol* 1977;61:202–208.

75. Coleman DJ. Role of vibrectomy in trauma. In: Gitter KA, ed. *Current concepts of the vitreous, including vitrectomy.* St. Louis: CV Mosby, 1966.

76. DeJuan E Jr, Sternberg P Jr, Michels RG. Penetrating ocular injuries: types of injuries and visual results. *Ophthalmology* 1983;90:1318–1322.

77. Benson WE, Machemer R. Severe perforating injuries treated with pars plana vitrectomy. *Am J Ophthalmol* 1976;81:728–732.

78. Cupples HP, Whitmore PV, Wertz FD III, Mazur DO. Ocular trauma treated by vitreous surgery. *Retina* 1983;3:103–107.

79. Ryan SJ, Allen AW. Pars plana vitrectomy in ocular trauma. *Am J Ophthalmol* 1979;88:483–491.

80. Cleary PE, Ryan SJ. Vitrectomy in penetrating eye injury: results of a controlled trial of vitrectomy in an experimental posterior penetrating eye injury in the rhesus monkey. *Arch Ophthalmol* 1981;99:287–292.

81. Vatne HO, Syrdalen P. Vitrectomy in double perforating eye injuries. *Acta Ophthalmologica* 1985;63:552–556.

82. Mieler WF, Mittra RA. The role and timing of pars plana vitrectomy in penetrating ocular trauma. *Arch Ophthalmol* 1997;113:1191–1192. Editorial.

83. Koenig SB, Ruttum MS, Lewandowski MF, Schultz RO. Pseudophakia for traumatic cataracts in children. *Ophthalmology* 1993;100:1218–1224.

84. Bienfait MF, Pameijer JH, Wildevanck de Blecourt-Devilee M. Intraocular lens implantation in children with unilateral traumatic cataract. *Int Ophthalmol* 1990;14:271–276.

85. Bloom SM, Wyszynski RE, Brucker AJ. Scleral fixation suture for dislocated posterior chamber intraocular lens. *Ophthalmic Surg* 1990;21:851–854.

86. Friedberg MA, Berler DK. Scleral fixation of posterior chamber intraocular lens implants combined with vitrectomy. *Ophthalmic Surg* 1992;23:17–21.

87. Hu BV, Shin DH, Gibbs KA, Hong YA. Implantation of posterior chamber lens in the absence of capsular and zonular support. *Arch Ophthalmol* 1988;106:416–420.

88. Pannu JS. A new suturing technique for ciliary sulcus fixation in the absence of posterior capsule. *Ophthalmic Surg* 1988;19:751–754.

89. Stark WJ, Goodman G, Goodman D, Gottsch J. Posterior chamber intraocular lens implantation in the absence of posterior capsular support. *Ophthalmic Surg* 1988;19:240–243.

90. Davis RM, Best D, Gilbert GE. Comparison of intraocular lens fixation techniques performed during penetrating keratoplasty. *Am J Ophthalmol* 1991;111:743–749.

91. Shapiro A, Leen MM. External transscleral posterior chamber lens fixation. *Arch Ophthalmol* 1991;109:1759–1760.

92. Chan CK. An improved technique for management of dislocated posterior chamber implants. *Ophthalmology* 1992;99:51–57.

93. Malinowski SM, Mieler WF, Koenig SB, et al. Combined pars plana vitrectomy/lensectomy and open loop anterior chamber lens implantation. *Ophthalmology* 1995;102:211–216.

94. Slusher MM, Greven CM, Yu DD. Posterior chamber intraocular lens implantation combined with lensectomy-vitrectomy and intraretinal foreign body removal. *Arch Ophthalmol* 1992;110:127–129.

95. Chan TK, Mackintosh G, Yeoh R, Lim ASM. Primary posterior chamber IOL implantation in penetrating ocular trauma. *Int Ophthalmol* 1993;17:137–141.

96. Lamkin JC, Azar DT, Mead MD, Volpe NJ. Simultaneous corneal laceration repair, cataract removal, and posterior chamber intraocular lens implantation. *Am J Ophthalmol* 1992;113:626–631.

97. Koenig SB, Mieler WF, Han DP, Abrams GW. Combined phacoemulsification, pars plana vitrectomy, and posterior chamber intraocular lens insertion. *Arch Ophthalmol* 1992;110:1101–1104.

98. Rubsamen PE, Irvine WD, McCuen BW II, et al. Primary intraocular lens implantation in the setting of penetrating ocular trauma. *Ophthalmology* 1995;102:101–107.

99. Pieramici DJ, MacCumber MW, Humayun MU, et al. Open-globe injury. Update on types of injuries and visual results. *Ophthalmology* 1996;103: 1798–1803.

100. DeBustros S. Intraoperative control of hemorrhage in penetrating ocular injuries. *Retina* 1990;10(suppl):55–58.

101. Han DP, Mieler WF, Abrams GW, Williams GA. Management of traumatic retinal incarceration with vitrectomy. *Arch Ophthalmol* 1988;106:640–645.

102. Brinton GS, Aaberg TM, Reeser FH, et al. Surgical results in ocular trauma involving the posterior segment. *Am J Ophthalmol* 1982;93:271–278.

103. Rosner M, Bartov E, Treister G, Belkin M. Prophylactic scleral buckling in perforating ocular injuries involving the posterior segment. *Ann Ophthalmol* 1988;20:146–149.

104. Haut J, Allagui M, Lepvrier N, Morec C. Preventive surgical scleral buckling of retinal detachment after severe ocular injuries. *J Francais D'Ophthalmologie* 1993;16:668–673.

105. Hermsen V. Vitrectomy in severe ocular trauma. *Ophthalmologica* 1984;189:86–92.

106. Jaccoma EH, Conway BP, Campochiaro PA. Cryotherapy causes extensive breakdown of the blood-retinal barrier: a comparison with argon laser photocoagulation. *Arch Ophthalmol* 1985;103:1728–1730.

107. Campochiaro PA, Cryan JA III, Conway BP, Jaccoma EH. Intravitreal chemotactic and mitogenic activity: implication of blood-retinal barrier breakdown. *Arch Ophthalmol* 1986;104:1685–1687.

108. Campochiaro PA, Gaskin HC, Vinores SA. Retinal cryopexy stimulates traction retinal detachment formation in the presence of an ocular wound. *Arch Ophthalmology* 1987;105:1567–1570.

109. The Silicone Oil Study Group. Vitrectomy with silicone oil or sulfur hexafluoride in eyes with severe proliferative vitreoretinopathy: results of a randomized clinical trial. Silicone study report #1. *Arch Ophthalmol* 1992;110:770–779.

110. The Silicone Oil Study Group. Vitrectomy with silicone oil or perfluoropropane gas in eyes with severe proliferative vitreoretinopathy: results of a randomized clinical trial. Silicone study report #2. *Arch Ophthalmol* 1992;110:780–792.

111. McCuen BW, Azen SP, Stern W, et al. Vitrectomy with silicone oil or perfluoropropane gas in eyes with proliferative vitreoretinopathy. Silicone study report #3. *Retina* 1993;13:279–284.

112. Barr CC, Mai MY, Lean JS, et al. Postoperative intraocular pressure abnormalities in the silicone study. Silicone study report #4. *Ophthalmology* 1994;100:1629–1635.

113. Hutton WL, Azen SP, Blumenkranz MS, et al. The effects of silicone oil removal. Silicone study report #6. *Arch Ophthalmol* 1994;112:778–785.

114. Abrams GW, Azen SP, Barr CC, et al. The incidence of corneal abnormalities in the silicone study. Silicone study report #7. *Arch Ophthalmol* 1995;113:764–769.

115. Antoszyk AN, McCuen BW, deJuan E Jr, Machemer R. Silicone oil injection after failed primary vitreous surgery in severe ocular trauma. *Am J Ophthalmol* 1989;107:537–543.

116. Skorpik C, Menapace R, Gnad HD, Paroussis P. Silicone oil implantation in penetrating injuries complicated by PVR: results from 1982 to 1986. *Retina* 1989;9:8–14.

117. Liggett PE, Mani N, Green RE, et al. Management of traumatic rupture of the globe in aphakic patients. *Retina* 1990;10(suppl):59–64.

118. Scott IU, Flynn HW Jr, Schiffman J, et al. Visual acuity outcomes among patients with appositional suprachoroidal hemorrhage. *Ophthalmology* 1997;104:2039–2046.

119. Brinton GS, Topping TM, Hyndiuk RA, et al. Post-traumatic endophthalmitis. *Arch Ophthalmol* 1984;102:547–550.

120. Rowsey JJ, Newsom DL, Sexton DJ, Harms WK. Endophthalmitis: current approaches. *Ophthalmology* 1982;89:1055–1065.

121. Parrish CM, O'Day DM. Traumatic endophthalmitis. *Int Ophthalmol Clin* 1987;27:112–119.

122. Roth DB, Flynn HW Jr. Antibiotic selection in the treatment of endophthalmitis: the significance of drug combinations and synergy. *Surv Ophthalmol* 1997;41:395–401.

123. Vinger PF: Eye injury resulting from violence: research and prevention. *Arch Ophthalmol* 1992;110:765–766.

124. Gilbert CM, Soong HK, Hirst LW. A two-year prospective study of penetrating ocular trauma at the Wilmer Ophthalmological Institute. *Ann Ophthalmol* 1967;19:104–106.

125. Cinotti AA, Matlzman BA. Prognosis and treatment of perforating ocular injuries. *Ophthalmic Surg* 1975;6:54–61.

126. Sternberg P Jr, deJuan E Jr, Michels RG, Auer C. Mulitvariate analysis of prognostic factors in penetrating ocular injuries. *Am J Ophthalmol* 1984;98:467–472.

127. Cherry PMH. Rupture of the globe. *Arch Ophthalmol* 1972;88:498–507.

128. Meredith TA, Gorden PA. Pars plana vitrectomy for severe penetrating injury with posterior segment involvement. *Am J Ophthalmol* 1987;103: 549–554.

129. Liggett PE, Gaudermann WJ, Moriera CM, et al. Pars plana vitrectomy for acute retinal detachment in penetrating ocular injuries. *Arch Ophthalmol* 1990;108:1724–1728.

130. Bonnet M, Fleury J. Management of retinal detachment after penetrating eye injury. *Graefe's Arch Clin Exp Ophthalmol* 1991;229:539–542.

131. Ramsey RC, Cantrill HL, Knobloch WH. Vitrectomy for double penetrating ocular injuries. *Am J Ophthalmol* 1985;100:586–589.

132. Punnonen E, Laatikainen L. Long-term follow-up and the role of vitrectomy in the treatment of perforating eye injuries without intraocular foreign bodies. *Acta Ophthalmologica* 1989;67:625–632.

133. Alfaro DV, Tran VT, Runyan T, et al. Vitrectomy for perforating eye injuries from shotgun pellets. *Am J Ophthalmol* 1992;114:81–85.

134. Williams DF, Mieler WF, Abrams GW, Lewis H. Results and prognostic factors in penetrating ocular injuries with retained intraocular foreign bodies. *Ophthalmology* 1988;95:911–916.

135. Mieler WF, Ellis MK, Williams DF, Han DP. Retained intraocular foreign bodies and endophthalmitis. *Ophthalmology* 1990;97:1532–1538.

136. Behrens-Baumann W, Praetorius G. Intraocular foreign bodies: 297 consecutive cases. *Ophthalmologica* 1989;198:84–88.

137. Armstrong MF. A review of intraocular foreign body injuries and complications in N Ireland from 1978–1986. *Int Ophthalmol* 1988;12:113–117.

138. Khani SC, Mukai S. Posterior segment intraocular foreign bodies. *Int Ophthalmol Clin* 1995;35:151–161.

139. Sen SC, Ghosh A. Gold as an intraocular foreign body. *Br J Ophthalmol* 1983;67:398–399.

140. Humayun M, de la Cruz Z, Maguire A, et al. Intraocular cilia: report of 6 cases of 6 weeks to 32 years' duration. *Arch Ophthalmol* 1993;111:1396–1401.

141. Fraser SC, Dowd TC, Bosanquet RC. Intraocular caterpillar hairs (setae): clinical course and management. *Eye* 1994;8:596–598.

142. Lambert HM, Sipperley JO. Intraocular foreign body from a nylon line grass trimmer. *Ann Ophthalmol* 1983;15:936–937.

143. Honda Y, Asayama K. Intraocular graphite pencil lead without reaction. *Am J Ophthalmol* 1985;99:494–495.

144. Duker JS, Fischer DH. Occult plastic intraocular foreign body. *Ophthalmic Surg* 1989;20;169–170.

145. Belkin M, Ivry M. Explosive intraocular foreign bodies. *Am J Ophthalmol* 1978;85:676–678.

146. Risco JM, Awad A. An unusual organic xenogenic intraocular foreign body. *Am J Ophthalmol* 1995;116:107–108.

147. Jaffe NS, ed. *Cataract surgery and its complications.* St. Louis: CV Mosby, 1972:305–306.

148. DeBustros S. Posterior segment intraocular foreign bodies. In: Shingleton BJ, Hersh PS, Kenyon KR, eds. *Eye trauma.* St Louis: Mosby-Year Book, 1991.

149. Ross WH, Tasman WS. The management of magnetic intraocular foreign bodies. *Can J Ophthalmol* 1975;10:168–173.

150. Coleman DJ, Lucas BC, Rondeau MJ, Chang S. Management of intraocular foreign bodies. *Ophthalmology* 1987;94:1647–1653.

151. Percival SBP. Late complications from posterior segment intraocular foreign bodies, with particular reference to retinal detachment. *Br J Ophthalmol* 1972;50:462–468.

152. Joondeph HC, Joondeph BC, Mulcahy T. Comparison of three permanent intraocular magnets. *Retina* 1992;12:270–272.

153. Coleman DJ. A suction tip for controlled removal of nonmagnetic intraocular foreign bodies. *Am J Ophthalmol* 1978;85:255–256.

154. McCarthy MJ, Pulido JS, Soukup B. The use of ureter stone forceps to remove a large intraocular foreign body. *Am J Ophthalmol* 1990;110:208–209.

155. Ahmadieh H, Sajjadi H, Azarmina M, et al. Surgical management of intraretinal foreign bodies. *Retina* 1994;14:397–403.

156. Slusher MM, Sarin LK, Federman JL. Management of intraretinal foreign bodies. *Ophthalmology* 1982;89:369–373.

157. Slusher MM. Intraretinal foreign bodies: management and observations. *Retina* 1990;10(suppl):50–54.

158. Ambler JS, Sanford MM. Management of intraretinal foreign bodies without retinopexy in the absence of retinal detachment. *Ophthalmology* 1991;98:391–394.

159. DeJuan E Jr, Sternberg P Jr, Michels RG, Auer C. Evauation of vitrectomy in penetrating ocular trauma: a case control study. *Arch Ophthalmol* 1984;102:1160–1163.

160. Peyman GA, Raichand M, Goldberg MF, Brown S. Vitrectomy in the management of intraocular foreign bodies and their complications. *Br J Ophthalmol* 1980;64:476–482.

161. Esmaeli B, Elner SG, Schork A, Elner VM. Visual outcome and ocular survival after penetrating trauma. *Ophthalmology* 1995;102:393–400.

162. Thompson JT, Parver LM, Engler CL, et al. Infectious endophthalmitis after penetrating injuries with retained intraocular foreign bodies. *Ophthalmology* 1993;100:1468–1474.

163. Boldt HC, Pulido JS, Blodi CF, et al. Rural endophthalmitis. *Ophthalmology* 1989;96:1722–1726.

164. Vastine DW, Peyman GA, Futh SB. Visual prognosis in bacterial endophthalmitis treated with intravitreal antibiotics. *Ophthalmic Surg* 1979;10:76–83.

165. Mieler WF, Glazer LC, Bennett SR, Han DP. Favourable outcome of traumatic endophthalmitis with associated retinal breaks or detachment. *Can J Ophthalmol* 1992;27:348–352.

166. Foster RE, Rubsamen PE, Joondeph BC, et al. Concurrent endophthalmitis and retinal detachment. *Ophthalmology* 1994;101:490–498.

167. Haymet T. Results in the treatment of bacterial endophthalmitis. *Aust NZ J Ophthalmol* 1985;13:401–409.

168. Laatikainen L, Tarkkanen A. Early vitrectomy in the treatment of postoperative purulent endophthalmitis. *Acta Ophthalmologica* 1987;65:455–460.

169. Diamond JG. Intraocular management of endophthalmitis: a systemic approach. *Arch Ophthalmol* 1981;99:96–99.

170. Thompson WS, Rubsamen PE, Flynn HW. Endophthalmitis after penetrating trauma: risk factors and visual acuity. *Ophthalmology* 1995;102:1696–1701.

171. Conway BP, Campochiaro PA. Macular infarction after endophthalmitis treated with vitrectomy and intravitreal gentamicin. *Arch Ophthalmol* 1986;104:367–371.

172. D'Amico DJ, Libert J, Kenyon KR, et al. Retinal toxicity of intravitreal genetamicin. *Invest Ophthalmol Vis Sci* 1984;25:565–572.

173. Campochiaro PA, Lim JI, Aminoglycoside Toxicity Study Group. Aminoglycoside toxicity in the treatment of endophthalmitis. *Arch Ophthalmol* 1994;112:48–53.

174. Endophthalmitis Vitrectomy Study Group. Results of the Endophthalmitis Vitrectomy Study. A randomized trial of immediate vitrectomy and of intravenous antibiotics for the treatment of post-operative bacterial endophthalmitis. *Arch Ophthalmol* 1995;113:1479–1496.

175. Foster RE, Martinez JA, Murray TG, et al. Useful visual outcomes after treatment of *Bacillus cereus* endophthalmitis. *Ophthalmology* 1996;103:390–397.

176. El Baba FZ, Trousdale MD, Gauderman WJ, et al. Intravitreal penetrating of oral ciprofloxacin in humans. *Ophthalmology* 1992;99:483–486.

177. El-Massry A, Meredith TA, Aguilar HE, et al. Aminoglycoside levels in the rabbit vitreous cavity after intravenous administration. *Am J Ophthalmol* 1996;122:684–689.

178. Mao LK, Flynn HW Jr, Miller D, Pflugfelder SC. Endophthalmitis caused by *Staphylococcus aureus*. *Am J Ophthalmol* 1993;116:584–589.

179. Meredith TA, Aguilar HE, Drews C, et al. Intraocular dexamethasone produces a harmful effect on treatment of experimental *Staphylococcus aureus* endophthalmitis. *Trans Am Ophthalmol Soc* 1996;94:241–252.

180. Aguilar HE, Meredith TA, Drews C, et al. Comparative treatment of experimental *Staphylococcus aureus* endophthalmitis. *Am J Ophthalmol* 1996;121:310–317.

181. Sneed SR, Weingeist TA. Management of siderosis bulbi 'due to retained ferrous containing intraocular foreign body. *Ophthalmology* 1990; 97:375–379.

182. Barr CC, Vine AK, Martonyi CL. Unexplained heterochromia. Intraocular foreign body demonstrated by computed tomography. *Surv Ophthalmol* 1984;28:409–411.

183. Talamo JH, Topping TM, Maumenee AE, Green WR. Ultrastructural studies of cornea, iris and lens in a case of siderosis bulbi. *Ophthalmology* 1985;92:1675–1680.

184. Monteiro MLR, Coppeto JR, Milani JAA. Iron mydriasis: pupillary paresis from occult intraocular foreign body. *J Clin Neuro-Ophthalmol* 1993;13:254–257.

185. Brunette JR, Wagdi S, Lafond G. Electroretinographic alterations in retinal metallosis. *Can J Ophthalmol* 1980;15:176–178.

186. Good P, Gross K. Electrophysiology and metallosis: support for an oxidative (free radical) mechanism in the human eye. *Ophthalmologica* 1998; 196:204–209.

187. Hope-Ross M, Mahon GJ, Johnston PB. Ocular siderosis. *Eye* 1993;7:419–425.

188. Rao NA, Tso MOM, Rosenthal AR. Chalcosis in the human eye. *Arch Ophthalmol* 1976;94:1379–1384.

189. Rosenthal AR, Marmor MF, Leuenberger P, Hopkins JL. Chalcosis: a study of natural history. *Ophthalmology* 1979;84:1956–1972.

190. Ahmadieh H, Soheilian M, Sajjadi H, et al. Vitrectomy in ocular trauma: factors influencing final visual outcome. *Retina* 1993;13:107–113.

191. Brown GC, Tasman WS, Benson WE. BB-gun injuries to the eye. *Ophthalmic Surg* 1985;16:505–508.

192. Sternberg P Jr, deJuan E Jr, Gren WR, et al. Ocular BB injuries. *Ophthalmology* 1984;91:1269–1277.

193. Conlon MR, Canney CLB. Favourable outcome in a patient with penetrating intraocular BB pellet injury. *Can J Ophthalmol* 1992;27: 251–253.

194. Lewis ML, Gass JDM, Spencer WH. Sympathetic uveitis after trauma and vitrectomy. *Arch Ophthalmol* 1978;96:263–267.

195. Lubin JR, Albert DM, Weinstein M. Sixty-five years of sympathetic ophthalmia. A clinicopathologic review of 105 cases (1913–1978). *Ophthalmology* 1980;87:109–121.

196. Green WR. The uveal tract. In: Spencer WH, ed. *Ophthalmic pathology*. Philadelphia: WB Saunders, 1986.

197. Reynard M, Riffenburgh RS, Maes EF. Effect of corticosteroid treatment and enucleation on the visual prognosis of sympathetic ophthalmia. *Am J Ophthalmol* 1983;96:290–294.

198. Kay ML, Yanoff M, Katowitz JA. Development of sympathetic uveitis in spite of corticosteroid therapy. *Am J Ophthalmol* 1974;78:90–94.

199. Dannenberg AL, Parver LM, Brechner JR, Khoo L. Penetrating eye injuries in the workplace: the National Eye Trauma System Registry. *Arch Ophthalmol* 1992;110:843–848.

200. Patel BCK, Morgan LH. Work-related penetrating eye injuries. *Acta Ophthalmologica* 1991;69:377–381.

Surgical Management of Infectious Retinitis

Thomas B. Connor, Jr.

Infectious retinitis may cause visual compromise via direct involvement of macula or optic nerve. Inflammation associated with the infection may lead to vitreous opacification or cystoid macular edema, either of which may affect visual acuity. Infected areas of retina may become necrotic, leading to the development of full-thickness retinal breaks and subsequent retinal detachment.

Agents responsible for infectious retinitis include bacterial, fungal, protozoal (primarily toxoplasma gondii), treponemal and viral (especially cytomegalovirus [CMV], varicella zoster virus [VZV], and herpes simplex virus [HSV]) sources. These retinal infections arise from hematogenous spread to the retina, where local infection may occur, and may spread to the choroid, vitreous, and other intraocular structures. While these infections may be observed in immunocompetent individuals, they are particularly noted in immunocompromised patients.

The primary therapy of infectious retinitis is usually the application of an antibiotic or anti-infective agent. Many of these agents may be delivered systemically, via oral or intravenous routes. However, if intraocular penetration via these routes is below desired therapeutic levels, or if adverse effects or intolerance are associated with systemic delivery, then intraocular delivery may be desirable.

The clinical diagnosis of infectious retinitis may require confirmation to ensure the institution of appropriate therapy. This confirmation may be particularly important in atypical presentations and when therapies carry risk of adverse reactions. In such cases, sampling of the vitreous or of the infected area of retina may yield needed diagnostic confirmation.

Surgical techniques may be applied to infectious retinitis for diagnostic and therapeutic purposes. Vitreous or endoretinal biopsy may be performed for diagnostic information in appropriate cases. Medications may be delivered via trans-pars plana routes as individual injections or in sustained-release form. Surgical techniques may also be used to address secondary effects of retinitis such as vitreous opacification, retinal breaks, or retinal detachment.

DIAGNOSTIC APPLICATIONS

Vitreous Sampling/Biopsy

Vitreous humor may be an important diagnostic tissue source in cases of infectious retinitis. Samples of vitreous may be examined for antigen or antibodies related to infectious agents, nucleic acid of infectious agents identified via polymerase chain reaction (PCR) testing, or even examined for the infectious agent by means of microbiologic culture (1–5). Appropriate handling of such specimens is crucial to success of desired testing. The small volume of sampled vitreous is usually sent to the diagnostic laboratory in undiluted, unpreserved form. In general, it is best to personally communicate with the microbiologic, diagnostic, or pathology laboratory that will be receiving the specimen so that it will be prepared and delivered in optimal condition. Additionally, suspected infectious agent(s) must be reviewed with the laboratory so that appropriate, focused testing may be done.

Preparation

Vitreous sampling may be performed under local anesthesia. The anesthetized eye is prepared with Betadine antiseptic solution. It may then be draped, and a speculum is placed between the lids. The superotemporal quadrant provides good exposure. A location 3.5 to 4.0 mm to the limbus is a site for trans–pars plana sampling.

Aspiration Sampling

A 27-gauge needle on a 1- to 3-mL syringe may be placed through this site trans-conjunctivally and trans–pars plana for manual aspiration/sampling of liquid vitreous. Fluid (0.1 to 0.3 mL) is removed, and a cotton-tip applicator is applied to the sampling site as the needle is withdrawn (6). Balanced salt solution may be injected through a separate site to reform the globe as needed. Obtained material is then delivered to the diagnostic laboratory. This technique may fail to yield sampling if formed vitreous occludes the bore in the needle. Indeed, such potential for traction on peripheral vitreous may precipitate a retinal break and subsequent retinal detachment.

Vitreous Biopsy

In theory, using a vitreous cutting instrument as a biopsy device may decrease the risk of traction on the peripheral vitreous. This biopsy may be performed separately as a single-port vitrectomy, or as part of a planned multi-port vitrectomy procedure (6–9). As a single-port technique, the eye is prepared as described above. A quadrantic peritomy may be performed with light cautery applied to the exposed episclera for surface hemostasis. A mark is made 3.5 to 4.0 mm from the limbus. The vitreous cutter is prepared. Its tubing should not be primed with fluid so that pure, undiluted vitreous sample is obtained. A 1- to 3-mL syringe is attached to the Luer lock of the aspiration side of the vitreous cutter tubing. This biopsy tubing adapter is typically 2.5 to 5.0 cm from the cutter handpiece. With microscope visualization, a sclerotomy is fashioned with a stiletto or MVR blade followed by placement of the vitreous cutter through the sclerotomy into the vitreous cavity. With automated cutting (>400 cuts per minute), vitreous is drawn into the unprimed tubing by means of syringe aspiration. Sample in the amount of 0.1 to 0.3 mL is removed. The cutter is removed, all specimen is aspirated from tubing dead space into the syringe, and the sample is sent to the appropriate diagnostic laboratory. The globe may be reformed with balanced salt solution or planned antibiotic injection, if needed. The 20-gauge sclerotomy may be closed with Vicryl or Dexon suture and the conjunctiva is similarly closed.

Vitreous biopsy may be obtained as part of a multi-port vitrectomy. Typically, an infusion line is placed first but is not turned on. Vitreous biopsy is described as above to obtain undiluted vitreous sample. Infusion line is then turned on to reform the globe, and vitrectomy proceeds.

Some smaller gauge sclerotomy/vitreous biopsy systems may be self-sealing and not require sclerotomy closure (10). A novel pneumovitrectomy device has been described for vitreous biopsy. It has a combined cutting/aspiration system and an infusion line that permits infusion of gas or air while undiluted vitreous sample is obtained (11).

Complications

Potential complications of vitreous sampling or biopsy include endophthalmitis, suprachoroidal hemorrhage, vitreous hemorrhage, retinal break, retinal detachment, wound leak, or lens damage. It is important to be vigilant for these events and manage them promptly if they occur. Vitreous sampling and biopsy may be associated with concurrent delivery of intraocular medications.

Endoretinal Biopsy

Diagnosis and management of infectious retinitis may require a tissue sampling of infected retina. The area of involved retina may be in attached or detached retina (12). Techniques involving scleral flap incisions to obtain chorioretinal biopsies have been described. We prefer combining pars plana vitrectomy with trans–pars plana retinal biopsy (10,13–15). As with all surgical biopsy specimens, it is important to communicate with the pathologist receiving the specimen so that proper tissue handling and preparation occurs.

Technique

A standard 3-port vitrectomy is performed. The site for biopsy is chosen, ideally containing areas of involved retina and adjacent uninvolved, normal appearing retina. If possible, any attached vitreous or membranes should be stripped from the biopsy site. Endocautery is used to delineate the area of biopsy, usually 2–4 mm by 2–6 mm (12–14). Infusion bottles are temporarily raised, and vertical intraocular scissors are used to cut the specimen free along the outline of the cautery marks. Intraocular forceps are used to gently grasp the specimen and remove it from the eye. Care is taken to avoid crushing the tissue. The specimen is then sent for examination. The biopsy site is inspected. Infusion bottles are lowered to normal height, and cautery is applied as needed. Vitrectomy and retinal reattachment techniques are continued, as needed. If the retina was attached at the time of biopsy, laser treatment is applied around the edges of the biopsy site, and tamponade of air, gas, or silicone oil is applied (14,16,17).

Complications

Complications that may accompany retinal biopsy include vitreous hemorrhage or choroidal hemorrhage; care with intraocular hemostasis and choosing areas of biopsy sites in detached retina away from the choroid may minimize these events (14,16,17). As with all intraocular procedures, endophthalmitis may occur. Subsequent retinal detachment and proliferative vitreoretinopathy (PVR) may occur, highlighting the importance of freeing the biopsy site from attached vitreous and membranes. In cases of retinal detachment with PVR following retinal biopsy, it is unclear whether the recurrent detachment with PVR was due to the biopsy procedure or to the underlying disease process.

THERAPEUTIC APPLICATIONS

Intravitreal Therapy

Central to treatment of infectious retinitis is the use of anti-infective agents. Therapeutic intraocular levels may be difficult to obtain through systemic administration of these agents; intraocular penetration may be limited via systemic or parenteral routes, or systemic use of these agents may be associated with adverse effects. Long-term intravenous therapy requires placement and maintenance of in-dwelling catheter, which itself may be associated with complications.

Intravitreal delivery of agents via trans-pars plana routes (through sclera or conjunctiva) provides rapid onset of high levels of agent without associated systemic intolerance (18,19). Agents may be delivered in this manner in an office setting or in the operating room. The technique described will be for office use, but it could easily be modified for use intraoperatively.

Surgical Technique

Anesthesia may be topical, subconjunctival, retrobulbar, or peribulbar. The patient may be reclined in a chair or placed on an examination/treatment table. Antibiotic drops and antiseptic solution (such as povidine-iodine) are placed in the conjunctival fornices. Medication for injection is prepared and now drawn up into a 1-mL syringe capped with a 30-gauge needle. Excess air and material is expelled from the syringe so the exact amount for appropriate dosing is ready in the syringe with needle. A sterilized speculum is placed. A measurement is made and marked 3.5 to 4.0 mm from the limbus; superior sites are preferred for ease of access. The globe may be fixated with toothed forceps in one hand while an injection is made through the marked site. The nonfixating hand places the needle through the sclera for about 2 to 3 mm aiming for the center of the globe, ideally visualizing the needle in the vitreous cavity with indirect ophthalmoscopy. With the needle bevel directed anteriorly, slow injection is made until the entire dose is delivered. A cotton-tip applicator is placed over the injection site as the needle is withdrawn, and the applicator is held there for 30 to 60 seconds.

Indirect ophthalmoscopy is performed to examine the injection site as well as to observe retinal perfusion. If perfusion is compromised, a separate 30-gauge needle on a 1-mL syringe is used at the limbus to perform anterior paracentesis, removing 0.05 to 0.1 mL of aqueous to accommodate the injected volume of medication. Alternatively, intermittent digital pressure to the globe or a Honan balloon manometer may be placed on the eye 15 minutes prior to injection to soften the eye to accommodate the injected volume of medication; these maneuvers may make anterior paracentesis unnecessary.

In patients who are aphakic, these agents may be delivered intraocularly via limbal injection, reducing the risk of peripheral retinal injury.

Agents Used

The agents below are used for viral or fungal retinitis. Other agents may be used for bacterial retinitis. However, such cases are often successfully managed with intravenous therapy. Bacterial retinitis that involves the vitreous is probably best managed as an infectious endophthalmitis.

Acyclovir The antiviral agent acyclovir has been used at doses 80–200 mcg/0.1 mL for varicella zoster and herpes simplex infections (20).

Ganciclovir The purine nucleotide analogue ganciclovir was demonstrated to be tolerable when administered intravitreally in 1985 (21). Dosing is 2 to 3 times per week for induction therapy for CMV retinitis, followed by weekly injections for maintenance therapy. Doses for injection are typically 200–400 mcg/0.1 mL (22–28). Toxicity in humans has been observed at 40 mg/0.1 mL (29).

Foscarnet Foscarnet injections are given 2 to 3 times per week for induction therapy for 2 weeks, followed by weekly injections for maintenance therapy of CMV retinitis. Typical doses for injection are 1200–2400 mcg/0.1 mL (30).

Cidofovir Cidofovir is a nucleotide analogue with increased potency and a narrow therapeutic window. A single 20 mcg/0.1 ml injection is effective for induction, with mean time to progression of CMV retinitis found to be 55 days. However, significant intraocular inflammation has been observed, with 71% of patients experiencing iritis, some with hypotony, following injection (31–35). Atrophy of the ciliary body has been observed histopathologically in eyes following injection (36). This amount was reduced to 18–26% by concurrent administration of oral probenecid as follows: 2 g PO 3 hours before injection, 1 g PO 2 hours post injection, 1 g PO 8 hours post injection. Probenecid presumably limits uptake of cidofovir by ciliary epithelium. Even with concurrent probenecid intake, intravitreal cidofovir use may be associated with uveitis in 18–26% of cases, managed with cycloplegia and topical or periocular steroids (35). Even with this regimen, permanent hypotony has been observed in 2% of eyes. Correct dilution is crucial when using this medication, as 10 mcg/0.1 mL may give no effect, while 40 mcg/0.1 mL may yield permanent hypotony (32).

Amphotericin Amphotericin is a macrolide antifungal agent. Doses are typically 2.5–5.0 mcg/0.1 mL per injection (37,38). Toxicities have been reported at higher doses (39,40).

Complications

Potential complications of trans-pars plana delivery of intravitreal agents include suprachoroidal injection of medication, subretinal injection of medication, peripheral retinal break or detachment, needle damage to crystalline lens or IOL, vitreous hemorrhage, endophthalmitis, or intraocular toxicity damage to ocular structures. Failure to inject into the vitreous cavity is rare, as is damage to peripheral retina if the site is chosen carefully and the injection performed with indirect ophthalmoscopic guidance. Late retinal breaks and detachment occur rarely (no cases of detachment in one series of 269 injections), and if they do occur they should be managed promptly and appropriately; patients with infectious retinitis are prone to areas of retinal necrosis and breaks, and detachments occur primarily from this mechanism. Endophthalmitis is a rare—1 case in 269 injections in one series—but potentially devastating complication best managed with vitreous sampling or vitrectomy and intraocular antibiotic injection. Vitreous hemorrhages may occur following therapeutic injection, and these hemorrhages typically clear spontaneously. Persistent, nonclearing, visually significant vitreous hemorrhage may be managed with vitrectomy techniques. Intraocular toxicity of injected agents is best avoided by careful monitoring of dilutions of injected agents. These dilutions may be supervised by the surgeon or performed by a pharmacist. We prefer to have standardized dilution protocols available for the agents we use. A copy of the protocol signed by the pharmacist performing the dilutions accompanies our medication for intraocular injection.

Ganciclovir Implant

Clinical Applications

First shown as efficacious in 1992 (41) and later approved in the United States for use in CMV retinitis in March 1996, the sustained-release ganciclovir implant ushered in a new era of therapy for vitreoretinal diseases (42). The sustained release implant provides a higher intraocular medication level than is possible by intravenous therapy, achieving these constant levels within 12 to 24 hours of implantation while avoiding systemic side effects and associated complications of chronic intravenous therapy. Initially used for patients with CMV retinitis who were intolerant of or unresponsive to systemic therapy, the ganciclovir implant has also been shown to be effective in recurrent retinitis (43,44) and even as primary therapy for newly diagnosed CMV retinitis. A comparison of intravenous ganciclovir to ganciclovir implant therapy as primary treatment for CMV retinitis demonstrated the risk of progression of CMV retinitis was 2.8-fold higher with intravenous therapy compared to implant therapy (45).

Surgical Technique

The implant is constructed as a 4.5-mg pellet of ganciclovir and polymer attached to a supporting tab or strut.

Primary placement or exchange and replacement of the implant is typically performed as an outpatient under monitored local anesthesia with optional supplemental sedation. After local anesthesia is administered, the surgical eye is prepared and draped (41,42).

The implant is prepared on a sterile field. Care is taken to minimize handling of the implant pellet; nonlocking needle holders or smooth, grooved forceps work well for this handling. Using spring action or Stevens scissors, 2.5 mm is trimmed from the distal end of the implant tab. Round tab corners with the same scissors. Use a sharp instrument (a 27G needle works well) to create a hole in the center of the trimmed tab, 0.5 mm from the distal end. Pass a double-armed 8-0 nylon suture (TG 175 needle) through the hole and tie down near the middle of the suture with small secure knot. The needles on the attached suture will then be used to secure the implant to the sclera later in the procedure.

Implant placement may be performed in any quadrant. We prefer placement inferotemporally or inferonasally. With placement inferiorly in the quadrant, we avoid areas that may be useful for possible future infusion cannula placement if vitrectomy is ever needed.

A limited quadrantic peritomy is performed; an optional traction suture through the horizontal rectus may be placed. Light episcleral cautery is applied to the region of planned scleral incision, excessive cautery may cause scleral shrinkage and weakening, and the incision site may need to be used for future implant exchange. Calipers are used to mark 4.0 mm from the limbus separated by a chord length of 5.5 to 6.0 mm. (This 5.5-mm length—parallel to the limbus—will be the site of scleral incision.) A sterile skin marker may be used to mark this site. Sclerotomy is then fashioned with blade of choice—an MVR or stiletto blade, a 15- or 30-degree blade, a keratome blade, etc.—making sure the entire length of the incision is through both sclera and uvea. This depth of penetration is confirmed via direct inspection; not uncommonly, the internal aspect of the wound needs enlargement. The vitrectomy handpiece is then used with cutting and suction to remove any prolapsed vitreous.

The prepared implant is then grasped securely by the tab near the tab/pellet junction. A lip of the scleral incision is grasped with fine-toothed forceps and spread wide, and the implant is inserted parallel to the limbus into the wound pellet first, with the pellet facing anteriorly. One end of the 8-0 nylon suture is placed, from the inside out, through the anterior lip of the center of the wound; the other end is placed in similar manner through the posterior lip. Careful indirect ophthalmoscopy is performed without pressure on the globe to confirm placement in the vitreous cavity and not in the suprachoroidal space.

Then the suture ends are tied securely, anchoring the implant; the purpose of this closure is to anchor the implant and not necessarily close the wound. Suture ends are left long. Any prolapsed vitreous is excised with the vitrectomy cutting instrument. The remaining free suture pieces of 8-0 nylon are used to close either end of the incision in running or "X" fashion on either side of the anchoring suture, placing the remaining limbs of the anchoring suture under the running or "X" closure. Care is taken so that passes through the posterior lip do not cause retinal perforation. Closure is made with the knots buried to reduce risk of erosion of overlying conjunctiva. Balanced salt solution is injected via a 30-gauge needle through the pars plana to reform the globe. The wound is inspected for water-tight closure. Indirect ophthalmoscopy is performed to inspect peripheral retina near the implant and to confirm proper implant placement. Conjunctiva is closed with suture (6-0 plain gut, 7-0 to 8-0 Vicryl or Dexon all work well). Subconjunctival antibiotic (such as cefazolin or vancomycin) and steroid (dexamethasone) injections may then be given. It is recommended that the surgeon make a drawing of the suture configuration of the wound closure so that the anchoring suture may be easily identified during subsequent removal or exchange of implant.

Implants may be exchanged when the medication is exhausted and reactivation of disease occurs. Alternatively, it may be exchanged at 32-week intervals, per previous study protocol (42). Options at time of exchange include 1) placing a new implant in the opposite inferior quadrant, 2) placing a new implant more inferiorly in the same quadrant through a new scleral incision, or 3) removing the previous implant and placing a new one through the original incision (46). I prefer option 1 for the first "exchange" followed by alternating sides for exchanges via option 3 at 32-week intervals. That is, first placement is inferotemporal: 32 weeks later, a second implant is placed inferonasally, 32 weeks after that, the inferotemporal implant is directly exchanged (18).

Implant exchanges at the same site of previous implantation are begun in a similar fashion to initial implantation (46). The new implant is prepared as described above. After the sclera is exposed, care is taken to remove adherent tissue from the old incision. The diagram of suture configuration from the previous surgery is consulted, and the anchoring suture is identified. Sutures on either side of the anchoring suture are removed. The old incision is then reopened with a 15-degree blade directed from either side of the anchoring suture and out toward the ends of the incision. The wound is then spread with toothed forceps, and the implant tab is exposed and grasped firmly. The anchoring suture is divided, and the implant is gently removed. Any prolapsed vitreous gel is removed with the vitrectomy cutting instrument. The procedure then continues as described above.

Postoperatively, cycloplegia, topical steroids, and antibiotics are administered for several weeks. Visual recovery, barring complications, typically returns to baseline within 2 to 4 weeks. Median acuity at 1 week postoperatively was 20/40 in one trial.

Implants may be left in place if future surgery is required, such as cataract surgery or retinal reattachment surgery. One should take care not to disturb the sutures anchoring and closing the implant incision.

Complications

Complications are infrequent, but they include vitreous hemorrhage, endophthalmitis, suprachoroidal implantation, wound dehiscence, and retinal tear or detachment (41,42,47,48). Suprachoroidal implantation is avoided by ensuring that the primary incision is completely open through sclera and choroid for the entire length of the incision. Placement in the vitreous cavity is confirmed prior to

tying down the anchoring suture. If suprachoroidal implantation is recognized, it is managed with repositioning.

Endophthalmitis is uncommon, having occurred in less than 1% of cases. It is managed with vitreous biopsy or vitrectomy and intraocular antibiotic injection and close monitoring to see if further intervention is needed.

Vitreous hemorrhage may occur in varying amounts postoperatively, and it is the most common cause for decreased vision in the immediate postoperative period. This hemorrhage typically clears over 2 to 4 weeks. Persistent, nonclearing, visually significant vitreous hemorrhage may be managed with vitrectomy, but this intervention is rarely needed.

Wound dehiscence is uncommon, but may present as unexplained redness or foreign-body sensation or surface discomfort. Hypotony may be observed as well as serous choroidal detachments; wound dehiscence should be suspected if either of these conditions arises in a patient with a ganciclovir implant. The wound dehiscence may be subtle, and as conjunctiva cover the scleral incision site, no direct leak may be observed, and the area may be Seidel test negative when, in fact, a wound dehiscence is present. Definitive management involves exploration and resuturing of the wound, as an open wound may present an avenue for the introduction of intraocular infection.

Retinal tears or retinal detachment can occur in any patient with CMV or other form of infectious retinitis. Retinal detachments were observed in 12% of patients post implant therapy compared with 5% of patients treated with intravenous therapy through 8 months' follow-up (42,45). A posterior vitreous separation frequently occurs 1 to 2 months postoperatively, and patients with implants should be counseled to alert the surgeon if such symptoms occur. Such patients should be promptly examined and treated appropriately.

While the implant delivers a high intraocular level of medication, it does not provide treatment for systemic CMV infection. The development of extraocular CMV infection has been observed in 10% to 30% of patients who were treated with only implant therapy (42,45). Any patient receiving intraocular therapy for CMV retinitis should be monitored for extraocular CMV infection; concomitant systemic therapy for such patients may be helpful.

MANAGEMENT OF COMPLICATIONS OF INFECTIOUS RETINITIS

Laser Demarcation of Retinal Breaks

The acute retinal necrosis (ARN) syndrome is a vasoocclusive necrotizing retinitis associated with varicella zoster or herpes simplex virus infection. This syndrome has a high incidence of retinal breaks and retinal detachment. Treatment is focused on systemic antiviral therapy to manage the infectious retinitis. Demarcating the areas of retinitis with laser photocoagulation treatment is used as a prophylactic treatment, ideally creating chorioretinal adhesion around areas of potential retinal breaks. Treatment may be performed with slit-lamp or indirect ophthalmoscope delivery using argon, krypton, or infrared diode wavelength. Three to four rows of at least 500 micron diameter spots are placed posterior to the areas of retinitis and as far anterior to the ora serrata as possible. Posterior areas within 2 disk diameters of the optic nerve or foveal center are avoided. Five such patients treated in this manner maintained retinal attachment, which is a favorable outcome (49) compared with the estimated 50% to 75% estimated occurrence of retinal detachment in untreated eyes with ARN.

Retinal detachment may complicate the course of CMV retinitis in 25% to 30% of HIV-infected patients. Photocoagulation of retinal tears and areas of limited retinal detachment may be useful in stopping or delaying the progression of detachment. Several series with limited follow-up reported success rates of 40% to 70% (50,51). One larger series with longer follow-up demonstrated success in 7 of 9 cases (79%) with laser demarcation of tears associated with CMV retinitis. Limited retinal detachments were successfully demarcated in this same series in 16 of 23 eyes (70%) (52).

Retinal Detachment

Retinal detachment may occur in association with infectious retinitis. The detachment may be tractional, encouraged by contraction directed on an inflamed/infected vitreoretinal region. Vitrectomy techniques may be applied to these areas if they are visually significant or vision threatening. More commonly, rhegmatogenous retinal detachments occur, with areas of infectious retinitis serving as a site of breaks developing in areas of necrotic retina. These detachments are typically complex and involve large areas of affected atrophic or necrotic retina with multiple breaks. These complex detachments are often best managed with vitrectomy techniques (53,54).

Cases of retinal detachment due to ARN and CMV retinitis in HIV-infected individuals require particular attention. Retinal detachment may occur in patients with ARN, estimated incidence being 50% to 75% (55). Retinal detachments may occur in 10% to 30% of HIV-infected patients with CMV retinitis (56,57). Management of these conditions includes addressing the infectious retinitis as well as any associated retinal detachment.

Surgical Technique
CMV Retinitis–Related Retinal Detachments While scleral buckling and pneumatic retinopexy may be used in limited cases of retinal detachment (51), the extensive areas of retinal involvement and the recurrent nature of the condition are often best managed with vitrectomy techniques and silicone oil tamponade (58–62). A standard 3-port pars plana vitrectomy is performed. Lensectomy is required only if significant lens opacity prevents accomplishing vitrectomy

goals. Removal of posterior cortical vitreous is attempted; if not possible, vitreous is trimmed back close to retinal surface anteriorly and around areas of retinitis. Subretinal fluid may be drained internally through a preexisting break or posterior retinotomy. Retina is reattached via fluid–air exchange or fluid–silicone exchange. Photocoagulation is placed via endoprobe or indirect ophthalmoscope delivery around breaks, retinotomies, with scatter treatment in the inferior midperiphery if this region was involved in the detachment and/or had active areas of retinitis. Silicone oil is injected, if not already done. Face-down position is maintained for 1 week postoperatively. With these techniques, total reattachment rates have been reported at 60% to 100%, and macular reattachment recorded at >70% with maintenance of ambulatory vision or better (50,57–65).

Scleral buckling may or may not be performed in conjunction with vitrectomy and silicone oil injection as described above (62). Some authors have suggested that placement of a scleral buckle prevents postoperative creeping inferior detachments by allowing broader area of inferior retina/silicone apposition (50,65). Lim et al (60) noted a higher success rate in total reattachment using vitrectomy with scleral buckle and laser demarcation than in cases without scleral buckle via historical comparison. Garcia et al (64) reported a reattachment rate of 85% both with and without scleral buckling; all patients had vitrectomy, removal of posterior cortical vitreous, fluid–gas exchange, photocoagulation around breaks, necrotic retina, retinotomies, and scatter treatment to the inferior midperiphery, and silicone oil tamponade.

Postoperative optic atrophy has been observed in these patients, possibly a consequence of low systemic perfusion with concomitant anemia and relative systemic hypotension due to compromised general health. Thus, these patients may be susceptible to intraocular ischemia with a moderate rise in intraocular perfusion pressure. Postoperative cataracts may be managed with modern phacoemulsification techniques. Care should be taken to keep the posterior capsule intact, and silicone intraocular lenses should be avoided. Ganciclovir implants may also be placed at the time of retinal reattachment surgery or cataract surgery, if needed.

ARN-Related Retinal Detachments ARN patients often have tractional and rhegmatogenous components to their retinal detachments. As such, they are often best managed with vitrectomy techniques combined with scleral buckling to support the vitreous base. Standard 3-port vitrectomy is performed. Lensectomy may be performed if lens opacity prevents achieving goals of posterior vitrectomy. If extensive vitreous base dissection is required, lensectomy may be required to gain access to this region. Epiretinal membranes and posterior cortical vitreous is stripped from the posterior retinal surface. Vitreous base dissection is performed with the help of scleral depression. After all traction has been relieved, retinal breaks are identified and marked with cautery, as needed. In some cases, relaxing retinectomy may be required to relieve retinal traction. Retinal reattachment may be achieved with perfluorocarbon liquid injection or fluid–gas exchange. Photocoagulation is applied via endoprobe or indirect ophthalmoscope delivery to areas of retinal breaks and surrounding areas of retinal necrosis. An encircling buckle supporting the vitreous base, in some cases supporting to the equator, is often advantageous. Photocoagulation may be applied to the region of buckle indentation. Long-acting gas or silicone oil tamponade is applied. With these techniques, retinal reattachment rates have risen from 22% to 88–100% (54,55,66,67). Postoperative acuity may be limited by the detachment as well as retinal and optic nerve involvement from the infectious agent.

Media Opacification

Vitritis associated with infectious retinitis may lead to opacification of the vitreous. While this opacification may clear with time, some patients may have nonclearing opacification—from inflammation or associated hemorrhage into the vitreous cavity—which may be visually significant and/or prevent fundus visualization to guide treatment. In such cases, vitrectomy may be beneficial in clearing ocular media as a form of visual rehabilitation (68). Stripping of the posterior hyaloid face may expose areas of retinal breaks in eyes with regions of retinal necrosis often associated with infectious retinitis. Such areas should be cautiously approached and carefully observed at the end of vitrectomy. Laser demarcation of such areas of retinal breaks is performed with laser photocoagulation via endoprobe or indirect ophthalmoscope delivery systems.

SUMMARY

Modern vitreoretinal techniques allow methods for the diagnosis and treatment of infectious retinitis as well as associated complications. While systemic therapies are quite useful for some cases of infectious retinitis, the application of long-acting intravitreal therapy is attractive for some disorders. High intraocular levels may be obtained for months without systemic adverse effects with intravitreal therapy.

REFERENCES

1. Cunningham ETJ, Short GA, et al. Acquired immunodeficiency syndrome–associated herpes simplex virus retinitis. Clinical description and use of a polymerase chain reaction–based assay as a diagnostic tool. *Arch Ophthalmol* 1996;114:834–840.
2. Davis JL, Feuer WJ, et al. Interpretation of intraocular and serum antibody levels in necrotizing retinitis. *Retina* 1995;15:233–240.
3. de Boer JH, Verhagen C, et al. Serologic and polymerase chain reaction analysis of intraocular fluids in the diagnosis of infectious uveitis. *Am J Ophthalmol* 1996;121:650–658.
4. Elkins BS, Holland GN, et al. Ocular toxoplasmosis misdiagnosed as cytomegalovirus retinopathy in immunocompromised patients. *Ophthalmology* 1994;101:499–507.
5. Stone RD, Irvine AR, et al. *Candida* endophthalmitis: report of an unusual case with isolation of the etiologic agent by vitreous biopsy. *Ann Ophthalmol* 1975;7:757.
6. Group EVS. Results of the endophthalmitis vitrectomy study group. A randomized trial of immediate vitrectomy and of intravenous antibiotics for the treatment of postoperative bacterial endophthalmitis. *Arch Ophthalmol* 1995;113:1479–1496.
7. Doft BH, Donnelly K. A single sclerotomy vitreous biopsy technique in endophthalmitis. *Arch Ophthalmol* 1991;109:465.
8. Scholda CD, Egger SF, et al. A system for obtaining undiluted intraoperative vitreous biopsy samples. *Arch Ophthalmol* 1996;114:1271–1272.
9. Tamai M, Nakazawa M. A collection system to obtain vitreous humor in clinical cases. *Arch Ophthalmol* 1991;109:465–466.
10. Peyman GA. A miniaturized vitrectomy system for vitreous and retinal biopsy. *Can J Ophthalmol* 1990;25:285–286.
11. Peyman GA. A pneumovitrector for the diagnostic biopsy of the vitreous. *Ophthalmic Surg Lasers* 1996;27:246–247.
12. Friedberg MA, Schwartz JC, et al. Systemic herpetic infection diagnosed by retinal biopsy. *Ophthalmic Surg* 1993;24:203–205.
13. Gross JG, Schneiderman TE, et al. Experimental endoretinal biopsy. *Am J Ophthalmol* 1990;110:619.
14. Freeman WR, Wiley CA, et al. Endoretinal biopsy in immunosuppressed and healthy patients with retinitis. *Ophthalmology* 1989;96:1559.
15. Knousse MC, Lorber B. Early diagnosis of *Nocardia* asteroides endophthalmitis by retinal biopsy: case report and review. *Rev Infect Dis* 1990;12:393.
16. Rutzen AR, Ortega-Larrocea G, et al. Clinicopathologic study of retinal and choroidal biopsies in intraocular inflammation. *Am J Ophthalmol* 1995;119:597–611.
17. Rutzen AR, Ortega-Larrocea G, et al. Retinal and choroidal biopsy in intraocular inflammation: a clinicopathologic study. *Trans Am Ophthalmol Soc* 1994;92:431–455.
18. Duker JS, Ashton P, et al. Long-term successful maintenance of bilateral cytomegalovirus retinitis using exclusively local therapy. *Arch Ophthalmol* 1996;114:881–882.
19. Freeman WR. Intraocular antiviral therapy. *Arch Ophthalmol* 1989;107:1737–1739.
20. Peyman GA, Goldberg MF, et al. Vitrectomy and intravitreal antiviral drug therapy in acute retinal necrosis syndrome. *Arch Ophthalmol* 1984;102:1618.
21. Pulido J, Peyman GA, et al. Intravitreal toxicity of hydroxyacyclovir (BW-B759U), a new antiviral agent. *Arch Ophthalmol* 1985;103:840–841.
22. Young SH, Morlet N, et al. High dose intravitreal ganciclovir in the treatment of CMV retinitis. *Med J Australia* 1992;157:370–373.
23. Ussery FM, Gibson SR, et al. Intravitreal ganciclovir in the treatment of AIDS-associated cytomegalovirus retinitis. *Ophthalmology* 1988;95:640–648.
24. Heery S, Hollows F. High-dose intravitreal ganciclovir for cytomegalovirus (CMV) retinitis. *Aus N Z J Ophthalmol* 1989;17:405–408.
25. Heinemann MH. Long term intravitreal ganciclovir therapy for cytomegalovirus retinopathy. *Arch Ophthalmol* 1989;107:1767–1772.
26. Henry K, Cantrill H, et al. Use of intravitreal ganciclovir (dihydroxypropoxymethyl guanine) for cytomegalovirus retinitis in a patient with AIDS. *Am J Ophthalmol* 1987;103:17–23.
27. Cochereau-Massin I, LeHoang P, et al. Efficacy and tolerance of intravitreal ganciclovir in cytomegalovirus retinitis in acquired immunodeficiency syndrome. *Ophthalmology* 1991;98:1348–1355.
28. Cantrill H, Henry K, et al. Treatment of cytomegalovirus retinitis with intravitreal ganciclovir: Long term results. *Ophthalmology* 1989;96:367–374.
29. Saran BR, Maguire AM. Retinal toxicity of high dose intravitreal ganciclovir. *Retina* 1994;14:248–252.
30. Diaz-Llopis M, Chipont E, et al. Intravitreal foscarnet for CMV retinitis in a patient with AIDS. *Am J Ophthalmol* 1992;114:742–747.
31. Kirsch LS, Arevalo JF, et al. Intravitreal cidofovir (HPMPC) treatment of cytomegalovirus retinitis in patients with acquired immune deficiency syndrome. *Ophthalmology* 1995;102:533–543.
32. Kirsch LS, Arevalo JF, et al. Phase I/II study of intravitreal cidofovir for treatment of cytomegalovirus retinitis in patients with the acquired immunodeficiency syndrome. *Am J Ophthalmol* 1995;119:466–476.
33. Rahal FM, Arevalo JF, et al. Intravitreal cidofovir for the maintenance treatment of cytomegalovirus retinitis. *Ophthalmology* 1996;103:1078–1083.
34. Rahal FM, Arevalo JF, et al. Treatment of cytomegalovirus retinitis with intravitreous cidofovir in patients with AIDS. *Ann Intern Med* 1996;125:98–103.
35. Taskintuna I, Rahhal FM, et al. Low-dose intravitreal Cidofovir (HPMPC) therapy of cytomegalovirus retinitis in patients with acquired immune deficiency syndrome. *Ophthalmology* 1997;104:1049–1057.
36. Chavez de la Paz E, Arevalo JF, et al. Anterior nongranulomatous uveitis after intravitreal HPMPC (cidofovir) for the treatment of cytomegalovirus retinitis. Analysis and prevention. *Ophthalmology* 1997;104:539–544.
37. Brod R, Flynn HW, et al. Endogenous *Candida* endophthalmitis. Management without intravitreal amphotericin B. *Ophthalmology* 1990;97:666–672.

38. Perraut LEJ, Perrault LE, et al. Successful treatment of *Candida albicans* endophthalmitis with intravitreal amphotericin B. *Arch Ophthalmol* 1981;99:1565.

39. Axelrod AJ, Peyman GA. Toxicity of intravitreal injection of amphotericin B. *Am J Ophthalmol* 1973;76:578–583.

40. Souri EN, Green WR. Intravitreal amphotericin B toxicity. *Am J Ophthalmol* 1974;78:77–81.

41. Sanborn GE, Anand R, et al. Sustained-release ganciclovir therapy for treatment of cytomegalovirus retinitis. Use of an intravitreal device. *Arch Ophthalmol* 1992;110:188–195.

42. Martin DF, Parks DJ, et al. Treatment of cytomegalovirus retinitis with an intraocular sustained-release ganciclovir implant: a randomized controlled clinical trial. *Arch Ophthalmol* 1994;1531–1539.

43. Marx JL, Kapusta MA, et al. Use of ganciclovir implant in the treatment of recurrent cytomegalovirus retinitis. *Arch Ophthalmol* 1996;114:815–820.

44. Kuppermann BD. Therapeutic options for resistant cytomegalovirus retinitis. *J Acquired Immune Deficiency Syndrome & Human Retrovirology* 1997;14(Suppl 1):S13–S21.

45. Musch DC, Martin DF, et al. Treatment of cytomegalovirus retinitis with a sustained-release ganciclovir implant. *N Engl J Med* 1997;337:83–90.

46. Morley MG, Duker JS, et al. Replacing ganciclovir implants. *Ophthalmology* 1995;102:338–342.

47. Anand R, Font RL, et al. Pathology of cytomegalovirus retinitis treated with sustained release intravitreal ganciclovir. *Ophthalmology* 1993;100:1032–1039.

48. Charles NC, Steiner GC. Ganciclovir intraocular implant—a clinicopathologic study. *Ophthalmology* 1996;103:416–421.

49. Han DP, Lewis H, et al. Laser photocoagulation in the acute retinal necrosis syndrome. *Arch Ophthalmol* 1987;105:1051–1054.

50. Irvine AR. Treatment of retinal detachment due to cytomegalovirus retinitis in patients with AIDS. *Trans Am Ophthalmol Soc* 1991;89:349–367.

51. Orellana J, Teich SA, et al. Treatment of retinal detachment in patients with the acquired immune deficiency syndrome. *Ophthalmology* 1991;98:939–943.

52. Davis JL, Hummer J, et al. Laser photocoagulation for retinal detachments and retinal tears in cytomegalovirus retinitis. *Ophthalmology* 1997;104:2053–2060.

53. Fish RH, Teeters VW, et al. Surgical management of the AIDS retinopathies. *Ophthalmol Clin N Am* 1994;7:101–111.

54. Krieger AE. *Management of combined inflammatory and rhegmatogenous retinal detachments (ARN and AIDS)*. St. Louis: Mosby-Year Book, 1989.

55. Clarkson JG, Blumenkranz MS, et al. Retinal detachment following the acute retinal necrosis syndrome. *Ophthalmology* 1984;91:1665.

56. Freeman WR, Friedberg DN, et al. Risk factors for development of rhegmatogenous retinal detachment in patients with cytomegalovirus retinitis. *Am J Ophthalmol* 1993;116:713–720.

57. Freeman WR, Henderly DE, et al. Prevalence, pathophysiology, and treatment of rhegmatogenous retinal detachment in treated cytomegalovirus retinitis. *Am J Ophthalmol* 1987;103:527–536.

58. Regillo CD, Vander JF, et al. Repair of retinitis-related retinal detachments with silicone oil in patients with acquired immunodeficiency syndrome. *Am J Ophthalmol* 1992;113:21–27.

59. Kuppermann BD, Flores-Aguilar M, et al. A masked prospective evaluation of outcome parameters for cytomegalovirus-related retinal detachment surgery in patients with acquired immune deficiency syndrome. *Ophthalmology* 1994;101:46–55.

60. Lim JI, Enger CS, et al. Improved visual results after surgical repair of cytomegalovirus-related retinal detachments. *Ophthalmology* 1994;101:264–269.

61. Freeman WR, Quiceno JI, et al. Surgical repair of rhegmatogenous retinal detachment in immunosuppressed patients with cytomegalovirus retinitis. *Ophthalmology* 1992;99:466–474.

62. Nassemann JE, Mutsch A, et al. Early pars plana vitrectomy without buckling procedure in cytomegalovirus retinitis–induced retinal detachment. *Retina* 1995;15:111–116.

63. Sandy SJ, Bloom PA, et al. Retinal detachment in AIDS-related cytomegalovirus retinitis. *Eye* 1995;9:277–281.

64. Garcia RF, Flores-Aguilar M, et al. Results of rhegmatogenous retinal detachment repair in cytomegalovirus retinitis with and without scleral buckling. *Ophthalmology* 1995;102:236–245.

65. Chuang EL, Davis JL. Management of retinal detachment associated with CMV retinitis in AIDS patients. *Eye* 1992;6:28–34.

66. Blumenkranz M, Clarkson JG, et al. Vitrectomy for retinal detachment associated with acute retinal necrosis. *Am J Ophthalmol* 1988;106:426.

67. McDonald HR, Lewis H, et al. Surgical management of retinal detachment associated with the acute retinal necrosis syndrome. *Br J Ophthalmol* 1991;75:455.

68. Belmont JB, Michelson JB. Vitrectomy in uveitis associated with ankylosing spondylitis. *Am J Ophthalmol* 1982;112:147–150.

Endophthalmitis

Dennis P. Han

Endophthalmitis is a potentially blinding condition involving infection of the vitreous cavity, usually associated with ocular surgery, trauma, or systemic disease. Severe, progressive, intraocular inflammation is the hallmark of endophthalmitis. Symptoms include loss of vision, ocular redness, and pain. Signs include lid edema, chemosis, corneal infiltrate, hypopyon (Fig. 49-1), relative afferent pupillary defect, vitritis, and loss of the red reflex. Advanced stages can lead to panophthalmitis, corneal perforation, and phthisis bulbi.

Timely diagnosis of endophthalmitis is critical to maximize preservation of visual function. Management consists of (1) acquisition of intraocular specimens for microbiologic studies, (2) elimination of the infecting agent with antimicrobial therapy, (3) selection of appropriate patients for pars plana vitrectomy, and (4) treatment of inflammation and secondary complications.

GENERAL MANAGEMENT

Preoperative Evaluation

Prior to surgical intervention, a detailed ocular history should be obtained. The examiner should inquire specifically about ocular surgery, trauma, systemic infection, and other predisposing conditions. The examination should detect significant anatomic abnormalities, such as wound leak, filtration bleb, vitreous wick syndrome, inflammatory capsular plaques, suture or wound abscess formation, corneal ulcer, penetrating injury, or intraocular foreign body. For suspected endogenous endophthalmitis, a systemic evaluation is warranted.

A- or B-scan ultrasound evaluation should be performed if significant media opacification prevents an adequate view of the fundus. Ultrasound findings include dispersed vitre-ous opacities from vitritis. In advanced cases, choroidal thickening and detachment may be detected (Fig. 49-2). The ultrasound examination should also rule out associated retinal detachment, dislocated lens material, or retained intraocular foreign bodies. If a metallic foreign body is suspected, a computed tomography scan with thin (1–2-mm) radiologic sections may be indicated. If a magnetic foreign body is suspected, magnetic resonance imaging is contraindicated because of the risk of uncontrolled movement of the foreign body within the eye.

For acute endophthalmitis, treatment must be initiated without delay to prevent severe and irreversible visual loss. In one study, delay of treatment for more than 24 hours was associated with a substantially higher risk of blindness compared to eyes treated sooner (1). When a clinical diagnosis of endophthalmitis is made, empiric therapy should be initiated as soon as possible. Since cultures require 1 or 2 days to show results, they cannot be relied on to determine the initial course of treatment.

Obtaining Intraocular Specimens for Microbiologic Study

Specimens for microbiologic study should be acquired immediately by anterior-chamber tap, by vitreous tap or vitreous biopsy, and by filtration of vitrectomy cassette washings. These should be obtained under sterile conditions prior to administration of intravitreal or subconjunctival antibiotics. If an emergent vitrectomy is planned (see below), the intraocular specimens can be obtained during the operative procedure. Otherwise, a more limited procedure is required. Preoperatively, two or three doses of topical cycloplegic agents (e.g., cyclopentolate 1%/phenylephrine 2.5%) are administered in the affected eye. Retrobulbar anesthesia may be necessary but must be administered cautiously in the

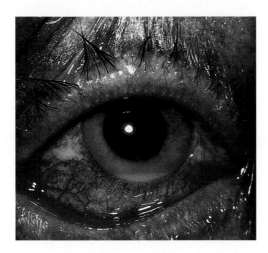

FIGURE 49-1.   *Hypopyon in an eye with postoperative endophthalmitis.*

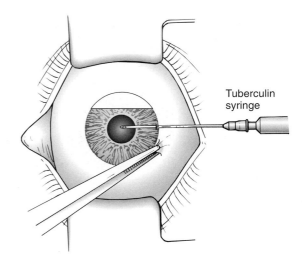

FIGURE 49-3.   *Anterior-chamber tap. The episclera is first grasped near the limbal insertion site with 0.12-mm toothed forceps, followed by insertion of a 27- to 30-gauge needle attached to a 1-mL (tuberculin) syringe into the anterior chamber. Aspiration of 0.1 to 0.2 mL of aqueous fluid into the syringe is performed manually. The limbal entry wound is usually self-sealing.*

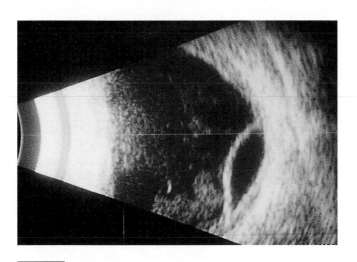

FIGURE 49-2.   *Ultrasound scan of the globe in an eye with postoperative endophthalmitis demonstrates vitreous opacities and choroidal detachment.*

presence of a recent ocular surgical wound. Currently, experience with peribulbar anesthesia in this setting is limited. Hyaluronidase (75–150 units) added to the anesthetic agent may facilitate adequate anesthesia in the inflamed eye. The eye is surgically prepared with povidone-iodine (Betadine 5%) solution and rinsed thoroughly with sterile balanced salt solution or normal saline solution to remove residual antiseptic from the ocular surface. A surgical drape, lid speculum, and operating microscope may be used.

Anterior-Chamber Tap

Although aqueous humor specimens have a lower microbiologic yield than do vitreous humor specimens (2,3), they may contribute to the overall rate of culture positivity. In the Endophthalmitis Vitrectomy Study (EVS), the aqueous

was the only source of a positive culture in 4% of eyes, and, considered alone, showed confirmed growth in 22% of eyes (4).

To obtain an aqueous specimen, a tuberculin syringe (1.0 mL) is attached to a ½-inch, 27- to 30-gauge needle. Larger needles may not create a self-sealing wound. The globe should be fixed with toothed forceps (0.12-mm Castroviejo forceps) near the limbus on the same side of the globe as the entry site, to facilitate atraumatic entry (Fig. 49-3). A temporal approach avoids the bridge of the nose and allows positioning of the needle parallel to the iris plane. Usually 0.1 mL of aqueous humor can be aspirated into the syringe without causing anterior-chamber collapse. If anterior-chamber collapse occurs, balanced salt solution can be injected to re-form the chamber.

Vitreous Tap and Vitreous Biopsy

A vitreous specimen can be obtained either by vitreous needle tap or by vitreous biopsy with a cutting/aspirating probe. To perform a vitreous biopsy, a 1-mL tuberculin syringe is directly attached to the suction tubing near the handpiece (5) (Fig. 49-4). To minimize dead space, the length between the handpiece and syringe is kept short (1–2 cm). A T-shaped conjunctival incision is made, and the vitrectomy cutter is inserted into the vitreous cavity through a sclerotomy incision placed 3.0 to 3.5 mm posterior to the limbus. Approximately 0.2 to 0.3 mL of vitreous can be removed from the anterior vitreous cavity using the automated cutting mechanism of the probe and slow, manual aspiration (Fig. 49-5A). Once the cutter is removed from the eye, the fluid is aspirated through the dead

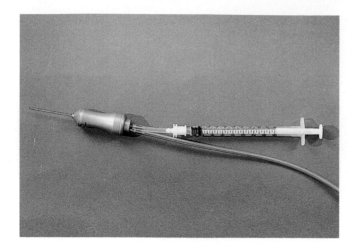

FIGURE 49-4. *Modification of the vitrectomy cutter assembly to allow vitreous biopsy. A 1-mL tuberculin syringe is attached to the aspiration tubing of the vitrectomy cutter via a female Luer lock microadapter. To minimize dead space, the tubing is kept short (1–2 cm).*

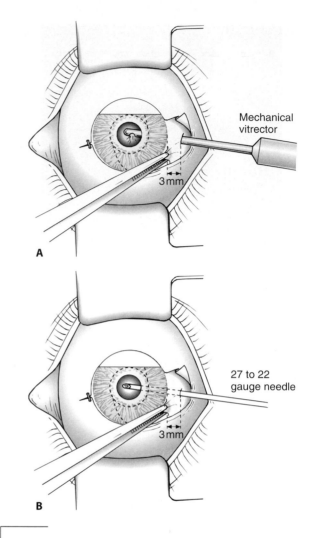

FIGURE 49-5. *A. Vitreous biopsy. A T-shaped conjunctival incision is made, and the vitrectomy cutter (modified as in Fig. 49-4) is inserted into the vitreous cavity through a sclerotomy incision placed 3 mm posterior to the limbus. Approximately 0.2 to 0.3 mL of vitreous is removed from the anterior vitreous cavity using the automated cutting mechanism of the probe and slow, manual aspiration of vitreous fluid. B. Vitreous needle tap. A T-shaped conjunctival incision is made and a 27- to 22-gauge needle attached to a 1-mL tuberculin syringe is inserted into the vitreous cavity through the sclera 3 mm posterior to the limbus. Approximately 0.2 to 0.3 mL is gently aspirated. If resistance is met and no fluid vitreous can be obtained, a vitreous biopsy must be performed instead to avoid aspirating formed vitreous.*

space into the syringe, or expelled onto culture media immediately.

Alternatively, a vitreous needle tap can be performed to obtain the specimen. A 22- to 27-gauge needle attached to a tuberculin syringe is inserted into the vitreous cavity through the pars plana and a similar volume of fluid vitreous is slowly aspirated (Fig. 49-5B). If resistance is met and no fluid vitreous can be obtained, a vitreous biopsy must be performed instead to avoid vitreous traction and secondary retinal tears.

Small (23-gauge) vitrectomy cutters have been designed and can be inserted transconjunctivally through correspondingly small pars plana incisions to obtain vitreous specimens (Fig. 49-6). In such cases, suture closure of both the smaller sclerotomy and the conjunctival incisions may not be necessary, as the smaller wound may be self-sealing.

After injection of intravitreal medications (see below), the pars plana entry sites and conjunctiva are closed with 7-0 or 8-0 absorbable suture. If the eye is hypotonous after these procedures, sterile balanced salt solution should be injected to normalize the intraocular pressure. Subconjunctival and topical antimicrobials and corticosteroids are also administered. Intravitreal and systemic corticosteroids can also be used (see section on Adjunctive Therapy later in this chapter).

Antimicrobial Therapy

Intravitreal administration of antimicrobial drugs has been accepted as the single most effective method of drug delivery for the treatment of acute bacterial endophthalmitis (3,6). Intravitreal drugs can be administered by injection of a specified dose directly into the vitreous cavity at the conclusion of vitrectomy or vitreous tap/biopsy, or by instillation in vitrectomy infusion fluid at a specified concentration in eyes undergoing vitrectomy (7). The former method has gained wider acceptance, and has the advantage of a potentially longer duration of antimicrobial activity in the vitreous cavity (8).

Because the vitreous cavity is an immune-privileged site, antimicrobial drugs chosen for intravitreal treatment should possess bactericidal or fungicidal capabilities (8). For

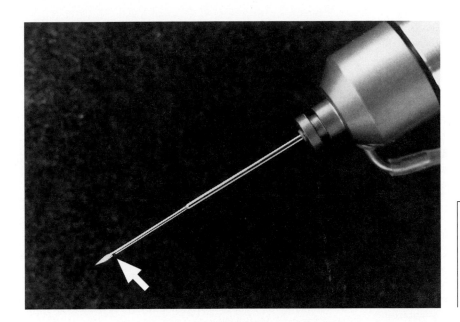

FIGURE 49-6. *Small (23-gauge) vitrectomy cutter. The sharpened tip of the cutter allows transconjunctival insertion of an instrument into the vitreous cavity and acquisition of vitreous biopsy material in a single step. A self-sealing wound may result. (Visitrec Vitreous Biopsy Probe, VISITEC, Sarasota, FL.)*

empiric therapy, broad-spectrum coverage effective against the potential infecting agents is desirable. Other desirable characteristics include low toxicity and adequate half-life to sustain levels capable of killing the infecting organisms. A list of useful antimicrobial agents and their respective dosages and methods of ocular delivery are listed in Table 49-1.

Topical, subconjunctival, and intravenous routes of antibiotic administration result in low intraocular levels of antibiotics relative to intravitreal delivery and have been largely ineffective in treating acute endophthalmitis. Topical and subconjunctival antibiotics are considered useful for the treatment of coexisting corneal or wound infections or for prophylaxis against infection when administered perioperatively. In the EVS, intravenous antibiotics were of no benefit in the treatment of acute postoperative bacterial endophthalmitis after cataract surgery (9). The role of systemic antibiotics for other forms of acute, exogenous endophthalmitis is not clear. Systemic antibiotics may play a role in *endogenous* endophthalmitis, particularly since distant, potentially life-threatening foci of infection may be present. (See section on Endogenous Endophthalmitis later in this chapter.)

Pars Plana Vitrectomy

Pars plana vitrectomy has been commonly used in the management of endophthalmitis, particularly in severe cases (10–13). Theoretical and practical advantages of vitrectomy include removal of bacteria and inflammatory debris from the eye, facilitation of antibiotic distribution throughout the vitreous cavity, and ability to obtain a large specimen for microbiologic studies. Animal studies suggest that vitrectomy, in concert with intraocular antibiotics, may be beneficial in reducing inflammation and culture positivity in the vitreous cavity (14,15).

Table 49-1. Topical, Subconjunctival, and Intraocular Dosages of Selected Antibiotics Used in the Treatment of Endophthalmitis

	Topical	Subconjunctival	Intravitreal
Amikacin	20 mg/mL	40 mg	400 µg
Amphotericin B	0.15%–0.50%	—	5–10 µg
Ampicillin	5 mg/mL	100 mg	5 mg
Cefamandole	50 mg/mL	75 mg	2 mg
Cefazolin	50 mg/mL	100 mg	2.25 mg
Ceftazidime	50 mg/mL	100 mg	2.25 mg
Clindamycin	—	30 mg	250 µg
Gentamicin	10–20 mg/mL	20 mg	200 µg
Methicillin	1% solution	100 mg	2 mg
Miconazole	10 mg/mL	5 mg	25 µg
Tobramycin	8–15 mg/mL	20 mg	200 µg
Vancomycin	50 mg/mL	25 mg	1 mg

Sources: Peyman GA, Schulman JA, eds. *Intravitreal surgery: principles and practice.* Norwalk: Appleton-Century-Crofts, 1986:407–455; Lee VHL, Pince KJ, Frambach DA, Martenhed B. Drug delivery to the posterior segment. In: Ryan SJ, ed. *Retina.* Vol. 1. 2nd ed. St. Louis: Mosby–Year Book, 1994:533–551; Parke DW II, Brinton GS. Endophthalmitis. In: Tabbara KF, Hyndiuk RA, eds. *Infections of the eye.* Boston: Little, Brown, 1986:563–585.

The EVS evaluated immediate pars plana vitrectomy for the treatment of acute bacterial endophthalmitis after cataract extraction or secondary intraocular lens (IOL) implantation (9). Immediate pars plana vitrectomy was beneficial for patients who presented with severe visual loss to the level of light perception only. However, there was no advantage to immediate vitrectomy over vitreous tap/biopsy in patients who could perceive hand motions or had better visual acuity. [In this study, patients who could perceive light but were unable to perceive hand motions at 2 feet (61 cm) were considered to have light perception only.] In the EVS, patients who had undergone initial vitreous tap/biopsy and appeared clinically worse for 36 to 60 hours after vitreous tap/biopsy (as indicated by increased hypopyon, persistent pain, worsening vitreous opacification, and visual acuity of less than 5/200) underwent delayed vitrectomy and reinjection of intravitreal antibiotics.

The EVS results regarding the role of vitrectomy for the treatment of acute postoperative endophthalmitis may not apply to other forms of endophthalmitis. Bleb-related, traumatic, or endogenous endophthalmitis may be associated with more virulent, toxin-producing organisms such as *Streptococcus* and *Bacillus* species (16–18), in which removal of toxins by vitrectomy may be important (17). In traumatic endophthalmitis, vitrectomy may be required for the management of retained intraocular foreign bodies, retinal tears or detachment, vitreous-lens admixture, vitreous incarceration into the wound, and vitreous hemorrhage.

Vitrectomy may not be possible if there are large choroidal detachments, or severe infiltration of anterior-segment structures with purulent material (Fig. 49-7). In such cases, management must consist of intravitreal injection of antibiotics without vitrectomy. The presence of large choroidal detachments may require that intraocular antibiotics be injected through the limbus rather than the pars plana to avoid retinal damage. The role of surgical drainage of choroidal detachments to facilitate vitrectomy or other intraocular procedures is not clear.

Objectives to be accomplished during vitreous surgery include (1) repair of wound leaks, if present; (2) removal of vitreous and inflammatory debris; (3) adequate clearing of the visual axis; (4) relief of vitreous incarceration into surgical or traumatic wounds; (5) management of coexisting problems (e.g., retinal detachment, retained lens material or foreign bodies); and (6) intravitreal antibiotic administration.

Technique of Pars Plana Vitrectomy

To maximize preoperative mydriasis, two or three doses of topical cycloplegic-mydriatic agents are administered in the affected eye. Retrobulbar or general anesthesia may be used. In some cases, general anesthesia may be required because of ineffectiveness of retrobulbar or peribulbar anesthesia.

The technique of pars plana vitrectomy can be carried out as either a two-port or a three-port procedure. The two-port vitrectomy is quicker and requires fewer conjunctival and scleral incisions than a three-port vitrectomy, and is ideal for limited vitrectomy procedures. However, if scleral buckling or multiple instrument exchanges are anticipated, a three-port system is recommended.

In the three-port procedure, an infusion cannula is inserted through a pars plana sclerotomy 3.0 to 3.5 mm posterior to the limbus and is sutured into place. Visualization of the cannula tip within the vitreous cavity is important to avoid inadvertent suprachoroidal infusion. A relatively long (4-mm) cannula will allow penetration through an edematous ciliary body, permitting immediate normalization of intraocular pressure after intraocular specimens are acquired. The cannula should be placed prior to obtaining the undiluted vitreous specimen, which is obtained as described for vitreous biopsy (see earlier text and Fig. 49-5). If possible, the infusion is not turned on until the specimens are obtained.

If the tip of the presutured infusion cannula cannot be visualized initially because of media opacification, the infusion should not be turned on. In this situation a secondary infusion line consisting of an angled 20-gauge cannula or bent needle can be inserted through the pars plana and its tip directed into the central vitreous cavity where it can be seen more easily. In aphakic or pseudophakic eyes, it can be directed into the pupillary space or immediately posterior to the IOL and posterior lens capsule (Fig. 49-8). This secondary infusion line may be used until the presutured infusion cannula can be visualized. A vitrectomy probe inserted through a third pars plana sclerotomy is then used to remove the media opacities interfering with visualization. Once the cannula is visualized, an endoilluminator is substituted for

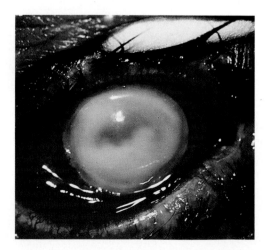

FIGURE 49-7. *Severe infiltration and opacification of the anterior segment in a patient with* Pseudomonas *endophthalmitis, making vitrectomy difficult.*

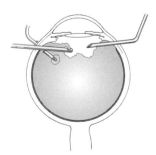

FIGURE 49-8. *Secondary infusion needle. If the sutured infusion cannula is obscured, an angled 20-gauge cannula or bent needle is inserted through the pars plana and its tip is directed into the central vitreous cavity where it can be seen more easily.*

the secondary infusion line and the vitrectomy procedure is completed. Posterior viewing may be obtained with indirect, noncontact biomicroscopy, or with a handheld or self-retaining contact lens (Fig. 49-9).

The goal of vitrectomy is to remove a large portion of the vitreous with the vitrectomy cutter. A posterior hypopyon, if present, can also be removed with a silicone-tip aspiration cannula to facilitate more rapid clearing of the vitreous cavity (Fig. 49-10). Attempts at removing an attached posterior hyaloid are unnecessary and dangerous because of the risks of a retinal break occurring.

Following the vitrectomy, careful indirect ophthalmoscopy is performed to rule out iatrogenic retinal tears or detachment.

In the two-port procedure, a handheld infusion-endoilluminator ("irrigating light pipe") is inserted through one of the superior sclerotomies and is used in place of a presutured infusion cannula throughout the procedure (Fig. 49-11). Instrument exchanges with the infusion-endoilluminator are minimized to avoid potentially traumatic reinsertion of instruments into a hypotonous eye. High suction should be avoided because of the lower infusion rate obtained through the infusion-endoilluminator relative to a conventional cannula. The infusion bottles can be raised slightly to speed the infusion rate, but caution should be used to avoid excessive elevation of intraocular pressure. If needed, fluid-air exchange is also possible by injecting air instead of irrigation fluid through the infusion-endoilluminator (Fig. 49-12). Once the infusion-endoilluminator is withdrawn and the sclerotomy sites are closed, air or gas must often be injected to restore intraocular pressure.

After pars plana vitrectomy, the sclerotomy sites are closed with 7-0 or 8-0 absorbable sutures. Intravitreal antibiotics are injected after sclerotomy closure. Prior to antibiotic injection, the intraocular volume is reduced slightly to avoid marked pressure elevation that may occur during injection. Following conjunctival closure with 7-0 or 8-0 absorbable sutures, subconjunctival antibiotics can be injected.

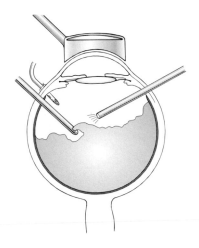

FIGURE 49-9. *Three-port vitrectomy with endoillumination. Once the tip of the sutured cannula is confirmed to be within the vitreous cavity, an endoilluminator is then substituted for the secondary infusion line and the vitrectomy procedure is completed.*

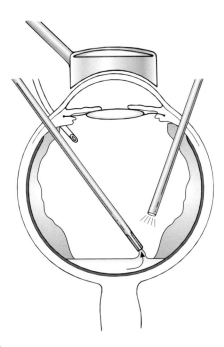

FIGURE 49-10. *Removal of posterior hypopyon during three-port vitrectomy, with a silicone-tip aspiration cannula.*

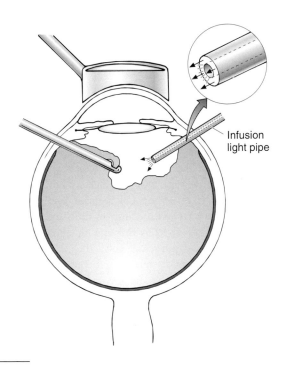

Infusion light pipe

FIGURE 49-11. *Two-port vitrectomy procedure. A handheld infusion-endoilluminator ("irrigating light piper") is inserted through one of the superior sclerotomies and is used in place of a presutured infusion cannula throughout the procedure.*

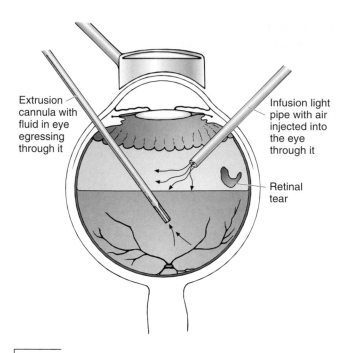

Extrusion cannula with fluid in eye egressing through it

Infusion light pipe with air injected into the eye through it

Retinal tear

FIGURE 49-12.   *Fluid-air exchange with an irrigating endoilluminator in an eye with a retinal tear. A silicone-tip extrusion cannula removes vitreous cavity fluid while air is injected through the irrigating endoilluminator, which is held anteriorly in the vitreous cavity.*

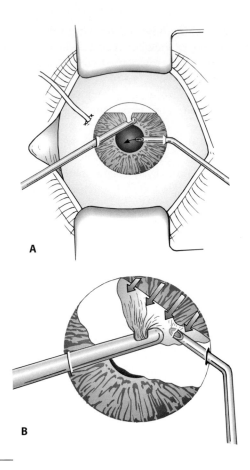

A

B

FIGURE 49-13.   A. *Removal of anterior-chamber opacities with a bimanual, limbal technique. A 20- to 23-gauge bent needle attached to infusion fluid and a 20-gauge vitrectomy cutter are inserted through the limbus into the anterior chamber at approximately the 2:30 and 9:30 meridians. If present, any layered, purulent material is removed, followed by mobilization of adherent membranes. B. Removal of adherent membranes in the anterior chamber. Membranes can be engaged initially with the needle or vitrectomy cutter, stripped from the surface of the iris, and subsequently excised with the cutter.*

Removal of Inflammatory Membranes

Inflammatory membranes are commonly adherent to the iris and IOL and may obscure the posterior segment. Removal of these membranes may be required to allow adequate visualization during pars plana vitrectomy. In the anterior chamber, these can be removed with a multifunction irrigation–cutting–aspiration probe inserted through the limbus. Alternatively, a bimanual technique, separating irrigation and cutting–aspiration into two entry sites, provides for greater flexibility in manipulating and excising these membranes through two smaller incision sites (Fig. 49-13). To perform the bimanual technique, a 20- to 23-gauge bent needle attached to infusion fluid and a 20-gauge vitrectomy cutter are inserted through the limbus into the anterior chamber at approximately the 2:30 and 9:30 meridians. After hypopyon removal, the membrane can be initially engaged with the needle or vitrectomy cutter and stripped from the surface of the iris (Fig. 49-13B). Subsequently, it can be excised with the cutter. Membranes at the posterior aspect of the iris and IOL can be removed in a similar fashion via the pars plana.

In pseudophakic or aphakic eyes, anterior-chamber membrane removal can be accomplished by inserting the vitrectomy cutter through the pars plana and creating a relatively large peripheral iridectomy with the cutter, through which it can gain access to the anterior chamber

(Fig. 49-14A). Additional access can be obtained by inserting the cutter through the pupil via the space between the IOL and the iris (Fig. 49-14B) (19). It is necessary for some type of intraocular infusion to be established prior to this maneuver, either with a secondary infusion needle (see Fig. 49-8) or by prior visualization of the sutured infusion cannula. If a posterior-chamber IOL is present, care is taken not to engage or damage the IOL haptics behind the iris. Gentle pressure against the posterior aspect of the iris may help to outline the haptics. Iris bleeding, IOL dislocation, and optical disturbances through a patent iridectomy are potential complications of this approach. Anterior-chamber collapse, Descemet's folds inhibiting subsequent posterior-segment viewing, and corneal endothelial damage are potential complications for any of the maneuvers attempting removal of anterior-chamber membranes.

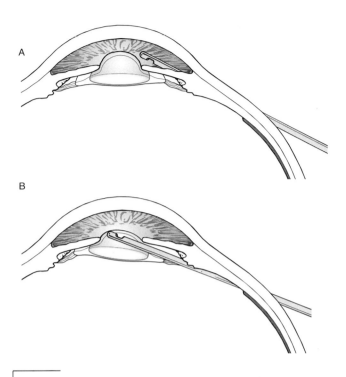

FIGURE 49-14.   A. *Pars plana approach to anterior-segment opacities. After safe infusion into the globe is established, a generous superior iridectomy is performed with the vitrectomy cutter, providing access to anterior-chamber opacities by the cutter.* B. *Additional access can be obtained by inserting the vitrectomy cutter through the pupil via the space between the intraocular lens and the iris.*

Pupillary Miosis

Pupillary miosis that interferes with visualization for vitrectomy is common because of severe inflammation, recent surgery, and the need for surgical manipulations to remove anterior-segment opacities. Iris retractors (20) may be helpful to achieve surgical mydriasis and to accomplish the goals of vitrectomy.

COMPLICATIONS

Retinal Breaks and Detachment

Retinal breaks and detachment can develop after endophthalmitis or following pars plana vitrectomy, vitreous tap, or vitreous biopsy. Reported retinal detachment rates vary widely, ranging from 3% to 21% after vitrectomy (9,13,21), and from 8% to 11% after vitreous biopsy or tap (EVS, unpublished data). Eyes with retinal detachment early in the course of endophthalmitis are at significant risk for proliferative vitreoretinopathy, owing to the development of inflammatory membranes in the vitreous cavity and on the retinal surface.

When a retinal detachment is recognized, surgical reattachment should be attempted. Standard vitreoretinal surgical techniques are used to repair retinal breaks or detachment, including scleral buckling, fluid-gas exchange, and retinal photocoagulation.

In eyes with both endophthalmitis and retinal detachment that require fluid-gas exchange, administration of intravitreal antibiotics may be problematic (22). Injection of antibiotic into a completely air-filled eye may reduce its distribution in the vitreous cavity and risk retinal toxicity due to concentration into a small fluid volume. A partial fluid-air exchange with reduction of the intraocular dosage proportional to the reduced fluid volume has been noted to be effective without clinical evidence of toxicity (23). In this manner, after an initial complete fluid-gas exchange to facilitate intraoperative retinal reattachment and endophotocoagulation, reinfusion of fluid is performed to fill half of the vitreous cavity, followed by intravitreal antibiotic injection using half the standard dose. Another method is the addition of antibiotics to the vitrectomy infusion fluid after intraocular culture specimens have been obtained but before the fluid-gas exchange (7,22). In this instance, the duration of antimicrobial activity in the vitreous cavity is likely to be short, given the very small amount of drug retained in the eye at the conclusion of surgery. In the event that immediate vitrectomy is not feasible, a recommended method is to initially treat with intravitreal antibiotics to cure the endophthalmitis, followed by standard retinal detachment repair at a later date. The visual prognosis in such cases is usually poor, however (22).

Hemorrhage

Intraoperative anterior-segment hemorrhage is noted commonly, often induced by transient hypotony in the presence of marked iris vascular congestion, especially occurring during the anterior-chamber or vitreous cavity tap. Elevation of infusion bottles or injection of balanced salt solution after ocular specimen acquisition to raise the intraocular pressure may be needed for hemostasis. If ineffective, intraocular diathermy can be directly applied to the bleeding sites.

Suprachoroidal hemorrhage is an uncommon, but feared complication with a potentially disastrous outcome. It can occur intraoperatively or postoperatively, often within 48 hours of the procedure. If observed intraoperatively, immediate sealing of all ocular wounds is critical and elevation of the infusion bottles to raise the intraocular pressure may help to obtain hemostasis. Drainage of suprachoroidal hemorrhage through external sclerotomies can be attempted. Because of the rapid clotting of blood in the suprachoroidal space, a delayed procedure with external drainage and adjunctive vitreoretinal procedures may be needed several days later, after clot lysis has occurred.

Macular Toxicity

Macular infarction and irreversible visual loss can result from intravitreal antibiotic therapy, most notably from the aminoglycosides (24,25). Its risk may increase with repetitive injection (26). Clinically, macular toxicity initially appears as a white-gray area in the posterior pole and eventually develops into an atrophic macula and optic disk. Compared to aminoglycosides, broad-spectrum, third-generation cephalosporins, such as ceftazidime, may be associated with a lower risk for this complication (27). Macular toxicity may result from inadvertent intravitreal injection of medications intended for subconjunctival use. This error can be prevented by waiting until intravitreal injections have been administered before introducing subconjunctival antibiotics into the operating environment. A standard protocol for mixing intravitreal antibiotics that is accessible both to the pharmacy and to the treating physician is highly recommended to reduce the risk of mixing errors.

Persistent Media Opacity

Persisting inflammatory vitreous debris, cataract, and posterior capsular opacification can interfere with subsequent visual recovery and require surgical intervention, such as pars plana vitrectomy, cataract extraction, and posterior capsulotomy.

Fibrin Formation

Massive fibrin formation can lead to the development of organized membranes in the vitreous and anterior segment, causing retinal detachment and pupillary block. In most instances, spontaneous dissolution of the fibrin membranes occurs. If severe, intraocular injection of recombinant tissue plasminogen activator (tPA) can rapidly dissolve these membranes (28) and may be useful to reverse complications from fibrin (Fig. 49-15). The effect of tPA on visual outcome is not known. An accepted dosage for intraocular injection is 6 to 12 μg/0.1 mL.

Macular Pucker

In a small percentage of eyes, contracting epiretinal membranes in the macula may produce macular pucker. Vitrectomy and membrane peeling may be beneficial in some cases.

Sympathetic Ophthalmia

Sympathetic ophthalmia can occur after pars plana vitrectomy for endogenous bacterial endophthalmitis (29).

ADJUNCTIVE THERAPY

Suppression of inflammation is important to minimize damage to the retina and optic nerve and to reduce other intraocular inflammatory sequelae. Once empiric antimicrobial therapy has been administered, intensive topical corticosteroid therapy should be initiated immediately. However, the role of systemic and intravitreal corticosteroid use for acute bacterial endophthalmitis is controversial. An accepted intraocular dosage of dexamethasone is 400 μg (0.1 mL of dexamethasone [Decadron] 4 mg/mL solution). An accepted regimen of systemic corticosteroid therapy is prednisone 1 mg/kg/day by mouth for approximately 5 to 7 days, followed by a tapering course over a few days, after which it is discontinued. Antacids or histamine blockers should be administered at the physician's discretion to reduce the risk of peptic ulcer disease. The corticosteroid medication should be discontinued if any systemic complications develop. Potential contraindications to systemic corticosteroid therapy include, but are not limited to, preexisting diabetes mellitus, peptic ulcer disease, congestive heart failure, immunosuppressed states, and infection elsewhere in the body.

The role of postoperative intensive topical and subconjunctival antimicrobial use for endophthalmitis is not clear,

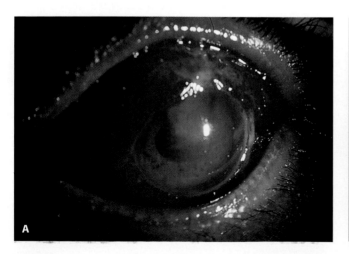
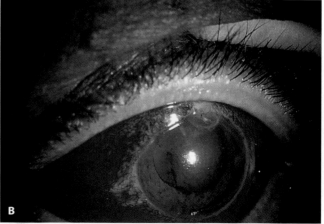

FIGURE 49-15. A. *An eye with bleb-related endophthalmitis and pupillary fibrin membrane obscuring the crystalline lens prior to intracameral injection of recombinant tissue plasminogen activator (tPA). B. Four hours after intracameral tPA injection. Fibrin membrane is dissolved and the intact crystalline lens is no longer obscured.*

given the poor intraocular penetration associated with these routes of administration. Topical treatment is generally recommended for 5 to 7 days, longer if clinical circumstances such as a wound infection or corneal infiltrate warrant. In such instances, material for cultures should be obtained from the wound or infiltrate prior to instituting topical antibiotic therapy. Initial therapy should cover both gram-positive and gram-negative organisms, but may be modified according to culture results. For most cases of endophthalmitis, adjunctive topical cycloplegia should be continued until inflammation has subsided.

POSTOPERATIVE CARE

A daily postoperative examination is appropriate until it is determined that the clinical course suggests stabilization or improvement, after which intervals between evaluations can be gradually increased. A significant reduction of pain, typically occurring within 24 hours after the initiation of therapy, may be an early sign of response to therapy. Signs of inflammation subside more gradually, often taking a period of 2 or 3 days to become appreciable. Worsening may be manifested as persistence or an increase in pain, a significant increase in hypopyon, or a loss of the red reflex. Anterior-chamber cell and flare and vitritis may appear somewhat worse on the first postoperative day, possibly relating to surgical intervention and a delay between the initiation of therapy and the reversal of inflammation. A more accurate assessment of treatment response may be possible on the second or third postoperative day. However, a rapidly worsening course may occur much sooner and justify repeated intervention.

In the event of a worsening course, reinjection of intravitreal antibiotics should be considered. Microbiology results may assist in the choice of antimicrobial therapy. A vitrectomy, if not already performed, should be strongly considered. The rationale for repeated vitrectomy in a previously vitrectomized eye is unclear, unless specific circumstances such as retinal detachment indicate otherwise.

MICROBIOLOGIC EVALUATION

Intraocular specimens should be submitted for aerobic, anaerobic, and fungal cultures, and inoculated on culture media with the greatest chance of successful yield. If unusual organisms are suspected, consultation with the microbiologist is important to choose the best technique available in the laboratory. Anaerobic cultures should be kept for at least 14 days to recover slow-growing species (e.g., *Propionibacterium acnes*). Fungal cultures should be kept for several weeks.

Culture results may determine subsequent intravitreal antimicrobial therapy in patients responding poorly to initial treatment. However, clinical parameters, not in vitro tests, should be used to decide further therapy, as the levels of antibiotics achieved with intravitreal injection may far exceed the laboratory thresholds used to judge resistance.

SPECIAL CONSIDERATIONS

Acute Postoperative Endophthalmitis

Acute postoperative endophthalmitis may occur after any type of intraocular surgery, or as a complication of inadvertent globe penetration during extraocular procedures. The incidence of endophthalmitis after cataract extraction is approximately 0.1% (30).

In acute postoperative endophthalmitis, gram-positive organisms predominate, including *Staphylococcus epidermidis*, other coagulase-negative staphylococci, *Staphylococcus aureus*, and streptococci. In endophthalmitis developing after cataract extraction, approximately 50% of eyes are infected with coagulase-negative micrococci, which may be associated with a good prognosis if treated appropriately. However, approximately 5% to 10% of eyes may harbor gram-negative organisms (31). Current antibiotic choices for empiric intravitreal therapy in acute postoperative endophthalmitis include combination therapy with vancomycin (1.0 mg) for gram-positive coverage and amikacin (400 μg) or ceftazidime (2.2 mg) for gram-negative coverage.

Chronic Postoperative Endophthalmitis

Chronic postoperative endophthalmitis is a low-grade inflammation that occurs following intraocular surgery due to infection with a variety of indolent microorganisms. Its exact incidence is unknown. It may result from infection with *P. acnes*, *Corynebacterium* species, gram-positive, coagulase-negative staphylococci, or fungi.

The presence of a white, indistinct plaque on the lens capsule in an eye with chronic inflammation after cataract extraction suggests possible infection with *P. acnes* (Fig. 49-16). Definitive management may require pars plana vitrectomy and capsulectomy to excise involved portions of the posterior capsule, accompanied by intraocular antibiotic injection (32). A currently accepted antibiotic for this purpose is vancomycin (1.0 mg). If there is no response to initial treatment, more aggressive intervention with repeat vitrectomy, complete capsulectomy, IOL removal, and reinjection of antibiotics may be required. In some instances, low-grade inflammation may be recalcitrant and require many weeks of topical anti-inflammatory therapy.

Filtering Bleb-Associated Endophthalmitis

Filtering bleb-associated endophthalmitis typically occurs months to years after glaucoma filtration surgery or development of an inadvertent filtration bleb. The incidence of late-onset, posttrabeculectomy endophthalmitis is estimated at 0.2% to 1.8% (16). Conjunctivitis and contact lens wear in the presence of a filtration bleb may be risk factors for endophthalmitis.

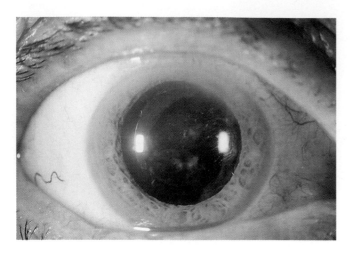

FIGURE 49-16. *A white, indistinct plaque on the lens capsule in an eye with chronic inflammation after cataract extraction indicative of chronic endophthalmitis due to* Propionibacterium acnes.

Eyes with bleb-associated endophthalmitis are typically infected with more virulent organisms than those associated with endophthalmitis following cataract extraction. Streptococci are especially common, and *Hemophilus influenzae* also was found with unusual frequency in one study (17). Current antibiotic choices for intravitreal injection are identical to those for acute postoperative endophthalmitis (see above).

Endogenous Endophthalmitis

Endogenous bacterial endophthalmitis can result from seeding of bacteria from any remote focus of bacterial infection, such as meningitis, endocarditis, urinary tract infection, gastrointestinal/abdominal infection, and pneumonia. It can also be associated with bacteremia without an identifiable focus of infection.

Common infecting agents include streptococci, *S. aureus*, *Bacillus cereus*, and fungi. There is a marked predominance of streptococci as a cause of endogenous bacterial endophthalmitis (33). Gram-negative organisms may be causative in patients with urinary tract or gastrointestinal infection, or in patients with meningitis due to *Neisseria meningitidis* or *H. influenzae*. Fungal endophthalmitis, especially from infection with *Candida albicans*, should be considered in premature infants, intravenous drug abusers, and patients with indwelling catheters or recent abdominal surgery. In most patients, the infecting organism must initially be presumed to be that causing the systemic infection. Culture results from systemic sources may determine the initial empiric antibiotic agents to use for ocular therapy.

Treatment of endogenous bacterial intraocular infection depends on the stage of involvement. Whereas focal chorioretinitis may respond to systemic antimicrobial therapy, pre-

sumably because of an existing blood supply to the infected site and localized blood-ocular barrier breakdown, progressive or significant vitreous opacification suggests infection of the vitreous cavity and the need for intravitreal antimicrobial therapy. For moderate to severe endophthalmitis, vitrectomy should be strongly considered, to assist in the elimination of potentially virulent organisms, such as streptococci and *B. cereus*, and their associated toxins.

For endogenous endophthalmitis due to fungi, vitrectomy may also be indicated (34,35). Until recently, intraocular penetration of most systemically administered antifungal agents has been poor, requiring intravitreal injection with agents such as amphotericin B (36). However, a newer, orally administered antifungal agent, fluconazole, has good vitreous cavity penetration and has been effective alone or in combination with vitrectomy in the management of endogenous fungal endophthalmitis (37). The accepted dosage of fluconazole is 100 to 200 mg/day orally for 2 or more months. In contrast to *endogenous* fungal endophthalmitis, systemic therapy with fluconazole has been ineffective in patients with *exogenous* fungal endophthalmitis who did not receive concurrent vitrectomy or intravitreal antifungal agents (37).

Traumatic Endophthalmitis

The incidence of endophthalmitis after penetrating trauma is about 5%. In eyes with retained intraocular foreign bodies it is about 10% (18,38). Gram-positive organisms are the most common infecting agents in traumatic endophthalmitis. *S. epidermidis*, *S. aureus*, and *Streptococcus* species account for about 45% of cases, while gram-negative organisms are found in 11% of affected eyes. *Bacillus* species are particularly common, infecting approximately 22% of eyes (18). Less commonly, infection with fungi or anaerobes may occur.

Intravitreal antibiotic should cover gram-positive organisms, including *B. cereus*. Intravitreal vancomycin (1 mg) is currently effective against both groups of organisms and is a rational choice for empiric intravitreal therapy. Intravitreal ceftazidime (2.2 mg) or amikacin (400 μg) should be considered for gram-negative coverage, particularly in cases involving contamination with organic matter (39). For fungal endophthalmitis, amphotericin B (5–10 μg) or other antifungal agents should be administered intravitreally.

For moderate to severe endophthalmitis following trauma, pars plana vitrectomy should be considered for reasons outlined previously (see earlier section on Pars Plana Vitrectomy). Vitrectomy may also be indicated for the management of retained intraocular foreign bodies, retinal detachment, vitreous-lens admixture, and other posterior-segment complications of ocular trauma.

The role of systemic antimicrobial therapy in established traumatic bacterial or fungal endophthalmitis is unclear, but agents such as oral ciprofloxacin (40,41), oral fluconazole (37), and intravenous vancomycin (42) can penetrate the vitreous cavity and may possibly be of benefit. These agents should be used as an adjunct to intravitreal antimicrobial delivery and pars plana vitrectomy, and should not supplant these more definitive measures.

Parasitic Endophthalmitis

Progressive vitritis may result from ocular infection with *Toxoplasma gondii*, *Toxocara canis*, *Taenia solium* (pork tapeworm), and other parasites. Vitrectomy may be useful to (1) obtain specimens for diagnostic study, (2) remove significant vitreous opacity, and (3) allow excision of intravitreal or subretinal parasites, such as those seen in intraocular cysticercosis (43) or gnathostomiasis (44). Diagnostic studies can include tests to detect intraocular antibodies (e.g., enzyme-linked immunosorbent assay titers) (45,46), polymerase chain reaction (47), and cytologic or histopathologic evaluation of surgically removed tissues. Definitive treatment depends on the causative agent and may include removal or destruction of the parasite surgically or pharmacologically or with photocoagulation.

CONCLUSIONS

Prompt intravitreal antibiotic therapy rapidly achieves bactericidal drug levels in the vitreous cavity and is the mainstay of treatment of infectious endophthalmitis. The choice of appropriate empirical antimicrobial therapy depends on the spectrum of possible infecting organisms and the therapeutic margin of available antimicrobial agents.

Pars plana vitrectomy is of proven benefit in eyes with endophthalmitis following cataract extraction and secondary IOL implantation that present with light-perception-only vision. Although its role is unclear in endogenous, bleb-related, or trauma-related endophthalmitis, pars plana vitrectomy should be considered of potential benefit because of the virulent organisms that are frequently encountered and the poor outcomes often associated with these conditions. Importantly, visual outcome may be optimized by additional measures, including suppression of inflammation and timely management of postsurgical or postinflammatory complications.

REFERENCES

1. Puliafito CA, Baker AS, Haaf J, Foster CS. Infectious endophthalmitis. *Ophthalmology* 1982;89:921–929.
2. Koul S, Philipson A, Arvidson S. Role of aqueous and vitreous cultures in diagnosing infectious endophthalmitis in rabbits. *Acta Ophthalmol (Stockh)* 1990;68:466–469.
3. Forster RK, Abbott RL, Gelender H. Management of infectious endophthalmitis. *Ophthalmology* 1980;87:313–319.
4. Barza M, Pavan PR, Doft BH, et al. Evaluation of microbiological diagnostic techniques in postoperative endophthalmitis in the Endophthalmitis Vitrectomy Study. *Arch Ophthalmol* 1997;115:1142–1150.
5. Doft BH, Donnelly K. A single sclerotomy vitreous biopsy technique in endophthalmitis. *Arch Ophthalmol* 1991;109:465. Letter.
6. Baum J, Peyman GA, Barza M. Intravitreal administration of antibiotic in the treatment of bacterial endophthalmitis. III. Consensus. *Surv Ophthalmol* 1982;26:204–206.
7. Peyman GA, Schulman JA, eds. *Intravitreal surgery: principles and practice*. Norwalk: Appleton-Century-Crofts, 1986:407–455.
8. Meredith TA. Vitrectomy for infectious endophthalmitis. In: Ryan S, ed. *Retina*. Vol. 3. 2nd ed. St. Louis: Mosby–Year Book, 1994:2525–2537.
9. The Endophthalmitis Vitrectomy Study group. Results of the Endophthalmitis Vitrectomy Study. A randomized trial of immediate vitrectomy and of intravenous antibiotics for the treatment of postoperative bacterial endophthalmitis. *Arch Ophthalmol* 1995;113:1479–1496.
10. Diamond JG. Intraocular management of endophthalmitis. A systematic approach. *Arch Ophthalmol* 1981;99:96–99.
11. Rowsey JJ, Newsom DL, Sexton DJ, Harms WK. Endophthalmitis. Current approaches. *Ophthalmology* 1982;89:1055–1066.
12. Driebe WT Jr, Mandelbaum S, Forster RK, et al. Pseudophakic endophthalmitis. Diagnosis and management. *Ophthalmology* 1986;93:422–448.
13. Olson JC, Flynn HW Jr, Forster RK, Culberston WW. Results in the treatment of postoperative endophthalmitis. *Ophthalmology* 1983;90:692–697.
14. Cottingham AJ Jr, Forster RK. Vitrectomy in endophthalmitis: results of study using vitrectomy, intraocular antibiotics, or a combination of both. *Arch Ophthalmol* 1976;94:2078–2081.
15. Meredith TA, Aguilar HE, Trabelsi A, et al. Comparative treatment of experimental *Staphylococcus epidermidis* endophthalmitis. *Arch Ophthalmol* 1990;108:857–860.
16. Katz LJ, Cantor LB, Spaeth GL. Complications of surgery in glaucoma. *Ophthalmology* 1985;92:959–963.
17. Mandelbaum S, Forster RK, Gelender H, Culbertson W. Late onset endophthalmitis associated with filtering blebs. *Ophthalmology* 1985;92:964–972.
18. Parrish CM, O'Day DM. Traumatic endophthalmitis. *Int Ophthalmol Clin* 1987;27:112–119.
19. Doft BH, Lobes LA, Rinkoff JS. A technique to clear the anterior chamber media to allow pars plana vitrectomy in endophthalmitis. *Ophthalmology* 1991;98:412–413. Letter.
20. deJuan E Jr, Hickingbotham D. Flexible iris retractor. *Am J Ophthalmol* 1991;111:776–777.
21. Nelsen PT, Marcus DA, Bovino JA. Retinal detachment following endophthalmitis. *Ophthalmology* 1985;92:1112–1117.
22. Foster RE, Rubsamen PE, Joondeph BC, et al. Concurrent endophthalmitis and retinal detachment. *Ophthalmology* 1994;101:490–498.
23. Mieler WF, Glazer LC, Bennett SR, Han DP. Favourable outcome of traumatic endophthalmitis with associated retinal breaks or detachment. *Can J Ophthalmol* 1992;27:348–352.
24. Campochiaro PA, Conway BP. Aminoglycoside toxicity: a survey of retinal specialists. *Arch Ophthalmol* 1991;109:946–950.
25. D'Amico DJ, Libert J, Kenyon KR. Comparative toxicity of intravitreal aminoglycoside antibiotics. *Am J Ophthalmol* 1985;100:264–275.
26. Oum BS, D'Amico DJ, Kwak HW, Wong KW. Intravitreal antibiotic therapy with vancomycin and aminoglycoside: examination of the retinal toxicity of repetitive injections after vitreous and lens surgery. *Graefes Arch Clin Exp Ophthalmol* 1992;230:56–61.
27. Irvine WD, Flynn HW Jr, Miller D, Pflugfelder SC. Endophthalmitis caused by gram-negative organisms. *Arch Ophthalmol* 1992;110:1450–1454.
28. Jaffe GJ, Abrams GW, Williams GA, Han DP. Tissue plasminogen activator for postvitrectomy fibrin formation. *Ophthalmology* 1990;97:184–189.
29. Croxatto JO, Galentine P, Cupples HP, et al. Sympathetic ophthalmia after pars plana vitrectomy-lensectomy for endogenous bacterial endophthalmitis. *Am J Ophthalmol* 1981;91:342–346.
30. Menikoff JA, Speaker MG, Marmor M, Raskin EM. A case control study of risk factors for postoperative endophthalmitis. *Ophthalmology* 1991;98:1761–1768.
31. Han DP, Wisniewski SR, Wilson LA, et al. Spectrum and susceptibilities of microbiologic isolates in the Endophthalmitis Vitrectomy Study. *Am J Ophthalmol* 1996;122:1–17.
32. Zambrano W, Flynn HW Jr, Pflugfelder SC, et al. Management options for *Propionibacterium acnes* endophthalmitis. *Ophthalmology* 1989;96:1100–1105.
33. Greenwald MJ, Wohl LG, Sell CH. Metastatic bacterial endophthalmitis. *Surv Ophthalmol* 1986;31:81–99.
34. Barrie T. The place of elective vitrectomy in the management of patients with *Candida* endophthalmitis. *Graefes Arch Clin Exp Ophthalmol* 1987;225:107–113.
35. Kroll P, Emmerick K-H, Fegeler W. *Candida albicans* endophthalmitis—results of pars plana vitrectomy without intraocular antimycotic therapy. *Klin Monatsbl Augenheilk* 1984;184:104–108.
36. Brod RD, Flynn HW Jr, Clarkson JG, et al. Endogenous *Candida* endophthalmitis. *Ophthalmology* 1990;97:666–674.

37. Akler ME, Vellend H, McNeely DM, et al. Use of fluconazole in the treatment of candidal endophthalmitis. *Clin Infect Dis* 1995;20:657–664.

38. Brinton GS, Topping TM, Hyndiuk RA, et al. Posttraumatic endophthalmitis. *Arch Ophthalmol* 1984;102:547–550.

39. Boldt HC, Pulido JS, Blodi CF, et al. Rural endophthalmitis. *Ophthalmology* 1989;96:1722–1726.

40. Lesk MR, Ammann H, Marcil G, et al. The penetration of oral ciprofloxacin into the aqueous humor, vitreous, and subretinal fluid of humans. *Am J Ophthalmol* 1993;115:623–628.

41. el Baba FZ, Trousdale MD, Gauderman WJ, et al. Intravitreal penetration of oral ciprofloxacin in humans. *Ophthalmology* 1992;99:483–486.

42. Meredith TA, Aguilar HE, Shaarawy A, et al. Vancomycin levels in the vitreous cavity after intravenous administration. *Am J Ophthalmol* 1995;119:774–778.

43. Steinmetz RL, Masket S, Sidikaro Y. The successful removal of a subretinal cysticercus by pars plana vitrectomy. *Retina* 1989;9:276–280.

44. Funata M, Custis P, De La Cruz Z, et al. Intraocular gnathostomiasis. *Retina* 1993;13:240–244.

45. Turunen HJ, Leinikki PO, Saari KM. Demonstration of intraocular synthesis of immunoglobulin G toxoplasma antibodies for specific diagnosis of toxoplasmic chorioretinitis by enzyme immunoassay. *J Clin Microbiol* 1983;17:988–992.

46. Biglan AW, Glickman LT, Lobes LA Jr. Serum and vitreous *Toxocara* antibody in nematode endophthalmitis. *Am J Ophthalmol* 1979;86:898–901.

47. Chan CC, Palestine AG, Li Q, Nussenblatt RB. Diagnosis of ocular toxoplasmosis by the use of immunocytology and the polymerase chain reaction. *Am J Ophthalmol* 1994;117:803–805.

Vitrectomy for Inflammatory Diseases

WILLIAM M. TANG   JOSE S. PULIDO   WILLIAM F. MIELER

Pars plana vitrectomy plays an important role in the diagnosis and management of uveitis. New indications for vitrectomy have recently emerged, especially in the setting of uveitis. The technique of vitrectomy has allowed the surgeon to perform a simple vitreous biopsy or a more complicated chorioretinal or endoretinal biopsy. New sophisticated testing methods such as immunocytochemical staining and the polymerase chain reaction (PCR) have shown promise to provide important diagnostic information even when only a very small biopsy specimen is available. Such methods may significantly increase the diagnostic yield of vitrectomy performed in uveitis patients.

Vitrectomy has numerous important applications in the management of uveitis as well. Pars plana vitrectomy may be performed for many vitreoretinal complications secondary to chronic uveitis. Because the vitreous cavity serves as a reservoir for many immunocompetent cells and inflammatory mediators, several investigators have postulated that mechanical removal of these agents may alter the course of inflammation and result in stabilization of the disease (1–7). In the surgical management of uveitic cataract, pars plana vitrectomy combined with pars plana lensectomy or anterior segment surgery can result in excellent visual outcome.

DIAGNOSTIC VITRECTOMY

Vitreous Biopsy

Principles

When presented with vitreous inflammation, the physician often relies on the ophthalmoscopic evaluation and ancillary blood studies to make a diagnosis and initiate treatment. In certain cases, however, the diagnosis remains uncertain and the treatment therefore may not be optimal. In addition, patients may be unresponsive or intolerant to therapy, or may develop significant ocular or systemic complications during therapy. In such situations, additional diagnostic information obtained from vitreous biopsy might be desirable.

For uveitic patients, vitreous biopsy is preferably performed by vitrectomy techniques rather than by fine-needle biopsy because vitrectomy provides a larger sample size and a more representative group of cells (8). Vitreous biopsy may be performed alone or during vitrectomy for a therapeutic purpose. The vitreous specimen can be subject to a variety of studies, including antibody analysis, cytologic analysis, and immunocytochemical studies. Because of the small sample size, culture for virus or other infectious agents is often unrewarding (9). The polymerase chain reaction (PCR) is a new technology that can allow the identification of a variety of infectious organisms even when only a very small specimen is available (10). It is likely that the use of PCR in analyzing vitreous biopsy specimen will increase in the future.

Indications

Vitreous biopsy may be indicated in uveitic patients when 1) the patient is unresponsive to medical therapy and alternative diagnoses are being considered; 2) the patient develops significant ocular or systemic complications during therapy and more diagnostic information is needed to guide therapy; 3) malignancy is suspected, especially in patients above the age of 60; and 4) a localized infection of intraocular contents is suspected.

Supported in part by an unrestricted grant from Research to Prevent Blindness, Inc., New York, New York.

Techniques

Antibody analysis and cultures require a vitreous specimen that is minimally diluted by infusate (11). To achieve this, the initial portion of the vitrectomy is generally conducted with the infusion line turned off, and the specimen is aspirated directly into a syringe through a three-way stopcock attached to the suction tubing. If an adequate specimen cannot be obtained without producing an unacceptable degree of hypotony, air may be infused through the infusion line. Next, the infusion line is opened, and approximately 10 mL of vitrectomy specimen is aspirated into a separate syringe through the three-way stopcock. This specimen is particularly suited for cytologic analysis, immunocytochemical studies, and culture. The remainder of the vitrectomy is completed in the standard fashion using automated suction. This specimen is then concentrated by centrifugation or filtration and may be used for additional studies such as PCR analysis.

Benefits and Complications

Numerous analyses can be performed on vitreous biopsy specimen to provide a more specific diagnosis in uveitis patients. Simple cytologic analysis by Giemsa or Gram stain can demonstrate tumor cells, bacteria, parasites, and fungi (11,12). Eosinophils and *Toxocara* larvae have been recovered from vitreous aspirate in one case (13) (Fig. 50-1).

Analysis of antibody levels can be useful in diagnosing infection with herpes simplex virus, varicella-zoster virus, cytomegalovirus, *Toxocara canis*, and *Toxoplasmosis gondii*. It is especially helpful in cases where the antibodies in serum cannot be detected or in cases where the antibody levels in the vitreous greatly exceed that in the serum (11,14). Baarsma et al (15) were able to use antibody analysis to make a diagnosis of HSV retinitis in one case and ocular toxoplasmosis in another case that were otherwise mis-

diagnosed. Demonstration of antilens antibodies can also confirm the diagnosis of lens-induced uveitis (9).

Immunocytochemical studies can provide information to divide the differential diagnoses of uveitis into three categories (12). Bacterial or fungal infections show prominent neutrophils and macrophages. Large cell lymphoma (reticulum cell sarcoma) most often demonstrates light chain restriction of the malignant B-lymphocytes (16–18). Autoimmune uveitis characteristically demonstrates a predominance of T-lymphocytes (Fig. 50-2) and HLA-DR activation (12).

Recently, PCR technology has allowed rapid and sensitive diagnoses of a variety of infections, including herpetic diseases, Whipple's disease, cat scratch disease, and toxoplasmosis. Table 50-1 lists infectious diseases that have been diagnosed by PCR. Further application of this technology to the diagnosis of uveitis will probably be forthcoming.

Complications after standard pars plana vitrectomy include the development of cataract, which is estimated to occur in 15% to 47% of cases within the first year after vitrectomy (19). Retinal detachment or other serious complications occur in less than 2% of patients undergoing pars plana vitrectomy (20). In a small series of 14 eyes undergoing vitreous biopsy reported by Davis et al (12), no postoperative complication related to the biopsy was observed. We agree with these researchers that if potentially important diagnostic information is anticipated, vitrectomy offers a relatively safe biopsy technique.

Chorioretinal Biopsy

Principles

In cases of retinochoroiditis of unclear etiology, vitreous biopsy alone may not provide useful information if the

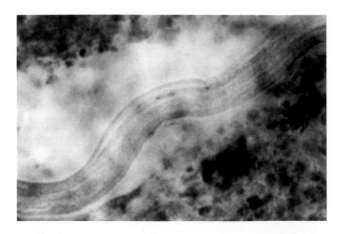

FIGURE 50-1.   *Second-stage larvae of* Toxocara canis *(original magnification, × 340). (Reproduced by permission from Maguire A, Green W, Michels R, Erozan YS. Recovery of intraocular* Toxocara canis *by pars plana vitrectomy.* Ophthalamology 1990; 97:675–680.)

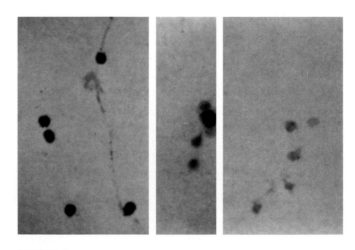

FIGURE 50-2.   *Microphotograph of vitreous specimen from autoimmune uveitides demonstrates majority of cells stained positively for T-helper/inducer marker (Leu 3a) (left), a few for macrophage marker (Leu M5) (center), and none for B-cell marker (Leu 14) (right) (avidin-biotin peroxidase stain; original magnification, × 400). (Reproduced by permission from Davis JL, Solomon D, Nussenblatt RB, et al. Immunocytochemical staining of vitreous cells.* Ophthalmology 1992;99:250–256.)

Table 50-1. Infectious Agents Identified by PCR

Bacteria
Rochalimaea henselae[1]
Tropheryma whippeli[2]
Mycobacterium tuberculosis[122]

Virus
Herpes simplex virus type 1 and type 2[123]
Varicella-zoster virus[124]
Cytomegalovirus[125]
Measles virus[126]

Spirochete
Borrelia burgdorferi[127]
Treponema pallidum[128]

Protozoa
Toxoplasma gondii[129]

Rickettsiae
Rickettsia rickettsii[3]

[1] Infectious agent in cat scratch disease.[130]
[2] Infectious agent in Whipple's disease.[131]
[3] Infectious agent in Rocky Mountain spotted fever.[132]

pathologic features are confined to the retina and the choroid (21–23). In such cases, direct biopsy of the retina and choroid might be desirable. Evaluation of chorioretinal biopsy specimens can help distinguish between an autoimmune, infectious, or neoplastic disorder. For an autoimmune disorder, immunohistochemical studies can help distinguish between different kinds of inflammatory processes by identifying the predominant type of lymphocytes. Such a distinction is important because therapeutic agents are now becoming available that target specific aspects of the immune system. For example, cyclosporine is an immunosuppressive agent which specifically blocks T-helper lymphocytes function by inhibiting the production of interleukin-2 (24). Cyclophosphamide, though less specific, has greater inhibitory action on B-lymphocytes than T-lymphocytes (25). Furthermore, immunohistochemical studies of chorioretinal biopsy specimens can provide important clues to elucidate the pathogenesis of various types of retinochoroiditis (26).

Indications

Biopsy of a chorioretinal lesion in the retinal periphery may be indicated when there is 1) macula-threatening lesions unresponsive to therapy, 2) suspicion of malignancy, or 3) suspicion of an infectious etiology. Information obtained from chorioretinal biopsy should be expected to assist in guiding therapy.

Techniques

The techniques of chorioretinal biopsy were first described by Peyman et al (27) and subsequently modified by Chan et al (26,28) (Fig. 50-3). Briefly, the conjunctiva is incised

for 360 degrees, the rectus muscles isolated on silk suture, and the quadrants inspected. A standard three-port pars plana vitrectomy is performed, and the vitreous specimen may be submitted for analyses. If preoperative visualization is adequate, laser photocoagulation is usually applied one to three days before surgery in a wide zone around the site to be biopsied. Otherwise, endolaser is applied at the time of vitrectomy. The site to be biopsied is marked on the external sclera, and markings for a 6 × 6-mm scleral flap are outlined beginning 5 to 6 mm posterior to the limbus. The infusion line is left in place, and a nearly full-thickness scleral flap, hinged posteriorly, is dissected. The flap is retracted exposing near-bare choroid with a few remaining thin fibers of overlying sclera. Penetrating diathermy surrounding the biopsy site is used for hemostasis. The infusion line is turned off and a 75 blade is used to make two incisions oriented parallel to the limbus, approximately 4 mm apart, through the choroid and retina. One blade of a 0.12 forceps is placed through the incision into the eye and full-thickness choroid and retina are grasped at one edge. The chorioretinal block is then completed by making two incisions, oriented perpendicular to the limbus, using Vannas scissors. A specimen with a size of 4 × 4 mm is preferred. A small amount of prolapsed vitreous is removed from the wound using a vitreous cutter, and the scleral flap is sutured closed with interrupted 9-0 nylon. Fluid-gas exchange is then performed.

The chorioretinal biopsy specimen should be immediately divided into three parts in a sterile manner under a dissecting microscope. One section is submitted for light and electron microscopy, the second section for tissue culture, and the third section for immunohistochemical examination. For immunohistochemical studies, antibodies directed against lymphocyte cell surface markers are used to determine the type of predominant immune response. Cell surface markers include CD3 (pan T-lymphocytes), CD4 (T-helper), CD8 (T-suppressor), CD56 (natural killer cell), CD22 (B-lymphocyte), CD11c/CD18 (macrophages), and major histocompatibility complex Class I and Class II antigens. Antibodies for herpes simplex virus, varicella-zoster virus, and cytomegalovirus may also be applied to rule out a viral etiology.

Benefits and Complication

Numerous infectious agents have been demonstrated on chorioretinal biopsy specimens from patients with posterior uveitis. In a series reported by Martin et al (30), two cases of acute retinal necrosis was confirmed by chorioretinal biopsy. In one case, herpes viral particles were seen on electron microscopic evaluation; in the other, herpes viral antigen was present in the retina by immunohistochemical study. Rutzen et al (28) reported a case of progressive outer retinal necrosis in which the diagnosis was confirmed by demonstration of herpes viral particles on electron microscopy. Moorthy et al (29) described a case in which *Toxoplasma gondii* organisms was demonstrated by electron microscopy in a patient with AIDS and negative *Toxoplasma*

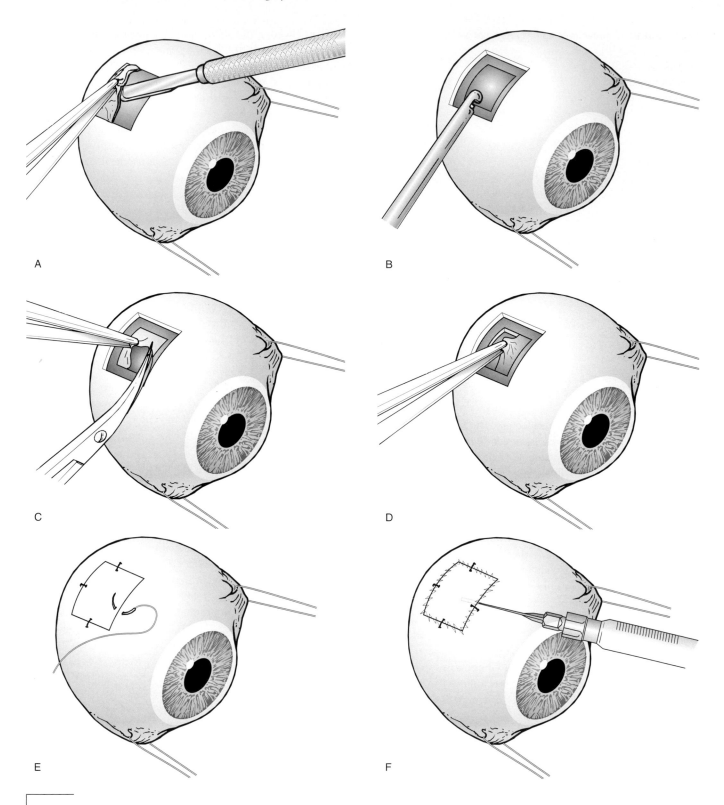

A

B

C

D

E

F

FIGURE 50-3.   *Chorioretinal biopsy techniques: (A) Near full-thickness scleral flap is dissected. (B) Penetrating diathermy is applied surrounding biopsy site for hemostasis. (C) Chorioretinal specimen is removed with scissors. (D) Vitrectomy is performed through biopsy site. (E) Scleral flap is sutured closed. (F) Fluid-gas exchange is then performed.*

titers, and appropriate therapy was instituted as a result of the biopsy findings.

The diagnoses of several autoimmune uveitides can also be made or confirmed by chorioretinal biopsy. The diagnosis of sarcoidosis was made in one case based on the finding of noncaseating granuloma in the retina and the predominance of T-lymphocytes and macrophages in the choroid (30). The diagnosis of multifocal choroiditis/progressive subretinal fibrosis syndrome was made in three cases, facilitated by the findings of B-lymphocytes in the choroid and the negative workup for an infectious agent (30) (Fig. 50-4). Fujikawa and Haugen found that positive immunochemical staining for T-helper lymphocytes and the HLA-DR antigen generally supports the diagnosis of autoimmune uveitis (9).

Intraocular neoplasms masquerading as posterior uveitis have also been diagnosed by chorioretinal biopsy. Kirmani et al (31) reported a case in which chorioretinal biopsy revealed the diagnosis of reticulum cell sarcoma even though vitreous biopsy was negative. Kumar et al (32) reported another case in which the diagnosis of HTLV-1 (Human T-cell lymphotrophic virus type-1) associated retinal T-cell lymphoma was made by chorioretinal biopsy (32) (Fig. 50-5). A case of bilateral diffuse uveal melanocytic proliferation was diagnosed in a patient with bilateral exudative retinal detachment when histologic examination demonstrated benign proliferation of densely pigmented melanocytes in the choroid (28).

When employed judiciously in selected cases, chorioretinal biopsy can provide crucial diagnostic information that may alter treatment options. In the series reported by Martin et al (30), therapy was altered in five out of seven patients as a result of biopsy findings.

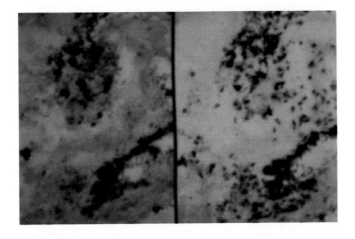

FIGURE 50-4. *Immunohistochemical staining of chorioretinal biopsy specimen in case of multifocal choroiditis demonstrates subretinal pigment epithelial infiltration by predominantly B-lymphocytes (left: CD22, right: CD3; original magnification, × 160). (Reproduced by permission from Chan CC, Palestine AG, Davis JL, et al. Role of chorioretinal biopsy in inflammatory eye disease. Ophthalmology 1991;98:1281–1286.)*

Complications related to chorioretinal biopsies have so far been relatively mild. Theoretical complications, such as expulsive hemorrhage and proliferative vitreoretinopathy, have not been observed (30). In the series of seven patients reported by Martin et al, the most common complication observed was progression of lens opacity. One eye that was extensively diseased preoperatively developed phthisis. One eye developed retinal neovascularization near the biopsy site. In another series of nine patients, one patient had a persistent retinal detachment, one had a recurrent retinal detachment, and two had a mild postoperative vitreous hemorrhage (28).

Endoretinal Biopsy

Principles

Endoretinal biopsy via the vitreous cavity is an alternative method for obtaining retinal tissue without performing a full-thickness resection of the retina and choroid. It can be particularly useful when the primary pathologic process involves the retina. In the case of viral retinitis, electron microscopy may demonstrate the presence of viral particles, especially if the biopsy site is at the border between involved and uninvolved retina (33). Newer techniques such as immunohistochemistry, in situ hybridization, and PCR can provide evidence to implicate a specific viral agent. In the case of noninfectious vasculitides, immunohistochemistry may provide evidence to corroborate an autoimmune process.

Indications

Endoretinal biopsy may be indicated for patients when less invasive diagnostic tests are unrevealing, especially if an etiologic diagnosis may assist the patient in selecting a specific and appropriate therapy.

Techniques

A core vitrectomy is first performed (33). A biopsy site, preferably in detached involved retina, is then chosen. A 20-gauge unimanual bipolar disposable endocautery (Mentor, Norwalk, MA) is used to cauterize visible retinal vessels at the posterior edge of the area to be biopsied. If the retina is attached, then after cauterizing the retina, a small bleb of fluid can be injected into the subretinal space to cause a small localized retinal detachment. A motorized 20-gauge vertical cutting scissors is inserted into the vitreous cavity and the lower blade is used to penetrate the retina at the site of a cautery burn. A rectangular piece of retina is then cut, one surface of which is along the previously cauterized area of retina. The strip varies from 2 to 4 mm wide and from 3 to 6 mm long. It is useful to leave a small (0.2-mm) area of attachment of the retinal biopsy to the remainder of the retina. When the scissors is removed from the area, the retinal biopsy has a tendency to slip posteriorly beneath the

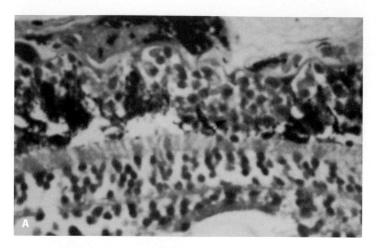

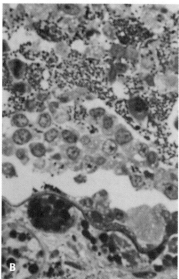

FIGURE 50-5. (A) *Chorioretinal biopsy specimen in case of HTLV-1 associate retina lymphoma: collections of mononuclear cells are noted in subretinal pigment epithelium region and retina (hematoxylin-eosin, original magnification, × 250). (B) Abnormal mitotic figures are seen in occasional cells (toluidine blue, original magnification, × 500). (Reproduced by permission from Kumar SR, Gill PS, Wagner DG, et al. Human T-cell lymphotropic virus type 1–associated retinal lymphoma.* Arch Ophthalmol *1994;112:954–959.)*

detached retina; however, the small area of attachment serves to anchor it in place. Intraocular forceps are then used to grasp the edge of the retinal biopsy, which is then moved into the center of the vitreous cavity, severing the small area of attachment in the process. The biopsy is guided toward the sclerotomies with a pick or pick forceps. The infusion bottle is raised to elevate the intraocular pressure and release the tissue. After the empty forceps are removed from the eye, the retinal biopsy is hydraulically directed into the sclerotomies site and allowed to plug the site. The tissue is gently teased out of the sclerotomies with a 0.12-mm forceps and spread over a piece of sterile paper on which it is cut.

The retinal tissue is cut into two or more small strips and each piece is placed onto a moistened piece of paper. After processing of the specimen, the eye is reentered and pneumohydraulic retinal reattachment is performed, removing subretinal fluid through the biopsy site. Endolaser treatment is placed around all breaks in eyes to be filled with a long-acting gas. In some eyes in which silicone oil is injected, endolaser is placed around breaks in the inferior half of the fundus. In most cases, the peripheral retina is encircled with either a scleral buckle or a band.

Benefits and Complications

Endoretinal biopsy has been helpful in distinguishing between viral retinitis, toxoplasma retinochoroiditis, and other types of intraocular infections when the clinical presentation is atypical. In one series, six out of ten patients with the clinical diagnosis of CMV retinitis demonstrated viral particles on biopsy specimens (28). On the other hand, two patients were found to have been misdiagnosed with CMV retinitis when retinal biopsy demonstrated the presence of *Toxoplasma gondii* cysts (34) (Fig. 50-6). In another case, retinal biopsy yielded an expected finding of *Candida* endophthalmitis in an otherwise healthy patient who was misdiagnosed with ocular toxoplasmosis (28).

Immunohistochemical staining on biopsy specimens can also assist in identifying an autoimmune process. Freeman et al (33) reported a case in which endoretinal biopsy revealed the presence of immune complex-mediated retinal vasculitis (33).

In a series reported by Rutzen et al (28), out of 24 patients who had undergone endoretinal biopsy, recurrent retinal detachment was observed in two patients; postoperative glaucoma was observed in one patient. Postoperative vitreous hemorrhage, endophthalmitis, choroidal hemor-

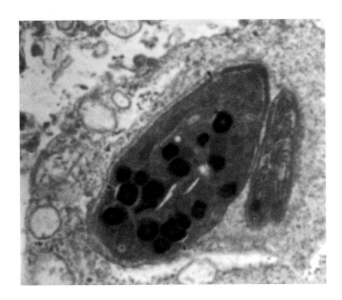

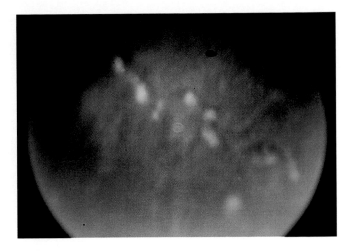

FIGURE 50-7. *Deep cortical inflammation overlying the viteous base in patient with pars planitis.*

FIGURE 50-6. *Endoretinal biopsy demonstrated* Toxoplasma gondii *cystozoite in patient with presumed CMV retinitis. (Reproduced by permission from Elkins BS, Holland GN, Opremcak M, et al. Ocular toxoplasmosis misdiagnosed as cytomegalovirus retinopathy in immunocompromised patients.* Ophthalmology *1994;101:499–507.)*

rhage, and proliferative vitreoretinopathy were not observed. In most cases, poor visual outcome was related to maculopathy from retinal detachment or progression of the disease into the macula.

THERAPEUTIC VITRECTOMY

Pars Planitis

Pars planitis is an inflammatory ocular condition that typically affects young healthy patients within the first three decades of life (35). The clinical picture is characterized by inflammatory cells and debris in the vitreous cavity (Fig. 50-7), varying degrees of cystoid macular edema, possible epiretinal membrane formation (Fig. 50-8), possible periphlebitis (Fig. 50-9), varying degrees of exudate and snowbank formation along the vitreous base region (Fig. 50-10), a relatively quiet anterior chamber, and the absence of chorioretinal infiltrates. The course is variable, ranging from a mild self-limited process to chronic disease with exacerbations and remissions (35).

Systemic Associations

Over the years, a number of underlying systemic conditions have been found to produce an ophthalmic picture of pars planitis (intermediate uveitis) (36,37). Appropriate management of patients with intermediate uveitis, therefore, depends not only on an understanding of this ophthalmic condition but also on an awareness of possible systemic associations. In a series reported by Zierhut and Foster (37), sarcoidosis and multiple sclerosis were each found in 10% of

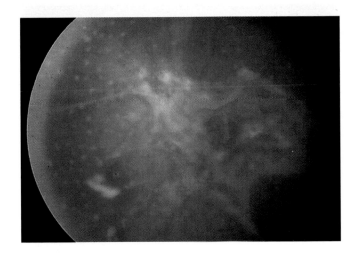

FIGURE 50-8. *Prominent, diffuse epiretinal membrane in patient with long-standing pars planitis.*

patients. Positive serology for *Borrelia burgdorferi* was found in an intermediate uveitis patient with bilateral pars plana exudate (38). Another recent study has shown a strong association between the human T-cell lymphotrophic virus type 1 and a type of intermediate uveitis without pars plana exudate (39). In addition, other conditions such as syphilis, tuberculosis, systemic amyloidosis, intraocular lymphoma, ocular toxocariasis, and Whipple's disease may produce a clinical picture mimicking pars planitis and should be considered (40–44).

Recently, Tang et al (45) have demonstrated a significant association between the HLA-DR15 specificity and intermediate uveitis. In this study, patients with HLA-DR15-positive intermediate uveitis were more likely to manifest another HLA-DR15-related disorder, such as multiple sclerosis and narcolepsy. The authors postulated that intermediate uveitis may belong to a constellation of HLA-DR15-related disorders.

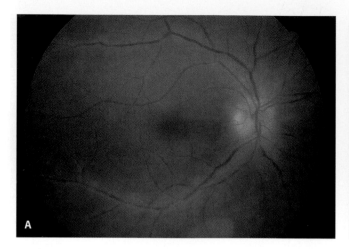

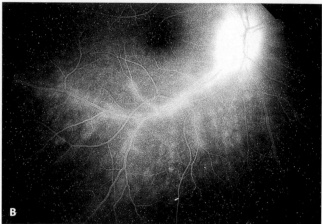

FIGURE 50-9.   (A) *Prominent periphlebitis.* (B) *Late frame flourescein angiogram showing diffuse staining along venules.*

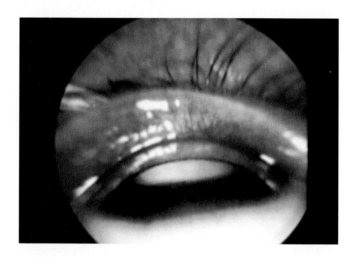

FIGURE 50-10.   *Dense vitreous base organization, seen through aid of external indentation with Q-tip.*

Ocular Complications

The most common anterior segment complication of pars planitis is the formation of a posterior subcapsular cataract (15% to 60%) (35,46). The incidence of glaucoma is quite low, reported to be 8% in one large series (46). The majority of glaucoma cases are corticosteroid-induced. Rarer anterior segment findings include band keratopathy (46), ectopia lentis (47), and autoimmune endotheliopathy (48).

Vitreous inflammation tends to be mild early in the course of disease, but the vitreous can later become organized and opacified (41,49). The finding of pars plana exudate has been considered a characteristic feature of pars planitis (50). However, many pars planitis patients do not demonstrate pars plana exudate (45). In patients with prominent pars plana exudate or the so-called snowbank formation (see Fig. 50-10), neovascularization of the vitre-

ous base (NVVB) may occur, resulting in vitreous hemorrhage in 3% to 9% of patients (35,51). NVVB may sometimes be difficult to visualize and may be surmised by observing large retinal vessels extending without attenuation to the ora serrata in the vicinity of a snowbank (41). In more severe cases, a vascularized membrane originating from the vitreous base region may proliferate along the anterior hyaloid face (52,53). Contraction of this membrane can result in ciliary body detachment, hypotony, funnel retinal detachment, and ultimately phthisis bulbi (53). Cystoid macular edema (CME) and macular degeneration secondary to CME are the most common causes for permanent decrease in vision and occur in 30% to 60% of patients. Retinal detachment occurs in approximately 5% to 22% of patients on an exudative, tractional, rhegmatogenous, or combined basis (35,41).

Medical Therapy

Topical corticosteroid therapy plays a minimal role in the therapy of pars planitis. Initial attempts to treat pars planitis should consist of subtenon corticosteroid injections (35). We preferred the technique described by Nozik (54). The conjunctiva is first touched with an applicator moistened with 4% cocaine in the superotemporal quadrant well back in the fornix. With the patient looking inferonasally, a five-eighths-inch needle (No. 25) attached to a tuberculin syringe is passed into the fornix through the conjunctiva without grasping it. The needle is to follow the curve of the globe posteriorly, with the tip of the needle moving side to side as it is passed posteriorly. We usually give monthly injections of 20 mg of triamcinolone acetonide (20 mg/0.5 cc), combined with Decadron (12 mg/0.5 cc), until the inflammation is controlled. The combination of a rapid-acting corticosteroid (Decadron) with a depot corticosteroid (triamcinolone) provides good control of inflammation. Alternatively, triamcinolone diacetate may be utilized with

Decadron, since some of its effect lasts only three months versus one year for the acetonide form (55,56).

Although systemic corticosteroids have been widely used for bilateral and recalcitrant cases, the physician needs to carefully consider and discuss with the patient the serious systemic side effects (41) and the possibility of developing a lifelong dependency on systemic corticosteroids. Death from disseminated opportunistic infection has been reported in a patient with intermediate uveitis treated with systemic corticosteroids for three months (57).

The use of immunosuppressive agents such as cyclosporine has been recommended in otherwise medically refractory cases (58). In one report, over 80% of patients treated with cyclosporine demonstrated improved visual acuity within three months. Once again, the potentially serious systemic side effects of these agents need to be considered. In some instances, we believe that locally invasive therapies, such as cryotherapy, peripheral scatter photocoagulation, or even pars plana vitrectomy, might be preferable to systemic immunosuppressive agents.

Cryotherapy

Principles and Indications

Cryoablation of peripheral retinal tissue for cases of inflammation intolerant or refractory to corticosteroids was first advocated by Aaberg et al (60,61). Cryotherapy is thought to reduce inflammation by eliminating the inflammatory stimulus in the peripheral retinal tissue (60,62). It has also been shown to be effective in the treatment of NVVB (61). Cryotherapy may reduce the neovascularization either by directly ablating the permeable neovascular tissue or by destroying the ischemic retinal tissue that serves as a stimulus for neovascularization (62,63). Cryotherapy may be performed in conjunction with pars plana vitrectomy in order to provide adequate control of the NVVB (49).

Techniques

Cryotherapy may be applied to the involved areas under direct visualization by indirect ophthalmoscopy using a double freeze-thaw technique (41,60). The ice ball should be seen to cover the exudative area. Uninvolved pars plana and retina are treated one probe width beyond the involved area. In areas where view of the ice ball is precluded, freezing should be continued for a time interval similar to that required in adjacent areas with adequate visualization. Retreatment is administered three to four months after the first ablative procedure if there is persistence of disease activity.

Benefits and Complications

Following the initial 1973 report on the use of cryotherapy by Aaberg et al (60), Devenyi et al (61) have reported on a series of 27 eyes with corticosteroid-resistant intermediate uveitis and NVVB treated with cryotherapy. Vitreous

inflammation was virtually eliminated in 78% of eyes, and visual acuity improved or remained unchanged in 89% of eyes. Cryotherapy eliminated the need for corticosteroid therapy in 90% of eyes. Eight-five percent of eyes required a single treatment. Complications of cryotherapy included transient decrease in accommodation, transient increase in vitreous turbidity, progression of cataract, and hyphema. In addition, cryotherapy has been associated with a possible increased risk of developing a rhegmatogenous retinal detachment, especially when cryotherapy is performed together with a pars plana vitrectomy (64). Rhegmatogenous retinal detachment has been noted in 5 of 11 eyes (45%) treated with cryotherapy and vitrectomy, compared with no retinal detachment in 10 eyes treated with vitrectomy alone. One possible cause for development of retinal tears and detachment may be the development of atrophic areas from cryoablation, especially if there is a certain amount of tractional proliferation in this region associated with the NVVB (64).

Peripheral Scatter Photocoagulation

Principles and Indications

Recently, peripheral scatter photocoagulation (PSP) has been investigated as an alternative treatment option besides cryotherapy for patients with NVVB (64). Similar to cryotherapy, PSP may cause regression of NVVB by ablating ischemic retinal tissue and reducing inflammation by destroying the inflammatory stimulus in peripheral retinal tissue. However, unlike cryotherapy, which has been associated with a possible increased risk for rhegmatogenous retinal detachment, PSP may actually create a barrier against the possible formation of retinal detachment. PSP may also potentially cause less breakdown of the blood-retinal barrier than cryotherapy (65). PSP may be performed in conjunction with pars plana vitrectomy.

Techniques

After a complete vitrectomy is performed, three rows of photocoagulation are delivered to the inferior retinal periphery, just posterior to the area of exudation, organization, and/or neovascularization. The area of photocoagulation treatment is extended approximately one clock hour beyond the margins of the neovascularization. Treatment may be carried out with either argon endophotocoagulation or with an indirect ophthalmoscopic delivery system utilizing argon or diode photocoagulation. Approximately 300 laser applications are placed (64) (Fig. 50-11).

Benefits and Complications

In the series of 10 eyes treated with PSP, all eyes demonstrated regression of NVVB, stabilization of inflammation, and at least partial resolution of cystoid macular edema (64). With a follow-up of 13.5 months, none of the eyes developed retinal detachment or any other major complication related to treatment. Visual improvement was noted in

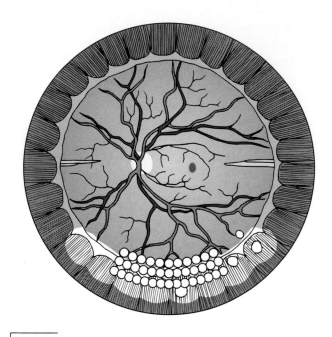

FIGURE 50-11. *Schematic diagram depicting technique of peripheral scatter photocoagulation for NVVB. Three rows of photocoagulation are delivered posterior to area of exudation, extending approximately one clock hour beyond margins of NVVB.*

70% of cases. Final visual acuity of 20/40 or less was generally due to cataract formation and/or mild cystoid macular edema.

Cataract Extraction and Intraocular Lens Implantation

Principles

The key factor in the surgical management of cataract is rigorous control of inflammation during the perioperative period (66,67). Eyes with cataracts and minimal posterior segment involvement often do well with anterior segment surgery alone. If vitreous opacification or another vitreoretinal complication exists, several approaches are possible. Pars plana lensectomy/vitrectomy is classically the procedure of choice (49). By excising the lens capsule and anterior hyaloid, pars plana lensectomy/vitrectomy eliminates the possibility of synechiae formation between the iris and lens capsule and reduces the likelihood of formation of cyclitic membranes (1–3,6,41,49,68,69). Despite excellent anatomic outcomes, however, visual rehabilitation for aphakic eyes may be problematic since many patients are either unable or unwilling to wear an aphakic contact lens (70).

Although intraocular lens (IOL) implantation in uveitis patients remains controversial, several reports of posterior chamber IOL implantation in intermediate uveitis patients have demonstrated that IOL implantation does not appear to have a deleterious effect on the visual outcome (70,71). Several techniques for IOL implantation exist. Sulcus fixation of a posterior chamber IOL is generally not rec-

ommended since the mechanical rubbing of the IOL on the iris and ciliary body may exacerbate inflammation (70,72). Implantation of an anterior chamber IOL is not recommended either (73). When implantation of an IOL is desirable, we advocate the combined procedure of phacoemulsification, pars plana vitrectomy, and endocapsular fixation of a posterior chamber IOL, which has been described by Koenig et al (70). Visual rehabilitation was rapid and excellent functional unaided vision was achieved in eyes after this procedure (68,70,74). On the other hand, if intraoperatively it is felt not to be feasible to insert the IOL into the capsular bag, we prefer to leave the patient aphakic (73).

Indications

Cataract extraction may be recommended when a sufficiently dense cataract either impairs the patient's vision or the surgeon's ability to visualize the posterior segment. In general, eyes should be free of inflammation for at least three to six months before cataract extraction (73). Occasionally, removal of a cataract may be indicated despite persistent dense vitreous inflammation, as in the case of a pars plana lensectomy/vitrectomy performed for a vitreoretinal complication (49). The decision to implant an intraocular lens after cataract removal may be difficult and should be based on whether inflammation has been effectively controlled by medical therapy and whether the patient is willing or able to undergo visual rehabilitation for aphakia (41,70). Even in quiet eyes, a brief course of systemic corticosteroids for three to five days preoperatively is generally warranted, with a tapering back to baseline levels in the early postoperative time frame.

Techniques

The surgical technique for pars plana lensectomy/vitrectomy is later described in the section Pars Plana Vitrectomy. Only the technique of combined phacoemulsification, pars plana vitrectomy, and posterior chamber IOL insertion is described here (70,75). Eyes are prepared for a three-port pars plana vitrectomy by placing 4-0 black silk sutures transconjunctivally beneath the horizontal recti muscles. A 180-degree fornix-based conjunctival flap is dissected superiorly. Sclerotomy sites are marked 3.0mm posterior to the limbus inferotemporally, superonasally, and superotemporally. A suture is preplaced for the inferotemporal sclerotomy site, and the vitreous cavity is entered with a 20-gauge myringotomy retinal blade. A 2.5-mm length infusion cannula is connected to a 50-mL bottle of irrigating solution, entered through the sclerotomy site, and sutured in place. Prior to initiation of irrigation, the tip of the cannula is directly inspected to ensure correct positioning.

Attention is then directed to the anterior chamber. A 6.5- to 7.0-mm partial-depth corneoscleral incision is made with a razor blade knife 1 to 2mm posterior to the superior limbus. A stab incision is made within the corneoscleral groove with a 3.0- or 3.2-mm keratome. The anterior chamber is filled with viscoelastic material. A 6-mm-diameter capsulorrhexis is made with a 25-gauge bent cystotome needle. The phacoemulsification needle is introduced into the anterior chamber and the lens nucleus emulsified in the posterior chamber. Residual cortical material is aspirated with the 0.3-mm tip of the irrigation-aspiration instrument. The wound is temporarily closed with a single 7-0 polyglactin (Vicryl) suture.

Attention is then directed back to the pars plana region. Two superiorly located sclerotomies are made with a 20-gauge myringotomy retinal blade, and the endoilluminator and vitrectomy instrument are introduced. After a complete pars plana vitrectomy, attention is then paid to removing any membranes or treating any vitreous base abnormalities. If there is vitreous base neovascularization, scatter photocoagulation treatment is applied throughout the inferior periphery as described earlier in this chapter. Next, the light pipe and vitrectomy instrument are removed from the eye and the sclerotomy sites temporarily closed with plugs. The retina is then inspected by indirect ophthalmoscopy. If the retina is anatomically intact, the previously placed polyglactin 9-0 suture is removed from the cataract wound and the capsular bag filled with viscoelastic material. The corneoscleral wound is enlarged to 6.5 to 7 mm using a corneoscleral scissors. A Sinskey-style posterior chamber lens implant is then placed in the capsular bag and centered with a Sinskey hook (Storz Instrument Co, St Louis, MO). The pupil is constricted with intracameral 0.01% carbachol, unless further posterior visualization is required. Any residual viscoelastic material is aspirated, and then the corneoscleral wound is closed with several interrupted 10-0 monofilament nylon sutures. The sclerotomy plugs are then removed and the sites closed with interrupted 7-0 polyglycolic acid (Dexan) sutures. The conjunctival flap is reapproximated with interrupted 7-0 polyglycolic acid sutures.

Benefits and Complications

Numerous reports on pars plana lensectomy/vitrectomy for pars planitis patients have documented good visual outcome (3,49,66,69,76,78). On average, 50% to 65% of patients achieved a visual acuity of 20/40 or better. The major limiting factor on visual recovery was cystoid macular edema (49).

Kaufman and Foster reported on a series of 18 patients who underwent the procedure of extracapsular cataract extraction with posterior chamber IOL implantation, combined with pars plana vitrectomy when indicated (67). The final visual acuity was equal to or better than 20/40 in 83% of patients. The excellent visual recovery appeared to be directly related to the control of inflammation before the development of cystoid macular edema. The factors that limited visual recovery were primarily macular and optic nerve pathology (cystoid macular edema, epiretinal membrane formation, and optic atrophy secondary to multiple sclerosis).

Another postoperative complication is the deposition of inflammatory debris on the anterior or posterior surfaces of the IOL. Occasionally, a cocoon-like dense fibrous membrane may envelop the IOL (70,77,78). One or more Nd:YAG laser procedures may be needed to remove the deposits, and occasionally the IOL needs to be removed (77). Michelson et al (77) reported on a series of 15 eyes that underwent this combined procedure and found that even mild chronic inflammation may be sufficient to result in a steady accumulation of IOL deposits and in the development of cystoid macular edema. They suggested that a chronic anti-inflammatory regimen might be beneficial after cataract extraction.

Pars Plana Vitrectomy

Principles

Pars plana vitrectomy may be performed for a vitreoretinal complication or to clear the visual axis in the case of dense vitreous organization and opacification (49). In the case of active vitreous inflammation refractory to corticosteroid therapy, pars plana vitrectomy may not only clear the visual axis, but by removing immunocompetent cells and inflammatory mediators from the vitreous cavity, vitrectomy may alter the course of inflammation and result in stabilization of the disease (1,2,6,68,69). Although the role of vitrectomy on improving cystoid macular edema (CME) remains unclear, vitrectomy may potentially reduce CME either by eliminating the contact between an inflamed vitreous body and the macula or by allowing better penetration or distribution of corticosteroids (2,49,64).

Indications

Indications for vitrectomy have included persistent, dense vitreous inflammation, vitreous hemorrhage, traction retinal detachment, and epiretinal membrane formation. CME refractory to medical therapy may be a relative indication, especially when another vitreoretinal complication exists. When a cataract is present as well, a pars plana lensectomy/vitrectomy may be performed (49). When active NVVB is present, cryotherapy or PSP should be performed in conjunction with pars plana vitrectomy, either preoperatively or intraoperatively (49,64).

Techniques

A standard three-port pars plana vitrectomy approach can be used in all cases (41,49,79). A limbal peritomy is performed to expose the pars plana region (Fig. 50-12). A pars plana infusion cannula is then sutured through the pars plana in the inferotemporal quadrant, 3.0 to 3.5 mm posterior to the limbus. Two additional sclerotomy sites are chosen, superonasally and superotemporally. If a pars plana lensectomy is performed, the myringotomy knife is entered through the pars plana superotemporally, and it is used to break any posterior synechiae and to disrupt the lens nucleus. A bent 20-gauge butterfly needle then replaces the

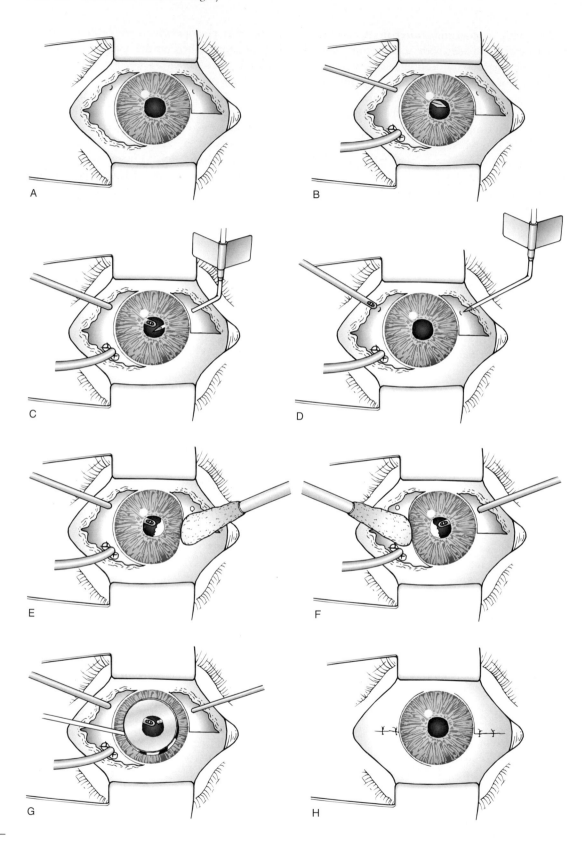

FIGURE 50-12.   (A) *Fornix-based peritomy used to expose sclera over pars plana region.* (B) *Infusion cannular sutured inferotemporal quadrant 3.0 mm posterior to limbus. Microvitreoretinal (MVR) blade disrupts nucleus and breaks posterior synechiae.* (C) *Secondary infusion line prepared for use. Instruments are shown outside pars plana sclerotomies.* (D) *Pars plana lensectomy performed with 20-gauge vitrectomy instrument and secondary infusion line.* (E) *Scleral plug inserted into superior nasal sclerotomy. Scleral depression is used nasally in order to expose peripheral lens material.* (F) *Similar scleral depression temporally with scleral plug in the superior temporal sclerotomy.* (G) *Posterior vitrectomy assisted by contact lens, using three-port approach.* (H) *Final closure of conjunctiva.*

myringotomy blade and is used as a secondary infusion line, entered directly into the lens through the equator (Fig. 50-13A). This secondary infusion cannula helps maintain eye pressure and also helps stabilize the position of the lens. Through the third and final superotemporal sclerotomy site, the nucleus is generally removed by ultrasonic fragmentation or, if the lens is soft, by cutting and aspiration with the standard 20-gauge vitrectomy instrument (Fig. 50-13B).

Once the lens has been removed, attention is directed to the vitreous cavity. The secondary infusion cannula and phacofragmenter are removed and replaced with an endo-illumination probe and the vitrectomy cutter. A complete vitrectomy is performed. Any retinal membranes are dissected or stripped from the retinal surface utilizing a combination of scissors, membrane picks, and forceps. If there is vitreous base exudation or neovascularization, it is treated with scatter photocoagulation, as previously described. Indirect ophthalmoscopy is utilized at the completion of the vitrectomy to search for any other retinal pathology, such as retinal tears. If present, they are treated with retinopexy. Eyes are restored to normal tension at the termination of the vitrectomy by injecting additional balanced salt solution if necessary after closure of all sclerotomies.

Benefits and Complications

The visual outcome in patients who underwent pars plana vitrectomy with or without lensectomy was excellent (49). The average improvement in visual acuity was five Snellen lines. Fifty percent of eyes attained a final visual acuity of 20/40 or better. The principal limiting factors in visual recovery were persistent CME and previous macula-off retinal detachment. Although the impact of vitrectomy on the course of inflammation was difficult to assess, the media

was clear at the last follow-up visit in all eyes and were not believed to limit the visual outcome. Postoperative complications may be quite frequent (58%) and may require additional surgeries. Reported complications include cataract formation, vitreous hemorrhage, tractional retinal detachment, rhegmatogenous retinal detachment, proliferative vitreoretinopathy, corticosteroid-induced glaucoma, and strabismus. Mieler et al (49) suggested that adequate control of active NVVB by either cryotherapy or PSP may reduce the frequency of postoperative complications.

JUVENILE RHEUMATOID ARTHRITIS

Clinical Features

Iridocyclitis related to juvenile rheumatoid arthritis (JRA) is an insidious childhood disease. Patients often experience little or no ocular symptoms while chronic inflammation slowly causes permanent ocular damage (24,80). In early stages, mild anterior chamber inflammation may be observed (24). Advanced stages are characterized by the presence of band keratopathy, posterior synechiae, cataract, glaucoma, and phthisis bulbi (Fig. 50-14). Wolf et al (80) reviewed a series of 51 patients with JRA-related iridocyclitis and identified two factors that might be predictive for a poor visual outcome: 1) the presence of posterior synechiae on initial evaluation and 2) the development of arthritis after the onset of uveitis.

Other factors that have been well correlated with poor visual outcomes include pauciarticular involvement (four or less joints affected), a young age at onset, female gender, and antinuclear antibody positivity (80). The course of JRA-related iridocyclitis is predominantly chronic. Sixty percent of patients have a relapsing and remitting course, while 20%

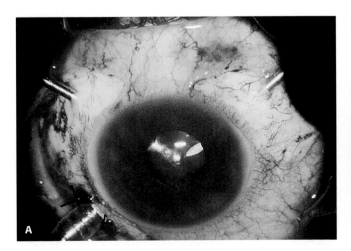
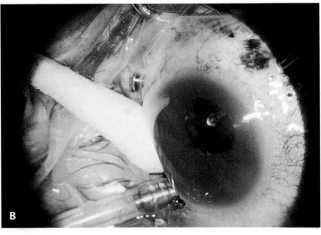

FIGURE 50-13. (A) *Color photograph. Pars plana lensectomy is being performed. A secondary infusion cannula has been placed into lens, while soft lens itself is being removed with vitrectomy cutter.* (B) *Remnants of lens capsule are removed through aid of external indentation with Q-tip.*

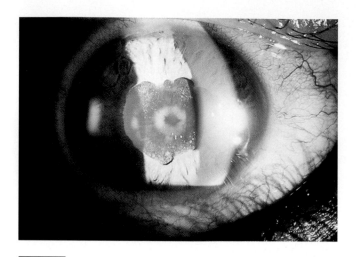

FIGURE 50-14.   *Cataract, anterior segment inflammation, and posterior synechiae in patient with juvenile rheumatoid arthritis.*

of patients have an unremitting course. Only 20% of patients have a single episode of intraocular inflammation (81).

Medical Therapy

Although topical and subtenon corticosteroid injections remain the mainstay in the therapy of anterior uveitis, up to 61% of patients with JRA-related iridocyclitis either do not respond to corticosteroid treatment or require prolonged therapy, with its attendant side effects (82). Patients who are unresponsive to topical corticosteroids generally show no benefit from systemic therapy (80). Moreover, systemic corticosteroid therapy is associated with an increased incidence of cataract and glaucoma, as well as other systemic side effects (80). Therefore, several investigators have advocated the concurrent use of nonsteroidal anti-inflammatory drugs (NSAIDs) and cytotoxic agents (83–85). The use of NSAIDs such as naproxen has allowed for reduction of corticosteroid dose (85).

Immunosuppressive agents such as methotrexate may also play a role in management. In one large study, virtually no toxicity was found in 127 patients in whom low-dose methotrexate was given in the management of JRA-related joint disease (83,86).

Cataract Extraction

Principles

Cataract surgery in patients with JRA may be technically challenging due to the frequent occurrence of posterior synechiae, miotic pupil, and corneal opacification (84). Standard extracapsular cataract extraction techniques have been met with complications, including posterior capsular opacification and cyclitic membrane formation, in as many as 70% of patients (87–90). Capsulectomy by the Nd:YAG

laser may be technically difficult in small children and inadequate in preventing subsequent proliferation of fibrous membranes (88). Cyclitic membranes require surgical removal to prevent the onset of chronic hypotony and phthisis bulbi (88,91). It has therefore been generally accepted that complete removal of the lens capsule and anterior hyaloid is important during cataract surgery to eliminate the scaffold on which cyclitic membrane can form (70,79,83,92).

The techniques of cataract extraction in JRA-related cataract may vary somewhat depending on the surgeon's preference. Pars plana lensectomy/vitrectomy has been advocated as the method of choice by Flynn et al and others (2,70,79,92–94). The advantages of this technique are that 1) it allows good surgical access for removal of peripheral lens material in the presence of small pupils and posterior synechiae, 2) it allows complete removal of the posterior capsule and anterior hyaloid, and 3) it allows removal of inflammatory debris in the central vitreous cavity to provide a clear visual access (79). An alternative procedure that has recently been advocated by Foster et al (83) is a combined phacoemulsification/pars plana vitrectomy. This technique allows for a relatively easy extraction of a lens with hard nucleus or calcified lenticular flakes (92).

The extent of posterior vitrectomy varies greatly among different investigators, from limited anterior vitrectomy to a complete vitrectomy with removal of the posterior hyaloid. A core vitrectomy, by mechanically removing immunocompetent cells and inflammatory mediators from the vitreous cavity, may result in stabilization of inflammation. It is also possible that vitrectomy with removal of the posterior hyaloid may help reduce CME, presumably by eliminating the contact between an inflamed vitreous body and the macula (95). However, the report by Flynn et al (79) has not shown this trend. Some eyes with removal of the posterior hyaloid demonstrate persistent CME, whereas some eyes with attached posterior hyaloid showed resolution of CME.

Indications

Visually significant cataract probably should be extracted as soon as possible in pediatric patients to minimize the risk of developing amblyopia. On the other hand, preoperative control of ocular inflammation is important to minimize the chance for postoperative complications such as secondary glaucoma and secondary pupillary membranes (92). A standard approach is to maintain the eye as free of inflammation as possible for at least three months prior to surgery. Another relative indication for performing pars plana lensectomy/vitrectomy is the presence of chronic hypotony. In such a case, the presence of a cyclitic membrane should be suspected preoperatively and assessed for via echography. Surgical excision of the cyclitic membrane may relieve ciliary body traction and result in normalization of intraocular pressure (24,88,96).

Techniques

The technique of pars plana lensectomy/vitrectomy has been previously described in the section entitled Pars Plana Vitrectomy, and the technique of combined phacoemulsification with pars plana vitrectomy has also been described in the section entitled Cataract Extraction. Therefore these techniques are not discussed here.

Benefits and Complications

Several large series on cataract extraction in JRA patients have demonstrated generally good visual outcomes. A five-year, long-term follow-up of eyes after pars plana lensectomy/vitrectomy documented a final visual acuity of 20/70 or better in 56% of eyes. Approximately 90% of patients experienced an overall improvement in visual acuity. A one-year follow-up of eyes after combined phacoemulsification/pars plana vitrectomy documented a visual acuity of 20/40 or better in 75% of eyes. The average improvement in visual acuity was 7.5 Snellen lines. Causes for reduced visual acuity at follow-up include progressive glaucoma, hypotony maculopathy, chronic CME, macular degeneration secondary to CME, macular pucker, amblyopia, and phthisis bulbi (79,92,95). Although it could not be ascertained whether pars plana lensectomy/vitrectomy altered the course of inflammation, all eyes were found to demonstrate a reduction of inflammation during postoperative follow-up (79).

OCULAR TOXOCARIASIS

Ocular *Toxocara canis* usually presents during childhood at an average age of 7½ years (97). The clinical manifestations of ocular *T. canis* may vary greatly, depending on the degree of intraocular inflammation and traction-related complications (Fig. 50-15). Typically, a retinal granuloma two disk

diameters or larger in size may be found in the posterior pole or the peripheral retina (Fig. 50-16) (98). The eye may be relatively quiet or chronically inflamed with CME as well as prominent exudate observed at the vitreous base. A more severely inflamed eye may present with an endophthalmitis-type picture mimicking retinoblastoma (98,99). Optic neuritis occurring in the setting of *T. canis* infection has also been reported (100–102).

Ocular complications secondary to *T. canis* are usually related to fibrous proliferation. Fibrous traction bands typically extend from the granuloma to the optic disk (see Fig. 50-15) or may involve large areas of the vitreous base. Traction-related complications, such as macular pucker, tractional retinal detachment, or combined tractional/rhegmatogenous retinal detachment, may develop and contribute to visual loss (Fig. 50-17) (103). Rhegmatogenous

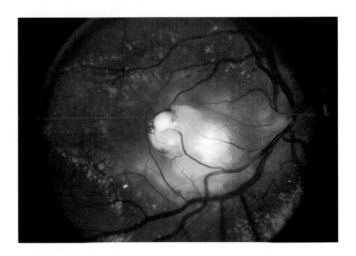

FIGURE 50-16. *Color photograph. Macular granuloma surrounded by exudate in patient with ocular toxocariasis.*

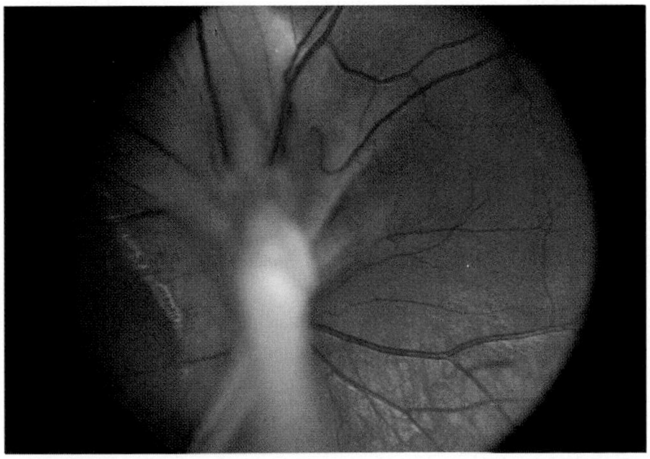

FIGURE 50-15. *Vitreous bands extending from optic disk and coursing inferiorly in patient with ocular toxocariasis. Localized tractional proliferation is noted superior to disk.*

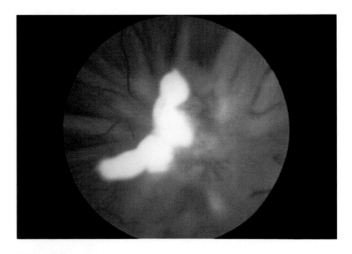

FIGURE 50-17. *Traction retinal detachment associated with posterior granuloma overlying optic disk in patient with ocular toxocariasis.*

retinal detachment with peripheral retinal tears or dialyses may also occur (98). Occasionally, an inoperable total retinal detachment or a cyclitic membrane may be found (98).

Serum antibodies to *T. canis* can be measured by enzyme-linked immunosorbent assay (ELISA). A dilution of 1:8 is considered positive (104). In cases in which the serum antibody titers are low, measurement of the antibody titer in the aqueous or the vitreous can be diagnostic (15). The presence of eosinophils in vitreous biopsy specimens also supports the diagnosis (105).

Medical Therapy

Medical therapy, including the use of anthelmintic and anti-inflammatory agents, has been met with variable success (105). Anthelmintics, such as thiabendazole and diethyl-carbamazine, by destroying viable nematodes, theoretically would eliminate any ongoing or potential injury caused by the motile larvae (106). However, ocular nematodes have been documented to be persistently motile despite anthelmintic treatment (107). In addition, death of a larvae may induce intense ocular inflammation (106). Topical, systemic, and peribulbar corticosteroid treatments can be used to suppress the inflammatory response (108). Laser photocoagulation of the intraocular larvae has also been successful in some cases when direct visualization is possible (109,110).

Surgical Therapy

Principles and Indications

Tractional macular detachment secondary to ocular *T. canis* are not amenable to medical therapy but can be approached with pars plana vitrectomy techniques. Treister and Machemer first reported the use of vitrectomy in ocular *T. canis*. Release of traction on the macula and restoration of a more normal anatomy to the macula may result in visual improvement or prevent progressive visual loss (111). Rhegmatogenous, tractional, or combined retinal detachments are other acceptable indications for surgical intervention. Vitrectomy may also be performed for severe vitreous inflammation and organization in order to clear the visual axis (112,113). In these situations, vitrectomy may help to remove inflammatory mediators and antigenic stimuli as well. Recovery of the intraocular larvae is usually not possible except in rare cases, possibly because of the small size of the organism or because of complete enzymatic digestion of the organism by inflammatory cells (105).

Techniques

For tractional macular detachment, pars plana vitrectomy and membrane peeling may be performed in a manner similar to that for other types of macular pucker (103). The fibrous membranes located between the peripheral granuloma and the optic disk usually have extensions into the underlying retina and need to be carefully lifted off from the retinal surface before they can be severed. These membranes usually remain tightly adherent to the optic disk and the peripheral granuloma, therefore they often need to be circumcised rather than delaminated or peeled. Because the granulomas appear to be an intimal part of the retina, attempts to extirpate the retinal granuloma are usually unsuccessful and may cause undesirable complications.

For eyes with rhegmatogenous retinal detachment without a significant tractional component, scleral buckling procedure may sometimes be performed alone without pars plana vitrectomy. For eyes with traction-related retinal holes, pars plana vitrectomy combined with scleral buckling procedure usually releases the retinal tension and closes the retinal holes.

Fibrous membranes over the pars plana area may be especially difficult to excise and may cause recurrent traction retinal detachment (113). For eyes with recurrent traction retinal detachment, Treister and Machemer (111) described a scleral resection procedure in which the eye wall was shortened to match the shrunken peripheral retina. A 5- to 6-mm wide scleral bed was first created and treated with diathermy. Subretinal fluid was then drained and a 3-mm silicone band was placed around the eye after cryotherapy.

Benefits and Complications

Small et al (103) reported a series in which 10 of the 12 eyes (83%) attained complete retinal reattachment after vitrectomy for tractional complications secondary to ocular *T. canis*. Recurrent retinal detachments occurred in 5 of the 12 eyes (42%) and were associated with fibrous proliferation. Visual acuity improved in seven eyes, remained unchanged in two eyes, and worsened in three eyes. Preoperative tractional retinal fold through the macula was associated with a poor visual outcome. Development of amblyopia is also an important limiting factor in a pediatric population (114).

Belmont et al (112) and Rodriguez et al (113) have reported on the benefits of vitrectomy performed for patients with dense vitreous opacification. Improvement in visual acuity was noted in most cases. Although it is debatable whether vitrectomy has any long-term impact on the course of inflammation, most eyes unresponsive to corticosteroids preoperatively demonstrated a dramatic reduction of intraocular inflammation postoperatively. In addition, clearing of the visual axis prevented the development of amblyopia in some cases.

A single case of complication was reported during attempted excision of a central macular granuloma. A large macular hole was created that eventually led to a persistent total retinal detachment (103).

MISCELLANEOUS UVEITIDES

Pars plana vitrectomy can have a therapeutic role in several other miscellaneous uveitides, especially when vitreous inflammation, opacification, and organization are prominent features. Vitrectomy performed to remove an opacified vitreous body secondary to ocular toxoplasmosis or ankylosing spondylitis-associated uveitis has been reported with good visual outcome (115,116). In rare instances, an intraocular larva may be identified, and vitrectomy may be performed to remove the larvae under direct visualization. Successful evacuations have been reported for tapeworm larva *Cysticercus cellulosae*, larva of roundworm *Porrocaecum*, and various fly larvae (117–121).

CONCLUSION

The use of pars plana vitrectomy and other advanced microsurgical techniques has allowed the surgeon to perform biopsy of the vitreous, retina, and choroid with an acceptable low frequency of complications. Numerous sophisticated analyses including polymerase chain reaction can be performed on biopsy specimens and can help to either identify a specific diagnosis or distinguish between an infectious, neoplastic, or autoimmune disorder (122–132). A more precise diagnosis can help the physician select the appropriate therapy and management.

Pars plana vitrectomy plays an integral role in the management of ocular inflammatory conditions such as pars planitis, JRA-related iridocyclitis, and ocular toxocariasis. Vitrectomy performed for dense vitreous inflammation may not only clear the visual axis but may also potentially alter the course of inflammation by mechanical removal of inflammatory mediators and antigenic stimuli. Other procedures may be combined with pars plana vitrectomy to provide optimal surgical management. Peripheral scatter photocoagulation may be performed together with pars plana vitrectomy to treat vitreous base neovascularization in patients with pars planitis. Pars plana lensectomy or anterior segment phacoemulsification may be combined with pars plana vitrectomy in the management of uveitic cataract. It is likely that as more adjunctive surgical procedures are developed for the management of uveitis, the number of indications for pars plana vitrectomy will increase accordingly, and the anatomic and visual results will continue to improve.

REFERENCES

1. Algvere P, Alanko H, Dickhoff K, et al. Pars plana vitrectomy in the management of intraocular inflammation. *Acta Ophthalmologica* 1981;59:727–736.
2. Diamond JG, Kaplan HJ. Uveitis: effect of vitrectomy combined with lensectomy. *Ophthalmology* 1979;86:1320–1327.
3. Girard LJ, Rodriguez J, Mailman ML, Romano TJ. Cataract and uveitis management by pars plana lensectomy and vitrectomy by ultrasonic fragmentation. *Retina* 1985;5:107–114.
4. Heiligenhaus A, Bornfeld N, Foerster MH, Wessing A. Long term results of pars plana vitrectomy in the management of complicated uveitis. *Br J Ophthalmol* 1994;78:549–554.
5. Kroll P, Romstock F, Grenzebach UH, Wiegand W. Fruhvitrektomie bei endogener juveniler uveitis intermedia-eine langzeitstudie. *Klin Monatsbl Augenheilkd* 1995;206:246–249.
6. Nolthenius PAT, Deutman AF. Surgical treatment of the complications of chronic uveitis. *Ophthalmologica* 1983;186:11–16.
7. Werry H, Honegger H. Pars-plana vitrektomie bei chronischer uveitis. *Klin Monatsbl Augenheilkd* 1987;191:9–12.
8. Laatikainen L, Tarkkanen A, Koivuniemi A. Vitrectomy: clinical data and cytologic findings of vitrectomy specimens. *Int Ophthalmol* 1985;7:215–222.
9. Fujikawa LS, Hauen JP. Immunopathology of vitreous and retinochoroidal biopsy in posterior uveitis. *Ophthalmology* 1990;97:1644–1653.
10. Eisenstein BI. The polymerase chain reaction. A new method of using molecular genetics for medical diagnosis. *N Engl J Med* 1990;322:178–183.
11. Hooper PL, Kaplan HJ. Surgical management of noninfectious endophthalmitis. In: Ryan SJ, Glaser BM, eds. *Retina*. 2nd ed. St. Louis: Mosby-Year Book, 1994:2539–2548.
12. Davis JL, Solomon D, Nussenblatt RB, et al. Immunocytochemical staining of vitreous cells. *Ophthalmology* 1992;99:250–256.
13. Maguire A, Green W, Michels R, Erozan YS. Recovery of intraocular *Toxocara canis* by pars plana vitrectomy. *Ophthalmology* 1990;97:675–680.
14. Biglan AW, Glickman LT, Lobes LA Jr. Serum and vitreous *Toxocara* antibody in nematode endophthalmitis. *Am J Ophthalmol* 1979;86:898–901.
15. Baarsma GS, Luyendijk L, Kijlstra A, et al. Analysis of local antibody production in the vitreous humor of patients with severe uveitis. *Am J Ophthalmol* 1991;112:147–150.
16. Kaplan HJ, Meredith TA, Aaberg TM, Keller RH. Reclassification of intraocular reticulum cell sarcoma (histiocytic lymphoma): immunologic characterization of vitreous cells. *Arch Ophthalmol* 1980;98:707–710.
17. Parver LM, Font RL. Malignant lymphoma of the retina and brain: initial diagnosis by cytologic examination of vitreous aspirate. *Arch Ophthalmol* 1979;97:1505–1507.
18. Engel HM, Green WR, Michels RG, et al. Diagnostic vitrectomy. *Retina* 1981;1:121–149.
19. de Bustros S, Thompson JT, Michels RG. Nuclear sclerosis after vitrectomy for idiopathic epiretinal membranes. *Am J Ophthalmol* 1988;105:160–164.
20. Lucke K, Laqua H. Netzhautkomplikationen bei der pars-plana-vitrektomie. *Klin Monatsbl Augenheilkd* 1985;187:17–20.
21. Ridley ME, McDonald HR, Sternberg P Jr, et al. Retinal manifestations of ocular lymphoma (reticulum cell sarcoma). *Ophthalmol* 1992;99:1153–1161.
22. Lopez JS, Chan CC, Burnier M, et al. Immunohistochemistry findings in primary intraocular lymphoma. *Am J Ophthalmol* 1991;112:472–474. Letter.
23. Constable IJ, Thompson D, van Bockxmeer F. The value of rational biopsy. Tissue culture of chorioretinal biopsies. *Trans Ophthalmol Soc UK* 1983;103:475–479.
24. Nussenblatt RB, Palestine AG. *Uveitis: fundamentals and clinical practice*. Chicago: Year Book Medical, 1989:145–184.
25. Buckley CE III, Gills JP Jr. Cyclophosphamide therapy of peripheral uveitis. *Arch Intern Med* 1969;124:29–35.
26. Chan CC, Palestine AG, Davis JL, et al. Role of chorioretinal biopsy in inflammatory eye disease. *Ophthalmology* 1991;98:1281–1286.
27. Peyman GA, Juarez CP, Raichand M. Full-thickness eye-wall biopsy: long-term results in 9 patients. *Br J Ophthalmol* 1981;65:723–726.
28. Rutzen AR, Ortega-Larrocea G, Dugel PU, et al. Clinicopathologic study of retinal and choroidal biopsies in intraocular inflammation. *Am J Ophthalmol* 1995;119:597–611.
29. Moorthy RS, Smith RE, Rao NA. Progressive ocular toxoplasmosis patients with acquired immunodeficiency syndrome. *Am J Ophthalmol* 1993;115:742–747.
30. Martin DF, Chan CC, deSmet MD, et al. The role of chorioretinal biopsy in the management of posterior uveitis. *Ophthalmol* 1993;100:705–714.
31. Kirmani MH, Thomas EL, Rao NA, Laborde RP. Intraocular reticulum cell sarcoma: diagnosis by choroidal biopsy. *Br J Ophthalmol* 1987;71:748–752.
32. Kumar SR, Gill PS, Wagner DG, et al. Human T-cell lymphotropic virus type 1-associated retinal lymphoma. *Arch Ophthalmol* 1994;112:954–959.
33. Freeman WR, Wiley CA, Gross JG, et al. Endoretinal biopsy in immunosuppressed and healthy patients with retinitis. *Ophthalmology* 1989;96:1559–1565.
34. Elkins BS, Holland GN, Opremcak M, et al. Ocular toxoplasmosis misdiagnosed as cytomegalovirus retinopathy in immunocompromised patients. *Ophthalmology* 1994;101:499–507.
35. Malinowski SM, Folk JC, Pulido JS. Pars planitis. *Curr Opin Ophthalmol* 1994;5:72–82.
36. Dinning WJ. Intermediate uveitis: history, terminology, definition of pars planitis: systemic disease associations. *Dev Ophthalmol* 1992;23:3–8.
37. Zierhut M, Foster CS. Multiple sclerosis, sarcoidosis, and other diseases in patients with pars planitis. *Dev Ophthalmol* 1992;23:41–47.

38. Breeveld J, Rothova A, Kuiper H. Intermediate uveitis and Lyme borreliosis. *Br J Ophthalmol* 1992;76:181–182.

39. Mochizuki M, Watanabe T, Yamaguchi K, et al. Uveitis associated with human T-cell lymphotropic virus type 1. *Am J Ophthalmol* 1992;114:123–129.

40. Barr CC, Green WR, Payne JW, et al. Intraocular reticulum cell sarcoma: clinicopathologic study of four cases and review of the literature. *Surv Ophthalmol* 1975;19:224–239.

41. Capone A Jr, Aaberg TM. Intermediate uveitis. In: Albert DM, Jakobiec FA, eds. *Principles and practice of ophthalmology: clinical practice.* 1st ed. Philadelphia: WB Saunders, 1994:423–442.

42. Knox DL, Bayles TM, Yardley JH, Charache P. Whipple's disease presenting with ocular inflammation and minimal intestinal symptoms. *Johns Hopkins Med J* 1968;123:175.

43. Wilkinson CP, Welch RB. Intraocular *Toxocara. Am J Ophthalmol* 1971;71:921–930.

44. Wong VG, McFarlin DE. Primary familial amyloidosis. *Arch Ophthalmol* 1967;78:208–213.

45. Tang WM, Pulido JS, Eckels DD, et al. The association of HLA-DR15 and intermediate uveitis. *Am J Ophthalmol* 1997;123:70–75.

46. Smith RE, Godfrey WA, Kimura SJ. Chronic cyclitis. I. Course and visual prognosis. *Trans Am Acad Ophthalmol Otolaryngol* 1973;77:760–768.

47. Belfort R, Nussenblatt RB, Lottemberg C, et al. Spontaneous lens subluxation in uveitis. *Am J Ophthalmol* 1990;110:714–716. Letter.

48. Khoudadoust AA, Karnama Y, Stoessel KM, Puklin JE. Pars planitis and autoimmune endotheliopathy. *Am J Ophthalmol* 1986;102:633–639.

49. Mieler WF, Will BR, Lewis H, Aaberg TM. Vitrectomy in the management of peripheral uveitis. *Ophthalmology* 1988;95:859–864.

50. Brockhurst RJ, Schepens CL, Okamura ID. Uveitis. II. Peripheral uveitis. Clinical description and differential diagnosis. *Am J Ophthalmol* 1960;49:1257.

51. Felder KS, Brockhurst RJ. Neovascular fundus abnormalities in peripheral uveitis. *Arch Ophthalmol* 1982;100:750–754.

52. Brockhurst RJ, Schepens CL. Uveitis. *Arch Ophthalmol* 1968;80:748–753.

53. Pederson JE, Kenyon KR, Green WR, Maumenee AE. Pathology of pars planitis. *Am J Ophthalmol* 1978;86:762–764.

54. Nozik RA. Results of treatment of ocular toxoplasmosis with injectable corticosteroids. *Trans Am Acad Ophthalmol Otolaryngol* 1977;83:811–818.

55. Goldstein DA, Fiscella RG, Tessler HH. Biochemical quantification of triamcinolone in subconjunctival depots. *Arch Ophthalmol* 1996;114:363–364.

56. Kalina PH, Erie JC, Rosenbaum L. Biochemical quantification of triamcinolone in subconjunctival depots. *Arch Ophthalmol* 1995;113:867–869.

57. Maumenee AE. Clinical entities in "uveitis": an approach to the study of intraocular inflammation. XXVI Edward Jackson Memorial Lecture. *Am J Ophthalmol* 1970;69:1–27.

58. de Vries J, Baarsma GS, Zaal MJ, et al. Cyclosporin in the treatment of severe chronic idiopathic uveitis. *Br J Ophthalmol* 1990;74:344–349.

59. Nussenblatt RB, Palestine AG, Chan CC. Cyclosporin A therapy in the treatment of intraocular inflammatory disease resistant to systemic corticosteroids and cytotoxic agents. *Am J Ophthalmol* 1983;96:275–282.

60. Aaberg TM, Cesarz TJ, Flickinger RR. Treatment of peripheral uveoretinitis by cryotherapy. *Am J Ophthalmol* 1973;75:685–688.

61. Devenyi RG, Mieler WF, Lambrou FH, et al. Cryopexy of the vitreous base in the management of peripheral uveitis. *Am J Ophthalmol* 1988;106:135–138.

62. Josephberg RG, Kanter ED, Jaffee RM. A fluorescein angiographic study of patients with pars planitis and peripheral exudation (snowbanking) before and after cryopexy. *Ophthalmology* 1994;101:1262–1266.

63. Phillips WB II, Bergren RL, McNamara JA. Pars planitis presenting with vitreous hemorrhage. *Ophthalmic Surg* 1993;24:630–631.

64. Park SE, Mieler WF, Pulido JS. Peripheral scatter photocoagulation for neovascularization associated with pars planitis. *Arch Ophthalmol* 1995;113:1277–1280.

65. Jaccoma EH, Conway BP, Campochiaro PA. Cryotherapy causes extensive breakdown of the blood-retinal barrier: a comparison with argon laser photocoagulation. *Arch Ophthalmol* 1985;103:1728–1730.

66. Foster CS, Fons LP, Singh G. Cataract surgery and intraocular lens implantation in patients with uveitis. *Ophthalmology* 1989;96:281–288.

67. Kaufman AH, Foster CS. Cataract extraction in patients with pars planitis. *Ophthalmology* 1993;100:1210–1217.

68. Dangel ME, Stark WJ, Michels RG. Surgical management of cataract associated with chronic uveitis. *Ophthalmic Surg* 1983;14:145–149.

69. Diamond JG, Kaplan HJ. Lensectomy and vitrectomy for complicated cataract secondary to uveitis. *Arch Ophthalmol* 1978;96:1798–1804.

70. Koenig SB, Mieler WF, Han DP, Abrams GW. Combined phacoemulsification, pars plana vitrectomy, and posterior chamber intraocular lens insertion. *Arch Ophthalmol* 1992;110:1101–1104.

71. Foster RE, Lowder CY, Meisler DM, Zakov ZN. Extracapsular cataract extraction and posterior chamber intraocular lens implantation in uveitis patients. *Ophthalmology* 1992;99:1234–1241.

72. Blankenship GW, Flynn HW, Kokame GT. Posterior chamber intraocular lens insertion during pars plana lensectomy and vitrectomy for complications of proliferative diabetic retinopathy. *Am J Ophthalmol* 1989;108:1–5.

73. Raizman MB. Cataract surgery in uveitis patients. In: Steinert RF, ed. *Cataract Surgery: Techniques, Complications, and Management.* 1st ed. Philadelphia: WB Saunders, 1995:243–246.

74. Foster RE, Lowder CY, Meisler DM, et al. Combined extracapsular cataract extraction, posterior chamber intraocular lens implantation, and pars plana vitrectomy. *Ophthalmic Surg* 1993;24:446–452.

75. Walker J, Rao NA, Ober RR, et al. A combined anterior and posterior approach to cataract surgery in patients with chronic uveitis. *Intl Ophthalmol* 1993;17:63–69.

76. Hooper PL, Rao NA, Smith RE. Cataract extraction in uveitis patients. *Surv Ophthalmol* 1990;35:120–144.

77. Michelson JB, Friedlaender MH, Nozik RA. Lens implant surgery in pars planitis. *Ophthalmology* 1990;97:1023–1026.

78. Tessler HH, Farber MD. Intraocular lens implantation versus no intraocular lens implantation in patients with chronic iridocyclitis and pars planitis. *Ophthalmology* 1993;100:1206–1209.

79. Flynn HW, Davis JL, Culbertson WW. Pars plana lensectomy and vitrectomy for complicated cataracts in juvenile rheumatoid arthritis. *Ophthalmology* 1988;95:1114–1119.

80. Wolf MD, Lichter PR, Ragsdale CG. Prognostic factors in the uveitis of juvenile rheumatoid arthritis. *Ophthalmology* 1987;94:1242–1248.

81. Rosenberg AM. Uveitis associated with juvenile rheumatoid arthritis. *Semin Arthritis Rheum* 1987;16:158–173.

82. Wakefield D, McCluskey P, Penny R. Intravenous pulse methylprednisolone therapy in severe inflammatory eye disease. *Arch Ophthalmol* 1986;104:847–851.

83. Foster CS, Barrett F. Cataract development and cataract surgery in patients with juvenile rheumatoid arthritis-associated iridocyclitis. *Ophthalmology* 1993;100:809–817.

84. O'Brien JM, Albert DM, Foster CS. Juvenile Rheumatoid Arthritis. In: Albert DM, Jakobiec FA, eds. *Principles and practice of ophthalmology: clinical practice.* 1st ed. Philadelphia: WB Saunders, 1994;233:2873–2886.

85. Olson NY, Lindsley CB, Godfrey WA. Nonsteroidal antiinflammatory drug therapy in chronic childhood iridocyclitis. *Am J Dis Child* 1988;142:1289–1292.

86. Giannini EH, Brewer EJ, Kuzmina N, et al. Methotrexate in resistant juvenile rheumatoid arthritis. Results of the U.S.A.-U.S.S.R. double-blind, placebo-controlled trial. *N Engl J Med* 1992;326:1043–1049.

87. Kanski JJ, Shun-Shin GA. Systemic uveitis syndromes in childhood: an analysis of 340 cases. *Ophthalmology* 1984;91:1247–1252.

88. Kanski JJ. Juvenile arthritis and uveitis. *Surv Ophthalmol* 1990;31:253–267.

89. Key SN, Kimura SJ. Iridocyclitis associated with juvenile rheumatoid arthritis. *Am J Ophthalmol* 1975;80:425–429.

90. Praeger DL, Schneider HA, Sakowski AD Jr, Jacobs JC. Kelman procedure in the treatment of complicated cataract of the uveitis of Still's disease. *Trans Ophthal Soc UK* 1976;96:108–171.

91. Puig-Llano Manuel, Irvine AR, Stone RD. Pupillary membrane excision and anterior vitrectomy in eyes after uveitis. *Am J Ophthalmol* 1979;87:533–535.

92. Kanski JJ. Lensectomy for complicated cataract in juvenile chronic iridocyclitis. *Br J Ophthalmol* 1992;76:72–75.

93. Nobe JR, Kokoris N, Diddie KR, et al. Lensectomy-vitrectomy in chronic uveitis. *Retina* 1983;3:71–76.

94. Petrilli AN, Belfort R Jr, Abreu MT, et al. Ultrasonic fragmentation of cataract in uveitis. *Retina* 1986;6:61–65.

95. Fox GM, Flynn HW, Davis JL, Culbertson W. Causes of reduced visual acuity on long-term follow-up after cataract extraction in patients with uveitis and juvenile rheumatoid arthritis. *Am J Ophthalmol* 1992;114:708–714.

96. Smith RE, Nozik RA. Surgery in uveitis patients. In: Smith RE, Nozik RA, eds. *Uveitis: a clinical approach to diagnosis and management.* Baltimore: Williams & Wilkins, 1989:113–114.

97. Brown DH. Ocular *Toxocara canis*: II. Clinical review. *J Pediatr Ophthalmol* 1970;7:182–191.

98. Hagler WS, Pollard ZF, Jarrett WH, Donnelly EH. Results of surgery for ocular *Toxocara canis. Ophthalmology* 1981;88:1081–1086.

99. Wilder HC. Nematode endophthalmitis. *Trans Am Acad Ophthalmol Otolaryngol* 1950;55:99.

100. Bird AC, Smith JL, Curtin VT. Nematode optic neuritis. *Am J Ophthalmol* 1970;69:72–77.

101. Molk R. Treatment of toxocaral optic neuritis. *J Clin Neuro Ophthalmol* 1982;2:109–112.

102. Philips CI, Mackenzie AD. Toxocaral larval papillitis. *Br Med J* 1973;1:154–155.

103. Small KW, McCuen BW II, de Juan E Jr, Machemer R. Surgical management of retinal traction caused by toxocariasis. *Am J Ophthalmol* 1989;108:10–14.

104. Shields JA, Felberg NT, Federmen JF. Discussion of ELISA for diagnosis of ocular toxocariasis. *Ophthalmology* 1979;86:750.

105. Maguire AM, Green WR, Michels RG, Erozan YS. Recovery of intraocular *Toxocara canis* by pars plana vitrectomy. *Ophthalmology* 1990;97:675–680.

106. Tabbara KF. Other parasitic infections. In: Tabbara KF, Hyndiuk RA, eds. *Infections of the eye.* Boston: Little, Brown, 1986.

107. Sorr EM. Meandering ocular toxocariasis. *Retina* 1984;4:90–96.

108. Molk R. Ocular toxocariasis: a review of the literature. *Ann Ophthalmol* 1983;15:216–231.

109. Fitzgerald CR, Rubin ML. Intraocular parasite destroyed by photocoagulation. *Arch Ophthalmol* 1974;91:162–164.

110. Siam AL. Toxocaral chorio-retinitis. Treatment of early cases with photocoagulation. *Br J Ophthalmol* 1973;57:700–703.

111. Treister G, Machemer RM. Results of vitrectomy for rare proliferative and hemorrhagic diseases. *Am J Ophthalmol* 1977;84:394–412.

112. Belmont JB, Irvine A, Benson W, O'Connor GR. Vitrectomy in ocular toxocariasis. *Arch Ophthalmol* 1982;100:1912–1915.

113. Rodriguez A. Early pars plana vitrectomy in chronic endophthalmitis of toxocariasis. *Graefe's Arch Clin Exp Ophthalmol* 1986;224:218–220.

114. Grand MG, Roper-Hall G. Pars plana vitrectomy for ocular toxocariasis. *Retina* 1981;1:258–261.

115. Belmont JB, Michelson JB. Vitrectomy in uveitis associated with ankylosing spondylitis. *Am J Ophthalmol* 1982;94:300–304.

116. Fitzgerald CR. Pars plana vitrectomy for vitreous opacity secondary to presumed toxoplasmosis. *Arch Ophthalmol* 1980;98:321–323.

117. Custis PH, Pakalnis VA, Klintworth GK, et al. Posterior internal ophthalmomyiasis. Identification of a surgically removed cuterebra larva by scanning electron microscopy. *Ophthalmology* 1983;90:1583–1590.

118. Goodart RA, Riekhof FT, Beaver PC. Subretinal nematode: an unusual etiology for uveitis and retinal detachment. *Retina* 1985;5:87–90.

119. Hutton WL, Vaiser A, Snyder WB. Pars plana vitrectomy for removal of intravitreous cysticercus. *Am J Ophthalmol* 1976;81:571–573.

120. Rapoza PA, Michels RG, Semeraro RJ, Green WR. Vitrectomy for excision of intraocular larva: (hypoderma species). *Retina* 1986;6:99–104.

121. Syrdalen P, Nitter T, Mehl R. Ophthalmomyiasis interna posterior: report of case caused by the reindeer warble fly larva and review of previous reported cases. *Br J Ophthalmol* 1982;66:589–593.

122. Donald PR, Victor TC, Jordaan AM, et al. Polymerase chain reaction in the diagnosis of tuberculous meningitis. *Scand J Infect Dis* 1993;25:613–617.

123. Kowalski RP, Gordon YJ, Romanowski EG, et al. A comparison of enzyme immunoassay and polymerase chain reaction with the clinical examination for diagnosing ocular herpetic disease. *Ophthalmology* 1993;100:530–533.

124. Hellinger WC, Bolling JP, Smith TF, Campbell RJ. Varicella-zoster virus retinitis in a patient with AIDS-related complex: case report and brief review of the acute retinal necrosis syndrome. *Clin Infect Dis* 1993;15:208–212.

125. Xu W, Sundqvist VA, Brytting M, Linde A. Diagnosis of cytomegalovirus infections using polymerase chain reaction, virus isolation and serology. *Scand J Infect Dis* 1993;25:311–316.

126. Mustafa MM, Weitman SD, Winick NJ, et al. Subacute measles encephalitis in the young immunocompromised host: report of two cases diagnosed by polymerase chain reaction and treated with ribavirin and review of literature. *Clin Infect Dis* 1993;16:654–660.

127. Pachner AR, Delaney E. The polymerase chain reaction in the diagnosis of Lyme neuroborreliosis. *Ann Neurol* 1993;34:544–550.

128. Hay PE, Clarke JR, Taylor-Robison D, Goldmeier D. Detection of treponemal DNA in the CSF of patients with syphilis and HIV infection using the polymerase chain reaction. *Genitourin Med* 1988;66:428–432.

129. Verhofstede C, Reniers S, Colebunders R, et al. Polymerase chain reaction in the diagnosis of Toxoplasma encephalitis. *AIDS* 1993;7:1539–1541.

130. Anderson B, Sims K, Regnery R, et al. Detection of *Rochalimaea henselae* DNA in specimens from cat scratch disease patients by PCR. *J Clin Microbiol* 1994;32:942–948.

131. Relman DA, Schmidt TM, MacDermott RP, Falkow S. Identification of the uncultured bacillus of Whipple's disease. *N Engl J Med* 1992;327:293–301.

132. Sexton DJ, Kanj SS, Wilson K, et al. The use of a polymerase chain reaction as a diagnostic test for Rocky Mountain spotted fever. *Am J Trop Med Hyg* 1994;50:59–63.

Management of Intraocular Tumors

J. William Harbour   Timothy G. Murray

The management of intraocular tumors has evolved dramatically in recent years. The ophthalmic surgeon who manages these tumors must now be aware of the wide variety of therapeutic options that are available. In this chapter, the principles and techniques of management for posterior uveal melanoma, retinoblastoma, melanocytic iris tumors, and intraocular vascular tumors will be discussed.

POSTERIOR UVEAL MELANOMA

Posterior uveal melanoma is the most common primary intraocular malignancy. The incidence in the United States is about 5 to 8 cases per million per year. Risk factors for uveal melanoma include light skin pigmentation, blue irides, and increasing age (101). Most patients are in their sixth or seventh decade at diagnosis, although younger individuals may be affected (20). There is a slight male predominance, and a possible link to sunlight exposure has been suggested by some studies (101).

Genetics

In contrast to retinoblastoma, uveal membranes are rarely multiple, bilateral, or familial. This suggests that acquired, rather than inherited, genetic abnormalities mainly are responsible for uveal melanoma. Nonrandom abnormalities on chromosomes 3, 6, and 8 have been reported (95), but no specific cancer genes have been linked to melanoma.

Diagnosis

Symptoms
Optimal management of intraocular tumors initially depends on establishing an accurate diagnosis. Posterior uveal melanomas are often asymptomatic, but they may present with visual changes, visual field abnormalities, photopsias, redness, or discomfort.

Clinical Appearance
The typical clinical appearance is of a pigmented choroidal mass, often with overlying orange lipofuscin pigment and subretinal fluid (Fig. 51-1). Thicker tumors (usually over 5 mm) may assume a "collar button" or "mushroom" configuration, indicating that the tumor has broken through Bruch's membrane (Fig. 51-2). Such tumors may develop retinal invasion, which may be recognized as a rough or velvety texture of the retinal surface overlying the tumor. About 30% of tumors are at least partially amelanotic. Subretinal or vitreous hemorrhage is occasionally seen in large tumors that have ruptured through Bruch's membrane. Hemorrhage associated with smaller masses suggests a simulating lesion. Lipid exudation is distinctly uncommon in melanoma and is more consistent with vascular leakage from a disciform process or retinal arterial macroaneurysm. Cystoid macular edema occasionally can be present. Panuveitis, gross extrascleral tumor extension, and orbital cellulitis can be seen in neglected cases, though rarely.

Due to their peripheral location, ciliary body melanomas may grow to a large size before clinical detection. Patients are usually asymptomatic but may have visual symptoms related to induced astigmatism, secondary cataract, exudative retinal detachment, or direct tumor obstruction of the visual axis. Clinical features may include sentinel vessels, a retropupillary mass, iridodialysis from tumor invasion into the anterior chamber, and extrascleral extension. Occult ciliary body melanomas may occasionally be detected during cataract surgery (89).

Ancillary Diagnostic Tests
Slit-lamp biomicroscopy and indirect ophthalmoscopy are essential in evaluating posterior uveal tumors, as are transil-

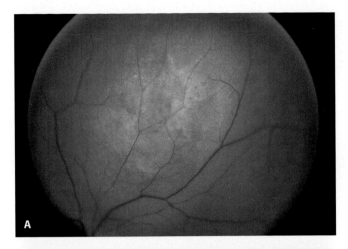

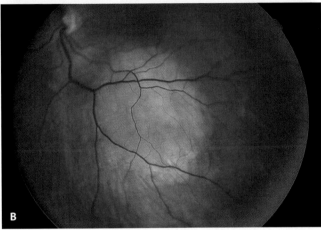

FIGURE 51-1.   A. *Pigmented choroidal melanoma with orange pigment and overlying subretinal fluid. B. Amelanotic choroidal melanoma.*

Table 51-1.   Diagnostic Tests for Posterior Uveal Melanoma

Ultrasonography, A- and B-scan
Fluorescein angiography
Magnetic resonance imaging (MRI)
Fine-needle aspiration biopsy
Computed tomography (CT)
Immunoscintigraphy
Color Doppler imaging

lumination and gonioscopy for tumors involving the ciliary body. In addition, a number of ancillary diagnostic tests are helpful in establishing the correct diagnosis (Table 51-1) (9,25,91). The most useful tests include ultrasonography, fluorescein angiography, and magnetic resonance imaging. Intraocular fine-needle biopsy occasionally is helpful when the diagnosis cannot be established by non-invasive means.

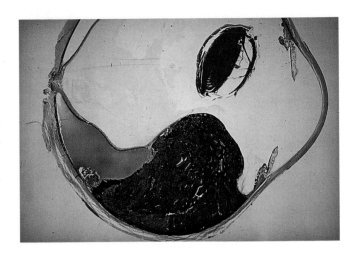

FIGURE 51-2.   *Histopathologic section of eye containing choroidal melanoma, demonstrating mushroom configuration.*

Ultrasonography   Ultrasound is the most useful ancillary diagnostic test in confirming the diagnosis of posterior uveal melanoma. A-scan ultrasonography typically shows low to medium internal reflectivity, decreasing spike amplitude, and spontaneous vascular spikes (Fig. 51-3A). B-scan imaging typically shows a dome- or mushroom-shaped mass, an internal acoustic "quiet zone," choroidal excavation, and orbital acoustic shadowing (Fig. 51-3B). Extrascleral foci of tumor extension as small as 0.5 mm can be detected.

Ultrasonography is particularly helpful in eyes with dense vitreous hemorrhage or other media opacity. High frequency ultrasound biomicroscopy may occasionally be helpful in ciliary body tumors to more clearly delineate anterior structures.

Fluorescein Angiography   The fluorescein angiographic pattern of posterior uveal melanoma is not diagnostic but can be helpful in ruling out simulating hemorrhagic lesions, such as retinal arterial macroaneurysms and disciform lesions, since blood will block choroidal fluorescence. The typical angiographic features of posterior uveal melanoma include early hypofluorescence with pinpoint areas of hyperfluorescence, intrinsic tumor vessels in larger tumors (the so-called "double circulation"), and late leakage (Fig. 51-4).

Magnetic Resonance Imaging (MRI)   MRI is not routinely performed for posterior uveal melanoma but can be helpful in ruling out simulating lesions, such as choroidal hemangiomas or hemorrhagic disciform lesions. The typical pattern for posterior uveal melanoma is a hyperintense signal on T1-weighting, hypointense signal on T2-weighting, and tumor enhancement with gadolinium (Fig. 51-5). This pattern is seen in up to 95% of posterior uveal melanomas (32). Fat-suppression technique on T1-weighted images may be helpful in juxtapapillary tumors to rule out optic nerve extension (32).

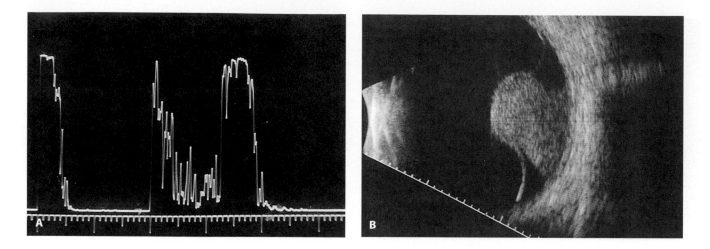

FIGURE 51-3. A. *A-scan ultrasonography of choroidal melanoma, demonstrating low to medium internal reflectivity and decreasing spike amplitude.* B. *B-scan ultrasonography of choroidal melanoma, demonstrating mushroom shape, internal acoustic "quiet zone," choroidal excavation, and orbital acoustic shadowing.*

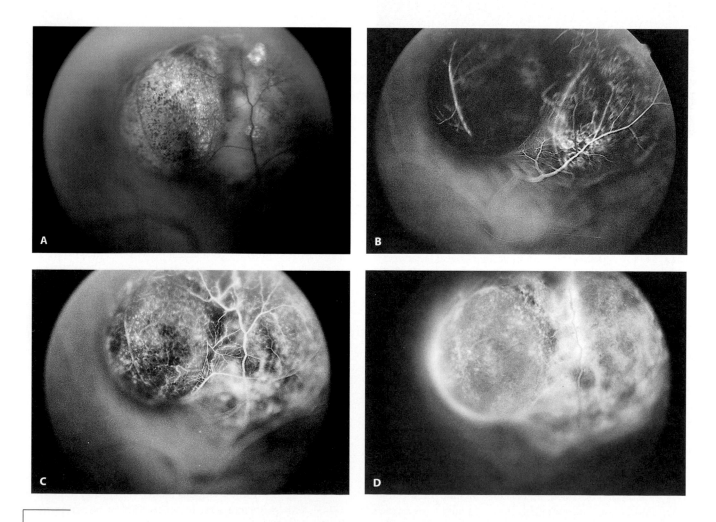

FIGURE 51-4. *Fluorescein angiography of choroidal melanoma.* A. *Early frames demonstrate lesional hypofluorescence with pinpoint areas of hyperfluorescence.* B. *and* C. *The intrinsic tumor vessels can be distinguished from normal choroidal vessels in larger tumors. This is the so-called "double circulation" sign.* D. *Late frames demonstrate leakage of fluorescein.*

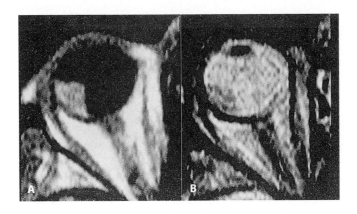

FIGURE 51-5. *MRI of choroidal melanoma. A. T1-weighted image demonstrating hyperintense tumor signal, relative to vitreous. B. T2-weighted image demonstrating hypointense tumor signal, relative to vitreous.*

Intraocular Fine-Needle Biopsy Fine-needle biopsy of intraocular tumors is occasionally indicated when the diagnosis of a posterior segment mass cannot reliably be established by noninvasive measures, and when the results of the biopsy will determine the subsequent treatment. Both transvitreal and transscleral approaches have been described (8,28). Both techniques have very low complication rates, and extraocular tumor seeding is extremely rare with either method when careful surgical technique is used.

Either local retrobulbar or general anesthesia can be used. A conjunctival peritomy is performed, the four rectus muscles are secured with 2-0 cotton sutures, and the tumor is localized by transillumination and indirect ophthalmoscopy. For the transscleral approach, a short 25- or 27-gauge beveled needle is passed through the sclera to a depth of 3 to 5 mm (usually to within 2 mm of the tumor apex), at a 30° to 45° angle to the scleral surface (Fig. 51-6). Moderate aspiration is applied while moving the needle tip back and forth slightly along the scleral track in a sawing motion. After three or four movements aspiration is released, the needle is removed, and a drop of cyanoacrylate tissue adhesive is immediately placed over the scleral entrance wound. If possible, the cytopathologist should be present in the operating room to prepare and analyze the specimen. In this way, the biopsy can be repeated if an inadequate specimen is obtained, and the appropriate surgical intervention can be initiated.

For the transvitreal approach, a long 25- or 27-gauge needle is connected by flexible tubing to a 5-cc syringe, passed through the pars plana 3.5 to 4.0 mm posterior to the limbus, and guided into the tumor mass using indirect ophthalmoscopy (or using the operating microscope and contact lens). The location of the scleral entry site should be 180° away from choroidal tumors and 45° away from ciliary body tumors. The surgeon employs a slight back-and-forth movement while the assistant applies moderate aspiration using the syringe (see Fig. 51-6). Although retinal

Uveal biopsy

transscleral

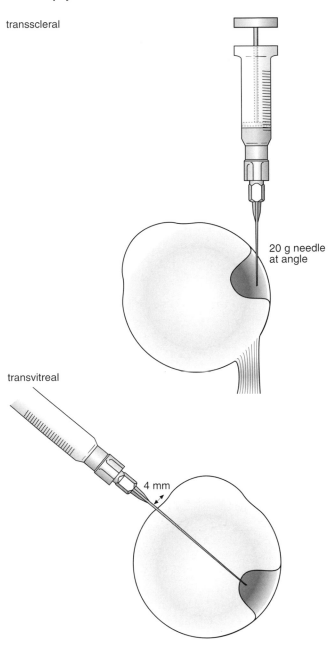

transvitreal

FIGURE 51-6. *Fine-needle aspiration biopsy techniques. A. Transscleral approach. B. Transvitreal approach.*

detachment following this procedure is rare, some surgeons prefer to treat the edges of the retinal break with laser photocoagulation.

Differential Diagnosis

A large number of benign and malignant processes can simulate posterior uveal melanoma (Table 51-2) (9,25,91). The ophthalmic surgeon who manages intraocular tumors

Table 51-2.   Conditions Considered in Differential Diagnosis of Posterior Uveal Melanoma

Choroidal nevus
Choroidal metastasis
Choroidal detachment
Choroidal hemangioma
Choroidal osteoma
Macular or extramacular disciform process
Retinal arterial macroaneurysm
Posterior scleritis
Congenital hypertrophy of the retinal pigment epithelium
Reactive hyperplasia of the retinal pigment epithelium
Combined hamartoma of the retina and retinal pigment epithelium
Bilateral diffuse uveal melanocytic proliferation
Retinal detachment
Retinoschisis
Melanocytoma

Table 51-3.   Treatment Considerations for Posterior Uveal Melanoma

Age
Overall health
Patient attitude toward treatment
Visual potential of the involved eye
Visual potential of the uninvolved eye
Metastatic workup
    Physical examination
    Liver function tests
    Chest x-ray
    Abdominal imaging studies (as indicated)
Features of the tumor
    Size
    Location
    Signs of activity

must be aware of the clinical features and distinguishing characteristics of these simulating lesions (19,25,91).

Treatment Considerations

Many factors must be considered in deciding on the best treatment for each individual patient (Table 51-3). Pretreatment metastatic workup (physical examination, liver function tests, and chest x-ray) is extremely important for treatment planning. If the results of this workup are suggestive of metastatic disease, further confirmation with thoracic or abdominal imaging studies are indicated before deciding on ocular treatment. The size and intraocular location of the tumor provide prognostic information regarding postoperative vision and survival and may influence the choice of treatment. The visual potential of the involved eye and the opposite eye must be considered, since most treatments are vision-threatening. Finally, the patient's age,

Table 51-4.   Clinical Risk Factors for Growth of Intermediate Choroidal Melanocytic Tumors

Increased thickness
Subretinal fluid
Overlying orange (lipofuscin) pigment
Visual symptoms
Pinpoint hyperfluorescence on fluorescein angiography
Internal acoustic quiet zone on B-scan ultrasonography

overall health, and attitude toward treatment are important management considerations.

Treatment Modalities

Observation

Observation is often indicated for melanocytic tumors with features intermediate between nevi and melanomas, or when a benign simulating lesion is suspected. Intermediate melanocytic tumors are generally less than 3 mm in thickness, less than 10 mm in largest basal dimension, and may demonstrate one or more risk factors for tumor growth (Table 51-4) (23). These tumors should be closely observed for evidence of growth, with the follow-up interval determined by the number of risk factors for growth that are present. If three or more risk factors (especially subretinal fluid and visual symptoms) are present, prompt treatment should be considered.

Observation consists of interval examination with indirect ophthalmoscopy, fundus drawing, ultrasonography, and fundus photography. There is no convincing evidence that short periods of careful observation of small to medium-sized melanomas for growth prior to treatment significantly increases the likelihood of systemic metastasis (18,23,43). About 10% per year of intermediate melanocytic tumors will grow substantially during observation (18), and most of these should be promptly treated.

Laser Therapy

Indications   Currently, there are four main indications for laser photocoagulation therapy: 1) ablation of thin marginal recurrences following radiation treatment (53), 2) primary ablative therapy (to avoid radiation-associated vision loss) for selected small posterior pole melanomas under 3 mm in height and located near the optic disk or fovea (67), 3) combined treatment with plaque radiotherapy (14,22), and 4) nonablative therapy of small juxtapapillary or juxtafoveal tumors to induce resorption of subretinal fluid and to inhibit progression of fluid into the fovea. In addition, diode laser hyperthermia increasingly is being advocated as a treatment for small melanomas and post-irradiation local recurrences (76).

Technique   The recommended laser settings for laser photocoagulation include a 100 to 500 μm spot size and 0.1 to 0.5 second duration. The energy (usually 200 to 600 mW) should be sufficient to produce moderately intense burns and will vary according to tumor pigmentation and the amount of subretinal fluid. Argon, krypton, or diode lasers can be used, although the latter two may achieve deeper tissue penetration. Either a slit-lamp or indirect ophthalmoscope system can be used. Confluent treatment is applied over the surface of the tumor. The desired end point is a chorioretinal scar with variable overlying RPE metaplasia (Fig. 51-7). Multiple treatments may be necessary and should be separated by 4 to 6 weeks to allow the full therapeutic effect. If the tumor does not respond after 5 or 6 treatments, alternative interventions should be pursued.

Similar settings are used for nonablative photocoagulation, except that light burns are applied in a nonconfluent pattern over the tumor surface. Alternatively, several rows of confluent burns can be applied to the posterior margin of subretinal fluid to induce chorioretinal adhesion and prevent progression of fluid into the fovea.

For laser hyperthermia, a diode laser is used in conjunction with a slit-lamp adapter that allows very large spot sizes (adapters are also available for the operating microscope and laser indirect ophthalmoscope). Currently, most centers are using a 3-mm spot size and 60-second treatments. The energy level initially is set very low (around 400 mW) and titrated up to the desired level (higher energy levels will be required in less pigmented tumors). The ideal energy level results in the appearance of a faint gray-white burn at around 50 seconds. Once this energy level is identified, overlapping spots should be applied to the entire tumor surface.

Complications Ablative treatment causes an absolute scotoma corresponding to the treated area. Occasional complications include subretinal or vitreous hemorrhage (usually self-limited), breaks in Bruch's membrane (which can lead to choroidal neovascular membrane or collar button formation), retinal breaks, cystoid macular edema, and retinal vascular occlusions. When hemorrhage is observed during treatment, momentary pressure with the contact lens will tamponade the bleeding. The complications associated with laser hyperthermia appear to be less severe than those associated with photocoagulation, but further study is needed in this area.

Results In our experience, the five-year control rate for laser photoablation of marginal recurrences is about 76% (53). When used as a primary therapy, however, laser photoablation is successful in only about half of the cases and requires multiple treatment sessions. Laser therapy combined with plaque radiotherapy causes a more rapid and complete tumor regression, but the long-term effect on survival is not known (17). Nonablative laser therapy causes substantial reduction of subretinal fluid in many tumors, but the malignant potential of the tumor is not significantly altered. Initial experience with laser hyperthermia has been promising (76), but further work is necessary to determine long-term results using this modality.

Episcleral Plaque Radiotherapy

Episcleral plaque radiotherapy is now one of the most common treatments for medium-sized posterior uveal melanomas.

Indications Patients with tumors up to 16 mm in largest basal dimension and up to 10 mm in thickness are the best candidates for plaque radiotherapy. Patients with larger tumors can be treated but have a very small chance of retaining useful vision. Relative contraindications to plaque radiotherapy include dense media opacities preventing accurate tumor localization, substantial extraocular extension, optic nerve invasion, and tumor-related glaucoma.

Technique Either local retrobulbar or general anesthesia can be used. A conjunctival peritomy is performed, the four rectus muscles are secured with 2-0 cotton sutures, and the tumor is localized by transillumination and/or indirect

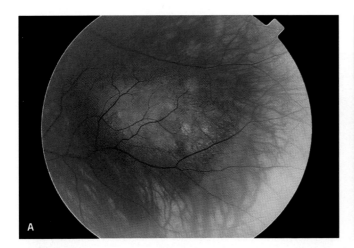
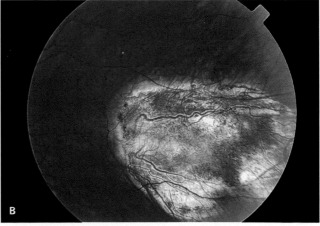

FIGURE 51-7. *Diode laser hyperthermia of posterior uveal melanoma. A. Prior to treatment. B. Successful treatment with residual atrophic chorioretinal scar.*

ophthalmoscopy with a fiberoptic light pipe (Fig. 51-8A, B). The margins of the tumor are marked with a sterile pen or diathermy tip. If access to the tumor is limited by a rectus muscle, the muscle should be secured with a double-armed 6-0 vicryl suture and temporarily severed.

A dummy plaque is temporarily sutured to the sclera with 5-0 nylon sutures, leaving a minimum border of 2 mm

around the tumor margins. Intraoperative B-scan ultrasonography is helpful in confirming accurate plaque localization, especially for posterior tumors (Fig. 51-8C) (54). The dummy plaque is removed, and the active plaque is secured to the sclera with the preplaced sutures. Prior to placement of the active plaque, it is inspected for the number and location of radioactive seeds. If an extraocular

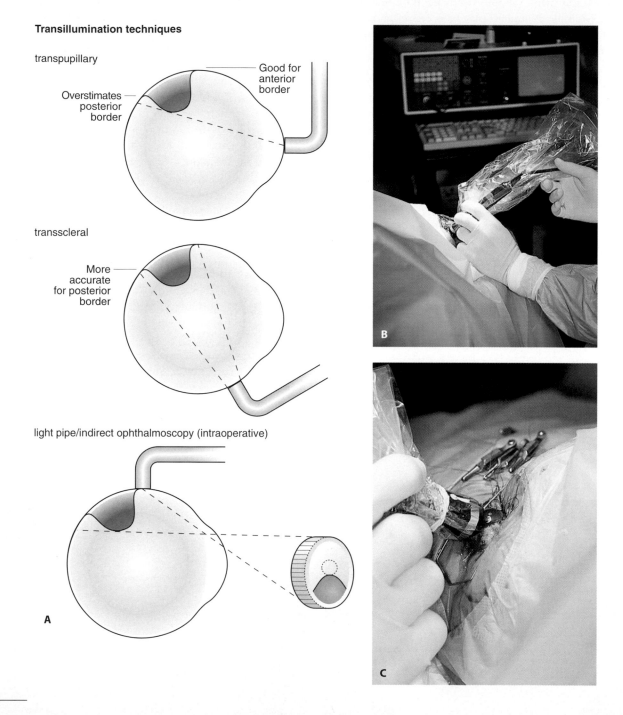

FIGURE 51-8.   *Techniques for localizing intraocular tumors. A. Transillumination: Transpupillary transillumination is best for identifying anterior tumor border but may overestimate posterior border by casting a tumor shadow posteriorly. Transscleral transillumination is least likely to overestimate posterior tumor margin, but it may be difficult to position the light source 180° away from the tumor. Indirect ophthalmoscopy and scleral indentation with fiberoptic light pipe. B. Intraoperative echography: A standard portable B-scan unit is used. C. The probe tip is covered with a sterile plastic sleeve.*

muscle was severed, it should be draped anteriorly and the sutures left long for later identification. The conjunctiva is then temporarily reapproximated with a 6-0 absorbable suture. An antibiotic/corticosteroid ointment is placed in the eye, followed by a sterile patch and lead shield over the eye.

Depending on local practice and laws, the patient is either admitted to the hospital for the duration of the plaque treatment as a public health measure, or discharged on topical antibiotics and corticosteroids.

The plaque is typically removed in 3 to 5 days, according to the calculations of the radiation physicist. The temporary conjunctival sutures are cut, the plaque is grasped with a toothed forceps, the scleral sutures are identified and cut with blunt-tipped scissors, and the plaque is removed. The plaque is inspected again to confirm the number of radioactive seeds. If a rectus muscle was previously severed, it is identified and secured to the sclera at its previous insertion. The conjunctiva is reapproximated with a 6-0 absorbable suture. Antibiotic/corticosteroid ointment and a patch are placed on the eye. Topical antibiotics and corticosteroids are used postoperatively for 7 to 10 days.

Complications Diplopia is common but usually is transient. Scleral penetration, infection, and intraocular hemorrhage can occur but are extremely rare with careful surgical technique. Radiation-induced complications are common and usually occur months or years after treatment. These include scleral necrosis, punctal occlusion and epiphora, keratoconjunctivitis sicca, anterior uveitis, retinopathy, optic neuropathy, neovascular glaucoma, and vitreous hemorrhage. Retinopathy and optic neuropathy usually begin to develop 12 to 36 months after treatment, with a mean posttreatment interval of 32 months before onset (42). After follow-up of 25 to 90 months following iodine-125 radiotherapy, the rate of radiation-induced cataract was 30%; retinopathy, 22%; optic neuropathy, 8%; and neovascular glaucoma, 6% (39). However, the risk for radiation-induced complications increases with longer follow-up and is influenced by tumor size and location, radiation dose and source, and patient-related factors.

Radiation Dosage and Isotopes There are no objectively derived guidelines for radiation dosage in the treatment of posterior uveal melanoma, but in most centers the currently accepted dosage to the tumor apex ranges from 75 to 100 Gy.

Several different radiation sources have been used for plaque radiotherapy, including radon-222 (68), cobalt-60 (96), ruthenium-106 (61), gold-198 (69), and palladium-103 (38). Iodine-125 is now the most commonly used isotope and was chosen for the Collaborative Ocular Melanoma Study (COMS) (36). The theoretical advantages of this isotope derive from the low-energy gamma particles, which can be shielded from orbital structures with a gold plaque, and which may cause less radiation-induced intraocular tissue damage. Repeated use of the radioactive seeds is limited, however, due to the short half-life of 60 days.

The COMS plaque is widely used and consists of a gold casing that is 0.4 mm thick, with scleral loops along its edge (Fig. 51-9). A silastic insert holds the seeds inside of the plaque at a distance of 1 mm from the scleral surface. This distance must be taken into account when calculating radiation dose to the tumor apex. Custom-designed notched plaques for juxtapapillary tumors are also available.

Results

Local Tumor Control. Successful treatment is characterized by gradual tumor shrinkage and the development of a grayish, shrunken, inactive mass, or a flat chorioretinal scar (Fig. 51-10). Appreciable tumor shrinkage usually begins 8 to 12 months after treatment. More rapid tumor regression may be associated with a higher metastatic death rate (12).

Local tumor recurrence has been reported in 3% to 17% of tumors treated with plaque radiotherapy (39,42,44, 61,77). The average time interval from plaque treatment to local recurrence is about 27 months (79). Local recurrence is a risk factor for metastatic death (102), and the risk appears to be stronger for vertical recurrences than for thin, marginal recurrences (53). Risk factors of tumor recurrence include large basal tumor dimensions and posterior or juxtapapillary location (53). Intraoperative echography for accurate plaque localization (54) and postoperative supplemental laser therapy (17) have been used in an attempt to reduce the risk for local recurrence, although a proven benefit has not been demonstrated for either intervention.

Visual Prognosis. Visual outcome following plaque radiotherapy depends on preoperative visual acuity, proximity of the tumor to the fovea and optic nerve, radiation dose, time interval after treatment, and patient-related factors. In general, at least 72% of patients will lose two or more lines of visual acuity in the treated eye (44,47). However, 19% to 23% of patients will retain 20/40 or better visual acuity (44,61), and 90% report no significant postoperative reduction in functional visual performance (13).

Systemic Prognosis. The prognosis for an individual patient depends on tumor size, location, patient age, and other patient-related factors (10). A large repository of retrospective, nonrandomized clinical data strongly suggest that the melanoma-specific mortality rate following plaque radiotherapy is not significantly different from that for enucleation (4,10,11). This question is currently being addressed prospectively by the COMS, a national, randomized, multicenter trial which is comparing iodine-125 plaque radiotherapy and enucleation for medium-sized choroidal melanomas (82).

Post-irradiation Follow-up Schedule Clinical follow-up after radiotherapy is critical in order to assess tumor response and detect tumor recurrence. In general, the patient should be reexamined every 3 to 4 months for the first two years, and every 6 months thereafter. Indirect ophthalmoscopy, fundus drawing, fundus photographs, and A- and B-scan

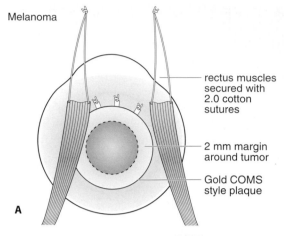

Melanoma

rectus muscles secured with 2.0 cotton sutures

2 mm margin around tumor

Gold COMS style plaque

A

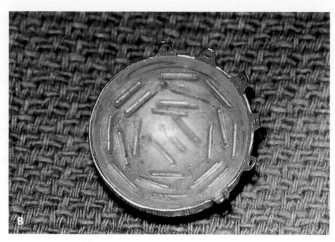

B

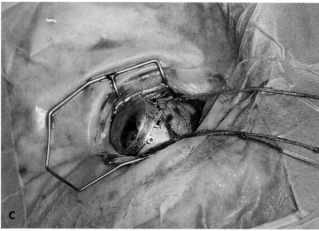

C

FIGURE 51-9. *Episcleral radioactive plaques. A. Surgical technique for application of episcleral plaque. Conjunctival peritomy is performed. The four rectus muscles are isolated with 2-0 cotton sutures. Tumor is localized and margins are marked with sterile pen or diathermy tip. Rectus muscle blocking access to tumor is secured with double-armed 6-0 vicryl suture and temporarily disinserted (as needed). Dummy plaque is secured to sclera (leaving a 2-mm border around the tumor margins) with 5-0 nylon sutures and a temporary knot. Accurate plaque localization is confirmed with indirect ophthalmoscopy, transillumination, and intraoperative ultrasonography (as needed). Dummy plaque is replaced with active plaque and secured to sclera. Any severed rectus muscle is draped anteriorly for later identification. B. COMS-type gold plaque with Iodine-125 seeds. (Courtesy of the COMS Study.) C. Plaque being sutured in place.*

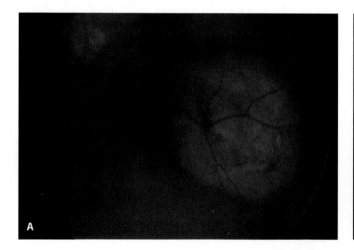

A

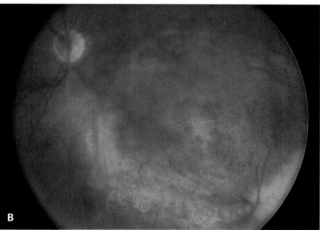

B

FIGURE 51-10. *Posterior uveal melanoma before treatment (A), and two years after plaque radiotherapy (B), demonstrating tumor shrinkage and early radiation retinopathy.*

ultrasonography should be performed at each visit. Tumor recurrence can develop at any time but is most common within the first 2 to 3 years after treatment (53). Flat marginal recurrences can usually be controlled with laser therapy, while vertical recurrences usually require enucleation (53). Metastatic workup, consisting of physical examination, liver function tests, and chest x-ray, should be performed at least once a year.

Charged Particle Radiotherapy

Charged particle radiotherapy using either protons or helium ions provides the theoretical advantages of a well-defined external radiation beam with minimal scatter, the Bragg peak effect (increased density of charged particles near the end of the treatment beam), and a more uniform delivery of radiation than plaque radiotherapy (49). However, some of the negative aspects of this modality include the high radiation complication rate, the high cost, and the limited number of centers with particle accelerators.

Indications, Technique, and Complications The indications are similar to those for plaque radiotherapy. Local tumor control may be better for posterior pole and juxtapapillary tumors using charged particle radiotherapy (29). The surgical technique is similar to that for placement of episcleral plaques, except that four tantalum rings are sutured to the sclera (25). The tantalum rings are nonmagnetic, radiopaque markers that are used by the radiation oncologist to target the radiation beam. Complications of charged particle radiotherapy are similar to those for plaque radiotherapy, except that cataract and neovascular glaucoma are more common with charged particle radiotherapy (29,59).

Results

Local Tumor Control. The actuarial five-year local control rate following proton beam radiotherapy is about 97% (50). In a randomized, prospective trial, the local tumor control rate was significantly higher for helium ion therapy than plaque radiotherapy, particularly for posterior pole tumors (29). Possible reasons for better local control with charged particles than with plaque radiotherapy are being investigated and include differences in relative biological effect of the radiation source, dosing schedule, technical difficulty in localizing posterior plaques, obstruction by retrobulbar structures, and plaque movement during treatment.

Visual Prognosis. One study using a median follow-up of 42 months showed that 47% of patients receiving helium ions retained 20/200 or better visual acuity (59). Visual prognostic factors are similar to those for plaque radiotherapy.

Systemic Prognosis. The overall five-year metastatic death rate after proton therapy was 20%, with a median time to metastasis of 2.1 years after treatment (51). After a mean follow-up of 66 months, the metastatic rate for helium ion therapy was 18% (26). No difference in survival was seen for charged particle radiotherapy compared to enucleation (84) or plaque radiotherapy (29).

Local Surgical Resection

With recent improvements in microsurgical techniques, the results of local resection for posterior uveal melanoma have improved (40,78,93). The most accepted technique currently is a partial lamellar sclerouvectomy using hypotensive anesthesia. The surgical procedure is time-consuming and technically challenging, but it may provide the best opportunity to retain good vision in selected patients.

Indications Tumors characteristics most suitable for local resection include nasal and anterior location, greater thickness, smaller basal dimensions, and subretinal fluid (15,31). Young, healthy patients are often good candidates because of their better general health and the potential for retaining long-term useful vision. Conditions that may preclude local resection with hypotensive anesthesia include cardiovascular or pulmonary disease, bleeding disorders, medically required use of anticoagulants, poor visual potential, optic nerve involvement, substantial retinal invasion, involvement of more than 30% to 40% of the ciliary body, substantial extraocular extension, or tumor-related intraocular inflammation or glaucoma.

Technique General anesthesia is administered. A 360° conjunctival peritomy is performed, the four rectus muscles are secured with 2-0 cotton sutures, episcleral blood vessels are thoroughly cauterized, and the tumor is localized by transillumination. The tumor margins are marked with a sterile pen or diathermy tip. If access to the tumor is limited by a rectus muscle, the muscle should be secured with a double-armed 6-0 vicryl suture and temporarily severed at the insertion. A supporting device for the globe is usually not necessary unless the tumor base is over 13 to 14mm in diameter. An octagonal or rectangular flap with 4 to 5mm margins around the tumor is drawn on the sclera, with the posterior edge serving as a hinge (Fig. 51-11). Using the operating microscope, a No. 67 Beaver is used to make a superficial scleral incision, which is carefully deepened to 80% scleral thickness. An angulated blade, such as a No. 57 Beaver blade, is used to develop a lamellar scleral flap.

Systemic hypotension (systolic blood pressure about 60mmHg) and reversed Trendelenburg positioning are then initiated. Removal of 1 to 2cc of vitreous to decompress the globe is achieved using the vitrectomy instrument inserted through a pars plana incision into the mid-vitreous cavity away from the tumor. The tumor margins are identified again with transillumination and marked with a sterile pen on the remaining inner sclera. Three rows of penetrating diathermy are then applied to the scleral bed around the tumor margin. A No. 75 blade is used to incise the scleral bed 3mm outside of the tumor margin. The scleral incision is continued for 360° around the tumor margins with Vannas scissors while cauterizing choroidal vessels as needed. The choroid is then freed and gently retracted away from the retina using fine-toothed forceps. The choroid is carefully perforated with a No. 75 blade, and the incision is extended for 360° with Vannas scissors while maintaining gentle traction on the choroid away from the retina. The tumor block is carefully removed from the eye by gently retracting the inner scleral lamella with a fine-toothed forceps while applying countertraction against the retina with a cyclodialysis spatula.

Any vitreous presenting at the scleral wound is removed with the vitrectomy instrument. If a small area of extrascleral tumor extension is found in the lamellar flap, this area is

A.   **Iridocyclectomy**

B.   **Choroidectomy**

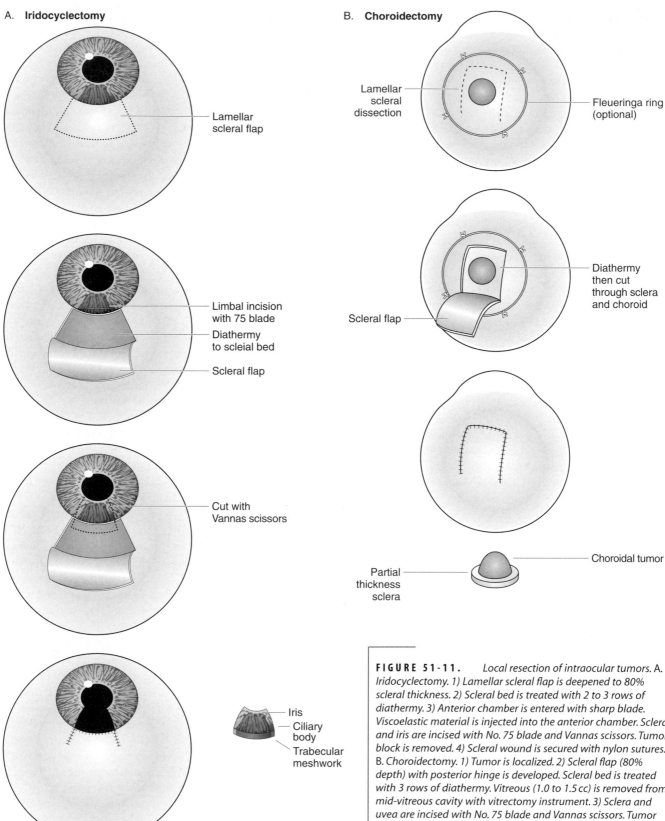

Lamellar
scleral flap

Lamellar
scleral
dissection

Fleueringa ring
(optional)

Limbal incision
with 75 blade

Diathermy
to scleial bed

Scleral flap

Diathermy
then cut
through sclera
and choroid

Scleral flap

Cut with
Vannas scissors

Choroidal tumor

Partial
thickness
sclera

Iris
Ciliary
body
Trabecular
meshwork

FIGURE 51-11.   *Local resection of intraocular tumors. A.
Iridocyclectomy. 1) Lamellar scleral flap is deepened to 80%
scleral thickness. 2) Scleral bed is treated with 2 to 3 rows of
diathermy. 3) Anterior chamber is entered with sharp blade.
Viscoelastic material is injected into the anterior chamber. Sclera
and iris are incised with No. 75 blade and Vannas scissors. Tumor
block is removed. 4) Scleral wound is secured with nylon sutures.
B. Choroidectomy. 1) Tumor is localized. 2) Scleral flap (80%
depth) with posterior hinge is developed. Scleral bed is treated
with 3 rows of diathermy. Vitreous (1.0 to 1.5 cc) is removed from
mid-vitreous cavity with vitrectomy instrument. 3) Sclera and
uvea are incised with No. 75 blade and Vannas scissors. Tumor
block is removed. Scleral wound is secured with nylon sutures.
Prophylactic encircling scleral buckle can be placed.*

removed full-thickness and replaced by a lamellar scleral patch graft. The scleral flap is then secured in place using 8-0 nylon sutures until the wound is watertight. Some surgeons routinely place a 360° scleral buckle (usually a 42-band) to support the vitreous base, while others will only do so if a retinal break or detachment is found during the procedure. If a rhegmatogenous retinal detachment is encountered, pars plana vitrectomy and fluid-gas exchange should be considered.

Any previously disinserted muscles are reattached, and the conjunctiva is reapproximated with 6-0 absorbable sutures. Routine subconjunctival corticosteroids and antibiotics are administered. The patient is placed on topical antibiotics, corticosteroids, and cycloplegics for 7 to 10 days. Postoperatively, 1 to 2 sessions of laser photoablation to the margins of the surgical coloboma are usually performed to reduce the risk of local tumor recurrence or retinal detachment.

Complications The most common complications include vitreous hemorrhage, retinal detachment, cataract, and residual or recurrent tumor (30,40). Vitreous hemorrhage usually clears spontaneously in a few weeks to months, but pars plana vitrectomy occasionally may be required. Retinal detachment can occur early or late and may be accompanied by proliferative vitreoretinopathy. Some surgeons are now routinely performing pars plana vitrectomy, fluid-gas exchange, and scleral buckling at the time of tumor resection to minimize this complication (30). Cataracts can usually be extracted using routine techniques. Residual or recurrent tumor is the main cause of severe vision loss and the main indication for enucleation following local resection (30). A histopathologic study of 30 eyes enucleated for posterior uveal melanoma found retinal invasion in 7 eyes (23%). However, it is not clear whether those tumors (which required enucleation) were similar in size, location, and other characteristics to those for which local resection is usually performed.

Results The eye is retained in 80% to 90% of cases, "count fingers" vision or better is achieved in approximately 80%, and residual or recurrent tumor occurs in 11% to 17% (40,78,93). In a retrospective, matched group comparison with plaque radiotherapy, local resection was more likely to cause early post-treatment severe visual loss but improved the chance of long-term useful vision (Fig. 51-12) (15). In the same study, no difference in five-year actuarial survival rate was found between local resection and cobalt-60 plaque radiotherapy.

Enucleation

The frequency of enucleation for posterior uveal melanoma has dropped in recent years due to increasing use of eye-sparing treatments. Hydroxyapatite orbital implants, which become integrated into the orbital tissues and provide improved prosthetic movement, are now widely used.

Indications The current indications for enucleation of posterior uveal melanomas include large tumor size (greater

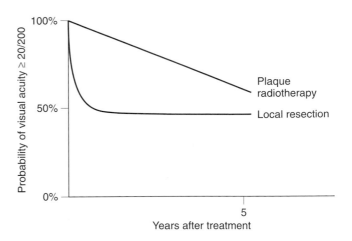

FIGURE 51-12. *Kaplan-Meier curve demonstrating probability of maintaining visual acuity of 20/200 or better following local resection versus cobalt plaque radiotherapy for posterior uveal melanoma. (Adapted from* Ophthalmic Surg *1990;21:682–688.)*

than 10 to 11 mm in thickness and 15 to 16 mm in basal diameter), tumor-related inflammation or glaucoma, substantial extraocular extension, and optic nerve invasion.

Technique Either general or retrobulbar anesthesia can be employed. A lid speculum is placed, and indirect ophthalmoscopy is performed to confirm that surgery is being performed on the correct eye. A 360° conjunctival peritomy is performed, conjunctiva and Tenon's capsule are bluntly dissected in all four quadrants, and the four rectus muscles are secured with muscle hooks. For all except the medial rectus muscle, a double-armed 6-0 vicryl suture is placed in a double-locking fashion through the muscle near the insertion. The muscle is temporarily clamped with a straight hemostat between the suture and the insertion, and the muscle is cut with Westcott scissors at the insertion. For the medial rectus, the procedure is the same, except that a long (3- to 4-mm) muscle stump is left attached to the globe. A small muscle hook is used to sweep inferoposteriorly along the globe and engage the inferior oblique muscle, which is temporarily clamped and then cut. A similar procedure is performed for the superior oblique muscle.

The medial rectus stump is securely clamped with a curved hemostat, which is then used to retract the globe anteriorly and place the optic nerve on stretch. With the other hand, the closed enucleation scissors are inserted medially into the orbit, and the blunt tip is used to identify the optic nerve using a strumming motion. The scissors are then opened around the optic nerve and tilted posteriorly to obtain a long nerve section (Fig. 51-13). The nerve is severed in one cut if possible, and the globe is lifted out of the orbit. A capped 10-mL sterile test tube immediately is placed in the orbit with moderate anteroposterior pressure for 5 to 10 minutes to achieve hemostasis.

Retinoblastoma

Enucleation with long stump

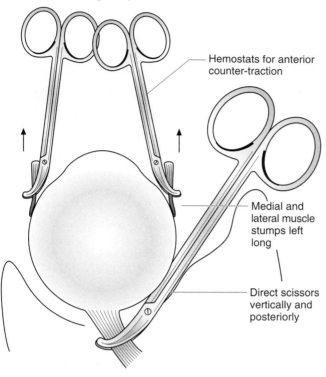

Hemostats for anterior counter-traction

Medial and lateral muscle stumps left long

Direct scissors vertically and posteriorly

FIGURE 51-13. *Enucleation for intraocular tumor. Conjunctival peritomy is performed. The four rectus muscles are secured with 2-0 cotton sutures. The two oblique muscles are identified and severed. Hemostat clamps are used to grasp the medial and lateral rectus stumps. Firm anterior traction is exerted. Enucleation scissors (closed position) are placed behind the globe and the optic nerve identified by strumming. The optic nerve is cut with the scissors oriented vertically and posteriorly to obtain a long optic nerve stump. Hydroxyapatite implant in sterile donor scleral shell is sutured to rectus muscles. Tenon's layer and conjunctiva are closed in three layers: 1) deep Tenon's closure with "purse string" or interrupted horizontal mattress sutures using 4-0 vicryl, 2) superficial Tenon's closure with vertical mattress sutures using 4-0 vicryl, and 3) conjunctival closure with a running 6-0 plain gut suture (without tension on sutures).*

The hydroxyapatite implant is wrapped in sterile donor sclera, which has been cut to size and snugly fitted to the implant using 6-0 vicryl sutures. Four windows are cut in the sclera at 90° apart, slightly anterior to the equator of the implant. The implant is then positioned in the orbit. The largest size that will fit should be used (usually 16 to 18 mm in children and 20 to 22 mm in adults). The muscle sutures are passed through the sclera anterior to the corresponding scleral window, and the muscle is drawn into the window (in contact with the implant) before securing the suture.

Tenon's capsule is closed with a 5-0 vicryl or chromic suture in two layers: a deep horizontal mattress closure (or a purse string) and a superficial vertical mattress closure. The conjunctiva is closed with a running 7-0 vicryl or plain gut

Table 51-5. Risk Factors for Melanoma-Related Death Following Enucleation

Clinical risk factors
  Age
  Anterior tumor location
  Tumor size
Histopathologic risk factors
  Callander cell type
  Pigmentation
  Extrascleral extension
  Intratumoral microvascular architecture
  Inverse standard deviation of nucleolar area
  Mitotic index
  BrDU uptake (marker of cycling cells)

suture. The purpose of this final closure is to bring the edges of conjunctiva into apposition and to avoid inclusion cysts. The conjunctival closure should not be under tension. A plastic conformer and antibiotic/corticosteroid ointment are placed in the eye, followed by a pressure patch. The pressure patch is re-applied the next day, and a light patch can be used thereafter. The patient can be fitted for a prosthesis at 6 to 8 weeks. If desired, the patient can have the implant drilled and fit with an integrated peg at 4 to 6 months to improve motility of the prosthesis. In our experience, most patients have acceptable motility without integration of the prosthesis with the orbital implant and choose not to undergo this additional procedure.

If a silicone sphere is used instead of the hydroxyapatite implant, a scleral shell is not used, and the rectus muscles are secured to the rectus muscle 180° away. Tenon's capsule and conjunctiva are closed in a similar manner.

Complications Potential complications of enucleation include conjunctival erosion, implant migration or extrusion, orbital infection, and orbital hemorrhage. All of these complications are uncommon.

Results In a meta-analysis of posterior uveal melanoma mortality data following enucleation, the five-year mortality rate was 16% for small tumors, 32% for medium tumors, and 53% for large tumors (34). Several clinical and histologic factors have been shown to be independent prognostic factors for melanoma-related death following enucleation (Table 51-5). Pre-enucleation external beam radiotherapy has not been demonstrated to improve survival following enucleation in retrospective studies (16), although the results of the COMS large tumor study (which addresses this issue) have not been published. External beam radiotherapy may have a role as an adjuvant to enucleation in selected patients with extraocular extension (57).

Exenteration

Orbital exenteration is rarely necessary in the treatment of posterior uveal melanoma. The primary indications include massive extraocular tumor extension and orbital recurrence following enucleation. A lid-sparing technique is usually employed (25).

Future Advances in Management

Investigators are exploring ways to improve the management of patients with posterior uveal melanoma through advances in local therapy, early detection of micrometastases, and more effective treatment of metastatic disease.

New local therapies under investigation include diode laser hyperthermia (76), photodynamic therapy (48), stereotactic radiosurgery (60), immunotherapy (58), gene therapy using "suicide genes" and radiosensitizing genes (21), and combined modality therapy (97). A potential approach for detecting micrometastases in peripheral blood involves a polymerase chain reaction–based assay for the tyrosinase gene product (preferentially expressed in melanocytes) (98). Improved treatments for disseminated metastases are being sought through advances in chemotherapy, vaccinations, cellular immunotherapy, and gene therapy (5,62,75).

RETINOBLASTOMA

Retinoblastoma is the most common primary intraocular cancer in children. The incidence is approximately one in 20,000 infants (70). Most patients present by two years of age, but retinoblastoma may also be diagnosed in older children and adults, though rarely.

Genetics

Understanding the distinctive genetics of retinoblastoma is critical for proper diagnosis, management, genetic counseling, and prognosis (3,70). Retinoblastoma tumors are thought to have mutations that inactivate both cellular copies of the retinoblastoma gene. About 60% to 65% of patients have a nonheritable (somatic) form of the disease in which the retinoblastoma gene mutations are only present within the tumor cells. These patients typically have unilateral, unifocal tumors and are not at risk for second cancers. About 35% to 40% of patients have a heritable (germline) form of the disease in which cells throughout the body carry the retinoblastoma gene mutation. Germline patients tend to present earlier, have a poorer prognosis, develop multifocal and bilateral retinoblastomas, develop other primary cancers throughout the body at a high rate, and pass on retinoblastoma to their children in an autosomal dominant fashion. Significantly, about 15% of unilateral patients actually harbor a germline mutation with all of the concomitant risks. Figure 51-14 shows the clinical distribution of genetic subtypes of retinoblastoma.

Diagnosis

Presenting Signs

The most common presenting signs are leukocoria and strabismus. Rarely, patients will present with ocular inflammation or orbital cellulitis.

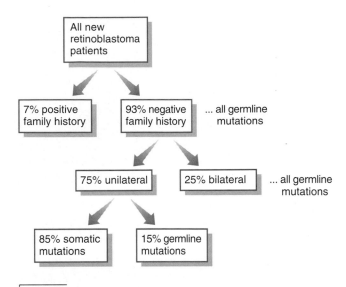

FIGURE 51-14. *Genetic subgroups of retinoblastoma patients.*

Clinical Appearance

The clinical appearance of retinoblastoma is extremely varied, but the tumors usually assume one of two basic growth patterns (both of which may be present in the same patient). The endophytic form grows into the vitreous with friable, loosely cohesive white tumors (Fig. 51-15A). The vitreous deposits are typically larger than the clumps of leukocytes seen in endophthalmitis or uveitis. Pseudohypopyon or tumor infiltrates on the iris may infrequently be seen.

The exophytic form predominantly grows toward the subretinal space, causing secondary retinal detachment that can be difficult to distinguish from Coats' disease (Fig. 51-15B). Small intraretinal tumors may resemble astrocytic hamartomas (Fig. 51-15C). Chalky white areas of intratumoral calcification, intrinsic capillary networks, and shunting of retinal vessels into the tumor are highly suggestive of retinoblastoma. Tumor-related glaucoma (due to secondary angle closure, tumor infiltration of meshwork, or neovascularization of the iris), buphthalmos, and hyphema may be seen. Cataract is uncommon in retinoblastoma and should suggest another diagnosis.

Ancillary Diagnostic Tests

Examination under anesthesia, including anterior segment examination and indirect ophthalmoscopy with scleral depression, are essential in the diagnostic evaluation for retinoblastoma.

The most important ancillary diagnostic test for retinoblastoma is computed tomography (CT). CT should be performed at presentation in all cases to detect intratumoral calcium (present in at least 80% of large retinoblastomas but extremely rare in simulating lesions in patients below the age of five), to evaluate the optic nerve and orbit, and to screen for midline intracranial primitive

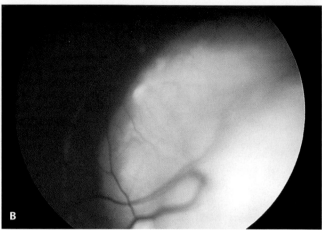

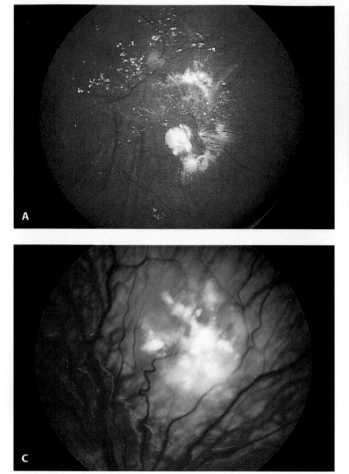

FIGURE 51-15.   *Clinical appearance of retinoblastoma.*
A. Endophytic form: Loosely cohesive tumor with seeding into the
vitreous cavity. B. Exophytic form: Large, white subretinal mass with
secondary retinal detachment. C. Small retinoblastoma: Intraretinal
tumor with fine capillary network and calcified intratumoral flecks.

neuroectodermal tumors (PNET), which are seen in 5% to 8% of bilateral patients (33).

Ultrasonography is used less often now that CT is widely available, but it is occasionally helpful in the diagnostic evaluation. With B-scan ultrasonography, retinoblastoma tumors may demonstrate intratumoral calcium flecks that appear as highly reflective interfaces with posterior shadowing. Simulating lesions without calcium usually do not have this feature. Ultrasonography may also be helpful in assessing optic nerve enlargement and scleral integrity when extraocular extension is suspected.

The fluorescein angiographic features of retinoblastoma have been described (25,91), but this modality is usually not necessary for accurate diagnosis.

Vitrectomy and subretinal fluid drainage should be avoided when retinoblastoma is suspected. However, intraocular fine-needle biopsy may be necessary, though very rarely, when a benign simulating lesion cannot be ruled out by noninvasive techniques (27). In such cases, a fine-needle biopsy can be performed as previously described, except that the needle is inserted through peripheral clear cornea and into the posterior segment through peripheral iris (see Fig. 51-6).

Differential Diagnosis

Retinoblastoma can be simulated by a wide range of ocular conditions (Table 51-6) (25,91). The ophthalmologist who manages retinoblastoma must be familiar with the clinical features of these disorders.

Treatment Considerations

A variety of clinical and genetic factors must be considered in determining the optimal treatment for each patient (Table 51-7) (25). In general, more conservative, vision-sparing treatments are employed in patients with bilateral tumors. Age, family history, and multifocality are important to assess in determining the potential for bilaterality. Examination of parents and siblings should be performed whenever possible to screen for undetected familial disease. Large tumor size, close proximity to the fovea and optic nerve, extraocular extension, optic nerve invasion, anterior chamber involvement, and tumor-related inflammation or glaucoma are poor prognostic factors for vision and survival and favor more aggressive therapy such as enucleation.

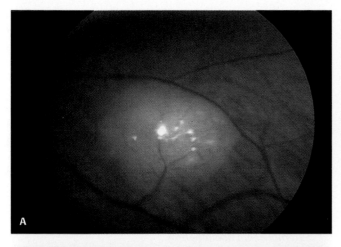

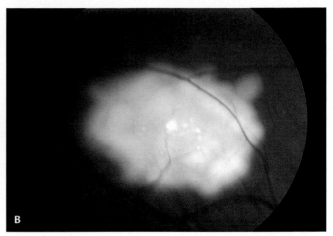

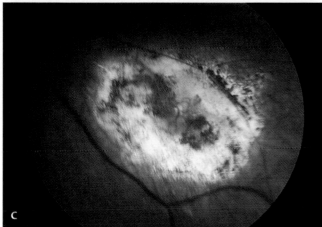

FIGURE 51-16. *Laser photoablation of retinoblastoma. A. Confluent laser burns over the tumor and one row around the tumor immediately after treatment. B. Residual chorioretinal scar two months after treatment.*

Treatment Modalities

Observation

Observation is virtually never appropriate when retinoblastoma is suspected, but a short period of close observation may be acceptable, though rarely, when the diagnosis is uncertain. Observation should only be considered if parent cooperation and reliability are certain.

Laser Therapy

Indications Laser photoablation is increasingly being used in the treatment of retinoblastoma. This modality can be used as primary treatment for small tumors up to 3.0 mm in thickness, and as supplementary treatment to cryotherapy or radiotherapy. Small tumors posterior to the equator that cannot easily be treated with cryotherapy are particularly suited for laser photoablation. Relative contraindications to laser treatment include vitreous seeding, macular or optic nerve involvement, and choroidal invasion.

Technique The argon laser indirect ophthalmoscope is most commonly used while the patient is under general anesthesia. Either continuous-mode or 0.1- to 0.2-second duration can be employed. The energy is initially set at 200 mW and gradually increased until the small tumor capillaries are seen to blanch on direct treatment. Confluent treat-ment is applied over the tumor and a 1-mm surrounding margin (Fig. 51-16). Photocoagulation of prominent feeder vessels can be facilitated by applying digital pressure to the globe, causing blood flow through the vessel to decrease, before commencing laser treatment. Typically, the patient is re-evaluated in 3 to 4 weeks to assess the treatment effect before considering further treatment. The desired end point is a chorioretinal scar. This may require 6 to 8 treatments.

Complications Breaks in Bruch's membrane and occlusions of small retinal vessels are fairly common but are rarely problematic. Retinal and vitreous hemorrhages are uncommon and are usually self-limited. A rare but potentially serious complication is tumor seeding into the vitreous. The risk of this complication can be minimized by avoiding high-energy and excessive treatment.

Results In one series, 76% of all tumors were controlled by laser therapy alone, and the best results were seen in tumors less than 3 mm in diameter and 2 mm in thickness without vitreous seeding (92).

Cryotherapy

Indications Tumors most suitable for cryotherapy are less than 3.5 mm in diameter, less than 3.0 mm in thickness,

Table 51-6.   Conditions Considered in Differential Diagnosis of Retinoblastoma

Congenital and developmental abnormalities
   Coats' disease (congenital retinal telangiectasis)
   Persistent hyperplastic primary vitreous
   "Morning glory" disk abnormality
   Retinopathy of prematurity
   Retinal dysplasia
   Chorioretinal coloboma
   Congenital cataract
   Myelinated nerve fibers
Inflammations or infections
   Toxocariasis
   Endophthalmitis
   Intermediate or posterior uveitis
Tumors
   Retinal astrocytic hamartoma
   Retinal capillary hemangioma
   Intraocular leukemia
   Medulloepithelioma
   Retinocytoma
Hereditary retinal diseases
   Familial exudative vitreoretinopathy
   Incontinentia pigmenti
   Norrie's disease
   Aicardi's syndrome
Rhegmatogenous retinal detachment
Orbital cellulitis

Table 51-7.   Treatment Considerations for Retinoblastoma

Age at presentation
Family history
Evidence of metastatic disease
Tumor characteristics
   Size
   Location
   Laterality
   Focality
   Optic nerve involvement
   Anterior chamber involvement
   Extraocular extension
   Intraocular pressure
   Neovascular glaucoma
   Orbital cellulitis

and anterior to the equator and have minimal vitreous seeding.

Technique   Under general anesthesia, the cryoprobe is localized over the tumor using scleral depression and indirect ophthalmoscopy. Each application is continued until ice begins to form on the tumor surface. The cryoprobe tip is thawed by irrigation with balanced salt solution before moving it from the sclera. The entire tumor should be treated with a triple freeze-thaw technique. If cryotherapy is used for posterior tumors, the probe can be passed through a small conjunctival peritomy.

Complications   Choroidal hemorrhage and exudative retinal detachment are uncommon complications of cryotherapy. These can be minimized by carefully thawing the probe tip between applications and avoiding excessive treatment. Generally, there is more postoperative discomfort with cryotherapy than with laser.

Results   About 70% to 79% of tumors can be controlled with cryotherapy (1,90). The factors limiting successful treatment are size, thickness, vitreous seeding, and location.

External Beam Radiotherapy

Indications   External beam radiotherapy (EBRT) is one of the most commonly used modalities for retinoblastoma. Indications include multiple tumors too large to treat with laser or cryotherapy, substantial vitreous seeding, and tumors within 2 mm of the fovea or within the papillomacular bundle. Contraindications include optic nerve invasion and extraocular extension.

Technique   Treatment planning is carefully coordinated with the radiation oncologist, who must be aware of the location and size of all tumors in the affected eye(s). The radiation dose typically is 35 to 40 Gy in divided fractions. Anterior ports treat the whole retina, but this technique results in a high rate of radiation cataracts (56). Lateral ports spare the crystalline lens, and cataract formation is much less likely (99). However, new tumors may continue to appear in the peripheral retina due to inadequate anterior treatment. These new tumors can usually be controlled with supplemental local therapies. Repeat EBRT after prior failure of a full course of radiotherapy should be avoided due to a high risk of radiation complications.

Complications   The most serious complications of EBRT are bony facial deformities (midfacial hypoplasia) and second primary tumors in the field of radiation. In a large retrospective study, the cumulative probability of death from second tumors in bilateral patients was 26% at 40 years after diagnosis (37). The second tumor risk in the field of radiation is dramatically increased by the use of EBRT and appears to be dose-related (100). Significant radiation retinopathy and optic neuropathy are uncommon at the doses typically used.

Results   Tumors usually begin to regress within 4 to 6 weeks and may demonstrate one of several distinct regression patterns. Type I has a chalky white appearance similar to cottage cheese, type II has a translucent quality likened to fish flesh (the most difficult to distinguish from active tumor), type III is a combination of the first two, type IV is a chorioretinal scar, and type 0 is complete disappearance of the tumor. The regression pattern appears to bear no prognostic significance (94). The overall cure rate with EBRT alone is about 72%, and with supplemental salvage therapies it is about 93% (99). Results may improve with the use of modified lateral beam and other new techniques (64). The Reese-Ellsworth classification system, which is based on prognosis for ocular salvage, does not take into account recent therapeutic advances but is still useful in estimating the stage of intraocular disease (Table 51-8) (80).

Episcleral Plaque Radiotherapy

Plaque radiotherapy for retinoblastoma has recently become more widely used in an attempt to decrease the radiation-related complications associated with EBRT.

Indications Plaque radiotherapy, either as a primary modality or following failure of other treatments, may be indicated for selected tumors that are less than 16 mm in diameter, less than 10 mm in thickness, and more than 2 to 3 mm from the optic disk or fovea. In addition, all other tumors in the eye must be controllable with other local therapies. Localized vitreous seeding over the tumor can be treated by plaque radiotherapy, but diffuse vitreous seeding is a contraindication.

Technique The surgical technique for applying radioactive plaques is similar to that used for posterior uveal melanoma patients (see Fig. 51-9), although the technical difficulty is greater in young children with smaller orbits. Iodine-125 is most commonly used, and the typical dose is 35 to 40 Gy to the tumor apex. Most tumors demonstrate regression within 4 to 6 weeks after treatment.

Complications General complications of plaque radiotherapy are similar to those for posterior uveal melanoma patients (see p. 689). The radiation dose to the orbit is much less than with EBRT. Longer follow-up data is required to determine whether plaque radiotherapy will be associated with a lower rate of radiation-induced cosmetic deformities and second primary orbital tumors.

Results In one series, 86% of tumors were controlled with one plaque application, and visual outcome was 20/400 or better in 62% (87). Frequent reexamination is important to detect local recurrence.

Systemic Chemotherapy

Systemic chemotherapy has been used extensively in the treatment of extraocular retinoblastoma (35), but now there is growing interest in its use for primary intraocular retinoblastoma in lieu of EBRT (41,103).

Indications Potential indications for chemotherapy include 1) primary intraocular retinoblastoma (indications are similar to those for EBRT), 2) following enucleation when there is gross or histopathologic evidence of extraocular extension or optic nerve invasion posterior to the lamina cribrosa, 3) to "sterilize" the orbit prior to enucleation or exenteration when there is evidence of extraocular extension, and 4) metastatic disease.

Technique The most commonly used agents are currently carboplatin, etoposide (VP-16), and vincristine. Some centers have found better results with the addition of cyclosporin-A, which is thought to be an inhibitor of the multidrug resistance conferred by P-glycoprotein in retinoblastoma cells (24). Treatments are given in 3 to 4 week cycles. The number of cycles that should be administered is controversial and depends on the tumor response, but at least 3 to 4 cycles are probably necessary in most cases. Hospitalization during treatments and frequent follow-up examinations under general anesthesia are required.

There is usually a dramatic tumor regression within 4 to 6 weeks following induction, but chemotherapy usually must be supplemented by focal therapy (laser or cyrotherapy) in order to achieve a sustained tumor response (41). One effect of adjuvant local therapy may be to break down the blood-retinal barrier and allow greater tumor penetration by chemotherapeutic agents. This may be particularly important when substantial vitreous seeding is present.

Complications Possible complications of chemotherapy include bone marrow suppression, sepsis, and second tumors. The doses used for all chemotherapeutic agents are relatively low, and the short-term complication rate has been low. Ostensibly, radiation-induced facial deformities and orbital malignancies are avoided with chemotherapy, but long-term follow-up will be necessary to determine the incidence of second primary cancers and other adverse effects with chemotherapy.

Results In a small, preliminary study of bilateral retinoblastoma patients, the tumor control rate was reported to be 76% with cyclosporin-A and 37% without cyclosporin-A (41). All patients required supplemental focal therapy.

Table 51-8. Reese-Ellsworth Classification of Retinoblastoma

Group	Description	Prognosis for Ocular Salvage
I	Solitary tumor less than 4 disk diameters in size, at or posterior to the equator	Very favorable
	Multiple tumors less than 4 disk diameters in size, at or posterior to the equator	
II	Solitary tumor 4 to 10 disk diameters in size, at or posterior to the equator	Favorable
	Multiple tumors 4 to 10 disk diameters in size, posterior to the equator	
III	Any tumor anterior to the equator	Doubtful
	Solitary tumor larger than 10 disk diameters, posterior to the equator	
IV	Multiple tumors, some larger than 10 disk diameters in size	Unfavorable
	Any tumor extending anterior to the ora serrata	
V	Massive tumors involving half of the retina	Very unfavorable
	Vitreous seeding	

Source: Reproduced with permission from Reese AB. Tumors of the eye. Hagerstown, MD: Harper & Row, 1976:90–132.

Further studies are needed to compare the long-term results of systemic chemotherapy versus EBRT.

Enucleation

Enucleation is still the treatment of choice for many retinoblastomas.

Indications Enucleation is indicated for large tumors occupying over half of the globe volume, or for massive vitreous seeding, anterior segment involvement, rubeosis iridis, tumor-related glaucoma, buphthalmos, or optic nerve involvement (determined clinically or by orbital imaging studies).

Technique The surgical technique for enucleation is similar to that for posterior uveal melanoma patients (see Fig. 51-13). The surgeon must be particularly careful to avoid globe penetration and to obtain a long segment of optic nerve (to minimize the risk of contiguous intracranial spread). The smaller, less curved Stevens scissors are superior to standard enucleation scissors for the small pediatric orbit. The scissors should be oriented as posteriorly in the orbit as possible to obtain a long segment of optic nerve. The hydroxyapatite implant is typically 16 to 18 mm in size, depending on the patient's age and size of the orbit.

Complications General complications of enucleation are similar to those for posterior uveal melanoma patients (see p. 694). The most serious complication in retinoblastoma eyes is penetration of the globe with orbital tumor seeding. This is uncommon with careful surgical technique.

Results The strongest prognostic factors for metastatic death include extraocular extension, optic nerve invasion, and massive choroidal invasion (63,66,85). Enucleated patients with any of these negative prognostic features should be considered for treatment with systemic chemotherapy.

Exenteration

Orbital exenteration may be indicated for orbital tumor involvement (25).

Follow-up Schedule

The risk for new intraocular tumors is greatest for children presenting under one year of age and decreases to a negligible level by age five (2,3). In general, patients should be examined under anesthesia at least every 1 to 3 months while under one year of age, every 2 to 4 months until age two, and every 4 to 6 months until age five. Beyond age five, most children can be adequately examined without anesthesia in the office. Follow-up intervals can be progressively lengthened to every 6 to 12 months, depending on disease activity. Nonfamilial unilateral patients may be seen less frequently beginning two years after the last treatment. More frequent examinations may be necessary in children with highly aggressive tumors or bilateral involvement.

Midline intracranial tumors (usually with histopathologic features consistent with PNET rather than pinealoblastomas)

occur in 5% to 8% of familial bilateral patients (33). The mean age at diagnosis is approximately two years. Since the likelihood of successful treatment of these tumors may be greater when diagnosed presymptomatically (33,74), some experts advocate contrast-enhanced MRI or CT of the brain every 6 to 12 months until age four or five in familial bilateral patients (33).

Familial bilateral patients are at risk for primary cancers throughout the body (inside or outside the field of radiation). These usually begin to appear in the teenage years but can occur at any age. Patients should undergo annual physical examinations throughout life for cancer screening (37,81).

Future Advances in Management

Research is ongoing in many laboratories to develop genetic testing methodology for accurately diagnosing patients with germinal mutations and those at risk for second tumors (70,105). In addition, new treatment modalities are being developed to improve local tumor control while reducing treatment-related visual loss and radiation-related complications.

Laser hyperthermia is a new technique that increasingly is being advocated as an adjunct to other modalities such as systemic chemotherapy (72). Hyperthermia may enhance the efficacy of other modalities through cytotoxic effects, vascular injury, increased tissue penetration of chemotherapeutic agents, or other mechanisms. The diode laser is mounted on the indirect ophthalmoscope or operating microscope. With the child under general anesthesia, the laser is delivered to the tumor with a large spot size (1 to 3 mm) for 15 to 30 minutes. The initial results from some centers have been promising (72), but further investigation is needed.

Other therapeutic approaches are being investigated, including systemic chemotherapy (41,103), local chemotherapy (55), immunotherapy (45), charged particle radiotherapy (71), and combined modality therapy (73).

MELANOCYTIC IRIS TUMORS

Iris melanocytic tumors include a spectrum of lesions ranging from benign nevi to malignant melanomas (25,91). Although derived from the uveal tract, iris melanocytic tumors tend to display more benign behavior than posterior uveal melanomas and are thus considered separately. The patient may notice changes in iris color or visual symptoms. Frequently, the lesion is found incidentally on ophthalmologic exam. Melanocytic iris tumors may range in color from deeply pigmented to amelanotic (Fig. 51-17). They may arise anywhere within the iris stroma, although the most common location is in the inferior half of the iris (presumably due to sunlight exposure). While the vast majority of these tumors are benign and never enlarge appreciably or

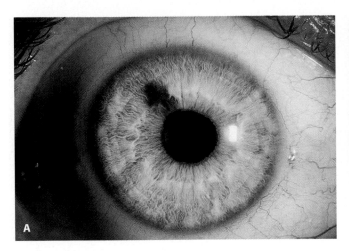
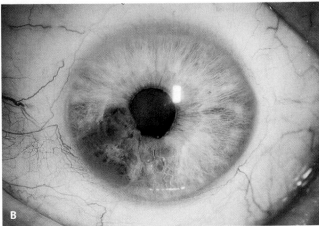

FIGURE 51-17.   *Clinical appearance of melanocytic iris tumors. A. Small, uniformly pigmented melanocytic iris tumor. Low probability of malignancy. B. Larger melanocytic iris tumor with elevation, pigment shedding into the angle and prominent intratumoral vessels. Higher probability of malignancy.*

metastasize, a subset of these tumors can be highly malignant (52).

Treatment

Observation

Most melanocytic iris tumors are initially managed by observation. Each office visit should include slit-lamp examination and measurements, gonioscopy, transillumination (as indicated), and dilated fundus examination. The size, appearance, and location of the tumor are further documented with slit-lamp photography of the iris and angle. Only about 6.5% of tumors that are initially managed by observation will grow within five years (52). The clinical feature that has been found to be most strongly predictive of growth is largest basal tumor diameter (52). There is no convincing evidence that observation for evidence of growth prior to treatment increases the risk of metastasis.

Local Resection (Iridocyclectomy)

Indications   Iridocyclectomy is the most common surgical treatment for iris tumors suspected of being malignant. While it is not possible to determine by clinical examination alone which tumors are malignant, several clinical features have been shown to correlate strongly with histopathologic malignancy and can serve as guidelines for determining treatment (Table 51-9) (52).

Technique   If the tumor is relatively small and does not involve the iris root, a partial iridectomy can be performed. For larger tumors and those involving the iris root and angle, an iridocyclectomy should be performed.

Either local or general anesthesia can be used. A 360° conjunctival peritomy is performed, and the four rectus muscles are secured with 2-0 cotton sutures. Using the operating microscope, a limbus-based scleral flap (80% scleral

Table 51-9.   Clinical Features Prognostic for Histopathologic Malignancy of Melanocytic Iris Tumors

Large basal tumor diameter
Pigment shedding into the angle
Prominent intratumoral blood vessels
Elevated intraocular pressure
Tumor-related ocular/visual symptoms

Source: Reproduced with permission from Harbour JW, Augsburger JJ, Eagle RC Jr. Initial management and follow-up of melanocytic iris tumors. *Ophthalmology* 1995;102:1987–1993.

thickness) is made (see Fig. 51-11). The flap should extend beyond the tumor by 1 to 2 mm on both sides and 2 to 3 mm posterior to the limbus to incorporate the anterior pars plicata in the resection. A more posterior flap should be made if the tumor extends into the ciliary body. Two rows of penetrating diathermy are applied around the periphery of the scleral bed. The scleral flap is then gently elevated, and a No. 75 blade is used to enter the anterior chamber at the limbus. Viscoelastic material is used to maintain the anterior chamber, and the limbal incision is extended in both directions with corneoscleral scissors. The No. 75 blade is then used to incise the scleral bed and underlying uvea within the area of diathermy. The uveoscleral incision is extended in both directions with Vannas scissors and carried into the iris to incorporate a 1-mm margin of normal iris around the tumor. If the tumor is encroaching on the pupillary margin, a sector iridectomy is performed. Otherwise, a peripheral iridectomy can be performed in order to preserve the pupil. The dissected tissue section is then removed with fine forceps.

Any vitreous presenting at the wound is removed with the vitrectomy instrument. The scleral flap is then secured with 8-0 nylon sutures on the sclera and 9-0 nylon sutures on the limbus until the wound is watertight. The conjunctiva is reapproximated with 6-0 absorbable sutures, and an antibiotic/corticosteroid ointment is placed in the eye, followed by a nonpressure patch and protective shield. The patient is treated with topical antibiotics, corticosteroids, and cycloplegics for 7 to 10 days.

Complications Vitreous hemorrhage and hyphema are common but usually resolve spontaneously. Rarely, a vitrectomy may be required if the vitreous hemorrhage does not clear within 4 to 6 months. Hypotony can occur if more than 4 to 5 clock hours of pars plicata are removed. Retinal detachment and endophthalmitis are rare.

Results The overall metastatic death rate from iris melanoma is about 3% (46). It is assumed that prompt excision of highly suspicious or growing tumors reduces the risk of metastasis, but this has not been proven.

Enucleation

Enucleation is indicated for tumor involvement of more than 4 to 5 clock hours of iris, extensive angle involvement, posterior segment extension, uncontrolled tumor-related glaucoma, or orbital extension. The technique for enucleation is similar to that for posterior uveal melanoma patients (see Fig. 51-13).

Radiotherapy

Episcleral plaque radiotherapy has been used in lieu of enucleation for iris melanomas that are not amenable to local resection (88). Further work is required to determine the role of this modality for iris melanoma. In rare cases, external beam radiotherapy is used as a palliative measure in terminally ill or incapacitated patients who are symptomatic from iris melanoma complications.

INTRAOCULAR VASCULAR TUMORS

Retinal Capillary Hemangioma

Clinical Considerations

Retinal capillary hemangiomas may be an isolated finding, or they may occur as part of the von Hippel-Lindau syndrome (autosomal dominant inheritance, multiple and/or bilateral retinal capillary hemangiomas, cerebellar hemangioblastomas, renal cell carcinomas, and pheochromocytomas) (47). The characteristic clinical features of these lesions include an elevated, vascularized retinal mass located anywhere in the retina, prominent feeder vessels, and lipid exudation (Fig. 51-18). Early tumors are small and flat and may be difficult to diagnose. The lipid exudates from peripheral tumors can accumulate in the macula, causing decreased vision. Exudative, rhegmatogenous, tractional, and complex retinal detachments can also occur.

Lesions with a similar appearance may be seen in patients with chronic retinal disease, such as retinitis pigmentosa, chorioretinitis, and retinal detachment. These "pseudoan-

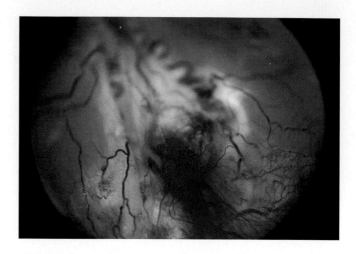

FIGURE 51-18. *Retinal capillary hemangioma with overlying gliosis, prominent feeder vessels, and lipid exudation.*

giomas" usually do not have prominent feeder vessels or lipid exudation into the macula, and they occur most commonly in the inferotemporal periphery (86).

Treatment

Retinal capillary hemangiomas have no malignant potential but may cause decreased visual acuity from subretinal lipid accumulation in the macula or exudative or traction retinal detachment. Since most of these tumors are progressive, even asymptomatic lesions usually should be treated. Triple freeze-thaw cryotherapy is often used for tumors over 3 mm in diameter, anterior tumors, and eyes with opaque media. Argon laser photocoagulation is often used for posterior tumors in eyes with clear media (7).

The tumor should be treated directly to induce shrinkage. The feeder vessels usually do not require direct treatment but will often diminish in caliber as the tumor regresses. Several treatment sessions may be necessary. Subretinal exudates gradually resolve following adequate treatment, often leaving a residual, yellow subretinal nodule. Tractional retinal detachments can often be repaired with vitrectomy and epiretinal membrane peeling techniques (65).

Choroidal Hemangioma

Clinical Considerations

Circumscribed choroidal hemangiomas occur sporadically and are not associated with any systemic syndromes. These lesions appear as an orange choroidal mass, often with overlying subretinal fluid, pigment clumping, and fibrous metaplasia of the overlying retinal pigment epithelium (Fig. 51-19). They are typically located in the posterior pole (6,104).

Diffuse choroidal hemangiomas are rare and are usually seen in association with Sturge-Weber syndrome (nonfa-

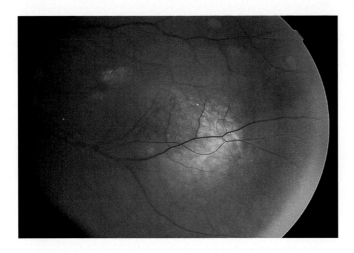

FIGURE 51-19. *Circumscribed choroidal hemangioma with characteristic orange color, overlying pigmentary changes, and subretinal fluid.*

milial ipsilateral hemangiomas of the facial skin, uveal tract, and meninges) (91). They are usually (but not always) unilateral and occupy the entire posterior uveal tract, producing a "tomato catsup fundus" due to the dark red choroidal color. These lesions may be overlooked unless the fundus color is compared with the uninvolved fellow eye. Exudative retinal detachment and glaucoma are the main causes of decreased visual acuity.

Treatment

Choroidal hemangiomas have no malignant potential and are not usually treated unless they are causing visual symptoms from subretinal fluid in the macula. Circumscribed choroidal hemangiomas are most commonly treated with the argon laser using light scatter treatment over the tumor surface. This may stimulate subretinal fluid resorption and chorioretinal adhesion (6). Low-dose plaque radiotherapy can also be effective and may be indicated for tumors involving the fovea or those resistant to laser therapy (106).

Bullous exudative retinal detachment associated with diffuse choroidal hemangiomas will often resolve with fractionated, low-dose (12 to 25 Gy) EBRT. Dramatic resolution of the retinal detachment may be seen (83).

REFERENCES

1. Abramson DH, Ellsworth RM, Rozakis GW. Cryotherapy for retinoblastoma. *Arch Ophthalmol* 1982;100:1253–1256.
2. Abramson DH, Gamell LS, Ellsworth RM, et al. Unilateral retinoblastoma: new intraocular tumours after treatment. *Br J Ophthalmol* 1994;78:698–701.
3. Abramson DH, Greenfield DS, Ellsworth RM. Bilateral retinoblastoma. Correlations between age at diagnosis and time course for new intraocular tumors. *Ophthalmic Paediatr Genet* 1992;13:1–7.
4. Adams KS, Abramson DH, Ellsworth RM, et al. Cobalt plaque versus enucleation for uveal melanoma: comparison of survival rates. *Br J Ophthalmol* 1988;72:494–497.
5. Albert DM, Niffenegger AS, Willson JK. Treatment of metastatic uveal melanoma: review and recommendations. *Surv Ophthalmol* 1992;36:429–438.
6. Anand R, Augsburger JJ, Shields JA. Circumscribed choroidal hemangiomas. *Arch Ophthalmol* 1989;107:1338–1442.
7. Annesley WH, Leonard BC, Shields JA, Tasman WS. Fifteen year review of treated cases of retinal angiomatosis. *Trans Am Acad Ophthalmol Otolaryngol* 1977;83:446–453.
8. Augsburger JJ. Fine needle aspiration biopsy of suspected metastatic cancers to the posterior uvea. *Tr Am Ophthalmol Soc* 1988;86:499–560.
9. Augsburger JJ. Diagnosis and management of posterior uveal tumors. In: Freeman WR, ed. Practical atlas of retinal disease and therapy. New York: Raven, 1993:103–124.
10. Augsburger JJ, Gamel JW, Sardi VF, et al. Enucleation vs cobalt plaque radiotherapy for malignant melanomas of the choroid and ciliary body. *Arch Ophthalmol* 1986;104:655–661.
11. Augsburger JJ, Gamel JW, Shields JA. Cobalt plaque radiotherapy versus enucleation for posterior uveal melanoma: comparison of survival by prognostic index groups. *Tr Am Ophthalmol Soc* 1989;87:348–361.
12. Augsburger JJ, Gamel JW, Shields JA, et al. Post-irradiation regression of choroidal melanomas as a risk factor for death from metastatic disease. *Ophthalmology* 1987;94:1173–1177.
13. Augsburger JJ, Goel SD. Visual function following enucleation or episcleral plaque radiotherapy for posterior uveal melanoma. *Arch Ophthalmol* 1994;112:786–789.
14. Augsburger JJ, Kleineidam M, Mullen D. Combined iodine-125 plaque irradiation and indirect ophthalmoscope laser therapy of choroidal malignant melanomas: comparison with iodine-125 and cobalt-60 plaque therapy alone. *Graefes Arch Clin Exp Ophthalmol* 1993;231:500–507.
15. Augsburger JJ, Lauritzen K, Gamel JW, et al. Matched group study of surgical resection versus cobalt-60 plaque radiotherapy for primary choroidal or ciliary body melanoma. *Ophthalmic Surg* 1990;21:682–688.
16. Augsburger JJ, Lauritzen K, Gamel JW, et al. Matched group study of preenucleation radiotherapy versus enucleation alone for primary malignant melanoma of the choroid and ciliary body. *Am J Clin Oncol* 1990;13:382–387.
17. Augsburger JJ, Mullen D, Kleineidam M. Planned combined I-125 plaque irradiation and indirect ophthalmoscope laser therapy for choroidal malignant melanoma. *Ophthalmic Surg* 1993;24:76–81.
18. Augsburger JJ, Schroeder RP, Territo C, et al. Clinical parameters predictive of enlargement of melanocytic choroidal lesions. *Br J Ophthalmol* 1989;73:911–917.
19. Augsburger JJ, Vrabec TR. Impact of delayed treatment in growing posterior uveal melanomas. *Arch Ophthalmol* 1993;111:1382–1386.
20. Barr CC, McLean IW, Zimmerman LE. Uveal melanoma in children and adolescents. *Arch Ophthalmol* 1981;99:2133–2136.
21. Blau HM, Springer ML. Gene therapy—a novel form of drug delivery. *N Engl J Med* 1995;333:1204–1207.
22. Boniuk M, Cohen JS. Combined use of radiation plaques and photocoagulation in the treatment of choroidal melanomas. In: Jakobiec FA, ed. Ocular and adnexal tumors. Birmingham, AL: Aesculapius, 1978:80–85.
23. Butler P, Char DH, Zarbin M, Kroll S. Natural history of indeterminate pigmented choroidal tumors. *Ophthalmology* 1994;101:710–716.
24. Chan HSL, Thorner P, Gallie BL. The multidrug-resistant phenotype in retinoblastoma correlates with P-glycoprotein expression. *Ophthalmology* 1991;98:1425–1431.
25. Char DH. Clinical ocular oncology. New York: Churchill Livingston, 1989.
26. Char DH, Castro JR, Kroll SM, et al. Five-year follow-up of helium ion therapy for uveal melanoma. *Arch Ophthalmol* 1990;108:209–214.
27. Char DH, Miller TR. Fine needle biopsy in retinoblastoma. *Am J Ophthalmol* 1984;97:686–690.
28. Char DH, Miller TR, Ljung BM, et al. Fine needle aspiration biopsy in uveal melanoma. *Acta Cytologica* 1989;33:599–605.
29. Char DH, Quivey JM, Castro JR, et al. Helium ions versus iodine 125 brachytherapy in the management of uveal melanoma. A prospective, randomized, dynamically balanced trial. *Ophthalmology* 1993;100:1547–1554.
30. Damato BE. Local resection of uveal melanoma. *Bull Soc Belge Ophthalmol* 1993;248:11–17.
31. Damato BE, Paul J, Foulds WS. Predictive factors of visual outcome after local resection of choroidal melanoma. *Br J Ophthalmol* 1993;77:616–623.
32. DePotter P, Flanders AE, Shields JA, et al. The role of fat-suppression technique and gadopentetate dimeglumine in magnetic resonance imaging evaluation of intraocular tumors and simulating lesions. *Arch Ophthalmol* 1994;112:340–348.

33. DePotter P, Shields CL, Shields JA. Clinical variations of trilateral retinoblastoma: a report of 13 cases. *J Pediatr Ophthalmol Strabismus* 1994;31:26–31.

34. Diener-West M, Hawkins BS, Markowitz JA, Schachat AP. A review of mortality from choroidal melanoma. II. A meta-analysis of 5-year mortality rates following enucleation, 1966 through 1988. *Arch Ophthalmol* 1992;110:245–250.

35. Doz F, Neuenschwander S, Plantaz D, et al. Etoposide and carboplatin in extraocular retinoblastoma: a study by the Societe Francaise d'Oncologie Pediatrique. *J Clin Oncol* 1995;13:902–909.

36. Earle J, Kline RW, Robertson DM. Selection of iodine 125 for the collaborative ocular melanoma study. *Arch Ophthalmol* 1987;105:763–765.

37. Eng C, Li FP, Abramson DH, et al. Mortality from second tumors among long-term survivors of retinoblastoma. *J Natl Cancer Inst* 1993;85:1121–1128.

38. Finger PT, Buffa A, Mishra S, et al. Palladium 103 plaque radiotherapy for uveal melanoma. Clinical experience. *Ophthalmology* 1994;101:256–263.

39. Fontanesi J, Meyer D, Xu S, Tai D. Treatment of choroidal melanoma with I-125 plaque. *Int J Radiat Oncol Biol Phys* 1993;26:619–623.

40. Foulds WS, Damato BE, Burton RL. Local resection versus enucleation in the management of choroidal melanoma. *Eye* 1987;1:676–679.

41. Gallie BL, Budning AS, Chan H, et al. New chemotherapy and focal therapy for intraocular retinoblastoma. *Ophthalmology* 1995;102(suppl.):109.

42. Garretson BR, Robertson DM, Earle JD. Choroidal melanoma treatment with iodine 125 brachytherapy. *Arch Ophthalmol* 1987;105:1394–1397.

43. Gass JDM. Observation of suspected choroidal and ciliary body melanomas for evidence of growth prior to enucleation. *Ophthalmology* 1980;87:523–528.

44. Gass JDM. Comparison of prognosis after enucleation vs cobalt 60 irradiation of melanomas. *Arch Ophthalmol* 1985;103:916–923.

45. Geer DC, O'Brien JM, Smith BJ, et al. Interleukin-12 treatment of retinoblastoma. *Invest Ophthalmol Vis Sci* 1995;36:S773.

46. Geisse LJ, Robertson DM. Iris melanomas. *Am J Ophthalmol* 1985;99:638–648.

47. Glenn GM, Choyke PL, Zbar B, Linehan WM. Von Hippel-Lindau disease. Clinical review and molecular genetics. *Probl Urol* 1990;4:312–330.

48. Gonzalez VH, Hu LK, Theodossiadis PG, et al. Photodynamic therapy of pigmented choroidal melanomas. *Invest Ophthalmol Vis Sci* 1995;36:871–878.

49. Gragoudas ES. The Bragg peak of proton beams for treatment of uveal melanoma. *Int Ophthalmol Clin* 1980;20:123–133.

50. Gragoudas ES, Egan KM, Seddon JM, et al. Intraocular recurrence of uveal melanoma after proton beam irradiation. *Ophthalmology* 1992;99:760–766.

51. Gragoudas ES, Seddon JM, Egan KM, et al. Metastasis from uveal melanoma after proton beam irradiation. *Ophthalmology* 1988;95:992–999.

52. Harbour JW, Augsburger JJ, Eagle RC Jr. Initial management and follow-up of melanocytic iris tumors. *Ophthalmology* 1995;102:1987–1993.

53. Harbour JW, Char DH, Kroll S, Quivey J. Metastatic risk for distinct patterns of post-irradiation local recurrence of posterior uveal melanoma. *Ophthalmology* 1997;104:1785–1793.

54. Harbour JW, Murray TG, Byrne SF, et al. Intraoperative echographic localization of I-125 episcleral radioactive plaques for posterior uveal melanoma. *Retina* 1996;16:129–134.

55. Harbour JW, Murray TG, Cicciarelli N, et al. Local carboplatin therapy in transgenic murine retinoblastoma. *Invest Ophthalmol Vis Sci* 1996;37:1892–1898.

56. Hungerford JL, Toma NMG, Plowman PN, Kingston JE. External beam radiotherapy for retinoblastoma: I. Whole eye technique. *Br J Ophthalmol* 1995;79:109–111.

57. Hykin PG, McCartney ACE, Plowman PN, Hungerford JL. Postenucleation orbital radiotherapy for the treatment of malignant melanoma of the choroid with extrascleral extension. *Br J Ophthalmol* 1990;74:36–39.

58. Ksander BR, Murray TG. Immunotherapy of ocular tumors using lymphokine gene transfer. *J Ophthalmic Photog* 1995;17:36–37.

59. Linstadt D, Castro J, Char D, et al. Long-term results of helium ion irradiation of uveal melanoma. *Int J Radiat Oncol Biol Phys* 1990;19:613–618.

60. Logani S, Helenowski TK, Thakrar H, Pothiawala B. Gamma knife radiosurgery in the treatment of ocular melanoma. *Stereotact Funct Neurosurg* 1993;61(suppl.):38–44.

61. Lommatzsch PK. Results after beta-irradiation (106-Ru/106-Rh) of choroidal melanomas: 20 years' experience. *Br J Ophthalmol* 1986;70:844–851.

62. Ma D, Niederkorn JY. Efficacy of tumor-infiltrating lymphocytes in the treatment of hepatic metastases arising from transgenic intraocular tumors in mice. *Invest Ophthalmol Vis Sci* 1995;36:1067–1075.

63. Magramm I, Abramson DH, Ellsworth RM. Optic nerve involvement in retinoblastoma. *Ophthalmology* 1989;96:217–222.

64. McCormick B, Ellsworth R, Abramson D, et al. Radiation therapy for retinoblastoma: comparison of results with lens-sparing versus lateral beam techniques. *Int J Radiat Oncol Biol Phys* 1988;15:567–574.

65. McDonald HR, Schatz H, Johnson RN, et al. Vitrectomy in eyes with peripheral retinal angioma associated with traction macular detachment. *Ophthalmology* 1996;103:329–335.

66. Messmer EP, Heinrich T, Hopping W, et al. Risk factors for metastases in patients with retinoblastoma. *Ophthalmology* 1991;98:136–141.

67. Meyer-Schwickerath G, Bornfeld N. Photocoagulation of choroidal melanomas: thirty years' experience. In: Lommatzsch PK, Blodi FC, eds. Intraocular tumors. Berlin: Akademie, 1983:269–276.

68. Moore RF. Choroidal sarcoma treated by intra-ocular insertion of radon seeds. *Br J Ophthalmol* 1930;14:145–152.

69. Moura RA, McPherson AR, Easley J. Malignant melanoma of the choroid: treatment with episcleral 198-Au plaque and xenon-arc photocoagulation. *Ann Ophthalmol* 1985;17:114–125.

70. Mukai S. Molecular genetic diagnosis of retinoblastoma. *Semin Ophthalmol* 1993;8:292–299.

71. Mukai S, Munzenrider JW, Jug EB, Gragoudas ES. Proton beam therapy of bilateral retinoblastoma. *Invest Ophthalmol Vis Sci* 1995;36:S488.

72. Murphree AL, Stout AU, Szirth B, et al. Carboplatin and laser generated hyperthermia: preliminary results in the treatment of focal intraocular retinoblastoma. *Invest Ophthalmol Vis Sci* 1992;34:S877.

73. Murray TG, O'Brien JM, Steeves RA, Albert DM. Interaction of ferromagnetic hyperthermia and external beam irradiation in the treatment of murine retinoblastoma. *Invest Ophthalmol Vis Sci* 1992;33:S877.

74. Nelson SC, Friedman HS, Oakes WJ, et al. Successful therapy for trilateral retinoblastoma. *Am J Ophthalmol* 1992;114:23–29.

75. Niederkorn JY, Mellon J, Pidherney M, et al. Effect of anti-ganglioside antibodies on the metastatic spread of intraocular melanomas in a nude mouse model of human uveal melanoma. *Curr Eye Res* 1993;12:347–358.

76. Oosterhuis JA, Journee-de Korver HG, Kakebeeke-Kemme HM, Bleeker JC. Transpupillary thermotherapy in choroidal melanomas. *Arch Ophthalmol* 1995;113:315–321.

77. Packer S, Stoller S, Lesser ML, et al. Long-term results of iodine 125 irradiation of uveal melanoma. *Ophthalmology* 1992;99:767–773.

78. Peyman GA, Juarez CP, Diamond JG, Raichand M. Ten years' experience with eye wall resection for uveal malignant melanomas. *Ophthalmology* 1984;91:1720–1725.

79. Quivey JM, Char DH, Phillips TL, et al. High intensity 125-iodine (125I) plaque treatment of uveal melanoma. *Int J Radiat Oncol Biol Phys* 1993;26:613–618.

80. Reese AB. Tumors of the eye. Hagerstown, MD: Harper & Row, 1976:90–132.

81. Roarty JD, McLean IW, Zimmerman LE. Incidence of second neoplasms in patients with bilateral retinoblastoma. *Ophthalmology* 1988;95:1583–1587.

82. Schachat AP, Hawkins BS. Collaborative ocular melanoma study. In: Ryan SJ, ed. Retina. 2nd ed. St. Louis: Mosby, 1994:828–831.

83. Scott TA, Augsburger JJ, Brady LW, et al. Low dose ocular irradiation for diffuse choroidal hemangiomas associated with bullous nonrhegmatogenous retinal detachment. *Retina* 1991;11:389–393.

84. Seddon JM, Gragoudas ES, Egan KM, et al. Relative survival rates after alternative therapies for uveal melanoma. *Ophthalmology* 1990;97:769–777.

85. Shields CL, Shields JA, Baez K, et al. Optic nerve invasion of retinoblastoma. Metastatic potential and clinical risk factors. *Cancer* 1994;73:692–698.

86. Shields CL, Shields JA, Barrett J, DePotter P. Vasoproliferative tumors of the ocular fundus. *Arch Ophthalmol* 1995;113:615–623.

87. Shields CL, Shields JA, DePotter P, et al. Plaque radiotherapy in the management of retinoblastoma. Use as a primary and secondary treatment. *Ophthalmology* 1993;100:216–224.

88. Shields CL, Shields JA, DePotter P, et al. Treatment of non-resectable malignant iris tumours with custom designed plaque radiotherapy. *Br J Ophthalmol* 1995;79:306–312.

89. Shields JA, Augsburger JJ. Cataract surgery and intraocular lenses in patients with unsuspected malignant melanoma of the ciliary body and choroid. *Ophthalmology* 1985;92:823–826.

90. Shields JA, Parsons H, Shields CL, Giblin ME. The role of cryotherapy in the management of retinoblastoma. *Am J Ophthalmol* 1989;108:260–264.

91. Shields JA, Shields CL. Intraocular tumors: a text and atlas, Philadelphia: WB Saunders, 1992.

92. Shields JA, Shields CL, Parsons H, et al. The role of photocoagulation in the management of retinoblastoma. *Arch Ophthalmol* 1990;108:205–208.

93. Shields JA, Shields CL, Shah P, Sivalingam V. Partial lamellar sclerouvectomy for ciliary body and choroidal tumors. *Ophthalmology* 1991;98:971–983.

94. Singh AD, Garway-Heath D, Love S, et al. Relationship of regression pattern to recurrence in retinoblastoma. *Br J Ophthalmol* 1993;77:12–16.

95. Sisley K, Cottam DW, Rennie IG, et al. Non-random abnormalities of chromosomes 3, 6, and 8 associated with posterior uveal melanoma. *Genes Chromosom Cancer* 1992;5:197–200.

96. Stallard HB. Malignant melanoblastoma of the choroid. *Mod Probl Ophthalmol* 1968;7:16–38.

97. Steeves RA, Murray TG, Moros EG, et al. Concurrent ferromagnetic hyperthermia and 125I brachytherapy in a rabbit choroidal melanoma model. *Int J Hyperthermia* 1992;8:443–449.

98. Tobal K, Sherman LS, Foss AJ, Lightman SL. Detection of melanocytes from uveal melanoma in peripheral blood using the polymerase chain reaction. *Invest Ophthalmol Vis Sci* 1993;34:2622–2625.

99. Toma NMG, Hungerford JL, Plowman PN, et al. External beam radiotherapy for retinoblastoma: II. Lens sparing technique. *Br J Ophthalmol* 1995;79:112–117.

100. Tucker MA, D'Angio GJ, Boice JD Jr, et al. Bone sarcomas linked to radiotherapy and chemotherapy in children. *N Engl J Med* 1987;317:588–593.

101. Tucker MA, Hartge P, Shields JA. Epidemiology of intraocular melanoma. *Recent Results Cancer Res* 1986;102:159–165.

102. Vrabec TR, Augsburger JJ, Gamel JW, et al. Impact of local tumor relapse on patient survival after cobalt 60 plaque radiotherapy. *Ophthalmology* 1991;98:984–988.

103. White L. Chemotherapy in retinoblastoma: current status and future directions. *Am J Pediatr Hematol Oncol* 1991;13:189–201.

104. Witschel H, Font RL. Hemangioma of the choroid. A clinicopathologic study of 71 cases and a review of the literature. *Surv Ophthalmol* 1976;20:415–431.

105. Yandell DW, Campbell TA, Dayton SH, et al. Oncogenic point mutations in the human retinoblastoma gene: their application to genetic counseling. *N Engl J Med* 1989;321:1689–1695.

106. Zografos L, Ludmila B, Chamot L, et al. Cobalt-60 treatment of choroidal hemangiomas. *Am J Ophthalmol* 1996;121:190–199.

Macular Surgery

Sandeep Saxena   Nancy M. Holekamp   Matthew A. Thomas

Modern vitreous surgery through the pars plana is now one of the most effective tools for treating posterior segment disease. Macular pucker, vitreomacular traction syndrome, macular hole, subfoveal choroidal neovascular membrane, and submacular hematoma comprise the spectrum of macular disease. Innovative and exciting developments in the field of macular surgery offer promise to patients with these conditions that were previously thought to be incurable.

MACULAR PUCKER

Epiretinal membranes are fine, nonvascular fibrotic membranes on the surface of the retina. They can cause a wrinkling or a puckering effect on the retinal surface, interfering with its function. These membranes can occur as a primary idiopathic disorder (Fig. 52-1), as a limited form of proliferative vitreoretinopathy after successful retinal reattachment surgery (Fig. 52-2), or as an associated finding in numerous other ocular disorders (1) (Fig. 52-3). The surgical removal of epiretinal membranes using pars plana vitrectomy was first described by Machemer (2). Surgical intervention has proved to be beneficial to patients who experience significant visual loss related to epiretinal membranes.

Pathogenesis

In idiopathic epiretinal membranes, Roth and Foos (3) proposed that glial cells of retinal origin proliferate through defects in the internal limiting membrane. Bellhorn and colleagues (4) demonstrated that glial cells from the neurosensory retina migrating through breaks in the inner lamina were responsible for producing epiretinal membranes. These breaks were usually associated with posterior vitreous sepa-

ration (5). Vitreous detachment might contribute to the development of these membranes through several mechanisms. Vitreous detachment can lead to retinal breaks, liberating retinal pigment epithelial (RPE) cells into the vitreous cavity, which can subsequently attach to the posterior retina and proliferate. Disruption of the internal limiting membrane at the time of posterior vitreous detachment could allow fibrous astrocytes access to the retinal surface to proliferate and create an extracellular matrix (4,5). Vitreous hemorrhage, inflammation, or both at the time of vitreous detachment might stimulate cellular proliferation. In cases of epiretinal membrane formation before the vitreous detaches, glial cells may grow into the vitreous cavity. As the epiretinal membrane extends over the retina, a layer of vitreous is trapped against the inner limiting lamina. This relationship between the membrane and vitreous explains one mechanism by which spontaneous separation of epiretinal membranes could occur with subsequent vitreous separation (6). Other cell types that contribute to epiretinal membrane formation include fibrocytes, myofibroblasts, macrophages, inflammatory cells, hyalocytes, retinal pigment epithelial cells, and vascular endothelial cells (7–10). Significant amounts of collagen are present in all surgically removed membranes (11). Once formed, both idiopathic and secondary epiretinal membranes behave similarly. After an initial period of growth and contraction, epiretinal membranes are morphologically and visually stable in approximately 90% of patients.

Clinical Features

Visual symptoms from epiretinal membranes manifest as a continuum from no symptoms to severe visual dysfunction and are usually related to the severity of the membrane. In fact the majority of patients with idiopathic epiretinal mem-

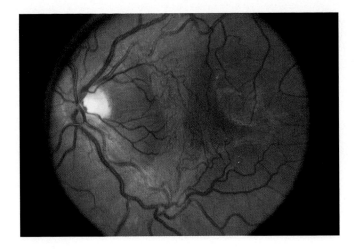

FIGURE 52-1.   *Idiopathic macular pucker.*

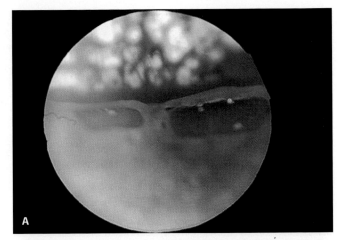

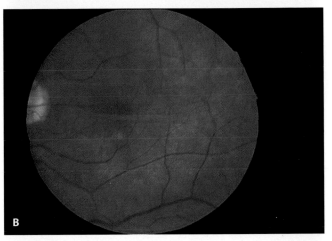

FIGURE 52-2.   A. *Open break on inferior buckle following successful retinal reattachment surgery.* B. *Macular pucker as a limited form of proliferative vitreoretinopathy.*

branes are asymptomatic (12). When minimally symptomatic, patients usually complain of mild metamorphopsia, and visual acuity remains 20/40 or better indicating that only the inner retinal surface is involved. In eyes with marked distortion of the retina patients may have severe metamorphopsia and visual acuity of less than 20/200 (13–18). Less commonly, central photopsia, macropsia, or diplopia is noted (19–23). The level of vision may also be related to preexisting retinal detachment (18). In fact, vision is usually reduced further in eyes with epiretinal membranes that occur after retinal detachment (24). Mechanisms for these symptoms include tissue covering or distorting macula, vascular leakage with cystoid macular edema, low-lying traction macular detachment, and obstructed axoplasmic flow (25,26).

The clinical characteristics vary according to the degree of the membrane. Gass (19) has proposed a classification scheme for epiretinal membranes. Translucent membranes unassociated with retinal distortion are grade 0 (cellophane maculopathy). Membranes that cause irregular wrinkling of the inner retina are grade 1 (crinkled cellophane maculopathy). Opaque membranes that cause obscuration of the underlying vessels and marked full-thickness retinal distortion are grade 2 (macular pucker).

An asymptomatic patient may have a glinting, irregular light reflex caused by a subtle epiretinal membrane. These "cellophane membranes" usually do not have a distinct edge. If the translucent membrane is more apparent, it can appear to cover the entire macula and even extend anteriorly beyond the vascular arcades. The full extent of an epiretinal membrane is best appreciated at the time of surgery, and sometimes idiopathic membranes can be stripped out past the equator (12). When internal membrane "contraction" or "shrinkage" is observed, there is an associated tractional effect on the entire inner retina, which produces fine retinal striae radiating from the center of the membrane, and tortuosity of

retinal vessels (Fig. 52-4). However, the membrane can extend beyond the area of retinal striae. In more severe and visually debilitating epiretinal membranes, vascular tortuosity with tethering and straightening of vessels occurs distal to the center of membrane contraction (12) (Fig. 52-5). If the membrane is centered distal to the macula, foveal ectopia can occur that causes complaints of diplopia. Occasionally, the epiretinal membrane lifts the sensory fovea off the retinal pigment epithelium in a subtle, shallow, table top manner. Cystoid macular edema may be present (Fig. 52-6). Pigmentation may also be present in the membrane. This may be caused by the presence of RPE cells and occurs mainly in eyes with peripheral retinal breaks or a history of prior retinal detachment (27–30).

Studies have shown an especially high incidence (75% to 93%) of posterior vitreous detachment in eyes with idiopathic epiretinal membranes (3,8,13–17,31–34). Partial or complete posterior vitreous detachment were also noted intraoperatively in 90% of eyes undergoing vitrectomy for idiopathic epiretinal membranes (32).

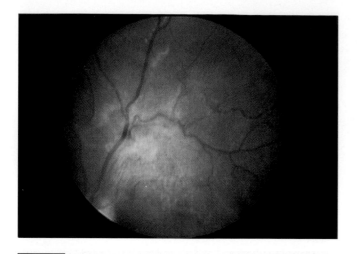

FIGURE 52-3.   *Macular pucker following branch retinal vein occlusion.*

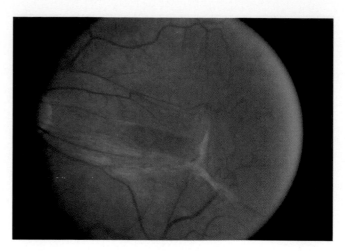

FIGURE 52-5.   *Tethering and straightening of retinal vessels occurs distal to the center of membrane contraction.*

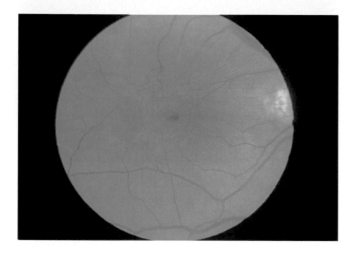

FIGURE 52-4.   *Red-free photograph demonstrates fine retinal striae radiating from center of membrane.*

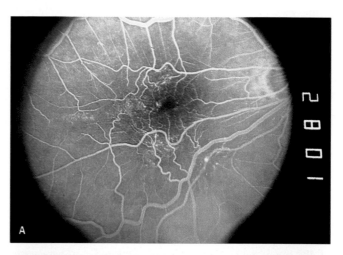

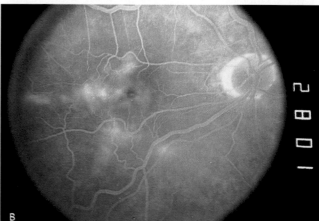

Natural History

The prevalence of epiretinal membranes varies with the underlying condition (1). The majority of patients with symptomatic idiopathic epiretinal membranes are older than 50 years. Bilateral involvement occurs in 10% to 20% of cases (14,16,34,35). Clinically significant epiretinal membranes affecting the macula occur in 4% to 8% of eyes after otherwise successful surgery for retinal detachment (36–38). Most epiretinal membranes are stable after an initial period of growth and contraction (21). Sidd and colleagues (15) in a study of 72 eyes with epiretinal membranes affecting the macula, found no change in the appearance of the membrane and the retina when reexamined an average of 31 months later. Seventy-three percent of the eyes maintained similar visual acuity during follow-up interval, and only rarely did vision improve or worsen markedly. Wiznia (16)

FIGURE 52-6.   *A. Retinal vascular tortuosity and capillary incompetence are seen in the early arteriovenous phase of fluorescein angiography. B. Late frames of the angiogram demonstrate cystoid macular edema.*

found visual loss of 2 or more Snellen lines, in 6 (12%) of 47 eyes, during a follow-up interval averaging 38 months. Occasionally, spontaneous separation of epiretinal membrane from the retinal surface can result in improvement in visual acuity (8,21,39–43). Such a phenomenon has been observed in eyes with idiopathic membranes (21,39), membranes after retinal detachment (42), retinal vascular disorders (43), and previous anterior segment surgery (39). The observation of spontaneous separation of epiretinal membranes stimulated thinking that vitreous surgery might be used to peel these membranes from the retinal surface in selected cases (2).

Surgical Case Selection

No absolute criteria exist for recommending vitrectomy for epiretinal membrane. Indications depend mainly on the visual needs of each patient (44,45). No form of treatment is known for mild epiretinal membranes (1). The optimal time for removal of epiretinal tissue is probably 6 to 8 weeks after the eye becomes symptomatic (1). Rapid progression is most common in cases with macular pucker after retinal detachment surgery. The epiretinal membrane is mature after 6 to 8 weeks and usually can be removed completely. In idiopathic cases, membrane growth is generally slow and surgery is recommended when the patient has substantial impairment of vision or severe metamorphopsia. The postoperative visual acuity may improve if the membrane has been present for a few months; however, the potential for improvement is reduced if the membrane has been present for an especially prolonged time (25,46,47). Other preoperative prognostic factors regarding final visual acuity include preoperative vision and the presence of cystoid macular edema. Although eyes with preoperative visual acuity of 20/70 or better have an improved postoperative visual acuity after vitrectomy for macular pucker, such eyes have been found to improve significantly fewer lines overall compared with those eyes with visual acuity of 20/80 or worse (47,48). Therefore, unless the patient is seriously hampered by symptoms of metamorphopsia, vitrectomy for macular pucker is often not advocated unless the visual acuity is in the range of 20/70 or worse (1,25,47). The presence of preoperative retinal vascular leakage and cystoid macular edema has been found to correlate with less visual improvement postoperatively (46,47,49). However, Margherio and colleagues (50) did not find any association between preoperative cystoid macular edema and lower postoperative vision. Removal of epiretinal membrane is usually associated with a later reduction in vascular leakage and retinal edema (19,51,52).

Surgical Technique

A conventional vitrectomy technique is used in the management of macular pucker. A complete posterior vitreous detachment is nearly always present. Sometimes the vitreous is not separated from the retina in young patients and in eyes with membranes associated with inflammatory conditions. The entire central vitreous gel is removed in aphakic and pseudophakic eyes. The anterior portion of central vitreous gel is spared in phakic eyes to decrease the possibility of trauma to the lens (50). Previously operated eyes with relatively high scleral buckles must be approached cautiously to avoid tearing the retina protruding over the buckle (48,50). The most accessible edge of the epiretinal membrane is engaged with a vitreoretinal pick. This is followed by a slight to-and-fro motion with gentle elevation (Fig. 52-7). If there is no preexisting elevation of the edge, the pick is used to apply centripetal traction on the membrane near its margin, until the edge becomes elevated (1). Often radiating striae, present in the inner retina central to the margin of the membrane, aid in the identification of the edge. A barbed microvitreoretinal blade is often used to create a plane between the epiretinal membrane and internal limiting membrane. After the edge is identified and dissection started, a vitreoretinal pick is used to avoid fragmentation of the membrane.

After a portion of the membrane has been separated from the retina, it is grasped with an intraocular forceps (Fig. 52-8). The membrane is usually removed as a single piece, although it may be necessary to engage it sequentially to tease it from the retinal surface. If an abnormally firm area of attachment to the retina is encountered, the membrane is amputated with an intraocular scissors or a vitrectomy probe. Once the epiretinal membrane is removed, the underlying retina may have an abnormal sheen, and the inner retinal surface may appear wrinkled. Prominent whitening probably represents obstruction of retrograde axoplasmic flow in the inner retinal surface and disappears in 48 to 72 hours after surgery (51). This change is important to recognize to avoid misinterpreting it intraoperatively as an additional layer of membrane. Petechial

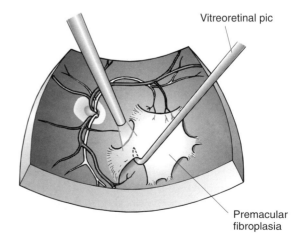

Vitreoretinal pic

Premacular fibroplasia

FIGURE 52-7. *A vitreoretinal pick is used to engage and elevate the edge of an epiretinal membrane.*

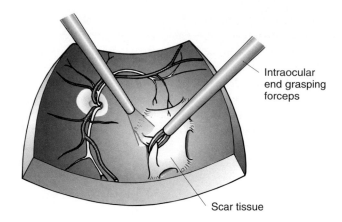

Intraocular
end grasping
forceps

Scar tissue

FIGURE 52-8.   *An intraocular forceps is used to grasp the elevated portion of the epiretinal membrane.*

hemorrhages commonly occur along the inner retinal surface as the membrane is removed (51), and denote that separation occurs at the level of the internal limiting membrane. Such minimal bleeding is usually self-limited, but may require temporarily increased intraocular pressure by elevation of the infusion bottle. Finally, at the close of each vitrectomy the retina must be carefully inspected by indirect ophthalmoscopy with peripheral scleral depression to rule out iatrogenic peripheral retinal breaks at the time of surgery.

Complications

Retinal breaks occur peripherally in 4% to 6% of eyes (26,32,47,53,54) and near the macula in fewer than 1% (14,29,35,37). Retinal detachment is reported to occur in 3% to 6% of cases (26,44,46,50). It appears to be more common in patients with macular pucker after prior retinal detachment (7%) (53) than in those with idiopathic epiretinal membranes (1%) (32). The incidence of postoperative nuclear sclerosis of the crystalline lens is reported to range from 12% to 68% (32,44,46,48,50,55). The rate of recurrent epiretinal membrane causing reduction in the best postoperative vision has been reported to range from 0 to 5% (11,25,26,46,50,56). Recurrent membranes occur in both idiopathic epiretinal membrane (5%) (55) and macular pucker after retinal detachment (2.5%) (53).

Results

In patients who underwent surgery for idiopathic epiretinal membranes, postoperative vision improved at least two Snellen lines in 78% to 87% of eyes (2,50,54,57). In the series of de Bustros and colleagues (53), vision was unchanged in 9% and worse in 4% of the eyes. In patients who underwent surgery for macular pucker after prior retinal tear or retinal detachment, vision improved at least two Snellen lines in 63% to 100% of eyes (3,31,57). In a

series of 119 eyes reported by Clarkson and colleagues (31), 104 eyes (88%) had visual improvement, 8 eyes (7%) had no change in vision, and 7 eyes (5%) had loss of vision. No difference was seen in the rate of improvement based on whether or not the macula had been damaged by the prior detachment, but the level of final visual acuity was substantially better if the macula had not been detached (1). Less frequently, vision returns to normal after surgical removal of epiretinal membrane. Margherio and colleagues (50), in their series of 184 eyes with idiopathic epiretinal membranes, reported final visual acuity of 20/30 or better in 14% of eyes and 20/50 or better in 44% of eyes. In the series of de Bustros and colleagues (53), only 2% of eyes achieved final visual acuity of 20/20, and 22% had final visual acuity of 20/40 or better. Fifteen (28%) of 51 eyes obtained final visual acuity of 20/40 or better if the macula was not detached previously, whereas 9 (16%) of 52 eyes achieved a similar level of visual acuity if the macula was involved by prior detachment.

McDonald and colleagues (44), in their series of 33 eyes, reported a mean preoperative visual acuity of 20/100 and a mean postoperative visual acuity of 20/50. Pesin and colleagues (45) reported the largest series of 270 eyes treated with pars plana vitrectomy and membrane peeling. Visual improvement of two or more lines was achieved in 58% of eyes at 3 to 5 years.

In addition to visual changes, metamorphopsia is frequently reduced postoperatively. This cannot be quantitated easily.

VITREOMACULAR TRACTION SYNDROME

Vitreomacular traction syndrome has been described as a distinct clinical entity (1). This syndrome comprises a broad spectrum of easily missed clinical findings, ranging from total peripheral vitreous separation with residual foveal attachment to multiple areas of subtle traction retinal detachment caused by persistent, focal, posterior, and peripheral vitreous attachment (8,18,20,58–63). The vitreomacular traction syndrome may represent a subset of idiopathic macular pucker (one without complete posterior vitreous detachment) and it may very well represent a premacular hole condition (albeit with low risk) (64). Because it has features that distinguish it from these entities, it deserves separate recognition (65).

The hallmark of vitreomacular traction syndrome is persistent anterior to posterior traction on the macula via a directly observable, persistent vitreoretinal attachment. The vitreous attachment margin can be observed because it is separated peripherally. This allows sharp contrast between the linear profile formed by the vitreous and optically clear postvitreous fluid. The attachment most commonly includes a one- to six-disk area zone centered on the fovea. It is usually contiguous with the optic nerve head, yielding a horizontally oriented oval or hourglass configuration of the margins. The zone of vitreous attachment also includes premacular tissue that mimics a macular pucker. The cystic macular changes stain with fluorescein and the extent of premacular tissue approximates the zone of persistent vitreous attachment (64).

Pathogenesis

The pathogenesis of vitreomacular traction syndrome is unknown. Two possible sequences may occur. Firstly, completion of subsequent vitreous separation may be prevented by epiretinal cellular proliferation. Secondly, an incomplete vitreous separation may lead to epiretinal membrane proliferation. The latter sequence seems more likely, because the visual loss tends to be progressive and the macular tissue has been observed in some cases to increase in size and extent with further follow-up (64). At the time of age-related vitreous syneresis and posterior vitreous detachment, the vitreous remains attached to the posterior pole. Some individuals have an unusually strong attachment between the posterior vitreous cortex, macula, and peripapillary retina (66–69). Vitreous cortex remnants have been found at the fovea after spontaneous vitreous detachment, which possibly indicates some degree of vitreoretinal adhesion that may not have been lysed during posterior vitreous separation (70). This supports the concept that during posterior vitreous detachment the cortical vitreous can remain attached to the posterior pole and cause traction on the macula. The occurrence of macular pucker after vitreous separation in the vitreomacular traction syndrome can result from traction-induced stimulation of proliferative cells or it may be caused by proliferation of hyalocytes stranded within persistent vitreous surface strands (8).

Transmission electron microscopy of removed epimacular tissue specimens has shown glial and contractile elements (68). Reese et al (71) demonstrated the cystic histopathologic macular changes associated with vitreomacular traction syndrome. Another histopathologic study reported a case of macular macrocystic changes in association with persistent vitreoretinal adhesion (72).

Clinical Features

The age, symptoms, and clinical appearance of patients with vitreomacular traction syndrome are similar to those with idiopathic macular pucker. The symptoms include decreased vision, metamorphopsia, and monocular diplopia. The visual symptoms may worsen gradually because persistent traction causes retinal vascular incompetence, leakage, and cystic degeneration. Alternatively, spontaneous release of the traction can occur, resulting in visual improvement. Reported cases of spontaneous peeling of an epiretinal membrane (41,43,73,74) may actually be cases in which the vitreous detachment progressed to completion and pulled the epiretinal tissue along with it.

Contact lens examination of the posterior pole may show subtle areas of traction retinal detachment, cystic macular

changes, retinal striae, a thickened posterior hyaloid face, an epiretinal membrane, and tractional changes on the optic nerve head (Fig. 52-9). Persistent posterior vitreous attachment is best seen at the posterior margin of the vitreous attachment. The characteristic area of residual posterior vitreous attachment and premacular tissue often involves a horizontally oriented, dumbbell-shaped area that encircles the macula and optic nerve head. Peripapillary vitreous traction appears as a ring of fibrous adherence lying on the optic nerve surface, the "fleshy doughnut" sign (75). McDonald and colleagues (75) categorized eyes anatomically as having either "classic" vitreomacular syndrome (eyes with 360° midperipheral vitreous detachment) or "variable" vitreomacular traction syndrome (eyes with a variety of midperipheral areas of vitreous separation). There is a variable amount of fibrous proliferation ranging from a diffuse cellophane-like macular appearance in mild cases to more discrete, heavy fibrous bands in more severe cases (64).

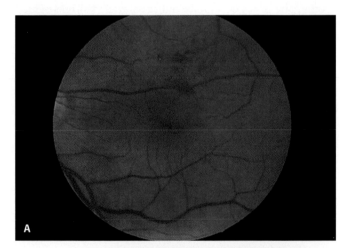

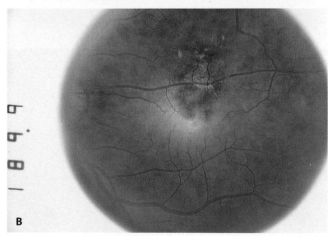

FIGURE 52-9. A. *Abnormal posterior vitreous attachment superior to the fovea produces mild tractional elevation, retinal striae, intraretinal hemorrhage, and cystic macular changes.* B. *A late frame of the angiogram confirms the presence of cystoid macular edema due to the vitreomacular traction syndrome.*

Although rare, persistent vitreomacular traction can lead to low-traction retinal detachment (Fig. 52-10). Two reported cases of idiopathic traction retinal detachment without posterior vitreous detachment may represent such a case of severe vitreomacular traction syndrome (76). Although the retina can be surgically attached in these cases, visual improvement may be limited by chronic detachment, premacular fibrosis, cystoid macular edema, or macular schisis (77). Cystic changes in the macula are seen more frequently than in idiopathic macular pucker. Fluorescein leakage has been observed more frequently than for idiopathic macular pucker (17,58) (Fig. 52-11). However, many cases may not show leakage (59). An association with vitreous cells and a higher prevalence in phakic patients has been noted (8,59).

Natural History

Jaffe (8,59) reported visual acuity that ranged from 20/25 to 20/70 in patients with the vitreomacular traction syndrome. The series of Smiddy and colleagues (58) represented patients who underwent surgery and thus their reported preoperative visual acuities were worse, ranging from 20/40 to 20/300. Two of the 16 fellow eyes had macular abnormalities, including epiretinal membrane and lamellar macular hole. Jaffe (59) reported spontaneous release of the vitreoretinal adhesion, with moderate improvement in vision and symptoms in 5 of 10 patients usually within 2 weeks, although it occurred in one patient 5 months after presentation. Recently, Hikichi and colleagues (78) reported the natural history of vitreoretinal traction syndrome in 53 consecutive symptomatic eyes. Of the 81% of eyes with cystoid macular changes at the initial diagnostic examination, 67% had cystoid changes that persisted during the median follow-up period of 60 months. In 64% of all eyes, visual acuity at the time of final examination decreased two Snellen lines or more from the initial measurement, and complete posterior vitreous detachment developed in 11% of eyes. The number of eyes with resolved cystoid changes or stable visual acuity was significantly higher when complete vitreomacular separation occurred.

Surgical Case Selection

Correctly diagnosing the vitreomacular traction syndrome allows the surgeon to inform the patient of prognosis and therapy. Idiopathic macular pucker can mimic vitreomacular traction syndrome because epiretinal membrane formation is common and vitreous insertion into the retinal surface may be difficult to observe. The relation of the vitreous to the retina, even in cases with epimacular proliferation, is the predominant feature that separates idiopathic macular pucker from vitreomacular traction syndrome (64).

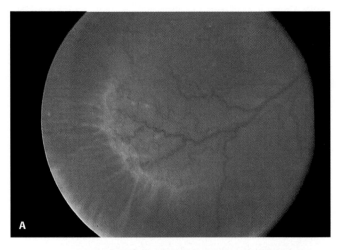

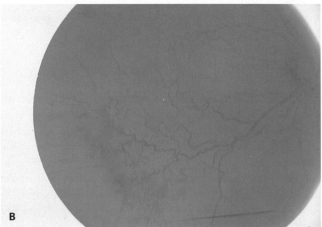

FIGURE 52-11.   A. *The margin of persistent vitreous attachment in the inferotemporal macula is easily seen. B. Fluorescein leakage is often observed at the margin of persistent vitreous traction.*

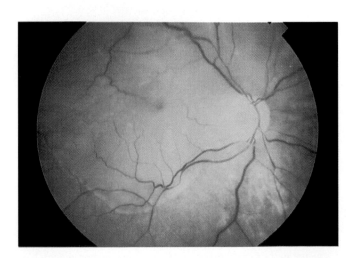

FIGURE 52-10.   *The vitreomacular traction syndrome with traction-induced macular detachment.*

In true epiretinal membranes, posterior vitreous separation is almost always present (79). Another diagnostic difficulty lies in differentiating vitreomacular traction syndrome from impending macular hole (61,80). The main distinguishing feature is observation of direct vitreomacular traction. Visual acuity is typically better in stage I macular hole than it is in vitreomacular traction syndrome, although patients with mild cases of vitreomacular traction syndrome may have good vision. Central serous chorioretinopathy and cystoid macular edema can also mimic vitreomacular traction syndrome. The distinguishing features between these clinical entities can usually be best observed with contact lens and biomicroscopy.

Surgical Technique

A standard three-port vitrectomy is performed to remove anterior to posterior vitreous traction. In cases with formed vitreous membranes, the posterior hyaloid is identified and elevated in an "en bloc" fashion using a vitreoretinal pick or a bent needle. Subsequently, the posterior hyaloid is removed along with any contiguous preretinal tissue. Special care is taken to avoid direct macular trauma. Frequently, it is impossible to determine the vitreoretinal relationship preoperatively. The vitreoretinal relationship can be determined intraoperatively using oblique intraocular illumination, noting the effect of gentle tractional forces on the macula. During surgery, Margherio and colleagues (60) divided the elements of vitreomacular traction into three types. Type 1 vitreomacular traction (noted in 73% of eyes) consists of tangential traction alone. Type 2 vitreomacular traction syndrome (noted in 19% of the eyes) is of anteroposterior variety. Type 3 (noted in 8% of eyes) is a combination of types 1 and 2. This classification has not been widely advocated, however.

Complications

Complications of vitreous surgery for vitreomacular traction syndrome include accelerated nuclear sclerosis (60,75), epiretinal membrane formation (75), retinal breaks (75), retinal detachment, and macular holes (60).

Results

Smiddy and colleagues (58) reported improvement in Snellen visual acuity by two lines or more in 10 of 16 eyes. The final visual acuity was 20/70 or better in 9 of 16 eyes. McDonald and colleagues (75) reported improvement in vision of two or more lines in 75% of eyes, with 40% obtaining 20/50 visual acuity or better. Recently, Melberg and colleagues (77) reported their experience with vitrectomy for vitreomacular traction syndrome with macular detachment. In seven of nine eyes (78%), the macula was attached after surgery. Visual acuity improved in four eyes and became worse in one eye.

IDIOPATHIC MACULAR HOLE

Recent advances in the pathogenesis, classification, and surgical intervention of idiopathic macular holes have generated a renewed interest in this entity. Better indicators of visual outcome as well as refinements in the surgical technique have led to improvements in the success of macular hole surgery.

Pathogenesis

Clinical characterization and theories on the pathogenesis of macular hole have continued to evolve (81). Although originally thought to be the result of trauma (82), it is now recognized that most macular holes occur in the absence of antecedent injury and are referred to as idiopathic. Theories for the pathogenesis of idiopathic macular holes have included progressive thinning of the foveal tissue (83) and prehole cyst formation (84,85). The primary pathogenic role of the vitreous was suggested by studies that indicated a low relative risk for macular hole formation in eyes with complete posterior vitreous detachment (83,84,86). Gass (61) and Gass and Johnson (80) proposed a theory whereby shrinkage of adherent cortical vitreous and subsequent tangential vitreous traction first cause a circumscribed foveolar detachment (stage I) followed by early retinal dehiscence (stage II), then enlargement of the macular hole with vitreofoveal separation (stage III) and finally complete posterior vitreous detachment (stage IV). Guyer and Green (87) proposed three mechanisms of tangential traction on the macula, including fluid movements and counter currents, cellular remodeling of cortical vitreous, and contraction of a cellular membrane on the inner surface of the tapered cortical vitreous.

Gass (61) emphasized the difficulty in distinguishing posterior vitreous detachment (PVD) from a zone of posterior vitreous liquefaction and attached posterior cortical vitreous over the macula. He also emphasized that unless the posterior cortical vitreous contains the vitreous condensation ring (Weiss's ring) over the optic nerve, an operculum, or a pseudo-operculum, the diagnosis of PVD is uncertain. Smiddy and colleagues (88) discovered the presence of a thin transparent structure adherent to the retina during vitrectomy for prevention of macular holes and provided a correlate to Gass' hypothesis. Results of histopathologic examination of the excised tissue confirmed its vitreous nature (89). Kishi and Shimizu (90) described a posterior precortical vitreous pocket in older patients with a layer of cortical vitreous over the macula. Kishi and colleagues (91) proposed tractional elevation of Henle's fiber layer with intraretinal cyst formation as the initial feature of macular hole development.

Recently, Gordon and colleagues (92) reported five cases of full-thickness macular hole formation in eyes with a preexisting, complete, posterior vitreous detachment and concluded that in these instances, some mechanism other than tangential traction by prefoveal vitreous cortex was responsible.

Clinical Features

Idiopathic macular holes occur most frequently in the sixth decade of life. Table 52-1 summarizes the biomicroscopic findings of various stages of macular hole (93). According to Gass (93), stage IA and IB lesions represent focal foveal detachments secondary to vitreous traction. A 100- to 200-μm diameter yellow spot is the earliest change observed. With progression, a 200- to 350-μm yellowish ring develops. Fine radiating striae are often seen surrounding the yellow ring. The vision is in the range of 20/25 to 20/70. Within several weeks to months, a full-thickness dehiscence develops. This dehiscence often starts eccentrically, then opens in a "can-opener" fashion to form a crescentic retinal defect, then a horseshoe-shaped hole, and finally a round hole with an operculum. In some cases, the dehiscence starts centrally, with gradual enlargement of the hole, and no operculum develops. A ring of retinal detachment usually surrounds the hole.

As the hole enlarges, the vision generally decreases and within several months it progresses to a fully developed hole that measures approximately 500 μm in diameter. When present, the operculum is suspended over the hole by the detached vitreous cortex. With time, round yellow deposits on the central retinal pigment epithelium, epiretinal membranes that cause contracture of the internal limiting membrane, depigmentation of the pigment epithelium under the cuff of retinal elevation, and a pigmentary demarcation ring defining the outer margin of the retinal detachment may be observed. Vision is usually in the range of 20/70 to 20/400. Posterior vitreous separation from the macula and disk develops in a small percentage of cases. Eyes with idiopathic macular hole lose vision secondary to tissue dehiscence, cystic changes, and retinal cuff elevation with photoreceptor degeneration. Clinical observations have led to the impression that the macular hole and cuff enlarge secondary to persistent tangential traction from the vitreous, tangential traction from epiretinal membranes, and the development of large cystic spaces within the surrounding cuff (94).

Natural History

The natural history of idiopathic macular hole is well established. Idiopathic macular holes usually lead to a decrease in visual acuity in the range of 20/100 to 20/400 (80,83,84,95–99). Histopathologic studies (100,101) have shown variable photoreceptor degeneration around the hole suggesting the inability to support good vision. However, characterization of visual status using scanning laser ophthalmoscope indicates that good visual function may persist at the edge of the hole. Aaberg (97) noted vision of 20/100

Table 52-1. Biomicroscopic Classification of Idiopathic Macular Hole

Stage	Biomicroscopic Findings	Anatomic Interpretation
IA (impending hole)	Central yellow spot Loss of foveolar depression No vitreofoveolar separation	Early serous detachment of foveolar retina
IB (impending or occult hole)	Yellow ring with bridging interface Loss of foveolar depression No vitreofoveolar separation	For small ring, serous foveolar detachment with lateral displacement of xanthophyll; for larger ring, central occult foveolar hole with centrifugal displacement of foveolar retina and xanthophyll, with bridging contracted prefoveolar vitreous cortex
II	Eccentric oval, crescent, or horseshoe retinal defect inside edge of yellow ring Central round retinal defect Rim of elevated retina with prefoveolar opacity Without prefoveolar opacity	Hole (tear) in contracted prefoveolar vitreous bridging round retinal hole, no loss of foveolar retina Hole with pseudo-operculum[a], rim of retinal detachment Hole, no posterior vitreous detachment from optic disk and macula
III	Central round ≥400 μm diameter No retinal defect Weiss's ring, rim of elevated retina With prefoveolar opacity Without prefoveolar opacity	 Hole with pseudo-operculum, no posterior vitreous detachment Hole with no posterior vitreous detachment from optic disk and macula
IV	Central round retinal defect, rim of elevated retina, Weiss's ring With prefoveolar opacity[b] Without prefoveolar opacity	 Hole with pseudo-operculum and posterior vitreous detachment from optic disk and macula Hole and posterior vitreous detachment from optic disk and macula

[a] Pseudo-operculum contains no retinal receptors.
[b] Prefoveolar opacity usually found near temporal border of Weiss's ring.
Source: Modified from Gass JDM. Reappraisal of biomicroscopic classification of stages of development of a macular hole. *Am J Ophthalmol* 1995;119:752–759.

to 20/400 in 80% of 73 eyes, with nearly half at a level of 20/200. McDonnell and colleagues (84) observed vision of 20/100 to 20/400 in most of their 17 eyes. Morgan and Schatz (83) reported vision of 20/100 to 20/400 in 60% of 132 eyes and 20/80 or better vision in 30%.

Yuzawa and colleagues (102) observed that the incidence of apparent disappearance of idiopathic full-thickness macular holes was low. Improvement in visual acuity was greater in those cases in which macular holes disappeared in a relatively short period of time. Kakehashi and colleagues (103) found that foveal detachment and macular break resolution seem to result from the release or weakening of vitreous traction on the fovea. Reattachment of the fovea preserves fair to good visual acuity.

Hikichi and colleagues (104) noted progression of stage II lesions to stage III and IV in 67% and 29% of eyes, respectively. They concluded that even though vitreomacular separation can improve the prognosis of a macular hole, stage II lesions usually will develop an enlarged hole and decreased visual acuity.

Fisher and colleagues (105) suggested that fellow eyes in patients with unilateral idiopathic macular holes have a relatively favorable natural history and that kinetic ultrasound examination can help determine which of these fellow eyes is at highest risk of full-thickness macular hole developing. Akiba and colleagues (106) found that 10 (37%) of 27 eyes that had an impending macular hole without vitreous separation from the fovea progressed to a fully developed macular hole. Akiba and colleagues (107) also reported that 14 fellow eyes (37%) of 38 eyes with stage I macular hole or unilateral full-thickness macular hole went on to development of full-thickness macular hole. Guyer and colleagues (108) reported that only 2 of 19 (10.5%) of the premacular hole lesions in their series progressed to macular hole formation. A resolved flat, reddish lesion was observed in 15 of 19 (79%) of their patients. Kokame and colleagues (109) found that eyes with stage I macular holes with best corrected visual acuity between 20/50 and 20/80 had a 66% risk of progression to full-thickness macular hole, whereas eyes with best corrected visual acuity between 20/25 and 20/40 had a 30% risk of progression to full-thickness macular hole.

The Vitrectomy for Macular Hole Study Group (110) has recently reported the baseline characteristics, natural history, and risk factors for progression in eyes with stage II macular holes. Forty-one eyes (37 patients) were analyzed; 19 eyes were randomized to observation (vs surgery). Mean Snellen visual acuity was 20/66 at baseline. Centric stage II holes usually had a small break (201 µm average diameter) with a dark yellow ring and without significant retinal elevation. Eccentric stage II holes had a high maximum/minimum diameter ratio and an incomplete cuff of subretinal fluid or yellow ring. Posterior vitreous detachment prevalence was 32% (8/25) and 0% (0/16) in the centric and eccentric hole groups, respectively. Progression rate to stage III or IV was 74%. Progression rate to stage III was 100% in eyes with

pericentral hyperfluorescence and 55% in eyes without pericentral hyperfluorescence. Enlargement occurred in 100% of eccentric holes and 60% of centric holes. This group concluded that eccentric and centric holes may have a different pathogenesis. In addition to purely tangential traction, some component of obliquely oriented anteroposterior vitreous traction component may be important for pathogenesis of senile macular holes, particularly stage II eccentric macular holes.

Surgical Case Selection

Many conditions that mimic macular holes have a favorable natural course and require different surgical maneuvers or are not amenable to surgical intervention. Premacular hole lesions are often misdiagnosed (111,112) and many conditions can masquerade as full-thickness macular holes (113). An epiretinal membrane with a pseudohole can be confused with a macular hole. The pseudohole usually allows better vision than does the macular hole. In addition, the pseudohole does not have a halo of fluid, an operculum, or yellow deposits at the level of retinal pigment epithelium. A foveal detachment due to central serous retinopathy (CSR) can be mistaken for a stage Ia macular hole. Both appear as a yellow spot; however, fluorescein angiography can distinguish these two entities. CSR occurs in young to middle-aged men, whereas idiopathic macular holes usually affect elderly women. Cystoid macular edema can also mimic the yellow spot of a stage I lesion. Fluorescein angiography and a history of cataract extraction can be useful in differentiating between these two conditions. The early yellow lesion of solar retinopathy can also appear similar to a stage I lesion. A central drusen or retinal pigment epithelium depigmentation with a small amount of subretinal fluid and a central fibrocellular epiretinal membrane with a macular detachment have been described as mimicking an impending macular hole. The vitreomacular traction syndrome can mimic an impending macular hole. Vitreous traction on the macula due to an incomplete vitreous detachment is responsible for this lesion. These disorders can be distinguished by examination of the vitreous.

A full-thickness macular hole is most accurately diagnosed clinically using a fundus contact lens and slit lamp biomicroscopy. Supplemental tests that can assist in or allow for more accurate diagnosis include Amsler grid testing (114), testing for a Watzke-Allen sign (115), and fluorescein angiography (97). Amsler grid testing is sensitive in detecting any form of macular abnormality, but is not specific enough to be useful in establishing a diagnosis of macular hole, and preoperative testing has not been standardized (116). The Watzke-Allen test and to a greater degree the laser-aiming beam test further improve the accuracy of diagnosis of full-thickness macular holes. The major advantage of these tests is that they are simple to perform, can be done in the office, and are easily accessible (116). Watzke-Allen sign testing in all patients with clinically defined macular holes shows a break or thinning of the slit beam. Thinning of the beam is seen in both macular hole and pseudomacular hole cases. Therefore, thinning is not as specific as a total break in the slit beam in full-thickness macular hole.

The laser-aiming beam test may yield similar diagnostic information, allowing the clinician to test focal areas of the retina for a scotoma. A 50-μ spot laser-aiming beam can be hidden in the macular lesion in all patients with clinically defined full-thickness macular hole. This contrasts with the finding in pseudohole eyes, which could detect the 50-μ spot. In addition, the inability to detect a 200- or 500-μ spot size is noted only by patients with macular holes. Thus, the absolute scotoma detected by the laser beam test is sensitive and specific for full-thickness macular holes.

Other ancillary tests, such as focal electroretinography (117), scanning laser ophthalmoscopy (118–120), confocal laser tomographic analysis systems (121), monochromatic photography (122), and laser biomicroscopy (123,124), have been applied to the study of macular holes with some success. These modalities are not available or feasible for many clinical practices, however.

Echographic features of idiopathic macular hole correlate reasonably accurately with clinical features (125,126). A pseudo-operculum is a focal condensation of the vitreous cortex suspended on detached invisible posterior hyaloid membrane, in front of either intact foveolar retina or full-thickness macular hole (81,127). It is demonstrable ultrasonographically (127). Its presence in front of intact foveolar retina indicates evidence of vitreofoveal separation and low risk of developing a macular hole.

Optical coherence tomography has been found effective in distinguishing full-thickness macular holes from partial-thickness holes, macular holes, and cysts. It has been successful in staging macular holes and providing a quantitative measure of hole diameter and the amount of surrounding macular edema. It can also detect small separations of the posterior hyaloid from the retina (128).

Careful patient selection is critical to a successful outcome. The ideal candidate would be a patient with bilateral holes of relatively recent onset, with vision in the better eye less than or equal to 20/100. Patients with unilateral symptomatic holes with recently reduced vision to 20/70 or worse are also good candidates (129).

As reported anatomic success rates for macular surgery increase, a method of accurately predicting postoperative visual acuity has increased clinical utility. Both laser interferometer and potential acuity meter have been found to be modestly accurate. Laser interferometer was found to be more accurate in predicting a visual acuity of 20/50 or better (130).

Management

Limited visual improvement in eyes with laser photocoagulation, in an effort to flatten the localized detachment around the hole, has been reported (131,132). This type of treatment could damage potentially viable photoreceptors at the margins of the macular hole.

The new understanding of the pathogenesis of this disorder led to the hypothesis that vision might stabilize or improve if it were possible to relieve the tangential traction, reduce the cystic changes, and reattach the cuff of detached retina surrounding the hole. The surgical objectives for repair of macular holes include relief of all tangential traction and retinal tamponade. Tangential traction is relieved by identification and removal of the cortical vitreous or posterior hyaloid and removal of fine epiretinal membranes around the hole. Tamponade is provided by total gas-fluid exchange with SF_6 or C_3F_8 and strict face-down positioning for at least one week (133).

Most eyes with macular hole have uniform intraoperative vitreous findings (134). A zone of collapsed vitreous fibers usually lies anterior to a posteriorly optically clear cavity. In most instances, the vitreous cortex or posterior hyaloid is invisible and remains attached to the underlying internal limiting membrane of the retina. In some cases, the presence of a focally detached vitreous is suggested by an operculum floating above the macular hole. After surgical removal of the central vitreous, it is necessary to develop and/or complete a PVD. Using active aspiration (150–250 mm Hg), a silicone-tipped suction cannula is gently swept over the retinal surface near the major arcades or the optic nerve. The area immediately around the hole is avoided. The silicone tip is noted to flex once the cortical vitreous is engaged (Fig. 52-12). This has been termed the "fish-strike sign" (135) or "divining rod sign." Once engaged, a PVD can be created by continuous suction with anterior-posterior-tangential traction while the tip is moved over the retinal surface (Fig. 52-13).

The dissection is carried from the area of initial detachment to adjacent attached areas in an attempt to complete the detachment from the posterior retina to the equatorial zone. The vitreous cortex or posterior hyaloid becomes visible as a translucent sheet, especially with oblique illumination. Occasionally, the disk attachments are so firm that the vitreous cutter on suction only, tissue forceps, or pick manipulation is required to complete the PVD in these areas. A 36-gauge subretinal pick can be useful in engaging the posterior hyaloid near the optic nerve and then pulling off Weiss's ring (Fig. 52-14). Frequently, an operculum is detected as a glial fragment attached to the vitreous cortex. Ryan and colleagues (136) described the use of intravitreal autologous blood to identify posterior cortical vitreous. We believe that this procedure is not necessary for the identification of posterior cortical vitreous. Once the vitreous is completely detached, vitrectomy is completed. If residual vitreous cortex is present, it becomes apparent during completion of the air-fluid exchange as a gelatinous substance on the surface of the retina.

Fifty percent of operated eyes have some degree of epiretinal membrane (ERM) proliferation (137). These ERMs, unlike typical ERMs, tend to be finer and more

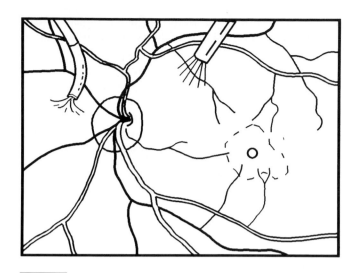

FIGURE 52-12. *A silicone-tipped suction cannula flexes once the cortical vitreous is engaged.*

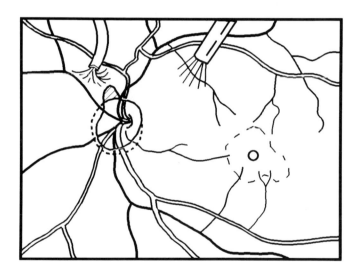

FIGURE 52-13. *With continuous suction and anterior-posterior-tangential traction, a posterior vitreous detachment can be created.*

friable, and at times are densely adherent to the retina. The ERMs may be present surrounding the hole or can involve only a few clock hours. A microbarbed myringotomy blade is used to create an edge in the ERM, which is grasped with tissue forceps and stripped. One disk area around the macular hole is checked and liberated from ERMs to ensure the relief of traction. During this maneuver, it is common to create small hemorrhages around the hole. Damage to the inner retina is avoided, an early sign of which may be the development of fluffy whitish areas.

Prolonged intense illumination from the light pipe near the macula is avoided to prevent phototoxicity. A total air-fluid exchange is performed and effort is made to dehydrate

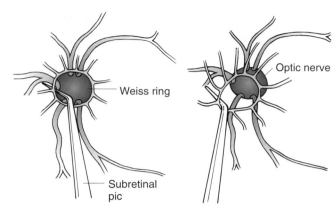

FIGURE 52-14. *A short-angled, 36-gauge subretinal pick can be useful in engaging the posterior hyaloid near the optic nerve and then pulling off Weiss's ring.*

the vitreous cavity. The shallow fluid in the base of the optic disk cup is aspirated repeatedly, with a soft-tipped cannula, until fluid no longer collects. A nonexpansive concentration of long-acting gas is exchanged for air. Postoperatively, strict prone positioning is prescribed. At the 1-week visit if the edges of the macular hole are flattened and imperceptible with flattening of the cuff of retinal detachment, anatomic success is assured. However, if the edges are still visible and the cuff elevated, anatomic failure is probable.

Results

Impending Macular Holes

Several studies have suggested that vitrectomy may be beneficial for patients with an impending macular hole. Smiddy and colleagues (88) reported arrest of progression of macular hole in 80% of eyes with premacular hole lesions. Improved vision was noted in 41% of these eyes. Jost and colleagues (138) reported arrest in progression of stage I macular hole in 90% of eyes at risk for formation of full-thickness macular hole. Improvement in vision, with 58% attaining a visual acuity of 20/25 or better, was reported. Four eyes were noted to have stage II macular holes at the time of vitrectomy. Two of these four eyes did not show progressive macular hole formation and had 20/25 visual acuity. Margherio and colleagues (60) reported a series of 106 consecutive symptomatic eyes considered to be at high risk of idiopathic macular hole formation that underwent vitrectomy with membrane peeling. Two eyes were found to have small microholes involving the fovea. Postoperatively, in both cases full-thickness holes continued to evolve, with further deterioration in visual acuity.

A prospective, multicentered trial was undertaken to study the role of vitreous surgery in impending macular holes (139,140). The study was conducted on patients with full-thickness macular holes in their first eye (stages III and

IV) and signs and symptoms of stage I macular holes in their fellow eye (study eye). Patients were randomized to surgery or observation. A full-thickness macular hole developed in 37% of the surgery group and in 40% of the observed group. Because of low recruitment the study was terminated before enough cases were enrolled to achieve statistical significance (141).

Stage II Macular Holes

Chambers and colleagues (142) reported a consecutive series treated with pars plana vitrectomy in which surgical manipulation of the prefoveal layer of cortical vitreous was avoided for stage I and stage II macular holes. The tangential and anteroposterior traction was relieved remote to the macula. No significant improvement in vision occurred in eyes with stage II macular holes, but visual acuity improved in 87% of the patients with stage I holes. Ruby and colleagues (143) reported the results for the treatment of stage II macular holes: 61% of the eyes had a visual acuity of 20/50 or better while only 18% had a visual acuity of 20/200 or worse. Seventy-five percent of the eyes showed a stable appearance of a very small hole, a decrease in the hole size, or a resolution of the full-thickness defect (Fig. 52-15).

Stages III and IV Macular Holes

Kelly and Wendel (134) reported the results of a pilot study for the treatment of stages III and IV full-thickness macular holes. Although 58% of their patients showed anatomic flattening of the macula and 73% of these improved by two or more Snellen lines of visual acuity, only 25% of all these patients had a visual acuity of 20/50 or better postoperatively, and 50% had 20/200 or worse. Subsequent follow-up study (144) on 152 consecutive eyes showed an improved anatomic success of 73%, but the percentage of patients with excellent central visual acuity has remained relatively

low, at 26%, with visual acuity of 20/40 or better. Ryan and Gilbert (145) reported the surgical treatment of recent-onset full-thickness idiopathic macular holes. In the early group (symptoms <6 months), 56% of the patients gained at least three lines of vision. Anatomic success rate was seen with one operation in 75% and with two operations in 87.5%. Stage II holes had a final anatomic success rate of 94.4%. In the late group (symptoms >6 months), closure of the hole with one operation was seen in 60% (Fig. 52-16).

Glaser and colleagues (146) used transforming growth factor β_2 (TGF β_2) as a pharmacologic adjuvant in surgery on macular holes. In the subset of patients given the highest dose of TGF β_2 (1330 ng), 91% improved two or more Snellen lines, but only 45% had visual acuity of 20/50 or better. In a subsequent study, Lansing and colleagues (147) reported a 96% anatomic success rate with 48% of the patients having visual acuity of 20/40 or better. Preliminary anatomic results of a multicenter, prospective study demonstrated that a single application of TGF β_2 had a statistically significant beneficial effect on resolution of the subretinal cuff surrounding a macular hole when used in conjunction with standardized vitrectomy for full-thickness macular holes (148). Thompson and colleagues (149) reported that a longer-duration intraocular gas tamponade from 16% C_3F_8 gives a much higher rate of successful closure of macular holes and improved visual acuity using vitrectomy and TGF β_2 than does air. Subsequently, a large, prospective randomized study sponsored by the pharmaceutical company that manufactures TGF β_2, found TGF β_2 to be no more efficacious in closing macular holes than placebo. Liggett and colleagues (150) have proposed the use of human autologous serum for treatment of full-thickness macular holes. In a small pilot study, all of the 11 eyes had resolution of the surrounding subretinal fluid and flattening of the macular hole, and showed improvement of at least two lines

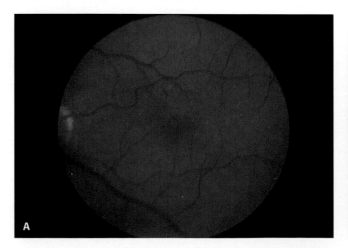
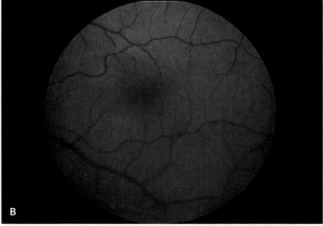

FIGURE 52-15.   A. *Preoperative stage II macular hole. Watzke-Allen sign is present.* B. *Postoperative fundus photograph shows closed macular hole. Visual acuity is 20/25-1. Watzke-Allen sign is absent.*

or more in visual acuity. A larger randomized, controlled trial has not been done.

The recovery of 20/20 visual acuity, the disappearance of focal hyperfluorescence corresponding with the macular hole angiographically, and the disappearance of absolute central scotomas observed in some patients after macular hole surgery suggest that centripetal movement of paracentral retinal receptors and their xanthophyll can occur after retinal reattachment (93,151,152). There does appear to be an inverse relationship between duration of symptoms and both anatomic success and visual improvement. Holes of shorter duration have better anatomic and visual results following surgery compared with long-standing holes. Visual results routinely lag 6 weeks behind anatomic success, with about 75% of the anatomically successful eyes improving by two lines or more of visual acuity (134). The release of macular traction creates the necessary environment for gas tamponade to reattach the cuff surrounding the macular hole in most cases. The role of chorioretinal and epiretinal proliferation in reattachment is unclear. The etiology of anatomic failure is uncertain. Patient noncompliance in postoperative prone positioning and subsequent inadequate tamponade, production of traction by residual ERMs, intrinsic retinal changes that cause stiffness, and prevention of retinal reattachment possibly play a role (137).

Experience with reoperation has been limited. If failure is believed to be secondary to residual ERMs, reoperation has been successful. If noncompliance with postoperative prone positioning is thought to be the cause of failure, newly motivated patients can be given a second chance. Macular holes can reopen after initial surgical repair. Those cells that can lead to the closure of an idiopathic macular hole can also contribute to its recurrence if the reparative process goes awry (153). Krypton laser photocoagulation and fluid gas exchange for recurrent macular hole have been reported (154).

Complications

The most common complication of a vitrectomy for impending macular hole and a full-thickness macular hole is the occurrence or progression of nuclear sclerotic cataracts. Of the patients treated for macular holes, 20% to 33% require cataract extraction postoperatively (134,144). Nuclear sclerotic cataracts progress substantially after macular hole surgery with a long-acting intraocular gas tamponade (155).

Park and colleagues (156) noted posterior segment complications in 23% of their cases. These included peripheral retinal breaks (3%), rhegmatogenous retinal detachment from a peripheral retinal break (14%), enlargement of the hole (2%), and late reopening of the hole (2%), retinal pigment epithelium loss under the hole (1%), photic toxicity (1%), and endophthalmitis (1%). Iatrogenic retinal breaks tend to be in the inferior and temporal retina, which establishes the need for greater intraoperative surveillance in these areas (157). Peripheral retinal tears may develop during stripping of cortical vitreous. The free edge of the macular hole is mobile and susceptible to incarceration during aspiration maneuvers, which can lead to tearing and enlargement of the hole (134). During membrane stripping or fluid aspiration care must be taken to avoid excessive traction and inadvertent damage to the edge of the macular hole and inner retina.

Retinal pigment epitheliopathy after macular hole surgery may portend a guarded visual prognosis in affected patients undergoing successful macular hole repair (Fig. 52-17). This may be the result of individual patient sensitivities to manipulation, direct trauma, or prolonged exposure to the endoilluminator (134). Poliner and Tornambe (158) hypothesized that combination of prolonged intraocular gas contact and light exposure exceeding threshold for an already compromised macula appear to be responsible for

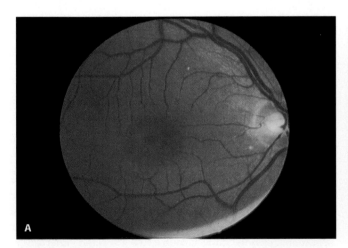
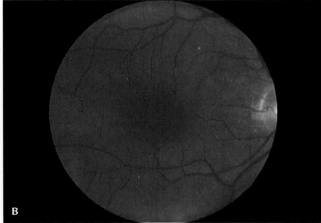

FIGURE 52-16. A. *Preoperative stage III macular hole. Visual acuity is 20/200.* B. *Postoperative fundus photograph shows closed macular hole. Visual acuity is 20/70.*

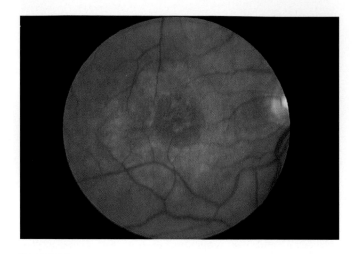

FIGURE 52-17. *Retinal pigment epitheliopathy following vitrectomy and gas-fluid exchange for stage IV macular hole. Although the hole is closed, the patient sees a ring scotoma, and visual acuity is 20/150.*

this pigmentary pattern. According to Charles (159), RPE changes seem more likely to be secondary to trauma to the RPE and photoreceptors and occur secondary to precipitous suction removal of thick subretinal fluid through macular holes. Duker (160) hypothesized that the persistence of subretinal fluid may be as important as individual susceptibility or overall light exposure for the development of this epitheliopathy.

Late reopening can complicate initially successful macular hole surgery and may occur in at least 4.8% of initially successful operations. Reopening has been documented to occur at between 2 and 22 months, and it has been hypothesized that the growth of an ERM plays a part in at least some of the eyes. Repeat vitrectomy with gas injection can result in reclosure of the hole and improvement in vision (161). Kokame (162) reported late recurrence of macular hole in an eye with impending macular hole, which initially resolved after surgical intervention. The mechanism of late recurrence may be similar in impending and full-thickness macular holes (162). Smiddy (163) also noted macular hole development after surgical peeling of epiretinal membrane over the macula. Thus macular holes can develop in certain situations in which the posterior cortical vitreous has been removed from the macula, either surgically or by natural posterior vitreous detachment (163).

SUBMACULAR SURGERY

In the last several years, a surge of interest has been seen in submacular surgery. Candidates for this surgery consist primarily of individuals with subfoveal choroidal neovascularization and those with submacular hemorrhage.

Subfoveal Choroidal Neovascularization

Choroidal neovascularization (CNV) is a principal cause of loss of central visual function in adults. Choroidal neovascular membranes disrupt normal macular anatomy (including the critical photoreceptor-retinal pigment epithelial interface); leak serum or formed blood elements, or both; and lead to irreversible loss of overlying photoreceptors (164). When fibrovascular membranes grow beneath the center of the foveal avascular zone (FAZ), the visual prognosis is generally poor. Choroidal neovascular membranes are most frequently caused by age-related macular degeneration (AMD) and presumed ocular histoplasmosis syndrome (POHS), although neovascularization may be observed as a complication of other ocular conditions (165–179).

Natural History

The visual prognosis is related to the underlying etiology of the subfoveal CNV. Bressler and colleagues (180) found that 70% of eyes with subfoveal membranes secondary to AMD had visual acuities of 20/200 or worse within 2 years. The Macular Photocoagulation Study Group (181) reported 3- and 4-year visual outcomes in eyes followed in two randomized clinical trials of laser photocoagulation for subfoveal CNV secondary to AMD. Four years after enrollment in the subfoveal new CNV study, 39 (47%) of 83 untreated eyes and 17 (22%) of 77 laser-treated eyes had lost six or more lines of visual acuity from baseline levels. At the 3-year examination in the subfoveal recurrent CNV study, 21 (36%) of 58 untreated eyes and 6 (12%) of the treated eyes had lost six or more lines of visual acuity from baseline levels. Eyes with POHS do better; as many as 14% may retain visual acuity of 20/40 despite subfoveal vessels (182,183). However, 90% of eyes with visual acuity of 20/200 or less still will have severely reduced visual acuity after 3 years. Only 7% of membranes in eyes with CNV secondary to POHS undergo spontaneous involution with improvement in visual acuity (184). Fibrovascular membranes, regardless of etiology, usually continue to grow without treatment. Vander and colleagues (185) documented an average growth rate of 9 μm a day in eyes with neovascular membranes in AMD. Enlarging membranes beneath the fovea often lead to disciform scars with poor visual function.

Management

The objective in treating CNV is to destroy the abnormal neovascular tissue and limit its damaging effects. Over the last 20 years, laser photocoagulation has been shown to be effective in the management of extrafoveal and juxtafoveal membranes of various etiologies (186–193). The Macular Photocoagulation Study Group (194–196) and other investigators (197,198) have demonstrated a marginal benefit of laser treatment compared with observation in certain eyes with AMD even when the neovascular tissue lies beneath the center of the fovea. One of the principal limitations of laser photocoagulation is the concomitant damage to overlying neurosensory retina (199). This is particularly harmful when the membrane is under the center of the fovea because central vision is almost always significantly reduced after treatment (195,196,200). Surgical removal is an alternative means of eradicating subfoveal CNV with potentially less damage to neurosensory retina and, in some cases, better visual function.

In 1988, de Juan and Machemer (201) reported four cases of submacular scar removal using modern vitrectomy techniques. Following vitrectomy, a large circumferential retinotomy was made on the temporal side of the macula, allowing direct access to and dissection of the submacular tissue. Because of a high incidence of proliferative vitreoretinopathy and retinal detachment, as well as discouraging visual results, this technique was not widely employed. Blinder and colleagues (202) proposed a similar technique creating large-flap retinotomies (between 200 and 260 degrees), modified by the preoperative administration of barrier photocoagulation treatment. Understanding the importance of subfoveal retinal pigment epithelium (RPE) integrity following subfoveal scar removal, they combined their technique with transposition RPE flaps and homologous RPE grafts with limited success (203).

In 1991, Thomas and Kaplan (204) reported a different approach to subfoveal neovascular membrane removal in POHS. The technique emphasized making a small retinotomy away from the center of the fovea; through this incision, the subfoveal neovascular complex was accessed and removed from the eye. A small retinotomy does not require laser photocoagulation at the conclusion of the procedure, thus preventing thermal damage to juxtafoveal retina, RPE, and choriocapillaris (205). The surgical technique has now become established (206–213). Emphasis has been placed on the design and development of smaller-gauge instruments to facilitate subretinal tissue manipulation while minimizing RPE and photoreceptor trauma. However, the principal limitations of the surgical technique arise from the concomitant damage to adjacent ocular structures associated with the CNV, especially in AMD. Thus case selection is of critical importance (214).

Case Selection

As with any new technique, the determination of appropriate case selection awaits the outcome of a randomized, prospective clinical trial that is currently under way. With our experience of the past 6 years, it appears that choroidal neovascular membranes anterior to the RPE seem to have the best surgical prognosis, as preservation of the RPE is a critical factor in the subsequent recovery of central visual function. If the goal of surgery is regaining central foveal function, then surgical removal of a subfoveal, choroidal neovascular membrane is advised if it appears to lie anterior

to the RPE. Contact lens examination of the macula combined with color-stereo views and stereoscopic fluorescein angiography helps in determining the membrane's location. The following clinical findings may suggest that the neovascular complex lies anterior to the RPE: 1) a well-defined edge with an abrupt transition to underlying RPE, 2) an anterior location apparent on stereoscopic viewing, 3) a thin layer of subretinal blood outlining the edges of a neovascular complex and the subjacent RPE, 4) a pigmented border (which corresponds to the rim of hypofluorescence occasionally seen angiographically) outlining the location of the membrane (Fig. 52-18). Some lesions that are indeed anterior to RPE may lack a sharp border perhaps because of their recent onset. Additionally, fibrin may obscure the border with underlying RPE (165). Angiographic findings suggestive of an anterior location of the membrane include the following: 1) a distinct boundary between the

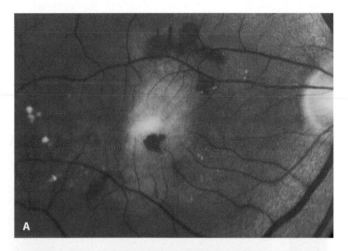

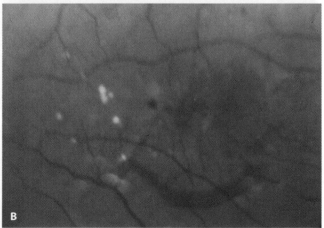

FIGURE 52-18. A. *This compact subfoveal neovascular membrane appears to lie anterior to the RPE, has a slightly pigmented border, and is partially outlined by a thin layer of subretinal blood. B. A one-day postoperative photograph confirms that the membrane was anterior to RPE and could be safely removed without damaging underlying structures.*

hyperfluorescence of the membrane and background choroidal fluorescence; 2) a rim of blocked fluorescence between the two; 3) compact angiographic appearance; 4) homogenous hyperfluorescence; 5) clearly visible lacy vascular pattern; 6) anterior location apparent on stereo-angiogram viewing; and 7) absence of late staining surrounding tissues (indicative of occult or sub-RPE neovascularization) (Fig. 52-19). Membranes posterior to the RPE tend to have clinical and angiographic findings that are the opposite of those for anterior membranes.

Instrumentation

Thomas and colleagues (215) have developed instruments that greatly facilitate subretinal removal of choroidal neovascular membranes and hematomas. Subsequently, Thomas and Ibanez (216) have developed a newer generation of subretinal instruments.

Angled Subretinal Pick   The angled pick, having a 20-gauge shaft, a 130-degree bend, and a flattened tip tapering to 0.305 mm (36 gauge) has been developed. The blade is used to perforate neurosensory retina to create the initial retinotomy, to push against and disconnect the neovascular complex and to dissect gently under the neovascular complex.

Subretinal Infusion Cannulas   The 20-gauge needle tapers to 33-gauge proximal to the 130-degree angle. The angled, slightly beveled 33-gauge tip measures 3.2 mm in length. A syringe filled with balanced salt solution is connected via a short piece of intravenous tubing to the hand piece and allows gentle infusion into the subfoveal space as opposed to refluxing into the vitreous cavity. Rarely (if retinotomies are large), subretinal fluid can be aspirated through a 30- or 33-gauge straight cannula. The smaller-caliber tip can facilitate aspiration of subretinal fluid with less risk of engaging neurosensory retina around the edges of a small retinotomy.

Subretinal Forceps   In many cases the trunk of vascular ingrowth from the choroid firmly tethers the subretinal membrane. In most cases, it is necessary to grasp this stalk to disconnect it. A 20-gauge, positive-action, horizontal forceps, with an angle of 130 degrees, narrow opposing blades (0.61 mm width of closed tips), and a tip length of 2.4 mm, has been designed. These forceps can be used to effectively pass behind the loosened membrane, grasp the stalk, and extract the membrane through the retinotomy. The current 20-gauge, horizontal subretinal forceps have been designed with blades that are slightly thinner yet grasp more firmly than earlier forceps. The superior grasping force is

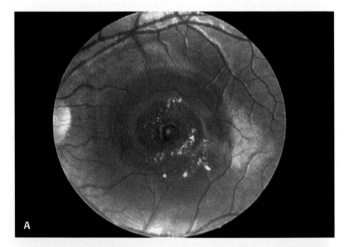

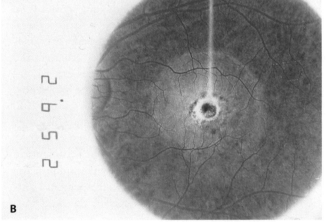

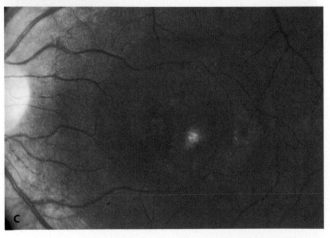

FIGURE 52-19.   A. *Compact, hyperpigmented subfoveal neovascular membrane with preoperative visual acuity of 20/200. B. The angiographic appearance is favorable for surgical removal. C. The membrane is completely removed without disturbing underlying RPE except for the focus of hypopigmentation at the ingrowth site. Visual acuity is 20/20-1.*

achieved by having the tips close first, so that the intrinsic spring of the metal tips gives additional force as the blades are pressed together. These have a 130-degree angle from the shaft and a length of 3.2 mm from the bend. Vertical action forceps are only occasionally useful in special situations. These narrow subretinal forceps have a fixed lower blade and an active anterior blade. When fully opened, the tips are separated by 1 mm. Peyman and Kwang (217) have designed a subretinal forceps consisting of a 25-gauge curved shaft housing a retractable, three-pronged tip resembling a rake in the open position. They believe this rake tip may be helpful in disconnecting CNV from surrounding RPE especially in AMD. In our experience, the neovascular complex usually breaks free from the surrounding, more normal subretinal tissue when traction is exerted on the main complex.

Subretinal Scissors   Horizontal subretinal scissors having a blade length of approximately 3 mm angled at 130-degree from the shaft have been developed. These scissors may be used to separate a laser scar from its overlying neurosensory retinal adhesion or to section recurrent membranes from their adjacent laser scars. Vertical subretinal scissors having a blade length of approximately 3 mm angled at 130-degree from the shaft have been developed. Rarely, one encounters a neovascular complex in which it is helpful to section the membrane into two pieces before extracting the tissue from the subretinal space.

Surgical Technique

Current surgical technique is most effective in those cases in which the membrane lies predominantly anterior to the RPE and thus can be removed without extracting large areas of RPE.

Sclerotomy Site   A standard three-port pars plana vitrectomy is performed. The placement of sclerotomies is critical. The surgeon should study the angiogram and decide preoperatively where the retinotomy is to be placed to avoid damaging major vessels and to provide adequate access to the subretinal membrane. These factors usually dictate that the retinotomy be created in a straight temporal location and thus the superotemporal sclerotomy should be made near the horizontal meridian. If a sewn-on ring system is used to hold a corneal contact lens, it is sometimes advantageous to rotate the fixation flanges superotemporally and inferonasally from the horizontal to allow a nearly horizontal placement of the temporal port. Occasionally, these horizontal sclerotomy sites bleed more than they do when placed more superiorly, but this has not proved to be a significant complication.

Removal of Posterior Hyaloid   Although there are no data to support the importance of removing the posterior hyaloid, its removal is attempted in every case, as described earlier.

Retinotomy   The placement of retinotomy takes into account 1) the exact location and extent of the membrane under the fovea, 2) the presence of presumed adhesions between the neurosensory retina and underlying tissue (previous photocoagulation scars and/or evidence of pigment migration into neurosensory retina or retinochoroidal vascular anastomoses), 3) the dimensions of the subretinal instruments (specifically, the length of the angled instrument tips that determines how far away from the fovea the retinotomy can be made and still allow the tips to reach the membrane), and 4) the topographic anatomy of the neurosensory retina and nerve fiber layer. In most cases, these factors dictate a straight temporal or slightly superotemporal location for the retinotomy (Fig. 52-20). However, a retinotomy can be created superonasal to the fovea (Fig. 52-21). With newer 33- and 36-gauge instruments, the retinotomies are small enough that no significant damage to the papillomacular bundle occurs.

Besides being in the most advantageous location, the retinotomy should be as small as possible. Initially, the retinal surface was lightly diathermized and then the microvitreoretinal blade was used to tease open a small hole. Currently,

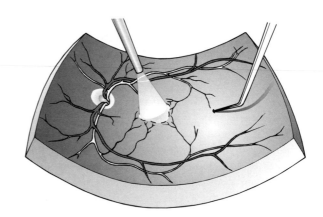

FIGURE 52-20.   *For a right-handed surgeon in a right eye, a straight temporal retinotomy is often best.*

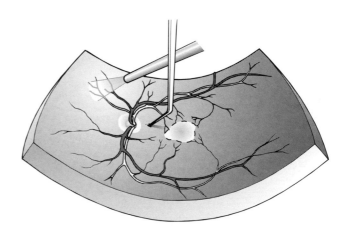

FIGURE 52-21.   *For a right-handed surgeon in a left eye, a retinotomy can be created superonasal to the fovea without significant damage to the papillomacular bundle.*

a 120-degree angled, sharply pointed 36-gauge subretinal pick is used to pierce undiathermized neurosensory retina. While intraocular pressure is raised, the tip can be pushed through neurosensory retina to achieve a very tiny retinotomy (Figs. 52-20 and 52-21). As the pick is obliquely advanced through the neurosensory retina, transient blanching of the choriocapillaris may be seen. Rarely, the local RPE underlying the retinotomy site may be scraped as the pick enters the subretinal space but this can be avoided by gently lifting the pick as the retina is perforated. A small hemorrhage can occur as retinal capillaries are cut, but this always responds to the increased intraocular pressure and is limited. Recently, Greve and colleagues (218) described a technique of retinotomy in nondiathermized retina. The direction of retinotomy is parallel to the nerve fiber layer. By incising the retina parallel to the nerve fiber layer, the directional forces on the surface of the retina created by the nerve fiber layer's inherent plasticity pull the walls of the retinotomy together, creating a self-sealing retinotomy.

Creation or Enhancement of Neurosensory Detachment   After retinotomy, an angled 33-gauge infusion cannula is introduced beneath the retina and the balanced salt solution is infused to elevate the neurosensory retina (Fig. 52-22). This is accomplished by gently pushing on the plunger of a syringe that is connected to the hub of the needle by a short piece of tubing. To avoid trapping air bubbles within the tip, balanced salt solution is gently infused as the instrument is entered into the eye and before the subretinal space is entered. Slow infusion is very important, as this step can lead to the development of a retinal break, especially in areas of strong chorioretinal adhesions. Excessive infusion pressure can tear the retina. A neurosensory detachment can also be created or enhanced by injecting balanced salt solution using a controlled infusion pump (219). As the fluid enters the subretinal space, attention is directed to edges of the laser scars or adhesions to the underlying membrane, or both.

Removal of Neovascular Membrane   The subretinal membrane is dislodged from the underlying RPE and the overlying neurosensory retina with the aid of a pointed, 36-gauge subretinal pick (Fig. 52-23). The sharp end of the pick is very helpful in engaging the edges of the neovascular complex, and facilitating its separation from the underlying RPE. The pick is moved in a pivoting or rotating manner to avoid stretching or enlarging the retinotomy. In most cases, the neovascular complex dislodges easily from the underlying subfoveal RPE but remains attached to the edge of a laser scar or to the stalk of choroidal vascular ingrowth. Occasionally, horizontal subretinal scissors are necessary to cut firm adhesions. If the retina is not mobilized over the entire photocoagulation scar, separation is achieved at least far enough into the scar to allow manipulation and extraction of the membrane without tearing adjacent retina. Trauma to foveal photoreceptors from either the pick or scissors is avoided.

A positive-action horizontal forceps is introduced (closed) through the retinotomy, which has usually enlarged during the subretinal manipulation. The opened blades are placed around the stalk or the adhesion, with the membrane in front of the blades. Gentle traction with the blades held closed breaks the connection (Fig. 52-24). If traction on the retina is seen, the membrane is released and further separation of the complex from neurosensory retina is accomplished. If excessive tugging and displacement of RPE are seen, consideration is given to using the subretinal scissors to cut the stalk rather than breaking it with the forceps. When the vascular connection from the choroid is about to be severed, the intraocular pressure is raised to approximately 80 mm Hg.

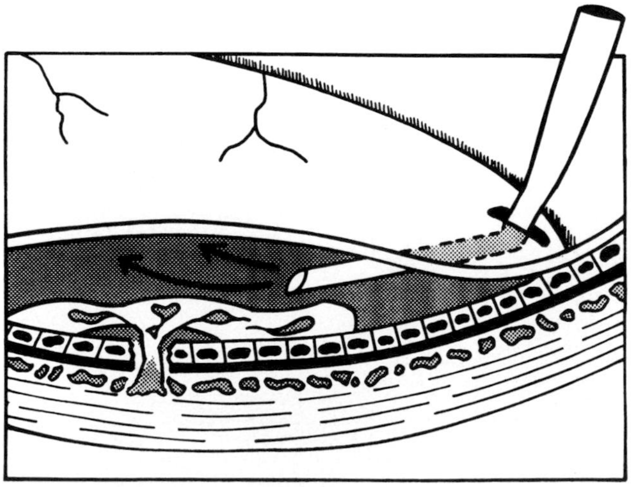

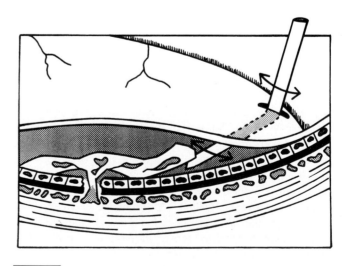

FIGURE 52-22.   *A gentle infusion of balanced salt solution through a 33-gauge cannula creates a small neurosensory retinal detachment.*

FIGURE 52-23.   *The neovascular tissue is dislodged from underlying RPE with the aid of a pointed, 36-gauge subretinal pick.*

Minimal hemorrhage is often encountered when the membrane is removed. The intraocular pressure is elevated for at least one minute and any evidence of rebleeding is observed while the pressure is slowly lowered. When these measures fail, hemostasis can be achieved by subretinal endophotocoagulation. Most membranes are easily grasped with horizontal subretinal forceps. Vertical action forceps may be needed to extract relatively thin disks of neovascularization that have been disconnected from the choroid.

Once hemostasis is achieved, the membrane is removed from the eye through the sclerotomy. Dividing a large membrane with intraocular forceps or a vitrector is preferable to enlarging the sclerotomy. Scleral plugs are placed and the retina is inspected with indirect ophthalmoscopy and scleral depression to verify that no peripheral tears have occurred. A complete air-fluid exchange is performed. Standard extrusion needles or silicone-tipped needles are used to aspirate over the optic nerve. The angled 33-gauge cannula can be used to aspirate subretinal fluid at the retinotomy. This generally everts the edges of the retinotomy, allowing for better closure. If the retinotomy is small and the surgeon desires a small gas tamponade, balanced salt solution is gently reinfused over the optic nerve after the vitreous cavity has been dry for a few minutes. The eye is almost completely filled with fluid and the patient is asked to be face down postoperatively. In early cases, endolaser photocoagulation of the retinotomy was done. Smaller-gauged instrumentation allows for the creation and preservation of a small retinotomy that does not require laser photocoagulation. This prevents thermal damage to neurosensory retina, RPE, and choriocapillaris, thus preserving extrafoveal retinal function and decreasing the size of a postoperative scotoma.

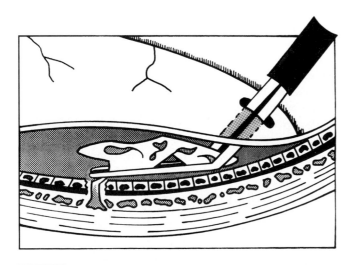

FIGURE 52-24. *Horizontal subretinal forceps are used to firmly grasp the neovascular tissue and slowly remove it from the subretinal space.*

Complications

Two changes in the milieu that occur in the setting of CNV have a practical impact on surgical technique and visual prognosis: cystoid macular edema and fibrin- or photocoagulation-related retinal adhesion to CNV (220). Cystoid changes render the fovea vulnerable to iatrogenic macular hole during fluid-assisted separation of the retina from the subjacent neovascular complex. Incomplete separation of the overlying retina from underlying CNV or prior photocoagulation scar places the fovea at risk of avulsion during membrane removal (220). Other intraoperative complications are subretinal hemorrhage, retinal tear, and retinal detachment (221,222).

Postoperative Management

Patients are examined at 24 hours and at 1 week after surgery for signs of infection, retinal detachment, or elevated intraocular pressure. Three weeks after surgery, the view is usually adequate to clinically detect the presence or absence of subfoveal RPE. Occasionally, residual subretinal blood will obscure the underlying tissues for a longer period of time. Within the first month, angiography is repeated to evaluate for recurrence of neovascularization. Not uncommonly, the site of the original choroidal ingrowth stalk demonstrates recurrent neovascularization. Often this site is not subfoveal and therefore slit lamp laser photocoagulation can be employed to ablate the recurrence. Since the membranes can recur in more than one third of cases within 6 months, close follow-up is essential.

Adjuncts to Surgery

Subretinal Endophotocoagulation Transretinal laser photocoagulation invariably damages the underlying RPE and the overlying neurosensory retina, thus minimizing the prospect for visual function in the treated site (223,224). Selected delivery of laser energy within the subretinal space could theoretically allow for the obliteration of a subretinal choroidal neovascular complex and reduce damage to the overlying photoreceptor layer. Subretinal endophotocoagulation in rabbits has shown that low- to moderate-intensity burns (<1.0 W) preserve the overlying retina, and high-laser energy powers (>1.0 W) will cause coagulative necrosis of the outer retinal layers (225).

Thomas and Ibanez (226) developed a subretinal laser delivery system as an adjunct to the surgical excision of subfoveal choroidal neovascular membranes. A 31-gauge subretinal endolaser probe is used; it takes advantage of the difference in the index of refraction between silica and balanced salt solution to produce a down and forward laser beam. Strong unrelenting adhesions to previous laser or inflammatory chorioretinal scars occasionally preclude safe excision of a neovascular complex. When this situation is encountered, the firm adhesion or stalk of neovascular ingrowth can be cut with subretinal scissors and photocoagulated (outside the fovea) with the subretinal endolaser probe, minimizing damage to subfoveal RPE, choriocapillaris, and the overlying neurosensory retina. In other instances, a small, subfoveal neovascular complex anterior to the RPE is found intraoperatively to have a larger sub-RPE component, the excision of which can lead to the development of a large RPE tear. In these cases, the anterior component of the neovascular complex can be reflected and photocoagulated in an extrafoveal location. Finally, subretinal endophotocoagulation also allows for the obliteration of a bleeding subretinal stump that has failed to respond to elevated intraocular pressure.

Pharmacologic Therapy   Given the limitations of photocoagulation and surgical intervention, many investigators have searched for drugs to control CNV. Interferon (INF) alfa-2a initially attracted widespread attention, but results have been discouraging. It is an endogenous glycoprotein with antiproliferative, immunoregulatory, antiviral, and antiangiogenic properties (227–232), and has been reported to be beneficial in the treatment of subretinal neovascularization (233,234). The early experience reported by Thomas and Ibanez (235) was disappointing. In a prospective study, patients with recurrent subfoveal neovascularization following surgical excision and patients with subfoveal choroidal neovascularization without previous surgical excision received INF alfa-2a in a dose of 3.0 to 6.0 million units/m^2 body surface area every other night for an average of 12 weeks. Use of INF alfa-2a did not improve visual acuity or fluorescein angiographic appearance of subfoveal neovascular membranes in 90% of cases and was associated with significant side effects, including fever, alopecia, leukopenia, thrombocytopenia, elevated liver enzymes, and suicidal tendencies.

Chan and associates (236) reported an efficacy and toxicity study on the treatment of choroidal, neovascular membranes by INF alfa-2a. The regression of choroidal neovascularization was minimal. Toxic effects that interfered with patients' performance status were associated with the treatment. It is possible that higher doses may achieve a therapeutic response.

In the future, better drug delivery systems may allow for the selective intraocular administration of high doses of INF alfa-2a, thus bypassing its toxicity. Unfortunately, a multinational, randomized, prospective study has revealed no treatment benefit (237). Other antineovascular agents that are being evaluated include thalidomide and peptide inhibitors of integrin molecules.

Tissue Plasminogen Activator   Tissue plasminogen activator (t-PA) is a fibrinolytic agent (238) that activates plasminogen specifically in the presence of fibrin and whose activity is enhanced in the presence of fibrin (239). Tissue plasminogen activator has been used as an adjunct to the surgical removal of subfoveal, choroidal neovascular membranes by Thomas et al (240). At a concentration of 6 μg/0.1 mL, t-PA was injected into the subretinal space and 30 to 40 minutes were allowed to elapse for fibrin breakdown to occur. t-PA dissolved the fibrin rim surrounding recent subfoveal membranes but was less effective on more mature

lesions. These authors proposed that enzymatic dissolution of the fibrin rim resulted in less shearing of surrounding photoreceptors and RPE when more recent subretinal neovascular membranes were grasped and removed. In contrast, with older membranes, the pseudopod-like strands of mature organized fibrin were more adherent and more manipulation was required for membrane removal. No increased bleeding occurred in these patients when the membranes were removed. Although t-PA may be a useful intraoperative tool, in our experience, gentle mechanical pressure against the edge of the neovascular complex usually "peels up" the fibrin rim without disturbing RPE (unless the complex has grown beneath the RPE).

Liquid Perfluorocarbons   Perfluoro-N-octane has been used to assist in the evacuation of subretinal hemorrhage and fluid, and to facilitate endophotocoagulation of the retinotomy site (241). Perfluoro-N-octane was injected after membrane removal to reattach the retina and tamponade bleeding. An air-fluid exchange with removal of the perfluoro-N-octane was performed before sclerotomy closure. Simple air-fluid exchange appears to achieve the same ends.

Results

Thomas and Kaplan (204) treated two patients with presumed ocular histoplasmosis subfoveal neovascular membranes and progressive visual acuity loss to 20/400. Visual acuity returned to 20/20 with 7 months follow-up in one patient and to 20/40 with 3 months follow-up in the other patient. Lambert and colleagues (241) reported the results of surgical excision of 10 consecutive, subfoveal choroidal neovascular membranes in patients with AMD. Six of these patients showed mixed visual improvement at 1-month and 3-month follow-up. Thomas and colleagues (221) reported surgical management of subfoveal CNV in 33 eyes with AMD, 20 eyes with POHS, and 5 eyes with miscellaneous etiologies. Five eyes also received subfoveal RPE patches. With limited follow-up, significant improvement in vision (defined as 2 Snellen lines) was achieved in 7 of 22 eyes with AMD CNV removal, 0 of 4 eyes with AMD CNV removal and RPE patches, and 1 of 7 eyes with AMD CNV disconnection. Significant improvement was achieved in 6 of 16 eyes with POHS removal and 0 of 4 eyes with POHS CNV disconnection. In 5 eyes with miscellaneous CNV, 2 improved. CNV recurred in 29%. Berger and Kaplan (242) reported their series of 15 patients with POHS and 19 patients with AMD followed for an average of 4 months postoperatively. Snellen visual acuity improved by two lines or more in 8 of 15 (53%) cases of POHS. Fourteen of 19 (74%) cases of AMD showed either slight improvement or stabilization of vision.

Thomas and colleagues (223) updated their surgical experience and explored possible correlations between preoperative characteristics and final postoperative visual acuity in 67 eyes with POHS, 41 eyes with AMD, 10 eyes with myopia, 9 eyes with multifocal choroiditis, 8 eyes with idiopathic CNV, 4 eyes with angioid streaks, and 8 eyes with miscellaneous etiologies for CNV. In eyes with POHS, mean follow-up was 10.5 months. Visual acuity was stable or improved in 56 (83%) eyes and was 20/40 or greater in 21 (31%) eyes. Mean interval to best visual acuity was 3 months. In eyes with AMD, mean follow-up was 15 months. Visual acuity was improved in only 5 (12%) eyes and was 20/40 or greater in only 2 (5%) eyes. The interval to best visual acuity was 5 months. Recurrence rates of 37% (POHS) and 27% (AMD) had no statistically significant effect on final visual outcome. Patients with focal disorders of the RPE–Bruch's membrane complex appear to have a better surgical outcome than do those with diffuse disease.

Adelberg and colleagues (219), in their retrospective analysis of surgical removal of CNV in myopia, angioid streaks, and other disorders, found visual acuity to be stable in 10 of 17 (59%) eyes, improved by two or more Snellen lines in 6 (35%) eyes, and decreased in 1 (6%) eye. Postoperative visual acuity of better than 20/80 was achieved in only a minority of eyes.

Ormerod and colleagues (243) reported long-term outcomes after the surgical removal of advanced neovascular membranes in age-related macular degeneration. The mean choroidal neovascular membrane size was 7 disk diameters. Surgically induced mean RPE defect was 14 standard disk areas in size. Eight of 10 patients improved one to two lines of Snellen visual acuity postoperatively. A 2-year recurrence rate of 40% was observed. Connor and colleagues (244) surgically removed extrafoveal fibrotic choroidal neovascular membrane in a patient with AMD. Visual acuity improved from 20/200 to 20/25.

Recently, Melberg and colleagues (245) reported their experience with recurrent neovascularization after subfoveal surgery in 120 patients with POHS. In 42% of all eyes, recurrence developed in an average time of 4.4 months. Recurrent CNV location was subfoveal in 66% of eyes.

Surgical excision of subfoveal neovascular membranes may result in recovery of excellent visual acuity in patients with POHS but not in patients with AMD. Gass (246) offered a rational explanation for these reported visual outcomes. He provided histopathologic evidence from autopsy eyes to propose a classification scheme. In type 1 CNV, as typically seen in individuals older than 50 years with AMD, the new vessels that arise in the choroid usually grow within the subpigment epithelial space and not in the subneurosensory retinal space. In type 2 CNV, typically seen in younger individuals with POHS, the new vessels are partly engulfed by a monolayer of proliferating RPE and lie anterior to normal RPE in the subneurosensory retinal space. Surgical excision of POHS membrane permits retention of intact normal RPE, reapproximation of the retinal receptors, and native pigment epithelium and may be associated with remarkable return of visual acuity (246).

Selected Cases

Case 1

An 82-year-old man had developed a fibrotic disciform scar in the left eye 3 years before presentation. Choroidal neovascularization developed in the right eye for which he underwent photocoagulation ×2. Recurrent neovascular tissue arose predominantly superior to the fovea, and best corrected visual acuity dropped to 20/300. Given the clinical appearance of the lesion (well-defined borders with blood apparently outlining a cleavage plane between the recurrent membrane and underlying retinal pigment epithelium), the referring retinal specialist believed that surgical removal of the complex might be preferable to additional laser (Fig. 52-25). Indeed during surgery, the membrane peeled up from underlying retinal pigment epithelium and came out in one piece with the prior laser scar. Within 3 months, visual acuity had improved to 20/40 (Fig. 52-26).

Case 2

A 57-year-old man presented with some drusen and pigment disturbance in both eyes, and an occult choroidal neovascular process was juxtafoveal in location in the right eye. He underwent laser photocoagulation; however, a subfoveal recurrence developed. Best corrected visual acuity was 20/400 before surgery (Fig. 52-27). During the vitrectomy, the recurrent neovascular complex could be reflected from the underlying foveal RPE, and the entire complex was removed. Postoperatively, a hyperpigmented reaction in the central RPE developed with a dark black appearance. Visual acuity improved to 20/20 and

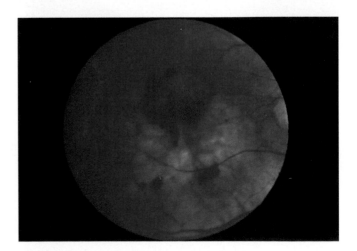

FIGURE 52-25. *Fundus appearance of the right eye of a recurrent neovascular membrane. Laser treatment had been applied two times elsewhere. Note the blood, which appears to outline a clear border between the neovascular complex and underlying tissue.*

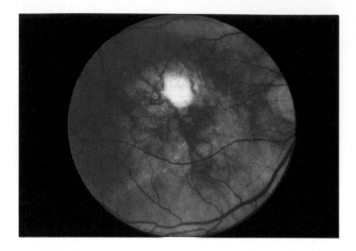

FIGURE 52-26.   *Postoperative clinical appearance. The atrophic white spot is the site of laser scar removal. The retinal pigment epithelium appears thinned where the membrane previously lay, but the tissue appears intact.*

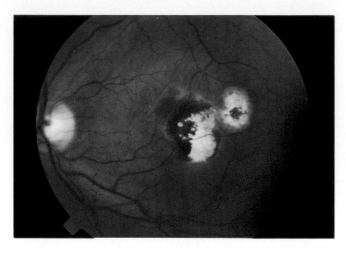

FIGURE 52-28.   *Four years after surgery, the subfoveolar retinal pigment epithelium has become densely pigmented, but vision remains 20/20. The atrophic scar temporal in the macula is the site of the retinotomy, which was lasered to create a chorioretinal adhesion. It is now understood that laser treatment of retinotomies is almost never required.*

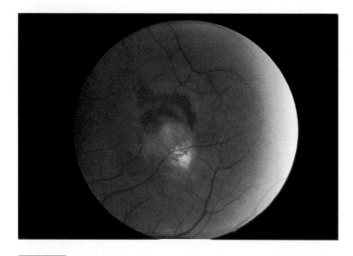

FIGURE 52-27.   *Preoperative appearance of recurrent subfoveal choroidal neovascularization (following laser). Best corrected visual acuity was 20/400.*

has remained at this level with 4 years follow-up (Fig. 52-28).

Experimental Studies

Within the last decade increasing attention has been focused on the problem of transplanting RPE onto Bruch's membrane (247–263). This attention has resulted from the observation that good postsurgical vision depends on intact subfoveal RPE, an infrequent occurrence in the removal of subfoveal AMD CNV. In humans, Peyman and colleagues (203) recognized that maculae left surgically devoid of RPE (following the excision of submacular scars) did not have good visual function. Thus they attempted to replace the

RPE intraoperatively through surgical techniques. Visual outcome remained poor.

Experiments have been performed in the nonhuman primate to address questions concerning repopulation of retinal pigment epithelial cells in situ and photoreceptor repair after submacular surgery (264). Subretinal fluid injection led to shortening of outer segments and occasional separation of RPE cells from Bruch's membrane, with no visible damage to the choriocapillaris (265). The photoreceptors regained their normal length by 9 months after the surgical procedure. Regeneration of RPE was observed only if Bruch's membrane was left intact (264). Morphologic effects of surgical debridement of RPE were also studied in the domestic pig (265). The choriocapillaris was intact in areas of Bruch's membrane that were repopulated by hypopigmented RPE. The RPE monolayer regenerates by division of RPE at the edges of the epithelial defect and subsequent cell migration (266,267). Clinically, there is a high correlation between areas of RPE dropout in atrophic age-related macular degeneration and corresponding areas of atrophy of the choriocapillaris in humans (268–271).

Atrophy of the choriocapillaris can also occur after the excision of choroidal neovascular membrane in humans (272–275). In vitro studies support the concept that RPE in tissue culture is capable of releasing factors that can influence cells arising from vascular tissue (276–278). If the RPE is removed or damaged during surgical excision of subfoveal neovascularization, it is unlikely to heal in the elderly human because senescent RPE has a limited ability to regenerate as demonstrated in tissue culture in comparison to young RPE (279). In addition, it is likely that the integrity of the underlying substrate is important for healing and determining the morphologic features of the RPE monolayer (280–282), and the RPE may not heal on the diseased Bruch's membrane after subfoveal surgery in elderly humans.

Future advances in the surgical management of choroidal neovascular membranes may involve stimulation of RPE growth factors to enhance RPE regeneration beneath the fovea (283,284). Alternatively, emerging technologies such as RPE and photoreceptor transplantation hold promise (283–285). For improving the visual prognosis after surgery in these patients, any new era will probably see the use of pharmacologic agents, retinal transplantation, and gene therapy to achieve therapeutic success (284).

The Submacular Surgery Trial

The safety and possible efficacy of submacular surgery have seen questioned (285,286). It is appropriate to proceed with a randomized, controlled, prospective multicenter clinical trial to further evaluate subfoveal surgery (214). A pilot study for the Submacular Surgery Trial is evaluating surgery in four categories (287): Group 1 includes eyes with AMD and subfoveal choroidal neovascular membranes in which the benefit of laser photocoagulation was minimal. Randomization is between surgery and observation. Group 2 includes eyes with AMD and recurrent subfoveal choroidal neovascular membranes that are deemed eligible for photocoagulation according to the Foveal Photocoagulation Study. Randomization is between surgery and laser photocoagulation. Group 3 includes eyes with AMD in which submacular hemorrhage comprises more than 50% of the macular lesion. Randomization is between surgery and observation. Group 4 includes eyes with POHS and idiopathic subfoveal CNV. Randomization is between surgery and observation. It is hoped that NIH funding will allow these pilot studies to expand into large multicenter studies. By carefully following the prospective protocol established in the submacular surgery trial data will be collected that will help define the appropriate role of submacular surgery in the management of patients with these difficult problems.

Submacular Hemorrhage

Blood beneath the neurosensory retina almost always originates from the choroidal circulation. Trauma to choroidal vessels can produce hemorrhage: from blunt or penetrating trauma, from inadvertent surgical trauma with a deep suture during scleral buckling, or from drainage of subretinal fluid either internally or externally (288,289). In the absence of trauma, hemorrhage can occur secondary to choroidal neovascularization (290,291). Small hemorrhages frequently accompany the ingrowth of vessels from the choroid through Bruch's membrane. Extensive hemorrhages are believed to occur as a result of rupture of large choroidal vessels that extend into fibrovascular complexes (221). Vessels in fibrovascular scars have been observed to have arterial and venous characteristics and are continuous with choroidal

arteries and veins, respectively (292). Leakage of blood or serous fluid from the neovascular tissue leads to detachment of the RPE and produces pressure on the artery and vein as they enter the fibrovascular scar. This pressure reportedly leads to necrosis of the artery and, when it ruptures, massive hemorrhage occurs with accumulation of blood under the RPE, under neurosensory retina, and in some cases in the vitreous cavity (292).

Mechanism of Retinal Injury

Subretinal blood is toxic to the outer retina and has been documented to cause irreversible photoreceptor damage (293,294). Laboratory animal studies have shown that the degree of retinal destruction is correlated with the duration of contact of the retina with hemorrhage. These animal studies show that damage can occur as early as 1 hour (295), with moderate to severe outer retinal destruction at 3 to 7 days and full-thickness retinal degeneration by day 14 (293,296,297). Subretinal blood clots form a mechanical barrier between the retina and the RPE. This can inhibit metabolic exchange between retina and RPE (293). Retinal toxicity can result from iron liberated from hemoglobin that is released from degenerating erythrocytes (294).

Glatt and Machemer (293) showed that subretinal blood clot adherence and retraction caused tractional forces on the photoreceptors, which led to outer retinal damage. The role of fibrin in causing retinal damage associated with subretinal hemorrhage was better defined by Toth and colleagues (295). They suggested that a fibrinolytic agent be used to dissolve the fibrin meshwork, thereby preventing the shearing effect on the photoreceptors.

Benner and colleagues (298) demonstrated that t-PA could be safely used in the subretinal space at concentrations of 2.5 to 200.0 mg/liter. Higher doses caused severe, irreversible toxic effects to the photoreceptor-RPE complex. The toxic effects of t-PA were attributable to the carrier vehicle. Recently, Coll and colleagues (299) reported the effect of intravitreal t-PA on experimental subretinal hemorrhage. Intravitreal t-PA 1 day after subretinal injection of blood in rabbits facilitated more rapid lysis of clotted blood; however, retinal damage was not prevented.

Natural History

The visual outcome of subretinal hemorrhage varies depending on the extent, location, and thickness of the hemorrhage (300). Gillies and Lahav (301) reported three patients with AMD, myopia, and trauma with neither thick nor large subretinal hemorrhages. Their initial visual acuities of counting fingers (2 eyes) and 20/400 improved to 20/40 in 6 months, 20/25 in 3 months, and 20/67 in 6 months, respectively. Bennett and associates (288) reviewed the cases of 29 patients with large subfoveal hemorrhages followed for an average of 3 years. Thicker hemorrhages had poorer final visual acuity than did thinner hemorrhages. Eyes with AMD had a worse final visual acuity than did non-AMD eyes. Eyes with choroidal rupture fared better than other eyes.

The presence of AMD, rather than the thickness of the hemorrhage, was the factor most predictive of poor outcome. Fekrat and associates (302) reviewed the natural history of 41 eyes with submacular hemorrhages and found a trend toward declining visual acuity over time. The median overall change between the initial and 3-year visual acuities was a loss of four lines. Eyes with larger and thicker hemorrhages had poorer visual acuity outcomes.

Management

In 1983, Dellaporta (303) described passing an endo-diathermy needle through retina, choroid, and sclera in a patient with a 10-week history of massive, posterior pole subretinal hemorrhage and a visual acuity of 3/200. The cauterized hole in the retina allowed the blood to spill into the vitreous cavity and vision returned to 20/25. Hanscom and Diddie (304) first used modern vitrectomy techniques, internal retinotomy, endodrainage of blood, and air-fluid exchange in the management of submacular hemorrhage. de Juan and Machemer (201) used vitrectomy and a combination of drainage and irrigation of subretinal clot and disciform scar removal. Early surgical intervention to avoid toxicity from subretinal hemorrhage was stressed by Slusher (305).

Case Selection

Multiple preoperative, intraoperative, and postoperative factors have an impact on the visual result following surgery for submacular hemorrhage. Preoperative factors, including the baseline health of the neurosensory retina and submacular RPE, the presence of choroidal neovascularization, disciform scarring, or previous foveal photocoagulation will determine the postoperative visual potential. The health status of the RPE and neurosensory retina can also influence the tolerance of these tissues to the noxious effects of subretinal blood. Eyes with AMD may have more extensive and diffuse photoreceptor/RPE dysfunction and less metabolic reserve than eyes without AMD (i.e., eyes with choroidal neovascular membranes due to POHS, macroaneurysm, or idiopathic causes). This may partially explain why eyes without AMD are more likely to have visual improvement following surgery than are eyes with AMD. The duration of submacular hemorrhage may also be an important factor. Progressive photoreceptor destruction has been observed to occur for up to 14 days following introduction of experimental subretinal hemorrhage. Postoperative visual function may also be affected by photoreceptor and/or RPE trauma induced by surgical manipulations in the subretinal space as well as intraoperative and postoperative complications.

In the absence of results from clinical trials, case selection remains unclear. The randomized, prospective Submacular Surgery Trial will compare surgical removal of large submacular hemorrhage secondary to AMD. No randomization trials have been proposed for hematomas of other etiologies. Hence, at the present time only impressions regarding case selection can be offered. Relatively thin hemorrhages unassociated with CNV often do well with observation. Thick hemorrhage without known CNV may be appropriate for removal. Thick hemorrhages with probable CNV remain controversial. Recent-onset hemorrhages probably have a better surgical result than do older hemorrhages and may be appropriate for t-PA use (Fig. 52-29).

Surgical Technique

Following a pars plana vitrectomy with removal of the posterior hyaloid, a retinotomy site is created adjacent to the clot. If the clot is less than 7 days old, t-PA is used. Following small retinotomy, 10 µg/0.1 mL recombinant t-PA is injected into the submacular clot. After a waiting period ranging from 20 to 40 minutes, the hemorrhage is drained with either a Lewis double-lumen subretinal irrigator-aspirator or a single 30-gauge subretinal cannula through the retinotomy site. Additional injections of t-PA (10 µg/0.1 mL) can be performed if clot lysis is incomplete. Kimura and colleagues (306) have reported removal of subretinal hemorrhage facilitated by preoperative intravitreal t-PA. Six µg (0.1 mL) t-PA is injected slowly into the midvitreous cavity through the pars plana with either topical or retrobulbar anesthesia 12 to 36 hours before surgery. A standard three-port pars plana vitrectomy is performed and an attempt is made to simply aspirate the liquefied hemorrhage with a soft-tipped cannula. If this is not completely successful, a balanced salt solution can be instilled subretinally to elevate the retina, and the aspiration is repeated.

If the clot is over 7 days old, the retina is elevated from the subretinal blood by gentle infusion of balanced salt solution through the retinotomy site. Aspiration of the clot can be attempted with a straight 30-gauge needle; occasionally clots are liquefied. In most cases, mechanical extraction is required, and horizontal subretinal forceps are introduced to grasp the clot. In a few cases, the silicone tip extrusion needle is used to actively aspirate the clot. Air-fluid exchange can also be helpful in evacuating residual subretinal hemorrhage. Depending on the size of retinotomy, an air bubble of 15% to 100% of the vitreous cavity can be used.

Complications

Substantial postoperative complications have been seen following surgical removal of subretinal hemorrhage. Postoperative retinal detachment, proliferative vitreoretinopathy, recurrent subretinal hemorrhage, subretinal fibrosis, cataract, and optic atrophy have been reported (202,209,289,290,291,292).

Results

Hanscom and Diddie (304) reported evacuation of subretinal hemorrhage of 1 week's duration from two patients (AMD and a ruptured macroaneurysm). Visual acuity improved from counting fingers and hand motions to

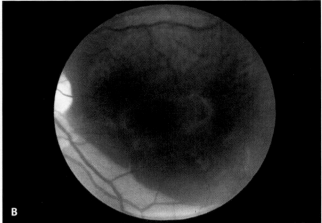

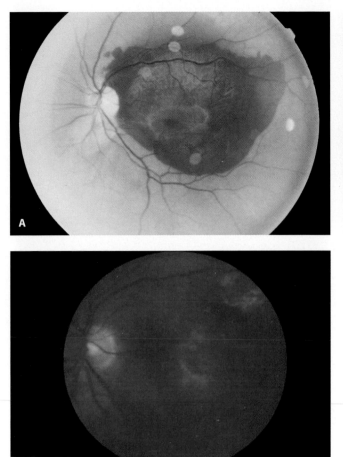

FIGURE 52-29. A. *Sixty-degree fundus photograph of large submacular hemorrhage.* B. *The thickness of submacular hemorrhage is better appreciated on higher magnification.* C. *Three months postoperatively, the macula is free of subretinal hemorrhage. The causative neovascular membrane was superotemporal. Visual acuity returned to 20/70.*

20/400 by 3 months and 20/80 at 1 month, respectively. De Juan and Machemer (201) obtained improved, though limited, visual acuity in three of four patients with exudative AMD and large submacular hemorrhage. These patients had subretinal hemorrhage for a greater than 1-week duration. Wade and colleagues (289) evacuated subretinal hemorrhage greater than five disk diameters in 14 patients. Five patients had massive subretinal hemorrhages associated with AMD. The other nine patients had hemorrhagic retinal detachments, scleral buckling complications that led to subretinal hemorrhage, traumatic retinal detachments, and sickle cell disease. All five AMD eyes had preoperative visual acuities of 20/200 or worse and postoperative visual acuities of 5/200 or less. Three other eyes had improved visual acuity postoperatively. AMD was associated with guarded recovery of visual acuity. Vander and colleagues (307) reported 11 patients, of whom 4 (36%) showed improved visual acuity after evacuation of the subretinal blood. However, retinal detachments with PVR developed postoperatively in 36% of patients and cataracts occurred postoperatively in another 36%. Because of the high rate of postoperative complications, the authors did not recommend evacuation of such large subretinal hemorrhages.

Peyman and colleagues (308) reported t-PA–assisted removal of subretinal hemorrhage. One (33%) of three eyes

had improved visual acuity and the other two eyes were stabilized. In the series of Lewis (309), only eyes with recently documented good vision before the hemorrhage in the affected eye underwent surgery. Twenty (83%) of these 24 eyes showed an improvement in visual acuity. Eight eyes (33%) had postoperative visual acuity of 20/200 or better. In the series of Lim et al (310), 5 (28%) of 18 eyes showed an improved visual acuity of two lines or more. The use of perfluoro-*N*-octane showed a trend toward better postoperative visual acuity outcomes. The perfluoro-*N*-octane served to tamponade the retinotomy site and keep the t-PA in the subretinal space during the waiting period. The subsequent use of perfluoro-*N*-octane to express blood from the subretinal space may limit the manipulation required and thus spare the underlying retinal pigment epithelium and the overlying retina from mechanical trauma and cellular loss. Ibanez and colleagues (311), in their 47 cases of submacular hemorrhage removal, noted that AMD eyes had a poor prognosis overall with or without use of t-PA. Recently, Kamei and colleagues (312) reported surgical removal of submacular hemorrhage using t-PA and perfluorocarbon liquid. Best postoperative corrected final visual acuity was 20/100 or better in 16 (73%) of the 22 eyes.

Despite the significant interest in the surgical removal of submacular hemorrhages, the visual outcomes in all reported series have been disappointing. However, the natural history of these eyes is often poor. Thus, a trial comparing surgery to observation appears to be warranted. The Submacular Surgery Trial (287) includes large AMD-associated hemorrhages in such a randomized comparison. The Submacular Surgery Trial currently is investigating the benefit of surgically evacuating massive submacular hemorrhage versus observing these eyes (313). In addition the recognition that preserving the RPE is related to better visual acuity outcomes will aid in selecting those cases with subretinal hemorrhage without associated subretinal pigment epithelial hemorrhage (310).

REFERENCES

1. Sjaarda RN, Michels RG. Macular pucker. In: Ryan SJ, ed. *Retina*. 2nd ed; vol. 3. St. Louis: Mosby, 1994:2301–2311.
2. Machemer R. Die chirurgische entfernung von epiretinalen makulamembranen (macular puckers). *Klin Monatsbl Augenheilkd* 1978;173:36–42.
3. Roth AM, Foos RY. Surface wrinkling retinopathy in eyes enucleated at autopsy. *Trans Am Acad Ophthalmol Otolaryngol* 1971;75:1047–1059.
4. Bellhorn MB, Friedman AH, Wise GN, Henkind P. Ultrastructure and clinicopathologic correlation of idiopathic preretinal macular fibrosis. *Am J Ophthalmol* 1975;79:366–373.
5. Foos RY. Vitreoretinal juncture—simple epiretinal membranes. *Graefes Arch Clin Exp Ophthalmol* 1974;189:231–250.
6. Wise GN. Macular changes after venous obstruction. *Arch Ophthalmol* 1957;58:544–557.
7. Green WR, Kenyon KR, Michels RG, et al. Ultrastructure of epiretinal membranes causing macular pucker after retinal re-attachment surgery. *Trans Ophthalmol Soc UK* 1979;99:63–77.
8. Jaffe NS. Macular retinopathy after separation of vitreoretinal adherence. *Arch Ophthalmol* 1967;78:585–591.
9. Kenyon KR, Michels RG. Ultrastructure of epiretinal membrane removed by pars plana vitreoretinal surgery. *Am J Ophthalmol* 1977;83:815–823.
10. Machemer R, van Horn DL, Aaberg TM. Pigment epithelial proliferation in human retinal detachment with massive periretinal proliferation. *Am J Ophthalmol* 1978;85:181–191.
11. Trese M, Chandler DB, Machemer R. Macular pucker. II. Ultrastructure. *Graefes Arch Clin Exp Ophthalmol* 1983;221:16–26.
12. McDonald HR, Schatz H, Johnson RN. Introduction to epiretinal membranes. In: Ryan SJ, ed. *Retina*. 2nd ed; vol. 3. St. Louis: Mosby, 1994:1819–1825.
13. Pearlstone AD. The incidence of idiopathic preretinal macular gliosis. *Ann Ophthalmol* 1985;17:378–380.
14. Scudder MJ, Eifrig DE. Spontaneous surface wrinkling retinopathy. *Ann Ophthalmol* 1975;7:333–341.
15. Sidd RJ, Fine SL, Owens SL, Patz A. Idiopathic preretinal gliosis. *Am J Ophthalmol* 1982;94:44–48.
16. Wiznia RA. Natural history of idiopathic preretinal macular fibrosis. *Ann Ophthalmol* 1982;14:876–878.
17. Hirokawa H, Jalkh AE, Takahashi M, et al. Role of vitreous in idiopathic premacular fibrosis. *Am J Ophthalmol* 1986;101:166–169.
18. Wise GN. Congenital preretinal macular fibrosis. *Am J Ophthalmol* 1975;79:363–365.
19. Gass JDM. *Stereoscopic atlas of macular diseases*. St. Louis: Mosby–Year Book, 1987:694–712.
20. McDonald HR, Aaberg TM. Idiopathic epiretinal membranes. *Semin Ophthalmol* 1986;1:189–195.
21. Schatz H. *Essential fluorescein angiography: a compendium of 100 classic cases*. San Francisco: Pacific Medical Press, 1982.
22. Wise GN. Preretinal macular fibrosis (an analysis of 90 cases). *Trans Ophthalmol Soc UK* 1972;92:131–140.
23. Wise GN. Congenital preretinal macular fibrosis. *Am J Ophthalmol* 1975;79:363–365.
24. Tanenbaum HL, Schepens CL, Elzeneiny I, Freeman HM. Macular pucker following retinal detachment surgery. *Arch Ophthalmol* 1970;83:286–293.
25. Michels RG. A clinical and histopathologic study of epiretinal membranes affecting the macula and removed by vitreous surgery. *Trans Am Acad Ophthalmol Soc* 1982;80:580–656.
26. Michels RG. Vitrectomy for macular pucker. *Ophthalmology* 1984;91:1384–1388.
27. Cherfan GM, Smiddy WE, Michels RG, et al. Clinicopathologic correlation of pigmented epiretinal membranes. *Am J Ophthalmol* 1988;106:536.
28. Dellaporta A. Macular pucker and peripheral retinal lesions. *Trans Am Ophthalmol Soc* 1973;71:329–340.
29. Laqua H. Pigmented macular pucker. *Am J Ophthalmol* 1978;86:56–58.
30. Robertson DM, Buettner H. Pigmented preretinal membranes. *Am J Ophthalmol* 1977;83:824–829.
31. Clarkson JG, Green WR, Massof D. A histopathologic review of 168 cases of preretinal membrane. *Am J Ophthalmol* 1977;84:1–17.
32. de Bustros S, Thompson JT, Michels RG, et al. Vitrectomy for idiopathic epiretinal membranes causing macular pucker. *Br J Trans Am Ophthalmol Soc* 1973;71:329–340.
33. Foos RY. Surface wrinkling retinopathy. In: Freeman HM, Hirose T, Schepens CL, eds. *Vitreous surgery and advances in fundus diagnosis and treatment*. New York: Appleton-Century-Crofts, 1977.
34. Spitznas M, Leuenberger R. Die primare epiretinale Gliose. *Kiln Montsbl Augenheilkd* 1977;171:410–420.
35. Wilson DJ, Green WR. Histopathologic study of the effect of retinal detachment surgery on 49 eyes obtained post mortem. *Am J Ophthalmol* 1987;103:167–179.
36. Hagler WS, Aturaliya U. Macular puckers after retinal detachment surgery. *Br J Ophthalmol* 1971;55:451–457.
37. Lobes LA, Jr, Burton TC. The incidence of macular pucker after retinal detachment surgery. *Am J Ophthalmol* 1978;85:72–77.
38. Francois-Cedilla J, Verbraeken H. Relationship between the drainage of the subretinal fluid in retinal detachment surgery and the appearance of macular pucker. *Ophthalmologica* 1979;179:111–114.
39. Allen AW Jr, Gass JDM. Contraction of a perifoveal epiretinal membrane simulating a macular hole. *Am J Ophthalmol* 1976;82:684–691.
40. Gass JDM. Photocoagulation of macular lesions. *Trans Am Acad Ophthalmol Otolaryngol* 1971;75:580–608.
41. Messner KH. Spontaneous separation of preretinal macular fibrosis. *Am J Ophthalmol* 1977;83:9–11.
42. Schwartz A. In: Dellaporta A. Discussion, Macular pucker and preretinal lesions. *Trans Am Ophthalmol Soc* 1973;71:329–340.
43. Sumers KD, Jampol LM, Goldberg FM, Huamonte FU. Spontaneous separation of epiretinal membranes. *Arch Ophthalmol* 1980;98:318–320.
44. McDonald HR, Verre WP, Aaberg TM. Surgical management of idiopathic epiretinal membranes. *Ophthalmology* 1986;93:978–983.
45. Pesin SR, Bovino JA. Macular pucker. In: Bovino JA, ed. *Macular surgery*. Norwalk, CT: Appleton & Lange, 1994:1–10.
46. Poliner LS, Olk RJ, Grand MG, et al. The surgical management of premacular fibroplasia. *Arch Ophthalmol* 1988;106:761–764.
47. Rice TA, de Bustros S, Michels RG, et al. Prognostic factors in vitrectomy for epiretinal membranes of the macula. *Ophthalmology* 1986;93:602–610.
48. Pesin SR, Olk RJ, Grand MG, et al. Vitrectomy for premacular fibroplasia. Prognostic factors, long term follow-up, and time course of visual improvement. *Ophthalmology* 1991;98:1109–1114.
49. Rowen RL, Glaser BM. Retinal pigment epithelial cell release: a chemoattractant for astrocytes. *Arch Ophthalmol* 1985;103:704–707.
50. Margherio RR, Cox MS Jr, Trese MT, et al. Removal of epimacular membranes. *Ophthalmology* 1985;92:1075–1083.
51. Michels RG. Vitreous surgery for macular pucker. *Am J Ophthalmol* 1981;92:628–639.
52. Shea M. The surgical management of macular pucker in rhegmatogenous retinal detachment. *Ophthalmology* 1980;87:70–74.
53. de Bustros S, Rice TA, Michels RG, et al. Vitrectomy for macular pucker after treatment of retinal tears or retinal detachment. *Arch Ophthalmol* 1988;106:758–760.
54. Michels RG, Gilbert HD. Surgical management of macular pucker after retinal reattachment. *Am J Ophthalmol* 1979;88:925–929.
55. de Bustros S, Thompson JT, Michels RG, et al. Nuclear sclerosis after vitrectomy for idiopathic epiretinal membranes. *Am J Ophthalmol* 1988;105:160–164.
56. Charles S. *Vitreous microsurgery*. 2nd ed. Baltimore: Williams & Wilkins, 1987.
57. Mittelman D, Green WR, Michels RG, de la Cruz Z. Clinicopathologic correlation of an eye after surgical removal of an epiretinal membrane. *Retina* 1989;9:143–147.

58. Smiddy WE, Michels RG, Glaser BM, de Bustros S. Vitrectomy for macular traction caused by incomplete vitreous separation. *Arch Ophthalmol* 1988;106:624–628.

59. Jaffe NS. Vitreous traction at the posterior pole of the fundus due to alterations in the vitreous posterior. *Trans Am Acad Ophthalmol Otolaryngol* 1967;71:642–652.

60. Margherio RR, Trese MT, Margherio AR, Cartright K. Surgical management of vitreomacular traction syndromes. *Ophthalmology* 1989;96:1437–1445.

61. Gass JDM. Idiopathic senile macular hole: its early stages and pathogenesis. *Arch Ophthalmol* 1988;106:629–639.

62. Michels RG. A clinical and histopathologic study of epiretinal membranes affecting the macula and removal by vitreous surgery. *Trans Am Ophthalmol Soc* 1982;80:580–656.

63. Carter JB, Michels RG, Glaser BM, de Bustros S. Iatrogenic retinal breaks complicating pars plana vitrectomy. *Ophthalmology* 1990;97:848–854.

64. Smiddy WE. Vitreomacular traction syndrome. In: Bovino JA, ed., *Macular surgery*. Norwalk, CT: Appleton & Lange, 1994:11–26.

65. Smiddy WE, Michels RG, Green WR. Morphology, pathology, and surgery for idiopathic macular disorders. *Retina* 1990;10:288–296.

66. Sebag J. Age-related differences in the human vitreoretinal interface. *Arch Ophthalmol* 1991;109:966–971.

67. Foos RY, Wheeler NC. Vitreoretinal juncture. Synchysis senilis and posterior vitreous detachment. *Ophthalmology* 1982;89:1502–1512.

68. Smiddy WE, Green WR, Michels RG, de la Cruz Z. Ultrastructural studies of vitreomacular traction syndrome. *Am J Ophthalmol* 1989;107:177–185.

69. Sebag J. Anatomy and pathology of the vitreo-retinal interface. *Eye* 1992;6:541–552.

70. Kishi S, Demaria C, Shimizu K. Vitreous cortex remnants at the fovea after spontaneous vitreous detachment. *Int Ophthalmol* 1986;9:253–260.

71. Reese AB, Jones IR, Cooper WC. Vitreomacular traction syndrome confirmed histologically. *Am J Ophthalmol* 1970;60:975–977.

72. Tolentino FI, Schepens CL. Edema of the posterior pole after cataract extraction. *Arch Ophthalmol* 1965;74:781–786.

73. Byer NE. Spontaneous disappearance of early postoperative preretinal traction. *Arch Ophthalmol* 1973;90:133–135.

74. Greven GM, Slusher MM, Weaver RG. Epiretinal membrane release and posterior vitreous detachment. *Ophthalmology* 1988;95:902–905.

75. McDonald HR, Johnson RN, Schatz HA. Surgical results in the vitreomacular traction syndrome. *Ophthalmology* 1994;101:1397–1403.

76. Thomas EL, Michels RG, Rice TA, et al. Idiopathic progressive unilateral vitreous fibrosis and secondary traction retinal detachment. *Retina* 1982;2:134–144.

77. Melberg NS, Williams DA, Balles MW, et al. Vitrectomy for vitreomacular traction syndrome with macular detachment. *Retina* 1995;15:192–197.

78. Hikichi T, Yoshida A, Trempe CL. Course of vitreomacular traction syndrome. *Am J Ophthalmol* 1995;119:55–61.

79. Smiddy WE, Maguire AM, Green WR, et al. Idiopathic epiretinal membranes. Ultrastructural characteristics in clinical pathologic correlation. *Ophthalmology* 1989;96:811–821.

80. Gass JDM, Johnson RN. Idiopathic macular holes. Observations, stages of formation, and implication for surgical intervention. *Ophthalmology* 1988;95:912–924.

81. Madreperala SA, McCuen BW II, Hickinbotham D, Green WR. Clinicopathologic correlation of surgically removed macular hole opercula. *Am J Ophthalmol* 1995;120:197–207.

82. Lister W. Holes in the retina and their clinical significance. *Br J Ophthalmol* 1924;8:1–20.

83. Morgan CM, Schatz H. Idiopathic macular holes. *Am J Ophthalmol* 1985;99:437–444.

84. McDonnell PJ, Fine SL, Hillis AI. Clinical features of idiopathic macular cysts and holes. *Am J Ophthalmol* 1982;93:777–786.

85. Kornzweig AL, Feldstein M. Studies of the eye in old age, II. Hole in the macula: a clinical-pathologic study. *Am J Ophthalmol* 1950;33:243–247.

86. Trempe CL, Weiter JJ, Furukawa H. Fellow eyes in cases of macular hole: biomicroscopic study of the vitreous. *Arch Ophthalmol* 1986;104:93–95.

87. Guyer DR, Green WR. Idiopathic macular holes and precursor lesions. In: Franklin RM, ed. Proceedings of the symposium on retina and vitreous, New Orleans Academy of Ophthalmology, New Orleans. New York: Kugler, 1993:135–162.

88. Smiddy WE, Michels RG, Glaser BM, de Bustros S. Vitrectomy for impending macular holes. *Am J Ophthalmol* 1988;105:371–376.

89. Campochiaro PA, Van Neil E, Vinores SA. Immunocytochemical labeling of cells in cortical vitreous from patients with premacular hole lesions. *Arch Ophthalmol* 1992;110:371–377.

90. Kishi S, Shimizu K. Posterior precortical vitreous pocket. *Arch Ophthalmol* 1990;108:979–982.

91. Kishi S, Kamei Y, Shimizu K. Traction elevation of Henle's fiber layer in idiopathic macular holes. *Am J Ophthalmol* 1995;120:486–496.

92. Gordon LW, Glaser BM, Darmakusuma Ie, et al. Full-thickness macular hole formation in eyes with a pre-existing complete posterior vitreous detachment. *Ophthalmology* 1995;102:1702–1705.

93. Gass JDM. Reappraisal of biomicroscopic classification of stages of development of a macular hole. *Am J Ophthalmol* 1995;119:752–759.

94. Smith RG, Hardman-Lea SJ, Galloway NR. Visual performance in idiopathic macular holes. *Eye* 1990;4:190.

95. Yaoeda H. Clinical observation on macular hole. *Nippon Ganka Gakkai Zasshi* 1967;71:1723–1736.

96. Margherio RR, Schepens CL. Macular breaks. I. Diagnosis, etiology, and observations. *Am J Ophthalmol* 1972;74:219–232.

97. Aaberg TM, Blair CJ, Gass JDM. Macular holes. *Am J Ophthalmol* 1970;69:555–562.

98. James M, Feman SS. Macular holes. *Graefes Arch Clin Exp Ophthalmol* 1980;215:59–63.

99. Bidwell AE, Jampol LM, Goldberg MF. Macular holes and excellent visual acuity. Case report. *Arch Ophthalmol* 1988;106:1350.

100. Frangieh GT, Green WR, Engel HM. A histopathologic study of macular cysts and holes. *Retina* 1981;1:311–336.

101. Guyer DR, Green WR, de Bustros S, Fine SL. Histopathologic features of idiopathic macular holes and cysts. *Ophthalmology* 1990;97:1045–1051.

102. Yuzawa M, Watanabe A, Takahashi Y, Matsui M. Observations of idiopathic full-thickness macular holes. *Arch Ophthalmol* 1994;112:1051–1056.

103. Kakehashi A, Schepens CL, Akiba J, et al. Spontaneous resolution of foveal detachments and macular breaks. *Am J Ophthalmol* 1995;120:767–775.

104. Hikichi T, Yoshida A, Akiba J, et al. Prognosis of stage II macular holes. *Am J Ophthalmol* 1995;119:571–575.

105. Fisher YL, Slakter JS, Yannuzzi LA, Guyer DR. A prospective natural history study and kinetic ultrasound evaluation of idiopathic macular holes. *Ophthalmology* 1994;101:5–11.

106. Akiba J, Yoshida A, Trempe CL. Risk of developing a macular hole. *Arch Ophthalmol* 1990;108:1088–1090.

107. Akiba J, Kakehashi A, Arzabe CW, Trempe CL. Fellow eyes in idiopathic macular hole cases. *Ophthalmic Surg* 1992;23:594–597.

108. Guyer DR, de Bustros S, Diener-West M, Fine SL. The natural history of idiopathic macular holes and cysts. *Arch Ophthalmol* 1992;110:1264–1268.

109. Kokame GT, de Bustros S, the Vitrectomy for Prevention of Macular Hole Study Group. Visual acuity as a prognostic indicator in stage I macular holes. *Am J Ophthalmol* 1995;119:112–114.

110. Kim JW, Freeman WR, El-Haig W, et al, the Vitrectomy for Macular Hole Study Group. Baseline characteristics, natural history, and risk factors to progression in eyes with stage II macular holes. Results from a prospective randomized clinical trial. *Ophthalmology* 1995;102:1818–1829.

111. Gass JDM, Joondeph BC. Observations concerning patients with suspected impending macular holes. *Am J Ophthalmol* 1990;109:638–646.

112. Fish RH, Anand R, Izbrand DJ. Macular pseudoholes. Clinical features and accuracy of diagnosis. *Ophthalmology* 1992;99:1665–1670.

113. Smiddy WE, Gass JDM. Masquerades of macular holes. *Ophthalmic Surg* 1995;26:16–24.

114. Amsler M. Quantitative and qualitative vision. *Trans Ophthalmol Soc UK* 1949;69:397.

115. Watzke RC, Allen L. Subjective slitlamp beam sign for macular disease. *Am J Ophthalmol* 1969;68:449–453.

116. Martinez J, Smiddy WE, Kim J, Gass JDM. Differentiating macular holes from macular pseudoholes. *Am J Ophthalmol* 1994;117:762–767.

117. Birch DG, Jost BF, Fish GE. The focal electroretinogram in fellow eyes of patients with idiopathic macular holes. *Arch Ophthalmol* 1988;106:1558–1563.

118. Sjaarda RN, Frank DA, Glaser BM, et al. Resolution of an absolute scotoma and improvement of relative scotoma after successful macular surgery. *Am J Ophthalmol* 1993;116:129–139.

119. Acosta F, Lashkari K, Reynaud X, et al. Characterization of functional changes in macular holes and cysts. *Ophthalmology* 1991;98:1820–1823.

120. Weinberger D, Stiebel H, Gaton H, et al. Three-dimensional measurements of idiopathic macular holes using a scanning laser tomograph. *Ophthalmology* 1995;102:1445–1449.

121. Bartsch DU, Intaglietta M, Bille JF, et al. Confocal laser tomographic analysis of the retina in eyes with macular hole formation and other focal macular diseases. *Am J Ophthalmol* 1989;108:277–287.

122. Oritz RG, Lopez PF, Lambert HM, et al. Examination of macular vitreoretinal interface disorders with monochromatic photography. *Am J Ophthalmol* 1992;113:243–247.

123. Ogura Y, Shahidi M, Mori MT, et al. Improved visualization of macular hole lesions with laser biomicroscopy. *Arch Ophthalmol* 1991;109:957–961.

124. Kiryu J, Ogura Y, Shahidi M, et al. Enhanced visualization of vitreoretinal interface by laser biomicroscopy. *Ophthalmology* 1993;100:1040–1043.

125. Dugel PU, Smiddy WE, Byrne SF, et al. Macular hole syndrome. Echographic findings with clinical correlation. *Ophthalmology* 1994;101:815–821.

126. Kokame GT. Clinical correlation of ultrasonographic findings in macular holes. *Am J Ophthalmol* 1995;119:441–451.

127. Van Newkirk MR, Gass JDM, Callanan D, et al. Follow-up and ultrasonographic examination of patients with macular pseudo-operculum. *Am J Ophthalmol* 1994;117:13–18.

128. Hee MR, Puliafito CA, Wong C, et al. Optical coherence tomography of macular holes. *Ophthalmology* 1995;102:748–756.

129. Sjaarda R. Macular hole. *Int Ophthalmol Clin* 1995;35:105–122.

130. Smiddy WE, Thomley M, Knighton RW, Feuer WJ. Use of the potential acuity meter and laser interferometer to predict visual acuity after macular hole surgery. *Retina* 1994;14:305–309.

131. Schocket SS, Lakhanpal V, Xiaoping M, et al. Laser treatment of macular holes. *Ophthalmology* 1988;95:574–582.

132. Makabe R. Kryptonlaserkoagulation bei idiopathischem makulaloch. *Klin Monatsbl Augenheilkd* 1990;196:202–204.

133. Melberg NS, Meredith TA. Success with macular hole surgery. *Ophthalmology* 1996;103:200–201. Letter.

134. Kelly NE, Wendel RT. Vitreous surgery for idiopathic macular holes. Results of a pilot study. *Arch Ophthalmol* 1991;109:654–659.

135. Mein CE, Flynn HW Jr. Recognition and removal of the posterior cortical vitreous during vitreoretinal surgery for impending macular holes. *Am J Ophthalmol* 1991;111:611–613.

136. Ryan EA, Lee S, Chern S. Use of intravitreal autologous blood to identify posterior cortical vitreous in macular hole surgery. *Arch Ophthalmol* 1995;113:822–823.

137. Wendel RT, Patel AC. Full-thickness macular hole. In: Bovino JA, ed. *Macular surgery*. Norwalk, CT: Appleton & Lange, 1994:49–60.

138. Jost BF, Hutton WL, Fullet DG, et al. Vitrectomy in eyes at risk for macular hole formation. *Ophthalmology* 1990;97:843–847.

139. de Bustros S. Early stages of macular holes. To treat or not to treat. *Arch Ophthalmol* 1990;108:979–982. Editorial.

140. de Bustros S. Vitrectomy for prevention of macular hole study. *Arch Ophthalmol* 1991;109:1057. Letter.

141. de Bustros S, the Vitrectomy for Prevention of Macular Holes Study Group. Vitrectomy for prevention of macular holes. Results of a randomized clinical trial. *Ophthalmology* 1994;101:1055–1060.

142. Chambers RB, Davidorf FH, Gresak P, Stief WC. Modified vitrectomy for impending macular holes. *Ophthalmic Surg* 1991;22:730–734.

143. Ruby AJ, Williams DF, Grand MG, et al. Pars plana vitrectomy for treatment of stage II macular holes. *Arch Ophthalmol* 1994;112:359–364.

144. Wendel RT, Patel AC, Kelly NE, et al. Vitreous surgery for macular holes. *Ophthalmology* 1993;100:1671–1676.

145. Ryan EH, Gilbert HD. Results of surgical treatment of recent-onset full-thickness idiopathic macular holes. *Arch Ophthalmol* 1994;112:1545–1553.

146. Glaser BM, Michels RG, Kupperman BD, et al. Transforming growth factor–beta 2 for the treatment of full-thickness macular holes. *Ophthalmology* 1992;99:1162–1173.

147. Lansing MB, Glaser BM, Liss H, et al. The effects of pars plana vitrectomy and transforming growth factor beta 2 without epiretinal membrane peeling on full thickness macular holes. *Ophthalmology* 1993;100:868–872.

148. Smiddy WE, Glaser BM, Thompson JT, et al. Transforming growth factor beta-2 significantly enhances the ability to flatten the rim of subretinal fluid surrounding macular holes. Preliminary anatomic results of a multicenter prospective randomized study. *Retina* 1993;13:296–301.

149. Thompson JT, Glaser BM, Sjaarda RN, et al. Effects of intraocular bubble duration in the treatment of macular holes by vitrectomy and transforming growth factor beta-2. *Ophthalmology* 1994;101:1195–1200.

150. Liggett PE, Skolik S, Horio B, et al. Human autologous serum for the treatment of full-thickness macular holes. A preliminary study. *Ophthalmology* 1995;102:1071–1076.

151. Funata M, Wendel RT, de la Cruz Z, Green WR. Clinicopathologic study of bilateral macular holes treated with pars plana vitrectomy and gas tamponade. *Retina* 1992;12:289–298.

152. Madreperla SA, Geiger GL, Funata M, et al. Clinicopathologic correlation of a macular hole treated by cortical vitreous peeling and gas tamponade. *Ophthalmology* 1994;101:682–686.

153. Fekrat S, Wendel RT, de la Cruz Z, Green WR. Clinicopathologic correlation of an epiretinal membrane associated with a recurrent macular hole. *Retina* 1995;15:53–57.

154. Del Priore LV, Kaplan HJ, Bonham RD. Laser photocoagulation and fluid-gas exchange for recurrent macular hole. *Retina* 1994;14:381–382.

155. Thompson JT, Glaser BM, Sjaarda RN, Murphy RP. Progression of nuclear sclerosis and long-term visual results of vitrectomy with transforming growth factor beta-2 for macular holes. *Am J Ophthalmol* 1995;119:48–54.

156. Park SS, Marcus D, Duker JS, et al. Posterior segment complications after vitrectomy for macular hole. *Ophthalmology* 1995;102:775–781.

157. Sjaarda RN, Glaser BM, Thompson JT, et al. Distribution of iatrogenic retinal breaks in macular hole surgery. *Ophthalmology* 1995;102:1387–1392.

158. Poliner LS, Tornambe PE. Retinal pigment epitheliopathy after macular hole surgery. *Ophthalmology* 1992;99:1671–1677.

159. Charles S. Retinal pigment epithelium abnormalities after macular hole surgery. *Retina* 1993;13:176. Letter.

160. Duker JS. Retinal pigment epitheliopathy after macular hole surgery. *Ophthalmology* 1993;100:1604–1605. Letter.

161. Duker JS, Wendel RT, Patel AC, Puliafito CA. Late reopening of macular holes following initial successful vitreous surgery. *Ophthalmology* 1994;101:1373–1378.

162. Kokame GT. Recurrence of macular holes. *Ophthalmology* 1995;102:172–173. Letter.

163. Smiddy WE. Atypical presentations of macular holes. *Arch Ophthalmol* 1993;111:626–631.

164. Gass JDM. Pathogenesis of disciform detachment of the neuroepithelium. III. Senile disciform macular degeneration. *Am J Ophthalmol* 1967;63:617–644.

165. Lopez PF, Grossniklaus HE, Lambert HM, et al. Pathologic features of surgically excised subretinal neovascular membranes in age-related macular degeneration. *Am J Ophthalmol* 1991;112:647–656.

166. Grossniklaus HE, Martinez JA, Brown VB, et al. Immunohistochemical and histochemical properties of surgically excised subretinal neovascular membranes in age-related macular degeneration. *Am J Ophthalmol* 1992;114:464–472.

167. Hotchkiss ML, Fine SL. Pathologic myopia and choroidal neovascularization. *Am J Ophthalmol* 1981;91:177–183.

168. Hampton GR, Kohen D, Bird AC. Visual prognosis of disciform degeneration in myopia. *Ophthalmology* 1983;90:923–926.

169. Avila MP, Weiter JJ, Jalkh AE, et al. Natural history of choroidal neovascularization in degenerative myopia. *Ophthalmology* 1984;91:1573–1581.

170. Singerman LJ, Hatem G. Laser treatment of choroidal neovascular membranes in angioid streaks. *Retina* 1981;1:75–83.

171. Clarkson JG, Altman RD. Angioid streaks. *Surv Ophthalmol* 1982;26:235–246.

172. Lim JI, Bressler NM, Marsh MJ, Bressler SB. Laser treatment of choroidal neovascularization in patients with angioid streaks. *Am J Ophthalmol* 1993;116:414–423.

173. Klein R, Lewis RA, Myers SM, Myers FL. Subretinal neovascularization associated with fundus flavimaculatus. *Arch Ophthalmol* 1978;96:2054–2057.

174. Miller SA, Bresnick GH, Chandra SR. Choroidal neovascular membrane in Best's vitelliform macular dystrophy. *Am J Ophthalmol* 1976;82:252–255.

175. Callanan D, Gass JDM. Multifocal choroiditis and choroidal neovascularization associated with the multiple evanescent dot syndrome and acute idiopathic blind spot enlargement syndrome. *Ophthalmology* 1992;99:1678–1685.

176. Morgan CM, Schatz H. Recurrent multifocal choroiditis. *Ophthalmology* 1986;93:1138–1147.

177. Beebe WE, Kirkland C, Price J. A subretinal neovascular membrane as a complication of endogenous *Candida* endophthalmitis. *Ann Ophthalmol* 1987;19:207–209.

178. Wysynski RE, Grossniklaus HE, Frank KE. Indirect chorodial rupture secondary to blunt ocular trauma: a review of eight eyes. *Retina* 1988;8:237–243.

179. Ruby AJ, Jampol LM, Goldberg MF, et al. Choroidal neovascularization associated with choroidal hemangiomas. *Arch Ophthalmol* 1992;110:658–661.

180. Bressler SB, Bressler NM, Fine SL, et al. Natural course of choroidal neovascular membranes within the foveal avascular zone in senile macular degeneration. *Am J Ophthalmol* 1982;93:157–163.

181. Macular Photocoagulation Study Group. Laser photocoagulation of subfoveal neovascular lesions of age-related macular degeneration. Updated findings from two clinical trials. *Arch Ophthalmol* 1993;111:1200–1209.

182. Olk RJ, Burgess DB, McCormick PA. Subfoveal and juxtafoveal subretinal neovascularization in the presumed ocular histoplasmosis syndrome. Visual prognosis. *Ophthalmology* 1984;91:1592–1602.

183. Kleiner RC, Ratner CM, Enger C, Fine SL. Subfoveal neovascularization in the ocular histoplasmosis syndrome. A natural history study. *Retina* 1988;8:225–229.

184. Campochiaro PA, Morgan KM, Conway BP, Stathos J. Spontaneous involution of subfoveal neovascularization. *Am J Ophthalmol* 1990;109:668–675.

185. Vander JF, Morgan CM, Schatz H. Growth rate of subretinal neovascularization in age related macular degeneration. *Ophthalmology* 1989;96:1422–1429.

186. Macular Photocoagulation Study Group. Argon laser photocoagulation for senile macular degeneration: results of a randomized clinical trial. *Arch Ophthalmol* 1982;100:912–918.

187. Macular Photocoagulation Study Group. Krypton laser photocoagulation for neovascular lesions of age-related macular degeneration: results of randomized clinical trial. *Arch Ophthalmol* 1990;108:816–824.

188. Macular Photocoagulation Study Group. Argon laser photocoagulation for neovascular maculopathy: three-year results from randomized clinical trials. *Arch Ophthalmol* 1986;104:694–701.

189. Macular Photocoagulation Study Group. Argon laser photocoagulation for ocular histoplasmosis: results of a randomized clinical trial. *Arch Ophthalmol* 1983;101:1347–1357.

190. Macular Photocoagulation Study Group. Argon laser photocoagulation for neovascular maculopathy: five year results from randomized clinical trials. *Arch Ophthalmol* 1991;109:1109–1114.

191. Macular Photocoagulation Study Group. Recurrent choroidal neovascularization after argon laser photocoagulation for neovascular vasculopathy. *Arch Ophthalmol* 1986;104:503–512.

192. Macular Photocoagulation Study Group. Persistent and recurrent neovascularization after krypton laser photocoagulation for neovascular lesions of age-related macular degeneration. *Arch Ophthalmol* 1990;108:825–831.

193. Macular Photocoagulation Study Group. Persistent and recurrent neovascularization after krypton laser photocoagulation for neovascular lesions of ocular histoplasmosis. *Arch Ophthalmol* 1989;107:344–352.

194. Macular Photocoagulation Study Group. Laser photocoagulation of subfoveal neovascular lesions in age-related macular degeneration. Results of a randomized clinical trial. *Arch Ophthalmol* 1991;109:1220–1231.

195. Macular Photocoagulation Study Group. Laser photocoagulation of subfoveal recurrent neovascular lesions in age-related macular degeneration. Results of a randomized clinical trial. *Arch Ophthalmol* 1991;109:1232–1241.

196. Macular Photocoagulation Study Group. Subfoveal neovascular lesions in age-related macular degeneration: guidelines for evaluation and treatment in the Macular Photocoagulation Study. *Arch Ophthalmol* 1991;109:1242–1257.

197. Sorensen JA, Yannuzzi LA, Shakin JL. Recurrent subretinal neovascularization. *Ophthalmology* 1985;92:1059–1074.

198. Coscas G, Soubrane G, Ramahefasolo C, Fardeau C. Perifoveal laser treatment for subfoveal choroidal new vessels in age-related macular degeneration: results of a randomized clinical trial. *Arch Ophthalmol* 1991;109:1258–1265.

199. Green WR. Clinicopathologic studies of treated choroidal neovascular membranes. A review and report of two cases. *Retina* 1991;11:328–356.

200. Fine SL, Wood WJ, Isernhagen RD. Laser treatment for subfoveal neovascular membranes in ocular histoplasmosis syndrome: results of a pilot randomized clinical trial. *Arch Ophthalmol* 1993;111:19–20. Letter.

201. de Juan E Jr, Machemer R. Vitreous surgery for hemorrhagic and fibrous complications of age-related macular degeneration. *Am J Ophthalmol* 1988;105:25–29.

202. Blinder KJ, Peyman GA, Paris CL, Gremillion CM Jr. Submacular scar excision in age-related macular degeneration. *Int Ophthalmol* 1991;15:215–222.

203. Peyman GA, Blinder KJ, Paris CL, et al. A technique for retinal pigment epithelium transplantation for age related macular degeneration secondary to extensive subfoveal scarring. *Ophthalmic Surg* 1991;22:102–108.

204. Thomas MA, Kaplan HJ. Surgical removal of subfoveal neovascularization in the presumed ocular histoplasmosis syndrome. *Am J Ophthalmol* 1991;111:1–7.

205. Dickinson JD, Aguilar HE, Thomas MA. Retinotomies in subfoveal surgery: neither laser nor long acting gas tamponade is required. Presented at American Academy of Ophthalmology meeting, 1994.

206. Thomas MA. The use of vitreoretinal surgical techniques in subfoveal choroidal neovascularization. *Curr Opin Ophthalmol* 1992;3:349–356.

207. Thomas MA, Williams DF, Grand MG. Surgical removal of submacular hemorrhage and subfoveal choroidal neovascular membranes. *Int Ophthalmol Clin* 1992;32:173–188.

208. Ibanez HE, Thomas MA. Surgical approach to subfoveal neovascularization and submacular hemorrhage. *Semin Ophthalmol* 1994;9:56–64.

209. Ibanez HE, Thomas MA. Surgical excision of subfoveal choroidal neovascularization. *Ophthalmol Clin North* 1994;7:51–57.

210. Thomas MA, Ibanez HE. Surgical excision of subfoveal neovascular membranes and subretinal strands. In: Tasman W, Jaeger EA, eds. *Duane's clinical ophthalmology*. Philadelphia: Lippincott, 1994:1–10.

211. Thomas MA. Surgical removal of subfoveal choroidal neovascular membranes. In: Ryan SJ, ed. *Retina*. 2nd ed; vol. 3. St. Louis: Mosby, 1994:2385–2393.

212. Thomas MA. Surgical removal of subfoveal choroidal neovascular membranes. In: Lewis H, Ryan SJ, eds. *Medical and surgical retina: advances, controversies, and management*. St. Louis: Mosby, 1994:63–81.

213. Thomas MA. Vitrectomy surgery for subfoveal choroidal neovascularization and submacular hemorrhage. In: Bovino JA, ed. *Macular surgery*. Norwalk, CT: Appleton & Lange, 1994:135–164.

214. Bressler NM. Submacular surgery. Are randomized trials necessary? *Arch Ophthalmol* 1995;113:1557–1560. Editorial.

215. Thomas MA, Lee CA, Pesin S, Lowe M. New instruments for submacular surgery. *Am J Ophthalmol* 1991;12:733–734.

216. Thomas MA, Ibanez HE. Instruments for submacular surgery. *Retina* 1994;14:84–87.

217. Peyman GA, Kwang KJ. A new subretinal forceps. *Retina* 1995;15:87–88.

218. Greve MDJ, Peyman GA, Millsap CM. Direction and location of retinotomy for removal of subretinal neovascular membranes. *Ophthalmic Surg* 1995;26:330–333.

219. Adelberg DA, Del Priore LV, Kaplan HJ. Surgery for subfoveal membranes in myopia, angioid streaks, and other disorders. *Retina* 1995;15:198–205.

220. Capone A Jr. Submacular surgical procedures. *Int Ophthalmol Clin* 1995;35:83–93.

221. Thomas MA, Grand MG, Williams DF, et al. Surgical management of subfoveal choroidal neovascularization. *Ophthalmology* 1992;99:952–996.

222. Thomas MA, Dickenson JD, Melberg NS, et al. Visual results after surgical removal of subfoveal choroidal neovascular membranes. *Ophthalmology* 1994;101:1384–1396.

223. Smiddy WE, Fine SL, Green WR, et al. Clinicopathologic correlation of krypton red, argon blue-green, and argon green photocoagulation in the human fundus. *Retina* 1984;4:15–21.

224. Thomas EL, Apple DJ, Swartz M, et al. Histopathologic and ultrastructure of krypton and argon laser lesions in human retina-choroid. *Retina* 1984;4:22–39.

225. Eldrini AA, Ogden TE, Ryan SJ. Subretinal endophotocoagulation. A model of subretinal neovascularization in the rabbit. *Retina* 1991;11:244–249.

226. Thomas MA, Ibanez HE. Subretinal endophotocoagulation in the treatment of choroidal neovascularization. *Am J Ophthalmol* 1993;116:279–285.

227. Baron S, Tyring SK, Fleischmann WR Jr, et al. The interferons. Mechanisms of action and clinical applications. *JAMA* 1991;266:1375–1383.

228. Spiegel RJ. Clinical overview of alpha interferon. Studies and future directions. *Cancer* 1987;59:626.

229. Volberding PA, Mitsuyasu RT, Golando JP, Spiegel RJ. Treatment of Kaposi's sarcoma with interferon alfa-2b (Intron A). *Cancer* 1987;59 (suppl 3): 620.

230. de Wit R, Schattenkerk JK, Boucher CA, et al. Clinical and virological effects of high-dosage recombinant interferon-alpha in disseminated AIDS-related Kaposi's sarcoma. *Lancet* 1988;2:1214.

231. Brouty-Boye D, Zetter BR. Inhibition of cell motility by interferon. *Science* 1980;208:516–518.

232. White CW, Wolf SJ, Korones DN, et al. Treatment of childhood angiomatous disease with recombinant interferon alpha-2a. *J Pediatr* 1991;118:59–66.

233. Fung WE. Interferon alpha-2a for treatment of age-related macular degeneration. *Am J Ophthalmol* 1991;112:349–350. Letter.

234. Spiegel RJ. Dosage and toxicity. Alpha interferon: dosage, toxicity and antibody formation. In: Silver HKB, ed. *Interferons in cancer treatment: biologic activity and clinical toxicity of interferons, clinical response to systemic interferons, alternate routes of administration*. Missiaugo, Ontario: MES Medical Education Services, 1986:17–27.

235. Thomas MA, Ibanez HE. Interferon alpha-2a in the treatment of subfoveal choroidal neovascularization. *Am J Ophthalmol* 1993;115:563–568.

236. Chan CK, Kempin SJ, Noble SK, Palmer GA. The treatment of choroidal neovascular membranes by alpha interferon. *Ophthalmology* 1994;101:289–300.

237. Pharmacological therapy for macular degeneration study group. Interferon alfa-2a is ineffective for patients with choroidal neovascularization secondary to age-related macular degeneration. *Arch Ophthalmol* 1997;115:865–872.

238. Collen D, Stassen JM, Marafino BJ, et al. Biological properties of human tissue-type plasminogen activator obtained by expression of recombinant DNA in mammalian cells. *J Pharmacol Exp Ther* 1984;231:146–152.

239. Tiefenbaum AJ, Robison AK, Kurnik PB, et al. Clinical pharmacology in patients with evolving myocardial infarction of tissue-type plasminogen activator produced by recombinant DNA technology. *Circulation* 1985;71:110–116.

240. Thomas JW, Lopez PF, Lambert HM. Tissue plasminogen activator in the surgical excision of subfoveal choroidal neovascular membranes. *Ophthalmic Surg* 1995;26:374–376.

241. Lambert HM, Capone A Jr, Aaberg TM, et al. Surgical excision of subfoveal neovascular membranes in age-related macular degeneration. *Am J Ophthalmol* 1993;115:563–568.

242. Berger AS, Kaplan HJ. Clinical experience with the surgical removal of subfoveal choroidal neovascular membranes: short-term post-operative results. *Ophthalmology* 1992;99:969–976.

243. Ormerod LD, Puklin JE, Frank RN. Long-term outcomes after the surgical removal of advanced subfoveal neovascular membranes in age-related macular degeneration. *Ophthalmology* 1994;101:1201–1210.

244. Connor TB, Wolf MD, Arrindel EL, Mieler WF. Surgical removal of an extra foveal fibrotic choroidal neovascular membrane with foveal serous detachment in age-related macular degeneration. *Retina* 1994;14:125–129.

245. Melberg NS, Thomas MA, Dickinson JD, Valluri S. Managing recurrent neovascularization after subfoveal surgery in presumed ocular histoplasmosis syndrome. *Ophthalmology* 1996;103:1064–1067.

246. Gass JDM. Biomicroscopic and histopathologic considerations regarding the feasibility of surgical excision of subfoveal neovascular membranes. *Am J Ophthalmol* 1994;118:285–298.

247. Brittis M, Lopez R, Gouras P, Kjeldbye H. Autotransplantation of cultured retinal pigment epithelium to Bruch's membrane in the rabbit eye. *Transplantation Procs* 1987;19:1133–1139.

248. Gouras P, Flood MT, Kjeldbye MK, et al. Transplantation of cultured human retinal pigment epithelium to Bruch's membrane of the owl monkey's eye. *Curr Eye Res* 1985;4:253–265.

249. Gouras P, Flood MT, Kjeldbye MK. Transplantation of cultured human retinal cells to monkey retina. *An Acad Bras Cienc* 1984;56:431–443.

250. Gouras P, Brittis M, Lopez R, et al. Transplantation of retinal pigment epithelium prevents photoreceptor degeneration in the RCS rat. In: La Vail M, Anderson RE, Holyfield JG, eds. *Inherited and environmentally induced retinal degenerations.* New York: Alan R. Liss, 1989:659–671.

251. Gouras P, Lopez R. Transplantation of retinal epithelial cells. *Invest Ophthalmol Vis Sci* 1989;30:1681–1683.

252. Lane C, Boulton M. Retinal pigment epithelium transplantation: technique and possible applications. *Adv Biosci* 1987;63:125–138.

253. Lane C, Boulton M, Bridgman A, Marshall J. Transplantation of retinal pigment epithelium in the miniature pig. *Invest Ophthalmol Vis Sci* 1988;29 (suppl):405.

254. Lane C, Boulton M, Marshall J. Transplantation of retinal pigment epithelium using a pars plana approach. *Eye* 1989;3:27–32.

255. Li L, Sheedlo HJ, Gaur V, Turner JE. Effects of macrophage and retinal pigment epithelial cell transplants on photoreceptor cell rescue in RCS rats. *Curr Eye Res* 1991;10:947–958.

256. Li L, Sheedlo HJ, Turner JE. Long-term rescue of photoreceptor cells in the retinas of RCS dystrophic rats by RPE transplants. *Prog Brain Res* 1990;82:179–185.

257. Li L, Turner JE. Transplantation of retinal pigment epithelium cells to immature and adult rat hosts: short- and long-term survival characteristics. *Exp Eye Res* 1988;47:771–785.

258. Li L, Turner JE. Inherited retinal dystrophy in the RCS rat: prevention of photoreceptor degeneration by pigment epithelial cell transplantation. *Exp Eye Res* 1988;47:911–917.

259. Liu Y, Silverman MS, Berger AS, Kaplan HJ. Transplantation of confluent sheets of adult human RPE. *Invest Ophthalmol Vis Sci* 1992;33 (suppl):1128.

260. Lopez R, Gouras P, Britts M, Kjeldbye H. Transplantation of cultured rabbit retinal epithelium to rabbit retina using a closed-eye method. *Invest Ophthalmol Vis Sci* 1987;28:1131–1137.

261. Lopez R, Gouras P, Kjeldbye H, et al. Transplanted retinal pigment epithelium modifies the retinal degeneration in the RCS rat. *Invest Ophthalmol Vis Sci* 1991;32:3167–3174.

262. Seaton AD, Turner JE. RPE transplants stabilize retinal vasculature and prevent neovascularization in the RCS rat. *Invest Ophthalmol Vis Sci* 1992;33:83–91.

263. Sheedlo HJ, Li L, Turner JE. Functional and structural characteristics of photoreceptor cells rescued in RPE–cell grafted retinas of RCS dystrophic rats. *Exp Eye Res* 1989;48:841–854.

264. Valentino TL, Kaplan HJ, Del Priore LV, et al. Retinal pigment epithelial repopulation in monkeys after submacular surgery. *Arch Ophthalmol* 1995;113:932–938.

265. Del Priore LV, Hornbeck R, Kaplan HJ, et al. Surgical removal of retinal pigment epithelium causes atrophy of the choriocapillaris and outer retina. *Invest Ophthalmol Vis Sci* 1995;36 (suppl):1142.

266. Del Priore LV, Hornbeck R, Kaplan HJ, et al. Debridement of the pig retinal pigment epithelium in vivo. *Arch Ophthalmol* 1995;113:939–944.

267. Del Priore LV, Glaser BM, Quigley HA, Green WR. Response of pig retinal epithelium to laser photocoagulation in organ culture. *Arch Ophthalmol* 1989;107:119–122.

268. Sarks SH, Van Driel D, Maxwell L, Killingsworth M. Softening of drusen and subfoveal neovascularization. *Trans Ophthalmol Soc UK* 1980;100:414–422.

269. Green WR, Key SN III. Senile macular degeneration: a histopathologic study. *Trans Am Ophthalmol Soc* 1977;75:180–254.

270. Friedman E, Smith TR, Kuwabara T. Senile choroidal vascular patterns and drusen. *Arch Ophthalmol* 1963;69:220–230.

271. Desai VN, Del Priore LV, Pollack JS, Kaplan HJ. Choriocapillaris atrophy after submacular surgery in the presumed ocular histoplasmosis syndrome. *Arch Ophthalmol* 1995;113:409–410.

272. Zarbin MA, Nasir M. Impaired choriocapillaris perfusion following subfoveal surgery for macular degeneration. *Ophthalmology* 1993;100(suppl):97.

273. Pollack JS, Kaplan HJ, Del Priore LV, Smith MS. Choriocapillaris atrophy following subfoveal membrane excision in exudative age-related macular degeneration. *Ophthalmology* 1993;100(suppl):122.

274. Nasir M, Zarbin MA. Choriocapillaris atrophy as a complication of surgical excision of choroidal neovascular membranes. *Invest Ophthalmol Vis Sci* 1993;34(suppl):834.

275. Pollack JS, Kaplan HJ, Del Priore LV, Smith MS. Choriocapillaris atrophy associated with exudative age-related macular degeneration. *Invest Ophthalmol Vis Sci* 1993;34(suppl):834.

276. Glaser BM, Campochiaro PA, Davis JL, Sato M. Retinal pigment epithelial cells release an inhibitor of neovascularization. *Arch Ophthalmol* 1985;103:1876–1880.

277. Campochiaro PA, Glaser BM. Endothelial cell release: a chemoattractant for retinal pigment epithelial cells in vitro. *Arch Ophthalmol* 1985;103:1876–1880.

278. Glaser BM, D'Amore PA, Michels RG, et al. Demonstration of vasoproliferative activity from mammalian retina. *J Cell Biol* 1980;84:298–304.

279. Del Monte MA, Maumenee IH. New techniques for in vitro culture of human retinal pigment epithelium. *Birth Defects* 1980;16:327–338.

280. Hay ED. In: Hay ED ed. *Cell biology of extracellular matrix.* New York: Plenum, 1981:379–409.

281. Reh TA, Nagy T, Gretton H. Retinal pigment epithelial cells induced to transdifferentiate to neurons by laminin. *Nature* 1987;330:68–71.

282. Song M-K, Lui GM. Propagation of fetal human RPE cells: preservation of original culture morphology after serial passage. *J Cell Physiol* 1990;143:196–203.

283. Del Priore LV, Kaplan HJ, Silverman MS, et al. Experimental and surgical aspects of retinal pigment epithelial cell transplantation. *Eur J Implant Ref Surg* 1993;5:128–132.

284. Kaplan H. Submacular surgery for choroidal neovascularization. *Br J Ophthalmol* 1996;80:101. Commentary.

285. Russell SR, Crapotta JA, Zerbolio DJ. Surgical removal of subfoveal neovascularization. *Ophthalmology* 1993;100:795–796. Letter.

286. Schachat AP. Should we recommend vitreous surgery for patients with choroidal neovascularization? *Arch Ophthalmol* 1994;112:459–461. Editorial.

287. *Submacular surgery trials manual of procedure,* September 1995. Baltimore: Johns Hopkins, 1995.

288. Bennett SR, Folk JC, Blodi CF, Klugman M. Factors prognostic of visual outcome in patients with subretinal hemorrhages. *Am J Ophthalmol* 1990;109:33–37.

289. Wade EC, Flynn HW, Olsen KR, et al. Subretinal hemorrhage management by pars plana vitrectomy and internal drainage. *Arch Ophthalmol* 1990;108:973–978.

290. Lewis H. Management of submacular hemorrhage. In: Lewis H, Ryan SJ, eds. *Medical and surgical retina: advances, controversies, and management.* St. Louis: Mosby, 1994:54–62.

291. Williams DF, Thomas MA. Vitrectomy for removal of submacular hemorrhage. In: Ryan SJ, ed. *Retina.* 2nd ed; vol. 3. St. Louis: Mosby, 1994:2557–2559.

292. El Baba F, Jarrett WH, Harbin TS, et al. Massive hemorrhage complicating age-related macular degeneration. *Ophthalmology* 1986;93:1581–1592.

293. Glatt H, Machemer R. Experimental subretinal hemorrhage in rabbits. *Am J Ophthalmol* 1982;94:762–763.

294. Koshibu A. Ultrastructural studies on absorption of experimentally produced subretinal hemorrhage: III. Absorption of erythrocyte breakdown products and retinal hemosiderosis at the late stage. *Nippon Ganka Gakkai Zasshi* 1979;83:386–400.

295. Toth CA, Morse LS, Hjelmeland LM, Landers MB. Fibrin directs early retinal damage after experimental subretinal hemorrhage. *Arch Ophthalmol* 1991;109:1731–1734.

296. Lewis H, Resnick SC, Flannery JG, Straasma BR. Tissue plasminogen activator treatment of experimental subretinal hemorrhage. *Am J Ophthalmol* 1991;111:197–204.

297. Johnson MW, Olsen KR, Hernandez E. Tissue plasminogen activator treatment of experimental subretinal hemorrhage. *Retina* 1991;11:250–258.

298. Benner JD, Morse LS, Toth CA, et al. Evaluation of a commercial recombinant tissue-type plasminogen activator preparation of the subretinal space of the cat. *Arch Ophthalmol* 1991;109:723–729.

299. Coll GE, Sparrow JR, Marinovic A, Chang S. Effects of intravitreal tissue plasminogen activator on experimental subretinal hemorrhage. *Retina* 1995;319–326.

300. Lim JI. Subretinal hemorrhage. *Int Ophthalmol Clin* 1995;35:95–104.

301. Gillies A, Lahav M. Absorption of retinal and subretinal hemorrhages. *Ann Ophthalmol* 1983;15:1068–1074.

302. Fekrat S, Avery RL, MacCumber M, Bressler NM. Natural history of subretinal hemorrhage in age related macular degeneration (AMD). *Invest Ophthalmol Vis Sci* 1993;34(suppl):1133.

303. Dellaporta A. Retinal damage from subretinal hemorrhage. *Am J Ophthalmol* 1983;95:568–570. Letter.

304. Hanscom TA, Diddie KR. Early surgical drainage of macular subretinal hemorrhage. *Arch Ophthalmol* 1987;105:1722–1723.

305. Slusher MM. Evacuation of submacular hemorrhage: technique and timing. In: Morris R, ed. *Vitreoretinal surgery and technology.* vol. 1. Thorofare, NJ: Slack, 1989:2,3,8.

306. Kimura AE, Reddy CV, Folk JC, Farmer SG. Removal of subretinal hemorrhage facilitated by preoperative intravitreal tissue plasminogen activator. *Retina* 1994;14:83–84.

307. Vander JF, Federman JL, Greven CL, et al. Surgical removal of massive subretinal hemorrhage associated with age-related macular degeneration. *Ophthalmology* 1991;98:23–27.

308. Peyman GA, Nelson NC Jr, Alturki W, et al. Tissue plasminogen activating factor assisted removal of subretinal hemorrhage. *Ophthalmic Surg* 1991;22:575–582.

309. Lewis H. Intraoperative fibrinolysis of submacular hemorrhage with tissue plasminogen activator and surgical drainage. *Am J Ophthalmol* 1994;118:559–568.

310. Lim JI, Drews-Botsch C, Sternberg P Jr, et al. Submacular hemorrhage removal. *Ophthalmology* 1995;102:1393–1399.

311. Ibanez HE, Williams DA, Thomas MA, et al. Surgical management of submacular hemorrhage. A series of 47 consecutive cases. *Arch Ophthalmol* 1995;113:62–69.

312. Kamei M, Tano Y, Maeno T, et al. Surgical removal of submacular hemorrhage using tissue plasminogen activator and perfluorocarbon liquid. *Am J Ophthalmol* 1996;121:267–275.

313. Capone A Jr, Sternberg P Jr. Advances in submacular surgery. *Am J Ophthalmol* 1994;118:659–663. Editorial.

Vitreoretinal Complications of Cataract Surgery

Saad El-Naggar   Frank L. Myers

In the era of intracapsular cataract extraction, the vitreous was a substance to be left undisturbed. The presence of vitreous in the cataract wound was greatly feared. Since the advent of vitrectomy surgical techniques, however, these complications can be dealt with in a number of ways with great success.

Vitreoretinal complications of cataract surgery can be classified according to their time relationship to the surgery (Table 53-1) and according to the type of complication (Table 53-2).

GLOBE PENETRATION BY ANESTHETIC INJECTION

Retrobulbar and peribulbar injections of anesthetic solutions are performed to induce anesthesia and akinesia before ocular surgery. Although rare, complications from these injections include needle penetration of the globe, central retinal artery and vein occlusions, Purtscher's retinopathy, optic nerve damage, respiratory arrest, seizures, and strabismus (1–10). Lincoff and associates (11) reported that intraocular injections of lidocaine 2%, lidocaine 2% with epinephrine 1:10,000, or hyaluronidase resulted in no detectable histologic damage to the retina. The intraocular complications of retinal breaks, vitreous hemorrhage, or retinal detachment that result from the needle trauma have been described (12,13). If needle penetration of the globe occurs, management options and final visual acuities are dependent on the site of the globe penetration.

Predisposing Factors

Predisposing factors to needle penetration of the globe include an uncooperative patient during the injection, injection by nonophthalmologists, and high myopia with axial length of 30 mm or greater (14). Morgan and associates (15) reported that a sharp, disposable 25-gauge needle is more likely to penetrate the globe and recommended the use of a blunt 23-gauge needle. In another series, needle entry into the eye occurred with both blunt and sharp needle with no statistically significant difference (16).

Prevention

A commonly used retrobulbar technique is to have the patient look up and in during entry of the needle into the inferior temporal orbital region. A recommended modification of this technique is to have the patient look straight ahead to avoid bringing the optic nerve into the path of the needle (17). Elevating the globe with an index finger has also been proposed as a technique to reduce the chance of needle penetration of the globe (18).

Alternatives to traditional retrobulbar anesthetic injections include the use of peribulbar anesthesia (19–23), subconjunctival anesthesia, topical anesthesia (24), and general anesthesia. In peribulbar anesthesia, the local anesthetic is injected outside the muscle cone and theoretically the chance of needle penetration of the globe should be reduced. However, Kimble and associates (25) reported cases of needle penetration of the globe that occurred with this technique. See Chapter 22 for more complete discussion of ocular anesthetic technique.

Symptoms and Signs

Symptoms of needle penetration of the globe include severe pain and sudden loss of vision. Signs of hypotony or sudden increase in intraocular pressure should warn the surgeon of the possibility of needle penetration. If globe perforation is suspected, the pupil should be dilated immediately, if this

Table 53-1. Time Relationship of Vitreoretinal Complications to Cataract Surgery

Preoperatively
Intraoperatively
Early postoperative (1 wk)
Delayed postoperative (2–6 wk)
Late

Table 53-2. Types of Vitreoretinal Complications of Cataract Surgery

Globe penetration during peribulbar or retrobulbar anesthesia
Posterior capsular rupture with vitreous loss
Intravitreal loss of lens material
Hemorrhage
   Vitreous
   Suprachoroidal
Aminoglycoside retinopathy
Intraocular lens dislocation
Cystoid macular edema
Retinal complications of Nd:YAG laser posterior capsulotomy
Retinal detachment
Endophthalmitis
   Acute
   Chronic
Acceleration of diabetic retinopathy
Light-induced retinopathy

has not been done previously, and the fundus examined carefully with the indirect ophthalmoscope. Perforation may be single or double, posterior or anterior. Vitreous, retinal, or choroidal hemorrhage and retinal detachment may be apparent. Retinal holes or tears may be difficult to see. Scleral depression can usually be performed if necessary without worry of additional damage.

Management

Management options depend on the nature and extent of the intraocular complications. If the intraocular pressure is high and no pulsation can be seen in the central retinal artery, an immediate paracentesis should be performed. If the media are clear, we generally recommend treatment of visible retinal breaks after needle penetration of the globe with either laser photocoagulation or cryopexy (26). Exploration of the sclera for penetration sites is generally not recommended since these holes are usually small and self-sealing.

POSTERIOR CAPSULAR RUPTURE DURING CATARACT SURGERY

Posterior capsular rupture during extracapsular cataract extraction with or without phacoemulsification is not

uncommon. Often it is not recognized until completion of the case or some time postoperatively. If associated with vitreous loss into the anterior chamber and to the wound, it can result in postoperative glaucoma, chronic iritis, or cystoid macular edema. Progressive intraocular lens dislocation can also develop.

Predisposing Factors

Hypermature, diabetic, and other complicated cataracts including pseudoexfoliation syndrome may have thin posterior capsules that are prone to rupture. Traumatic cataracts may have an already ruptured capsule. Inexperience with phacoemulsification techniques and excessive suction or infusion may play a role. A large brow or deep orbit that requires a more posterior angle of the phaco instrument tip can also be contributory. Not infrequently, sudden patient movement from sedation techniques that results in patient confusion can occur and produce capsule rupture from the instrument tip.

Symptoms and Signs

Posterior capsular rupture may be difficult to recognize. If the anterior hyaloid face remains intact, it may not present a problem, especially if the rent is small and does not extend into the anterior capsule. Distortion of the iris is an indication that vitreous may be present in the anterior chamber. Loss of lens material posteriorly is an obvious sign that rupture has occurred.

Prevention

Awareness of predisposing factors and careful technique with avoidance of high infusion pressures are important in these cases. The use of iris retraction (27) can be helpful in allowing a safer and more complete phacoemulsification when pupil size is small. With a prominent brow or deep-set eyes, utilization of a temporal incision rather than the usual 12 o'clock incision should be considered in order to reduce pressure on the posterior capsule by flattening the instrument angle.

Management

If vitreous is noted in the anterior chamber, it is important to remove all remaining lens material as completely as possible utilizing the phaco instrument. Then a limited anterior vitrectomy should be performed using a standard, disposable, guillotine vitreous suction cutter instrument through the corneoscleral wound. If an infusion sleeve is used, pressure should be kept low. Vitreous should be aspirated and cut until iris distortion is eliminated and the vitreous can be seen to fall in back of the iris plane. The posterior chamber should then be rigorously inspected to make sure no lens fragments remain. This can be facilitated by the use of iris retractors or scleral depression, or both, especially superiorly. If anterior vitrectomy cannot be adequately performed through the corneoscleral wound and if no lens fragments have fallen back into the posterior vitreous, consideration should be given to an anterior pars plana approach with incisions 2.5 mm posterior to the limbus (Fig. 53-1). The corneoscleral wound should be temporarily closed and a separate infusion terminal inserted inferotemporal through the pars plana. This should be inspected to make sure the tip is through the ciliary epithelium cleanly. A second incision, superior temporal or nasal, is made for the suction cutter. Another incision for an endoilluminator is usually not required, although residual vitreous is often seen better by the retroillumination that a light pipe provides. Iris retraction can again be of great help in visualization. While all lens fragments and vitreous should be carefully removed, as many anterior and posterior capsular elements as possible should be retained to act as support for a sulcus-placed intraocular lens (IOL).

At the conclusion of the vitrectomy, whether by corneoscleral or pars plana approach, and before placement of the IOL, the retina should be inspected with the indirect ophthalmoscope to make sure that no lens fragments are present posteriorly and that no retinal breaks are seen anteriorly. If either is noted, appropriate referral to a vitreoretinal surgeon should be made. At this point a decision must be made as to the type of IOL to be utilized.

Assuming that all vitreous and lens fragments have been removed anteriorly, a decision must be made as to the placement of the IOL and the type and size to be utilized. If sufficient anterior capsule remains for support, a lens with a larger optic (6.5–7.0 mm) can be placed into the

sulcus. If large, anterior capsular tears are present, a posterior chamber lens can be inserted with sulcus fixation using two scleral fixation sutures 180 degrees apart. Alternatively, an open-loop, flexible, all–polymethylmethacrylate (PMMA) Kelman-style anterior chamber lens can be placed (28).

LOSS OF LENS MATERIAL INTO THE VITREOUS DURING CATARACT SURGERY

Dislocation of fragments of the crystalline lens into the vitreous cavity is a potentially serious complication of cataract surgery. The incidence is dependent on the level of experience of the cataract surgeon and on the technique. Phacoemulsification is associated with a greater incidence than are other forms of cataract extraction (29–36).

Predisposing Factors

Although occasionally zonular rupture results in loss of the entire intact lens into the vitreous, most cases of lens loss are associated with rupture of the posterior capsule during an extracapsular procedure. Thus one or more factors mentioned previously that predispose to posterior capsule rupture are generally present. Eyes that have previously undergone vitrectomy surgery are also predisposed to have weak zonules or posterior capsules, or both.

Prevention

Awareness of those factors associated with weak zonules, such as pseudoexfoliation or the presence of phacodenesis, or both, should make one consider an intracapsular, rather than extracapsular, extraction. Being alert for signs of posterior capsular rupture, avoiding high infusion pressure, and utilizing low vacuum and low emulsification power during phacoemulsification are important. Hydrodissection should be avoided in marked brunescent cataracts, which tend to have thin posterior capsules. Creation of sharp edges on the lens should be avoided since this can rupture the capsule if they begin to tumble.

Signs and Symptoms

Radial tears that extend from the anterior capsule posteriorly are often associated with lens loss. Sudden partial subluxation of the nucleus posteriorly is an indication that this has occurred. Vibration of the entire lens is a sign of zonular rupture and may precede posterior dislocation. If these signs are noted during phacoemulsification it is generally best to remove the phaco tip and convert to a different technique.

The dislocated lens fragments, both nuclear and cortical, can produce uveitis, increased intraocular pressure, corneal edema, vitreous opacification, and cystoid macular edema. This is very stressful for both the patient and cataract surgeon since expectations for immediate improvement in

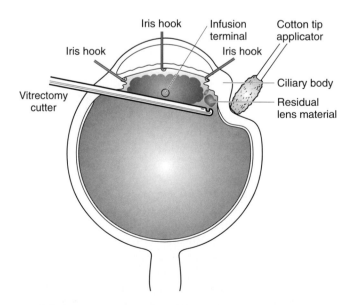

FIGURE 53-1. *Removal of residual cortical lens material via anterior pars plana approach after posterior capsular rupture. Scleral depression is used to bring fragments into view.*

vision are high. Usually the loss of lens fragments into the vitreous is recognized immediately by the surgeon. However, occasionally residual cortical or nuclear fragments, or both, will dislocate through unrecognized capsular rents during surgery or in the early postoperative period. Careful examination of the fundus with the indirect ophthalmoscope should be performed in all cases of increased intraocular pressure, uveitis, or cystoid macular edema to rule out the presence of retained lens fragments in the inferior vitreous. It should be kept in mind that endophthalmitis can occur in association with retained intravitreal lens fragments (37).

Management

If only partial subluxation of the nucleus has occurred, it may be possible to make an incision in the pars plana, insert a spatula to prolapse the cataract anteriorly, and then insert a Sheets glide to prevent further loss. If the lens has sunk too posteriorly to attempt this, it is tempting for the anterior segment surgeon to try to float the lens back up by irrigation. This should be avoided because of danger of retinal injury (38). Unless the surgeon has extensive posterior segment and pars plana vitrectomy experience, he or she should proceed to clean up any remaining cortical remnants and if necessary perform an anterior vitrectomy. However, no attempt to perform a deep posterior vitrectomy should be made via a limbal approach. If enough posterior capsule is visible to provide support, a posterior chamber IOL can be placed and the eye closed. If not, an anterior chamber lens can be placed. Referral then should be made to an experienced vitreoretinal surgeon.

If a vitreoretinal surgeon is immediately available, a pars plana vitrectomy and removal of the lost lens material can be performed at this time; however, this is not an emergency and the vitrectomy can be done at some later convenient time. In fact, unless glaucoma that cannot be controlled medically occurs, the procedure can be postponed for a considerable period. If the fragments are small and made up of lens cortex, they may absorb out spontaneously. However, nuclear fragments will usually not absorb and must eventually be removed.

Patients with increased intraocular pressure should be treated with systemic and topical antiglaucoma medications as well as topical steroids. Uveitis should be aggressively treated by frequent topical and, if necessary, systemic corticosteroids. Occasionally it may be necessary to wait for surgical removal until the cornea has cleared.

Pars plana vitrectomy is the most effective means of removing retained lens fragments and obtaining resolution of persistent uveitis and glaucoma (39).

Indications and Timing of Vitrectomy

As noted previously small fragments of cortical material will usually absorb out spontaneously and, if glaucoma and inflammation can be controlled medically, they can be observed.

The indications for vitrectomy are prominent uveitis, uncontrolled glaucoma, and cystoid macular edema (35,36). The timing of surgery has not been shown to affect significantly the ultimate visual outcome (40). However, prompt vitrectomy produces rapid resolution of uveitis and improved control of glaucoma as well as a more immediate restoration of vision (41).

Surgical Technique

A three-port pars plana vitrectomy with aspiration of the retained lens fragments is the most successful method except when nuclear fragments are extremely dense (38,42–47). A careful vitrectomy should be performed initially to completely free the retained lens fragments and to avoid peripheral vitreous traction during aspiration. Next, the vitreous cutter can be used to remove softer cortical material. Larger cortical and nuclear fragments can then be aspirated using a phacofragmentor tip to emulsify the material (Fig. 53-2). The instrument should be used to initially aspirate the material from the surface of the retina, with the emulsification performed in the midvitreous cavity only to avoid retinal injury. It is important to use the lowest emulsification energy possible, as high power levels will blow away the fragment. The fiberoptic light pipe or light pipe with pick may be helpful in holding and/or stuffing the lens fragment into the cutter port or fragmetome opening. Both cutter and fragmetome may have to be removed periodically and flushed of thick lens material.

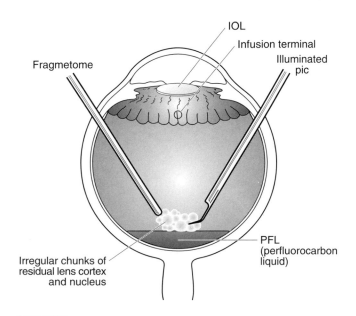

FIGURE 53-2. *Removal of cortical and nuclear lens fragments from the vitreous utilizing ultrasonic fragmentation and aspiration, illuminated pic, and perfluorocarbon liquid.*

The use of perfluorocarbon liquids can also be helpful to elevate fragments away from the retina and prevent impingement on the retina with subsequent tear formation posteriorly. However, only small volumes should be used since the fragments may migrate peripherally resulting in possible vitreous base traction during aspiration.

If the nucleus is so hard that posterior phacoemulsification cannot be accomplished the fragment may have to be elevated into the anterior chamber and removed through the limbus or through the pars plana if an IOL is in place. If a posterior chamber IOL has been implanted, attention should be given to the removal of residual lens material from under the iris and surrounding the IOL without removal of capsular material, which might destabilize the IOL. If an anterior chamber IOL has been implanted, removal of the lens capsule remnant should be performed.

INTRAOCULAR LENS DISLOCATION INTO THE VITREOUS

Dislocation of an intraocular lens into the vitreous can happen at any time but usually occurs in the late postoperative phase. It can occur precipitously or gradually, in which case it is referred to as the "sunset syndrome."

Predisposing Factors

Rupture of the posterior capsule during cataract surgery is the most common predisposing factor. Other factors are pseudoexfoliation, improper sulcus fixation, improper implant size, and trauma (48).

Prevention

Recognition of posterior capsular rupture, use of an anterior chamber IOL when indicated, and use of proper sulcus fixation technique can help to prevent this complication (49).

Signs and Symptoms

Diplopia, intermittent or sudden monocular blurring, or positional blurring of vision in a patient with previously good postoperative vision may indicate subluxation or dislocation of the IOL. Slit lamp examination will reveal a decentered or missing IOL and if complete dislocation has occurred it may be seen floating in the vitreous on fundoscopic examination. It may be hinged at its inferior pole and only seen by indirect ophthalmoscopy on the inferior pars plana.

Management

Numerous techniques have been described for retrieval and either removal, IOL exchange, or replacement with or without suture of the old posterior chamber (PC) IOL in place (50–57). In some instances it may be better to leave the implant undisturbed and to fit the patient with an aphakic correction or contact lens, or to leave the patient uncorrected if the other eye is good. Implantation of an anterior chamber lens without removal of the dislocated posterior lens has also been done. If the subluxation is partial, then repositioning can be accomplished by an anterior segment approach. However, if the lens is hinged backward or totally free in the vitreous, a posterior approach is indicated to prevent retinal tractional complications. If dislocation occurred during or immediately after cataract surgery, a period of at least 2 to 3 weeks should elapse before repositioning is attempted in order to allow fibrosis of the residual posterior capsular ring to occur.

Using a three-port vitrectomy technique, any vitreous in the anterior chamber and to the wound is removed but the capsular remnants are left to serve as support. Residual cortical lens material is removed if necessary, however. The vitreous around the lens is aspirated and cut and the lens completely freed, using scleral depression if necessary to free the lens where it is hinged at six o'clock. Perfluorocarbon liquids can be used to float the lens away from the retinal surface (58). The IOL is then grasped with forceps and brought anteriorly. If the haptics are of the flexible type, an attempt can be made to place one of the haptics into the ciliary sulcus at 6 o'clock, and while compressing it, to slip the other haptic into the sulcus superiorly. If the lens is a one-piece, rigid polymethylmethacrylate type, this may not be possible.

In order to allow manipulation of the lens without it falling posteriorly, transfixion with a 27-gauge $1\frac{1}{4}$-in. needle placed from 12 to 6 o'clock through the pars plana behind the lens may be useful. Reverse Sinskey hooks can then be placed through the sclerotomy incision to rotate the lens into position behind the iris and anterior to residual lens capsule. If posterior capsular support is not judged to be adequate and the lens is unstable, then one or both haptics can be fixated either to iris or sclera. Scleral fixation is generally preferred and can be done either internally as described by Campo et al (59) or externally as described by Chan (60). The external method is easier and more secure (Fig. 53-3). Additional sclerotomes are made 1.0 to 1.5 mm posterior to the limbus at 3 and 9 o'clock and the haptics are externalized through these incisions with the intraocular forceps. Double-armed 9-0 Prolene sutures are tied around the haptics at the distal one half to one third and the haptics are replaced inside the eye. The sutures are gently snugged up and then inverted bites are taken in the lips of the sclerotomy; next the sutures are tied, automatically closing the sclerotomy and burying the knots.

HEMORRHAGE ASSOCIATED WITH CATARACT SURGERY

Hemorrhagic complications of cataract surgery include vitreous hemorrhage, choroidal hemorrhage, suprachoroidal

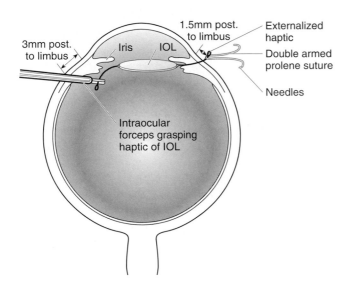

FIGURE 53-3. *External scleral fixation of dislocated intraocular lens utilizing intraocular forceps via the pars plana.*

hemorrhage (SCH), and explusive hemorrhage. The latter, either during or after cataract surgery, can be a catastrophic complication (61–65). Intraoperative SCH can result in a massive degree of hemorrhage and the expulsion of intraocular contents through the surgical wound. If SCH develops in the postoperative period, it is usually not associated with expulsion of intraocular contents. The overall incidence of expulsive SCH has been widely regarded to be about 0.2% (66). This figure appears to be independent of the type of cataract extraction method (intracapsular, extracapsular, or phacoemulsification) (67).

Predisposing Factors

Diabetes, anticoagulation, blood dyscrasias, and hypertension have all been associated with intra- and postoperative hemorrhage. Sclerosis and fragility of choroidal vessels associated with age and arteriosclerosis have frequently been described as predisposing factors. Tachycardia with an intraoperative pulse rate above 90 per minute has also been found to be associated with expulsive hemorrhage. Various ocular conditions, including glaucoma, elevated intraocular pressure, axial myopia, and inflammation, have been linked to SCH. Intraoperative hypotony appears to be a major precipitating factor, resulting in rupture of a long or short posterior ciliary artery. Coughing, straining, nausea and vomiting, and Valsalva-type maneuvers have all been implicated as contributing factors (68–73).

Prevention

Preoperatively patients should avoid the use of aspirin or other nonsteroidal anti-inflammatory agents. Diabetic patients should be under satisfactory blood glucose control.

The use of phenylephrine as a preoperative dilating drop should be limited to avoid provoking systemic hypertension. In patients with hypertension or tachycardia, or both, consideration should be given to performing surgery under local monitored anesthesia, and efforts should be made at the time of operation to lower heart rate and blood pressure. Labetalol, a rapidly acting intravenous agent with alpha- and beta-adrenergic antagonist activity, has been suggested for use in such high-risk patients. Intraocular pressure should be controlled before the eye is opened in order to avoid sudden hypotony. Intravenous carbonic anhydrase inhibitors and hyperosmotic agents should be used if necessary. With the use of small self-sealing incisions, phacoemulsification, and foldable lenses, expulsion of intraocular contents is unlikely to happen.

Postoperatively the patient must be instructed to avoid any eye trauma or pressure on the eye and Valsalva maneuvers should be avoided. Laxatives and antiemetics are therefore recommended in high-risk patients. Postoperative inflammation should be vigorously controlled because it can contribute to serous fluid accumulation in the suprachoroidal space, thereby starting the cascade of events that leads to SCH.

Signs and Symptoms

Early signs of intraoperative SCH include a sudden increase in intraocular pressure with firming of the globe, loss of red reflex, shallowing of the anterior chamber with forward displacement of the iris and lens or lens implant, and vitreous prolapse.

Postoperative SCH more often presents after uncomplicated glaucoma-filtering surgery and less frequently after cataract surgery. Typically, the patient experiences a sudden onset of severe ocular pain accompanied by marked loss of vision and often nausea and vomiting. On slit lamp examination shallowness of the anterior chamber is seen, with loss of the red reflex. Vitreous prolapse into the anterior chamber may be noted. Intraocular pressure may be markedly elevated. On fundoscopic examination dark, elevated, dome-shaped masses may be seen to arise in the peripheral retina. In the presence of opaque media, SCH may be difficult to diagnose. Corneal edema, breakthrough vitreous hemorrhage, or a kissing configuration of choroidal detachments may make adequate visualization of the posterior chamber impossible. Standardized A and B scan echography can be extremely useful in establishing an accurate diagnosis and in differentiating between hemorrhagic choroidal detachment and serous choroidal effusion (74–76).

Management

Intraoperative Suprachoroidal Hemorrhage

Suprachoroidal hemorrhage requires rapid recognition and management. If intraoperative SCH is suspected, immediate tamponading of the open globe is required. This can be accomplished by direct digital pressure or by rapid suturing of the wound. If intraocular contents are noted to be expelling, they should be reposited as quickly as possible. Reformation of the anterior chamber by saline or air injection is recommended. Decreasing systolic blood pressure, intravenous hyperosmotic agents, and sedation for agitated patients may be helpful. Removal of the lid speculum and bridle suture can also decrease direct pressure on the globe, preventing further extrusion of intraocular contents.

Making either a "blind" stab wound through the sclera at or anterior to the equator temporally, or in the quadrant where loss of the red reflex was initially noted, has been suggested in the past as a desperate measure to relieve the pressure of the SCH by draining the blood externally. While this has been reported to be successful, it should only be attempted as a last resort (77).

Postoperative Suprachoroidal Hemorrhage

If the intraocular pressure is elevated, aggressive medical therapy with topical and systemic medication is indicated, as well as medication to control pain. Topical and oral steroids may be necessary to control inflammation.

Indications for Surgical Management

The decision to reoperate on patients with SCH is controversial. Many reports have advocated early surgical intervention in the management of SCH (78,79). In analyzing these reports, we must distinguish expulsive from delayed SCH, because their long-term prognosis may differ. Regardless of the cause of SCH, however, several indications for early surgical drainage have been proposed (78,79). Particular concerns include retinal detachment, central retinal apposition, vitreous incarceration into a surgical wound, breakthrough vitreous hemorrhage, increased intraocular pressure (IOP), retained lens material during cataract surgery, and intractable eye pain.

Surgical Techniques

When reoperation is considered in patients with SCH, the surgical approach can be one of two choices: drainage procedures, to remove the SCH and re-establish normal IOP, or vitreoretinal surgery in combination with a drainage procedure, to remove vitreous hemorrhage or retained lens material, relieve vitreoretinal traction, and re-establish the normal anatomic configuration of the posterior segment. Even when performing only a surgical drainage procedure, the cataract surgeon should consult a vitreoretinal surgeon. Commonly, posterior segment complications such as retinal dialysis and retinal detachment can arise during drainage of SCH (77,80,81).

Drainage Procedures

Mean clot lysis time has been reported to be between 7 and 14 days. Attempts to drain this type of hemorrhage before colt lysis are typically unsuccessful. The surgical principles of all these methods are essentially the same. Drainage sclerotomies are created in the quadrant or quadrants of the involved SCH. The IOP is then maintained by continuously injecting a vitreous substitute into the globe. Usually, an anterior chamber approach is recommended, as most of these eyes are aphakic or pseudophakic.

Several vitreous substitutes have been recommended for re-establishing IOP, all with advantages and disadvantages. Balanced salt solution and viscoelastic solutions have been advocated as vitreous substitutes (82). Drainage sclerotomies are created posteriorly in a radial fashion before engagement of the infusion system. The sclerotomies are then held open with forceps, allowing drainage of the suprachoroidal space as the eye is reformed with solution. A cyclodialysis spatula can also be gently introduced into the suprachoroidal space to facilitate removal of persistent blood clots.

Vitreoretinal Surgical Approaches

As mentioned above, when retinal detachment, vitreoretinal traction, vitreous hemorrhage, or dislocated lens fragments are present in the setting of SCH, vitreoretinal surgery at the time of the SCH drainage procedure is usually advisable (83). Drainage of hemorrhage from the suprachoroidal space is initially required before the creation of any pars plana incisions. The choice of the vitreous substitute used to re-establish IOP during this drainage procedure is usually limited to clear liquid solutions, to enable good visualization during vitrectomy. Balanced salt solution and viscoelastic agents can be used to accomplish drainage of suprachoroidal blood, as outlined in the previous section (78,81,82,84).

Perfluorocarbon liquids (PFLs) have been recommended as a surgical adjunct in cases of complex vitreoretinal pathology (84). These agents are clear liquids with a specific gravity that is higher than that of water. When instilled into the vitreous cavity, these liquids sink to the posterior pole of the eye, forcing all other ocular fluids, both within the vitreous cavity (i.e., aqueous, vitreous, and saline) and within the suprachoroidal space (i.e., hemorrhage), anteriorly. These physiochemical properties make them ideally suited for use in drainage of SCH. Indeed, perfluoroperhydrophenanthrene, a PFL, has been used successfully in the drainage of SCH (84). Unlike the above methods, when using a PFL, the drainage sclerotomies should be placed anteriorly, about 4 mm posterior to the limbus. A 30-gauge needle attached to a syringe that contains PFL is then introduced through the limbus. PFL is then slowly injected, and it immediately moves posteriorly. As it fills the posterior chamber, the PFL flattens the posterior pole while forcing suprachoroidal blood anteriorly, thereby allowing complete removal of this blood through anteriorly placed sclerotomies (Fig. 53-4). An added benefit of PFL in these circumstances is that this liquid tamponades the retina against the inner wall of the eye, while forcing vitreous and vitreous debris anteriorly. This allows for easier removal of vitreous or lens components during vitrectomy, while protecting the retina from iatrogenic damage. After the SCH is drained using PFL, a conventional three-port pars plana vitrectomy configuration can be created. Vitreous strands that cause vitreoretinal traction can be severed. If a rhegmatogenous retinal detachment is present, the retinal break can be treated with retinopexy (photocoagulation or cryopexy). Finally, the PFL can be removed using either a fluid-fluid exchange with infusion fluid or a PFL-air exchange. A scleral buckling procedure can then be performed if residual vitreoretinal traction persists or if support to areas of retinal breaks is required. Internal tamponade with a long-acting intraocular gas or silicone oil may also be required.

AMINOGLYCOSIDE RETINAL TOXICITY

Accidental injection of intracameral gentamicin sulfate has been reported as a complication of cataract surgery that results in acute retinal toxic effects, and devastating ocular consequences. McDonald et al (85) reported five cases of retinal toxic effects secondary to intraocular gentamicin injection, each resulting in a final visual acuity of 20/400 or worse. Early findings include retinal vascular nonperfusion, intraretinal hemorrhages, and retinal edema. Late

findings include optic atrophy, rubeosis iridis, neovascular glaucoma, and retinal pigmentary changes. DeMaro and Oliver (86) recently reported a single patient with presumed retinal toxic effects from gentamicin injection following phacoemulsification and posterior lens implantation who recovered with a visual acuity of 20/70 over 7 months.

Prevention

Strict precautions, including the labeling of all injectable solutions and adherence to systematic procedures for administering medications, should be employed to prevent inadvertent injections.

Signs and Symptoms

Profound loss of vision on the first postoperative day in the absence of pain or other evidence of endophthalmitis should make one suspicious. Fluorescein angiography will show marked capillary and arteriolar nonperfusion in the posterior pole (Fig. 53-5).

Management

In the laboratory, Chu et al (87) performed immediate pars plana vitrectomy and lavage in rabbit eyes after high-dose intracameral injection of gentamicin and demonstrated decreased retinal toxic effects. Daily et al (88) reported a patient who recovered visual acuity of 20/30 following an inadvertent injection of a toxic dose of gentamicin. Immediate anterior chamber washout, pars plana vitrectomy, and lavage of the vitreous cavity were carried out. Every effort should be made to remove as much antibiotic, which may pool in the posterior pole, as possible. Therefore, in addition to immediate lavage of the anterior chamber, immediate vitrectomy should be considered when possible.

CYSTOID MACULAR EDEMA

In 1953, Irvine (89) described a syndrome occurring after cataract extraction that included vitreous and macular changes. In 1966, Gass and Norton (90) first described aphakic eyes with characteristic fluorescein angiographic features, which they called cystoid macular edema. Thus, cystoid macular edema that occurs after cataract surgery has become known as the Irvine-Gass syndrome.

Macular edema is defined as increased fluid within the sensory retina of the macula. Cystoid macular edema is almost always associated with disruption of the blood-retinal barrier, as detected with high sensitivity by leakage on fluorescein angiography. In fact, in clinical practice, the diagnosis of cystoid macular edema is commonly made if fluorescein leakage is seen. However, the amount of leakage

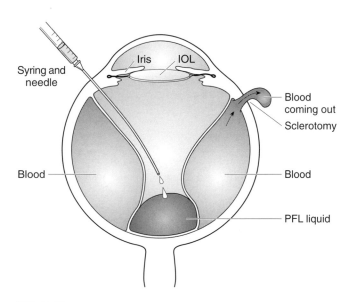

FIGURE 53-4. *Drainage of suprachoroidal hemorrhage with intravitreal instillation of perfluorocarbon fluid to anteriorly displace blood.*

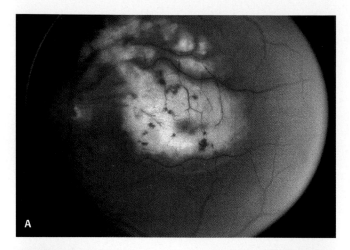

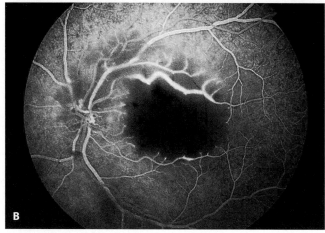

FIGURE 53-5. A. *Fundus photograph of gentamicin-induced retinal toxicity.* B. *Fluorescein angiogram of same eye showing nonperfusion of posterior pole.*

on fluorescein angiography and the degree of macular thickening do not correlate completely (91).

Three categories of cystoid macular edema have been defined. Angiographic cystoid macular edema is present when there is leakage of fluorescein angiography with no symptoms. Clinically significant cystoid macular edema is present if the patient has reduced vision. Chronic cystoid macular edema is present if clinically significant cystoid macular edema persists for 6 months or more (92,93).

Incidence

Several early, large retrospective studies found an incidence of cystoid macular edema of approximately 1% (94–96). Prospective studies using angiography in patients undergoing extracapsular surgery have shown an incidence of approximately 10% to 20% (97,98). The incidence of clinically significant cystoid macular edema must be less than 10%, and that of chronic cystoid macular edema is even lower, about 1% (91,99).

Predisposing Factors

It is generally believed that if cystoid macular edema has developed in one eye, the other is at increased risk for its development after surgery (100,101). Cystoid macular edema occurs more commonly among older patients (101). Most investigators have found a reduced incidence after extracapsular surgery as opposed to intracapsular procedures (102,103). Cystoid macular edema is more common in the presence of vitreous loss, interruption of the anterior hyaloid membrane, adherence of the vitreous to the inner surface of the operative wound, poor positioning of an intraocular lens, or chronic inflammation (102).

Symptoms

Cystoid macular edema is more likely to develop when surgical complications have occurred. Typically, the patient has excellent visual acuity immediately following surgery but then days to months later notes increasing blurring. With clinically significant cystoid macular edema the chief symptom is usually reduced central vision, with visual acuity occasionally as low as 20/200. Patients may also complain of photophobia and floaters (102,104,105).

Signs

Anterior chamber flare and cells may be seen, while the intraocular pressure is usually normal. Sometimes a rupture of the anterior hyaloid face occurs. The frequency of vitreomacular adhesions with partial, posterior vitreous detachment is controversial (90,92,94,106).

The foveal area may appear translucent with a granular surface and loss of the foveal reflex. A deep, soft, yellow-white spot in the fovea may be present. Intraretinal cystoid spaces demarcated by a stellate pattern of refractile lines may be seen. In chronic cases, atrophic or hyperpigmentary changes in the pigment epithelium may develop (107).

Fluorescein Angiography

Early fluorescein angiography shows punctate points of hyperfluorescence in both deep and superficial layers of the retina (Fig. 53-6A) that represent localized areas of breakdown of the blood-retinal barrier in the perifoveal capillaries (105). Later, the dye fills the intraretinal cystoid spaces (Fig. 53-6B), giving the classic pattern of hyperfluorescence resembling the petals of a flower (90,91). There may also be leakage from the optic nerve head (108,109).

Differential Diagnosis

Hypotony retinopathy, various types of optic neuropathy, preexisting age-related macular degeneration, and rhegmatogenous retinal detachment are among the other causes

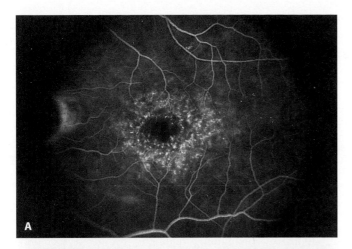

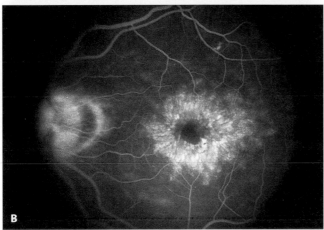

FIGURE 53-6.   A. *Early-phase fluorescein angiogram of aphakic cystoid macular edema showing perimacular capillary dilatation. B. Late-phase fluorescein angiogram of aphakic cystoid macular edema showing leakage of dye from capillaries into cystoid spaces surrounding the macula.*

of reduced vision in the postoperative period (110). The fundus findings of cystoid macular edema in some cases may be confused with a stage 1 macular hole. Sometimes one must differentiate macular edema related to the surgery from that caused by diabetes. Cystoid macular edema related to surgery tends to be located symmetrically around the fovea, whereas areas of diabetic macular edema tend to be located in patches scattered throughout the macula in association with leaking microaneurysms and hard exudate.

Course

Cystoid macular edema usually occurs 4 to 12 weeks postoperatively. Rarely it may occur months or years later (111). Most cases of cystoid macular edema resolve spontaneously within a few weeks to months. However, chronic cystoid macular edema occurs in about 1% of cases (90,99). Optic disk leakage appears to be a risk factor for the development

of chronic cystoid macular edema and for a poorer visual outcome (112).

In the Vitrectomy Aphakic Cystoid Macular Edema Study (92), which was a national, prospective, randomized investigation of 115 eyes with chronic cystoid macular edema and vitreous adherent to the corneoscleral wound, each eye had reduced vision for 6 months to 4 years, and each was followed for at least 6 months. Of the 47 eyes observed without surgery, 27% attained a visual acuity of 20/50 or better if the vision had never fallen to 20/80 or worse. If the vision fell to this level, only 8% of the eyes spontaneously improved to at least 20/50. No systemic vascular factors were identified that correlated significantly with the prognosis. Furthermore, the investigators were not able to show that improvement occurred after a short course of systemic antiprostaglandins, or systemic or topical steroids.

Management

The natural course of the disease is to improve spontaneously in most cases. Therefore, the majority of untreated eyes eventually recover about the same visual level as do treated eyes.

Pharmacologic Approaches

Many studies found that when cyclo-oxygenase inhibitors were given both preoperatively and for varying periods after surgery, they were effective in reducing the incidence of angiographic cystoid macular edema (113,114), but were not effective in improving visual acuity or providing sustained benefit. Most studies of patients in whom treatment was started after the development of cystoid macular edema have shown no benefit.

An exception is the double-masked, randomized, placebo-controlled study of Flach and associates (93,98) that used topical ketorolac tromethamine. They showed a highly significant visual improvement attributable to the drug. Large, collaborative trials may be necessary to enroll enough patients to demonstrate conclusively a meaningful therapeutic benefit of cyclo-oxygenase inhibitors.

Miyake and coworkers (115) showed benefit from topical indomethacin in patients who underwent surgery for retinal detachment. Cox and associates (116) used acetazolamide to treat cystoid macular edema associated with several conditions, and patients who had undergone cataract surgery tended to respond.

Surgical Approaches

Vitreous adhesions to the cataract incision are associated with cystoid macular edema, regardless of the mechanism. Investigators in the Vitrectomy Aphakic Cystoid Macular Edema Study (92) found a statistically significant improvement in visual acuity in the eyes that underwent surgery. They recommended 1) delaying intervention until the visual acuity was stable for 2 or 3 months, 2) considering vitrectomy before the visual acuity was 20/80 or less, 3) performing vitrectomy before the visual acuity was 20/80 or less for 2 years, and 4) performing vitrectomy via the pars plana approach or via a combination of pars plana and limbal approaches (Fig. 53-7).

The neodymium (Nd):YAG laser has also been used to cut the vitreous strands to the wound in patients with cystoid macular edema, with encouraging visual results (117,118).

RETINAL COMPLICATIONS OF NEODYMIUM:YAG LASER POSTERIOR CAPSULOTOMIES

Several studies of Nd:YAG laser posterior capsulotomies document the incidence of the complications of cystoid macular edema and retinal detachment after this procedure (119–121). The incidence of cystoid macular edema was noted to be between 0.55% and 4.9% and that of retinal detachments to be between 0.17% and 3.6% (122–126).

Mechanism of Complications

The precise mechanisms for the development of these retinal complications after Nd:YAG capsulotomy remain unclear. Retention of the posterior capsule has been shown to decrease the incidence of cystoid macular edema and retinal detachment (102,127). Investigators generally believe that these complications result from the capsulotomy opening itself and not from factors intrinsically related to the Nd:YAG laser technique (104,125,128).

Risk Factors

Stark and associates (104) concluded that the longer the interval between cataract surgery and capsulotomy, the lower

the risk of cystoid macular edema. In another study (129) with a mean time of 21.9 months from surgery to laser, a lower incidence rate for cystoid macular edema was not found, compared to previous reports with shorter surgery to laser intervals. The same study suggests that patients in whom cystoid macular edema develops may have had a greater inflammatory reaction to their cataract operation than do most cataract patients.

Potential risk factors for the development of a retinal detachment were also studied. Koch and associates (130) reported myopia to be a risk factor for postcapsulotomy retinal detachment. In another study Steinert and associates (129) reported three of eight patients in whom a retinal detachment developed more than one year after capsulotomy. This finding highlights the need for long-term surveillance of patients after this procedure and suggests that the laser energy does not directly cause the detachment.

Management

The Nd:YAG laser is a practical method for improving vision that has been decreased by an opacified posterior capsule. Opening of the posterior capsule does, however, carry a low risk of serious complications. Clinicians should be alert to the development of complications. Cystoid macular edema, or retinal detachment, should be treated accordingly.

RETINAL DETACHMENT AFTER CATARACT EXTRACTION

An increased incidence of retinal detachment has long been known to be associated with cataract extraction. Intracapsular cataract extraction has the highest incidence, variously reported to be around 2% to 4% (127,131). With the reintroduction of extracapsular techniques, the incidence has dropped to 1% to 2% (121,132,133). Most detachments occur within the first 4 to 6 months after cataract extraction, but can develop up to several years postoperatively.

Predisposing Factors

Ocular factors, such as high myopia with lattice retinal degeneration, subluxated lenses, Sticker's syndrome, and other developmental and hereditary abnormalities as well as a history of trauma, are risk factors for retinal detachment after cataract surgery (119,134). Operative complications, including vitreous loss, loss of lens fragments, and suprachoroidal hemorrhage, also increase the risk. Postoperative endophthalmitis, IOL dislocation, and trauma are all associated with an increased incidence of retinal detachment.

Prevention

Gentle, atraumatic, extracapsular cataract extraction with or without phacoemulsification to help reduce intraoperative

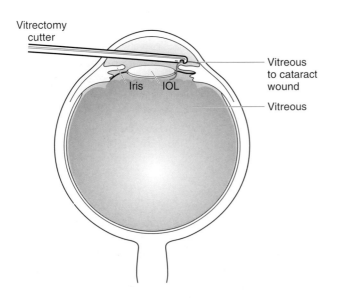

FIGURE 53-7. *Removal of vitreous bands to old cataract wound with vitrectomy cutter via a limbal approach.*

complications and vitreous loss is important. Preoperative prophylactic cryo or laser treatment to areas of lattice degeneration has been shown to reduce the incidence of postoperative detachment in eyes with these findings. Aggressive treatment of postoperative inflammation is also important.

Signs and Symptoms

All patients who undergo cataract extraction should be warned about the possible complication and the symptoms of flashes and floaters and peripheral field loss. They should be instructed to check each eye individually daily. Detachments may be asymptomatic early, and the cataract surgeon should check the peripheral retina with the indirect ophthalmoscope at each postoperative visit.

Management

Retinal breaks in aphakic and pseudophakic eyes tend to be small, peripheral, at or anterior to the vitreous base, and difficult to find. Unless considerable vitreous loss, proliferation, or traction is present, a scleral buckling technique with an encircling band is generally the procedure of choice. Vitrectomy may be necessary where PVR is extensive. Pneumatic retinopexy has a reduced success rate in the aphakic or pseudophakic eye and is not generally recommended, especially when an open posterior capsule is present (135,136).

In the scleral buckling technique, all definite and suspicious breaks including small tented-up areas and meridional complexes are marked and treated with cryoretinopexy. If the breaks are small and located the same distance posterior to the ora serrata, a small-width grooved section of silicone can be used along with a narrow encircling band, or a wider band can be utilized alone as long as it is placed over or slightly posterior to the breaks. Perforation for drainage of subretinal fluid is often necessary, but if perforation is carried out at or anterior to the equator, the risk of incarceration is greater because of the tendency of these detachments to flatten anteriorly. Consideration should be given to perforating posteriorly outside of the bed of the buckle (Fig. 53-8). Excessive hypotony should be avoided in these eyes because of a tendency toward development of choroidal detachment or suprachoroidal hemorrhage. Drainage should be intermittent with snugging up of the scleral sutures or encircling band between periods of drainage to keep the eye relatively firm. Often these eyes have considerable subretinal fluid and after drainage the buckle may have to be very high in order to maintain intraocular pressure. Consideration should then be given to intraocular saline or air injection with loosening of the encircling tape and reduction in buckle height. If intraocular air or gas is used or a pneumatic retinopexy is performed, every effort should be made to keep the patient in the prone or head-forward position to prevent the bubble from entering the anterior chamber and resulting in pupil block and elevated intraocular pressure.

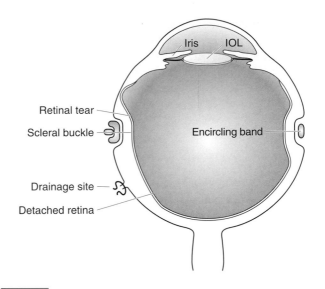

FIGURE 53-8. *Scleral buckling of pseudophakic retinal detachment with drainage of subretinal fluid posterior to the bed of the buckle via sclerotomy.*

ENDOPHTHALMITIS FOLLOWING CATARACT EXTRACTION

Infectious endophthalmitis after cataract surgery is a rare but devastating complication. The incidence of endophthalmitis following cataract surgery was evaluated by Allen and Mangiaracine (137) and was found to be 0.086%. Koul and coworkers (138) reported an incidence that ranged from 0.33% (clinically) down to 0.06% (culture positive) including cataract surgery and other procedures. The prognosis has improved in recent years with prompt diagnosis, intravitreal antibiotic therapy, and vitreous surgery. However, only 39% to 73% of affected eyes have visual acuity outcomes of 20/400 or better (139–143).

Predisposing Factors

Preoperative blepharitis and conjunctivitis are obvious sources of infection, but inadequate lid and conjunctival preparation, contamination by operating room personnel, contaminated instruments or solutions, air-borne contaminants, or a contaminated IOL are all possible sources of infection (144).

Prevention and Prophylaxis

Meticulous attention to treatment of blepharitis preoperatively as well as presurgical prep and intraoperative aseptic technique are required to keep the incidence at an acceptable level. The spread of infection from the anterior chamber to the vitreous appears to be restricted if the posterior capsule is intact (145). One third of postoperative endophthalmitis cases reportedly follow vitreous loss, unplanned extracapsular cataract extraction, or a problem with cataract wound closure (141).

The routine use of subconjunctival antibiotics at the end of surgery does not completely prevent postoperative endophthalmitis. In one series of 62 culture-positive cases, 90% of a subgroup of patients who received subconjunctival antibiotics at the end of cataract surgery were infected with an organism that was sensitive to the antibiotic administered (141).

Symptoms and Signs

Pain is the earliest symptom of endophthalmitis. With early improved vision after cataract surgery, decreased vision as the initial symptom of endophthalmitis may also be reported by the patient (146).

Signs of endophthalmitis include conjunctival hyperemia, chemosis, cells and flare in the anterior chamber, hypopyon, vitritis, scattered retinal hemorrhages, and, in extreme cases, corneal opacification (147). The postoperative use of topical steroid may minimize hyperemia as well as delay hypopyon formation (148,149).

Diagnosis

Typically, bacterial endophthalmitis has its onset within 24 to 48 hours of surgery and progresses rapidly (150,151). However, infection caused by less virulent organisms can delay clinical presentation to 4 days or longer. Infection by indolent organisms such as *Propionibacterium* may be delayed for several months or years before clinical signs are apparent (148,149).

The diagnosis of bacterial endophthalmitis must be suspected on the basis of inflammation that is out of proportion of the clinical setting. In certain cases, ultrasound examination may be helpful in diagnosis. Accurate diagnosis ultimately rests with the demonstration of infectious organisms within the eye by appropriate cultures and stains.

Diagnostic Cultures

It is important to obtain specimens for bacterial culture in order to identify causative organisms and to direct therapy. Approximately 64% of eyes with a clinical diagnosis of infectious endophthalmitis will have a positive culture result (138,141,152).

Several studies have confirmed the necessity of vitreous culture as well as anterior chamber culture in endophthalmitis, as the anterior chamber culture result is negative in the face of a positive vitreous culture result in a substantial number of cases. On the other hand, a negative vitreous culture result may be accompanied by a positive anterior chamber culture (137,141,153). The value of a conjunctival specimen culture is quite limited.

Specimens should be cultured on blood agar at 25°C and at 37°C, on thioglycolate, and on Sabouraud's agar, and on an anaerobic medium such as cooked meat medium. In cases of suspected fungal endophthalmitis, evaluation with Calcofluor white may allow rapid identification of fungal infection. Smears should be examined by microscopy with Gram's and Giemsa's stains.

Approximately 56% to 90% of isolates in postoperative patients are gram positive, 7% to 29% are gram negative, and 3% to 13% are fungal (137,141,154). An incidence of mixed gram-positive infections of as high as 33% has been reported (140). Of the gram-positive isolates, 30% to 50% are *Staphylococcus epidermidis*, 10% to 30% are *Staphylococcus aureus*, and 15% to 30% are *Streptococcus* species. *Staphylococcus epidermidis* is the predominant organism encountered in postoperative cases of endophthalmitis (155).

Management of Early Acute-Onset Endophthalmitis

Medical

Intravitreal antibiotic therapy has improved the possibility of saving vision in endophthalmitis (156,157). Intravitreal agents are selected in advance of culture results, and coverage with a combination of drugs directed against gram-positive and gram-negative organisms is required. Review of the most common organisms encountered after cataract extraction indicates that coverage for staphylococci is most critical. Intravitreal cephalosporin or methicillin has been widely used with success (158). With the increasing development of methicillin-resistant staphylococci, vancomycin has been the intravitreal drug of choice for gram-positive coverage. In several studies, 100% of the gram-positive organisms tested were sensitive to vancomycin (141,142,155,159–161).

Regarding gram-negative coverage, the aminoglycoside antibiotics continue to be effective against the majority of organisms (162). The retinal toxicity of these drugs has been the subject of considerable study (see Aminoglycoside Retinal Toxicity) (163–169). Although the intravitreal injection of 100 μg gentamicin is widely employed for gram-negative coverage, the growing occurrence of gentamicin-resistant strains in ocular infections (160,170,171) suggests that amikacin should be considered the aminoglycoside of choice for intravitreal drug therapy (172).

The half-life of gentamicin injected into the vitreous has been studied and was found to be 32 hours in control phakic rabbit eyes compared with 12 hours aphakic eyes (173). Extrapolations of these data suggested that therapeutic vitreous levels are maintained for 24 to 48 hours after intravitreal injection of 100 μg gentamicin in humans. In a clinical series, in all cases, the specimen taken just before the second intravitreal injection was culture negative, indicating the efficacy of a single intravitreal injection in most instances of endophthalmitis therapy. Also, 2 of 12 patients who received repeat injections of gentamicin displayed retinal atrophy and pigment clumping suggestive of drug toxicity (174). Because of the possibility of aminoglycoside toxicity, the use of ceftazidine, 2.0 mg, for gram-negative coverage should be considered (175).

Antibiotics are usually administered by topical, subconjunctival, and systemic routes for a period of 5 to 10 days. Topical and subconjunctival injection of gentamicin produces antibacterial levels in the aqueous but not in the vitreous (174,176,177). Intravenous or intramuscular injection does not produce therapeutic levels in the aqueous or the vitreous (174,177).

Intravitreal steroid therapy is recommended in the treatment of endophthalmitis, although the exact indications and dosages require further study (143,163). Experimental study confirmed the beneficial effects of an intravitreal injection of 400 μg dexamethasone in experimental endophthalmitis in the rabbit; in addition, no retinal toxicity was observed with this dose, as evaluated by light microscopy and electroretinography (178).

Vitrectomy

Vitrectomy for endophthalmitis is associated with advantages and disadvantages. The advantages would include obtaining an adequate vitreous sample for culture with the vitrectomy instrument, clearing of the ocular media, removal of potentially toxic bacterial products and debris, and permitting ease of intravitreal drug therapy and drug circulation throughout the eye. Potential disadvantages include the iatrogenic creation of retinal holes or detachments or choroidal hemorrhage (138).

Puliafito and colleagues (140) compared visual results in endophthalmitis between cases in which vitrectomy was performed within the first 24 hours and those with later vitrectomy. Improved visual results were observed with early vitrectomy. Diamond (143) reported 20/400 or better visual acuity in 10 of 12 culture-positive cases treated with intravitreal antibiotics and steroids only, compared with 9 of 14 cases also treated with vitrectomy. However, he clearly stated that vitrectomy was offered in those cases that had a delay in diagnosis, nonsurgical trauma, vitreous opacities on ultrasound, or failure to respond to intravitreal drug therapy alone after 3 hours; these selection criteria inevitably worsen the prognosis for patients who receive vitrectomy.

The accumulated data suggest that vitrectomy is beneficial in the restoration of media clarity. Coupled with the known advantages of obtaining definitive culture, vitrectomy therapy continues to be a mainstay of treatment.

Data have recently become available from the Endophthalmitis Vitrectomy Study (EVS) (179). This randomized controlled trial of 420 patients with clinical evidence of bacterial endophthalmitis within 6 weeks of cataract or secondary lens implantation surgery showed that amikacin and ceftazidime given intravenously made no difference in final outcome. In addition, in eyes with hand motion or better vision at presentation, no difference was seen in final outcome between immediate vitrectomy with intravitreal antibiotics or immediate vitreous tap with intravitreal antibiotics. However, in eyes with vision of light perception only at presentation, better visual results were obtained with immediate vitrectomy and intravitreal antibiotics than with vitreous tap and intravitreal antibiotics.

Delayed Endophthalmitis

Postoperative endophthalmitis caused by indolent organisms such as *Propionibacterium acnes* has recently been described (148,149). These patients present with a chronic, recurring, steroid-responsive uveitis that occurs months or even years after cataract extraction.

Symptoms and Signs

Symptoms of delayed endophthalmitis include a decrease in vision and pain. Signs include conjunctival hyperemia, keratic precipitates, a variable anterior chamber reaction, and vitritis. These eyes typically display a white plaque within the equator of the remaining lens capsule. The patient is often initially diagnosed with idiopathic uveitis and treated with topical steroids with subsequent improvement. However, with several episodes, the possibility of chronic endophthalmitis should be considered.

Diagnosis

The diagnosis is established by culture of aqueous specimens. Anaerobic culture is most important, and cultures must be maintained for at least 14 days in order to maximize the recovery of these organisms. The most common cause of this syndrome is *P. acnes*, but *S. epidermidis*, *Propionibacterium granulosum*, *Achromobacter*, *Corynebacterium*, and fungi have also been reported.

Therapy

The optimal therapy for *P. acnes* endophthalmitis is unknown; intravitreal injection of vancomycin has been reported, but recurrences are common with this therapy. Current recommendations for initial therapy include a vitrectomy with a posterior capsulectomy and intravitreal injection of vancomycin. For recurrent cases removal of the IOL, residual lens capsule, and equatorial material, with repeat injection of intravitreal vancomycin, is recommended (148,180).

Fungal Endophthalmitis

Postoperative endophthalmitis is infrequently caused by fungi, with *Candida* species predominating in reported cases (141,181). A well-documented epidemic of *Candida parapsilosis* endophthalmitis caused by contaminated intraocular irrigating solution has been described (181).

Diagnosis

The use of Cellufluor or Calcofluor white techniques for the identification of fungal elements in a smear of fresh vitreous is a significant advance in the rapid diagnosis of fungal endophthalmitis (182).

Treatment

Intravitreal therapy with amphotericin B as well as vitrectomy is advocated. Some experts now advocate the use of systemic ketoconazole as an alternative to amphotericin B (183). *Candida* endophthalmitis does not require routine IOL removal for successful sterilization, although recurrences are possible (181).

RETINAL COMPLICATIONS OF CATARACT EXTRACTION IN DIABETICS

Cataract is more common in diabetic patients than in the general population and may require surgical intervention both to improve the vision and to better visualize the fundus for follow-up and treatment of the retinopathy. Cataract surgery in diabetics may be complicated by progression of the retinopathy, anterior segment neovascularization, and postoperative endophthalmitis. There is also a higher incidence of cystoid macular edema (184–187).

Predisposing Factors

Progression of Diabetic Retinopathy and Development of Cystoid Macular Edema

Alpar (188) prospectively studied the risk of progression of retinopathy in patients who underwent either extracapsular or intracapsular surgery. He found the lowest incidence of progression of retinopathy in the group undergoing extracapsular extraction but did not differentiate on the basis of preoperative retinopathy, which appears from other studies to be an important factor.

Jaffe and Burton (189) described eight patients who progressed from background diabetic retinopathy to severe exudative maculopathy after extracapsular cataract extraction, with diffuse retinal thickening and fluorescein leakage.

Cheng and Franklin (186) studied 28 eyes in 21 patients with diabetes who did not have diabetic retinopathy preoperatively. Most patients had extracapsular surgery with posterior chamber lens implantation. Although two patients acquired background diabetic retinopathy postoperatively, the corrected visual acuities were 20/40 or better in 88% of the patients 12 months after operation. On the other hand, in 18 eyes of 15 patients with retinopathy preoperatively the outcome was poorer, with one third of the patients having postoperative visual acuities of less than 20/200. Cystoid macular edema developed in 8 of 18 eyes (186).

Rubeosis Iridis and Neovascular Glaucoma

Aiello et al (187) retrospectively studied 154 diabetic patients who had undergone routine intracapsular cataract extraction unilaterally. Neither eye received laser photocoagulation before surgery or during the first year after operation. All of the patients, regardless of the degree of preoperative retinopathy, had a statistically significantly increased risk of rubeosis iridis and neovascular glaucoma in the operative eye (8 vs. 0%). In patients with active proliferative diabetic retinopathy preoperatively, the risk was even higher (40 vs. 0%).

Prevention

It is speculated that an intact lens capsule or anterior hyaloid face acting as a semipermeable barrier between the anterior and the posterior chambers can reduce the risk of postoperative complications, both neovascular and inflammatory.

Management

Because of the increased risks associated with cataract surgery in patients with diabetic retinopathy, special consideration should be made both preoperatively and postoperatively (190).

Preoperatively

When a cataract is developing in a diabetic patient, effort should be made to perform focal or scatter photocoagulation as indicated before the density of the cataract obscures the view. Diabetic patients scheduled to undergo cataract surgery should be examined carefully preoperatively for the presence of any treatable lesions, which should be treated as indicated before surgery.

Operatively

All surgical effort should be made toward keeping the posterior capsule intact. Wounds should be sutured well since wound healing is slower in diabetics. This also allows laser photocoagulation with a contact lens postoperatively, if this proves to be necessary.

Postoperatively

Because of the increased rate of cystoid macular edema postoperatively in diabetic patients, it may be worth considering topical or oral nonsteroidal anti-inflammatory agents as well as topical steroids. In addition, the use of mydriatics, especially atropine, should be considered in order to reduce postoperative inflammation, prevent posterior synechiae, and maintain an adequate pupillary size should retinal treatment be required. Close follow-up postoperatively is essential, with examination of the iris for neovascularization and a dilated examination of the fundus for macular edema or progression of retinopathy. Any progression of the retinopathy should be handled accordingly. Surgeons should recall that diabetics have a higher incidence of endophthalmitis than nondiabetics and appear to have a poorer visual outcome (184).

LIGHT-INDUCED RETINOPATHY FROM THE OPERATING MICROSCOPE

Tso (191) demonstrated a photic maculopathy in rhesus monkeys after exposure to the light of an indirect ophthalmoscope for 1 hour. In 1983, McDonald and Irvine (192) described a light-induced macular lesion in a group of patients who had undergone recent cataract extraction and intraocular lens placement. Robertson and Feldman, in 1986 (193), demonstrated that a 60-minute exposure to light from an operating microscope can cause a retinal lesion in humans. In a review of 135 consecutive patients who had undergone cataract extraction, retinal changes suggestive of photic retinopathy were found in 10 patients (7.4%) (194).

Photic retinopathy by the operating microscope is believed to be caused by photochemical damage from the focusing of high-intensity coaxial light on the retina (192,195,196). Much of the damage may be due to short-wavelength blue light and ultraviolet (UV) light (197,198).

Predisposing Factors

The most significant risk factor in the development of photic retinopathy from the operating microscope is a prolonged operating time. Khwarg and associates (194) found that the mean operating time in affected patients was significantly higher at 124 minutes, compared with 73 minutes in unaffected patients. No significant difference in the rate of retinopathy in patients with and without intraocular lenses has been shown. Lack of UV filters in intraocular lenses and operating room microscopes is a contributing factor (199,200).

Studies in pseudophakic rhesus monkeys demonstrate that the threshold exposure with the high-intensity setting of the coaxial illumination of the Zeiss OpMi-6 30-W operating microscope for an ophthalmoscopically visible lesion is between 4.0 and 7.5 minutes. The intensity of the light beam is also an important factor. Berler and Peyser (196) found that increased intensity of the operating microscope is associated with decreased postoperative visual acuity in patients who have undergone cataract surgery.

Symptoms and Signs

In most instances, patients are asymptomatic, and a lesion is noted postoperatively on examination. Patients may note decreased vision or paracentral scotoma, usually on the first or second postoperative day. Vision generally returns to normal after several months. In some cases, a paracentral scotoma may persist.

The retinal lesion consists of an oval area of light-yellow to white, deep retinal lesion with a size that varies from 0.8 to 2.5 disk diameters. One study found that the lesions are usually located inferior to the fovea (194) and another study noted a tendency for lesions to be in the temporal macula (201). Mottled pigmentation of the lesion occurs over the following few weeks. In the late stages, the lesion changes to a sharply outlined area of retinal pigment epithelial atrophy (Fig. 53-9A).

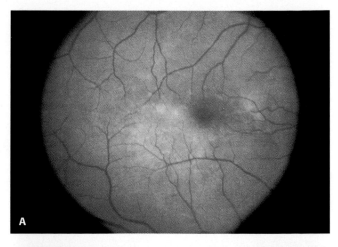

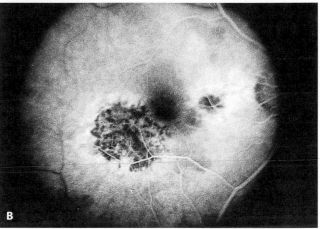

FIGURE 53-9. A. *Fundus photograph of light-induced chorioretinal lesions nasal and inferotemporal to the macula following vitrectomy. B. Fluorescein angiogram of same lesion showing retinal pigment epithelial changes.*

Fluorescein angiography demonstrates intense staining of the acute lesion. Irregular window defects corresponding to the retinal pigment epithelial changes are noted in the presence of late-stage lesions. Leakage is not a characteristic finding (Fig. 53-9B).

Prevention

It is recommended that filtration to cut off wavelengths less than 450 nm be incorporated into the operating microscope illumination system (201). The avoidance of intense illumination by reducing the brightness as much as possible is recommended (202–204). Oblique illumination during wound closure may help to place the intense image of the beam in the retinal periphery (199). Pupil constriction and the use of corneal covers and eclipse filters to limit retinal illumination during prolonged operation are also recommended.

REFERENCES

1. Sullivan KL, Brown GC, Forman AR, et al. Retrobulbar anesthesia and retinal vascular obstruction. *Ophthalmology* 1983;90:373–377.
2. Kraushar MF, Seelenfreund MH, Freilich DB. Central retinal artery closure during orbital hemorrhage from retrobulbar injection *Trans Am Acad Ophthalmol Otolaryngol* 1974;78:65–70.
3. Feibel RM. Current concepts in retrobulbar anesthesia. *Surv Ophthalmol* 1985;30:102–110.
4. Erie JC. Acquired Brown's syndrome after peribulbar anesthesia. *Am J Ophthalmol* 1990;109:349–350.
5. Friedberg HL, Kline OR. Contralateral amaurosis after retrobulbar injection. *Am J Ophthalmol* 1986;101:688–690.
6. Goldsmith MO. Occlusion of the central retinal artery following retrobulbar hemorrhage. *Ophthalmologica* 1967;153:191–196.
7. Hersch M, Baer G, Dieckert JP, et al. Optic nerve enlargement and central retinal artery occlusion secondary to retrobulbar anesthesia. *Ann Ophthalmol* 1989;21:195–197.
8. Lemange JM, Michiels X, van Causenbroeck S, Snyers B. Purtscher-like retinopathy after retrobulbar anesthesia. *Ophthalmology* 1990;97:859–861.
9. Beltranena HP, Vega MJ, Garcia JJ, Blankenship G. Complications of retrobulbar Marcaine injection. *J Clin Neurol Ophthalmol* 1982;2:159–161.
10. Pautler SE, Grizzard WS, Thompson LN, Wing GL. Blindness from retrobulbar injection into the optic nerve. *Ophthalmic Surg* 1989;17:334–337.
11. Lincoff HE, Zweifach P, Brodie S, et al. Intraocular injection of lidocaine. *Ophthalmology* 1985;92:61–64.
12. Ramsay RC, Knobloch WH. Ocular perforation following retrobulbar anesthesia for retinal detachment surgery. *Am J Ophthalmol* 1978;86:61–64.
13. Cibis PA. General discussion. In: Schepens CL, Regan CDJ, eds. Controversial aspects of retinal detachment. Boston: Little, Brown, 1965:222–223.
14. Grizzard WS, Kirk NM, Pavan PR, et al. Perforating ocular injuries caused by anesthesia personnel. *Ophthalmology* 1991;98:1011–1016.
15. Morgan CM, Schatz H, Vine AK, et al. Ocular complications associated with retrobulbar injections. *Ophthalmology* 1988;95:660–665.
16. Hay A, Flynn HW, Hoffman JI, Rivera AH. Needle penetration of the globe during retrobulbar and peribulbar injections. *Ophthalmology* 1991;98:1017–1024.
17. Unsold R, Stanley JA, deGroot J. The CT topography of retrobulbar anesthesia: anatomic-clinical correlation of complications and suggestion of a modified technique. *Graefes Arch Clin Exp Ophthalmol* 1988;217:125–136.
18. Schneider ME, Milstein DE, Oyakawa RT. Ocular perforation from a retrobulbar injection. *Am J Ophthalmol* 1988;106:35–40.
19. Bloomberg LB. Administration of periocular anesthesia. *J Cataract Refract Surg* 1980;12:677–679.
20. Gills JP, Loyd TL. Extracapsular cataract extraction with intraocular lens insertion. *J Am Intraocular Implant Soc* 1979;5:9–12.
21. Davis DB, Mandel MR. Posterior peribulbar anesthesia: an alternative to retrobulbar anesthesia. *Geriatr Ophthalmol* 1987;3:27–28.
22. Weiss JL, Deichman CB. A comparison of retrobulbar and periocular anesthesia for cataract surgery. *Arch Ophthalmol* 1989;107:96–98.
23. Davis DB, Mandel MR. Periocular anesthesia: a review of technique and complications. *Ophthalmol Clin North Am* 1990;3:101–110.
24. Mein CE, Woodcock MG. Local anesthesia for vitreoretinal surgery. *Retina* 1990;10:47–49.
25. Kimble JA, Morris RE, Witherspoon CD, Feist RM. Globe perforation from peribulbar injection. *Arch Ophthalmol* 1987;105:749.
26. Rinkoff JS, Doft BH, Lobes LA. Management of ocular penetration from injection of local anesthesia preceding cataract surgery. *Arch Ophthalmol* 1991;109:1421–1425.
27. de Juan EJ, Hiskingbotham D. Flexible iris retractor. *Am J Ophthalmol* 1991;111:776–777.
28. Malinowski SM, Mieler WF, et al. Combined pars plana vitrectomy-lensectomy and open loop anterior chamber lens implantation. *Ophthalmology* 1995;102:211–215.
29. Emery JM, Wilhelmus KA, Rosenberg S. Complications of phacoemulsification. *Ophthalmology* 1978;85:45–51.
30. Emery JM, McIntyre DJ. Extracapsular cataract surgery. St. Louis: Mosby, 1983.
31. Fung WE. Phacoemulsification. *Ophthalmology* 1978;1978:45–51.
32. Hurite FG. The contraindications to phacoemulsification and summary of personal experience. *Trans Am Acad Ophthalmol Otolaryngol* 1974;78:OP14–17.
33. Kelman CD. Symposium: phacoemulsification. Summary of personal experience. *Trans Am Acad Ophthalmol Otolaryngol* 1974;78:OP35–38.
34. Chern S, Yung C. Dislocation of the nucleus during phacoemulsification. *Ophthalmic Surg* 1995;26:114–116.
35. Hutton WL, Snyder WB, Vaiser A. Management of surgically dislocated intravitreal lens fragments by pars plana vitrectomy. *Ophthalmology* 1978;85:176–189.
36. Michels RG, Shacklett DE. Vitrectomy technique for removal of retained lens material. *Arch Ophthalmol* 1977;95:1767–1773.
37. Kim JE, Flynn HWJ, Rubsamen PE, et al. Endophthalmitis in patients with retained lens fragments after phacoemulsification. *Ophthalmology* 1996;103:575–578.
38. Daily M. How to deal with a dropped nucleus. *Rev Ophthalmol* 1996;3:100–102.
39. Epstein DL. Diagnosis and management of lens-induced glaucoma. *Ophthalmology* 1982;89:227–230.
40. Bourne MJ, Tasman W, Regillo C, et al. Outcomes of vitrectomy for retained lens fragments. *Ophthalmology* 1996;103:971–976.
41. Kapusta MA, Chen JC, Lam W-C. Outcomes of dropped nucleus during phacoemulsification. *Ophthalmology* 1996;103:1184–1187.
42. Gillialand GD, Hutton WF, Fuller DG. Retained intravitreal lens fragments after cataract surgery. *Ophthalmology* 1992;99:1263–1269.
43. Blodi BA, Flynn HW, Blodi CF, et al. Retained nuclei after cataract surgery. *Ophthalmology* 1992;99:41–44.
44. Peyman GA, Raichand M, Goldberg MF, Rittaca D. Management of subluxated and dislocated lenses with the vitreophage. *Br J Ophthalmol* 1979;63:771–778.
45. Shapiro MJ, Resnick KI, Kim SH, et al. Management of the dislocated lens with a perfluorocarbon liquid. *Am J Ophthalmol* 1991;112:401–405.
46. Lambrou FHJ, Steward MW. Management of dislocated lens fragments after cataract surgery. *Ophthalmology* 1992;99:1260–1262.
47. Fastenberg DM, Schwartz PL, Shakin JL, et al. Management of dislocated nuclear fragments after phacoemulsification. *Am J Ophthalmol* 1991;112:535–539.
48. Smith SG, Lindstrom RL. Malpositioned posterior chamber lenses. Etiology, prevention, and management. *J Am Intraocul Implant Soc* 1985;2:584.
49. Hamilton RS. Prevention and management of the sunset syndrome. *Trans Am Ophthalmol Soc* 1983;81:276–279.
50. Flynn HW Jr. Pars plana vitrectomy in the management of subluxed and posteriorly dislocated intraocular lenses. *Graefes Arch Clin Exp Ophthalmol* 1987;225:169–172.
51. Eifrig DE. Two principles for repositioning intraocular lenses. *Ophthalmic Surg* 1986;17:486–489.
52. Sternberg P Jr, Mihels RG. Treatment of dislocated posterior chamber intraocular lenses. *Arch Ophthalmol* 1986;104:1391–1393.
53. Anland R, Bowman RW. Simplified technique for suturing dislocated posterior chamber intraocular lenses to the ulray sulcus. *Arch Ophthalmol* 1990;108:1205–1206. Letter.
54. Shapiro A, Leen MM. External transcleral posterior chamber lens fixation. *Arch Ophthalmol* 1991;109:1759–1760.
55. Panton RW, Sulewski ME, Parker TS, et al. Surgical management of subluxed posterior-chamber intraocular lenses. *Arch Ophthalmol* 1993;111:919–926.
56. Maquire AM, Blumenkranz MS, Ward TG, et al. Scleral loop fixation for posteriorly dislocated intraocular lenses. *Arch Ophthalmol* 1991;109:1754–1758.
57. Smiddy WE, Flynn HW Jr. Needle assisted scleral fixation suture technique for relocated posterior dislocated intraocular lenses. *Arch Ophthalmol* 1993;111:161–162.
58. Lewis H, Sanchez G. The use of perfluorocarbon liquids in the repositioning of posteriorly dislocated intraocular lenses. *Ophthalmology* 1993;100:1055–1059.
59. Campo RV, Chung KD, Oyakawa RT. Pars plana vitrectomy in the management of dislocated posterior chamber lenses. *Am J Ophthalmol* 1989;108:529–534.
60. Chan CK. An improved technique for management of dislocated posterior chamber implants. *Ophthalmology* 1992;99:51–57.
61. Brubaker RF, Pederson JE. Ciliochoroidal detachment. *Surv Ophthalmol* 1983;27:281–289.
62. Maumenee AE, Schwartz MF. Acute intraoperative choroidal effusion. *Am J Ophthalmol* 1985;100;147–154.
63. Manschot WA. The pathology of expulsive hemorrhage. *Am J Ophthalmol* 1955;19:344–349.
64. Wolter JR. Expulsive hemorrhage: a study of histopathological details. *Graefes Arch Clin Exp Ophthalmol* 1982;219:155–158.
65. Wolter JR, Garafinkel RA. Ciliochoroidal effusion as precursor of suprachoroidal hemorrhage: a pathologic study. *Ophthalmic Surg* 1988;19:344–349.
66. Taylor DM. Expulsive hemorrhage. *Am J Ophthalmol* 1978;78:961–966.

67. Speaker MG, Guerriero PN, Met JA, et al. A case control study of risk factors for intraoperative suprachoroidal expulsive hemorrhage. *Ophthalmology* 1991;98:202–209.

68. Davison JA. Acute intra-operative suprachoroidal hemorrhage in extracapsular cataract surgery. *J Cataract Refract Surg* 1986;12:606–622.

69. Hoffman P, Pollack A, Oliver M. Limited choroidal hemorrhage associated with intracapsular cataract extraction. *Arch Ophthalmol* 1984;102:1761–1765.

70. Purcell JJ. Expulsive hemorrhage in penetrating keratoplasty. *Ophthalmology* 1982;89:41–43.

71. Straatsma BR, Khwarg SG, Rajcich GM, et al. Cataract surgery after expulsive choroidal hemorrhage in the fellow eye. *Ophthalmic Surg* 1986;17:400–403.

72. Cantor LB, Katz KJ, Spaeth GL. Complications of surgery in glaucoma: suprachoroidal expulsive hemorrhage in glaucoma patients undergoing intraocular surgery. *Ophthalmology* 1985;92:1266–1270.

73. Ruderman JM, Harbin T Jr, Campbell DG. Postoperative suprachoroidal hemorrhage following filtration procedures. *Arch Ophthalmol* 1986;104:201–205.

74. Chu TG, Cano MR, Green RL, et al. Massive suprachoroidal hemorrhage with central retinal apposition—a clinical and echographic study. *Arch Ophthalmol* 1991;109:1575–1581.

75. Campbell JK. Expulsive choroidal hemorrhage and effusion—a reappraisal. *Ann Ophthalmol* 1980;12:332–342.

76. Nasr A, Wingeist TA. The importance of standardized echography in the assessment of postsurgical choroidal detachments. Dordrect, the Netherlands: Martinus Nijhoff, 1987. (Ossoining KC, ed. Ophthalmic echography.)

77. Duehr PA, Hogenson CD. Treatment of subchoroidal hemorrhage by posterior sclerotomy. *Arch Ophthalmol* 1947;38:365–367.

78. Abrams GW, Thomas MA, Williams CA, Burton TI. Management of postoperative suprachoroidal hemorrhages with continuous infusion air pump. *Arch Ophthalmol* 1986;104:1455–1458.

79. Labrou F, Meredith TA, Kaplan HJ. Secondary surgical management of expulsive choroidal hemorrhage. *Arch Ophthalmol* 1987;105:1195–1198.

80. Davidson JA. Vitrectomy and fluid infusion in the treatment of delayed suprachoroidal hemorrhage after combined cataract and glaucoma filtration surgery. *Ophthalmic Surg* 1987;18:334–338.

81. Vail D. Posterior sclerotomy as a form of treatment in subchoroidal expulsive hemorrhage. *Am J Ophthalmol* 1938;21:256–260.

82. Baldwin LB, Smith TJ, Hollins JL, Pearson PA. The use of viscoelastic substances in the drainage of postoperative suprachoroidal hemorrhage. *Ophthalmic Surg* 1989;20:504–507.

83. Welch JC, Spaeth GL, Benson WE. Massive suprachoroidal hemorrhage. Follow up and outcome of 30 cases. *Ophthalmology* 1988;95:1202–1206.

84. Desai UR, Peyman GA, Chen AJ, et al. Use of perfluoroperhydrophenanthrene in the management of suprachoroidal hemorrhages. *Ophthalmology* 1992;99:1542–1547.

85. McDonald HR, Schatz H, Alien AW, et al. Retinal toxicity secondary to intraocular gentamicin injection. *Ophthalmology* 1986;93:871–877.

86. DeMaio R, Oliver GL. Recovery of useful vision after presumed retinal and choroidal toxic effects from gentamicin administration. *Arch Ophthalmol* 1994;112:736–738.

87. Chu TG, Fenceiva M, Aber RR. Immediate pars plana vitrectomy in the management of inadvertent intracameral injection of gentamicin. *Retina* 1994;14:59–64.

88. Daily M, Kachmeryk M, Foody R. Successful prevention of visual loss with emergency management following inadvertent intracameral injection of gentamicin. *Arch Ophthalmol* 1995;113:855–856.

89. Irvine SR. A newly defined vitreous syndrome following cataract surgery. *Am J Ophthalmol* 1953;39:599.

90. Gass JDM, Norton EWD. Cystoid macular edema and papilledema following cataract extraction: a fluorescein fundoscopic and angiographic study. *Arch Ophthalmol* 1966;76:646.

91. Nussenblatt RB, Kaufman SC, Palestine AG, et al. Macular thickening and visual acuity measurement in patients with cystoid macular edema. *Ophthalmology* 1987;94:1143.

92. Fung WE. Vitrectomy for chronic aphakic cystoid macular edema. Results of a national, collaborative, prospective randomized investigation. *Ophthalmology* 1985;92:1102.

93. Flach AJ, Dolan BJ, Irvine AR. Effectiveness of ketorolac trimethamine 0.5% ophthalmic solution for chronic aphakic and pseudophakic cystoid macular edema. *Am J Ophthalmol* 1987;103:479.

94. Tolentino FF, Schepens CL. Edema of the posterior pole after cataract extraction: a biomicroscopic study. *Arch Ophthalmol* 1965;74:781.

95. Welch RB, Cooper JC. Macular edema, papilledema, and optic atrophy after cataract extraction. *Arch Ophthalmol* 1958;59:665.

96. Keerl G. Maculaodem nach Kataraktoperation. *Klin Monatsbl Augenheilkd* 1970;156:850.

97. Kraft MC, Sanders DR, Jampol LM, et al. Prophylaxis of pseudophakic cystoid macular edema with topical indomethacin. *Ophthalmology* 1982;89:885.

98. Flach AJ, Stegman RC, Graham J, et al. Prophylaxis of aphakic cystoid macular edema without corticosteroids. *Ophthalmology* 1990;97:1253.

99. Jampol LM. Cystoid macular edema following cataract surgery. *Arch Ophthalmol* 1988;106:894.

100. Gass JDM, Norton EWD. Followup study of cystoid macular edema following cataract extraction. *Trans Am Acad Ophthalmol Otolaryngol* 1969;73:665.

101. Meredith TA, Kenyon KR, Singerman LJ, et al. Perifoveal vascular leakage and macular edema after intracapsular cataract extraction. *Arch Ophthalmol* 1976;60:765.

102. The Miami Study Group. Cystoid macular edema in aphakic and pseudophakic eyes. *Am J Ophthalmol* 1979;88:45.

103. Jaffe NS, Clayman HM, Jaffe MS. Cystoid macular edema after retinal detachment surgery and the use of topical indomethacin. *Ophthalmology* 1982;89:25.

104. Stark WJ, Worthen DM, Holladay JT, et al. The FDA report on intraocular lenses. *Ophthalmology* 1983;90:311.

105. Gass JDM, Norton EWD. Fluorescein studies of patients with macular edema and papilledema following cataract extraction. *Trans Am Ophthalmol Soc* 1966;64:232.

106. Schepens CL, Avila MP, Jalkh AE, et al. Role of the vitreous in cystoid macular edema. *Surv Ophthalmol* 1984;28(suppl):499.

107. Bovino JA, Kelly TJ, Marcus DF. Intraretinal hemorrhages in cystoid macular edema. *Arch Ophthalmol* 1984;102:1151.

108. Kottow M, Hendrickson P. Iris angiography in cystoid macular edema after cataract extraction. *Arch Ophthalmol* 1975;82:487.

109. Salzman J, Seiple W, Carr R, et al. Electrophysiological assessment of aphakic cystoid macular edema. *Br J Ophthalmol* 1986;70:819.

110. Lakhapal V, Schocket SS. Pseudophakic and phakic retinal detachment mimicking cystoid macular edema. *Ophthalmology* 1987;94:785.

111. Mao LK, Holland PM. "Very late onset" cystoid macular edema. *Ophthalmic Surg* 1988;19:633.

112. Barbera LG, Kung JS, Kimmel AS, et al. Optic disc leakage as a prognostic indicator in aphakic cystoid macular edema. *CLAO J* 1988;14:51.

113. Mishima H, Masuda K, Miyake K. The putative role of prostaglandins in cystoid macular edema. *Prog Clin Biol Res* 1981;312:251.

114. Jampol LM. Pharmacologic therapy of aphakic and pseudophakic cystoid macular edema. 1985 update. *Ophthalmology* 1985;92:807.

115. Miyake K, Miyake Y, Maekubo K, et al. Incidence of cystoid macular edema after retinal detachment surgery and the use of topical indomethacin. *Am J Ophthalmol* 1983;95:451.

116. Cox SN, Hay E, Bird AC. Treatment of chronic macular edema with acetazolamide. *Arch Ophthalmol* 1988;106:1190.

117. Katzen LE, Fleischman JA, Trokel S. YAG laser treatment of cystoid macular edema. *Am J Ophthalmol* 1983;95:589.

118. Steinert RF, Wasson PJ. Neodymium:YAG laser anterior vitreolysis for Irvine-Gass cystoid macular edema. *J Cataract Refract Surg* 1989;15:304.

119. Tielsch JM, Legro MW, Cassard SD, et al. Risk factors for retinal detachment after cataract surgery: a population based case control study. *Ophthalmology* 1996;103:1537–1545.

120. Powell SK, Olson RJ. Incidence of retinal detachment after cataract surgery and neodynium:YAG laser capsulotomy. *J Cataract Refractive Surg* 1995;21:132–135.

121. Javitt JC, Tielsch JM, Canner JK, et al. The cataract patient outcomes research team. Natural outcomes of cataract extraction. Increased risk of retinal complications associated with Nd:YAG laser capsulotomy. *Ophthalmology* 1992;99:1487–1497.

122. Rickman-Barger L, Florine CW, Earson RS, Lindstrom RL. Retinal detachment after neodymium:YAG laser posterior capsulotomy. *Am J Ophthalmol* 1989;107:531.

123. Shah GR, Gills JP, Durham DG, Asmus WH. Three thousand YAG lasers in posterior capsulotomies. An analysis of complications and comparison to polishing and surgical discission. *Ophthalmology* 1986;93:473.

124. Winslow RL, Taylor BC. Retinal complications following YAG capsulotomy. *Ophthalmology* 1985;92:785.

125. Liesengang TJ, Bourne WM, Listrup DM. Secondary surgical and neodynium-YAG laser discissions. *Am J Ophthalmol 100* 1985;100:510.

126. Johnson S, Kratz R, Olson P. Clinical experience with the Nd:YAG laser. *Am J Intraoc Implant Soc* 1984;10:452.

127. Percival SPB, Anand V, Das SK. Prevalence of aphakic retinal detachment. *Br J Ophthalmol* 1983;67:43.

128. Ficker LA, Steel AD. Complications of Isld-YAG laser posterior capsulotomy. *Trans Ophthalmol Soc UK* 1985;104:529.

129. Steinert RF, Puliafito CA, Kumar SR, et al. Cystoid macular edema, retinal detachment and glaucoma after Nd:YAG laser posterior capsulotomy. *Am J Ophthalmol* 1991;112:373–380.

130. Koch DD, Liu JF, Gill EP, Parke DW. Axial myopia increases the risk of retinal complications after neodymium-YAG laser posterior capsulotomy. *Arch Ophthalmol* 1989;107:986.

131. Francois J, Verbraeken H, Stranskki T. Aphakic retinal detachment. *Ophthalmology* 1977;175:181–184.

132. Javitt JC, Vitale S, Canner JK. Natural outcome of cataract extraction. 1. Retinal detachment after in patient surgery. *Ophthalmology* 1991;98:895–902.

133. Ninn-Pedersen K, Bauer B. Cataract patients in a defined Swedish population, 1986–1990. V. Postoperative retinal detachments. *Arch Ophthalmol* 1996;114:382–386.

134. Yoshida A, Ogasawara H, Jalkh AE, et al. Retinal detachment after cataract surgery. Predisposing factors. *Ophthalmology* 1992;99:453–459.

135. Chen JC, Robertson JE, Coonan P, et al. Results and complications of pneumatic retinopexy. *Ophthalmology* 1988;95:601–608.

136. McAllister IL, Meyers SM, Zegarra H, et al. Comparison of pneumatic retinopexy with alternative surgical techniques. *Ophthalmology* 1988;95:877–883.

137. Allen HF, Mangiaracine AB. Bacterial endophthalmitis after cataract extraction. II. Incidence in 36,000 consecutive operations with special reference to preoperative topical antibiotics. *Arch Ophthalmol* 1974;91:3–7.

138. Koul S, Philipson A, Philipson BT. Incidence of endophthalmitis in Sweden. *Acta Ophthalmol* 1989;67:499–503.

139. Rowsey JJ, Newsom DL, Sexton DJ. Endophthalmitis: Current approaches. *Ophthalmology* 1982;89:1055–1066.

140. Puliafito CA, Baker AS, Haaf J, Foster CS. Infectious endophthalmitis. *Ophthalmology* 1982;89:921–929.

141. Driebe WT, Mandelbaum S, Forster RK, et al. Pseudophakic endophthalmitis: diagnosis and management. *Ophthalmology* 1986;93:442–448.

142. Bohigian GM, Olk RJ. Factors associated with a poor visual result in endophthalmitis. *Am J Ophthalmol* 1981;101:332–334.

143. Diamond JG. Intraocular management of endophthalmitis. *Arch Ophthalmol* 1981;99:96–99.

144. Sherwood DR, Rich WJ, Jacob JS, et al. Bacterial contamination of intraocular and extraocular fluids during extracapsular cataract extraction. *Eye* 1989;3:308–312.

145. Beyer TL, Vogler G, Sharma D, O'Donnell FE. Protective barrier effect of the posterior lens capsule in exogenous bacterial endophthalmitis: an experimental primate study. *Invest Ophthalmol Vis Sci* 1984;25:108–112.

146. Deutsch TA, Goldberg MF. Painless endophthalmitis after cataract surgery. *Ophthalmic Surg* 1984;15:837–840.

147. Packer AS, Weingeist TA, Abrams GW. Retinal periphlebitis as an early sign of bacterial endophthalmitis. *Am J Ophthalmol* 1983;96:66–71.

148. Ficker L, Meredith TA, Wilson LA, et al. Chronic bacterial endophthalmitis. *Am J Ophthalmol* 1987;103:745–748.

149. Jaffe GJ, Whiteher JP, Biswell R, Irvine AR. *Propionibacterium acnes* endophthalmitis seven months after extracapsular cataract extraction and intraocular lens implantation. *Ophthalmic Surg* 1986;17:791–793.

150. Forster RK. Etiology and diagnosis of bacterial postoperative endophthalmitis. *Ophthalmology* 1978;85:320–326.

151. Maylath FR, Leopold IH. Study of experimental intraocular infections. *Am J Ophthalmol* 1984;40:86–101.

152. Forster RK, Zachary IG, Cottingham AJ, Norton EWD. Endophthalmitis: diagnostic cultures and visual results. *Arch Ophthalmol* 1974;92:387–392.

153. Forster RK, Zachary IG, Cottingham AJ, Norton EWD. Further observation on the diagnosis, cause, and treatment of endophthalmitis. *Am J Ophthalmol* 1976;81:52–56.

154. Smith MA, Sorenson JA, Lowy FD, et al. Treatment of experimental methicillin-resistant *Staphylococcus epidermidis* endophthalmitis with intravitreal vancomycin. *Ophthalmology* 1986;93:1328–1335.

155. Mandelbaum S, Forster RK, Gelender H, Culbertson WW. Late onset endophthalmitis associated with filtering blebs. *Ophthalmology* 1985;92:964–972.

156. Duglid JP, Ginsberg M, Fraser IC, et al. Experimental observations on the intravitreal use of penicillin and other drugs. *Br J Ophthalmol* 1947;31:193–211.

157. Sorsby A, Ungar J. Intravitreal injection of penicillin. Study of the levels of concentrations reached and therapeutic efficacy. *Br J Ophthalmol* 1948;32:857–864.

158. Olson JC, Flynn HW, Forster RK, Culbertson WW. Results in the treatment of postoperative endophthalmitis. *Ophthalmology* 1983;90:692–699.

159. Affeldt JC, Flynn HW, Forster RK, et al. Microbial endophthalmitis resulting from ocular trauma. *Ophthalmology* 1987;94:407–413.

160. Lambert SR, Stern WH. Methicillin- and gentamicin-resistant *Staphylococcus epidermidis* endophthalmitis after intraocular surgery. *Am J Ophthalmol* 1985;99:725–726.

161. Kervick GN, Flynn HW, Alfonso E, Miller D. Antibiotic therapy for *Bacillus* species infections. *Am J Ophthalmol* 1990;110:683–687.

162. Peyman GA, Paque JT, Meisels HI, Bennett TO. Postoperative endophthalmitis: a comparison of methods for treatment and prophylaxis with gentamicin. *Ophthalmic Surg* 1975;6:45–55.

163. Peyman GA, Herbst R. Bacterial endophthalmitis: treatment with intraocular injection of gentamicin and dexamethasone. *Arch Ophthalmol* 1974;91:416–418.

164. Peyman GA, May DR, Ericson ES, Apple D. Intraocular injection of gentamicin: toxic effects and clearance. *Arch Ophthalmol* 1974;92:42–47.

165. D'Amico DJ, Caspers-Velu L, Libeft J, et al. Comparative toxicity of intravitreal aminoglycoside antibiotics. *Am J Ophthalmol* 1985;100:264–275.

166. Zachary IG, Forster RK. Experimental intravitreal gentamicin. *Am J Ophthalmol* 1976;82:604–611.

167. Conway BP, Campochiaro PA. Macular infarction after endophthalmitis treated with vitrectomy and intravitreal gentamicin. *Arch Ophthalmol* 1986;104:367–371.

168. Brown GC, Eagle RC, Shakin EP, et al. Retinal toxicity of intravitreal gentamicin. *Arch Ophthalmol* 1990;108:1740–1744.

169. D'Amico DJ, Liberr J, Kenyon KR, et al. Retinal toxicity of intravitreal gentamicin: an electron microscopic study. *Invest Ophthalmol Vis Sci* 1984;25:564–572.

170. Insler MS, Cavanaugh HD, Wilson WA. Gentamicin-resistant *Pseudomonas* endophthalmitis after penetrating keratoplasty. *Br J Ophthalmol* 1985;69:189–191.

171. Majerovics A, Tanenbaum HL. Endophthalmitis and pars plana vitrectomy. *Can J Ophthalmol* 1984;19:25–28.

172. Talamo JH, D'Amico DJ, Kenyon KR. Intravitreal amikacin in the treatment of bacterial endophthalmitis. *Arch Ophthalmol* 1986;104:1483–1485.

173. Cobo LM, Forster RK. The clearance of intravitreal gentamicin. *Am J Ophthalmol* 1981;92:59–62.

174. Furgiuele FP. Ocular penetration and tolerance of gentamicin. *Am J Ophthalmol* 1967;64:421–426.

175. Fisher JP, Civiletto SE, Forster RK. Toxicity, efficacy and clearance of intravitreally injected cefazolin. *Arch Ophthalmol* 1982;100:650–652.

176. Ellerhorst B, Golden B, Jarudi N. Ocular penetration and tolerance of gentamicin. *Am J Ophthalmol* 1975;64:421–426.

177. Litwack KD, Pettit T, Johnson BL. Penetration of gentamicin: administered intramuscularly and subconjunctivally into aqueous humor. *Arch Ophthalmol* 1969;82:687–693.

178. Graham RO, Peyman GA. Intravitreal injection of dexamethasone: treatment of experimentally induced endophthalmitis. *Arch Ophthalmol* 1974;92:149–154.

179. Endophthalmitis Vitrectomy Study Group. Results of the Endophthalmitis Vitrectomy Study. A randomized trial of immediate vitrectomy and of intravenous antibiotics for the treatment of postoperative bacterial endophthalmitis. *Arch Ophthalmol* 1995;113:1479–1496.

180. Fox GM, Joondeph BC, Flynn HW, et al. Delayed-onset pseudophakic endophthalmitis. *Am J Ophthalmol* 1991;111:163–173.

181. Stern WH, Tamura E, Jacobs RA, et al. Epidemic postsurgical *Candida parapsilosis* endophthalmitis: clinical findings and management of 15 consecutive cases. *Ophthalmology* 1985;92:1701–1709.

182. Sutphin JE, Robinson NM, Wilhelmus KR, Osato MS. Improved detection of oculomycoses using induced fluorescence with Celluquor. *Ophthalmology* 1986;93:416–417.

183. Pflugfelder SC, Flynn HW, Zwickey TA, et al. Exogenous fungal endophthalmitis. *Ophthalmology* 1988;95:19–30.

184. Phillips WBN, Tasman WS. Post operative endophthalmitis in association with diabetes mellitus. *Ophthalmology* 1994;101:508–518.

185. Sebestyn JG. Intraocular lenses and diabetes mellitus. *Am J Ophthalmol* 1986;101:425–428.

186. Cheng H, Franklin SL. Treatment of cataract in diabetics with and without retinopathy. *Eye* 1988;2:607.

187. Aiello LM, Wand M, Liang G. Neovascular glaucoma and vitreous hemorrhage following cataract surgery in patients with diabetes mellitus. *Ophthalmology* 1983;90:814.

188. Alpar JJ. Cataract extraction and intraocular lenses. *J Cataract Refract Surg* 1987;13:43.

189. Jaffe GJ, Burton TC. Progression of nonproliferative diabetic retinopathy following cataract extraction. *Arch Ophthalmol* 1988;106:745.

190. Lischwe TD, Ide CH. Predicting visual acuity after cataract surgery using the blue field entoptoscope and projected slides. *Ophthalmology* 1988;95:256.

191. Tso MOM. Photic maculopathy in rhesus monkey. A light and electron microscopic study. Invest Ophthalmol 1973;12:17–34.

192. McDonald HR, Irvine AR. Light-induced maculopathy from the operating microscope in extracapsular cataract extraction and intraocular lens implantation. *Ophthalmology* 1983;90:945–951.

193. Robertson DM, Feldman RB. Photic retinopathy from the operating room microscope. *Am J Ophthalmol* 1986;101:561–569.

194. Khwarg S, Linstone FA, Daniels SA, et al. Incidence, risk factors, and morphology in operating microscope light retinopathy. *Am J Ophthalmol* 1987;103:255–263.

195. Irvine AR, Wood I, Morris BW. Retinal damage from the illumination of the operating microscope: an experimental study in pseudophakic monkeys. *Trans Am Ophthalmol Soc* 1984;82:239–260.

196. Berler DK, Peyser R. Light intensity and visual acuity following cataract surgery. *Ophthalmology* 1983;90:933–936.

197. Noell WK, Walker VS, Kang BS, Berman S. Retinal damage by light in rats. *Invest Ophthalmol* 1966;5:450–473.

198. Ham WT, Mueller HA, Ruffolo JJ, et al. Action spectrum for retinal injury from near-ultraviolet radiation in the aphakic monkey. *Am J Ophthalmol* 1982;93:299–306.

199. McIntyre DJ. The eclipse filter. *Ophthalmology* 1985;92:361–365.

200. Henry MM, Henry LM. A possible cause of chronic cyclic maculopathy. *Ann Ophthalmol* 1977;9:455–457.

201. Keates RH, Armstrong PF. Use of a short-wavelength filter in an operating microscope. *Ophthalmic Surg* 1985;16:40–41.

202. Sliney DH. Eye protective techniques for bright lights. *Ophthalmology* 1983;90:937–944.

203. Byrnes GA, Mazur DO, Maller S. Retinal light damage and eye surgery. *Ophthalmology* 1996;103:546–547. Letter.

204. Minckler D. Retinal light damage and eye surgery. *Ophthalmology* 1995;102:1741–1742.

Surgical Pathology of the Retina

Jose A. Sahel   Alfred Brini   Daniel M. Albert

This chapter discusses the surgical pathology of the various retinal diseases and conditions discussed in this section. A complete review of the pathology of the retina was recently published (1).

RETINAL DETACHMENT

Retinal detachment is a separation between the retinal pigment epithelium (RPE) and the neuroepithelium at the embryonic cavity between the two layers of the optic vesicle.

Except at the optic disk and ora serrata, attachment of the neurosensory retina to the RPE is dependent on several mechanisms including intraocular pressure, vitreous support and pressure, gravity, interdigitation of photoreceptor outer segments and RPE apical microvilli, interphotoreceptor matrix and adhesion molecules, the subretinal space, and RPE-dependent active transport of fluids, ions, and molecules from the subretinal space to the choroid (2–5).

Rhegmatogenous retinal detachment is the most common type of retinal detachment. It results from accumulation of vitreous fluid beneath the neural retina through a tear or a hole, and is most often secondary to degenerative retinal changes linked to vitreous alterations with vitreous traction. Equatorial lattice-type perivascular vitreoretinal adhesions, degenerative retinoschisis, white without pressure, or peripheral cystoid degeneration are among the vitreoretinal changes associated with retinal detachment. Vitreous traction may lead to hole formation when vitreous adheres to the inner limiting membrane.

Following retinal detachment, the principle changes occur in the outer layers of the sensory retina, presumably as a consequence of separation from the blood supply and interruption of the normal shedding of photoreceptor outer

segments by the RPE. Research in owl monkeys showed disruption and disorganization of the outer segments with separation of phagosomes from the RPE to be among the earliest pathologic changes. The RPE undergoes degenerative hyperplasia at the posterior limit of the detached retina. After 3 months, a demarcation line develops with fibrous metaplasia. Proliferation of the RPE at the ora serrata results in a large, pigmented plaque (ringschwiele). Cystic changes appear in the outer layers of the neurosensory retina. With long-standing inferior detachments, intraretinal macrocystoid spaces may develop in the equatorial area (6–8).

Two postmortem studies of eyes with successfully treated retinal detachment showed photoreceptor atrophy in approximately one-fourth of the eyes, an unexpectedly high incidence of epiretinal membranes, macular pucker, and cystoid macular edema (9,10). These findings may explain the reduced vision after successful retinal reattachment surgery and the incidence and role of epiretinal proliferations (Figs. 54-1 and 54-2).

Tractional retinal detachment results when the neuroepithelium is pulled by intravitreal membranes. This may result from trauma (spontaneous or surgical) with vitreous incarceration in the wound or proliferative retinopathies such as diabetic retinopathy, sickle cell disease, retinopathy of prematurity (ROP), and proliferative vitreoretinopathy (PVR) following rhegmatogenous retinal detachment. In these entities, secondary retinal holes can occur.

Other types of retinal detachment are exudative, transudative, and hemorrhagic. These result from an accumulation of subretinal fluid from the choroidal or retinal vessels. Many diseases manifest these accumulations, including choroidal melanomas (and other tumors), inflammatory conditions (Harada's disease, scleritis, sympathetic ophthalmia), and vascular disease (hypertension, eclampsia).

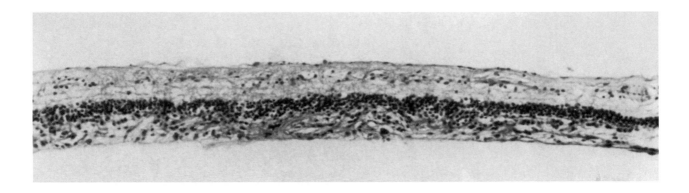

FIGURE 54-1. *Midperipheral retina. Patient had total retinal detachment. Postoperative visual acuity was 20/200. Note absence of photoreceptors and atrophy of outer plexiform and outer nuclear layers (H&E, original magnification ×100). (Reprinted with permission from Barr CC. The histopathology of successful retinal detachment.* Retina *1990;10:189.)*

PVR is a major cause of failure of retinal detachment surgery. On histopathologic examination, migration and proliferation of retinal, subretinal, and intravitreal cells are seen on both surfaces of the neural retina as well as on the vitreous base and posterior surface. Tractional retinal detachments result from the growth and subsequent contraction of the cellular membranes. Formerly described as massive vitreous retraction or massive periretinal retraction, PVR is now recognized as a separate entity (11–19).

The first cellular event is the release and dispersion of RPE cells into the vitreous cavity during retinal tearing, separation, cryotherapy, or scleral depression (20–24). The RPE cells migrate in the vitreous cavity and attach preferentially to the inferior part of the retina. Fibronectin and platelet-derived growth factor, both normal serum components that may enter the vitreous cavity as a consequence of cryotherapy-induced breakdown of the normal blood–ocular barrier, mediate the migration and chemotaxis of RPE cells to collagen and sodium hyaluronate. The interaction of RPE cells with the matrix components induces a morphologic change from an epithelial to a fibroblastic type, then active engagement and dragging of vitreous fibrils, with subsequent contraction of the vitreous gel. Production of a chemoattractant to astrocytes and a growth factor follows. This factor appears to be transforming growth factor-β (TGF-β), a chemoattractant to fibroblasts. In addition, monocytes stimulate fibroblast proliferation and production of collagen and fibronectin, a multifunctional glucoprotein of the extracellular matrix that stimulates cell proliferation and migration. Other extracellular matrix components such as tenascin, decorin, laminin, and vitronectin play a role at various stages, vitronectin acting as a modulator of adhesion mechanisms in established membranes (25,26). The role of inflammatory breakdown of the blood–retinal barrier in the release of serum growth factors [platelet-derived growth factor (PDGF), TGF-β], complement, immunoglobulins, and fibronectin has been thoroughly investigated (27–30).

In several studies of membranes obtained during vitrectomy, inflammatory cells and components [e.g., CD4 and CD8 T lymphocytes, macrophages, activated complement components (C1q, C4, C3, C3c, C3d), immunoglobulins] were identified (31). Expression of the major histocompatibility complex (MHC) class II antigen HLA-DR is consistently documented in the membranes (32,33). The primary or reactive role of inflammation at various stages of the disease remains to be determined.

Although RPE cells are a major factor in the formation of PVR membranes, the glial and monocytic cell types as well as the normal (type I) and newly formed collagen fibrils (types II and III) have a key role in membrane development and contraction. Many fibroblasts and fibroblast-like cells of these membranes assume a myofibroblastic morphology with cytoplasmic strands of contractile intermediate filaments, such as the myofibroblasts involved in wound contraction during the normal healing process. This finding, as well as a recent demonstration of the very early proliferative response (days 2–4) of every nonneuronal cell type to retinal detachment (34), supports the view that PVR may simply be an exaggerated and mislocated healing process with devastating consequences (35,36).

Although the proportions of cellular types may vary from one case to another (37–40), collagen development and dragging as well as myofibroblastic properties appear to be the common denominator of PVR membranes that accounts for their contraction. Cellular invasion, proliferation, and membrane contraction may occur at various locations on the posterior vitreous surface, producing a taut transvitreal membrane close to the equator and extending from the vitreous base and the anterior cortex to the pars plana, ciliary processes, or iris. This membrane causes an anterior PVR with consecutive circumferential retinal folds, peripheral radial folding, reopening of retinal breaks (41), and on the inner retinal surface, distortion and "star folding" (Fig. 54-3) (42–44).

The subretinal space is another site of membrane formation where subretinal proteins cause the induction of early RPE migration and attachment to the retina. This is followed by proliferation of fibrocytes, macrophages, fibrous

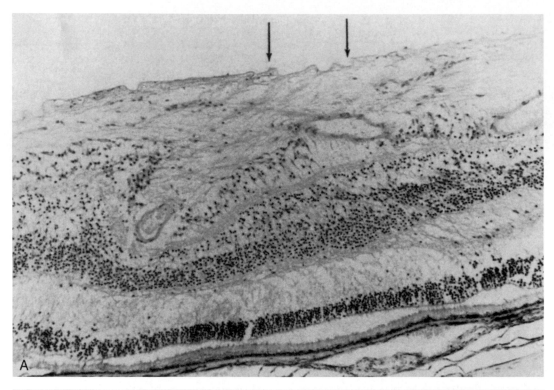

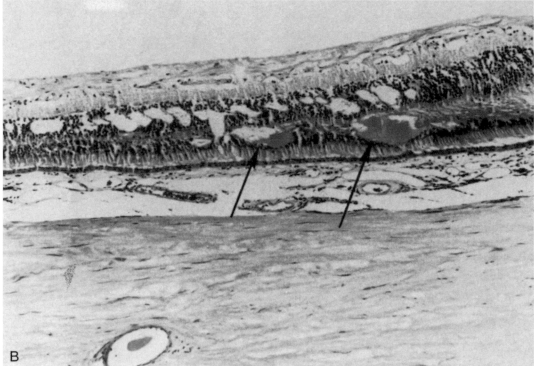

FIGURE 54-2. A. *Macular area demonstrating retinal folding and edema from epiretinal membrane (arrows). Final visual acuity was 5/200. (H&E, original magnification ×100). B. Macular area. Visual acuity as 20/25. Note cystoid spaces in the outer plexiform layer and the outer nuclear layer as indicated by arrows (H&E, original magnification ×100). (Reprinted with permission from Barr CC. The histopathology of successful retinal detachment.* Retina *1990;10:189.)*

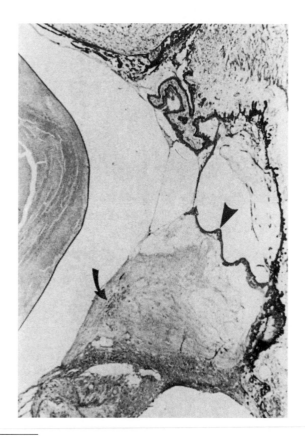

FIGURE 54-3. *Densely organized vitreous at vitreous base in anterior proliferative vitreoretinopathy tissue is tightly adherent to the retina surface, where prominent glial proliferation is noted. Most of the organized vitreous contains proliferated metaplastic pigment epithelial cells (arrow) embedded in fibrous extracellular matrix. Attachments to pars plana and pars plicata have caused tractional separation of nonpigmented and pigmented neuroepithelial layers (arrowhead) (PAS, ×7.88). (Reprinted with permission from Elner SG, Elner VM, Diaz-Rohena R, et al. Anterior PVR II: clinicopathologic, light microscopic and ultrastructural findings. In: Freeman HM, Tolentino FI, eds. Proliferative vitreoretinopathy (PVR). New York: Springer-Verlag, 1989.)*

astrocytes, and myofibrocytes associated with fibrin and collagen deposition. Simple subretinal membranes with little extracellular material are distinguished from taut subretinal membranes with a prominent contractile RPE and type I to IV collagen components (45–48). The role of these membranes in retinal detachment surgery failure is still disputed (43,45–49).

The international classification of PVR and its recent updates are well correlated with the previously mentioned clinicopathologic studies pioneered by Machemer et al in the 1970s (12–17,20).

VITREOUS DETACHMENT

Vitreous aging and detachment are widely recognized as crucial factors in the pathogenesis of retinal detachment, whether rhegmatogenous or tractional, as well as in the development of idiopathic vitreoretinal macular disorders.

The vitreoretinal interface is where the inner limiting membrane of the retina meets the posterior vitreous cortex forming the posterior hyaloid. The posterior vitreous cortex is composed of densely packed vitreous collagen and presents with some important anatomic variations (50–52). It is lacking at the surface of the optic nerve, and should there be posterior vitreous detachment (PVD), this prepapillary hole forms a well-identified structure seen with biomicroscopy termed the *Weiss ring* (52). In the area of the macula, the vitreous cortex is thinned and adherent. With age, it separates the macular surface from the precortical vitreous pocket described by Kishi and Shimizu (53). This pocket is independent from the degree of vitreous liquefaction.

Vitreous body aging is initially characterized by the formation of thickening fibers and the progression of central liquefaction (syneresis). It is likely that the aging process involves degradation of the glycosaminoglycans, especially hyaluronic acid, and of their interactions with vitreous collagen types II, XI, and IX (54–56). Vitreous liquefaction is accelerated in myopic eyes and by inflammation (e.g., uveitis and trauma) (57). Foos (58) detected 25% vitreous liquefaction in autopsy studies of eyes from subjects in their third decade. PVD was detected in at least one eye in 10% of subjects younger than 50 years, 27% of subjects between 60 and 69, and 63% of those older than 70. In the same study, a significant correlation was found between the degree of vitreous syneresis and the prevalence of PVD. Both phenomena are age related (58,59). According to Eisner (60,61), PVD occurs acutely as a consequence of posterior cortical vitreous tearing. The liquefied vitreous gel empties through the premacular gap in the retrovitreal space, inducing vitreous collapse and PVD (62,63). Eisner suggested differentiating this type of rhegmatogenous vitreous detachment from vitreous detachments occurring without identifiable cortical vitreous breaks, as in proliferative diabetic retinopathy. This view is not unanimously accepted and has been challenged by the increasing recognition of the role of the premacular pocket in the pathogenesis of vitreomacular disorders (43).

As the vitreous separates from the retina, complications may be induced either by traction on preexisting vitreoretinal adhesions with subsequent intravitreal or retrovitreal hemorrhage and retinal tearing, or by incomplete separation of the cortical vitreous. Pathogenetic mechanisms involve a combination of 1) partial or complete PVD, 2) sagittal or tangential tractional forces exerted by active contraction of proliferative membranes, or 3) passive movements.

In the case of traction or retrocortical adhesions, peripheral retinal breaks may evolve to retinal detachment. The pathogenesis of macular holes and their relationship to PVD are still debated. In 1987 and 1988, Gass (64,65) proposed that posterior vitreous alterations occurring before the development of PVD are the cause of macular holes. He suggested that contraction of prefoveal vitreous induces traction detachment of the fovea at early stages. In this hypothesis, traction over the thin premacular cortical layer at the posterior pole of Shimizu's pocket could result either from mechanical fluid movements or from hypocellular traction. In his first description, Gass suggested that prolonged traction causes the development of macular holes, with formation of an operculum. PVD occurs later, with the operculum remaining adherent anteriorly to the posterior hyaloid membrane. In 1995, Gass, in view of clinical and pathologic recent findings, suggested that the first stage of foveal elevation and detachment with a cystic yellowish appearance is followed with distribution of the xanthophilic pigment around a central foveal opening hidden by vitreous cortex. At later stages, enlargement of the hole, intraretinal edema, and retinal detachment around the hole occur. The presence of an operculum in front of the hole can indicate partial PVD or total PVD, corresponding clinically to an observation of the prepapillary Weiss ring with cortical densification facing the hole. Other hypotheses include choroidal ischemia with involutional mechanisms (66) and sagittal vitreous traction (67–69). Smiddy et al (70) found associated epiretinal membranes in 16 (73%) of 22 eyes. Recent histopathologic studies of surgical specimens provided important but still preliminary information including the presence of indigenous vitreous collagen on the posterior part of the retina (71,72). Opercula removed surgically contained only cortical vitreous and some glial cells (73). Ezra et al (73a) showed that 39% of opercula contain neuronal elements, such as cones, and that this finding is related to a poorer functional result. Postmortem study of a successfully treated stage III macular hole showed a 16-μm defect in the inner limiting membrane, sealed by expansions of Müller's cell (74,75). At the base of the hole, nodular proliferation of the RPE overlies eosinophilic material, which is visible as yellow deposits (64).

The pathogenesis of idiopathic epiretinal macular membranes is still debated. The once widely mentioned finding of PVD in such cases now is questioned in view of the frequent perioperative finding of a large, empty intravitreal space mistaken for the retroretinal space (53). In a series of 84 eyes, total PVD was seen in 36 (43%), no or partial PVD in 48 (57%) (53). Moreover, in eyes with total PVD, a round or oval defect in the posterior hyaloid corresponding to the epiretinal membrane was described. Contraction of the thin layer of cortical vitreous tissue remaining in front of the macula is implicated in the development of some premacular idiopathic membrane (76). It is likely that as suggested by Sebag et al (77), at least two subtypes of epiretinal membranes can occur: hypocellular with intracortical vitreoschisis or thick, proliferative, contractile cells with cortical remnants after PVD. Smiddy et al (72) found PVD in 101 eyes of their series on surgically excised idiopathic macular pucker. Almost all nonneuronal cell types in the macular region have been implicated and detected in epiretinal membranes, including hyalocytes (78), glial cells (79,80), and RPE cells (Fig. 54-4) (76,78–81). New collagen is present in these membranes. The RPE cells predominate in most series

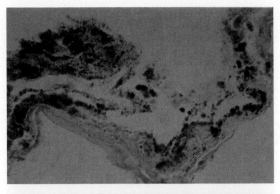

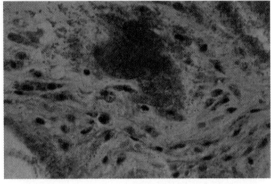

FIGURE 54-4.   A. *Epiretinal membrane; predominance of retinal pigment epithelium-derived pigmented cells in epiretinal membrane (H&E, ×10).* B. *Epiretinal membrane: fibroblast-like partially pigmented cells with collagen formation (H&E, ×40). (Reprinted with permission from Sahel JA, Brini A, Albert DM. Pathology of the retina and vitreous. In: Albert DM, Jakobiec FA, eds.* Principles and practice of ophthalmology. *Philadelphia: WB Saunders, 1994:2247.)*

(76,81–84). The pathogenetic significance of this finding is not yet understood; it may represent migration of RPE cells through subclinical or self-healed retinal breaks, transretinal migration of RPE cells, and even transformation of glial cells. Myofibroblastic differentiation of migrating and proliferating cells is a common finding, accounting for membrane retraction (76).

In an experimental model of epiretinal membranes, Russell and Hageman (85) showed that intravitreal injection of chondroitin sulfate induces a glial proliferation in the rabbit after 3 weeks, with formation of a mature complex membrane after 6 weeks. These experiments confirmed the role of Müller's cells and of the extracellular matrix. In another model, Kono et al (86) induced a glial and macrophagic proliferation 2 weeks after intravitreal injection of autologous blood followed by the formation of a mature glial membrane within 6 months. Linder (87) observed minor intravitreous bleeding considerably after PVD developed in 13% to 19% of cases. This high incidence is not surprising in view of the strong vitreovascular adherences described by several authors (88,89).

In cases of vitreomacular traction syndrome, surgically excised specimens contain new collagen, predominantly fibrous astrocytes, and some myofibroblasts. Cell migration to the vitreoretinal junction is thought to be either a consequence of incomplete PVD or a preexisting event causing vitreoretinal adhesion and limiting PVD (84).

Therefore, it should be emphasized that despite the reservations expressed about the role of PVD in the pathogenesis of some vitreomacular diseases, its role in vitreoretinal disorders should not be overlooked (37,38,70,90–92).

VITREOUS OPACITIES

Asteroid Hyalosis

Asteroid hyalosis is a common degenerative process usually occurring unilaterally in patients older than 60 years. Asteroid bodies are attached to the collagenous vitreous frame and may arise from vitreous fibril degeneration (93). Asteroid bodies consist of an amorphous basophilic substance that stains positively with periodic acid–Schiff (PAS) and lipid and acid mucopolysaccharide stains. Birefringent crystals are embedded in this substance. These characteristics (94) support Verhoeff's suggestion that asteroid hyalosis represents a calcium-containing lipid (probably phospholipid) (Fig. 54-5) (95).

Cholesterosis Bulbi

After intravitreal hemorrhage, cholesterol crystals may accumulate and move freely inside the vitreous cavity.

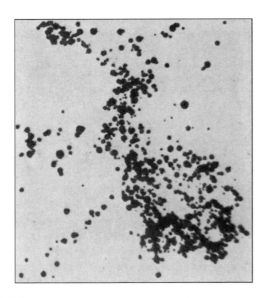

FIGURE 54-5. *Group of asteroid opacities as seen by transmitted light. (Reprinted from Verhoeff FH. Microscopic findings in a case of asteroid hyalitis. Am J Ophthalmol 1921;4:155.)*

Histologically, cholesterol crystals are dissolved by routine alcohol dehydration and appear as empty slit-like spaces. Other sequelae of vitreous hemorrhages include hemosiderosis, ghost cells, hemoglobin spherulosis (96), and macrophages containing blood breakdown products.

Systemic Primary Amyloid

Systemic primary amyloid can induce early bilateral vitreous opacification. Excised vitreous shows the usual staining reactions characteristic of amyloid. Doft et al (97) showed immunocytochemically that the major amyloid constituent resembles prealbumin.

Diabetic Retinopathy

The main anatomic lesions of diabetic retinopathy with their clinical correlates and presumed pathogenesis are discussed here (98–103).

Clinically, diabetic retinal lesions are usually divided into background (intraretinal vascular changes) and proliferative phases, initially incipient and later preretinal. The pathologic process can be studied as a microangiopathy characterized by capillary microaneurysm formation, dilation and hyperpermeability with exudates, hemorrhages, and edema; capillary occlusion resulting in microinfarctions; shunts and neovascularization within and at the retinal inner surface and optic nerve; and vitreous hemorrhage, traction, and tractional retinal detachment.

Capillary basement membrane thickening is the earliest change in the retinal, cerebral, and renal capillaries observed in diabetic humans and in animal models (104). Various biochemical processes (e.g., sorbitol and aldose-reductase pathway, altered basement membrane collagen, critical protein glycosylation, and decrease in heparin sulfate proteoglycan production) take part in the pathogenesis of this early change. The structural and functional role of basement membrane thickening in the alteration of the capillary retinal bed, the breakdown of the blood-retina barrier, the regulation of pericytes, and endothelial cell proliferation are not fully understood (101,102,105–110). In the early 1960s, Cogan et al (110) first demonstrated loss of capillary pericytes using an original technique of trypsin digestion of formalin-fixed retinal specimens. In the retina of normal young adults, the pericyte–endothelial cell ratio is 1:1. Pericyte dropout is detected by the presence of balloon-like spaces or pericyte "ghosts" in trypsin digest preparations. Loss of intramural pericytes is considered a specific characteristic of diabetic retinopathy and is not detectable in the other organs involved in diabetic vascular complications. Explanations for such a specificity remain putative (e.g., selective presence of the sorbitol pathway in retinal pericytes). The loss of pericytes has an important impact on the regulation of microvascular blood flow, the formation of microaneurysms, and the inhibition of endothelial cell proliferation (107–109).

Microaneurysms are the earliest ophthalmoscopically detectable change in diabetic retinopathy, although more of them are observed microscopically or by fluorescein angiography. They commonly are considered to be the result of pericyte loss with focal weakening of the microvessel wall and focal dilation (110). Most microaneurysms appear in the posterior part of the retina in areas of ischemia. This led some investigators (103) to speculate that microaneurysms might represent an early intraretinal microvascular anomaly produced by bidimensional endothelial cell proliferation, probably as a consequence of loss of inhibition by the normal basal membrane and pericytes (101,107). At the early stage of microaneurysms, the line between so-called background and proliferative retinopathy appears to be rather arbitrary. Whether induced by localized weakening of the vascular wall or by early vascular proliferation, microaneurysms cause a breakdown of the inner blood-retina barrier and predispose to edema, exudates, and hemorrhage. Some microaneurysms may not hyperfluoresce on fluorescein angiography because of occlusion by their increased basement membrane elaboration.

In conjunction with or secondary to microaneurysm formation, arteriolar-venular shunts with capillary dilation, decrease in capillary blood flow, and capillary atrophy occur consecutively (111,112). Other related abnormalities are capillary acellularity, intraluminal basement membrane thickening, and swelling of the arteriolar wall (as in hypertensive retinopathy). As a result, a significant part of the microvascular bed is destroyed, providing a basis for retinal ischemia (103,112).

The breakdown of the blood-retina barrier is a functional event that occurs early in diabetic retinopathy and is produced by various intricate mechanisms at the inner and outer levels of the blood-retina barriers. These include microaneurysms, vascular dilation, increased intraluminal and transmural pressures, opening of the tight junctions between endothelial cells, and endothelial fenestration. The RPE is also involved by the metabolic alterations and biochemical processes described earlier, including alterations in the aldose reductase–dependent pathways. Increased infolding of the basal plasmic membrane of RPE cells also contributes to early breakdown of the blood-retina barrier (113).

Intraretinal hemorrhages may assume various shapes according to retinal location. Dot and blot hemorrhages spread from the inner nuclear layer into the outer plexiform layer. Flame hemorrhages are located between the axons of the nerve fiber layer. Larger hemorrhages may involve several or all retinal layers, the latter often appearing globular. Localized hemorrhages probably originate from aneurysms or altered capillaries. Larger hemorrhages are often significant features of severe "background" retinopathy and may break into the vitreous space (Fig. 54–6).

Macular edema is the main cause of visual loss in patients with background retinopathy. Macular edema usually is classified into focal and diffuse edema, whether cystoid or not. Extravascular fluid leakage results from the structural

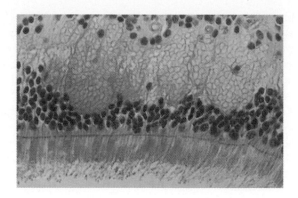

FIGURE 54-6.   Intraretinal hemorrhage with thickening of the outer plexiform layer in diabetic retinopathy (H&E, ×40). (Reprinted with permission from Sahel JA, Brini A, Albert DM. Pathology of the retina and vitreous. In: Albert DM, Jakobiec FA, eds. Principles and practice of ophthalmology. Philadelphia: WB Saunders 1994:2259.)

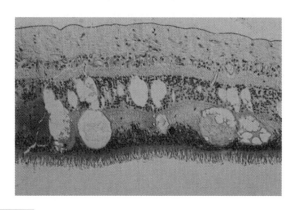

FIGURE 54-7.   Cystoid retinal edema in diabetic retinopathy (H&E ×40). (Reprinted with permission from Sahel JA, Brini A, Albert DM. Pathology of the retina and vitreous. In: Albert DM, Jakobiec FA, eds. Principles and practice of ophthalmology. Philadelphia: WB Saunders, 1994:2259.)

and functional alterations described earlier at the capillary level. Some studies showed that moderate amounts of fluid initially accumulate in Müller's cells (114–117). Further accumulation leads to excessive ballooning and degeneration of Müller's cells and formation of multiple cystoid spaces in the outer plexiform and inner nuclear layers (Fig. 54-7). The lesions at this stage are often irreversible and may evolve toward macular retinoschisis or hole (Fig. 54-8).

In focal edema, the leakage diffuses from foci of microaneurysms in a circinate pattern. The aqueous content of the exudate pools is progressively reabsorbed in the outer plexiform layer. The insoluble lipoproteins form hard exudates that accumulate at some distance from the leaking zone in complete or partial rings, separating the edematous zone from the surrounding nonedematous retina. If the leak is appropriately treated by photocoagulation, the edema is

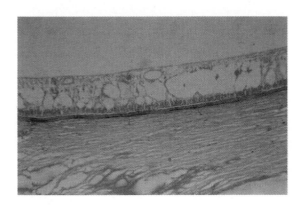

FIGURE 54-8. *Cystoid retinal degeneration following long-standing cystoid macular edema in diabetic retinopathy (H&E, ×10). (Reprinted with permission from Sahel JA, Brini A, Albert DM. Pathology of the retina and vitreous. In: Albert DM, Jakobiec FA, eds. Principles and practice of ophthalmology. Philadelphia: WB Saunders, 1994:2260.)*

transported through the RPE and adjacent capillaries. However, the exudates cannot follow this path and are progressively removed by macrophages. These can be observed histopathologically as lipid-laden macrophages and are particularly numerous in the outer plexiform layer (64,112,118). Cystoid macular edema is uncommon in focal circinate retinopathy.

In contrast, diffuse macular edema often is associated with macular cystoid pooling. Diffuse leakage through a dilated capillary bed and an altered outer blood-retina barrier is often bilateral. Lipid accumulation is theoretically unlikely in this process because large molecules remain intravascular. The imbalance between the intracapillary hydrostatic and tissue osmotic pressures on the one hand and the plasmatic osmotic and tissue hydrostatic pressures on the other may be enhanced by a capillary dilation to compensate for capillary occlusion and widening of intercapillary spaces. For this reason, diffuse macular edema and macular ischemia may coexist and contribute to central visual loss.

An intermediate or preproliferative stage between background and proliferative retinopathy is characterized by the addition or exacerbation of the following changes: 1) larger, darker hemorrhages; 2) intraretinal microvascular anomalies (i.e., irregular segmental dilatations of the capillary bed that developed as new vessels originating from the venous side of the microvascular bed and produced at the border of areas of arteriolar nonperfusion) (119); 3) multiple cotton-wool spots reflecting acute extensive hypoxia (120); and 4) venous dilation and beading. All of these "transitional" findings related to increasing retinal ischemia contribute to poor visual prognosis, because in the macular region irreversible and untractable visual loss ensues. These changes are probably not just forerunners but actually part of the proliferative phase.

Proliferative Diabetic Retinopathy

Proliferative diabetic retinopathy is thought of as a vision-threatening response to retinal ischemia (121–123). The mechanisms involved in the development of this major complication include breakdown of the inner blood-retina barrier, leading to retinal edema and liberation of cytokines and of inflammatory cells (77); strong vitreoretinal adherences provoked by gliovascular proliferation (124); and partial vitreous detachment (125) with formation of a strong and wide adhesion at the posterior wall of Shimizu's pocket, where vigorous traction forces can exert. These modifications are consequences of collagen alterations (e.g., cross-linking, nonenzymatic glycation forming early products such as glucitallysine, glucytallylhydroxylysine) (77,124,126). The presence of acidic and basic fibroblast growth factor and its synthesis has been demonstrated using immunocytochemistry and in situ hybridization in many retinal cell types. Vascular endothelial growth factor (VEGF) and insulin-like growth factor I have also been implicated (127,128). Loss of inhibition of new vessel formation by pericytes and normal basement membrane and putatively by the RPE suggests an imbalance between neovascularization promoting and inhibiting factors in the onset of proliferative diabetic retinopathy (100–102,107,129).

New vessels initially proliferate intraretinally from the venous side of the microcirculation. After having broken through the inner limiting membrane, they spread parallel to the inner retinal surface. As they grow toward the vitreous, they become densely attached to the posterior hyaloid if it is not detached (125). Because of their lack of tight junctions and the presence of fenestrations between endothelial cells, these new vessels are extremely leaky. In parallel or as a consequence of the neovascular network leakage and proteolytic activity, vitreous syneresis and collapse occur. Among vitreous alterations at the proliferative stage, changes in the extracellular matrix include accumulation of fibronectin and vitronectin (103,118,130,131), tinascin, and decorin, inducing modifications of cellular adhesion and proliferation. Vitreous retraction is limited by the strong neovascular tufts that are accompanied by a fibroglial component (originating from Müller's cells or astrocytes, hyalocytes, pericytes, RPE) forming preretinal membranes adherent to the retinal surface and the posterior hyaloid (Fig. 54-9) (103,118,130,131). Therefore, funnel-shaped contraction of the posterior hyaloid, a major evolutive event, provokes bleeding, retinal traction, or rhegmatogenous detachment, all causes of severe visual loss. Conversely, PVD prior to gliovascular proliferation appears to be protective.

This contraction is not only a consequence of biochemical or mechanical events. Intracellular contraction occurs in contractile cells such as myofibroblasts identified in proliferative diabetic retinopathy pathology specimens. Elaboration of neocollagen stabilizes contractile structures. Focal or plurifocal adherences can be either punctiform, at the level

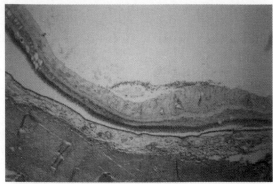

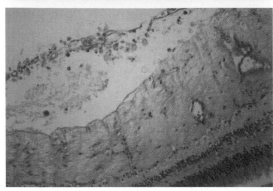

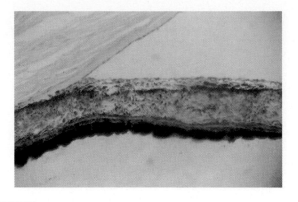

FIGURE 54-10. *Proliferative diabetic retinopathy. Angle-closure with synechiae rubeosis iridis (H&E, ×10). (Reprinted with permission from Sahel JA, Brini A, Albert DM. Pathology of the retina and vitreous. In: Albert DM, Jakobiec FA, eds.* Principles and practice of ophthalmology. *Philadelphia: WB Saunders, 1994:2261.)*

FIGURE 54-9. A. *Cystoid retinal edema and intraretinal gliosis in the ganglion cell layer with preretinal proliferation (H&E ×10).* B. *Thickening of the inner retina secondary to gliosis. Preretinal proliferation (H&E, ×40). (Reprinted with permission from Sahel JA, Brini A, Albert DM. Pathology of the retina and vitreous. In: Albert DM, Jakobiec FA, eds.* Principles and practice of ophthalmology. *Philadelphia: WB Saunders, 1994:2260.)*

of a neovascular pedicle, or diffuse, corresponding to epiretinal membranes. Most often, diffuse adherences are associated with retinal folding. They are formed by coalescence and retraction of a thickened and gliotic posterior hyaloid between multiple fibrovascular epicenters. Retinal detachments occur as a consequence of vitreous detachment. This event can start near temporal vessels at the posterior pole, near the optic nerve or macula, or in the midperiphery. According to studies (132,133) on 70 autopsy eyes, it can be absent (24%), total (7%), or partial (69%), stopped by the adherences. These detachment and adhesions concur to produce tractional forces, both tangential and anteroposterior. Most detachments can remain extramacular, with a rate of progression toward the macula of 14% at 1 year and 23% at 3 years (134). In some instances, the proliferation, mostly glial and fibroblastic, predominates at the temporal arcades, inside the limits of Shimizu's pocket, forming a contractile ring uniting these arcades. At this level, concentric contraction with a papillary epicenter provokes macular edema, detachment, or heterotopia (135). Other sites of neovascularization include the optic nerve and the iris (rubeosis iridis) (Fig. 54-10).

CHOROIDORETINAL MANIFESTATIONS OF TRAUMA

Direct Injury to Ocular or Periocular Tissue

Traumatic Retinopathy

Usually occurring after severe direct blunt ocular trauma, this condition is often termed *commotio retinae* or *Berlin's edema*, in recognition of its first description by Berlin in 1873 (136). The main feature of commotio retinae is whitening of the outer layer of the retina involving either the macular area only or extending to the peripheral area. This clinical picture is sometimes asymptomatic but may be associated with transient or permanent visual loss. The histopathologic features underlying the gray-white retinal opacity and its visual consequences were better understood after the studies by Berlin (136), Blight and Hart (137), Sipperly et al (138), Cogan (139), and Hart et al (140) all attributed this deep retinal opacity to extracellular or intracellular edema (Fig. 54-11). Histologic findings in animal models correlated this opacity with fragmentation of the photoreceptor outer segments and early damage to the photoreceptor cells. This disruption is followed after 24 hours by phagocytosis of fragmented outer segments by RPE cells. After 48 hours, the RPE cells begin to migrate into the neural retina, and with severe trauma these cells may be found throughout the entire retinal tissue. Disappearance of photoreceptor outer segments, in conjunction with RPE hyperplasia and migration, may result in direct apposition of multilayered RPE cells to photoreceptor inner segments and in diffuse thinning of the entire outer layer of the retina (137,138). A clinicopathologic study by Mansour (141) showed in the peripheral part of the retina, a disruption of the photoreceptors, subretinal accumulation of outer-segment debris and pigment granules, and alterations of the apex of RPE cells with remarkable preservation of the inner layer of the retina and Müller's cells. Cogan (139)

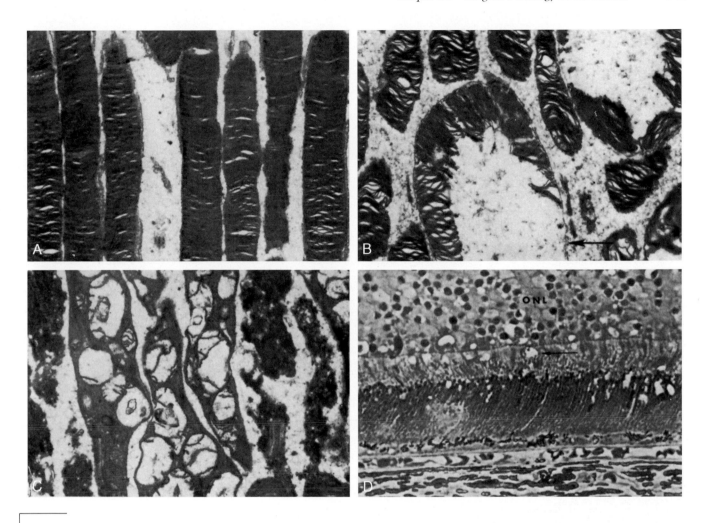

FIGURE 54-11. *A. Electron micrographs of normal photoreceptor outer segments of owl monkey (×9000). B. Compared with damaged outer segments (bottom) 4 hours after trauma. Note marked disruption of lamellar pattern and frank ruptures of plasma membrane (arrow) (×12,000). C. Electron micrograph of inner segments of photoreceptors 21 hours after trauma shows marked disruption of mitochondria (×12,000). D. Electron micrograph 40 hours after trauma. Note vacuolation of inner segment layer of photoreceptors (arrow) and marked number of pyknotic nuclei in outer nuclear layer (ONL) (paraphenylenediamine, ×140) (Reprinted with permission from Sipperly JO, Quigley HA, Gass JDM. Traumatic retinopathy in primates: the explanation of commotio retinae.* Arch Ophthalmol *1978;96:2267.)*

also found selective outer retinal damage simulating retinitis pigmentosa. In their animal model of traumatic retinopathy, Blight and Hart (137) described in addition to photoreceptor outer-segment disruption, transient damage to the RPE cell membranes associated with intracellular edema.

Traumatic Retinal Holes, Tears, Dialysis, and Detachment

The effects of direct or indirect trauma on the vitreoretinal interface may result in various types of retinal damage, including subretinal, intraretinal, or intravitreous hemorrhage; macular hole caused by vitreoretinal traumatic separation (67); retinal dialysis, giant tears, or horseshoe-shaped tears with opercula, which can be classified according to associated vitreoretinal relationships; and avulsion of the vitreous base (142,143).

Indirect Ocular Injury

Purtscher's retinopathy was first described in 1912. This retinopathy is characterized by peripapillary retinal hemorrhages and multiple patches of superficial whitening occurring after severe head trauma (144). However, similar fundus findings are encountered after the development of fat emboli and a rapid increase of nontraumatic intravascular pressure, most often caused by strenuous activities. These ophthalmoscopic features are associated with fluorescein leakage from the retinal arterioles, capillaries, and venules, as well as with arteriolar obstruction. Pathogenetic hypotheses include trauma-related acute endothelial damage predisposing the retinal vessels to intravascular coagulopathy or granulocytic aggregation, as well as air or fat embolism following chest compression or long-bone fracture, respectively (64,145). These presumptive mechanisms are supported by histopathologic and experimental results that are compatible with retinal arteriolar occlusion (146,147).

Shaken baby syndrome includes various ophthalmic findings involving mainly the retina that are present in association with neurologic and neurovegetative symptoms (64,148). The clinical picture is similar to Purtscher's retinopathy or retinal central vein occlusion (64). Histopathologic findings include intraretinal hemorrhage as well as submeningeal bleeding around the optic nerve (Fig. 54-12) (64,149).

Most posttraumatic choroid ruptures involve only Bruch's membrane and the underlying choriocapillaris. Direct ruptures occur anteriorly at the site of impact. Indirect ruptures occur as a consequence of coexisting lateral forces and the stabilizing effect of the optic nerve on adjacent structures and are generally posterior and display crescent shapes concentric to the optic nerve (145,150,151). Histopathologic findings at early stages include acute subretinal hemorrhage often associated with serous detachment of the macula and juxtapapillary region (Fig. 54-13) (64,151). As early as 6 to 14 days after injury, hemorrhage is followed by fibroblastic proliferation, resulting in the for-

mation of mature scar tissue after 3 to 4 weeks. RPE hyperplasia at the margins of the rupture and choroid neovascularization are part of the healing process. The latter most often regresses spontaneously without sequelae. However, in some instances subretinal or intravitreal new vessels may persist or develop at later stages and induce visual loss as a consequence of bleeding or exudation. Chorioretinal anastomoses also were reported by Goldberg (152). The role of Bruch's membrane breaks in the induction of choroid neovascularization is still debated (64,150).

Intraocular foreign bodies may be organic (vegetable or hair) or inorganic (lead, iron, copper, or gold). Intraocular iron may become oxidized and produce localized siderosis if the foreign body lodges in the sclera, or siderosis bulbi when the foreign body is intravitreally diffuse (153,154). The iron concentrates mainly in intraocular epithelial cells (e.g., iris and ciliary body epithelium, RPE, and inner limiting membrane neurosensory retina) (155). Accumulation of intracellular iron leads to inner retinal and RPE degeneration followed by full-thickness retinal degeneration and secondary gliosis (Fig. 54-14). A similar clinical picture is encountered after long-standing intraocular hemorrhage

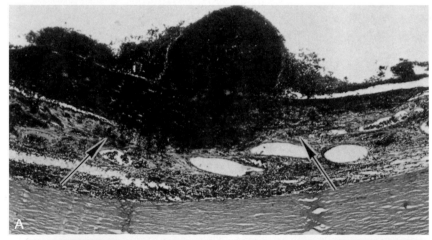

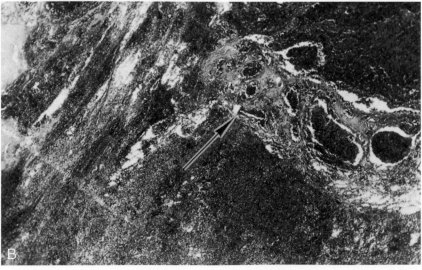

FIGURE 54-12.   *Examples of recent indirect choroidal ruptures. A. There is discontinuity of retinal pigment epithelium and Bruch's membrane (between arrows), with hemorrhage extending into the subretinal space (H&E, ×49, EP 55725). B. Area shows one margin (arrow) of choroid rupture (H&E, ×30, EP 46627). (Reprinted with permission from Spencer WH, ed. Ophthalmic pathology: an atlas and textbook. Vol. 3. Philadelphia: WB Saunders, 1986:1792.)*

(hemosiderosis bulbi) (64,118). Chalcosis differs because staining is primarily in the "glass membranes" of the eye, as is also seen in Wilson's disease (130,156,157). Chalcosis is also marked by an inflammatory reaction involving leukocytes, macrophages, and Müller's cells.

VIRAL INFECTIOUS RETINITIS

Herpes Simplex and Zoster Viruses

These viruses can cause, in healthy or immune-compromised patients, unilateral or bilateral acute and often necrotizing retinal lesions [acute retinal necrosis (ARN)] characterized by vitritis, retinal vasculitis, and pale yellow-white confluent retinal lesions. Herpes simplex virus type 1 (HSV-1) and less commonly, herpes zoster virus (HZV) infections can induce exudative retinal detachment and pro-

gressive outer retinal necrosis (PORN). Histopathologic studies, most often performed in patients who died from encephalitis, demonstrated acute and chronic inflammatory lesions of the optic nerve, RPE, and retina (158–162), providing both light and electron microsopic evidence for direct herpsevirus infection. In eyes with ARN, Culbertson et al (163) observed widespread full-thickness retinal necrosis sharply demarcated from adjacent areas, where eosinophilic cytoplasmic inclusions predominate in the inner layers. Inflammatory cells, mainly lymphocytes, are numerous in areas of vasculitis, choroiditis, and papillitis. In the late stages, Rummelt et al (164) noticed glial scarring, chronic granulomatous choroiditis, periarteriolar cellular infiltration, and ischemic optic atrophy. In eyes with active PORN, Margolis et al (165) found mostly multifocal necrotic areas, with minimal inflammation, and occasional vascular and optic nerve lesions.

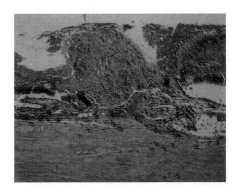

FIGURE 54-13. *Choroid rupture. Retinal hemorrhage and scar formation. (Reprinted with permission from Sahel JA, Brini A, Albert DM. Pathology of the retina and vitreous. In: Albert DM, Jakobiec FA, eds. Principles and practice of ophthalmology. Philadelphia: WB Saunders, 1994:2256.)*

Cytomegalovirus

In acquired adult disease, mostly in patients with acquired immunodeficiency syndrome (AIDS) or other immunodeficiency states, the lesions are often restricted to the neural retina and RPE (166). Choroidal lesions are either moderate or subjacent to retinal necrotic areas without viral antigens in the choroid (160). Retinal necrosis with disruption of all retinal layers is observed in multiple areas, either sharply demarcated or separated by a transition zone from normal retina. Viral antigens are identifiable in the retinal tissue (160). The inflammatory response is mild (167), comprising mostly lymphocytes with a reversal of the normal helper T-cell to cytotoxic T-cell ratio and some neutrophils (160). Consecutive to retinal necrosis, retinal holes predisposing to retinal detachment and gliotic membranes occur at late stages.

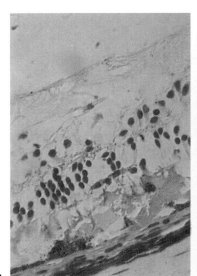
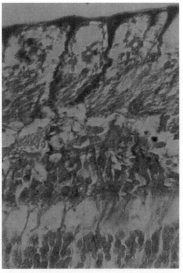

FIGURE 54-14. A. *Retinal degeneration and thinning following siderosis (H&E, ×40).* B. *Iron stain showing deposits in the retina (×63). (Reprinted from Sahel JA, Brini A, Albert DM. Pathology of the retina and vitreous. In Albert DM, Jakobiec FA, eds. Principles and practice of ophthalmology. Philadelphia: WB Saunders, 1994:2257.)*

A

B

RETINAL RADIATION AND DRUG TOXICITY

The literature on retinal radiation and drug toxicity has increased dramatically during the past two decades as physicians have gained a better understanding of the role and side effects of radiation in the treatment of ocular tumors and the lengthening list of potentially retina-toxic drugs used in therapy and industry.

Radiation retinopathy can be observed after brachytherapy or external irradiation and should be considered a "tissue-limiting toxicity of treatment" rather than a complication (168). Comparison of data between series is difficult because large variations in retinal cell sensitivity exist as a consequence of both the total dose and dose rate (mean, 50 Gy in weeks) and the length of follow-up and the association of chemotherapy or retinal vascular disease such as diabetes (169–171). Pathologic changes including dilatation, microaneurysm formation, loss of endothelial cells, endothelial proliferation, and capillary closure predominate on retinal vessels (172). Most of the changes induced in the neural retina can be considered merely as consequences of vascular lesions, as retinal neurons and photoreceptors, like the central nervous system, are resistant to radiation.

Photic retinopathy is a general term that describes various types of light-related damage to retinal cells resulting from photochemical, photodynamic, photocoagulative, or even mechanical processes. Light toxicity is widely quoted as a major pathogenetic mechanism in the etiology of age-related macular degeneration (ARMD), surgical microscope–induced lesions, and cystoid macular edema (173,174). Noell et al (175) showed that low levels of light, far too low to induce a thermal lesion, could, through cumulative effects, damage directly the photoreceptors at the level of the rhodopsin chromophore. Ham et al (176) showed that short wavelengths are more harmful and emphasized the protective role of melanin granules. Solar retinopathy is characterized by focal coagulation necrosis of photoreceptor cell nuclei and outer segments in the foveal area associated with focal necrosis, thinning, and depigmentation of the surrounding foveal RPE cells (64,177–181).

Several drugs have deleterious effects on the retina. Chloroquine is correlated histopathologically with degeneration of RPE cells, subretinal pigment clumping, and photoreceptor cell elements (182). Electron microscopy has disclosed inclusions in the ganglion cell layer and curvilinear intracytoplasmic bodies within the RPE; experimental studies demonstrated chloroquine deposition in ganglion cells, photoreceptors, and RPE cells; the primary site of toxicity is probably at the level of the RPE (183,184). Phenothiazines also accumulate at the level of the RPE and uvea within pigment granules (185) with secondary inhibition of enzymatic activity and phototoxicity. Yet, other study results are suggestive of a lesion of photoreceptor outer segments with accompanying or subsequent lesions of the RPE (186).

COATS' DISEASE

Coats' disease is characterized by vascular alterations, intraretinal exudates, and massive subretinal exudation or hemorrhage with cholesterol clefts and lipid-laden macrophages. Vascular changes include peripheral telangiectases, arteriovenous anastomosis, aneurysms of various sizes, and obliterative changes such as sheathing, sclerosis, perivasculitis, and fibrin deposition (135). Occlusion of the vascular lumen can result from endothelial swelling or proliferation and thickening of the wall by intramural fibrillar deposits (Fig. 54-15).

Intraretinal exudation usually occurs within the outer retina and is often associated with hemorrhage leading to the accumulation of fibrin, PAS-positive deposits, cholesterol clefts, and lipid-laden macrophages. The retina is usually detached, with subretinal exudates containing albumin, cholesterol clefts, macrophages, epithelioid cells, and ghost or foamy cells. The latter are derived from the RPE or histiocytes and glial cells. At later stages, the subretinal space is replaced by connective tissue, with fibrosis and fibrous metaplasia of RPE cells (135,187–193).

RETINOBLASTOMA

Retinoblastoma is the most common malignant eye tumor of childhood and the second most common primary intraocular malignancy of the eye. Approximately 1% of all deaths due to cancer before the age of 15 years have been attributed to retinoblastoma (194,195). The cell of origin has been the topic of debate since the Scottish surgeon Wardrop first recognized retinoblastoma as a discrete tumor, distinct from "fungus haematodes" or soft cancers that arose from the breast and limbs (196,197). His astute observations, published in 1809, were based on dissections and made without benefit of the microscope and convinced him that the tumor arose from the retina. Various pathologists of the nineteenth century, including Robin and Langenbec (198), confirmed these observations. Virchow named it a "glioma of the retina" (199,200), supporting glial cells as the cell of origin of the tumor. Flexner (201) and later Wintersteiner (202) suggested the use of the term *neuroepithelioma*, believing that the tumor was of neuroepithelial origin, and regarded rosettes that bear their names as an attempt to form photoreceptors. Verhoeff (201–203) concluded that the tumor was derived from undifferentiated embryonic retinal cells called *retinoblasts*, comparable to the neuroblasts originating from the medullary epithelium, and proposed the term *retinoblastoma* (204–206). The American Ophthalmological Society adopted this term in 1926 (207). Mawas in France proposed the term *retinoblastoma* for undifferentiated tumors in 1922 to 1924 (207). Zimmerman proposed to restrict the name *retinocytoma* to differentiate tumors displaying benign features under thorough histologic sampling, for which Gallie et al preferred the term *retinoma* (207,208). The most widely held concept of histogenesis of

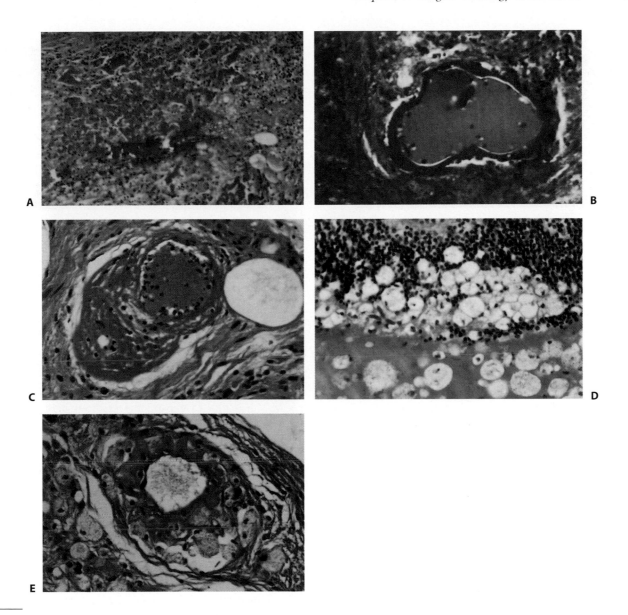

FIGURE 54-15. A. *Coats' disease. Exudative areas are better seen after staining with PAS. B. Telangiectasis and thickening of vascular wall. C. Telangiectasis; leaking of vascular wall, perivascular exudates. D. Lipid-containing macrophages. Foam cells in the retina and subretinal fluid. E. Perivascular foam cells. (Reprinted with permission from Brini A, Dhermy P, Sahel J.* Oncology of the eye and adnexa: atlas of clinical pathology. *Dordrecht: Kluwer Academic, 1990:127.)*

retinoblastoma holds that it generally arises from a multipotential precursor cell that could develop into almost any type of inner or outer retinal cell. This heterogeneity of the histopathologic, ultrastructural, and immunohistochemical features of retinoblastoma has been described (207,209–211).

By light microscopy, undifferentiated retinoblastoma is composed of small round cells with a large hyperchromatic nucleus of various shapes and scanty cytoplasm. Differentiated areas are found within many, most commonly as rosettes, first described by Flexner and Wintersteiner in the 1890s (Fig. 54–16) (201,202). These structures consist of clusters of cuboidal or short columnar cells around a central

lumen. The nuclei are displaced away from the lumen, which by light microscopy appears to have a limiting membrane resembling the external limiting membrane of the retina. Photoreceptor-like elements protrude through the membrane, and some taper into fine filaments (203,207). The lumen of these rosettes contains hyaluronidase-resistant acid mucopolysaccharides similar to those found between normal photoreceptors and the pigment epithelium (212). Homer Wright–type rosettes are seen less frequently than Flexner-Wintersteiner–type rosettes. These are composed of radial arrangements of cells around a central tangle of fibrils (213) and are identical to the rosettes found in neuroblastomas and medulloblastomas.

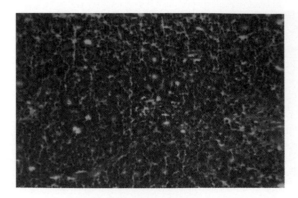

FIGURE 54-16. *Flexner-Wintersteiner rosettes. The aspect under low power has been compared to a flower bud. They differ from Homer Wright rosettes, which present a fibrillar center and are less distinctive. (Reprinted with permission from Brini A, Dhermy P, Sahel J.* Oncology of eye and adnexa: atlas of clinical pathology. *Dordrecht: Kluwer Academic, 1990:127.)*

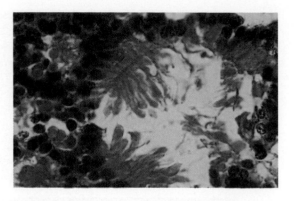

FIGURE 54-17. *Clusters of well-differentiated visual cells (Tso's "fleurettes"). The outer segments of the photoreceptors converge toward large cavities. (Reprinted with permission from Brini A, Dhermy P, Sahel J.* Oncology of the eye and adnexa: atlas of clinical pathology. *Dordrecht: Kluwer Academic, 1990:127.)*

An additional differentiated structure is the fleurette, first described by Tso et al (Fig. 54-17) (214). The fleurette is thought to represent a higher degree of photoreceptor differentiation. The term was applied to denote the fleur-de-lis–like arrangement of the apparently abortive photoreceptor structures characterized by larger cells with abundant eosinophilic cytoplasm and less hyperchromatic nuclei than the surrounding areas. Tso (215) suggested that tumors containing such benign components might be less radioresponsive. A few tumors are exclusively composed of benign-appearing cells exhibiting photoreceptor differentiation with almost no mitoses. These tumors represent the retinomas or retinocytoma (208) and may be the most benign end of the spectrum of malignant possibilities induced by the genetic mechanisms of retinoblastoma formation. Malignant transformation of this variant has been reported, however (216).

In widespread retinoblastoma with necrosis, the diagnosis may be confused by the degree of inflammation present. Areas of tumor necrosis are common in large tumors. Common findings include collars of viable tumor cells in uniform thickness surrounding the remaining blood vessels, often designated inappropriately as "pseudorosettes"; beyond these collars, ischemic areas of necrosis are prominent. Areas of intracellular and extracellular calcification are often present. In other areas of necrosis, large numbers of lymphocytes are observed, and hyperplasia of the vascular endothelium is seen, possibly including the lumen of vessels in some areas (217–219). Precipitated DNA tumor cells are occasionally evident, both surrounding and within the wall of the vessels and other structures at a distance from the tumor (220). It should be noted that areas of photoreceptor cell differentiation are devoid of necrosis. Probably related to necrosis, numerous inflammatory cells may be present, and in some cases, secondary endophthalmitis may occur (207,221,222). Rubeosis iridis accompanied by

ectropion uveae may develop, with resultant glaucoma or hyphema (222).

Early ultrastructural investigations of retinoblastoma served primarily to expand the previous light microscopic descriptions of the tumor (209,223–227). More noteworthy contributions gave evidence of the presence of photoreceptor cell elements in retinoblastoma (203,214,215,228), and a strong resemblance of retinoblastoma to human fetal retina has been demonstrated (229,230).

Retinoblastoma cells have been examined in some detail using transmission electron microscopy (231). Photoreceptor cell elements occur within Flexner-Wintersteiner rosettes, and fleurettes represent photoreceptor cell differentiation. Triple membrane structures involving both the nuclear and cytoplasmic membranes are extremely common in retinoblastoma and fetal retina. Annulate lamellae, cytomembranes that structurally resemble a nuclear envelope, occur in a high percentage of tumor cells. Cilia are plentiful and appear in longitudinal, oblique, and transverse planes. In the latter planes, nine double tubules with no central pairs are seen. This "9 + 0" pattern is characteristic of the photoreceptor cell. Microtubules can be identified in most retinoblastoma cells, most commonly in Golgi's area, but may be diffusely distributed throughout the cytoplasm. These cytoplasmic components have an outside diameter of 15 to 27 nm, a wall thickness of approximately 5 nm, and an indefinite length. The microtubules are often clumped together and on occasion may appear in the nucleus. The tubular structures in rod fibers observed by Fine (232) and by Sheffield (233) behave in a similar manner. Bristle-coated vesicles are found free in the cytoplasm, budding from the cell membrane, and in the intercellular spaces. These are believed to form at the cell surface by a pinocytic invagination of the apical membrane and subsequently to move toward and fuse with multivesicular bodies that serve to transport protein. Occasional retinoblastoma cells contain numerous dense-core granules structurally similar to those in cells of sympathetic innervation. Zonula adherens–like cell attachments occur and are similar to the junctions between normal photoreceptor cells. Giant cells have occasionally been demonstrated in retinoblastoma. Their significance is not clear (234). The surface morphology of retinoblastoma has been observed by scanning electron microscopy (231,235). Two distinct populations of retinoblastoma cells have been noted, one with abundant distinctive surface characteristics and the second relatively featureless. The first type of cell exhibits surface projections that are continuous with the plasma membrane and of various lengths (microvilli), spherical extensions of the cell surface representing transient extrusions of cytoplasm (zeiotic blebs), and ruffle-like structures (lamellipodia) on the free margin of the cell. Long, slender projections (filopodia) also develop. The second population of cells are spherical and smooth and are thought to represent cells in mitosis.

Most immunohistochemical studies aim at determining whether retinoblastomas derive from a common progenitor cell capable of differentiation into either glial or neuronal cells or from neuron-committed cells (236–239). Variables in these studies include tissue fixation, staining procedures, specific areas taken into consideration, tumor cell differentiation, antigen expressivity, and age of the tumor. Consequently, caution is required when interpreting most immunohistochemical results (240–244). A related controversy surrounds the interpretation of proliferating glial cells, seen occasionally. Whether they represent tumor cells or reactive stroma has not been fully resolved.

Neuronal Markers

Many studies demonstrated neuron-specific enolase (NSE) tumor cell lines (241,245–247). NSE has been detected in undifferentiated areas, well-differentiated areas, well-differentiated Flexner-Wintersteiner rosettes, and fleurettes (241,246). Synaptophysin, a neural membrane glycoprotein of presynaptic vesicles, has been detected immunohistochemically in 45 to 54 formalin-fixed and paraffin-embedded retinoblastoma specimens (248).

As described, strong evidence supports the presence of photoreceptor cell elements in retinoblastoma. Since the compelling studies by Felberg and Donoso (249), many antigens attributed to photoreceptor cells in the retina have been under scrutiny (250). Rhodopsin monoclonal antibodies have been demonstrated in fleurettes and Flexner-Wintersteiner rosettes. S antigen (arestin) monoclonal and polyclonal antibodies have been detected (251) in the same differentiated structures, in diffuse areas of differentiated retinoblastoma, in trilateral retinoblastoma, and in cell lines. S antigen could not be identified in undifferentiated retinoblastomas. Donoso et al (237,252) further demonstrated that monoclonal antibodies to rhodopsin and S

antigen bind to the same areas. They also mentioned a personal observation of retinoblastoma staining positively for α-transducin. This can be related to Bogenmann et al's finding of transcripts for L-transducin, as well as to the red- or green-cone cell photopigment in retinoblastoma cell lines (253,254). Genes to rod cell marker genes were not expressed, leading these researchers to suggest a cone lineage.

In the lumen of Flexner-Wintersteiner rosettes, Rodrigues et al (255–257) noted interphotoreceptor cell–binding protein (IRBP), which is secreted by the rod photoreceptor cells into the extracellular matrix. The amount of IRBP in tumor samples correlated with the degree of tumor differentiation.

Bridges et al (258,259) investigated retinoid-binding proteins in fresh tumors and in cell lines using a combination Western blot, Northern blot, and radiolabeled ligand-binding techniques. They found expression to be variable in tumor cells. The only retinoid-binding protein that was consistently expressed by both types of cells was IRBP, which was present at a level similar to that in a normal retina at 22 weeks of gestation, suggesting that these findings are consistent with the embryonic origin of the cells. These investigators suggested that the tumor did not arise earlier than the 22-week stage, but this remains speculative.

Tarlton and Easty (260) tested a panel of 18 monoclonal antibodies against six retinoblastomas and compared the reactivity of the tumor with adult and fetal retinas. They found that the closest normal cell type is a 13- to 16-week outer retinal cell. They noted, however, that the tumor expressed antigens detected in both inner and outer layers (260). Because of the potential of the precursor cell to differentiate into photoreceptor cells as well as "inner" retinal cells, they speculated a tumor origin from a primitive multipotential cell type that predominated before the eighth week of gestation and declined in parallel with later retinal development.

Conclusions are difficult to draw from such contradictory data. Tissue culture studies were first attempted to determine the cell of origin and differentiation patterns of retinoblastoma (261–263). Both *plasticity* and multipotentiality were demonstrated, thus contradicting many studies providing evidence for a neuronal nature and differentiation.

Complete spontaneous regression of retinoblastoma is an unusual but well-documented entity. Twenty-two histopathologic reports of 39 such tumors have been published (217,264–271). It is usually characterized by a severe inflammatory reaction followed by phthisis bulbi. Most researchers ascribe this to complete intraocular ischemic necrosis of the tumor after a central retinal vessel obstruction (217,272). Histopathologic study demonstrated dense calcification, necrotic tissue, fossilized tumor cells, massive proliferation of the RPE, inflammatory reaction, and various degrees of ossification. The constant finding of extensive calcification of these tumors led Verhoeff to speculate that necrosis may result from calcification (219). He proposed the therapeutic value of hypervitaminosis D, a hypothesis that recently found some support in vitro and in animal studies (273). Marcus et al (274) emphasized that a reliable distinction has not been made between spontaneous necrosis and retinomas-retinocytomas in nonphthisical eyes. These investigators concurred with Zimmerman (207) and others who view such tumors as benign variants of retinoblastoma. Each of these lesions differs from the patterns of tumor observed after irradiation (274) (i.e., formation of a glial scar with complete destruction of the tumor and associated atrophy of surrounding choroid and vessels after treatment).

LYMPHOMA

Except for the so-called reticulum cell sarcoma, vitreoretinal involvement by tumor cells in Hodgkin's or non-Hodgkin's lymphoma has rarely been documented pathologically (275–285). Therefore, when hemorrhage or exudate is seen, other mechanisms of retinal involvement should be suspected. Nonetheless, it must be borne in mind that actual retinal infiltrates by tumor cells may occasionally occur.

Diffuse large-cell lymphomas are often referred to as *reticulum cell sarcomas* or *histiocytic lymphomas* and *microgliomatosis* (281–284). Immunohistochemical and in vitro lymphocyte function studies demonstrated that these tumors are composed of transformed B and T lymphocytes (285). The misnomer *reticulum cell sarcoma* continues to be used because of the lack of a fully accepted definitive classification of non-Hodgkin's lymphomas and the relative paucity of information on intraocular involvement by lymphomas. *Large-cell B-lymphocytic malignant lymphoma* is the preferred term (286,287). This tumor occurs most frequently between the ages of 37 and 82 years, with a mean age at diagnosis of 61 years. Once a rare diagnosis, more than 120 cases have been reported in the past decade (270,288–303). Published case reports and pathology societies' presentations have declined, leading to a lack of accumulation of epidemiologic data. It appears, however, that there is no clear sexual or racial predisposition. Eighty percent of reported cases appeared bilaterally but were frequently asymmetric. The mean interval between diagnosis and death was 39 months (292).

Pathology

Vitreous samples are routinely processed with a Millipore filter and stained with the Papanicolaou stain (281,296). The tumor cells typically are large pleomorphic cells with scant cytoplasm and round, oval, or indented nuclei with prominent, eccentrically located nucleoli (282,302,304,305). Characteristic finger-like outpouchings are seen in some nuclei.

On cytopathologic examination, the presence of an intense inflammatory element may be confusing, and finding only normal-appearing lymphocytes in an aspirate does not rule out the diagnosis. Immunocytochemical identification of a monoclonal strain of B cells suggests neoplasia (306,307). Electron microscopy may demonstrate intranuclear inclusions, cytoplasmic crystalloids, and occasional pseudopodial extensions and cytosomes, as well as autophagic vacuoles (308). When a high level of clinical suspicion exists, some practitioners advocate the use of retinochoroid biopsy, arguing that the uvea is more densely infiltrated through the vitreous (221). Studies of enucleated eyes showed that tumor cells have a perivascular pattern in the retina and brain, whereas uveal involvement consists of diffuse infiltration usually occurring as placoid masses of closely packed cells. The cells characteristically form a mass between the RPE and Bruch's membrane (282). This uveal infiltration differs from lymphoid uveal infiltrates with low-grade small lymphoplasmocytic lymphomas that do not involve the retina and vitreous and were formerly termed *reactive lymphoid hyperplasia* (309,310).

RETINAL METASTASES

In contrast to the uvea, metastases to the retina are rare. Leys et al (311) reported two cases and compiled a review of the literature. This survey found 11 cases of retinal metastasis from carcinoma and 11 cases from skin melanoma. It is likely, however, that the actual incidence is higher because 1) prospective autopsy series should demonstrate foci of metastatic cells, as indicated by Fishman et al (312), who found two patients with retinal metastases in a series of 15 consecutive patients with skin melanomas; 2) the use of diagnostic vitreous aspiration or vitrectomy should improve detection of these cases (313–315); and 3) the length of survival of patients with carcinomas is increasing.

The primary tumor is usually a carcinoma of the lung, breast, stomach, retrosigmoid, or uterus or a skin melanoma (312,313,315–332). Tumor cells gain access to the retina by the internal carotid artery (319), possibly accounting for the frequent association with brain metastases (318). Uveal metastases, which represent the most common intraocular malignancy, are frequent and vitreous invasion may be associated with retinal metastases after infiltration of the superficial retina and retinal vessels (315,319,332).

In some patients with a known primary malignancy and metastases, tissue diagnosis may not be necessary. In other instances, vitreous surgery or aspiration (311,314,315, 328,333–335) is necessary and will facilitate the planning and treatment. A modified Papanicolaou stain and cytologic analysis by an experienced pathologist using immunocytochemistry techniques or electron microscopy may be required.

AGE-RELATED MACULAR DEGENERATION

Aging of the RPE is correlated histopathologically with an increase in size and content of lipofuscin parallel to a decrease in the number of melanin granules. The bases of RPE cells lose their digitations, and the cells become less cuboidal and regular in shape (62,336–338). The cells are separated from their basal membrane by membranous debris and basal laminar deposits. Degeneration of RPE cells can occur in several patterns, including lipoidal degeneration and apoptosis, while neighboring cells phagocytose the pigment released by degenerating cells and migrate in an attempt to maintain cell-to-cell contact. Pigment changes and atrophy result from exhaustion of these compensating processes (Fig. 54-18) (339).

On ultrastructural examination, Bruch's membrane is an acellular membrane composed of five layers (i.e., basal membrane of the RPE, inner collagen layer, elastic layer, outer collagen layer, and the basement membrane of the choriocapillaris). All are progressively altered with increasing age (340). Debris accumulates in Bruch's membrane in the inner collagen layer during the second decade of life and later on in the elastic layer, the outer collagen layer, and the choriocapillaris (341). Early light microscopy studies showed thickening, increased basophilia, and calcification of Bruch's membrane (342–344) corresponding at the ultrastructural level to an accumulation of coated membrane-bound bodies containing granular and vesicular material, and membranous debris along with a segment of long-spacing collagen (342–344). Changes in Bruch's membrane collagen affect initially the inner portions of the membrane, and in older age the outer layers. Collagen type I accumulates in the choriocapillaris and inner capillary region (345). Loss of hyaluronic acid (346) and progressive mineralization of Bruch's membrane, particularly the elastic layer, account for the loss of elasticity and the increased fragility.

During the seventh decade of life, as demonstrated by Sarks et al (337,338), a fine granular material accumulates between the RPE and its basement membrane. These basal laminar deposits are a major feature of age-related RPE impairment and are considered an abnormal secretory product elaborated by RPE cells, with subsequent deposition of collagen and fibronectin and later formation more internally of a hyalinized PAS-positive deposit (338–344).

Drusen are localized deposits of extracellular material between the basement membrane of the RPE and the inner collagen layer of Bruch's membrane. They are classified clinically and pathologically into several subtypes: hard, soft, diffuse, basal, nodular, mixed, and calcified regressing drusen. Hard drusen are correlated histopathologically with the accumulation of a hyaline PAS-positive material in the collagenous zones of Bruch's membrane. Data from ultrastructural studies (338,347–349) support the hypothesis that hard drusen develop either by extrusion of the basal portion of RPE cells (apoptosis) with its content of membranous debris (e.g., bristle-coated vesicles, tube-like structures) or by lipidization and lipoid degeneration of single cells (350,351). Soft (serous) drusen consist of amorphous material that stains lightly with PAS and contains ultrastructurally membranous debris located between the thickened basement membrane of the RPE and the other layers of Bruch's membrane (352). The actual difference between soft drusen and serous detachments of RPE may be only a matter of size. Moreover, some investigators consider these drusen to be merely an "intra-Bruch's membrane separation" as a consequence of an ill-defined localized accentuation of the continuous layer of membranous debris called *diffuse drusen* (353,354) or *basal linear deposits* (337,338). Therefore, soft drusen, like basal linear deposits, reflect a diffuse and severe dysfunction of the RPE that is likely to predispose to vascularization.

In contrast, hard drusen are considered representative of a more localized degenerative process, akin to dominant drusen. A correlation between hard drusen, reticular degeneration of the RPE, and geographic atrophy has been reported (338).

Other types of drusen have been described; most represent either mixed or evolving patterns [e.g., mixed (soft) drusen and calcified drusen]. Some degree of confusion exists about the terminology of drusen as a result of disagreement among pathologists regarding the precise definition of certain terms and the clinicopathologic correlations that they denote.

Visual loss in age-related macular degeneration results from photoreceptor degeneration and death as a consequence of geographic atrophy of the RPE and choriocapillaris or the complications of subretinal neovascularization.

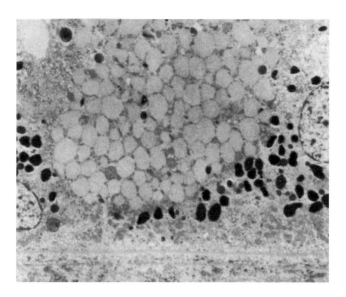

FIGURE 54-18. *A single retinal epithelial pigment cell with marked accumulation of lipid inclusion in an eye of a 40-year-old woman who had systemic lupus erythematosus and who had an orbital exenteration because of a squamous cell carcinoma of the lid (EP 4227, paraphenylenediamine ×3790). (Reprinted with permission from Green WR. Clinicopathologic studies of senile macular degeneration. In: Nicholson DH, ed. Ocular pathology update. New York: Masson, 1980:115–140.)*

Choroidal Alterations and Atrophic Form (Geographic or Areolar Atrophy)

Atrophy of the choriocapillaris is a common finding in age-related macular degeneration, as shown by Kornzweig (355) and confirmed by others (356,357). The extremely high rate of oxidative metabolism of photoreceptors is impaired, with subsequent photoreceptor degeneration and death in the areas of RPE atrophy (358). Sclerosis of the choriocapillaris underlying RPE atrophy in a lobular pattern, with thickening of the intercapillary septa and ultimately total choriocapillaris atrophy, has often been interpreted as an argument for a vascular pathogenesis of age-related macular degeneration. However, Green and Key (353) emphasized that such choroidal ischemia should have induced retinal lesions reaching to the inner nuclear layer (359), whereas retinal lesions in age-related macular degeneration are limited at early stages to the RPE and photoreceptor layer. Moreover, Henkind and Gartner (360) showed experimentally that destruction of the RPE induces *secondary* atrophy of the choriocapillaris. Geographic atrophy also can follow serous detachment of RPE or can coexist with subretinal neovascularization.

The pathogenesis of subretinal neovascularization is still disputed. Green (361,362) provided comprehensive descriptions. Neovascularization is located initially within Bruch's membrane and invades the sub-RPE space. As reviewed elsewhere (362), many authors emphasized that subretinal neovascularization is more clinically underestimated. Preservation of a good vision and masking of the new vessels by the RPE could explain this discrepancy. The use of indocyanine green angiography allows better visualization of occult new vessels, whether included in a fibrovascular tissue or in a RPE detachment. The subretinal capillaries are fenestrated, like their choroidal precursors, and induce subretinal transudates, exudates, and hemorrhage. Cystoid macular edema may be produced by subfoveolar new vessels (64). Invasion of the subretinal space occurs later, as shown by Green and Enger (363). Histopathologic findings include 1) breaks in Bruch's membrane, either secondary to thickening and increased fragility or produced by the neovascular ingrowth; 2) a granulomatous inflammatory pattern with macrophages, lymphocytes, and fibroblasts (364); 3) capillary-like vessels becoming at later stages arteries and veins; 4) basal laminar deposits and soft drusen; and 5) RPE depigmentation, hypertrophy and hyperplasia, and folding (337,338,353,365,366).

The interpretation of these findings remains uncertain. Yet, the sub-RPE location of most vessels and sources of neovascularization are rarely unique [average 2.2 per eye in the series of Green and Enger (363)]; they account for the poor functional results of submacular surgery in this condition (367). Among several histopathologic studies of specimens removed surgically, the one by Hsu et al (368) showed removal to be successful, with subsequent repopulation of the surgical area by RPE but the presence of neovascular tissue (persistence or recurrence) and marked photoreceptor loss.

RPE tears, which are actually intra–Bruch's membrane tears, most often are related to subretinal neovascularization (64,353,369). Disciform scars with a thickened vascular component and proliferation of the RPE are associated with photoreceptor atrophy, cystoid macular degeneration, and often choroidoretinal anastomosis (337,353,370).

In cases of submacular hemorrhage complicating subretinal new vessels, dramatic visual loss occurs as a consequence of sub-RPE hemorrhage, often followed by subretinal, intraretinal, and intravitreal breaking-through. Severe photoreceptor damage occurs if the blood is not removed within 7 days (371).

REFERENCES

1. Sahel J, Brini A, Albert D. Pathology of the retina. In: Albert D, Jakobiec F, eds. *Principles and practice of ophthalmology.* 2nd ed. Philadelphia: WB Saunders, 1998.
2. Marmor MF. Mechanisms of normal retinal adhesion. In: Glaser BM, Michels RG, eds. *Retina.* 2nd ed. Vol. 3. St. Louis: Mosby, 1994:1931–1953.
3. Zauberman H, Berman ER. Measurement of adhesive forces between the sensory retina and the pigment epithelium. *Exp Eye Res* 1969;8:276.
4. Zauberman H, de Guillebon H. Retinal traction in vivo and postmortem. *Arch Ophthalmol* 1972;87:549.
5. Hollyfield JG, Varner HH, Rayborn MF, Osterfeld AM. Retinal attachment to the pigment epithelium: linkage through and extracellular sheath surrounding photoreceptor. *Retina* 1989;9:59.
6. Machemer R. Experimental retinal detachment in the owl monkey. II: histology of retina and pigment epithelium. *Am J Ophthalmol* 1968;66:388.
7. Kroll AJ, Machemer R. Experimental retinal detachment in the owl monkey: photoreceptor protein renewal in early retinal reattachment. *Am J Ophthalmol* 1971;72:356.
8. Marcus DF, Aaberg TM. Intraretinal macrocysts in retinal detachment. *Arch Ophthalmol* 1979;97:1273.
9. Wilson DJ, Green WR. Histopathologic study of the effect of retinal detachment surgery on 49 eyes obtained postmortem. *Am J Ophthalmol* 1987;103:179.
10. Barr CC. The histopathology of successful retinal detachment. *Retina* 1990;10:189.
11. Guerin CJ, Anderson DH, Fariss SK. Retinal reattachment of the primate macula. *Invest Ophthalmol Vis Sci* 1989;30:1708.
12. Laqua H, Machemer R. Glial cell proliferation in retinal detachment (massive periretinal proliferation). *Am J Ophthalmol* 1975;80:602.
13. Laqua H, Machemer R. Clinical pathological correlation in massive periretinal proliferation. *Am J Ophthalmol* 1975;80:913.
14. Kroll AJ, Machemer R. Experimental retinal detachment in the owl monkey. II: Electron microscopy of retina and pigment epithelium. *Am J Ophthalmol* 1968;66:410.
15. Machemer R, Laqua H. Pigment epithelial proliferation and retinal detachment (massive periretinal proliferation). *Am J Ophthalmol* 1975;80:1.
16. Machemer R, VanHorn D, Aaberg TM. Pigment epithelial proliferation in human retinal detachment with massive periretinal proliferation. *Am J Ophthalmol* 1977;85:181.
17. Machemer R. Pathogenesis and classification of massive periretinal proliferation. *Br J Ophthalmol* 1978;62:737.
18. The Retina Society Terminology Committee. The classification of retinal detachment with proliferative vitreoretinopathy. *Ophthalmology* 1983;90:121.
19. The Retina Society Terminology Committee. An updated classification of retinal detachment with proliferation vitreoretinopathy. *Am J Ophthalmol* 1991;112:159.
20. Mandelcorn MS, Machemer R, Finberg R, et al. Proliferation and metaplasia of intravitreal retinal pigment epithelium cell autotransplants. *Am J Ophthalmol* 1975;80:227.

21. Glaser BM, Cardin A, Biscoe B. Proliferative vitreoretinopathy: the mechanism of development of vitreoretinal traction. *Ophthalmology* 1987;94:320.

22. Glaser BM, Lemor M. Pathobiology of proliferative vitreoretinopathy. In: Glaser BM, Michels RG, eds. *Retina*. 2nd ed. Vol. 3. St. Louis: Mosby, 1994:2249–2263.

23. Campochiaro PA, Kaden IH, Vidaurri-Leal J, Glaser BM. Cryotherapy and intravitreal dispersion of viable retinal pigment epithelial cells. *Arch Ophthalmol* 1985;103:434.

24. Singh AK, Michels RG, Glaser BM. Scleral indentation following cryotherapy and repeat cryotherapy enhances release of viable retinal pigment epithelial cells. *Retina* 1986;6:176.

25. Hagedorn M, Esser P, Wiedemann P, Heimann K. Tenascin and decoverin in epiretinal membranes of proliferative vitreoretinopathy and proliferative diabetic retinopathy. *German J Ophthalmol* 1993;2:28–31.

26. Marano RPC, Vilaro S. The role of fibronectin, laminin, vibronectin and their receptors on celular adhesion in proliferative vitreoretinopathy. *Invest Ophthalmol Vis Sci* 1994;35:2791–2803.

27. Grisanti S, Heimann K, Wiedemann P. Origin of fibronectin in epiretinal membranes of proliferative vitreoretinopathy and proliferative diabetic retinopathy. *Br J Ophthalmol* 1993;77:238–242.

28. Jaccoma EH, Conway BP, Campochiaro PA. Cryotherapy causes extensive breakdown of the blood-retinal barrier: a comparison with argon laser photocoagulation. *Arch Ophthalmol* 1985;103:1728.

29. Campochiaro PA, Jerdan JA, Glaser BM, et al. Vitreous aspirates from patients with proliferative vitreoretinopathy stimulate retinal pigment epithelial cell migration. *Arch Ophthalmol* 1985;103:1403.

30. Yamada KM, Olden K. Fibronectins—adhesive glycoproteins of cell surface and blood. *Nature* 1978;275:179–184.

31. Esser P, Heimann K, Wiedemann P. Macrophages in proliferative vitreoretinopathy and proliferative diabetic retinopathy: differentiation of subpopulation. *Br J Ophthalmol* 1993;103:1728.

32. Baudouin C, Fredj-Reygrobellet D, Gordon WC, et al. Immunohistologic study of proliferative vitreoretinopathy. *Am J Ophthalmol* 1989;108:387.

33. Charteris DG, Hiscott P, Robey HL, et al. Inflammatory cells in proliferative vitreoretinopathy subretinal membranes. *Ophthalmology* 1993,100. 43–46.

34. Fisher SK, Erickson PA, Lewis GP, Anderson DH. Intraretinal proliferation induced by retinal detachment. *Invest Ophthalmol Vis Sci* 1991;32:1739.

35. VanHorn DL, Aaberg TM, Machemer R, Fenzl R. Glial cell proliferation in human retinal detachment with massive retinal periretinal proliferation. *Am J Ophthalmol* 1977;84:383.

36. Fisher SK, Anderson DH. Cellular effects of detachment on the retina and the retinal pigment epithelium. In: Glaser BM, Michels RG, eds. *Retina*. 2nd ed. Vol. 3. St. Louis: Mosby, 1994:2035–2061.

37. Johnson RN, Gass JDM. Idiopathic macular holes: observations, stages of formation, and implications for surgical intervention. *Ophthalmology* 1988;95:924.

38. Kampik A, Green WR, Michels RG, Nase PK. Ultrastructural features of progressive idiopathic epiretinal membrane removed by vitreous surgery. *Am J Ophthalmol* 1980;90:797.

39. Clarkson JG, Green WR, Massaf D. A histopathologic review of 168 cases of preretinal membrane. *Am J Ophthalmol* 1977;84:1.

40. Kenyon KR, Michels RG. Ultrastructure of epiretinal membranes removed by pars plana vitreoretinal surgery. *Am J Ophthalmol* 1977;83:815.

41. Elner SG, Elner VM, Diaz-Rohena R, et al. Anterior PVR. II: clinicopathologic, light microscopic, and ultrastructural findings. In: Freeman HM, Tolentino FL, eds. *Proliferative vitreoretinopathy (PVR)*. New York: Springer, 1988:34–45.

42. Green WR. Retina. In: Spencer WH, ed. *Ophthalmic pathology*. Vol. 2. 4th ed. Philadelphia: WB Saunders, 1996:780–799.

43. Michels RG, Wilkinson CP, Rice TA. *Retinal detachment*. St. Louis: Mosby, 1990.

44. Lindsey PS, Michels RG, Luckenbach M, Green WR. Ultrastructural epiretinal membrane causing retinal starfold. *Ophthalmology* 1983;90:578.

45. Wilkes SR, Mansour AM, Green WR. Proliferative vitreoretinopathy: histopathology of retroretinal membranes. *Retina* 1987;7:94.

46. Trese MT, Chandler DB, Machemer R. Subretinal strands: ultrastructural features. *Graefes Arch Clin Exp Ophthalmol* 1985;223:35.

47. Hiscott P, Grierson I. Subretinal membranes of proliferative vitreoretinopathy. *Br J Ophthalmol* 1991;75:53.

48. Lewis H, Aaberg TM, Abrams GW. Subretinal membranes in proliferative vitreoretinopathy. *Ophthalmology* 1989;96:1403.

49. Schwartz D, De La Cruz Z, Green WR, et al. Proliferative vitreoretinopathy: ultrastructural study of 20 retroretinal membranes removed by vitreous surgery. *Retina* 1988;8:275.

50. Balazs EA. Molecular morphology of the vitreous body. In: Smelser GK, ed. *The structure of the eye*. New York: Academic, 1961:293–310.

51. Theopold H, Faulborn T. Scanning electron microscopic aspects of the vitreous body. *Mod Probl Ophthalmol* 1979;20:92–95.

52. Streeten RA, Wilson AJ. Disorders of the vitreous. In: Garner A, Klintworth GK, eds. *Pathobiology of Ocular Disease: A Dynamic Approach*. 2nd ed. New York: Dekker, 1994:700–742.

53. Kishi S, Shimizu K. Posterior precortical vitreous pocket. *Arch Ophthalmol* 1990;108:979.

54. Van der Rest M. Type IX collagen. In: *Structure and function of collagen types*. New York: Academic, 1987;195–221.

55. Seery CM, Davison PF. Collagens of the bovine vitreous. *Invest Ophthalmol Vis Sci* 1991;32:1540.

56. Spencer WH. *Ophthalmic pathology, an atlas and textbook*. Philadelphia: WB Saunders, 1996.

57. Akiba J, Veno N, Chakrabarti B. Molecular mechanisms of posterior vitreous detachment. *Graefes Arch Clin Exp Ophthalmol* 1993;231:408–412.

58. Foos RY. Posterior vitreous detachment. *Trans Am Acad Ophthalmol Otolaryngol* 1972;76:480.

59. O'Malley P. The pattern of vitreous detachment: a study of 800 autopsy eyes. In: Irvine AR, O'Malley C, eds. *Advances in vitreous surgery*. Springfield, IL: Charles C Thomas, 1976.

60. Eisner G. *Biomicroscopy of the peripheral fundus: an atlas and textbook*. New York: Springer, 1973.

61. Eisner G. Clinical anatomy of the vitreous. In: Jakobiec FA, ed. *Ocular anatomy, embryology, and teratology*. New York: Harper & Row, 1982:391–424.

62. Sebag J. Aging of the vitreous. *Eye* 1987;1:254.

63. Foos RY, Whielter NC. Vitreoretinal juncture synechiasis, senilis and posterior vitreous detachment. *Ophthalmology* 1982;89:1502.

64. Gass JDM. *Stereoscopic atlas of macular diseases: diagnosis and treatment*. 3rd ed. St. Louis: Mosby, 1987.

65. Gass JDM. Idiopathic senile macular hole: its early stages and pathogenesis. *Arch Ophthalmol* 1988;106:629.

66. Morgan CM, Schatz H. Involutional macular thinning: a pre-macular hole condition. *Ophthalmology* 1986;93:153.

67. Margherio RR, Schepens CL. Macular breaks: diagnosis, etiology and observations. *Am J Ophthalmol* 1972;74:219.

68. Franjieh GT, Green WR, Engel HM. A histopathologic study of macular cysts and holes. *Retina* 1981;1:311.

69. McDonnel PJ, Patel A, Green WR. Comparison of intracapsular and extracapsular cataract surgery: histopathologic study of eyes obtained post-mortem. *Ophthalmology* 1985;92:1208.

70. Smiddy WE, Michels RG, Green WR. Morphology, pathology and surgery of idiopathic vitreoretinal macular disorders. *Retina* 1990;10:288.

71. Smiddy WE, Michels RG, DeBustros S, et al. Histopathology of tissue during vitrectomy for impending idiopathic macular holes. *Am J Ophthalmol* 1989;108:360.

72. Smiddy WE, Maguire AM, Green WR, et al. Idiopathic epiretinal membranes, ultrastructural characteristics, clinicopathologic correlation. *Ophthalmology* 1989;96:811.

73. Madreperla SA, McCuen BW, Hickingbotham D, Green WR. Clinicopathologic correlation of surgically removed macular hole opercula. *Am J Ophthalmol* 1995;20:197–207.

73a. Ezra E, Munro PMG, Charteris DG, et al. Macular hole opercula. Ultrastructural features and clinico-pathological correlation. *Arch Ophthalmol* 1997;115:1381–1387.

74. Funata M, Wendel RT, de la Cruz Z, Green WR. Clinicopathologic study of bilateral macular holes treated with pars plana vitrectomy and gas tamponade. *Retina* 1992;12:289–298.

75. Madreperla SA, Geiger GL, Funata M, et al. Clinicopathologic correlation of a macular hole treated by cortical vitreous peeling and gas tamponade. *Ophthalmology* 1994;101:682–686.

76. Jaffe NS. Macular retinopathy after separation of the vitreoretinal adherence. *Arch Ophthalmol* 1967;78:585.

77. Sebag J, Buckingham B, Charles A, Reiser K. Biochemical abnormalities in vitreous of humans with proliferative diabetic retinopathy. *Arch Ophthalmol* 1992;110:1472–1476.

78. Green WR, Kenyon KR, Michels G, et al. Ultrastructure of epiretinal membranes causing macular pucker after retinal reattachment surgery. *Trans Ophthalmol Soc UK* 1979;99:63.

79. Foos RY. Vitreoretinal juncture, epiretinal membranes and vitreous. *Invest Ophthalmol Vis Sci* 1977;16:416.

80. Foos RY. Vitreoretinal juncture—simple epiretinal membranes. *Graefes Arch Clin Exp Ophthalmol* 1974;189:231.

81. Maguire AM, Smiddy WE, Nanda SK, et al. Clincopathologic correlation of recurrent epiretinal membranes after previous surgical removal. *Retina* 1990;10:213.

82. Grierson I, Hiscott PS, Hitchins CA, et al. Which cells are involved in the formation of epiretinal membranes? *Semin Ophthalmol* 1987;2:99.

83. Hiscott PS, Grierson I, McLeon D. Retinal pigment epithelial cells in epiretinal membranes: an immunohistochemical study. *Br J Ophthalmol* 1984;68:708.

84. Smiddy WE, Green WR, Michels RG, et al. Ultrastructural characteristics of vitreoretinal traction syndrome. *Am J Ophthalmol* 1989;107:177.

85. Russell S, Hageman G. Chondroitin sulfate-induced generation of epiretinal membranes. *Arch Ophthalmol* 1992;110:1000–1006.

86. Kono T, Kohno T, Inomata H. Epiretinal membrane formation. Light and electron microscopic study in an experimental rabbit model. *Arch Ophthalmol* 1995;113:359–363.

87. Linder B. Acute posterior vitreous detachment and its retinal complications: a clinical biomicroscopic study. *Acta Ophthalmol* 1966;87(suppl):1–108.

88. Mutlu F, Leopold IH. Structure of the human retinal vascular system. *Arch Ophthalmol* 1964;71:93.

89. Spencer LM, Foos RY. Paravascular vitreoretinal attachments. *Arch Ophthalmol* 1970;84:557–564.

90. Zarbin MA, Michels RG, Green WR. Epiretinal membrane contracture associated with macular prolapse. *Am J Ophthalmol* 1990;110:610.

91. Guyer DR, Green WR, de Bustros S, Fine SL. Histopathologic features of idiopathic macular holes and cysts. *Ophthalmology* 1990;97:1045.

92. Kampik A, Kenyon KR, Michels RG, et al. Epiretinal and vitreous membranes, comparative study of 56 cases. *Arch Ophthalmol* 1981;99:1445.

93. Rodman HI, Johnson FB, Zimmerman LE. New histopathological and histochemical observation concerning asteroid hyalitis. *Arch Ophthalmol* 1961;66:552.

94. Miller H, Miller B, Rabinowitz H. Asteroid bodies—an ultra-structural study. *Invest Ophthalmol Vis Sci* 1983;24:133.

95. Verhoeff FH. Microscopic findings in a case of asteroid hyalitis. *Am J Ophthalmol* 1921;4:155.

96. Grossniklaus HE, Frank KE, Farhi DC, et al. Hemoglobin spherulosis in the vitreous cavity. *Arch Ophthalmol* 1988;106:961.

97. Doft BH, Rubinow A, Cohen AS. Immunocytochemical demonstration of prealbumin in the vitreous in heredofamilial amyloidosis. *Am J Ophthalmol* 1984;97:296.

98. Kishi S, Tso MOM, Hayreh SS. Fundus lesions in malignant hypertension: a pathologic study of experimental hypertensive choroidopathy. *Arch Ophthalmol* 1985;103:1189.

99. Yanoff M. Ocular pathology of diabetes mellitus. *Am J Ophthalmol* 1969;67:21.

100. Merimme TJ. Diabetic retinopathy: a syneresis of perspectives. *N Engl J Med* 1990;322:978.

101. Frank RN. Etiologic mechanisms in diabetic retinopathy. In: Ryan SJ, ed. *Retina*. 2nd ed. Vol. 2. St. Louis: Mosby, 1994:1243–1276.

102. Frank RN. On the pathogenesis of diabetic retinopathy: a 1990 update. *Ophthalmology* 1991;98:586.

103. Garner A. Pathogenesis of diabetic retinopathy. *Semin Ophthalmol* 1987;2:4.

104. Yamashita T, Becker B. The basement membrane in the human diabetic. *Diabetes* 1961;10:167.

105. Joyce NC, Decamilli P, Boyles J. Pericytes, like vascular smooth muscle cells, are immunohistochemically positive for cyclic GMP-dependent protein kinase. *Microvasc Res* 1984;28:206.

106. Joyce NC, Haire MF, Palade GE. Contractile proteins in pericytes. Part 1. *J Cell Biol* 1985;100:1379.

107. Antonelli-Orlidge A, Saunders KB, Smith SR, D'Amore PA. An activated form of transforming growth factor beta is produced by cocultures of endothelial cells and pericytes. *Proc Natl Acad Sci USA* 1989;86:4544.

108. de Venecia G, Davis M, Engerman R. Clinicopathologic correlations in diabetic retinopathy. *Arch Ophthalmol* 1976;94:1766.

109. Bloodworth JMB Jr, Molitor DL. Ultrastructural aspects of human and canine diabetic retinopathy. *Invest Ophthalmol* 1965;4:1037.

110. Cogan DG, Toussaint D, Kuwabara T. Retinal vascular patterns. IV: diabetic retinopathy. *Arch Ophthalmol* 1961;66:366.

111. Bresnick GH, Davis MD, Myers FL, et al. Clinicopathological correlations in diabetic retinopathy. II: clinical and histologic appearances of retinal capillary microaneurysms. *Arch Ophthalmol* 1977;95:1215.

112. Bresnick GH. Non-proliferative diabetic retinopathy. In: Ryan SJ, ed. *Retina*. 2nd ed. Vol. 2. St. Louis: Mosby, 1994:1277–1318.

113. Grimes PA, Laties AM. Early morphological alteration of the pigment epithelium in streptozotocin-induced diabetes: increased surface area of the basal cell membrane. *Exp Eye Res* 1980;30:631.

114. Fine BS, Brucker AJ. Macular edema and cystoid macular edema. *Am J Ophthalmol* 1981;92:466.

115. Wolter JR. The histopathology of cystoid macular edema. *Graefes Arch Clin Exp Ophthalmol* 1981;216:85.

116. Tso MOM. Pathology of cystoid macular edema. *Ophthalmology* 1982;89:902.

117. Schatz H, Patz A. Cystoid maculopathy in diabetes. *Arch Ophthalmol* 1976;94:761.

118. Green WR. Pathology of the macula. In: Spencer WH, ed. *Ophthalmic pathology: an atlas and textbook*. Vol. 2. Philadelphia: Saunders, 1996:1124–1128.

119. Muraoka K, Schimizu K. Intraretinal neovascularization in diabetic retinopathy. *Ophthalmology* 1984;91:1440.

120. Ashton N. Studies of the retinal capillaries in relation to diabetic and other retinopathies. *Br J Ophthalmol* 1963;47:521.

121. Michaelson IC. The mode of development of the retinal vessels and some observations of its significance in certain retinal disease. *Trans Ophthalmol Soc UK* 1948;68:137.

122. Michaelson IC. *Retinal circulation in man and animals*. Springfield, IL: Charles C Thomas, 1954.

123. Patz A. Retinal neovascularization: early contributions of Professor Michaelson and recent observations. *Br J Ophthalmol* 1984;68:42.

124. Faulborn J, Bowland S. Microproliferations in diabetic retinopathy and their relation to the vitreous: corresponding light and electron microscopic studies. *Graefes Arch Clin Ophthalmol* 1985;223:103–108.

125. Foos RY, Krieger AE, Forsythe AB, et al. Posterior vitreous detachment in diabetic subjects. *Ophthalmology* 1980;87:122.

126. Augustin AJ, Breipohl W, Boker T, et al. Increased lipid peroxide levels and myeloperoxidase activity in the vitreous of patients suffering from proliferative diabetic retinopathy. *Graefes Arch Clin Exp Ophthalmol* 1993;231:647–650.

127. Grant M, Caballero S, Millard W. Inhibition of IGF-1 and b-FGF stimulated growth of human retinal endothelial cells by the somatostatin analogue, octreotide: a potential treatment for ocular neovascularization. *Regul Peptides* 1993;48:267–278.

128. Smith L, Kopchick J, Chen W, et al. Essential role of growth hormone in ischemia induced retinal neovascularization. *Science* 1997;276:1706–1709.

129. Baird A, Esch F, Gospodarowicz D, Fuillemin R. Retina- and eye-derived endothelial cell growth factors: partial molecular characterization and identity with acidic and basic fibroblast growth factors. *Biochemistry* 1985;24:7855.

130. Yanoff M, Fine BS. *Ocular pathology: a text and atlas*. 3r ed. Philadelphia: JB Lippincott, 1989.

131. Baudouin C, Fredj-Reygrobellet D, Lapalus P, Gastaud P. Immunohistopathologic finding in proliferative diabetic retinopathy. *Am J Ophthalmol* 1988;105:383.

132. Packer AJ. Vitrectomy for progressive macular traction associated with proliferative diabetic retinopathy. *Arch Ophthalmol* 1987;105:1679–1682.

133. Bresnick GH, Haight B, de Venecia G. Retinal wrinkling and macular heterotropia in diabetic retinopathy. *Arch Ophthalmol* 1979;97:1890.

134. Lewis H, Abrams GW, Blumenkranz MS, Campo RV. Vitrectomy for diabetic macular traction and oedema associated with posterior hyaloid traction. *Ophthalmology* 1992;99:753–759.

135. Coats G. Ueber retinitis exudativa (retinitis haemorrhagica externa). *Graefes Arch Clin Exp Ophthalmol* 1912;81:275.

136. Berlin R. Zur sogenannten commotio retinae. *Klin Monastsbl Augenheilkd* 1873;1:42.

137. Blight R, Hart JCD. Structural changes in the outer retinal layers following blunt mechanical non-perforating trauma to the globe. *Br J Ophthalmol* 1977;61:573.

138. Sipperly JO, Quigley HA, Gass JDM. Traumatic retinopathy in primates: the explanation of commotio retinae. *Arch Ophthalmol* 1978;96:2267.

139. Cogan DG. Pseudoretinitis pigmentosa: report of two traumatic cases of recent origin. *Arch Ophthalmol* 1969;81:45.

140. Hart JCD, Blight R, Cooper R. Electrophysiological and pathological investigation of concussional injury. *Trans Ophthalmol Soc UK* 1975;95:326.

141. Mansour AM, Green WH, Hogge C. Histopathology of commotio retinae. *Retina* 1992;12:24–48.

142. Cox MS, Schepens CL, Freeman HM. Retinal detachment due to ocular contusion. *Arch Ophthalmol* 1966;76:678.

143. Goffstein R, Burton TC. Differentiating traumatic from nontraumatic retinal detachment. *Ophthalmology* 1982;89:361.

144. Purtscher O. Angiopathia retinae traumatica: Lymphorrhagien de Augengrundes. *Graefes Arch Clin Exp Ophthalmol* 1912;82:347.

145. Williams DF, Mieler WF, Williams GA. Posterior segment manifestations of ocular trauma. *Retina* 1990;10:S35.

146. Pratt MV, De Venecia G. Purtscher's retinopathy: a clinicohistopathological correlation. *Surv Ophthalmol* 1970;14:417.

147. Ashton N, Henkind P. Experimental occlusion of retinal arterioles (graded glass ballotini). *Br J Ophthalmol* 1965;49:225.

148. Friendly DS. Ocular manifestations of physical child abuse. *Trans Am Acad Ophthalmol Otolaryngol* 1971;75:318.

149. Ober RR. Hemorrhagic retinopathy in infancy: a clinicopathologic report. *Pediatr Ophthalmol Strabismus* 1980;17:17.

150. Wyszinski RE, Grossniklaus HE, Frank KE. Indirect choroidal rupture secondary to blunt ocular trauma. *Retina* 1988;8:237.

151. Aguilar LP, Green WR. Choroidal rupture: a histopathological study of 47 cases. *Retina* 1984;4:269.

152. Goldberg MF. Choroidoretinal vascular anastomoses after blunt trauma to the eye. *Am J Ophthalmol* 1976;82:892.

153. Cibis PA, Yamashita T, Rodriguez F. Clinical aspects of ocular siderohemosiderosis. *Arch Ophthalmol* 1959;62:180.

154. Burch PG. Transcleral ocular siderosis. *Am J Ophthalmol* 1977;84:90.

155. Tawara A. Transformation and cytotoxicity of iron in siderosis bulbi. *Invest Ophthalmol* 1986;27:226.

156. Rosenthal AR, Appelton H. Histochemical localization of intraocular foreign bodies. *Am J Ophthalmol* 1975;79:613.

157. Rosenthal AR, Marmor MF, Leuenberger P, et al. Chalcosis: a study of natural history. *Ophthalmology* 1979;86:1956.

158. Minckler DS, et al. Herpes virus hominis encephalitis and retinitis. *Arch Ophthalmol* 1976;94:89–95.

159. Johnson BL, Wisotzkey HM. Neuroretinitis associated with herpes simplex encephalitis in an adult. *Am J Ophthalmol* 1977;83:481–489.

160. Pepose JS, et al. Immunocytologic localization of herpes simplex type I viral antigens in herpetic retinitis and encephalitis in an adult. *Ophthalmology* 1985;92:160–166.

161. Pepose JS, et al. Herpes virus antibody levels in the etiologic diagnosis of the acute retinal necrosis syndrome. *Am J Ophthalmol* 1992;113:248–256.

162. Holland GN, Tufail A, Jordan MC. Cytomegalovirus diseases. In: Pepose JS, Holland GN, Wilhelmus KR, eds. *Ocular Infection and Immunity*. St. Louis: Mosby, 1996:1088–1128.

163. Culbertson WW, Atherton SS. Acute retinal necrosis and similar retinitis syndromes. *Ophthalmology* 1993;33:129–143.

164. Rummelt V, et al. Detection of varicella zoster virus DNA and viral antigen in the late stage of bilateral acute retinal necrosis syndrome. *Arch Ophthalmol* 1992;110:1132–1136.

165. Margolis TP, et al. Varicella-zoster virus retinitis in patients with the acquired immunodeficiency syndrome. *Am J Ophthalmol* 1991;112:119–131.

166. De Venecia G, Zu Rhein GM, Pratt MV, Kisken W. Cytomegalic inclusion retinitis in an adult. *Arch Ophthalmol* 1971;86:44–57.

167. Jensen OA, Gerstoft J, Thomsen HK, Marner K. Cytomegalovirus retinitis in the acquired immunodeficiency syndrome (AIDS): light-microscopical, ultrastructural and immunohistochemical examination of a case. *Acta Ophthalmol (Copen)* 1984;62:1–9.

168. Maguire AM, Schachat AP. Radiation retinopathy. In: Ryan SJ, ed. *Retina*. St Louis: Mosby, 1996:1509–1514.

169. Brown GC, Shields JA, Sanborn G, et al. Radiation retinopathy. *Ophthalmology* 1982;89:1494–1501.

170. Lopez PF, Sternberg P, Dabbs CK, et al. Bone marrow transplant retinopathy. *Am J Ophthalmol* 1991;112:635–646.

171. Nakissa H, Rubin P, Strohl R, Keys H. Ocular and orbital complications following radiation therapy of paranasal sinus malignancies and review of literature. *Cancer* 1983;51:980–986.

172. Archer DB, Amoaku WMK, Gardner TA. Radiation retinopathy—clinical, histiopathological, ultrastructural and experimental correlations. *Eye* 1991;5:239–251.

173. Bord RD, Olsen KR, Ball SF, Packer AJ. The site of operating microscope induced light injury on the human retina. *Am J Ophthalmol* 1989;107:390–397.

174. Kraff MC, Sanders DR, Jampol LM, Lieberman HL. Effect of an ultraviolet-filtering intraocular lens on cystoid macular edema. *Ophthalmology* 1985;92:366–369.

175. Noell WK. Possible mechanisms of photoreceptor damage by light in mammalian eyes. *Vision Res* 1980;20:1163–1171.

176. Ham WT Jr, Mueller HA, Sliney DH. Retinal sensitivity to damage from short wavelength light. *Nature* 1976;260:153–155.

177. Tso MOM. Photic maculopathy in rhesus monkey: a light and microscopic study. *Invest Ophthalmol* 1973;12:17.

178. Tso MOM. Recovery of the rod and cone cells after photic injury. *Trans Am Acad Ophthalmol Otolaryngol* 1972;76:1247.

179. Tso MOM. The human fovea after sungazing. *Trans Am Acad Ophthalmol Otolaryngol* 1975;79:788.

180. Tso MOM. Effect of photic injury on the retinal tissues. *Ophthalmology* 1983;90:952.

181. Weiter J. Phototoxic changes in the retina. In: Miller D, ed. *Clinical light damage to the eye*. New York: Springer, 1987.

182. Wetterholm D, Winter FC. Histopathology of chloroquine retinal toxicity. *Arch Ophthalmol* 1964;71:82.

183. Ramsey MS, Fine BS. Chloroquine toxicity in the human eye: histopathologic observations by electron microscopy. *Am J Ophthalmol* 1972;73:229.

184. Rosenthal AR, Kolb H, Bergsma D, et al. Chloroquine retinopathy in the monkey. *Invest Ophthalmol Vis Sci* 1978;17:1158.

185. Weekley RD, Potts AM, Reboton J, May RH. Pigmentary retinopathy in patients receiving high doses of a new phenothiazine. *Arch Ophthalmol* 1960;64:65–76.

186. Miller FS III, Bunt-Millam AH, Kalina RE. Clinical-ultrastructural study of thioridazine retinopathy. *Ophthalmology* 1982;89:1478–1488.

187. Woods AC, Duke Jr. Coats' disease. I: review of the literature, diagnostic criteria, clinical findings and plasma lipid studies. *Br J Ophthalmol* 1963;17:385.

188. Ishikawa T. Fine structure of subretinal fibrous tissue in Coats' disease. *Jpn J Ophthalmol* 1976;20:63.

189. Henkind P, Morgan G. Peripheral retinal angioma with exudative retinopathy in adults (Coats' lesion). *Br J Ophthalmol* 1996;50:2.

190. Hada K. Clinical and pathological study of Coats' disease. I: clinical and histopathological observation. *Acta Soc Ophthalmol Jpn* 1973;77:438.

191. Givner J. Coats' disease (retinitis exudativa): a clinicopathologic study. *Am J Ophthalmol* 1954;38:852.

192. Bonnet M. Le syndrome de Coats. *J Fr Ophthalmol* 1980;3:57.

193. Archer D, Krill AE. Leper's miliary aneurysms and optic atrophy. *Surv Ophthalmol* 1971;15:384.

194. Devesa SS. The incidence of retinoblastoma. *Am J Ophthalmol* 1875;80:263.

195. Miller RW. Fifty-two forms of childhood cancer: United States mortality experience 1960–1966. *J Pediatr* 1969;75:685.

196. Albert DM. Historic review of retinoblastoma. *Ophthalmology* 1987;94:654.

197. Wardrop J. *Observations on the fungus Haematodes*. Edinburgh: Constable, 1809.

198. Dunphy EB. The story of retinoblastoma. *Trans Am Acad Ophthalmol Otolaryngol* 1964;68:249.

199. Virchow R. *Die Kranklaften Gesswuelste*. Vol. 2. Berlin: August Hirschwals, 1864.

200. Hemes GD. Untersuchung nach dem Vorkommen von Glioma Retinae bei Verwandte von mit dieser Krankheit Behafteten. *Klin Monatsbl Augenheilkd* 1931;82:331.

201. Flexner S. A peculiar glioma (neuroepithelioma) of the retina. *Bull Johns Hopkins Hosp* 1891;2:115.

202. Wintersteiner H. *Die Neuroepithelioma Retinae. Etine Anatomische und Klinische Studie*. Leipzig: Dentisae, 1897.

203. Tso MOM. The Flexner-Wintersteiner rosette in retinoblastoma. *Arch Pathol* 1969;88:664.

204. Herm RL, Heath P. A study of retinoblastoma. *Am J Ophthalmol* 1956;41:22.

205. Verhoeff FH. A rare tumor arising from the pars ciliaris retinae (teratoneuroma) of a nature hitherto unrecognized and its relation to the so-called glioma retinae. *Trans Am Ophthalmol Soc* 1904;10:351.

206. Verhoeff FH, Jackson E. Minutes of the proceedings. Sixty-second Annual Meeting of Trans Am Ophthalmol. *Trans Am Ophthalmol Soc* 1926;24:33.

207. Zimmerman LE. Retinoblastoma and retinocytoma. In: Spencer WH, ed. *Ophthalmic pathology*. Vol. 2. Philadelphia: Saunders, 1985.

208. Margo C, Hidayat A, Kopelman J, Zimmerman LE. Retinocytoma: a benign variant of retinoblastoma. *Arch Ophthalmol* 1983;101:1519.

209. Allen RA, Latta H, Straatsma BR. Retinoblastoma. *Invest Ophthalmol* 1962;1:728.

210. Macklin MT. A study of retinoblastoma in Ohio. *Am J Hum Genet* 1960;12:1.

211. Mafee WF, Goldberg MF, Cohen SB, et al. Magnetic resonance imaging versus computed tomography of leukocoric eyes and use of vitro proton magnetic resonance spectroscopy of retinoblastoma. *Ophthalmology* 1989;96:965.

212. Zimmerman LE. Application of histochemical methods for the demonstration of acid mucopolysaccharides to ophthalmic pathology. *Trans Am Acad Ophthalmol Otolaryngol* 1958;62:697.

213. Wright JH. Neurocytoma or neuroblastoma: a kind of tumor not generally recognized. *J Exp Med* 1910;12:556.

214. Tso MOM, Zimmerman LE, Fine BS, Ellsworth RM. A cause of radioresistance in retinoblastoma: photoreceptor differentiation. *Trans Am Acad Ophthalmol Otolaryngol* 1970;74:959.

215. Tso MOM. The nature of retinoblastoma. I: photoreceptor differentiation: a clinical and histopathologic study. *Am J Ophthalmol* 1970;89:339.

216. Eagle RC, Shields JA, Donoso L, Miller R. Malignant transformation of spontaneously regressed retinoblastoma, retinoma/retinocytoma variant. *Ophthalmology* 1989;96:1389.

217. Albert DM, Sang DN, Craft JL. Clinical and histopathologic observations regarding cell death and tumor necrosis in retinoblastoma. *Jpn J Ophthalmol* 1978;22:358.

218. Kremer I, Hartmann B, Haviv D, et al. Immunohistochemical diagnosis of a totally necrotic retinoblastoma: a clinicopathological case. *J Pediatr Ophthalmol Strabismus* 1988;25:90.

219. Verhoeff FH. Retinoblastoma undergoing spontaneous regression: calcification agent suggested in treatment of retinoblastoma. *Am J Ophthalmol* 1966;62:573.

220. Mullaney J. DNA in retinoblastoma. *Lancet* 1968;2:918.

221. Char DH. *Clinical ocular oncology.* New York: Churchill Livingstone, 1989.

222. Shields JA. *Diagnosis and management of intraocular tumors.* St. Louis: Mosby, 1983.

223. Bierring F, Egeberg J, Jensen OA. A contribution to the ultrastructural study of retinoblastoma. *Acta Ophthalmol* 1967;45:424.

224. Francois J, Hanssens M, Lagasse A. The ultrastructure of retinoblastoma. *Ophthalmologica* 1965;149:53.

225. Matsuo N, Takayama T. Electron microscopic observations of visual cells in a case of retinoblastoma. *Folia Ophthalmol Jpn* 1965;16:574.

226. Tokunaya T, Nakamura S. Electron microscopic features of retinoblastoma. *Acta Soc Ophthalmol Jpn* 1963;67:1358.

227. Ikui H, Tominaya Y, Konomi I, Ueono K. Electron microscopic studies on the histogenesis of retinoblastoma. *Jpn J Ophthalmol* 1966;10:282.

228. Tso MOM, Zimmerman LE, Fine BS. The nature of retinoblastoma. II: photoreceptor differentiation: an electron microscopic study. *Am J Ophthalmol* 1970;89:350.

229. Popoff N, Ellsworth RM. The fine structure of nuclear alterations in retinoblastoma and the developing human retina: in vivo and in vitro observations. *J Ultrastruct Res* 1969;29:535.

230. Popoff N, Ellsworth RM. The fine structure of retinoblastoma: in vivo and in vitro observations. *Lab Invest* 1971;25:389.

231. Albert DM, Craft JL, Sang DN. Ultrastructure of retinoblastoma: transmission and scanning electron microscopy. In: Jakobiec FA, ed. *Ocular and adnexal tumors.* Birmingham, AL: Aesculapius, 1978:157–172.

232. Fine BS. Observations on the axoplasm of neural elements in the human retina. *Proceedings of the Third European Regional Conference on Electron Microscopy.* Prague: Publishing House of Czechoslovak Academy of Science, 1964:319.

233. Sheffield JB. Microtubules in the outer layer of rabbit retina. *J Microsc* 1966;5:173.

234. Howard MA, Dryja TP, Walton DS, Albert DM. Identification and significance of multinucleated cells in retinoblastoma. *Arch Ophthalmol* 1989;107:1025.

235. Craft JL, Robinson NL, Roth NA, Albert DM. Scanning electron microscopy of retinoblastoma. *Exp Eye Res* 1978;27:519.

236. Bonnin JM, Rubenstein LJ. Immunohistochemistry of central nervous system tumors: its contributions to neurosurgical diagnosis. *J Neurosurg* 1984;60:1121.

237. Donoso LA, Shields CA, Lee E. Immunohistochemistry of retinoblastoma. *Ophthalmic Paediatr Genet* 1989;10:3.

238. Molnar ML, Stefansson K, Marton LS, et al. Immunohistochemistry of retinoblastoma in humans. *Am J Ophthalmol* 1984;97:301.

239. Sasaki A, Ogawa A, Nakazato Y, Ishido Y. Distribution of neurofilament protein and neuron-specific enolase in peripheral neuronal tumors. *Virchows Arch (A)* 1985;407:33.

240. Campbell M, Chader G. Retinoblastoma cells in tissue culture. *Ophthalmic Paediatr Genet* 1988;9:171.

241. Kivela T. *Antigenic properties of retinoblastoma tissue.* Helsinki: University of Helsinki, 1987.

242. Kivela T, Tarkkanen A. S-100 protein in retinoblastoma revisited. *Acta Ophthalmol* 1986;64:664.

243. Roberts DF, Duggan-Keen M, Aherene GES, Long DR. Immunogenetic studies in retinoblastoma. *Br J Ophthalmol* 1986;70:686.

244. Garrido CM, Arra A. Studies of ocular retinoblastoma with immunoperoxidase technique. *Ophthalmologica* 1986;193:242.

245. Abramson DH, Greenfield DS, Ellsworth RM, et al. Neuron specific enolase and retinoblastoma: clinicopathologic correlations. *Retina* 1989;9:148.

246. Kivela T. Neuron-specific enolase in retinoblastoma: an immunohistochemical study. *Acta Ophthalmol* 1986;64:19.

247. Kobayashi M, Sawada T, Mukai N. Immunohistochemical evidence of neuron specific enolase (NSE) in human adenovirus-12 induced retinoblastoma-like tumor cells in vitro. *Acta Histochem Cytochem* 1985;18:551.

248. Virtanen I, Kivela T, Bugnoli M, et al. Expression of intermediate filaments and synaptophysin show neuronal properties and lack of glial characteristics in Y79 retinoblastoma cell. *Lab Invest* 1988;59:649.

249. Felberg NT, Donoso LA. Surface cytoplasmic antigens in retinoblastoma. *Invest Ophthalmol Vis Sci* 1980;19:1242.

250. Vrabec T, Arbizo V, Adamus G, et al. Rod cell-specific antigens in retinoblastoma. *Arch Ophthalmol* 1989;107:1061.

251. Donoso LA, Hamm H, Dietzschold B, et al. Rhodopsin and retinoblastoma. *Arch Ophthalmol* 1986;104:111.

252. Donoso LA, Rorke LB, Shields JA, et al. S-Antigen immunoreactivity in trilateral retinoblastoma. *Am J Ophthalmol* 1987;103:57.

253. Bogenmann E. Retinoblastoma cell differentiation in culture. *Int J Cancer* 1986;38:833.

254. Bogenmann E, Lochrie MA, Simon MI. Cone cell specific genes expressed in retinoblastoma. *Science* 1988;240:76.

255. Rodriques MM, Wilson ME, Wiggert B, et al. Retinoblastoma: a clinical, immunohistochemical, and electron microscopic case report. *Ophthalmology* 1988;93:1010.

256. Rodriques MM, Wiggert B, Shields J, et al. Retinoblastoma: immunohistochemistry and cell differentiation. *Ophthalmology* 1987;94:378.

257. He W, Hashimoto H, Tsuneyoshi M, et al. A reassessment of histological classification and an immunohistochemical study of 88 retinal blastomas. *Cancer* 1992;70:2901.

258. Bridges CDB, Fong SL, Landers RA, et al. Interstitial retinal binding protein (IRBP) in retinoblastoma. *Neurochem Int* 1985;7:875.

259. Fong SL, Balakier H, Canton M, et al. Retinoid-binding proteins in retinoblastoma tumors. *Cancer Res* 1988;48:1124.

260. Tarlton JF, Easty DL. Immunohistological characterization of retinoblastoma and related ocular tissue. *Br J Ophthalmol* 1990;74:144.

261. Herman MM, Perentes E, Katsetos CD, et al. Neuroblastic differentiation potential of the human retinoblastoma cell lines Y-79 and WERI-Rb-1 maintained in an organ culture system. *Am J Pathol* 1989;134:115.

262. Kyritsis AP, Tsokos M, Triche TJ, Chader GJ. Retinoblastoma: origin from a primitive neuroectodermal cell? *Nature* 1984;307:471.

263. Lemieux N, Leung T, Michaud J, et al. Neuronal and photoreceptor differentiation of retinoblastoma in culture. *Ophthalmic Paediatr Genet* 1990;11:109.

264. Boniuk M, Zimmerman LE. Spontaneous regression of retinoblastoma. *Int Ophthalmol Clin* 1962;2:525.

265. Boniuk M, Girard LJ. Spontaneous regression of bilateral retinoblastoma. *Trans Am Acad Ophthalmol Otolaryngol* 1969;73:194.

266. Karsgaard AT. Spontaneous regression of retinoblastoma: a report of 2 cases. *Can J Ophthalmol* 1971;6:218.

267. Lindley-Smith JS. Histology and spontaneous regression of retinoblastoma. *Trans Ophthalmol Soc UK* 1974;94:953.

268. Morris WE, LaPiana FG. Spontaneous regression of bilateral retinoblastoma with preservation of normal visual acuity. *Am J Ophthalmol* 1974;6:1192.

269. Nehen JH. Spontaneous regression of retinoblastoma. *Acta Ophthalmol* 1975;53:647.

270. Reese AB. *Tumors of the eye.* 3rd ed. New York: Harper & Row, 1976.

271. Stewart JK, Smith JLS, Arnold EL. Spontaneous regression of retinoblastoma. *Br J Ophthalmol* 1956;40:449.

272. Sang DN, Albert DM. Recent advances in the study of retinoblastoma. In: Peyman GA, Apple DJ, Sanders DR, eds. *Intraocular tumors.* New York: Appleton-Century-Crofts, 1977:172–180.

273. Cohen SM, Saulenas AM, Sullivan CR, Albert DM. Further studies of the effect of vitamin D on retinoblastoma: inhibition with 1,25 dihydroxycholecalciferol. *Arch Ophthalmol* 1988;106:541.

274. Marcus DM, Craft JL, Albert DM. Histopathologic verification of Verhoeff's 1918 irradiation cure of retinoblastoma. *Ophthalmology* 1990;97:221.

275. Gartner J. Mycosis fungoides mit Beteiligung der Aderhaut. *Klin Monatsbl Augenheilkd* 1957;131:61.

276. Karp LA, Zimmerman LE, Payne T. Intraocular involvement in Burkitt's lymphoma. *Arch Ophthalmol* 1971;85:295.

277. Keltner JL, Fritsch E, Cykiert RC, Albert DM. Mycosis fungoides, intraocular and central nervous system involvement. *Arch Ophthalmol* 1977;95:645.

278. Nelson CC, Hertzberg BS, Klintworth GK. Histopathologic study of 716 unselected eyes in patients with cancer at the time of death. *Am J Ophthalmol* 1983;95:788.

279. Schachat AP. Leukimas and lymphomas. In: Ryan SJ, ed. *Retina*. Vol. 1. St. Louis: Mosby, 1989:775–793.

280. Fisher D, Mantell BS, Urich H. The clinical diagnosis and treatment of microgliomatosis: report of a case. *J Neurol Psychiatry* 1969;81:591.

281. Fisher ER, Davis ER, Lemmen LJ. Reticulum cell sarcoma of the brain (microglioma). *Arch Neurol Psychiatry* 1959;81:591.

282. Mann RB, Jaffee ES, Berard CW. Malignant lymphoma: a conceptual understanding of morphologic diversity. *Am J Pathol* 1979;94:105.

283. Russell DS, Rubenstein LJ. *Pathology of the nervous system*. Vol. 1. 4th ed. Baltimore: Williams & Wilkins, 1977.

284. Schaumburg HH, Plank CR, Adams RD. The reticulum cell sarcoma microglia group of brain tumors: a consideration of their clinical features and therapy. *Brain* 1972;95:199.

285. Portlock CS. The non-Hodgkin's lymphomas. In: Wyngaarden JB, Mith LH, eds. *Cecil's textbook of medicine*. Philadelphia: Saunders, 1988:994–999.

286. Harris NL, Jaffe ES, Stern H, et al. A revised European-American classification of lymphoid neoplasm: a proposal from the International Lymphoma Study Group. *Blood* 1994;84:1361–1392.

287. Green W. The uveal tract, lymphomas. In: Spencer W, ed. *Ophthalmic pathology: a text and atlas*. Vol. 3. 4th ed. Philadelphia: Saunders, 1996:1741–1774.

288. Allen RA, Straatsma BR. Ocular involvement in leukemia and allied disorders. *Arch Ophthalmol* 1961;66:490.

289. Barr C, Green WR, Payne JE, et al. Intraocular reticulum cell sarcoma: clinicopathologic study of four cases and review of the literature. *Surv Ophthalmol* 1975;19:224.

290. Cooper EL, Riker JL. Malignant lymphoma of the uveal tract. *Am J Ophthalmol* 1951;34:1153.

291. Currey TA, Deutsch AR. Reticulum cell sarcoma of the uvea. *South Med J* 1965;58:919.

292. Freeman LN, Schachat AP, Knox DL, et al. Clinical features, laboratory investigation, and survival in ocular reticulum cell sarcoma. *Ophthalmology* 1987;94:1631.

293. Givner I. Malignant lymphoma with ocular involvement. *Am J Ophthalmol* 1955;239:29.

294. Green WR. The retina. In: Spencer WH, ed. *Ophthalmic pathology: an atlas and textbook*. Vol. 2. 4th ed. Philadelphia: Saunders, 1996:1133–1141.

295. Klingele TC, Hogan MJ. Ocular reticulum cell sarcoma. *Am J Ophthalmol* 1975;79:39.

296. Michels RG, Knox DL, Erozan YS, Green WR. Intraocular reticulum cell sarcoma: diagnosis by pars plana vitrectomy. *Arch Ophthalmol* 1975;93:1331.

297. Mincker DS, Font RL, Zimmerman LE. Uveitis and reticulum cell sarcoma of the brain with bilateral neoplastic seeding of vitreous without retinal or uveal involvement. *Am J Ophthalmol* 1975;80:433.

298. Nevins RC Jr, Frey WW, Elliott JH. Primary solitary intraocular reticulum cell sarcoma (microgliomatosis): a clinicopathologic case report. *Trans Am Acad Ophthalmol Otolaryngol* 1968;72:867.

299. O'Connor GR. The uvea. *Arch Ophthalmol* 1973;89:505.

300. Babel J, Owens G. Sarcome reticulaire intra-oculaire et cerebral. *Arch Ophtalmol (Paris)* 1975;35:409.

301. Sullivan SF, Dallow RL. Intraocular reticulum cell sarcoma: its dramatic response to systemic chemotherapy and its angiogenic potential. *Ann Ophthalmol* 1977;9:401.

302. Vogel MH, Font RL, Zimmerman LE, Levine RA. Reticulum cell sarcoma of the retina and uvea: report of six cases and review of the literature. *Am J Ophthalmol* 1968;66:205.

303. Guyer DR, Schachat AP, Vitale S, et al. Leukemic retinopathy: relationship between fundus lesions and hematologic parameters at diagnosis. *Ophthalmology* 1988;96:860.

304. Cravioto H. Human and experimental reticulum cell sarcoma (microglia of the nervous system). *Acta Neuropathol (Berl)* 1975;4(suppl):135.

305. Polack M. Microglioma and/or reticulosarcoma of the nervous system. *Acta Neuropathol (Berl)* 1975;6(suppl):115.

306. Corriveau C, Esterbrook M, Payne D. Lymphoma simulating uveitis (masquerade syndrome). *Can J Ophthalmol* 1986;21:144.

307. Kaplan HJ, Meredith TA, Aaberg TM, Keller RH. Reclassification of intraocular reticulum cell sarcoma (histiocytic lymphoma): immunologic characterization of vitreous cells. *Arch Ophthalmol* 1980;98:707.

308. Horvat B, Pen C, Fisher ER. Primary reticulum cell sarcoma (microgliosis) of the brain. *Arch Pathol* 1969;87:609.

309. BenEzra D, Sahel JA, Harris NL, et al. Uveal lymphoid infiltrates: immunohistochemical evidence for lymphoid neoplasia. *Br J Ophthalmol* 1989;73:846.

310. Jakobiec FA, Sacks E, Kronish HW, et al. Multifocal static creamy choroidal infiltrates: an early sign of lymphoid neoplasia. *Ophthalmology* 1987;94:397.

311. Leys AM, VanEyck LM, Nuttin BJ, et al. Metastatic carcinoma to the retina: clinicopathologic findings in two cases. *Arch Ophthalmol* 1990;108:1448.

312. Fishman ML, Tomaszewski MM, Kuwabara T. Malignant melanoma of the skin metastatic to the eye: frequency in autopsy series. *Arch Ophthalmol* 1976;94:1309.

313. Char DH, Schwartz A, Miller TR, Abels JS. Ocular metastases from systemic melanoma. *Am J Ophthalmol* 1980;90:702.

314. Engel HM, Green WR, Michels RG, et al. Diagnostic vitrectomy. *Retina* 1981;1:121.

315. Robertson DM, Wilkinson CP, Murray JL, Gordy DD. Metastatic tumor to the retina and vitreous cavity from primary melanoma of the skin: treatment with systemic and subconjunctival chemotherapy. *Ophthalmology* 1981;88:1296.

316. Adamuk V. Ein fall von metastatischem melanosarcom der uvea. *Z Augenheilkd* 1909;21:505.

317. Albert DM, Lahav M, Troczynski E, Bahr R. Black hypopion: report of two cases. *Graefes Arch Clin Exp Ophthalmol* 1975;193:81.

318. Albert DM, Rubenstein RA, Scheie HG. Tumor metastasis to the eye. I: incidence in 213 adult patients with generalized malignancy. *Am J Ophthalmol* 1967;63:723.

319. Albert DM, Zimmerman AW Jr, Zeidman I. Tumor metastasis to the eye. II: fate of circulating tumor cells to the eye. *Am J Ophthalmol* 1963;67:733.

320. Boente R. Metastatische Melanoblastome in der Retina. *Klin Monatsbl Augenheilkd* 1929;82:732.

321. DasGupta T, Brasfield R. Metastatic melanoma. *Cancer* 1964;17:1323.

322. DeBustros S, Augsburger JJ, Shields JA, et al. Intraocular metastases from cutaneous malignant melanoma. *Arch Ophthalmol* 1985;103:937.

323. Font RL, Naumann G, Zimmerman LE. Primary malignant melanoma of the skin metastatic to the eye and orbit. *Am J Ophthalmol* 1967;63:738.

324. Letson AD, Davidorf FH. Bilateral retinal metastases from cutaneous malignant melanoma. *Arch Ophthalmol* 1982;100:605.

325. Liddicoat JA, Wolter JR, Wilkinson WC. Retinal metastasis of malignant melanoblastoma: a case report. *Am J Ophthalmol* 1959;48:177.

326. Osterhuis JA, DeKeiser RJN, De Wolff-Rovendaal D. Ocular and orbital metastases of cutaneous melanoma. *Int Ophthalmol* 1987;10:175.

327. Riffenburgh RS. Metastatic malignant melanoma to the retina. *Arch Ophthalmol* 1961;66:487.

328. Schachat AP. Tumor involvement of the vitreous cavity. In: Ryan SJ, ed. *Retina*. Vol. 1. St. Louis: Mosby, 1989:805–818.

329. TerDoesschatte G. Uber metastatische Sarkom de Auges. *Lin Monatsbl Augenheilkd* 1921;66:766.

330. Uhler EM. Metastatic malignant melanoma of the retina. *Am J Ophthalmol* 1940;23:158.

331. Wagenmann D. Ein fall von multipler melanosarkomen mit eigenartigen komplikationen beider augen. *Dtsch Med Wochenschr* 1900;25:262.

332. Young SE. Retinal metastases. In: Ryan SJ, ed. *Retina*. Vol. 1. St. Louis: Mosby, 1989:591–596.

333. Eide N, Syrdalen P. Intraocular metastasis from cutaneous malignant melanoma. *Acta Ophthalmol* 1990;68:102.

334. Piro P, Pappos HR, Erozan YS. Diagnostic vitrectomy in metastatic breast carcinoma in the vitreous. *Retina* 1982;2:182.

335. Sahel JA. Vitreous metastasis from cutaneous malignant melanoma. Presented at the European Ophthalmic Pathology Society/Verhoeff Society Meeting, Nuremberg, 1991.

336. Marshall J. The aging retina: physiology or pathology. *Eye* 1987;1:282.

337. Sarks SH. Aging and degeneration in the macular region: a clinicopathological study. *Br J Ophthalmol* 1976;60:324.

338. Sarks JP, Sarks SH, Killingsworth MC. Evolution of geographic atrophy of the retinal pigment epithelium. *Eye* 1988;2:552.

339. Sarks SH, Sarks JP. Age-related macular degeneration: atrophic form. In: Ryan SJ, 4th ed. *Retina*. Vol. 2. St. Louis: Mosby, 1996:1071–1104.

340. Hogan MJ, Alvarado JA, Weddell JE. *Histology of the human eye*. Philadelphia: Saunders, 1971.

341. Feeney-Burns L, Ellersieck MR. Age-related changes in ultrastructure of Bruch's membrane. *Am J Ophthalmol* 1985;100:686.

342. Spencer WH. Symposium: macular diseases. Pathogenesis: light microscopy. *Trans Am Acad Ophthalmol Otolaryngol* 1965;69:662.

343. Hogan MJ. Bruch's membrane and disease of the macula: role of elastic tissue and collagen. *Trans Ophthalmol Soc UK* 1967;87:113.

344. Hogen MJ, Alvarado J. Studies on the human macula. IV: aging changes in Bruch's membrane. *Arch Ophthalmol* 1967;77:410.

345. Newsome DA, Hewitt AT, Huh W, et al. Detection of specific extracellular matrix molecules in drusen, Bruch's membrane, and ciliary body. *Am J Ophthalmol* 1987;104:373–381.

346. Tate DJ Jr, Oliver PD, Miceli MV, et al. Age-dependent change in the hyaluronic acid content of the human chorioretinal complex. *Arch Ophthalmol* 1993;111:963–967.

347. Hogan MJ. Role of the retinal pigment epithelium in macular disease. *Trans Am Acad Ophthalmol Otolaryngol* 1972;76:64.

348. Sarks SH, Van Driel D, Maxwell L, Killingsworth M. Softening of drusen and subretinal neovascularization. *Trans Ophthalmol Soc UK* 1980;100:414.

349. Burns RP, Reeney-Burns L. Clinico-morphologic correlations of drusen of Bruch's membrane. *Trans Am Ophthalmol Soc* 1980;78:206.

350. Fine BS. Lipoidal degeneration of retinal pigment epithelium. *Am J Ophthalmol* 1981;91:469.

351. El Baba F, Green WR, Fleischmann J, et al. Clinicopathological correlation of lipidization and detachment of retinal pigment epithelium. *Am J Ophthalmol* 1986;101:576.

352. Frank RN, Green WR, Pollack IP. Senile macular degeneration. Clinicopathologic correlations of a case in the predisciform stage. *Am J Ophthalmol* 1973;75:587.

353. Green WR, Key SN. Senile macular degeneration: a histopathological study. *Trans Am Ophthalmol Soc* 1977;75:180.

354. Green WR, MacDonnell PJ, Yeo JH. Pathologic features of senile macular degeneration. *Ophthalmology* 1985;92:615.

355. Kornzweig AL. The eye in old patients. V: diseases of the macula: a clinicopathologic study. *Am J Ophthalmol* 1965;60:835.

356. Verhoeff FH, Grossman HP. Pathogenesis of disciform degeneration of macula. *Arch Ophthalmol* 1937;18:561.

357. Ramrattan RS, van der Schaft TL, Mooy CM, et al. Morphometric analysis of Bruch's membrane, the choriocapillaris, and the choroid in aging. *Invest Ophthalmol Vis Sci* 1994;35:2857–2864.

358. Young RW. Pathophysiology of age-related macular degeneration. *Surv Ophthalmol* 1987;31:291.

359. Okun E. Gross and microscopic pathology in autopsy eyes. II: perichorioretinal atrophy. *Am J Ophthalmol* 1960;50:574.

360. Henkind P, Gartner S. The relationship between retinal pigment epithelium and choriocapillaris. *Trans Ophthalmol Soc UK* 1983;103:444.

361. Green WR. Clinicopathologic studies of treated choroidal neovascular membranes. A review and report of two cases. *Retina* 1991;11:328–356.

362. Green WR, ed. *The retina*. In: Spencer WH, ed. *Ophthalmic pathology*. Philadelphia: Saunders, 1996:973–1108.

363. Green WR, Enger C. Age-related macular degeneration. Histopathologic studies. The 1992 Lorenz E. Zimmerman lecture. *Ophthalmology* 1993;100:1519–1535.

364. Dastgheib K, Green WR. Granulomatous reaction to Bruch's membrane in age-related macular degeneration. *Arch Ophthalmol* 1994;112:813–818.

365. Sarks SH. New vessel formation beneath the retinal pigment epithelium in senile eyes. *Br J Ophthalmol* 1973;57:951.

366. Kenyon KR, Maumenee AE, Ryan SJ, et al. Diffuse drusen and associated complications. *Am J Ophthalmol* 1985;100:119.

367. Thomas MA, Ibanez HE. Subretinal endophotocoagulation in the treatment of choroidal neovascularization. *Am J Ophthalmol* 1993;116:279–285.

368. Hsu JK, Thomas MA, Ibanez H, Green WR. Clinicopathologic studies of an eye after submacular membranectomy for choroidal neovascularization. *Retina* 1995;15:43–52.

369. Hoskin A, Bird AC, Sehmi K. Tears of detached retinal pigment epithelium. *Br J Ophthalmol* 1981;65:417.

370. Green WR, Gass JDM. Senile disciform degeneration of the macula: retinal arterialization of the fibrous plaque demonstrated clinically and histopathologically. *Arch Ophthalmol* 1971;86:487.

371. Thomas MA. The use of vitreoretinal surgical techniques in subfoveal choroidal neovascularization. *Curr Opin Ophthalmol* 1992;3:349–356.

Index

Note: Page numbers in *italics* refer to illustrations; page numbers followed by t refer to tables.